Pharmacologic Basis of Nursing Practice

FIFTH EDITION

Pharmacologic Basis of Nursing Practice

JULIA B. FREEMAN CLARK, PH.D.
Health Scientist Administrator
National Institutes of Health
Bethesda, Maryland

SHERRY F. QUEENER, PH.D.
Professor of Pharmacology
Indiana University School of Medicine
Indianapolis, Indiana

VIRGINIA BURKE KARB, R.N., PH.D.
Associate Dean and Associate Professor
School of Nursing
University of North Carolina at Greensboro
Greensboro, North Carolina

with 115 illustrations

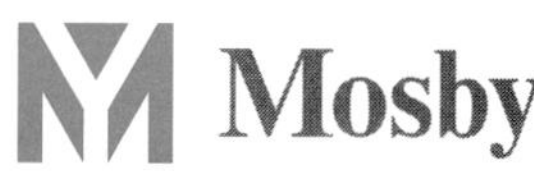

St. Louis Baltimore Boston Carlsbad Chicago Naples New York Philadelphia Portland
London Madrid Mexico City Singapore Sydney Tokyo Toronto Wiesbaden

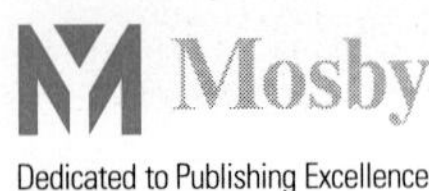

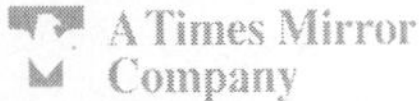

Publisher: Nancy L. Coon
Editor: Robin Carter
Developmental Editor: Gina Wright
Project Manager: Carol Sullivan Weis
Project Specialist: Pat Joiner
Manufacturing Supervisor: Karen Lewis
Editing and Production: Top Graphics
Design Manager: Sheilah Barrett
Design: Jeanne Wolfgeher Design
Cover Illustrator: Linda Frichtel

FIFTH EDITION

A NOTE TO THE READER
The author and publisher have made every attempt to check dosages and nursing content for accuracy. Because the science of pharmacology is continually advancing, our knowledge base continues to expand. Therefore we recommend that the reader always check product information for changes in dosage or administration before administering any medication. This is particularly important with new or rarely used drugs.

Printed in the United States of America
Composition by Top Graphics
Printing/binding by Von Hoffmann Press

Mosby–Year Book, Inc.
11830 Westline Industrial Drive
St. Louis, Missouri 63146

International Standard Book Number 0-323-00655-8

96-24743
CIP

98 99 00 01 02 / 9 8 7 6 5 4 3 2

Preface

Pharmacology is a rapidly changing field. The dynamic nature of drug therapy and health care presents continual challenges. The role of the nurse becomes increasingly sophisticated as new drugs and new strategies are applied to patient care.

CONTENT AND FEATURES

Pharmacologic Basis of Nursing Practice effectively presents pharmacology in an understandable format. Emphasizing clear rationales for drug therapy, it relates the physiologic factors of disease processes to drug mechanisms. This fifth edition of *Pharmacologic Basis of Nursing Practice* contains ***more than 60 new drugs*** that have been introduced during the 4 years since the last edition was published.

We have thoroughly revised specific content to include these new drugs in the tables and to integrate discussion of these agents in the text. The entire text has been reviewed, revised, and in many instances entirely reformatted to keep up with current knowledge on drug mechanisms and therapeutic uses of agents.

In addition, we have included four new chapters. Chapter 2, *Effects of Life Span, Genetics, and Medical Conditions on Drug Therapy,* highlights important variations in drug action and drug therapies specific to special populations. Chapter 8, *Issues of Drug Abuse,* provides perspective and guidance in treating the patient who is abusing drugs. Chapter 32, *Management of the Patient in Pain,* presents a practical overview of an issue related to all body systems and one that the nurse encounters on a daily basis. Chapter 35, *Immunomodulators and Care of the Patient With Altered Immune Function,* helps students prepare for the special challenges of treating immunocompromised patients and keep abreast of the latest drug therapies. To help students become more proficient in calculating dosages and to ensure proper drug administration, we have thoroughly revised Chapter 6, *Calculating Drug Dosages,* by focusing it more directly on clinical situations.

The fifth edition also contains the following new features to facilitate use of the book and to integrate more fully the nursing-related aspects of pharmacology with the text:

- **Key Drugs.** Prototypical or important drugs in a class are given thorough treatment and are highlighted with a special symbol ✚ for quick identification.
- **Patient Outcomes.** This new stage of the nursing process, presented within the Nursing Process Overview section, focuses care on the desired outcome of therapy.
- **Critical Thinking Questions.** At the end of every chapter both application and critical thinking are emphasized in this review of important content.
- **Research Highlights.** These special boxes directly relate recent pharmacologic research to its application in nursing practice.

Several content features have been retained from the previous edition:

- **Key Terms** highlight important terminology and concepts for review.
- **Special Boxes** emphasize various topics of special concern to the nurse. The fifth edition includes special boxes in the following areas:
  - Geriatric Considerations
  - Pediatric Considerations
  - Drug Abuse Alerts
  - Dietary Considerations
  - Patient Problems
  - Research Highlights
  - Home Health

GOALS

Our goal remains to provide an up-to-date, scientifically based pharmacology book that assists nursing students in studying drugs. Specifically, we seek to (1) present clearly the concepts of pharmacology that guide all drug use, (2) discuss the major drug classes with an emphasis on mechanisms of action, and (3) detail the nursing implications for drug administration throughout the nursing process. Our approach is to emphasize the rationale for drug therapy by relating the physiologic factors of disease processes to drug mechanisms. In addition to presenting a more thorough description of the scientific basis of drug action than most textbooks for nursing students do, this book carefully reviews pertinent physiologic fact so that students can readily see how drugs modify physiologic processes and apply this knowledge to nursing practice.

Because students often express frustration about trying to remember the large number of drugs they must learn, we have adopted a key drug approach, highlighting the drugs that are most important in a particular drug class. We also strive to minimize students' difficulty by dealing with drug classes first and then emphasizing the similarities between drugs of a single drug class. Chapters are focused on the grouping of drugs according to their mechanism of action.

For the instructor, our goal is to provide a book that can be adapted to various curricula. This book is divided into 16 sections. Each section contains two or more chapters, and the chapters include distinct segments for different therapeutic situations. For example, antianginal drugs are covered in a section of the chapter on drugs to improve circulation, *Antianginals and Other Vasodilators.* This chapter is one of seven chapters in the section titled *Drugs Affecting the Cardiovascular and Renal Systems.* This organization allows the instructor to rearrange the order in which material is presented and gives students succinct sections to master.

ORGANIZATION

Section I, *How Drugs Work in the Body,* Section II, *Nursing Care Related to Drug Therapy,* and Section III, *How the Nervous System Controls Body Functions,* provide a solid foundation for applying pharmacologic principles and knowledge of medication administration to nursing management. Sections IV through XVI are devoted to drug category discussions, which are grouped by body system.

Each chapter begins with objectives, a chapter overview, and key terms and ends with a series of critical thinking questions that directly apply chapter content to nursing practice. Drug category chapters are presented in a streamlined, consistent format. First, the Therapeutic Rationale discussion provides a detailed review to set the stage for why certain drugs are used in the treatment of a specific disorder or disease and what these agents are supposed to do. Next, the Therapeutic Agents discussion presents individual drugs and explores them in detail. *Key (or prototypical) drugs* are clearly identified. Key drugs are especially useful in programs in which pharmacology is integrated with another course in the curriculum. The key drug approach can be used to help students prioritize their study and compare the most important agents used within a drug class. Individual drugs are presented in a consistent drug monograph format that includes the following subheadings: mechanism of action, pharmacokinetics, uses, adverse reactions and contraindications, toxicity, and interactions. The Therapeutic Agents section may be repeated within a chapter if more than one category of drugs is used to treat the disease or disorder under discussion.

The Nursing Process Overview immediately follows the Therapeutic Agents discussion. This overview directly applies the nursing process to the content in the chapter with the five-step format of assessment, nursing diagnoses, patient outcomes, planning/implementation, and evaluation. The patient outcomes section focuses care on the desired outcome of therapy. In this way students can relate knowledge of medications to the overall plan of care for the patient.

At the end of every chapter a Nursing Implications Summary, highlighted in color, presents general guidelines for drug groups or specific therapies and provides detailed, specific nursing implications for each therapeutic agent, with emphasis on drug administration and patient and family education. Next, a series of Critical Thinking Questions engage and develop students' higher analytical processes. The questions are divided into two areas. First, application questions help students test their comprehension of pharmacologic principles related to nursing. Next, more complex critical thinking questions challenge students to conceptualize how pharmacologic principles are applied in nursing practice.

NURSING CONTENT

Much attention is given to emphasizing the relevant nursing information for the drugs discussed. The Nursing Process Overview provides a framework for applying pharmacologic knowledge to nursing practice. It is not meant to supplant the use of additional nursing textbooks or current nursing literature. The focus is on the pharmacologic factors rather than on the disease process itself within the five-step nursing process format of assessment, nursing diagnoses, patient outcomes, planning/implementation, and evaluation.

Assessment briefly summarizes the key aspects of the assessment database. The nursing diagnoses section presents examples of appropriate nursing diagnoses. These diagnoses reflect common side effects, drug interactions, serious potential complications, or anticipated major lifestyle changes that most patients will need to make. Patient outcomes describe the desired outcomes, or goals, of drug therapy and provide the rationale for the plan of care. Planning/implementation identifies the type of data that should be monitored throughout therapy and some of the nursing activities needed to promote the drug activity or foster patient well-being. The evaluation stage relates measurable criteria to the assessment data, nursing diagnoses, and plan of care to help the nurse establish whether goals are met or further planning and implementation are required.

ACKNOWLEDGMENTS

The production of this textbook has involved several able and experienced members of the editorial staff at Mosby. We wish to thank Robin Carter and Gina Wright for their special editorial contributions. We also thank Pat Joiner, Carol Sullivan Weis, and Carlotta Seely for production and Sheilah Barrett and Jeanne Wolfgeher for design.

Special thanks to Lynne Pearcey, R.N., Ph.D., Dean of the School of Nursing at the University of North Carolina at Greensboro, for her encouragement and support. Henry R. Besch, Jr., Ph.D., Chairman of the Department of Pharmacology and Toxicology at Indiana University School of Medicine, deserves special mention for the support he has given us during the development of all editions of this book. Mrs. Janie Siccardi, Administrative Assistant in the Department of Pharmacology and Toxicology, has greatly aided us in this effort. The continued contribution of Dr. Lynn R. Willis, Professor of Pharmacology at Indiana University School of Medicine, is also much appreciated.

Finally, we would like to thank two special colleagues who have lived with the book as long as we have. They are Dr. Stephen W. Queener, Research Scientist, Eli Lilly and Company; and Dr. Kenneth S. Karb, Medical Oncologist, Greensboro, North Carolina.

Julia B. Freeman Clark
Sherry F. Queener
Virginia Burke Karb

Contributors

Sandra Handley, R.N., Ph.D., C.A.R.N.
School of Nursing
University of Kansas
Kansas City, Kansas

Lynn R. Willis, Ph.D.
Vice-Chair and Professor
Department of Pharmacology and Toxicology
Indiana University School of Medicine
Indianapolis, Indiana

Eleanor J. Sullivan, Ph.D., R.N., F.A.A.N.
Professor, School of Nursing
University of Kansas
Kansas City, Kansas
Moog Visiting Professor, Barnes College of Nursing
University of Missouri–St. Louis
St. Louis, Missouri

Reviewers

Ann Bello, M.A., R.N.
Professor of Nursing
Norwalk Community–Technical College
Norwalk, Connecticut

Shari L. Clarke, M.S.N., F.N.P., R.N.C.
Family Nurse Practitioner
Fayetteville, Georgia

Gloria Fazio, M.S.N., R.N.C.
Professor of Nursing
Norwalk Community–Technical College
Norwalk, Connecticut

Barbara K. Polacsek, M.A., R.N.
Professor of Nursing
Norwalk Community–Technical College
Norwalk, Connecticut

Janis Waite, R.N., M.S.N.
Associate Professor
Illinois Central College
East Peoria, Illinois

Contents

SECTION III
How the Nervous System Controls Body Functions

SECTION IV
Drugs Affecting the Cardiovascular and Renal Systems

SECTION V
Drugs Modifying the Blood

SECTION XIII
Drugs for the Neurologic System

SECTION XIV
Drugs Affecting the Endocrine and Reproductive Systems

SECTION XV
Drugs for the Patient Receiving Anesthesia

SECTION XVI
Ophthalmic Drugs

SECTION I

How Drugs Work in the Body

CHAPTER 1 *Drugs in the Body* covers the principles that govern the action of all drugs in the body. These basic concepts and related terms recur repeatedly throughout the study of pharmacology. Initial study of these concepts will help the student approach the study of individual drugs and rationalize the manner in which they are used clinically.

CHAPTER 2 *Effects of Life Span, Genetics, and Medical Conditions on Drug Therapy* illustrates how drug effects can be influenced by age or genotype. The influence of organ impairment or failure on drug responses is also explored.

CHAPTER 3 *Legal Implications of Drug Therapy* places the legal status of modern drugs in perspective. It also introduces the Schedule of Controlled Substances and the Drug Efficacy Study Implementation (DESI) rating—topics that recur at appropriate points throughout the text. Canadian drug classifications are covered in this chapter and are referred to elsewhere in the text.

CHAPTER 4 *Application of the Nursing Process to Drug Therapy* discusses the use of the nursing process with patients receiving drug therapy. The chapter also discusses patient education; medication errors; the roles of the nurse, physician, and pharmacist; and patient compliance.

CHAPTER 1

Drugs in the Body

OBJECTIVES

After studying this chapter, you should be able to do the following:

- *Describe the three principles of drug action.*
- *Describe three ways in which drugs interact with the body.*
- *Discuss mechanisms that produce unwanted drug reactions.*
- *Explain how drug dissolution, the lipid solubility of the drug, and the presence of gastric contents can influence enteral absorption of drugs.*
- *Discuss the advantages and disadvantages of common routes of administration.*
- *Explain how the elimination half-life of a drug influences the time required to attain a steady-state concentration of drug given at fixed intervals.*

CHAPTER OVERVIEW

Pharmacology is the study of the interaction of chemicals with living organisms to produce biologic effects. This book presents chemicals that produce therapeutically useful effects, chemicals referred to as *drugs*. This chapter explains how groups or classes of drugs act in the body. This information forms the basis for understanding the actions of specific drugs discussed in later chapters of the book.

KEY TERMS

affinity
agonist
anaphylaxis
antagonists
bioavailability
biotransformation
duration
efficacy
enterohepatic circulation
first-pass effect
half-life
lipid soluble
onset
pharmacodynamics
pharmacokinetics
receptor
serum sickness
side effects
time to peak effect
urticaria

MECHANISMS OF DRUG ACTION

Drug Action Is Determined by How a Drug Interacts With the Body

Most drugs produce biologic effects by interacting with specific targets at the drug's site of action. The magnitude of the biologic effect produced by a drug is related to the concentration of the drug present at the site of action and the strength of interaction of the drug with the target. **Pharmacodynamics** is the study of drug action at the level of the drug target.

Drugs differ in their intrinsic ability to produce an effect, in their ability to penetrate to the site of action, and in their rate of removal from that site. **Pharmacokinetics** is the study of how drugs enter the body, reach their site of action, and are removed from the body. Both the pharmacokinetics and the pharmacodynamics of a drug determine how a drug is administered, how often it is given, and what the dose is.

Drugs May Chemically Alter Body Fluids

Drugs that chemically alter body fluids directly enter a body fluid or compartment. An example is an antacid, which enters the stomach and neutralizes excess stomach acid. Alteration of gastric pH is the only intended action of this drug. Other examples are drugs that accumulate in urine and alter urinary pH. By acidifying the urine with ammonium chloride or alkalinizing the urine with sodium bicarbonate, ion flow in the kidney is altered and drug excretion patterns are changed.

Drugs May Chemically Alter Cell Membranes

Drugs that chemically alter cell membranes interact nonspecifically. The interaction is a chemical attraction usually based on the lipid nature of the cell membrane and the lipid attraction of the drug. General anesthetic gases may act in this way by dissolving in lipid-rich membranes and thereby altering properties of the cells involved.

Drugs May Act Through Specific Receptors

The biologic activity of most drugs is determined by the ability of the drug to bind to a specific **receptor;** the ability to bind is determined by the chemical structure of the drug. The interaction of a drug with a specific receptor is similar to a lock-and-key fit (Figure 1-1). Only a certain critical portion of the drug is usually involved in binding, not the entire molecule. Drugs that have similar critical regions but differ in other parts of the molecule might also be expected to have similar biologic activity *(drugs D, E,* and *F* in Figure 1-1).

The ability to bind to the receptor and the capability of stimulating an action by the receptor are two different aspects of drug action. The ability to bind to the receptor is known as **affinity.** Drugs with high affinity have a strong attraction to the receptor. The capability of stimulating the receptor to some action is called **efficacy.**

When receptors are highly specific and have high affinity for the compounds that bind to them, very low concentrations of these compounds may show biologic activity. For example, hormones naturally present in the body act through specific receptors. Some of these hormones are found in the blood at concentrations of less than 1 picomole, or less than one part per trillion. Nevertheless, these tiny amounts are biologically effective because hormones are detected and bound by specific receptors.

Receptors also allow localization of drug effects to certain tissues. Each tissue or cell type possesses a unique array of specific receptors. For example, certain cells in the kidney possess specific receptors for antidiuretic hormone (see Chapter 59). These cells therefore have the capacity to respond to this hormone. Cells in other tissues that lack these receptors cannot respond to antidiuretic hormone.

The idea of drug receptors is a key concept in pharmacology. The specific receptors called *drug receptors* are actually natural components of the body intended to respond to some chemical normally present in blood or tissues. For example,

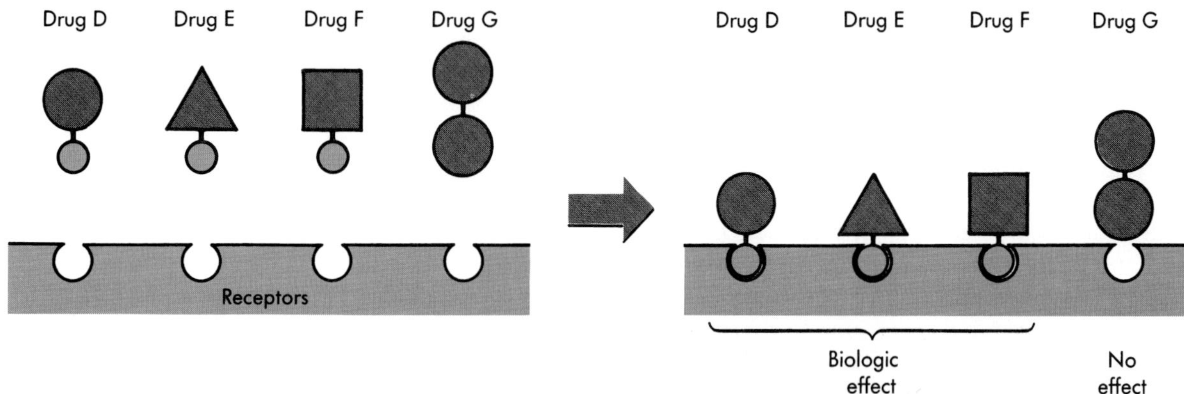

FIGURE 1-1
Lock-and-key fit between drugs and receptors through which they act. Site on receptor that interacts with drug has definite shape. Those drugs conforming to that shape can bind and produce biologic response. In example, only shape along lower surface of drug molecule is important in determining whether drug will bind to receptor.

opioid receptors within the brain respond to morphine and related compounds from the opium poppy, but the natural function of these receptors is to bind to *enkephalins* and *endorphins.* These compounds found in the brain are more potent than morphine in producing analgesia (see Chapter 31).

Any compound, either natural or synthetic, that binds to a specific receptor and produces a biologic effect by stimulating that receptor is called an **agonist.** For example, the hormone norepinephrine binds to specific sites in the heart called *beta-1 adrenergic receptors.* Stimulation of these receptors causes the heart to beat faster. The synthetic drug isoproterenol acts on the same cardiac receptors and produces the same effects. Both norepinephrine and isoproterenol are therefore called *agonists* for the beta-1 adrenergic receptor (see Chapter 10). Agonists have both affinity for receptors and efficacy (because they cause some action by the receptor).

Some drugs produce their action not by stimulating receptors but by preventing natural substances from stimulating receptors. These drugs are called **antagonists.** For example, the drug propranolol blocks beta-1 adrenergic receptors and prevents agonists such as norepinephrine from stimulating the receptor normally. Propranolol therefore is classed as an antagonist of the action of norepinephrine. Antagonists have affinity for receptors but lack efficacy. When the receptor is occupied by an antagonist, the receptor cannot carry out its normal function.

Drugs Do Not Create Functions but Modify Existing Functions Within the Body

Drugs must always be considered in terms of the physiologic functions they alter in the body. In no case do drugs *create* a function in a tissue or organ. For example, digitalis is a drug used to strengthen the action of the heart. Digitalis produces this effect by altering the existing pattern of ion flow into and out of heart cells; it does not create a new way for the heart to contract. Digitalis simply alters the natural process.

To emphasize this principle, subsequent chapters on drug families start with a brief description of the normal physiology influenced by that group of drugs.

No Drug Has a Single Action

The desired action of a drug is an expected, predictable response. Ideally, each drug would have the desired effect on one physiologic process and produce no other effect. However, all drugs have the potential for altering more than one function in the body. These unwanted actions are known as **side effects.** For example, the desired action of digitalis is to strengthen a failing heart, but at the same time it may cause erratic heartbeats, which is an undesirable side effect.

Predictable reactions arising from known pharmacologic actions of drugs account for between 70% and 80% of all drug reactions. For example, barbiturates put a patient to sleep because they depress the central nervous system, but excessive depression of the central nervous system is lethal because the brain centers that control breathing are also depressed. Respiratory depression would therefore be an expected side effect when barbiturates are used at doses that allow the drug to accumulate in the body. Other predictable side effects may occur at normal therapeutic doses and are related to the secondary actions of the drug. For example, at normal therapeutic doses barbiturates increase the drug-metabolizing activity of the liver. This ability is unrelated to the therapeutically desired activity of these drugs and actually leads to a number of interactions with other drugs.

Unpredictable reactions to drugs account for 20% to 30% of all drug reactions. Although experience shows that a certain percentage of the population may be expected to react to a drug in an unusual manner, it is often not possible to predict which individual will show the reaction. The unpredictable drug reactions are of two types: idiosyncratic and allergic. Idiosyncratic reactions have no immediately obvious cause and may relate to an undetected genetic difference from the majority of the population. Allergic reactions to drugs account for between 6% and 10% of all drug reactions. The allergic reaction may be triggered by the drug in its original form or by a metabolite of the drug formed in the body.

Drug allergies can be divided into four types, based on the mechanism of the immune reaction. Type I reactions occur soon after exposure and commonly produce **urticaria,** also called *hives.* These raised, irregularly shaped patches on the skin are frequently accompanied by severe itching. Although allergic reactions involving the skin are annoying, they are not usually serious; they can, however, progress to a severe acute allergic reaction that involves the cardiovascular and respiratory systems. This rare but dangerous reaction is called **anaphylaxis** or *anaphylactic shock.* Anaphylaxis is marked by sudden contraction of the bronchiolar muscles and frequently by edema of the mouth and throat. Anaphylactic reactions may completely cut off airflow to the lungs. In addition, blood pressure falls and the patient may go into shock. These violent reactions may occur within a very short time, and aggressive therapy is required to save the patient's life.

Symptoms of type I reactions are caused by immunoglobulin E (IgE) antibodies, which are released in response to the drug and prompt target cells to discharge immune modulators such as histamine (see Chapters 28 and 33). Drugs associated with type I reactions include penicillins, cephalosporins, and iodides.

Type II reactions to drugs involve immunoglobulin M (IgM) or immunoglobulin G (IgG) antibodies, which can trigger lysis of specific blood cells under the appropriate conditions. These delayed reactions are sometimes called *autoimmune responses.* Examples include hemolytic anemia induced by methyldopa and thrombocytopenic purpura induced by quinidine. Procainamide and hydralazine can induce a condition resembling systemic lupus erythematosus.

Type III reactions are often described as **serum sickness.** Symptoms include urticaria, pain in the joints, swollen lymph nodes, and fever. Penicillins, iodides, sulfonamides, and phenytoin can cause this type of delayed reaction, which may involve IgE, IgM, or IgG antibodies.

The type IV reaction is contact dermatitis, which is caused by topical application of drugs.

Any patient can suffer an allergic reaction in response to any drug, but certain drugs are more prone to cause reactions.

Patients receiving these agents should be closely monitored to detect early signs of allergic responses and thereby to protect them from injury.

Allergic reactions do not occur during the first exposure to a drug because time is required for the immune system to develop antibodies that cause these reactions. Documenting prior exposure to a drug is helpful but is not always easy. Patients do not always know the names of drugs they have received and are not always reliable sources of information on prior reactions to drugs. Moreover, persons may be unknowingly exposed to antibiotics or other drugs through food or milk if the drugs have been improperly used in animal medicine.

HOW DRUG DOSE RELATES TO DRUG ACTION

Pharmacokinetics

Factors Controlling Drug Absorption by Enteral Routes

To be effective systemically, a drug must be present in body fluids or tissues in a free or available form. For most medications less than the total amount of administered drug is ultimately available to produce effects on target tissues. The term **bioavailability** describes what proportion of the administered drug is available to produce systemic effects. If a drug has low bioavailability, most of the administered dose of the drug is lost or destroyed, never reaching the blood in a form that can be effective. Drugs that are freely and rapidly absorbed have a high bioavailability. The many factors that can influence bioavailability are discussed in the following sections.

Drug dissolution. About 80% of drugs used in clinical practice are administered orally, primarily because of the ease and convenience of administration by this route. The drug may be given in liquid form or in a solid form such as a tablet or capsule (Table 1-1). To achieve this solid form, the drug is usually mixed with other compounds that serve various functions. Starches and other compounds may be added as inert fillers, especially when the actual amount of drug required per dose is too small to be conveniently handled. Adhesive substances called *binders* may also be added to allow a tablet to hold together after it is compressed in manufacture. Other compounds called *disintegrators* may be required to allow a tablet to absorb water and to break apart in the body. Lubricants are frequently added to prevent tablets from sticking to machinery during manufacture. These additions to the dosage form may make up the bulk of the tablet. For example, in tablets containing 100,000 units of penicillin the active ingredient, potassium penicillin, makes up only 11% of the tablet mass.

To be effective, the solid dose of a drug must break apart in the gastrointestinal tract and allow the drug to go into solution. Only dissolved drug is absorbed from the gastrointestinal tract into the blood. Because breakdown of the solid dosage form is required for absorption of the drug, any variability in this process can affect how rapidly and completely the drug is absorbed. The formulation of a tablet or capsule affects dissolution rates. Tablets from different manufacturers that contain the same amount of active ingredient but different types and amounts of inert ingredients may not be identical in clinical action because each formulation may have different dissolution properties. Tablets may also change with age and conditions of storage. Older tablets tend to dry out and are harder to disintegrate, which leads to reduced bioavailability of the drug.

Gastrointestinal tract. The presence of food influences the dissolution and absorption of drugs. For example, the antibiotic tetracycline should be given on an empty stomach because food blocks absorption of the drug. In contrast, a drug like griseofulvin is best absorbed when taken with fatty foods.

Stomach acidity also influences absorption. For example, penicillins are not stable in acid, and part of the dose is destroyed rather than absorbed. There is considerable variation from person to person in gastric emptying times and, therefore, in the length of time a drug spends in stomach acid. In addition, the amount of acid in the stomach varies with the individual and the time of day. The very young and older adults have less stomach acid than middle-aged persons. Lower acidity may mean less drug is degraded and more is available to be absorbed.

Chemical properties of the drug. In addition to the physical state of the drug, its chemical nature determines how satisfactory oral administration will be. To pass through membranes lining the gastrointestinal tract, a drug must be relatively **lipid soluble** because the membranes themselves contain a high concentration of lipid. Ionic (charged) forms of drugs do not easily pass through these membranes. Many drugs can exist in an ionic state or in an uncharged lipid-soluble state, depending on the pH of the environment. This environment changes throughout the gastrointestinal tract (Figure 1-2). Stomach fluid is highly acidic. A drug such as aspirin, which is a weak acid, is converted from a charged to an uncharged form by the strong acid in the stomach. Because the uncharged form of the drug can readily diffuse through the lipid membranes of the stomach cells, the drug is rapidly absorbed.

Enteric coatings on tablets or capsules protect some drugs that are sensitive to stomach acid (see Table 1-1). These coatings are inert at low (acidic) pH but soluble at higher (alkaline) pH. Therefore the drug passes through the stomach and is released in the intestine. Enteric coatings are also used for drugs that are highly irritating to the gastric mucosa.

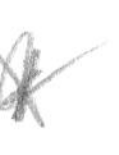

Fluids in the small intestine are slightly alkaline. This higher pH favors absorption of weakly basic drugs because at this pH range weak bases are uncharged (see Figure 1-2). The small intestine also has an enormous surface area for drug absorption, which makes it a major site of absorption. However, some drugs, particularly proteins such as insulin or growth hormone, are destroyed in the small intestine by the action of digestive enzymes from the pancreas.

Drugs that are absorbed from the small intestine are transported by portal circulation directly to the liver before being circulated to the rest of the body (Figure 1-3). The liver may metabolize much of the drug before it can enter general cir-

TABLE 1-1 Forms of Medication

FORM	DESCRIPTION
Capsules	Solid dosage forms for oral use in which medication is enclosed in gelatin shell that dissolves in stomach or intestine. Gelatin of capsules is colored to aid in product identification. Manufacturers use distinctive shapes for identifying their capsules.
Douche	Aqueous solution used as cleansing or antiseptic agent for part of body or body cavity. Douches are usually sold as powder or liquid concentrate to be dissolved or diluted before use.
Elixirs	Clear fluids for oral use that contain water and alcohol with glycerin and sorbitol or another sweetener sometimes added. Alcohol content of these preparations varies.
Glycerites	Solutions of drugs in glycerin for external use. Solution must be at least 50% glycerin.
Patches	Inner surface of the patch contacts skin and allows transdermal absorption of lipid-soluble drugs. The total amount of drug on the patch is very large, but typically only a small fraction is absorbed.
Pills	Solid dosage forms for oral use in which drug and various vehicles are formed into small globules or ovoids. True pills are rare; most have been replaced by compressed tablets.
Solution	Liquid preparations, usually in water, containing one or more dissolved compounds. Solutions for oral use may contain flavoring and coloring agents. Solutions for intravenous injection must be sterile and particle free. Other injectable solutions must be sterile. Solutions of certain drugs may also be used externally.
Suppositories	Solid dosage forms to be inserted into body cavity where medication is released as solid melts or dissolves. Suppositories often contain cocoa butter (theobroma oil), which is solid at room temperature but liquid at body temperature, or glycerin, polyethylene glycol, or gelatin, which dissolves in secretions from mucous membranes.
Suspension	Finely divided drug particles that are suspended in suitable liquid medium before being injected or taken orally. Suspensions must not be injected intravenously.
Sustained-action drugs	Form of medication altered so that dissolution is slow and continuous for extended period. Total dosage in sustained-action medication is greater than for regular formulations because drug is not all released at once.
Syrups	Medication dissolved in concentrated solution of sugar such as sucrose. Flavors may be added to mask unpleasant taste.
Tablets	Solid dosage forms shaped like disks or cylinders that contain, in addition to drug, one or more of following ingredients: binder (adhesive that allows tablet to stick together), disintegrators (substances promoting tablet dissolution in body fluids), lubricants (required for efficient manufacturing), and fillers (inert ingredients to make tablet size convenient).
Enteric-coated drugs	Solid dosage forms for oral use. Medication in tablet form is coated with materials designed not to dissolve in stomach but to dissolve in intestine, where medication may be absorbed.
Press-coated or layered drugs	Preformed tablet that has another layer of material pressed on or around it. This practice allows incompatible ingredients to be separated and causes them to be dissolved at slightly different rates.
Tincture	Alcoholic or water-alcohol solutions of drugs.
Transdermal creams	Relatively lipid-soluble drugs that may be absorbed transdermally. Dosage is usually measured in inches of cream extruded from tube.
Troches (also called *lozenges* or *pastilles*)	Solid dosage forms often shaped like disks or cylinders that contain drug, flavor, sugar, and mucilage. Troches dissolve or disintegrate in mouth, releasing medication such as antiseptic or anesthetic for action in mouth or throat. Troches dissolve more slowly than tablets.

culation. The term **first-pass effect** refers to this process. Liver metabolism often inactivates drugs; when this happens, the first-pass effect lowers the amount of active drug released into the systemic circulation. For example, morphine is very rapidly extracted from blood and metabolized by the liver; therefore to achieve the same level of pain relief, it is necessary to administer six times more morphine orally than intramuscularly. In contrast, the related drug codeine is much less affected by the first-pass effect; therefore it takes only two times more codeine orally than intramuscularly to produce the same degree of pain relief. In these examples the larger doses compensate for the drug lost through inactivation by the liver.

The first-pass effect may be avoided by using other routes of administration, such as sublingual (drug dissolved under the tongue), buccal (drug dissolved between the cheek and gum), and rectal routes (see Figure 1-3). Drugs taken by these routes are absorbed directly across the mucous membranes and rapidly enter the systemic circulation. The sublingual and buccal routes are useful when a palatable, highly lipid-soluble

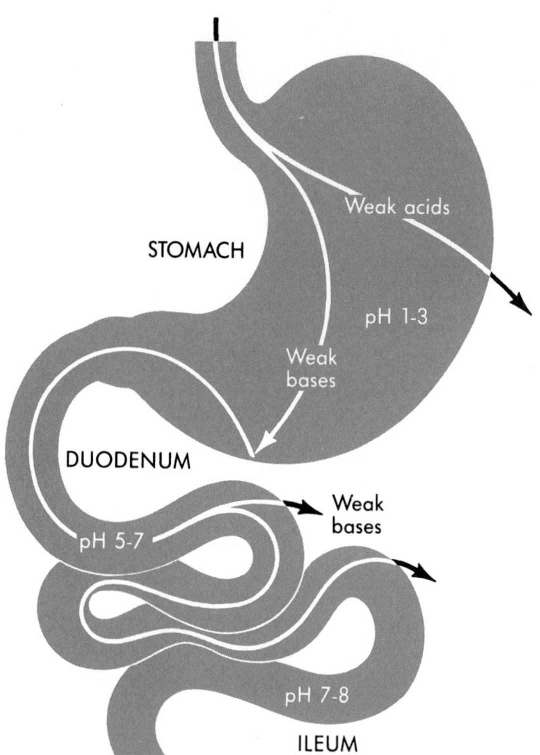

FIGURE 1-2
Effect of pH on ability of drugs to cross gastrointestinal membranes. Strongly acidic environment of stomach (pH 1 to 3) maintains weak acids in uncharged form, which is more easily absorbed. Weak bases remain charged in stomach but are converted to uncharged forms as pH approaches neutrality (pH 7) or becomes slightly alkaline (pH 7 to 8).

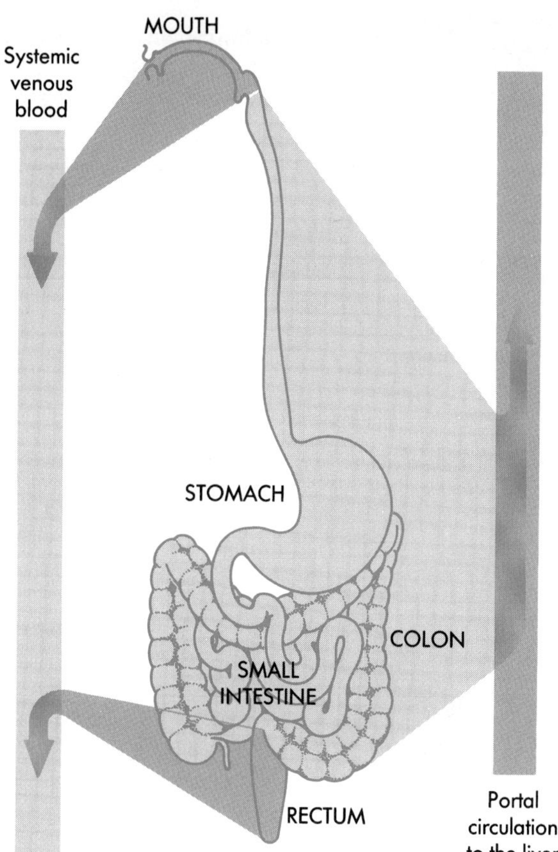

FIGURE 1-3
Two circulatory pathways for materials absorbed from gastrointestinal tract. Materials absorbed from stomach, small intestine, or colon enter portal circulation, which perfuses liver before returning to heart. Materials absorbed from these sites are exposed first to action of liver microsomal enzymes and then are circulated to rest of body. In contrast, absorption through membranes lining mouth or rectum deliver material directly to systemic circulation.

drug is involved. The rectal route is especially useful for unconscious patients. The best physical form for rectal use is a suppository that will melt at body temperature and release the drug for absorption (Table 1-2).

Factors Controlling Drug Absorption by Parenteral Routes

Parenteral routes of drug administration require injection of drug into the skin, muscle, or blood (see Chapter 5). Injection necessarily involves breaking the skin, and sterile technique must be used to prevent bacteria or viruses from gaining entry (see Table 1-2). Special precautions often must be taken to avoid producing undue tissue damage from irritating drugs. These precautions may involve preventing the drug from contacting skin; some drugs require dilution before administration.

Subcutaneous injection. Subcutaneous injection (under the skin) is appropriate for small drug volumes and for drugs intended to be slowly absorbed (e.g., insulin). When very slow absorption is desired, drugs may be formulated as solid inserts that release the drug over prolonged periods. An example is the insert that releases hormones and provides birth control for months (see Chapter 65).

Intramuscular injection. Intramuscular injection (into a muscle) is appropriate when large volumes of drug must be injected. Absorption from intramuscular sites is faster than from subcutaneous sites because muscles have a better blood supply than does skin. Absorption from subcutaneous or intramuscular sites can be hastened by applying heat or massage to the site to accelerate blood flow. Absorption can be slowed by decreasing blood flow to the injection site by applying ice packs or by the simultaneous injection of a drug such as epinephrine, which constricts blood vessels.

The forms of drugs intended for intramuscular or subcutaneous injection may be relatively insoluble. Some drugs are formulated specifically to dissolve slowly and therefore to be absorbed slowly from injection sites. These dosage forms are called *depot injections.*

Intravenous injection. Intravenous injection (directly into a vein) requires special precautions. Drugs for intravenous use must always be in solution and can contain no particulate

TABLE 1-2 Summary of Major Routes for Administration of Drugs

DESCRIPTION	ADVANTAGES	DISADVANTAGES
Aerosol Fine particles or droplets are breathed in.	Direct delivery to lung	Irritation of lung mucosa may occur. Special equipment is required. Patient must be conscious.
Buccal Drug is dissolved between cheek and gum and absorbed across mucous membrane.	Convenient Sterility not needed Direct delivery to general circulation	Not useful for drugs with unpleasant taste. Irritation to oral mucosa may occur. Patient must be conscious. Useful only for highly lipid-soluble drugs.
Inhalation Drug is inhaled as a gas.	Continuous dosing Patient may be unconscious.	Useful only for drugs that are gases at room temperature. Irritation of mucosa may occur.
Intramuscular Drug is injected into muscle mass.	Rapid absorption Soluble or insoluble drug forms Patient may be conscious or unconscious.	Sterile procedures are necessary. Minor pain is common. Irritation and local reactions may occur.
Intravenous Drug is injected directly into vein.	Direct control of drug concentration in blood Rapid attainment of effective blood levels	Sterile procedures are necessary. Risk of transient high drug concentrations is possible if injected too rapidly.
Oral Drug is swallowed and absorbed from stomach or small intestine.	Convenience Sterility not needed Economical	Unpleasant taste may cause noncompliance. Irritation to gastric mucosa may induce nausea. Patient must be conscious. Digestive juices may destroy drug. Absorbed drug enters portal circulation to liver, where it may be metabolized.
Subcutaneous Drug is injected under skin.	Patient may be conscious or unconscious.	Sterile procedures are necessary. Pain and irritation at site may occur.
Sublingual Drug is dissolved under tongue and absorbed across mucous membrane.	Convenient Sterility not needed Direct delivery to general circulation	Not useful for drugs with unpleasant taste. Irritation to oral mucosa may occur. Patient must be conscious. Useful only for highly lipid-soluble drugs.
Transdermal Drug is absorbed directly through skin.	Continuous dosing Sterility not needed Direct delivery to general circulation	Effective only for lipid-soluble drugs. Local irritation can occur. Discarded patches may pose danger of poisoning.

matter. Some drugs irritate the veins and cause thrombophlebitis if administered at too high a concentration. Other drugs must be injected slowly to avoid toxic concentrations of drug from reaching the heart or other vital organs. The intravenous route is valuable when drug concentrations must be maintained continuously, but potential harm to the patient is significant by this invasive route.

Special injection routes may be used in certain circumstances. For example, local anesthetics may be injected into the spinal column to produce certain types of anesthesia. Other drugs may be injected directly into body cavities or joints. Such routes are used when conventional routes of injection do not allow high enough drug concentrations to be achieved at the desired site of drug action.

Factors Controlling Drug Persistence in the Blood

After a drug has entered the blood, its ultimate fate is determined by the chemical properties of the drug and the way it is affected by blood and the tissues it contacts. Some drugs are metabolized by enzymes in blood. An example is succinylcholine. Drugs that persist in the blood are usually bound to blood proteins rather than being simply dissolved directly in plasma.

The most important carrier protein is albumin, which is formed in the liver and released into the blood. Drugs bound to albumin or other carrier proteins remain in the blood because these proteins do not diffuse easily through capillary walls. Drug binding to albumin is a reversible process, and an equilibrium is established between drug that is bound to protein and drug that is free in solution. Only free drug is able to diffuse into tissues, interact with receptors, and produce biologic effects. The same proportion of bound and free drug is maintained in the blood at all times. Thus when free drug leaves the blood, some drug is released from protein binding to reestablish the proper ratio between bound drug and free drug.

The anticoagulant dicumarol is an example of a drug that binds to plasma protein. In blood 99% of this drug is bound to plasma albumin. Therefore only 1% of the blood content of dicumarol is free to diffuse to its site of action or to its sites of elimination. The net effect of binding to albumin is to create a reservoir of drug that is released to replenish free drug removed to other sites. In general, drugs that do not bind to plasma albumin remain in the body for shorter periods than do drugs that are tightly bound. A drug such as dicumarol, which is very strongly bound to albumin, remains in the body for up to 3 days. Drugs that are bound to plasma proteins are thus characterized by longer duration of action.

Factors Controlling Drug Distribution Throughout the Body

High lipid solubility and low protein binding favor diffusion of a drug through membranes. All transport into tissues involves passing through lipid-containing membranes, a process that is difficult for water-soluble compounds but easy for lipid-soluble agents. High concentrations of free drug in blood also favors diffusion into tissues; high protein binding lowers free drug concentrations in blood and impedes diffusion into tissues.

Factors Controlling Drug Metabolism in the Body

Biotransformation is the ability of living organisms to modify the chemical structure of compounds. Most drugs are metabolized by the liver, specifically by the microsomal enzyme system. These enzymes allow the body to metabolize potentially toxic compounds. Many types of chemical transformations are carried out, but in general these reactions create water-soluble compounds that are more easily eliminated from the body by the kidneys. These enzymes have two important properties. First, the enzymes are relatively nonspecific, and therefore many drugs may be metabolized by the same enzyme system. Second, the liver can synthesize more enzyme if it is chronically exposed to certain drugs. This property means that the liver can increase its capacity to destroy a drug over a period of a few days. This increase in microsomal enzyme content in the liver is called *enzyme induction.*

Biotransformation often inactivates drugs, but there are exceptions. For example, drugs such as codeine, diazepam, and amitriptyline are all converted by the liver into metabolites that are also active. A few drugs are not active until they are biotransformed by the liver. For example, the anticancer drug cyclophosphamide is inactive, but one of its metabolites produced in the liver is a highly reactive alkylating agent that is effective against cancer cells.

The liver is by far the most important site for biotransformation of drugs, but it is not the only one. The kidney is another important site for biotransformation of certain types of drugs. Biotransformation may also be carried out by bacteria within the colon. This process may limit absorption of drug from the bowel after oral administration, or drug may diffuse from the blood into the bowel and be destroyed.

Factors Controlling Drug Elimination

The three main routes by which drugs may be eliminated from the body involve the liver, kidney, and bowel.

Elimination in feces. The first route involves uptake of drug by the liver, release into bile, and elimination in feces. For some drugs, such as erythromycin and penicillins, the concentration of drug in bile may be much higher than its concentration in blood. Because between 600 and 1000 ml of bile is formed each day, this route of elimination may dispose of significant amounts of drug. However, drugs in bile enter the small intestine, where they may be reabsorbed into the blood, returned to the liver, and again secreted into bile. This secretion and reabsorption process is called **enterohepatic circulation.** Drugs that are extensively reabsorbed from the intestinal tract after biliary secretion persist in the body much longer than drugs that remain in the lumen of the intestine and pass out with feces. If the reabsorbed drug is in an active form, the duration of action is prolonged.

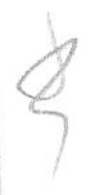

Elimination in urine after metabolism by the liver. The second route of elimination involves both liver and kidneys. Common biotransformations of drugs by the liver include formation of glucuronides, hydroxylations, and acetylations. The kidney is also capable of forming glucuronides and sulfates. All these reactions tend to form polar compounds, which can be more efficiently excreted by the kidneys. For example, a drug such as the antibiotic chloramphenicol normally enters glomerular fluid by passive diffusion but is reabsorbed from the tubules and reenters the blood. In the liver, however, chloramphenicol is transformed into chloramphenicol glucuronide. In this form the drug enters glomerular fluid, cannot be reabsorbed from the tubules, and hence is excreted in urine.

Various factors may influence the ability of the liver to metabolize drugs. For example, premature infants and neonates have immature livers that are incapable of carrying out certain biotransformations (see Chapter 2). Therefore these patients may accumulate drugs that must be metabolized in the liver before they can be excreted renally. Patients who have suffered hepatic damage, such as those who suffer from chronic alcoholism, may also accumulate drugs normally excreted by this route.

Elimination in urine without metabolism by the liver. Some drugs are not extensively metabolized anywhere in the body and are excreted unchanged in urine. This excretion may take place in one of two ways. Some drugs are excreted by passive diffusion into glomerular fluid. Other drugs are actively secreted by specific systems in the renal tubule. These active processes lead to more rapid drug elimination and allow much higher urinary concentrations of drug to be achieved. The antibiotic penicillin G is a good example of a drug that is actively secreted by the renal tubule. Half of an intravenous dose of penicillin G can be eliminated in about 20 minutes by active tubular secretion. In contrast, an antibiotic such as tetracycline, which is eliminated primarily by passive diffusion in the kidneys, persists in the body for several hours.

Drugs that are normally excreted unchanged in urine accumulate in the body when there is a loss of renal function (see Chapter 2). Patients with renal disease often must have drug dosages lowered to compensate for the reduced ability of the kidneys to excrete the drug. Renal function declines with age even in healthy persons, and older adult patients may show a reduced ability to excrete drugs in their urine. Certain drugs such as aminoglycoside antibiotics are nephrotoxic and may directly damage the kidneys and thereby interfere with their own excretion.

Pharmacodynamics

Dose-Response Curve

The relationship between the dose of drug and the response produced is described by an S-shaped (sigmoid) curve called the *dose-response curve* (Figure 1-4). This curve is obtained by plotting the observed response (on a linear scale) against the dose of the drug used to elicit that response (on a logarithmic scale).

The dose-response curve illustrates several important quantitative properties about drugs. First, there is a threshold for each drug-induced response. Doses of drug below that threshold will produce no observable effect. Second, the drug-induced response will reach a plateau rather than increase indefinitely. For example, the drug shown in Figure 1-4 produces its maximum response at a dose of about 512 units. Doubling the dose produces no detectable further effect. Even beginning at lower drug concentrations, doubling the dose still does not double the effect. In this example the 50% maximum response to this drug is produced by a dose of 16 units, but twice that dose (32 units) produces only about 70%, not 100%, of the maximum response. In summary, the dose-response curve demonstrates that a finite dose is required to see a response and that doubling the dose does not necessarily double the response.

The dose-response curve in Figure 1-4 shows the effect of a drug on an individual (or average responses from several individuals). The same type of curve is produced when the drug response is instead defined as an all-or-none phenomenon (e.g., asleep vs. awake) and the logarithm of the drug dose is plotted against the percentage of patients who show the drug effect at that given dose. The plateau for this curve is the drug dose at which all patients respond, and the threshold is the drug dose below which no patients respond. The recommended therapeutic dose of the drug is a dose at which most patients respond to the drug. Figure 1-5 shows this second type of dose-response curve.

Drugs produce multiple predictable biologic effects, and for each of these effects a dose-response curve may be drawn. For example, the drug digitalis increases the force of contraction of a failing heart, but it also produces nausea, headaches,

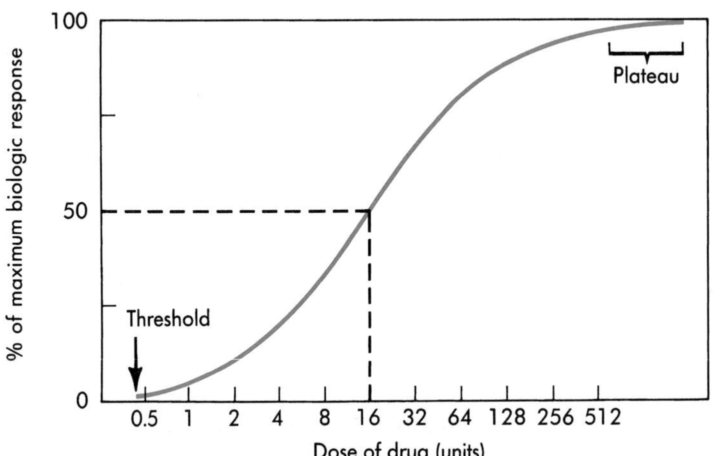

FIGURE 1-4
Log dose-response curve. Percent of maximum biologic response is plotted on linear scale on vertical axis. Dose of drug is plotted on logarithmic scale on horizontal axis. Threshold is dose of drug required to cause measurable response. Plateau is region of curve where increasing drug dose does not increase biologic response.

visual disturbances, and cardiac arrhythmias and ultimately triggers ventricular fibrillation. Each of these responses can be plotted as a dose-response curve (see Figure 1-5). The dose-response curve for nausea lies close to the dose-response curve for the therapeutic effect; therefore many patients receiving therapeutic doses of digitalis also experience nausea. With increasing doses of the drug, more and more patients suffer visual disturbances and arrhythmias. At drug concentrations well above normal therapeutic doses, ventricular fibrillation occurs. These predictable drug reactions become an important part of patient care. For digitalis the visual disturbances are a warning that the concentration of drug in the patient is approaching toxic levels, which can cause cardiac arrhythmias and ventricular fibrillation.

Each drug may be described as relatively safe or relatively dangerous, based on dose-response curves such as those in Figure 1-5. For example, nausea is frequently associated with the use of digitalis because doses that produce nausea are only slightly greater than those that increase the force of contraction of the heart. Doses of digitalis that produce more serious reactions are only slightly higher than those that cause nausea. Digitalis therefore is a drug with a narrow margin of safety; doses must be rigorously controlled, and great care must be taken to keep blood levels of the drug within a very narrow range. In contrast, a drug with a wide margin of safety, such as penicillin G, may be given in does greatly exceeding normal therapeutic doses without much danger of producing direct toxic effects.

Therapeutic index. The relative safety of drugs is also sometimes expressed as a therapeutic index. The therapeutic index (TI) is the ratio of the dose of the drug lethal in 50% of a tested population (LD_{50}) to the dose of the drug therapeutically effective in 50% of the tested population (ED_{50}), or TI = LD_{50}/ED_{50}. These figures come from tests conducted in animals. A drug with a high therapeutic index has a wide safety margin; the lethal dose greatly exceeds the therapeutic dose. A drug with a low therapeutic index is more dangerous for patients because small increases over normal doses may be sufficient to induce toxic reactions.

Time Course of Drug Action

Drugs may enter the body by a number of routes, but, except for the intravenous route, some time will be required for the drug to enter the blood after administration. There is also a delay between the time the drug enters the blood and the time it reaches its site of action. If the response to a single dose of a drug is measured as a function of time, the pattern shown in Figure 1-6 is observed. The time for the **onset** of drug action is the time it takes after the drug is administered to reach a concentration that produces a response. As the drug continues to be absorbed, higher concentrations of drug reach the site of action, and the response increases. As the drug is being absorbed, it is also subject to influences that tend to eliminate it from the body. Ultimately elimination dominates, and the concentration of drug in the body begins to fall. As a result the response will also begin to diminish. The **time to peak effect** is the time it takes for the drug to reach its highest effective concentration. The **duration** of action of a drug is the time during which the drug is present in a concentration large enough to produce a response. Onset and duration are determined by the rates of absorption and elimination.

Insulins are good examples of drugs for which an understanding of onset and duration of action is critical for successful drug therapy. Insulin lowers blood sugar levels, and the peak drug action must be planned to coincide with the absorptive period after meals when blood sugar levels rise rapidly. If insulin is injected at the proper dose but at the wrong time, a serious hypoglycemic (low blood sugar) reaction may endanger the patient.

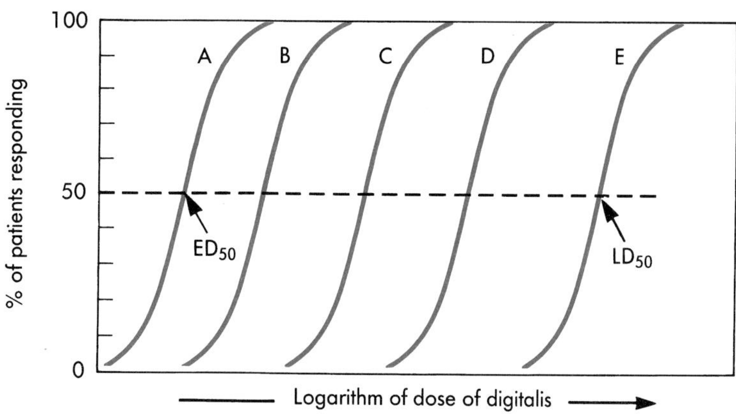

FIGURE 1-5

Log dose-response curves for effects of digitalis. Percent of patients responding to digitalis is plotted on vertical axis, and dose of digitalis is plotted on logarithmic scale on horizontal axis. These undesirable effects are all dose-related responses to digitalis. *Curve A,* strengthened force of contraction of heart produced by digitalis; *curve B,* nausea; *curve C,* visual disturbances; *curve D,* cardiac arrhythmias; *curve E,* ventricular fibrillation and death.

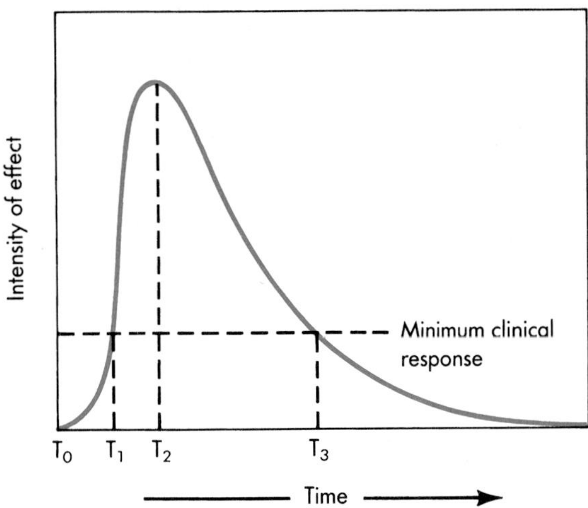

FIGURE 1-6
Time course of action of single dose of drug. Drug is administered at *T0*. Time interval between *T0* and *T1* represents time of onset of action of drug. Peak action occurs at *T2*. Time interval between *T0* and *T2* represents time for peak action. At *T3*, drug response falls below minimum required for clinical effectiveness. Time interval between *T1* and *T3* represents duration of action of drug.

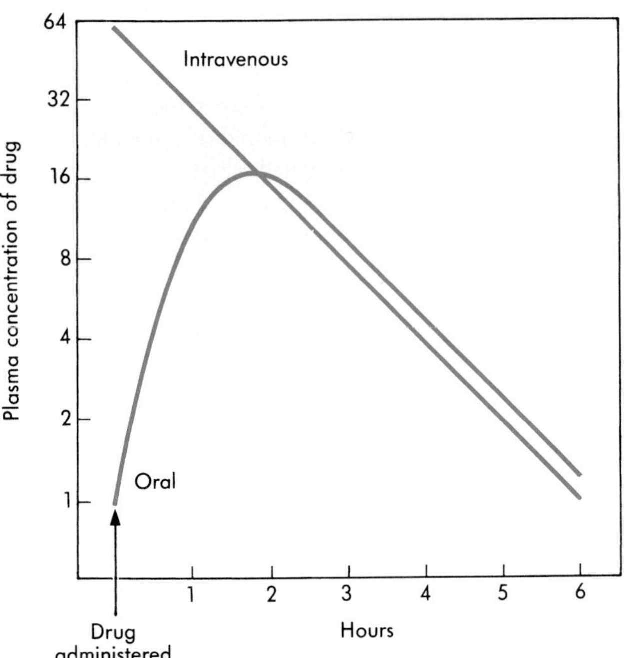

FIGURE 1-7
Absorption and elimination rates for drug administered by oral or intravenous route. Plasma concentration of drug is plotted on logarithmic scale on vertical axis.

Half-life. The concepts of onset and duration of drug action are also important for understanding the proper timing of administration of drugs given repeatedly for a course of therapy. The drug **half-life,** or elimination half-time, is how long it takes for elimination processes to reduce the blood concentration of drug by half. For example, the peak concentration of penicillin G in blood occurs a few moments after the drug is administered intravenously. Thereafter penicillin is rapidly excreted by the kidneys and disappears from blood. The length of time required for these processes to decrease the blood concentration of penicillin by 50% is the drug half-life, or elimination half-time, which for penicillin G is about 20 minutes. Therefore 20 minutes after an intravenous dose of penicillin, only one half of the initial concentration of drug remains in the blood. After 40 minutes only one quarter of the initial concentration remains, and after 60 minutes only one eighth remains. During each succeeding 20-minute period the remaining concentration decreases by half.

When drug absorption is not instantaneous, elimination processes compete with absorptive processes, delaying the appearance of peak blood concentrations of drug. The example shown in Figure 1-7 is for a drug with a half-life of 1 hour. When the drug is given intravenously, the highest concentration is achieved on administration and decreases thereafter because of elimination processes. When the same dose is given orally, the drug is absorbed relatively slowly so that drug elimination is responsible for lowering the peak drug concentration that can be achieved. Once in the general circulation, however, the drug is eliminated in the same way, no matter what the initial route of administration.

Plateau principle. When a drug is given repeatedly for therapy at fixed dosage intervals, its concentration in blood reaches a plateau and is maintained at that level until the dose or the frequency of administration is changed. An example is shown in Figure 1-8, in which a rapidly absorbed drug is given at fixed intervals. The concentration of drug in blood fluctuates around a mean value, which approaches a plateau after four elimination half-times have passed; this leveling off happens regardless of the dose or frequency of administration, as long as these factors are constant. The actual dose of drug and frequency of dosage determine the plateau concentration of drug in the blood, but they do not determine how long it will take to reach that plateau.

As an example of this plateau principle, consider a patient who is given a drug with a half-life of 24 hours. The patient takes 1 tablet at 8 AM every day. In 4 days the amount of drug being taken in each dose roughly equals the amount of drug being eliminated each day; the plateau has been reached (Figure 1-9, *patient A*). The dose in this case is sufficient to produce clinically effective blood levels but is below the level that produces toxicity. On day 6 the patient decides to take 2 tablets instead of 1 tablet each morning. As a result the mean concentration of the drug in the blood rises, and after 4 days (four elimination half-times) a new plateau concentration is reached. At this new higher level some drug toxicity is seen. When the patient returns to the old dosage schedule of 1 tablet daily, the mean drug concentration returns to the original plateau concentration after 4 days (four elimination half-times) and is maintained until the dosage amount or intervals change.

Patient B in Figure 1-9 receives the same drug as patient A, but patient B takes 1 tablet every 12 hours instead of once daily. As a result the plateau concentration of drug in the blood is higher in patient B than when patient A took 1

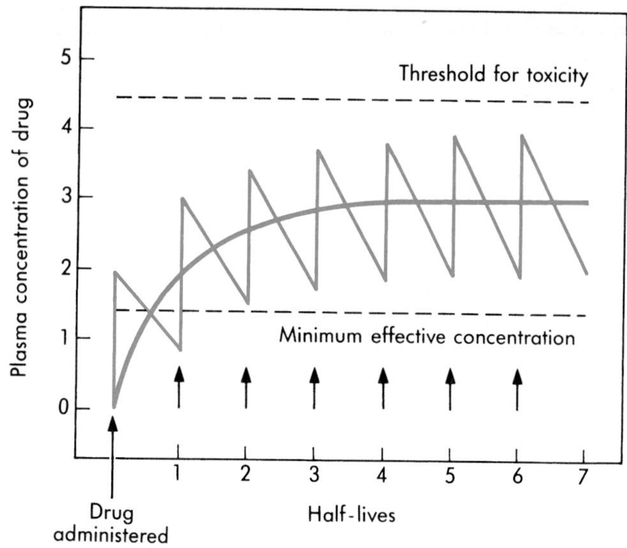

FIGURE 1-8

Plateau principle. In example, drug is administered once every elimination half-time for drug. Plasma concentration of drug rises and falls as drug doses are rapidly absorbed and slowly eliminated. Drug accumulates over time so that after four elimination half-times average plasma concentration of drug has reached steady state. By adjusting dose, average plasma concentration of drug may be adjusted.

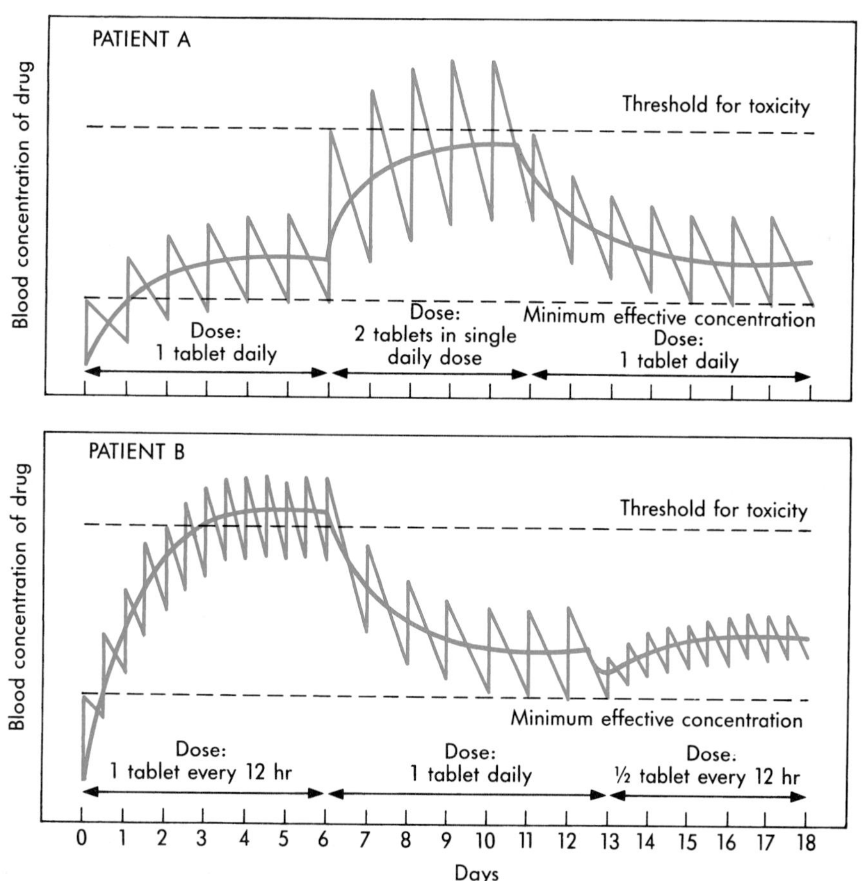

FIGURE 1-9

Plateau principle in practice. Patient A receives drug with half-time of 24 hours. Increasing dose of drug from 1 to 2 tablets in single daily dose increases plateau concentration of drug. In contrast, patient B illustrates that, by dividing dose (taking ½ tablet every 12 hours rather than 1 tablet once daily), fluctuations in drug concentration are minimized.

tablet every 24 hours. Note, however, that it still takes 4 days (four elimination half-times) to reach the plateau concentration. After 3 days of therapy patient B mentions some unusual symptoms, which the nurse recognizes as toxic reactions to the drug. On the basis of this report the physician reduces the frequency of drug dosing to 1 tablet daily. After 5 days on this dosage schedule the patient complains that the medication effect wears off by early morning. The physician therefore advises the patient to take a ½ tablet every 12 hours. This dosage regimen minimizes fluctuations in drug concentration in blood, but the mean plateau concentration is ultimately the same.

These examples illustrate the importance of maintaining regular dosage schedules and adhering to prescribed doses and dosage intervals. If the total dose of drug administered during each drug half-life is held constant, the average concentration of drug in the blood stays constant. Timing of the dose (single dose or divided doses) affects the peak concentration and the minimum concentration of the drug in blood. For some drugs these variations may not be critical, but for many drugs the difference between a safe dose and a toxic dose is not great.

Monitoring levels of certain drugs in blood is a routine part of patient care in many settings. Direct assays for drugs allow physicians to adjust doses to ensure safe and effective blood levels of such drugs as gentamicin, amikacin, digitoxin, and phenytoin, which have a low therapeutic index. The nurse's responsibility in dealing with patients being monitored in this way may include drawing blood samples at specific times or adjusting the dosage or timing of doses in response to the physician's instructions.

NURSING PROCESS OVERVIEW

Drugs in the Body

Assessment

The material presented in this chapter forms the framework for subsequent specific information about drugs. Study the mechanism of action of each drug class presented. Does this drug operate through specific receptors? Does it alter a body fluid or cell membranes? What are the anticipated effects? How does the typical patient manifest these effects?

Planning/Implementation

Consider the possible side effects of the action of the drug in tissues. For example, does the drug affect receptors in more than one organ or tissue? Note whether experience has indicated that allergies or idiosyncratic reactions are common with the drug. How might the drug's half-life influence the patient's response? What is the drug's dosing schedule?

Evaluation

Consider the balance between the positive effects of the drug and the negative reactions to understand what place a drug has in clinical practice. For example, some highly effective drugs have limited clinical use because the side effects that they produce are unacceptable for most patients. Understanding the pharmacology of individual drugs thus becomes a rational process and is much more easily accomplished. Chapter 4 deals with the application of the nursing process to drug therapy.

CRITICAL THINKING

APPLICATION

1. What is the difference between a drug action and a side effect?
2. What are the two major types of unpredictable reactions to drugs that the nurse may encounter?
3. What are the four types of allergic reactions to drugs that the nurse may encounter?
4. What are the three general mechanisms by which drugs interact with a patient's body to produce a biologic effect?
5. What is an agonist?
6. What is a drug antagonist?
7. How does affinity differ from efficacy?
8. How are pharmacodynamics and pharmacokinetics helpful to the nurse in understanding the clinical use of drugs?
9. Describe how a drug in tablet form enters the blood after oral administration. What factors may influence absorption?
10. What is the first-pass phenomenon? Does it apply to all routes of administration?
11. How does the binding of drugs to proteins in the blood influence the effect of the drug?
12. What is biotransformation?
13. What is enterohepatic circulation?
14. What information is expressed in a log dose-response curve?
15. What is the therapeutic index of a drug?
16. What is the onset time for a drug, and how does it differ from the duration of action of a drug? What is the elimination half-time of a drug?
17. What is the plateau principle?

CRITICAL THINKING

1. What are the advantages and disadvantages of subcutaneous, intramuscular, and intravenous routes of drug administration?

CHAPTER 2

Effects of Life Span, Genetics, and Medical Conditions on Drug Therapy

OBJECTIVES

After studying this chapter, you should be able to do the following:

- *Explain why fetuses and neonates may be more sensitive to drugs than are adults.*
- *Discuss why certain drugs such as tetracyclines should be avoided in children.*
- *Explain why older adults may need reduced doses of drugs.*
- *Discuss why glucose-6-phosphate dehydrogenase deficiency increases the risk of hemolysis with certain drugs.*
- *Discuss what adjustments in drug therapy may be necessary for patients with renal or hepatic impairment.*
- *Explain how drugs may interact in the body.*
- *Discuss the effects of alcohol or smoking on drug effects.*

KEY TERMS

creatinine clearance
disulfiram reaction
drug interaction
hemolysis
iatrogenic
induction
potentiation
synergism

CHAPTER OVERVIEW

Not all patients respond to a particular drug dosage in the same way. Moreover, it is usually not possible to predict which patients will be more sensitive or less sensitive to a drug than normal. The term *normal* in this context means average.

Biologic variability is based on subtle physiologic differences among people. For example, absorption of oral drug doses can be greatly influenced by stomach acidity, gastrointestinal motility, pancreatic function, and gastrointestinal bacteria. These parameters vary greatly in most people. Likewise, individuals vary in the sensitivity of certain tissues to drugs. This variability may result from differences in the number or type of drug receptors, differences in permeability barriers, and many other factors. These factors are all difficult to assess and yet greatly influence the magnitude of drug effects in patients.

In the clinical setting the causes of biologic variation are not usually known for certain. Patients are observed for proper response to a drug, and dosages are usually adjusted on the basis of clinical assessment of progress. Although the exact causes of biologic variation are not known for an individual, factors such as age, gender, genetic background, and overall health status can influence patient responses to medications.

EFFECTS OF AGE ON DRUG RESPONSE

Embryos and Fetuses

Developing embryos and fetuses are unintended targets of drugs and chemicals taken by their mothers. The effects of many drugs are benign or at least cannot be proved to be harmful, but a few drugs pose grave risks to the unborn. The degree of damage may be related to dose and length of exposure, but it is often also associated with the developmental stage of the fetus at the time of exposure. Table 2-1 summarizes the potential adverse effects of representative drugs.

Drugs that are absorbed systemically have been labeled by the Food and Drug Administration (FDA) according to the level of risk to a fetus. These FDA pregnancy categories are summarized in Table 2-2, along with examples of drugs in each category. Discussions of individual drugs throughout the text also refer to the FDA pregnancy category.

Neonates

Premature infants and neonates may respond to medications quite differently from adults or older children. Many of these different responses are caused by immaturity of the liver and kidneys in infants. At birth the liver lacks many of the metabolizing enzymes that enable an adult liver to biotransform various types of compounds. Before these metabolizing enzymes increase to adult levels during the first weeks or months of life, neonates are more vulnerable than adults to chemicals requiring detoxification in the liver.

The kidney is also less efficient at birth than in adult life. Therefore excretion of many compounds takes longer in neonates than in adults. Failure to take into account this reduced excretory capacity when calculating drug dosage can be important when certain drugs are administered to a neonate.

The antibiotic chloramphenicol illustrates the clinical effect of reduced detoxification and excretion in neonates. This potentially toxic drug is detoxified in the adult liver by the formation of chloramphenicol glucuronide, a metabolite that is efficiently excreted by adult kidneys. Unable to form the glucuronide or excrete the drug efficiently, neonates quickly accumulate chloramphenicol and suffer potentially lethal toxicity. This deadly outcome is prevented by reducing the dose of drug to take into account the reduced routes of elimina-

TABLE 2-1 Adverse Drug Effects During Pregnancy*

EFFECT OF DRUG	DRUGS KNOWN TO PRODUCE THE EFFECT IN HUMANS
First-Trimester Effects on Embryonic Development	
Abortion	Isotretinoin, quinine
Multiple anomalies involving craniofacial development	Dicumarol, ethanol, isotretinoin, methotrexate, paramethadione, phenytoin, quinine, trimethadione
Neural tube defects	Valproate
Goiter	Iodide, methimazole, propylthiouracil
Abnormalities of reproductive organs	Androgens, diethylstilbestrol, estrogens, progestins
Inhibition of growth	Methotrexate, tetracycline, tobacco smoke
Second- and Third-Trimester Effects on Fetal Development	
Abortion, mortality	Heroin, isotretinoin, tobacco smoke
Mental retardation	Dicumarol, ethanol
Altered cardiovascular function	Anticholinergic drugs, propranolol, terbutaline
Hearing loss and loss of balance	Aminoglycoside antibiotics
Hyperbilirubinemia	Nitrofurantoin, sulfonamides
Hemolytic anemia	Nitrofurantoin
Goiter	Iodide, methimazole, propylthiouracil
Abnormalities of reproductive organs	Androgens, diethylstilbestrol, estrogens, progestins
Inhibition of growth	Dicumarol, ethanol, heroin, methotrexate, tetracycline, tobacco smoke
Labor, Delivery, and Perinatal Period	
Increased mortality	Tobacco smoking, cocaine abuse
Altered cardiovascular function	Anticholinergic agents, caffeine, heroin, lidocaine, meperidine, propranolol, terbutaline
Gray-baby syndrome	Chloramphenicol
Respiratory depression	Diazepam, meperidine, morphine, phenobarbital, ethanol, tobacco smoking
Respiratory distress	Reserpine
Bleeding	Aspirin, dicumarol, indomethacin
Hypoglycemia	Chlorpropamide, propranolol, tolbutamide
Hyperbilirubinemia	Nitrofurantoin, sulfonamides
Hemolytic anemia	Nitrofurantoin
Hyperirritability	Cocaine

*This list does not include all drugs that affect fetal and neonatal function but is intended to give representative examples. The nurse should check sources of specific information about individual agents when drugs are administered to pregnant patients.

TABLE 2-2 FDA Pregnancy Categories

CATEGORY	LEVEL OF RISK WITH DRUG EXPOSURE	EXAMPLES
A	Controlled studies in women fail to demonstrate risk in the first trimester (and there is no evidence of risk in later trimesters), and possibility of fetal harm appears remote.	Thyroid hormones
B	Animal reproduction studies have not demonstrated fetal risk, but there are no controlled studies in pregnant women. Animal reproduction studies have shown adverse effect (other than decreased fertility) that was not confirmed in controlled studies on women in first trimester. There is no evidence of risk in later trimesters.	Amoxicillin, buspirone, cimetidine, fluoxetine, hydrochlorothiazide, metronidazole, piperacillin
C	Studies in animals have revealed adverse effects on fetus, and there are no controlled studies in women. In some cases, studies in women and animals are not available. Drugs in this category should be given only if potential benefit justifies risk to fetus.	Alteplase, captopril, ciprofloxacin, codeine, enalapril, gentamicin, isoproterenol, lisinopril, morphine, nizatidine, reserpine, tubocurarine
D	There is positive evidence of human fetal risk, but the benefits for pregnant women may be acceptable despite the risk, as in life-threatening diseases for which safer drugs cannot be used or are ineffective. An appropriate statement must appear in the "warnings" section of the labeling of drugs in this category.	Amikacin, midazolam, netilmicin, tobramycin
X	Studies in animals or humans have demonstrated fetal abnormalities, there is evidence of fetal risk based on human experience, or both. The risk of using the drug in pregnant women clearly outweighs any possible benefit. The drug is contraindicated in women who are or may become pregnant. An appropriate statement must appear in the "contraindications" section of the labeling of drugs in this category.	Isotretinoin, lovastatin, methotrexate

tion. The result is that less drug is required per kilogram of body weight to maintain effective concentrations of chloramphenicol in neonates than in adults.

Infants and Children

It is not safe to assume that any drug used in adults can also be used at adjusted doses in children. Many drugs have not been adequately tested in children, and therefore safe doses have not been established. This situation occurs frequently with new drugs. As more experience is gained, the drug may be made available for children and recommended dosages may be published, or the drug may be contraindicated in children. For example, tetracycline antibiotics are used safely by most adults, but these drugs should not be used in children. This class of antibiotics binds tightly to bones and may impede bone growth in very young children. Tetracycline antibiotics also bind to calcium salts in teeth and become permanently incorporated in teeth that are forming. Since children younger than 12 years old are constantly forming teeth, their teeth may become permanently discolored by tetracycline. These problems are avoided by limiting the use of tetracycline antibiotics to adults or children older than 12 years.

Children can be sensitive to drugs because development of some tissues is not complete until adulthood. For example, the fluoroquinolone antibiotics are known to damage cartilage in young animals, which leads to deformities and changes in gait. The risk of this effect, which is specific for young mammals whose cartilage is still developing, is sufficient reason to avoid using these drugs in children.

Children can also have special sensitivity to certain drugs. For example, aspirin is used safely by millions of adults, but this drug can cause a dangerous reaction in children who are suffering from a viral infection such as chickenpox. Although this reaction is uncommon, it is sufficient cause to avoid administering aspirin to children with fever.

Older Adults

Older adults are also especially at risk from many drugs. Several factors may be involved. Altered central nervous system function may mask signs of drug toxicity. Reduced renal function and changes in ratios of body water, body fat, and lean muscle mass can influence the distribution of a drug in the body and change rates of excretion. Older adult patients are more likely to be malnourished, which may alter serum albumin levels and influence drug binding. Older adults often suffer from chronic diseases, and therefore they may be receiving more than one drug, which increases their risk of drug interactions. For these reasons older adults need special attention to detect early signs of drug interactions or drug toxicity related to diminished excretory capacity, altered drug sensitivity, or altered drug distribution.

The aminoglycoside antibiotic gentamicin exemplifies the type of drug likely to cause troublesome reactions in older adults. Aminoglycosides are excreted almost exclusively by the kidneys. Since renal function decreases with age, older adult patients excrete aminoglycosides at reduced rates. If the physician does not reduce doses to take this effect into account, aminoglycosides will accumulate. One of the early signs of toxicity may be partial loss of hearing or equilibrium, but loss of hearing or an unstable gait in an older adult patient may be mistaken for a sign of aging. Therefore the older patient may suffer toxicity for a longer time than a younger patient would because in the younger patient the same signs would be recognized immediately as **iatrogenic** (caused by a drug). Moreover, if an older person is taking an aminoglycoside and also receiving a drug such as furosemide for hypertension, the risk of ototoxicity is increased because both aminoglycosides and furosemide cause this side effect.

Nursing Process Overview

Life Span

Assessment

Assess the patient's age and weight. If the patient is an infant, was the child premature? Assess the patient's ethnic background. Take a family health history and check for allergies. Check renal function and liver function tests. Assess the patient's history of smoking or alcohol use.

Nursing Diagnoses

There are no diagnoses based solely on the patient's age or background, but this information combined with an individualized assessment may provide the foundation for a nursing diagnosis.

Patient Outcomes

Information about the patient's age, gender, ethnic background, history of smoking or alcohol use, and existing medical problems will be reflected, if appropriate, in the dose and choice of drug prescribed. The patient will improve without serious adverse effects.

Planning/Implementation

Monitor the patient's vital signs and weight. Calculate dosages carefully, especially if the doses are small for infants and children. Monitor intake and output if necessary to monitor renal function. Encourage the patient to limit smoking or stop if possible. Monitor parameters that would indicate improvement in the patient's condition, and consult with the physician when there are indications that the dose of medication may be inappropriate for a specific patient situation. Develop and implement a teaching plan appropriate for the age of the patient.

Evaluation

Ideally, there will be improvement in the patient's health status, with few side effects. Any side effects that do occur will be minor and will be diagnosed early. Adjustments in dose or drug will be made based on regular evaluation of the patient's condition.

EFFECTS OF GENETIC TRAITS ON DRUG THERAPY

Gender of the Patient

Men and women may respond differently to drugs. For example, metabolism of a drug such as propranolol occurs much more quickly in men than in women. As a result, when similar doses are used, the levels of drug in blood are about twice as high in women as in men. Whether such differences exist for the vast majority of drugs is not known because specific trials to show differences based on gender have not been performed.

Men and women also respond differently to small amounts of ingested ethanol. In men a high level of the enzyme alcohol dehydrogenase exists in the stomach; this enzyme rapidly destroys significant amounts of the alcohol before it can be absorbed. In women the level of this enzyme is reduced and as a result more ethanol is absorbed, producing a higher blood level of the drug than the same dose produces in men.

Specific Traits Related to Ethnicity

Different ethnic groups may respond differently to some drug classes. For example, blockers of the beta-adrenergic receptors are frequently used to control blood pressure, but African-American patients tend to respond less well to beta-blockers than do Caucasians; Chinese patients are much more sensitive to these drugs than either Caucasian or African-American patients. The causes of these differences are not well understood, but they may involve dietary factors and differences in drug metabolism.

Glucose-6-Phosphate Dehydrogenase Deficiency

Some drug reactions are clearly linked to a particular genetic trait that is more prevalent in certain ethnic groups. For example, the enzyme glucose-6-phosphate dehydrogenase (G6PD) is abundant in the tissues of most people. In red blood cells this enzyme plays a role in generating reduced nicotinamide-adenine dinucleotide phosphate (NADPH), a compound required to maintain active hemoglobin. As a result of a genetic alteration, some persons lack adequate concentrations of this enzyme in their red blood cells. Therefore NADPH is generated slowly. Under normal circumstances this alteration would not be critical, but if a person with this trait is exposed to chemicals that enhance the conversion of hemoglobin to methemoglobin (a relatively inactive form of hemoglobin), serious problems can arise. Because of the lack of G6PD, too little NADPH is present to fully reform active hemoglobin. When too much methemoglobin accumulates, the red blood cell is destroyed.

G6PD deficiency is important for pharmacology because many drugs accelerate methemoglobin formation. Sulfonamides, antimalarial medications, and analgesic-antipyretic drugs (including aspirin) fall into this category. In a person lacking adequate G6PD activity, these drugs can cause life-threatening **hemolysis** (rupture of the red blood cells). The same drugs are relatively innocuous in most people who possess adequate G6PD activity.

Certain populations have a high proportion of the gene that causes G6PD deficiency. For example, 13% of African-American men and 20% of African-American women may carry this gene. Sardinians also have an incidence of approximately 14%. More than half of Kurdish Jewish populations show G6PD deficiencies. This genetic difference from the majority of the American population places patients from these special populations at greater risk for serious reactions with certain drugs. When these patients receive medications, they should be observed carefully for signs of toxicity.

Acetylation

The rate of drug acetylation in the liver is another genetically determined trait that may affect the incidence of certain drug reactions. About one half of Americans, both African-Americans and Caucasians, possess liver enzyme systems that acetylate drugs and other chemicals slowly, at rates less than half of those of the rest of the population. In contrast, slow acetylation is very rare in Eskimos and persons of Japanese ancestry.

Isoniazid, a drug used to treat tuberculosis, illustrates how the genetically determined ability to acetylate a drug can influence unwanted reactions. Isoniazid is inactivated primarily by acetylation and is eliminated in urine entirely as metabolites. In slow acetylators the half-life of the drug is about 3 hours, but in rapid acetylators it is only about 1 hour. Liver damage may be more common in rapid acetylators because the concentration of a hepatotoxic acetylated metabolite is high. Slow acetylation may be more closely associated with dose-related toxicity (neuropathy, depression of liver biotransformation enzymes) because the untransformed drug may accumulate in persons with this trait. Therefore doses may need to be lowered for slow acetylators.

Pseudocholinesterase Deficiency

Not all differences in drug handling are related to observable traits such as gender or ethnicity. Unsuspected genetic differences can produce unexpected reactions to drugs. For example, a small percentage of the population lacks pseudocholinesterase, an enzyme usually found in blood. Persons lacking this enzyme show no signs of this difference until they are exposed to drugs such as succinylcholine. Succinylcholine is a paralyzing agent used before surgery to relax the muscles and allow easy tracheal intubation. In most persons the drug is very short acting because it is destroyed by pseudocholinesterase. In persons lacking this enzyme, succinylcholine stays in the bloodstream, and the drug is very long acting. These patients require artificial ventilation until the paralyzing effects of succinylcholine wear off, whereas most people recover within a minute and require no assistance.

EFFECTS OF MEDICAL CONDITIONS ON DRUG THERAPY

Renal Impairment

Renal function decreases with age, but it can also be diminished in younger persons as a result of progressive hypertension, diabetes mellitus, or other causes. For many drugs excreted primarily through renal processes, doses must be adjusted to compensate for reduced renal excretion. For example, cephalosporin antibiotics such as ceftazidime are excreted renally, and blood levels of the antibiotic are influenced by the degree of renal impairment. If reduced renal excretion is not taken into account, the drug may accumulate to toxic levels.

To adjust dosage to compensate for renal impairment, some measure of renal function must be made. A common measure of renal function is **creatinine clearance,** expressed in milliliters per minute (ml/min) or milliliters per second. Creatinine clearance is 100 to 120 ml/min when renal function is normal. Table 2-3 shows information from the package insert for the antibiotic ceftazidime. Note that if creatinine clearance is >50 ml/min, no dosage adjustment is needed with this drug; the normal adult dose of 1 gm every 8 hours can be given. If renal function is impaired, lower creatinine clearances are noted, and the dosage interval must be increased and/or the dose must be decreased. Note that if renal function is lost and the patient is undergoing hemodialysis, the dose is given only once in the interval between hemodialyses. Without renal excretion, blood levels of the drug persist for prolonged periods.

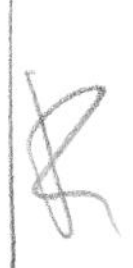

If direct measurement of creatinine clearance cannot be made, this value can be estimated from creatinine concentrations in the serum according to the following formula:

$$\text{Creatinine clearance (men)} = \frac{(140 - \text{Age}) \times (\text{Body weight in kg})}{72 \times \text{Serum creatinine}}$$

The creatinine clearance for women is 85% of the value calculated by this equation. This formula is not as accurate as a direct determination of clearance, but measuring serum cre-

TABLE 2-3 Adjustment of Ceftazidime Dosage Based on Renal Function

CREATININE CLEARANCE (ML/MIN)	DOSAGE
>50	Usual adult dose (1 gm q8h)
31-50	1 gm q12h
16-30	1 gm q24h
6-15	500 mg q24h
<5	500 mg q48h
Hemodialysis patients:	1 gm after each hemodialysis period

atinine is much easier than measuring clearances and the accuracy of this calculation is adequate for most situations.

Alterations of Hepatic Function

Liver function may be diminished by drugs, infectious agents, or chronic alcohol consumption. These factors may make a patient much more sensitive than normal to toxicity from specific drugs. For example, the antituberculosis agent isoniazid causes clinical hepatitis in about 0.3% of healthy young adults who receive it for prophylaxis. In contrast, the incidence of acute hepatitis is 2.6% in patients who drink alcohol daily or who have significant liver disease.

Certain chemicals cause the liver to make more drug-metabolizing enzymes. This process, called **induction,** allows the liver to metabolize drugs more efficiently. For example, the anticonvulsant phenytoin can stimulate hepatic metabolism of the bronchodilator theophylline. As a result the therapeutic effects of theophylline may be lost or diminished.

As a rule drug dosage is not adjusted based strictly on measures of hepatic function. The common strategy is to monitor blood levels of the drug in question and adjust dosage accordingly. In the example just given, for a patient receiving both phenytoin and theophylline, serum concentrations of both drugs should be monitored and the doses should be adjusted to maintain therapeutic concentrations.

Drug Interactions

Patients frequently have more than one condition for which they receive medical attention, and therefore they often take more than one medication at a time (see box). This situation creates the possibility for the drugs to interact. A **drug interaction** is any modification of the action of one drug by another drug. Interactions may either increase or decrease the action of the drugs involved. Drug **synergism** is a special interaction in which the effect of two drugs combined is greater than the effect expected if the individual effects of the two drugs independently were added together.

Drug interactions are commonly encountered in clinical practice and are sometimes planned as part of a therapeutic program. An excellent example is the treatment of chronic moderate hypertension, which frequently involves several

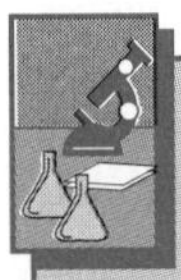

Research Highlight

Drug Combinations and Potential for Risk of Adverse Drug Reaction Among Community-Dwelling Elderly

— RL Pollow, EP Stoller, LE Forster, TS Duniko: Nurs Res 43(1):44, 1994.

PURPOSE

Research has shown repeatedly that older adults take large numbers of prescription and over-the-counter (OTC) medications. These medications place patients at risk for adverse drug reactions (ADRs), some serious enough to result in hospitalization. Older adults are at risk because of the physiologic changes associated with aging, multiple chronic health problems, and the number of medications they take. It is recognized that some categories of drugs, including analgesics, antiarthritics, anticoagulants, and antihypertensives, place older adults, in comparison to other groups, at greater risk for ADR. What is the incidence of drug use and the potential for ADRs in community-based older adults?

SAMPLE

Subjects included people older than age 65 who were selected through probability sampling in northeastern New York state. There were 667 participants. All lived in a community setting. The living environment for the sample included rural areas (12%), rural villages (22%), communities with a population of 2500 to 25,000 (50%), and urban areas with a population greater than 25,000 (16%). The mean age was 74.1 years.

METHODOLOGY

A structured personal interview was held with each participant. Patients who were unsure of the names of the medications they were taking were asked to show their medications to the interviewer. Respondents were also asked about alcohol consumption.

FINDINGS

The most frequently reported prescription medication category was antihypertensives (35.4%), followed by diuretics (27%), antiarthritics (18.9%), antianginals (12.3%), cardiac drugs (11.2%), and psychoactive drugs (10.6%). Almost one quarter (24.7%) took no prescription medications. Only 4.5% were taking no medications at all. Over half of the participants (57.1%) sometimes drank alcohol.

Data indicated that 65.8% took at least one potentially risky combination. Possible adverse outcomes associated with drug-drug or drug-alcohol combinations included hypotension, cognitive impairment, bleeding, counteractive effects (caused by two or more drugs with opposing actions), potentiation of diabetic medications, and potentiation of diuretics.

IMPLICATIONS

Older adult patients take many medications. Although many of these patients manage their drug regimens without difficulty, the number of medications places them at risk for potential problems. Nurses must anticipate the need for thorough and repeated teaching.

drugs, each amplifying the action of the others to lower the blood pressure.

The negative aspect of drug interaction is that expected therapeutic results from a drug can be greatly affected by other drugs. This negative influence can be diminished if health care personnel are aware of major drug interactions, are thorough in determining which over-the-counter or prescription drugs a patient is taking, and give careful instruction to patients about drugs that interact with their prescribed medication.

Comprehensive lists of drug interactions have been published.

Pharmacokinetic Interactions

Drug interactions may arise when one drug alters the pharmacokinetics of another drug. For example, one drug may alter the dissolution, absorption, protein-binding activity, metabolism, or elimination of another drug. Pharmacokinetic interactions change the concentration of drug in the blood and at its site of action. For instance, if one drug decreases the absorption of a second drug, the concentration of the second drug is diminished and therefore the usual dose does not give the expected result. The same effect is produced if the metabolism or elimination of the second drug is increased by the first drug.

Some drugs also increase the concentration of other drugs, producing **potentiation.** Pharmacokinetic potentiation may arise because one drug increases the absorption or decreases the protein-binding activity, metabolism, or elimination of a second drug. The second drug is therefore present in higher concentrations than would be anticipated for the dose.

Pharmacodynamic Interactions

Drug interactions may also arise when one drug alters the pharmacodynamics of a second drug. If two drugs have the same action, drug potentiation results. An example is seen with vasodilators, which can lower blood pressure. A vasodilator such as hydralazine might be part of a therapeutic program for control of hypertension. Nitroglycerin is another vasodilator, but it is used to relieve angina. Patients who take hydralazine for hypertension and also take nitroglycerin for angina should anticipate a severe hypotensive response to nitroglycerin; they may need to lie down when taking the nitroglycerin to avoid fainting.

Drugs that are antagonists often produce pharmacodynamic interactions that diminish the response of both drugs at the usual therapeutic doses. An example is the beta-receptor antagonist propranolol, often prescribed for patients with hypertension. If such a patient were to develop asthma, a beta-receptor agonist such as albuterol would be indicated. Although in this example the therapeutic target for propranolol is the heart and that for albuterol is the bronchioles, the two drugs would antagonize each other at all organs with beta-adrenergic receptors and neither drug would give the desired therapeutic effect. (In fact, propranolol would make the asthma worse and could not be used.)

ENVIRONMENTAL FACTORS AFFECTING DRUG THERAPY

Smoking

In addition to medications, environmental chemicals increasingly are being recognized as agents that cause significant drug interactions in some patients. For example, polycyclic hydrocarbons in cigarette smoke and chlorinated hydrocarbons in pesticides are active inducers of liver metabolic enzymes. Persons chronically exposed to these chemicals metabolize drugs such as the antiasthmatic medication theophylline more rapidly than normal. In these persons the blood concentration of theophylline may be lower than desired unless dosage adjustments are made (see Chapter 27).

Alcohol

Alcohol (ethanol) is a common cause of pharmacodynamic drug interactions. As a central nervous system depressant, alcohol acts synergistically with other drug classes that depress the central nervous system: antihistamines, sedative-hypnotics, antianxiety drugs, antidepressants, antipsychotics, general anesthetics, and narcotic analgesics. At low doses the drowsiness characteristic of these drug classes is exaggerated by alcohol, but at higher doses respiration can be dangerously depressed.

Alcohol may also interact with certain drugs to cause an intense reaction, including flushing of the face, palpitations, rapid heart rate (tachycardia), and low blood pressure (hypotension). This set of symptoms is called the **disulfiram reaction,** named for the chemical first shown to cause the reaction in persons drinking alcohol. This reaction is occasionally observed in patients who ingest alcohol while receiving certain antibiotics, the sedative chloral hydrate, oral hypoglycemic agents, and other drugs (see patient problem box on alcohol use and disulfiram on p. 635).

Food

Foods may interact with drugs and alter the effect of therapy, most obviously by altering the absorption of an orally administered drug. A few drugs are better absorbed or tolerated on a full stomach, but most drugs are absorbed more slowly or less completely when taken with food (see box, p. 22). A few of these interactions may significantly diminish the clinical usefulness of the drug. For example, the antibiotic tetracycline forms insoluble precipitates with calcium and magnesium in food. This interaction lowers absorption of the drug so that insufficient amounts of the antibiotic enter the blood and therapy fails.

Some food-drug interactions directly antagonize the action of the drug in the body. For example, patients receiving a coumarin anticoagulant may lose the action of the drug if they ingest large amounts of leafy green vegetables and other foods high in vitamin K. Vitamin K directly antagonizes the action of the coumarins.

Conversely, chronic administration of a drug may interfere with normal vitamin metabolism (Table 2-4). For exam-

ORAL ADMINISTRATION OF SELECTED DRUGS

Normally Taken on Empty Stomach With Full Glass of Water

Acetaminophen
Aspirin
Cephalosporins
Erythromycin*
Isoniazid
Penicillins
Propantheline
Quinidine*
Rifampin
Sulfonamides
Tetracyclines*
Theophylline*

Normally Taken With Food to Improve Absorption

Carbamazepine
Cimetidine
Griseofulvin†
Hydralazine
Indomethacin*
Lithium
Nitrofurantoin*
Propranolol
Spironolactone

*Gastric irritation may require that the drug be taken with food, but absorption is delayed or diminished
†This drug is taken with foods rich in fat for best absorption.

ple, long-term use of the antituberculosis drug isoniazid can deplete vitamin B_6 and cause neuritis. This complication can be prevented by administering vitamin B_6 supplement during isoniazid therapy.

Other food-drug interactions may arise when drugs interfere with normal mechanisms for removing noxious compounds from the body. For example, patients receiving monoamine oxidase inhibitors have a diminished ability to metabolize catecholamines and related compounds such as tyramine. When these patients eat foods with high concentrations of tyramine, such as aged cheese or red wine, they cannot eliminate the tyramine rapidly and it may accumulate, causing headache and hypertension.

TABLE 2-4 Drug Effects on Vitamin Metabolism

EFFECT	DRUGS
Interferes with absorption or action of folic acid, which can cause folate deficiency.	Aminopterin, antibiotics, anticonvulsants, aspirin, clofibrate, cycloserine, ethanol, methotrexate, oral contraceptives
Depletes vitamin B_6.	Hydralazine, isoniazid, oral contraceptives
Interferes with absorption or action of vitamin B_{12}.	Aminopterin, antibiotics, anticonvulsants, clofibrate, colchicine, ethanol, oral hypoglycemic agents
Interferes with absorption or action of vitamin D.	Antacids, anticonvulsants, mineral oil
Interferes with synthesis or absorption of vitamin K.	Antibiotics, mineral oil

NURSING IMPLICATIONS SUMMARY

General Guidelines: Drug Therapy

- Include questions about alcohol consumption and tobacco use in the health history.
- Obtain a family history. What is the family's place of origin? Are the parents and grandparents still living? If not, what was the cause of death? Are siblings of the parents and siblings of the patient still living? Any chronic health problems? Causes of death (if applicable)? Can the patient identify any chronic health problems in the family?

Neonates and Infants

- Monitor vital signs.
- Monitor fluid intake and output and body weight. Monitor laboratory work, including complete blood count (CBC), serum creatinine, blood urea nitrogen (BUN), and liver function tests.
- Double-check dosage calculations, especially if your math skills are not good or the dose is unusually small.
- Use equipment that reduces the possibility of overdose or overload, such as minidrip tubing, volume-control devices in intravenous tubing, and rate-controlling devices.
- Have a colleague double-check intravenous drug doses and volumes before administration.

Older Adults

- Monitor vital signs. Routinely check weight. Be alert to changes in mental status. Assess gait and balance.
- Monitor CBC, BUN, serum creatinine, liver function tests, serum drug levels, and other tests appropriate to the patient's medical history and medications.
- Ask the patient to bring all medications to the physician or nurse at each visit, or on a regular basis, so they can be checked. Are all these medications still needed? Are there any nonprescription drugs that the patient is also taking?

CRITICAL THINKING

APPLICATION

1. What consideration should the nurse be aware of in administering drugs that require hepatic detoxification to a premature infant?
2. Why should the use of aspirin be avoided in a child with fever?
3. What major organ system involved in drug elimination is likely to have diminished function in normal older adults?
4. Why must biologic variability be considered in drug therapy?
5. What are some of the possible reasons for the observed differences in drug response seen among patients?
6. Why are persons of African or Mediterranean ancestry more likely to suffer drug-induced hemolysis than most other American populations?
7. When is dosage adjustment needed in patients with impaired renal function?
8. How may chronic alcohol consumption influence drug therapy?
9. What are drug interactions? What are the two major mechanisms by which they occur?
10. How can smoking, environmental chemical exposure, or dietary patterns influence the response of a patient to a drug?

CRITICAL THINKING

1. Many years ago mixed racial or ethnic marriages were more unusual, so most people were born of parents of the same general background. Today children of mixed backgrounds are more common, but this fact often cannot be determined by the child's appearance. What kinds of questions can the nurse ask while taking a patient history to help alert the health care team to possible genetic traits that may be important to consider regarding medication use by the patient?
2. Consider the major industries in your local area. To what environmental hazards are people who work in these industries exposed? Are there known health problems associated with these agents? What are the signs and symptoms? How can you find out about these risks?
3. Some patients deny alcohol consumption even if they drink alcohol regularly; others report less alcohol intake than is true. Some patients may do the same when asked about smoking. When taking a health history, how can the nurse phrase questions to increase the likelihood of eliciting an accurate history of smoking or alcohol consumption?

CHAPTER 3

Legal Implications of Drug Therapy

OBJECTIVES

After studying this chapter, you should be able to do the following:

- *Discuss how drugs are tested for safety.*
- *Explain how a drug is determined to be effective for use in patients.*
- *Explain what controlled substances are.*
- *Discuss the role of the nurse in drug testing.*

KEY TERMS

double-blind design
generic names
orphan drugs
physical addiction
placebo effect
trade names

CHAPTER OVERVIEW

This chapter discusses the legal implications of drug therapy for nurses. Patients receiving medications have always faced certain risks, which include the possibility that the medication (1) will not produce the beneficial effect claimed by those who make and sell the drug, (2) may be directly harmful, or (3) may be improperly administered. Modern drug legislation is designed to reduce or eliminate these risks to patients.

ESTABLISHMENT OF SAFETY AND EFFICACY OF DRUGS

History of Drug Development

The earliest form of medical practice involved the use of various natural products that, by trial and error, were discovered to have certain effects on the body. For example, the ancient Egyptians knew that parts of the poppy plant could be used to relieve pain. This remedy was already well established when it was recorded in the Ebers papyrus in 1500 BC. Equally ancient is the use of parts of the ephedra shrub by the Chinese, who called the preparation *ma huang.* In the New World, South American Indians used the bark of the cinchona tree to relieve the symptoms of malaria. Even in more recent times natural products were used for medical practice. For example, in 1785 a British physician named Withering described the use of the leaf of the foxglove plant to relieve a certain type of edema that had previously resisted all therapy.

Until the last hundred years, natural products such as those discussed here were the only medicinal agents available. The most common medications, made from plants, were called *botanicals.* Most botanicals have been replaced as chemists have analyzed these crude products and identified their active ingredients. The active ingredients are the chemicals in the crude preparation that are responsible for producing the biologic effect of the medicinal agent. For example, the poppy plant relieves pain because it contains opium. *Ma huang* produces its effects on the heart, lungs, and other organs because it contains ephedrine, an agent that stimulates the sympathetic nervous system. Similarly, the quinine in cinchona bark relieves the symptoms of malaria, and the digitalis in foxglove leaves relieves the edema associated with heart failure.

Identification of the active ingredient in a crude medicinal agent has two benefits. First, the amount of active ingredient can be measured in the crude preparation, and the dose of the active ingredient can be adjusted for the content of the medicinal product. For example, the digitalis content of foxglove leaves varies from plant to plant. A dosage based on the amount of leaf taken may actually contain a variable amount of digitalis and may therefore have variable biologic effects. Because the biologic activity of a drug is related to the dose of the active ingredient, dosages based on the weight of pure digitalis should have a more predictable biologic effect.

The second benefit of identifying the active ingredient of a medicinal agent is that the chemical structure and properties of the active drug are revealed. This knowledge can lead to better ways of isolating the active material from natural sources. Alternatively, after the structure of an active agent is known, chemists may be able to synthesize the material. Ephedrine is an example of a drug that is currently chemically synthesized in a simple, economical process that has replaced the more complicated procedure of isolating the drug from plant materials.

Standardization of Agents

Recognizing the relationship between drug dose and biologic effect produced, most nations of the world have attempted to adopt codes for standardizing the content of medicinal agents. Drugs sold in the United States must comply with the standards established in the *United States Pharmacopeia (USP)* and the *National Formulary (NF).* The *USP* contains chemical, physical, and biologic information on all active ingredients used in medications. To qualify as a standard, or official, medication, the preparation must conform to the information listed in this source. The latest editions, *USP 23* and *NF 18,* became official January 1, 1995. The volume is updated continuously by way of published supplements.

As an example of the type of information found in the *USP,* we may consider aspirin. The *USP* classifies aspirin as an antipyretic (fever-reducing) analgesic (pain-reducing) agent. A variety of tablet sizes is described, containing amounts of aspirin ranging from 65 to 650 mg. To meet *USP* standards, tablets must contain between 95% and 105% of the amount of aspirin indicated on the label. Thus an aspirin tablet labeled 500 mg must contain between 475 and 525 mg of aspirin. The aspirin used in these tablets must meet the chemical and physical standards listed for that compound in the *USP.* Although drug doses for adults and children are listed, the *USP* is less useful for clinical personnel than for persons in pharmaceutical manufacture or pharmacy.

Some drugs used in medical practice cannot be standardized easily by chemical analysis because the drug preparations are relatively complex. These products can be standardized by measuring a biologic effect. Complex pharmaceutical preparations, such as sera, vaccines, and human blood products, are tested and licensed by the Food and Drug Administration (FDA) Center for Biologic Evaluation and Research.

Standards for medicinal agents vary from country to country. Several pharmacopeias and other references may apply. In Canada the current *Compendium of Pharmaceuticals and Specialties (CPS)* indexes agents available and contains monographs on specific drugs. The *British Pharmacopoeia 1993* is the current standard reference for the United Kingdom. It also includes information from the *European Pharmacopoeia* and is updated yearly with published addenda. The *International Pharmacopoeia* published by the World Health Organization (WHO) includes drug methods and standardizations for reference use in any country.

The information in these references is indexed by **generic,** or nonproprietary, **names.** The generic name applies to the drug, no matter who manufactures or markets it. **Trade,** or proprietary, **names** belong to a specific company. For example, cefuroxime sodium is the nonproprietary name for a specific antibiotic; this single compound is sold under the trade names of Zinacef by Glaxo, Inc., and Kefurox by Eli Lilly & Co.

Legislation

Drug manufacturing and sale are regulated by state and federal agencies. For federal laws to apply, a drug must enter interstate commerce. A drug totally manufactured within a single state and sold only in that state would not be subject to the federal drug laws. Very few drugs fall into this category.

The first effective federal law concerning drugs in the United States was passed in 1906 (Table 3-1). This law was intended to protect citizens from adulterated medicines and medications that contain harmful ingredients not listed on the label. Each new law passed since that time has been intended to overcome specific problems that have arisen. For example, in the early 1900s a certain patent medicine was advertised as a cure for cancer. The federal government sought to force the manufacturer to stop using the false advertisement. However, the drug label on the bottle was accurate in naming the contents of the medicine. Under the 1906 law, accurate labeling of the contents was all the government could require. When the Sherley Amendment was added in 1912, both advertising claims and contents of the drug label could be controlled.

Drug legislation passed in 1938 added the requirement that a drug sold in the United States be shown as safe before it could be marketed. Before this law became effective, a pharmaceutical company was not responsible for the safety of the drugs it manufactured and sold. For example, in 1937 more than 100 people died from taking a product that was sold as an "elixir of sulfanilamide." The cause of death was not the sulfanilamide but the propylene glycol used to dissolve the drug. The amazing fact is that no one had tested the toxicity

TABLE 3-1 Federal Drug Legislation in the United States

DATE	TITLE OF LAW	MAJOR PROVISIONS
1906	Pure Food and Drug Act	Established *USP* and *NF* as official standards. Set standards for proper drug labeling.
1912	Sherley Amendment	Prohibited fraudulent claims for therapeutic effects of drugs.
1914	Harrison Narcotic Act	Legally defined term *narcotic.* Regulated importation, manufacture, sale, or use of opium, cocaine, marijuana, and other drugs likely to produce dependence.
1938	Food, Drug, and Cosmetic Act	Maintained major provisions of previous laws. Required that a drug be proven safe before it was marketed.
1941-1945	Amendments to Pure Food and Drug Act	Required that biologic products used as drugs (e.g., insulin) be certified on a batch-by-batch basis by a government agency.
1952	Durham-Humphrey Amendment	Designated certain drugs as legend drugs (must be marked "Caution: Federal Law prohibits dispensing without prescription"). Restricted right of pharmacist to distribute legend drugs.
1962	Kefauver-Harris Amendment	Required proof of efficacy for a drug to remain on market. Authorized FDA to establish official names for drugs.
1970	Comprehensive Drug Abuse Prevention and Control Act (or Controlled Substances Act)	Defined *drug dependency* and *drug addiction.* Classified drugs by abuse potential and medical usefulness. Established methods for regulating manufacture, distribution, and sale of controlled substances.
1983	Orphan Drug Act	Offered tax relief to companies marketing orphan drugs. Protected companies for 7 years against competition on nonpatentable orphan drugs.
1984	Drug Price Competition and Patent Term Restoration Act	Drugs first marketed after 1962 are eligible for shortened drug application. Generic drugs are more easily introduced. Established guidelines for bioequivalence. Restored up to 5 years of patent protection for time used in drug development.
1986, 1988	National Childhood Vaccine Injury Act	Private health care providers are required to keep records on adverse events following immunization. Covers diphtheria, measles, mumps, pertussis, poliomyelitis, rubella, and tetanus toxoids or vaccines.
1987	Prescription Drug Marketing Act	Bans diversion of prescription drugs from legitimate channels. Restricts reimportation of drugs from other countries.
1988	Food and Drug Administration Act	Establishes the FDA within the Department of Health and Human Services. Sets mechanism for appointing the Commissioner of Food and Drugs.

of propylene glycol before using it in this medication. Under the law in 1937, however, the company responsible for this disaster could be charged only with mislabeling the drug because an elixir is by definition an alcohol solution.

One major provision of legislation currently controlling drug marketing and use in the United States is that a drug must be effective in treating the medical condition for which it is recommended (see Table 3-1). The requirement for proving effectiveness and safety has increased the amount of drug testing done by companies that develop new drugs. As a result fewer new drugs enter the market, and more time and money are required to place a drug on the market. On the other hand, drugs that do enter the market are much more reliable medications than they were in the past.

One class of drugs especially affected by the great cost of drug development is known as orphans. **Orphan drugs** are medicines that have not been profitable to develop and market, either because the market is too small (e.g., drugs used for treatment of rare diseases) or because patent protection has expired on the drug. Under provisions of the Orphan Drug Act (1983), companies can recover much of their development costs for orphan drugs. Companies that develop and market nonpatentable orphan drugs are also protected from competition by an FDA policy that limits approval for an orphan drug to one company for the first 7 years. Orphan drugs are listed in an appendix of *Drug Information for the Health Care Professional.*

Another current provision of drug legislation is that pharmaceuticals be produced by *good manufacturing practices.* Under this provision of the Food and Drug Act, the FDA inspects manufacturing facilities and oversees the production of medications. Good manufacturing practices are general procedures, not specific processes. Indeed, the methods employed to produce the same medication can vary widely from company to company. Such variation is acceptable as long as all procedures are in accordance with good manufacturing practices.

Legislation adopted in 1984 set guidelines for bioequivalence of drugs and streamlined application processes so that approval of generic drugs was facilitated. When a drug is first introduced, it is sold only by the company that developed it or by others licensed to sell it. The developer's control of the drug is protected for 17 years by patents. After that time other companies can manufacture the drug and sell it if they have met FDA requirements for good manufacturing processes and have satisfied bioequivalence standards. For example, the antibiotic clindamycin was discovered by Upjohn and sold under the trade name Cleocin. Sales were protected by Upjohn's patent rights to the compound, but when the patent expired, several other companies applied for the right to manufacture and market the drug. These companies cannot use the trade name Cleocin, but they can sell the generic compound clindamycin. These generic preparations of clindamycin currently share the market with the original drug.

Under the existing drug laws, several federal agencies are involved in regulating drug trade. In addition to official government agencies, a number of private organizations contribute advice or expertise to the government on matters concerning medicines. These organizations are listed and described in Table 3-2.

DRUG TESTING

The development of new drugs and biologicals is a major industry in the United States. To meet the current standards set by drug legislation, a detailed format is followed to test drugs as they are developed for market. This format is described in this section. The final stage of this drug development is testing in humans. Nurses play an important role in drug testing trials.

Assessment of Safety of Drugs

All medications intended for human use must undergo extensive toxicity testing in at least two species of animals. The toxicity tests must include acute and chronic studies. Acute toxicity tests assess the short-term effects of extreme doses of the drug. The intent of these tests is to identify organs or tissues that may be sensitive to the drug. The acute tests also allow researchers to determine how dangerous the drug might be in cases of overdose in humans.

Chronic toxicity tests assess the effects of prolonged dosage with the experimental agent. Several exposure levels are usually tested, with at least one group of animals receiving doses far in excess of those expected to be used in humans. After prolonged exposure to the test drug, the animals undergo extensive pathologic and histologic examinations to detect any effects on organs or tissues. Significant toxicity observed in animals is usually sufficient cause for abandoning development of a drug.

Chronic toxicity tests are the stage at which a drug is usually tested for carcinogenic (cancer-inducing) effects. The carcinogenic effects of compounds may also be assessed by the Ames test, which measures mutagenicity in bacteria. Because many chemicals that are mutagens are also carcinogens, this test can help predict which drugs may be carcinogenic. This bacterial test is less expensive and faster than chronic toxicity tests in animals, which may last months or years.

Drugs are also tested for their effects on pregnant animals and on fetuses. Drugs that cause fetal abnormalities are called *teratogens.* Some drugs are very dangerous to fetuses at certain stages in embryonic development but relatively harmless to adult animals or more mature fetuses. The stage of fetal development in which the fetus is most sensitive to drugs or toxins is the first third of fetal life. A tragic example of this sensitivity occurred with the drug thalidomide. Thalidomide is a sleep medication that was widely marketed in Europe during the 1960s. The drug was not dangerous to adults, but when used by women in the early stages of pregnancy, it inhibited proper development of fetal limb buds. The result was a number of babies born with tiny nonfunctional limbs—a tragedy that could have been prevented by more extensive drug testing. Thalidomide was, in fact, never marketed in the United States because insufficient information was available to satisfy FDA guidelines for new drugs.

TABLE 3-2 Organizations Involved in Drug Regulation in the United States

NAME	COMMON ABBREVIATION	FUNCTION
Department of Health and Human Services	HHS	The secretary of HHS is a cabinet-level officer whose duties include designating the official names for drugs sold in the United States and overseeing the Public Health Service.
Drug Enforcement Administration	DEA	This agency within the Department of Justice is the sole drug enforcement arm of the U.S. government, under the Controlled Substances Act of 1970.
Federal Trade Commission	FTC	This federal agency regulates advertisement of medications aimed at the general public (not medical personnel).
Food and Drug Administration	FDA	This federal agency is responsible for guaranteeing the safety, purity, effectiveness, and reliability of drugs sold in the United States. In addition, this agency regulates the advertising of medications to medical personnel.
National Academy of Sciences–National Research Council	NAS–NRC	The NAS is a private organization composed of scientists in the United States. The NRC is the research arm of the NAS and is involved in evaluating the efficacy of drugs for the FDA in the Drug Efficacy Study Implementation.
Public Health Service	PHS	This federal agency funds clinical research and is responsible for maintaining basic research programs under the National Institutes of Health. Biologicals used as drugs are also certified by this agency.
Pharmaceutical Manufacturers Association	PMA	This private organization representing the companies where most drugs are developed functions as an advisory group to the FDA and as a lobbying group to Congress.
United States Adopted Names Council	USAN	This private group contains members from government, private industry, the medical profession, and research institutions whose function is to advise the secretary of HHS as to the appropriate official name for each new drug introduced.
United States Pharmacopeial Convention	USP	This group of experts sets standards for medications (published in the *USP*) and establishes consensus on drug uses (published in the *USP Drug Information* volumes).

Efficacy of Drugs

After an experimental drug has been tested for toxicity in animals, the manufacturer may file with the FDA a "notice of claimed investigational exemption for a new drug (IND)." The chemical structure of the new drug is included, partly to prove that the drug really is new. All the toxicity data in animals, data on drug absorption and metabolism, and data on the expected biologic activity of the drug must be included. The manufacturer or licenser must justify the tests that will be conducted in human subjects.

Phase I, the first testing of a drug in humans, is carried out on a small number of healthy volunteers. The purpose of this phase is to identify a safe dosage range for the drug in most persons and to establish how well the animal studies correlate with the results in humans. For example, drug absorption in humans may be different from that observed in certain animal species. Therefore it may be necessary to repeat certain studies in humans. Occasionally an unexpected side effect may appear at this stage of testing. For example, alterations of mood may not be easily recognized in experimental animals and yet may be severe enough in humans to prevent further development of an experimental drug.

Phase II, the second stage of testing in humans, involves clinical trials on patients. Clinical trials may take many forms, but all are designed to answer the question, "Is this drug an effective treatment for a defined medical condition?" To answer this question, a relatively large number of patients must be studied, and the results must be analyzed in an objective manner, usually with statistical methods.

The **double-blind design** is one highly effective format for a clinical trial. In this type of study patients are randomly assigned to treatment groups or are assigned so that groups have the same average age, the same proportion of men and women, or some other desired characteristic. One group receives the drug to be tested. Another group receives a placebo (a dosage form containing no pharmacologically active ingredient). The drug and the placebo should be in the same form so that they cannot be told apart by sight or taste. The placebo-treated group of patients serves as a control and allows the researcher to assess how many patients would improve without therapy. The term *double-blind* refers to the fact that during the experiment neither the patients nor the medical personnel dispensing the medication know which patients are receiving the test drug and which are receiving the placebo. In some studies the control group receives the therapy that is currently accepted as the best available for the condition being tested rather than a placebo. This type of control allows researchers to compare the efficacy of a new drug to that of existing therapy.

Patients who receive placebo in clinical trials and show clinical improvement may be of two types. The first type includes patients whose disease has gone into spontaneous remission during the course of the clinical trial. For example, spontaneous remission is commonly observed in some depressive diseases and in certain types of arthritis. The second type includes patients who improve while receiving placebo simply as a result of receiving medical attention rather than an effective drug. For example, as many as 30% of patients suffering mild pain report significant relief when they are given a placebo. With drugs affecting mood, the response to placebo is observed in an even higher percentage of patients.

The **placebo effect** (clinical improvement in response to placebo) is a complication in clinical trials and makes the task of clearly evaluating the role of a particular drug in therapy more difficult. The existence of such an effect, however, emphasizes the importance of sympathetic human contact in relieving a patient's suffering. A patient who responds to placebo should by no means be considered to have been suffering from an imaginary complaint. We now understand the normal mechanisms by which the body produces analgesia (see Chapter 32) and realize that these internal mechanisms may be regulated by the central nervous system and affected by emotional states. Therefore the attention and support given to patients may alter their emotional state and allow the natural mechanisms of the body to improve the patient's clinical condition.

After a drug has been proved effective in controlled clinical trials, the manufacturer may request the FDA to release the drug for testing at several sites on large numbers of patients. This is *phase III* of the evaluation process. During the first round of clinical trials the total number of patients tested may be small. When the drug is released into limited circulation, it may be tested in a few thousand patients. This larger number of patients allows assessment of rare complications of drug therapy that could not be predicted from more limited trials. Before a tested drug is finally released for interstate marketing, its developer must file a new drug application (NDA) with the FDA. The NDA includes all data available on toxicity of the new drug, its use in patients, and results of the clinical trials. If the FDA rules that the drug has been proved safe and effective and that the claims made for the drug in the package insert and other professional advertising are supported by the results of clinical trials, the drug may be released for sale in interstate commerce.

The procedure for testing drugs as outlined in the preceding discussion was a careful, conservative approach that often took many years to complete. In 1985 the FDA streamlined procedures to bring new drugs into the marketplace more rapidly. The agency reduced the number of case reports required in the application but increased requirements for postmarketing surveillance. All serious adverse effects must be reported to the FDA within 15 days; all adverse effects must be reported every 3 months for the first 3 years and yearly thereafter. Forms for reporting these reactions are published regularly as part of the *FDA Drug Bulletin* and other publications.

Further pressure for more rapid movement of drugs into clinical tests arose as the acquired immunodeficiency syndrome (AIDS) epidemic began. Without treatment, AIDS patients live a very short time. For these patients and for others with conditions for which no effective therapy exists, a new procedure was created to allow experimental agents to be used on a wider scale than was previously possible. This process releases drugs for use in patients who meet set criteria, even though the drug is not yet on the market. For example, while didanosine was in trials against human immunodeficiency virus (HIV), it was available under the treatment IND for use in AIDS patients more than 12 years of age who had symptomatic HIV infection, were intolerant to the standard drug zidovudine, and were unable to enroll in a phase II trial because of geographic location.

Drug Efficacy Study Implementation

All drugs introduced after the Kefauver-Harris Amendment in 1962 needed to go through the extensive testing just described and had to be proved effective and safe before they could be sold. Drugs already on the market in 1962 posed a special problem because they had been tested primarily for safety and not efficacy. To bring all drugs up to the same standard, the FDA contracted the National Research Council of the National Academy of Sciences to evaluate all medications being sold in the United States. This project was the Drug Efficacy Study Implementation (DESI). To carry out this project, scientific and clinical experts were called to study data from clinical trials. Based on this information, drugs were rated according to the system shown in Table 3-3. Drugs rated as ineffective were removed from the market. Drugs listed as possibly effective or probably effective required reformulation or retesting to stay on the market.

Rights of the Patient in Drug Testing

Anyone involved in assessing the clinical usefulness of a new drug is bound by certain moral and legal constraints. No one may be coerced into receiving a drug that is under investigation. All drug studies must be done on volunteers who have read, understood, and signed informed consent forms. The law requires that all potential hazards associated with use of the drug be clearly explained to the patient. The patient or volunteer must not be promised unrealistic benefits from

TABLE 3-3 DESI Rating System

RATING	DESCRIPTION
Effective	Substantial evidence exists to show that drug is effective treatment for defined medical condition.
Probably effective	Some evidence exists, but more is needed to prove drug effective.
Possibly effective	Minimum evidence exists to suggest that drug may be effective.
Ineffective	Controlled trials failed to show that drug is more effective than placebo.
Ineffective as a fixed combination	Individual components of medication might be effective alone at appropriate doses, but no evidence suggests that all components of medication are necessary to effect.
Effective but	Qualification to use of drug is made, which must be added to labeling.

therapy. The patient must also be free to withdraw from the study at any time without fear that his or her level of medical care received will be compromised.

Although compliance with these constraints may seem a simple matter, there are complications in practice. For example, some people believe that experimental drugs are always better than currently used drugs. These people may not have realistic expectations, in spite of having been told the properties of the drug being tested. Another problem concerns patients who are intimidated by medical personnel and are afraid to refuse to participate in a drug study. These patients may confide their fears to an accessible and sympathetic nurse. It is the duty of the nurse to assist such patients in making their true feelings known.

Nurses assist patients in many ways throughout drug testing, including acting as an advocate for the patient. The nurse assesses whether the patient understands the possible benefits and limitations of the drugs being tested and the testing protocol. During testing the nurse assesses the patient for benefits, fears, drug side effects, and changes in the underlying health problem. Finally, the nurse supports the patient's decisions regarding participation in drug testing. This may be a difficult process because the nurse may disagree with the patient's decision but must support it.

NURSING PROCESS OVERVIEW

Nurses and Drug Testing

Laws governing the role of the nurse in drug testing vary among countries. In the United States each state's nurse practice act regulates all aspects of nursing practice for that state. Examine the appropriate laws governing practice to determine the extent to which nurses are allowed to participate in drug testing in your state, province, or country.

Assessment

Assess all patients in a thorough, individualized manner, whether or not the patient is involved in a drug testing program.

Nursing Diagnoses

Nursing diagnoses are based on individualized patient assessment. In the early stages of drug testing, the major focus may be to identify and describe frequently encountered drug side effects.

Planning/Implementation

Patient management in a drug testing study may differ from that in a normal clinical situation. For example, the nurse should be certain that the institution where the study is taking place permits the nurse to administer investigational drugs. Some institutions require that the person conducting the experiment (study) actually administer the experimental drugs. The nurse should also determine whether a nurse is legally allowed to obtain informed consent. Some institutions do not permit anyone but the principal investigator to obtain informed consent from the patient.

Evaluation

Evaluation of patients receiving experimental drugs may be a major component of the research in a drug testing program. In many cases thorough evaluation is carried out by the physician or researcher, including detailed patient histories, laboratory tests, and radiographic evaluation. Nevertheless, the nurse should continue to evaluate patients in a manner consistent with good nursing practice. The extent to which nursing evaluations become part of the permanent record of the experiment depends on the institution and the protocols established by the investigator.

CONTROLLED SUBSTANCES

Addiction

Certain substances can alter normal functions of the human body so profoundly that the body becomes dependent on that substance and suffers physical harm if it is withdrawn. This condition is **physical addiction** or *dependence* (see Chapter 8). Other substances, although not producing clear evidence of physical addiction, cause psychologic addiction. Examples of compounds that produce each of these types of addiction are listed in Table 3-4.

Regulation of Controlled Substances

Because substances that produce physical or psychologic addiction clearly have the capacity to harm their users, they have been regulated extensively in the United States and Canada, and throughout the world. The original legislation in the United States was the Harrison Narcotic Act of 1914. This law restricted importation of many of these addictive substances. One of the major aims of the Pure Food and Drug Act of 1906 and the Harrison Act was to prevent the sale of patent medicines that contained no active ingredient except one of these addicting agents.

The Harrison Act did not eliminate the problem of illicit drug use and addiction. This legislation was replaced by a more comprehensive law in 1970, the Controlled Substances Act. In addition to supplying guidelines for defining drug dependency and establishing education and treatment programs, this law clearly classifies drugs based on abuse potential and clinical usefulness and specifies the restrictions that apply to each type of controlled drug. The drug schedules are described in Table 3-5.

Drugs in each schedule defined by the Controlled Substances Act are regulated by rules appropriate to them. For example, schedule I substances have no approved medical use and are therefore banned. Schedule II drugs are controlled at every stage from initial manufacture through distribution and final use. By law, no prescription for a schedule II drug may be refilled. Physicians must be licensed to prescribe these medications and must keep accurate records to ensure that the drugs are used strictly for legitimate purposes. Likewise, pharmacies must be specially licensed and keep accurate records for schedule II drugs.

Drugs in schedules III, IV, and V are considered less dangerous than those in schedule II. For the most part this greater safety results from inherent properties of the chemi-

TABLE 3-4 Compounds That Produce Dependence With Continued Use

TYPE OF DEPENDENCE	DRUG CATEGORY	SPECIFIC DRUGS
Physical and psychologic	Narcotic analgesics	Morphine, heroin, codeine, paregoric, methadone
Physical and psychologic	General depressants	Ethanol, barbiturates, glutethimide, methaqualone
Psychologic	Psychomotor stimulants*	Amphetamines, cocaine, methylphenidate
Psychologic	Hallucinogens	Lysergic acid diethylamide (LSD), mescaline (peyote), *N,N*-dimethyltryptamine (DMT), 2,5-dimethoxy-4-methyl amphetamine (STP), phencyclidine
Psychologic	Cannabis	Marijuana, hashish

*Physical dependence has been suggested for certain of these drugs but remains controversial.

TABLE 3-5 Classification of Controlled Substances

CLASSIFICATION	DESCRIPTION	SPECIFIC SUBSTANCES
Schedule I	Drugs that have high potential for abuse and no accepted medical use. Containers are marked C-I.	Heroin, LSD, peyote, marijuana
Schedule II	Drugs that have high potential for abuse but have accepted medical use. Dependence may include strong physical and psychologic dependence. Containers are marked C-II.	Amobarbital, amphetamine, codeine, dextroamphetamine, meperidine, methadone, hydromorphone, morphine, opium, pentobarbital, phenazocine, methylphenidate, secobarbital
Schedule III	Medically accepted drugs that may cause dependence but are less prone to abuse than drugs in Schedules I and II. Containers are marked C-III.	Codeine-containing medications, butabarbital, paregoric
Schedule IV	Medically accepted drugs that may cause mild physical or psychologic dependence. Containers are marked C-IV.	Chloral hydrate, chlordiazepoxide, diazepam, meprobamate, phenobarbital
Schedule V	Medically accepted drugs with very limited potential for causing mild physical or psychologic dependence. Containers are marked C-V.	Drug mixtures containing small quantities of narcotics, such as over-the-counter cough syrups containing codeine

cals in these schedules, but some chemicals appear in more than one schedule. For example, codeine used alone as an antitussive is a schedule II drug. However, medications that contain codeine compounded with aspirin, acetaminophen or other agents are schedule III drugs, even when the total dose of codeine is the same as that used in schedule II preparations. One reason that these compounded forms of codeine are less likely to be abused is that adverse symptoms from overdoses of the other ingredients discourage abuse of these mixtures. Codeine also appears in several cough syrups that are schedule V drugs. The recommended single dose of codeine for adults in these schedule V medications is 5 or 10 mg, whereas the doses found in schedule II or III forms are 15 to 60 mg. This lower dose in the cough medications is responsible for the schedule V classification.

NURSING PROCESS OVERVIEW

Controlled Substances

Because of the addictive potential of many controlled substances, legal restraints have been placed on the use of these drugs in medical practice. These regulations, as well as the special nature of the drugs, add a special burden and responsibility for the nurse.

Assessment

Research has shown repeatedly that when patients use controlled substances for legitimate medical reasons, drug addiction is extremely rare. Observe whether an individual displays signs and symptoms that make the use of the controlled substance appropriate. Be alert to signs of drug abuse in patients. Patients may have obtained prescriptions from several physicians to acquire excessive amounts of controlled substances. Be alert not only to physical signs of excessive drug use but also to the psychologic signs pointing to this problem. For example, a patient who is dependent on drugs obtained under false pretenses may be reluctant to enter the hospital for even the most routine testing, fearing that the drug dependency will be discovered in the closely regulated hospital environment.

Nursing Diagnoses

- Constipation related to frequent use of narcotic analgesics
- Altered comfort: nausea related to narcotic use

Planning/Implementation

When dealing with controlled substances, the nurse has legal and nursing responsibilities. The legal responsibilities include ensuring that controlled substances (schedules II through IV, United States) are kept under lock and key. These substances are available only to authorized personnel. Since all the material must be accounted for, records on the use of these substances must be kept. Any unauthorized use of controlled substances must be reported to the proper authority.

The nurse must also be aware of institutional policies regarding the use of these drugs, such as standing orders for controlled substances. For example, for schedule II drugs (United States) the physician's order may require renewal every 48 hours. A nurse who administers the drug after the 48-hour period without obtaining a renewal order is in violation of institutional policy. There are comparable national and institutional restrictions related to Canadian narcotics and schedule G drugs.

On the other hand, patients with a legitimate need for controlled substances should not be refused the medications they need. See Chapter 31 for guidelines for patients requiring narcotics for pain relief. Patients receiving controlled substances may express concern about possible drug dependence. The use of the medication should be explained in terms of the patient's own condition, and the patient should be appropriately reassured.

Evaluation

For controlled substances, patient evaluation is a two-level process. First, the patient evaluation should be performed as for any other type of drug. Ascertain whether the medication is successfully controlling the signs and symptoms for which it was given. Second, evaluate the patient for psychologic response to addictive drugs. Note signs of drug dependence and excessive fears of addiction. These observations may dictate changes in the therapeutic program.

CANADIAN DRUG LEGISLATION

Food and Drugs Act

Drug regulation is carried out through the Health Protection branch of the Canadian government. Under this branch the Drugs Directorate oversees the bureaus that deal with specific areas of regulation. For example, the Bureau of Human Prescription Drugs deals with new drugs for human use. Separate bureaus deal with veterinary products, nonprescription drugs, biologicals, drug research, and control of drug quality.

Under the Food and Drugs Act of 1953, drugs are divided into categories (Table 3-6). When approved for sale, all Canadian drugs are assigned a six-digit number preceded by the letters GP (proprietary drug) or DIN (over-the-counter drug). In addition, each prescription drug must be well marked with a symbol to identify the schedule to which it belongs. Regulations covering the various schedules of drugs differ, making the clear identification system important. Drugs listed in schedule F are sold only by prescription, with refills limited to 6 months. Drugs in schedule G are called *controlled drugs* and have more stringent controls regulating

TABLE 3-6 Canadian Drug Classifications

CLASSIFICATION	DESCRIPTION	SPECIFIC SUBSTANCES
Nonprescription Drugs		
Proprietary medicines	Drugs that may be widely purchased for self-treatment of symptoms of minor self-limiting diseases; identified by six-digit code preceded by letters *GP*	Cough drops, medicated shampoos, minor pain relievers
Over-the-counter drugs	Drugs available through a pharmacy and used on advice of a health professional for control of symptoms of minor self-limiting diseases; identified by six-digit code preceded by letters *DIN*	Laxatives, cough syrups, cold remedies, sinus preparations, certain vitamins
Prescription Drugs		
Schedule F	Over 200 drugs that may not be used except after professional consultation; identified by symbol *Pr* on label	Hormones, antibiotics, tranquilizers
Schedule G	Drugs that affect central nervous system (e.g., stimulants, sedatives); identified by symbol *C* on label	Amphetamines, barbiturates
Narcotics	Drugs used primarily for relief of pain but also possessing significant psychotropic activity; identified by letter *N* on label	Cannabis (marijuana), cocaine, codeine, morphine, opium, phencyclidine
Restricted Drugs		
Schedule H	Drugs with no recognized medical use and significant danger of physiologic and psychologic side effects; available only to institutions for research	Lysergic acid diethylamide (LSD), *N,N*-diethyltryptamine (DET), *N,N*-dimethyltryptamine (DMT), 4-methyl-2, 5-dimethoxyamphetamine (STP, DOM)

the number and timing of refills for prescriptions. Certain controlled drugs are called *designated drugs* because their use is restricted to specific conditions described by law. For example, dextroamphetamine is designated for use in narcolepsy in adults or attention-deficit hyperactivity disorder in children, but it must not be used for other conditions without special permission.

The Food and Drugs Act in Canada also protects citizens from contaminated, adulterated, or unsafe drugs. To ensure drug quality, the law requires inspection of manufacturing facilities, calls for analysis of drug samples by government laboratories, and maintains an active monitoring system to detect adverse reactions to drugs. Drug labeling is also closely controlled so that false, misleading, or deceptive labels are prohibited. Drugs may not be advertised to the general public as cures for alcoholism, cancer, heart disease, infectious diseases, and other specific conditions. No prescription drug may be advertised to the general public.

Narcotic Control Act

The Narcotic Control Act (1961) regulates the manufacture, distribution, and sale of narcotic drugs, establishing this group as separate from drugs regulated under the Food and Drugs Act. Regulations with the force of law spell out specific provisions of this act and are frequently revised in response to changing needs.

All steps in the manufacture, distribution, and sale of drugs on schedules G and H and of narcotics are subject to stringent regulation. Possession of these drugs for any reason other than those related to medical use as described in the legislation is an offense subject to severe penalties. Dispensers of these drugs must be licensed by the government and must maintain extensive records documenting the sources of and recipients for all drugs and the amounts and dates for all transactions. As in the United States, nurses may be in possession of narcotics or controlled and restricted drugs only when authorized by a physician's order to administer the drug to a patient or when authorized to act as official custodian of drugs for a specific unit of a health care facility.

Development of New Drugs in Canada

New drugs are evaluated in Canada by a sequence of tests similar to those used in the United States. Promising drugs undergo preclinical testing in three mammalian species, including one nonrodent species, to determine threshold doses that produce toxicity or death. The next stage is a clinical pharmacology trial similar to phase I trials in the United States. During clinical pharmacology trials the drug is given to healthy human volunteers to establish safety for doses that might be used clinically. If the drug is proved safe and if manufacturing processes produce a pure and uniform preparation for human use, the manufacturer may apply for permission to distribute the drug to qualified investigators who will test it in patients. This stage of testing is similar to phase II in the United States. Before the drug can be released for general use, extensive documentation concerning formulation, labeling, packaging, clinical data on humans, and test data on animals must be filed and evaluated. All new drugs are monitored after being placed on the market. Only after extensive information has been accumulated to document the safety of a new drug when used in normal medical practice is the drug released from the controls required for a new drug.

NURSING IMPLICATIONS SUMMARY

General Guidelines: Legal Implications of Drug Therapy

- Be familiar with the nurse practice acts that govern practice in your setting. Since these acts are written in legislative language, ask questions as needed to clarify the meaning of all components.
- Stay informed of agency policies related to dispensing, administering, and accounting for drugs. Observe deadlines and expiration dates of orders. Maintain vigilance in working with controlled and scheduled drugs.
- Consult the current literature, the pharmacist, and the physician to learn about new drug preparations. Ask questions as needed to clarify changes in protocols for administration of drugs.
- Assess each patient individually, and ask "Is this the right drug in the right dose for this patient?" See Chapter 4 for additional information.
- Be familiar with policies regarding the role of the nurse with investigational drugs. Serve as the patient's advocate in working with patients involved in drug studies.

CRITICAL THINKING

APPLICATION

1. What is the "active ingredient" of a medicinal preparation?
2. What is the purpose of the *United States Pharmacopeia* and the *National Formulary?*
3. Outline the steps involved in getting a new drug approved in the United States or Canada.
4. What is a clinical trial? Describe a clinical trial following the double-blind design.
5. What is the placebo effect?
6. What is the purpose of the informed consent form?
7. What is a treatment IND?
8. What is the purpose of the Drug Efficacy Study Implementation?
9. What are controlled substances? What are some nursing implications related to administering a controlled substance?
10. What special precautions are required in handling controlled substances?

CRITICAL THINKING

1. Suggest two explanations for the placebo effect observed in drug trials. How might the nurse use knowledge of the placebo effect to attempt to improve the patient's response to a medication?

CHAPTER 4

Application of the Nursing Process to Drug Therapy

OBJECTIVES

After studying this chapter, you should be able to do the following:

- *Discuss the use of the nursing process with patients receiving medications.*
- *Explain the five rights of drug administration.*
- *Describe the factors that influence patient compliance with drug therapy.*
- *Discuss legal constraints on the administration of drugs.*
- *Describe the nurse's role when medication errors occur.*

KEY TERMS

assessment
evaluation
five rights of drug administration
implementation
nursing diagnosis
nursing process
patient outcomes
planning

CHAPTER OVERVIEW

The focus of this chapter is the use of the nursing process in administering drugs. The chapter includes a discussion of the classic steps in the nursing process. In addition, it elaborates on the issues that the nurse should consider in preparing and administering drugs. This chapter complements Chapter 3 *(Legal Implications of Drug Therapy)*, Chapter 5 *(Drug Administration)*, and Chapter 7 *(Over-the-Counter Drugs and Self-Medication)*.

THE NURSING PROCESS AND PHARMACOLOGY

Assessment

Assessment involves gathering data about the patient. This database is important in the treatment of the patient. The assessment forms the baseline against which changes will be compared. It also allows the nurse to develop an individualized care plan for the patient.

The physical assessment should be complete yet tailored to the patient's needs and the severity of the presenting health problems. The history of the present health problems includes a drug history (Figure 4-1). Information from the drug history helps the nurse better understand the patient's previous drug use, attitudes about drugs, and knowledge about drugs. In addition, the nurse can learn about any over-the-counter (OTC) drugs the patient may be using and his or her current lifestyle, including smoking, drinking alcoholic beverages, and dietary habits.

Another component of the assessment comes from laboratory results, radiology reports, and results of other diagnostic testing. These data may confirm existing health problems or provide a baseline against which the nurse can later check for deviations or improvement, possibly related to the drugs administered.

Nursing Diagnoses

A **nursing diagnosis** is a statement of a health problem or potential problem that a nurse is licensed and competent to treat. The nurse derives nursing diagnoses by analyzing the data obtained in the patient assessment. There are no nursing diagnoses that apply solely to drug administration. The diagnoses reflect an analysis of the entire patient and the patient's needs, which may include aspects of drug administration.

The wording of the nursing diagnoses is specific, established by the North American Nursing Diagnoses Association (NANDA). NANDA has met regularly since 1973 to refine the list of NANDA-approved nursing diagnoses. The most recent listing is published when it is updated. With regard to medication administration, several points about nursing diagnoses should be made. The only nursing diagnosis that can be applied in all situations of drug administration is that of "knowledge deficit." Most patients who are to receive a new drug therapy have some knowledge deficit, but it may be minimal. Careful assessment may reveal that other diagnoses are more appropriate.

A nursing diagnosis that encompasses an entire health problem may be more appropriate than one that focuses on the drug therapy alone. For example, for the patient with diabetes, who must take insulin, a nursing diagnosis of "Risk for altered health maintenance related to lack of knowledge of diabetes mellitus, management, and signs and symptoms of complications" would allow for a more detailed plan than a diagnosis that focuses on insulin alone would.

Side effects that are frequently encountered or are very serious may form the basis for some nursing diagnoses. For example, narcotic analgesics cause constipation. When these narcotics are used for only 2 or 3 doses, the constipation may be minimal. When narcotics are used in high doses for extensive periods, as for some patients with cancer, it would be appropriate to include in the plan a nursing diagnosis that comes from knowledge of the drug and the side effect of constipation. Thus for a patient with cancer who is receiving frequent or high doses of narcotics, a nursing diagnosis of "Risk for constipation related to narcotic use for pain relief" may be appropriate. For a patient on a diuretic known to contribute to potassium loss, "Risk for electrolyte abnormalities (hypokalemia) related to furosemide therapy" may be appropriate.

Nursing diagnoses may describe a problem for which additional data are needed. Consider the patient who must take moderate to large doses of corticosteroids. These drugs have the side effects of weight gain and development of a characteristic round face (moon face). A nursing diagnosis might be "Possible self-concept disturbance related to physical changes secondary to prednisone therapy."

It would be easy to develop extensive lists of "risk for" and "possible" diagnoses related to any known side effect of drug therapy. However, it is more prudent to use such diagnoses for serious or frequently encountered problems. Remember that each patient is unique and therefore a problem for one patient will not necessarily be the same for another.

Sometimes patients are at risk for a potential complication that cannot be prevented or treated with nursing measures alone. In such a situation the patient may have, instead of or in addition to nursing diagnoses, one or more collaborative problems. Consider an acutely ill patient with diabetes. The patient may have the potential complication (PC) of hypoglycemia/hyperglycemia.

Patient Outcomes

Patient outcomes describe the goal(s) of therapy in terms of the patient. The outcomes should be objective or measurable so that it will be possible to determine if the outcomes have been achieved. For example, an outcome for the patient receiving regular morphine might be: "The patient will have a bowel movement at least every 48 hours." Each nursing diagnosis should have at least one patient outcome. Patient outcomes should be developed with the patient and family. Such collaboration helps the patient understand what the health care team is trying to achieve and allows an opportunity to teach the patient.

If the patient has one or more potential complications that are collaborative problems, the goals may be worded in terms of the nurse: "The nurse will manage and minimize episodes of hypoglycemia or hyperglycemia."

Planning/Implementation

Planning involves developing an outline of nursing interventions needed to treat the nursing diagnoses. The plan should spell out the nursing interventions that should be used by members of the team. These interventions may be carried out

Name ______________________________

Age ______________ Date ______________

Major health problems: ______________________________

____

Other health problems requiring medications: ______________________________

____

1. Medications used for major health problems

   These questions are only a guide. The patient's comments may lead the examiner to pursue certain topics in more detail.

   What medicines are you currently taking?

Medicine	Dose	Frequency	Comments

   Are you having problems with any of these medicines? *Go through each medicine, asking the following questions:*

   a. Are you able to take this drug the way it is ordered? What time(s) each day do you take it?
   b. Are you having any side effects? *Use words that the patient can understand, such as "Are there reasons you cannot take this medicine?" or "Are there any problems with taking this medicine?"*
   c. Do you think this drug is helping? *For example, "Is your blood pressure pill helping your blood pressure?"*
   d. If appropriate, ask about cost: *"Some patients find that this medicine is very expensive. Has the cost of this drug been a problem?"*
   e. If appropriate, ask about ability to obtain refills: *"Do you have any problems getting refills for this drug?" "Do you have any problems picking up your refills at the drugstore?"*

Note anything that might be important in teaching this patient about medications: drugs that should be refrigerated or left at room temperature, dangers of putting drugs in unlabeled containers, importance of storing drugs out of reach of small children, etc.

2. General drug use

   How do you take care of the following problems/conditions? What medicines do you use for them?

   "How often do you take the medicine?" "Does it work?" "When did you last take it?"

   a. Pain: headache, muscle pains, toothaches? *Expand as needed for each patient.*
   b. Gastrointestinal system: constipation, diarrhea, upset stomach, heartburn?
   c. Skin conditions: psoriasis, athlete's foot, dry skin? *Ask about special shampoos and creams.*
   d. Nervous, mental, or emotional disorders: nervousness, being unable to sleep, upset?
   e. Reproductive system: birth control pills, female hormones, menstrual pain, backache?
   f. Nutritional deficiencies: iron, vitamins, bran, yeast, etc.?
   g. Upper respiratory tract, eye, and nose: What do you do for a cold? Cough? Stuffy nose? Sinus problem? Do you take nosedrops? Use nasal spray? Eyedrops?
   h. Other: special teas, liniments, plasters, soda, drugs made from roots? *Knowledge of local custom is helpful in this category.*

3. General health habits

   a. Do you smoke? How much?
   b. How much whiskey (beer, wine) do you drink? (Response may not be accurate.)
   c. How often do you do drugs on a recreational basis? (Response may not be accurate. Remain nonjudgmental.)
   d. Do you follow any special diet (low salt, diabetic, low protein, etc.)? Are you a vegetarian? *In some cases a complete diet history might be warranted.*
   e. Where do you work? What kinds of work have you done in the past? Have you lived anywhere else in the country?
   f. Are you allergic to anything? Are there any medicines you cannot take? Why?
   g. Which immunizations have you received? When did you last have a tetanus shot?

FIGURE 4-1

Sample drug history.

on a daily timetable, or deadlines for accomplishing components of the plan may be identified. Thus an intervention to "Check the stool for occult blood" should be done each time a patient has a bowel movement. Another intervention might be to "Increase ambulation by walking 10 feet more each time the patient is up; by Tuesday the patient should be able to walk to the end of the hall and back." This intervention includes a goal within the intervention.

The **implementation** phase is the carrying out of the plan. In this phase the nurse must incorporate the steps of the plan in the patient's daily routine. It is often during this phase that the nurse or the patient begins to identify changes that need to be made. For example, the nurse may see that the plan is unreasonable, the goal (patient outcome) is not realistic, or the patient is not ready for such detailed instruction.

Evaluation

Evaluation, although listed as the final step of the nursing process, takes the nurse back to the first step of assessment. During evaluation the nurse determines whether the plan is working. Is the patient displaying the desired patient outcomes? What should be modified in the plan? What additional data are needed? Are the drugs working as planned? Are side effects developing? What new problems have occurred?

The nursing process is often *presented* in a linear fashion:

Assessing → Diagnosing →
Planning/implementing → Evaluating

However, it often *occurs* in a circular fashion (Figure 4-2). Working closely with the patient, the nurse may assess the patient and begin to develop nursing diagnoses. As more information is needed, the nurse obtains additional assessment data. In developing the plan and implementing it, the nurse constantly evaluates its feasibility and success. While evaluating the plan, the nurse continues to assess. The **nursing process** is a systematic, organized way of approaching the patient and developing a plan for health care.

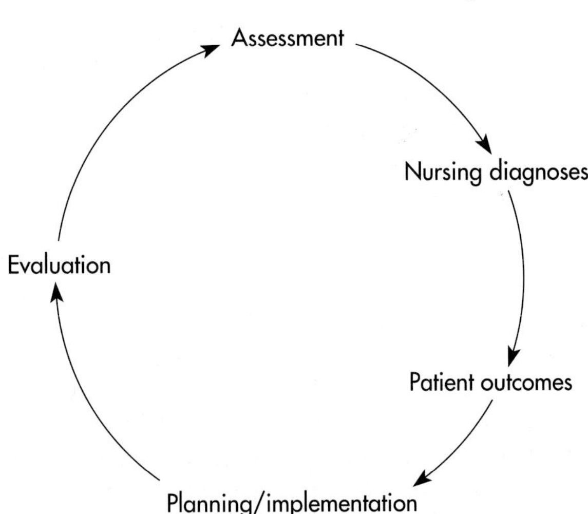

FIGURE 4-2
The nursing process as a continuous activity.

THE FIVE RIGHTS OF DRUG ADMINISTRATION

Traditionally, the teaching of principles of drug administration has centered around the **five rights of drug administration** (see box): the right drug, via the right route, in the right dose, at the right time, and to the right patient. Although at first glance it might seem that these rights should be easy to achieve, the day-to-day practice of nursing requires thoughtful attention to these rights at all times.

The Right Drug

The right drug suggests that the patient not only receive the prescribed drug but also the right drug for the specific health problem being treated. The nurse must pay careful attention to drug orders and medication labels while preparing drugs and be familiar with each patient and his or her health care problems. To know if a prescribed drug is appropriate, the nurse must know and understand the patient's health problems and be current in pharmacologic knowledge. The rest of this book provides basic material about drugs, but in practice the nurse must also regularly consult printed materials and other health care professionals for additional information. Some of these sources are discussed in Chapters 3 and 7.

The Right Route

To ensure that the patient receives prescribed medications via the right route, the nurse must know each medication that is administered. The student may have difficulty understanding how or why a nurse could administer a medication via the wrong route, but in a busy nurse's day errors can occur easily. For example, an experienced nurse who usually works in the coronary care setting was asked to work for a day in the surgical intensive care unit. The nurse, accustomed to administering morphine intravenously for cardiac pain, administered all parenteral pain medications intravenously in the surgical intensive care setting, even those ordered via the intramuscular route. Fortunately, in this true incident the nurse discovered the errors and reported them, and no harm came to the patients.

THE FIVE RIGHTS OF DRUG ADMINISTRATION

The right *drug*
The right *route*
The right *dose*
The right *time*
The right *patient*

The Right Dose

Administering the right dose of medication is extremely important. Not only must the nurse double-check calculations for mathematic accuracy; the nurse also must ask, "Is this dose appropriate for the size and age of the patient?" This responsibility emphasizes the need for current knowledge about drugs and usual dosage ranges. Although the administration of an incorrect dose is serious for any patient, it can be especially serious in the pediatric patient, for whom prescribed doses are often small. A review of dosage calculations can be found in Chapter 6.

The Right Time

Ensuring that the patient receives drugs at the right time may be difficult. Often the health care team must weigh the information available about the pharmacokinetics and pharmacodynamics of drugs (see Chapter 1) against the patient's lifestyle and potential for compliance. In the critical care setting, where one nurse may care for one or two patients, drugs are administered at evenly spaced intervals throughout a 24-hour period. The nurse, although usually very busy, can concentrate on administering medications to a few patients. However, on a busy general care unit the nurse may have 20 or more patients who must receive drugs, and these patients may be coming and going to the radiology department, physical or occupational therapy, or surgery. In addition, most patients would prefer not to be wakened at night to receive medications. In the home it is even easier for the patient to forget to take a dose or to be less careful about the interval between doses. Another factor in the home setting is general lifestyle. For example, patients who work a night shift and sleep during the day may need help determining the right time to take drugs.

Other factors that influence the right dosage time include whether the patient is receiving multiple drugs, whether a drug can be taken on an empty or full stomach, and whether a prescribed drug can be taken with other medications. To ensure that a patient receives drugs at the right time, the nurse must know about the patient, the health care problems, and the drugs.

The Right Patient

Finally, the right patient must receive the drug. The nurse must check the patient's identity *each time* a drug is administered. Not only should the patient be Ms. Smith, but it must be the right Ms. Smith. The right patient also means that the right drugs were prescribed for the right patient, and thus the nurse is back to the first of the five rights of drug administration.

PATIENT EDUCATION AND MEDICATIONS

One of the major goals of nursing care in drug administration is preparing the patient and family for a return to independent functioning in the home or community. The patient, when able, will take over the role of self-administration of medications. No one can guarantee that the patient will take a medication exactly as directed and derive the expected benefits of drug therapy. However, careful patient assessment, planning, and teaching by the nurse can help the patient to better understand prescribed medications and how to use them safely.

Attitudes About Medications

All patients come to the health care system with preexisting ideas and attitudes about who should take medications, whether or not medications are generally helpful, what the meaning of sickness and health is, and what to expect of the health care team. Additional factors include personally held beliefs, attitudes and opinions of family and friends, religious and cultural beliefs, and the influence of the media about certain kinds of medications. The public may not even use the same vocabulary as the health care team. For example, a nurse or physician may use the words *drug, medicine,* or *medication* interchangeably; but these words may have different connotations to the patient.

To be successful in preparing the patient for self-management, the nurse needs to assess the patient's attitudes about medicines. This is done by asking questions or developing an assessment tool, by remaining attuned to the patient's response to medications in the health care setting, and by attempting to validate these impressions with the patient. The nurse in the hospital or institution is generally in control of the medication situation, and the patient can avoid becoming very involved in the self-medication plans. The nurse in the home is given many more clues about patient attitudes regarding medication administration. Any plan for teaching patients about drugs will be more successful if it is compatible with the patient's existing beliefs and attitudes. It is possible to change attitudes and beliefs, but doing so requires careful planning and is difficult.

General Principles to Teach About All Medications

Regardless of the specific drugs prescribed for a patient, there are some general principles about drugs to teach all patients (see box, p. 40). Instruct patients to keep all drugs out of reach of children and to keep the drugs in the original labeled containers. Decorative pill boxes are attractive, but many patients fill them with several different types of drugs. This practice provides great potential for error and may hasten decomposition of some drugs. Remind patients to use child-proof caps unless the patient cannot remove them without assistance. Even so, children must be protected from access to drugs. Explain that, ideally, all drugs should be stored in a locked container, out of reach of children.

Emphasize that medications should be taken only as ordered. Patients should not double up on medication to catch up when a dose has been missed. Remind patients not to share medications with family or friends. Warn patients that altering the dose amount does not improve the effect; two pills are not better than one. Explain that if any medication is

SAFE MEDICATION USE: POINTS TO REVIEW WITH ALL PATIENTS

Take drugs prescribed for you; do not borrow drugs from others or share your drugs with others.

Take only the dose prescribed. If you feel the dose is too high or too low, check with the physician before adjusting the dose or frequency of doses.

When a new drug is prescribed, find out what to do if a dose is missed. Usually, do not double-up for missed doses. Take a missed dose as soon as it is remembered, unless it is within 2 hours of the next regularly scheduled dose. Resume the regular dose schedule.

When a new drug is prescribed, find out how to take it in relation to meals or other drugs you may be taking. Some drugs should be taken with meals or food, whereas others should be taken on an empty stomach.

Each time a new drug is prescribed, find out why you are taking it and what the common side effects are. Never hesitate to call the doctor if an unexpected sign or symptom develops; it may be related to the medications you are taking.

Store your medications properly. Usually, this means in a dry place—not in the bathroom, where steam and moisture may cause medicines to deteriorate and lose strength. Do not mix different pills in the same container, such as a pill box for your pocket or purse. This may cause the medicines to lose their strength, and without labels, you may take the wrong drug by accident.

Write down the names of the drugs you are taking, and take this list whenever you visit the doctor, nurse, dentist, podiatrist, ophthalmologist, osteopathic physician, chiropractor, or clinic. Keep all your health care providers informed of all the drugs you are taking, even those you purchase over the counter.

Keep drugs out of the reach of children. Use childproof caps if there are children in your home. Never refer to medications as candy.

Read the label each time you take a dose of medicine to make sure you are taking the drug you think you are taking. Sometimes two different drugs look alike.

Wear a medical identification tag, bracelet, or necklace listing your chronic health problems and medication allergies.

Keep track of your prescription drugs. Try not to run out of them on the weekend or during holidays, when it may be difficult to get a prescription refilled. If your drug supply is getting low, call the physician's office. Be prepared to give the nurse the name of the drug and dose and the name of the pharmacy and its telephone number where you wish to have the prescription filled.

Keep the telephone number of the local poison control center near your telephone. Keep ipecac in your home but out of the reach of children. This drug can be used to make a person vomit if a drug was taken that should not have been. Never use ipecac unless the poison control center or your doctor says you should.

left after a health problem has been treated, it should be discarded. Emphasize that drugs purchased over the counter should be treated with the same degree of respect as other medications; they are not to be considered less seriously because they have not been prescribed by a physician or dispensed by a pharmacist.

Instruct patients to keep all health care providers informed of all drugs they are taking. Patients taking multiple drugs should keep a list of drugs and dosages, preferably with them at all times, and check it regularly to see if it is current. Encourage patients with chronic conditions or severe allergies to wear a medical identification bracelet or necklace listing the allergy, medical condition, or type of medication used.

Teach all individuals, especially parents of young children, to keep the number of the local poison control center near the phone in the event of ingestion of a toxic amount of drugs or exposure to or ingestion of other toxic substances. Teach children that drugs are not for playing and that they are not candy. This rule applies to all drugs, including vitamins, birth control pills, laxatives, and other prescription and nonprescription substances (see accompanying box and boxes on p. 41).

Information About a Specific Drug

To teach a patient about a specific drug, the instructional approach should be tailored to the needs and abilities of the patient. Careful patient assessment and analysis form the foundation of the teaching plan. Figure 4-1 illustrates a sample drug history that may provide data for use in developing a teaching plan. It could also be incorporated into the general health history recorded for all patients. The drug history questions should be modified as needed.

Teach the patient what the name and dosage of the prescribed drug are, why the drug is being used, and what the anticipated benefits of the drug are. Discuss the potential side effects in sufficient detail so that the patient will be able to list the most frequently encountered side effects. Whether the more serious (sometimes fatal, but also more rare) side effects should be discussed in detail depends on the patient and the situation. Instruct all patients and caregivers about whom to call (e.g., physician or nurse practitioner) if anything unexpected occurs.

If there are any management decisions that the patient must make, review them carefully with the patient. Examples include changes in dose strength or frequency, depending on

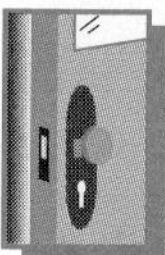

HOME HEALTH

Assessment of Medication Use in Homes With Young Children

- Where are medications kept in the house? The kitchen? The bathroom? On the kitchen table?
- Are there prescription or OTC medications that are out of date? Can you work with the family to discard them?
- Ask the caregiver to demonstrate preparing medications. Can the caregiver manipulate the equipment? Are oral suspensions shaken before the dose is poured? Are medications that should be refrigerated stored in the refrigerator?
- Is the caregiver able to monitor and record the patient's weight, pulse, blood glucose, or other parameters appropriate to the health condition?
- Is there anything about the general environment that might place the patient at risk?
- Are there medications within easy reach of a young child?
- Does the family have ipecac in the house? Do they know what it is for and how to use it? Is the number of the nearest poison control center posted near the telephone?

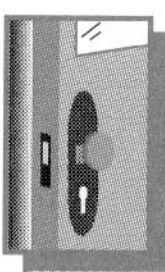

HOME HEALTH

Assessment of Medication Use in Older Adult Patients

- How does the patient keep track of when medications are due and whether they have been taken each day?
- Ask the patient to tell you how he or she manages medications each day.
- Where are medications kept in the house? The kitchen? The bathroom? On the nightstand?
- Are there OTC medications in the home that the patient uses regularly but forgot to mention?
- Are there prescription or OTC medications that are out of date? Can you work with the patient to discard them?
- Ask the patient to demonstrate preparing medications. Can the patient manipulate the equipment? Can the patient see the syringe or medicine dropper well enough to prepare the correct dose? Can the patient see well enough to test blood glucose?
- Is the patient able to monitor and record his or her weight, pulse, or other parameters appropriate to the health condition?
- Consider the medications the patient is supposed to take. Is there anything about the general environment that might place the patient at risk? For example, are there small bottles of ear medicine, glue, or other items kept close to the place where eyedrops are kept? If the patient taking a diuretic gets up at night to urinate, is the way to the bathroom uncluttered? Is there a night-light or hall light that can be left on so the patient can see?
- If possible, look in the refrigerator and the kitchen cabinets. Is the patient's diet adequate?

the patient's response to the medication, or home treatment of frequently encountered side effects. Have the patient practice any measurements that would be made at home (e.g., taking and recording pulse and checking blood glucose).

Inform the patient of any special considerations related to the dose, such as whether to take the drug on an empty or full stomach, whether to avoid milk, or whether to avoid taking two particular drugs simultaneously. If a new drug administration technique is involved, ascertain that the patient can demonstrate how to do this safely and accurately. Include appropriate general principles related to drug use.

Finally, provide the patient with information about how and when follow-up will occur and how to call for help or additional information. It is often advisable and helpful to have one or more family members present if the instruction is lengthy and complicated. In addition, provide written instructions whenever possible. It also may be helpful to refer the patient to a community-based nursing agency for follow-up in the home.

Patient Compliance

Even when the nurse has developed and implemented what seems to be a complete and individualized teaching plan, patient compliance may be poor. The many possible reasons for this include the following:

- The patient or family misunderstands the directions.
- Poor vision or hearing leads to errors in understanding or reading medication labels.
- The patient cannot get the prescription refilled because it must be renewed by the physician, the patient cannot get to the pharmacy, or the patient cannot afford the cost.

- The patient becomes confused by the number of medications being taken and takes the drugs in incorrect amounts and at wrong times.
- The patient cannot manage the new route of administration in the home without help (e.g., self-injection).
- The patient is unable to accept a particular diagnosis (e.g., the teenager with diabetes who does not check blood glucose in the morning before insulin administration or who injects insulin too late in the day).
- Intolerable side effects occur, and the patient is too embarrassed to mention them to anyone (e.g., sexual impotence).
- Side effects occur that cause the patient to feel worse than the health problem alone did. This is a common problem with some drugs, such as antihypertensives.

The nurse who is in the patient's home may find clues to noncompliance. For example, too many pills may remain in the bottle at the end of the month, or the patient may not be able to describe how to take the prescribed medications. In the office or hospital setting it may be more difficult for the nurse to find these clues. Only the lack of congruence between objective data and subjective response (e.g., the patient describes taking the antihypertensive, but the blood pressure remains high) may give the nurse a clue. The nurse must use careful nonjudgmental questioning to find out if there is a problem and to help the patient find a way to better manage the health problem (i.e., by taking the drug).

The nurse must be creative in finding ways to help patients (see box). Some frequently tried methods include making a special calendar with items that the patient must check off when the dose is taken or putting the pills into color-coded cups or containers that correspond to a specific mealtime. The doses of a medication may be prepared for 7 days and left with the patient who has difficulty preparing the dosage form. Pill containers with an alarm are also available; these can be set to go off each time a patient is scheduled to take a dose of drug. In other situations compliance can be improved by adjusting the dose, changing the time the drug is to be taken, or even changing the drug. Consult the physician about such adjustments. Finally, remember that patients have the right to choose whether or not and how they will take their medications. Some simply choose not to comply.

INABILITY TO READ

If a patient cannot read, the standard written instructions will not be helpful. Some patients who cannot read are frank about this limitation and will let the nurse know immediately. Others have managed to keep this information secret from friends and family and may be reluctant to tell the nurse. Actions that *may* indicate that the patient cannot read include the following:

- Not filling out the menu when in the hospital
- Not reading the newspaper, if available
- Professing fatigue and asking family members present to read instructions or the menu
- When asked if instructional materials have been read, indicating fatigue or forgotten glasses or stating something like: "I'll read them after my husband [wife] gets here"
- Not recording weight or pulse or blood glucose results at home

If the nurse suspects that the patient cannot read, or has limited reading skills, the nurse should include pictures or icons of some kind on instructional materials. A medication chart that combines pictures that represent times of the day, with a drawing of the medication, will be more helpful to the patient. The pharmacist may be able to help by providing one dose of each medication that can be pasted onto the instruction sheet.

REGULATIONS AND DRUG ADMINISTRATION

Personnel: Who Does What?

Many people may be involved in the prescription, preparation, and administration of a drug to a patient. Generally, physicians prescribe drugs. Their authorization to prescribe is granted through licensing and medical practice acts. Other individuals do prescribe, including dentists and oral surgeons, osteopathic physicians, podiatrists, nurse practitioners, midwives, and physician's assistants. However, the degree of independence of practice that these and other health care practitioners may exercise varies with the laws of the state, province, or nation. This issue introduces the first of many points that the nurse must consider before administering a drug: Who has prescribed the drug, and does that person have the legal right to do so in that setting?

In the institutional setting safeguards are often created to prevent unauthorized prescription of drugs. For example, to be granted privileges to practice in a hospital, a physician must present appropriate credentials, proof of licensure, and other documents required by that hospital.

After a nurse has worked on a nursing unit for several weeks, he or she will know the physicians, which also helps reduce the chance of errors related to who may prescribe. Even in the hospital, the nurse ascertains the role of each person on the health care team. For example, in some teaching hospitals it is customary for medical students to be acting interns with rotations (they may have other titles also). Although these individuals are not yet licensed, they may be caring for patients under the supervision of licensed preceptors (physicians). The nurse must be clear about the legal ramifications of administering drugs prescribed by a nonlicensed individual.

When looking for guidance about who may prescribe and whose prescriptions must be administered, the nurse can consult the nurse practice act (or comparable professional practice act) for that state, province, or nation. The written policies of the employing agency or institution also provide guidance. Finally, nurses must consider their own moral and ethical codes of conduct in deciding whether to administer a specific drug to a patient. The nurse always has the personal right to refuse to administer a medication. For example, a nurse may refuse to give an ordered medication if the nurse's professional judgment indicates that the dose is excessively high. The nurse must notify the physician and the nurse in charge about the decision not to administer the medication.

It is important to remember that the legal constraints the nurse must consider may have little meaning to the patient. This situation is faced more often in the home, where the patient may wish to have the nurse administer a medication or home remedy prescribed or recommended by someone not recognized by the nurse practice act.

Pharmacists, who usually dispense medication, are licensed to do so and are governed by legal statutes. Pharmacies often employ aides or technicians to help fill prescriptions, but these individuals function under the supervision of the registered pharmacist. The pharmacist is an excellent source of information about drugs for the nurse or the patient but is often underused in this role.

Registered nurses can administer medications within the legal framework of the nurse practice act. Licensed practical nurses and licensed vocational nurses also have practice acts that regulate the role they play in drug administration. In some areas pharmacists, medication technicians, medical students, emergency medical technicians, or others may administer drugs as employees of an institution or agency. Various students may be permitted to administer drugs in an agency, institution, or other setting if they are supervised. This category includes students participating in nursing, medical, physician assistant, emergency medical technician, and other educational programs. As the health care system changes, the responsibilities of individuals in various settings may also change. Therefore nurses must stay current with the various roles of members of the health care team. In the home the patient and family administer drugs.

Institutional Policies and Practices

The nurse practices within not only the legal framework of the nurse practice act but also the policies and procedures of the employing agency. The nurse is responsible for reading carefully any written information that defines restrictions or expectations of practice within the employing agency structure. The nurse should not blindly adhere to policy that is in direct conflict with legal guidelines or reasonable ethical and moral standards, but neither should the nurse practice outside the role defined by the agency.

In some agencies verbal orders for drugs may be taken only by registered nurses. Students, licensed practical nurses, and others may not take these orders (see box). Some institutions prohibit the nurse from obtaining the patient's informed consent for investigational drugs; they may require this consent to be obtained only by the physician. In other settings the physician alone may administer investigational drugs. Medication orders written by medical students may be administered only after they are co-signed by a licensed physician. Such policies often develop as an interpretation of the law or to prevent anticipated problems.

VERBAL MEDICATION ORDERS

Steps you should follow when taking a verbal medication order include the following:

1. If possible, have the patient's chart and medication records at hand.
2. Write down the order as it is dictated by the physician. (This may be done on scrap paper.)
3. Have the physician spell any unclear words.
4. Clarify any unclear part of the order.
5. Read the order back to the physician, including the patient's name and room number; the drug, dose, frequency, route of administration, and any other information given in the order; and the physician's name.
6. Glance at the other medications that the patient is receiving. If a question arises about the new medication ordered and the other medications the patient is currently receiving, ask the physician at that time.
7. Transcribe the order to the patient's record, noting the physician's name, your name, the date, and the time of day. Also note whether the order was given in person or by telephone.

Certain procedures in an agency are often developed in response to previous problems or errors. Examples include the requirements that all heparin and insulin doses be checked by two nurses before they are administered, that any parenteral drugs administered to pediatric patients be checked by two nurses before being administered, and that narcotics be counted at the end of each shift by two nurses, one from the ending shift and one from the beginning shift.

It may not be necessary for the nurse to know exactly *why* a policy or procedure has been developed. It *is* important for the nurse to practice within policy and procedure guidelines and, if the guidelines need to be changed, to work through the appropriate channels to change them. The beginning nurse may view these *dos* and *donts* as time-consuming, and some probably are not as important as others. However, all were designed to ensure safe patient care. Careless nursing practice can result in harm to the patient and malpractice suits. Failure to adhere to stated policies and procedures may weigh against the nurse in determination of legal liability.

Medication Errors

All medications are ordered, prepared, and administered with the best intentions. However, errors do occur with surprising frequency.

What Is an Error?

Defining an error is not always easy. It is clear that an error has occurred if a patient receives the wrong drug, if a patient is overmedicated, or if a prescribed drug is omitted. Other situations may be less clear-cut but also involve an error. Consider the following examples. A patient receives tetracycline with a glass of milk (tetracycline should not be administered with milk). A patient in the radiology department receives his 10 AM drugs at noon. Through an error in calculation, another patient receives the correct drug at the correct time but in half the ordered dose.

Some institutions differentiate between an *error* and an *incident.* Others define any deviation from policy and procedure as an *error.* This variability emphasizes the need for the nurse to know and adhere to the standards of practice defined by the nurse practice act, the policies and procedures of the employing agency and institution, and common sense.

The times at which drugs are administered in a hospital or institution are established by that setting; they are usually part of the policies and procedures. In addition, there is usually an explicit definition of what is meant by administering a drug on time. For example, a drug to be administered at 10 AM is considered to be on time if it is administered any time between 9:30 AM and 10:30 AM. The way a particular patient unit or entire institution handles deviations from the "half hour before to half hour after" rule influences whether the time at which a particular drug is administered is called an error. Since the times for qid, bid, and qd are set by custom or policy, they also can be readjusted.

Another factor that affects the time is the drug itself and how frequently it is ordered. Consider the following situations. A vitamin ordered for qd, customarily given at 10 AM, is forgotten and given at 2 PM. Most agencies would not consider this an error and would not notify the physician. Insulin ordered for qd is administered at 10 AM instead of before breakfast (when it should be given). This is an error. Another drug is ordered to be given qid. On a particular unit, that schedule is customarily 10 AM, 2 PM, 6 PM, and 10 PM. A nurse misreads the medications record and administers it at 8 AM. Depending on the medication, the nurse's action may not be considered an error since the dosage times could be readjusted to 8 AM, 12 noon, 4 PM, and 8 PM.

Causes of Errors

There are many causes of the errors associated with administering medications. The following situations are examples:

- A drug is ordered for the wrong patient (i.e., written on the wrong patient's chart).
- The wrong dose is ordered.
- The correct drug or dose is ordered, but because of poor penmanship the wrong drug or dosage is dispensed.
- An error in calculating the dose is made, so the patient receives the wrong dose.
- A drug is given via the wrong route.
- The patient's identity is not checked, and the wrong patient receives the drug.
- The first person who administers a drug fails to record it immediately afterward. A second person, checking the patient's chart, thinks that the drug has not been administered and so administers a dose. The patient has received a double dose.

What to Do if an Error Occurs

A professional accepts responsibility for his or her actions. If you think an error in drug administration has occurred, take the following steps. First, check the patient. Obtain any subjective or objective data appropriate to the patient's condition. If the patient received the wrong drug or the wrong dose, assess the individual for the effects of the drug. For example, if too large a dose of antihypertensive was administered, take the patient's blood pressure, and then put the patient to bed. Notify the nurse in charge and the physician. Fill out any error forms required by the institution. Continue to monitor the patient. Modify your personal nursing practice, if needed, to help avoid the error in the future.

Two points need to be emphasized. The student or beginning practitioner may lack experience in handling an error or in deciding what is an error. If unsure, the practitioner should always report any problem associated with drug administration to the nurse in charge and to the physician. There are students and nurses in practice who want to avoid filling out incident forms or medication error forms because they believe that admitting that an error has occurred will be detrimental to their employment or student status with the institution or agency. However, records of errors help institutions develop new policies, procedures, and systems that will reduce the overall incidence of errors. No hospital or agency wants to continue to employ nurses who make repeated errors, especially of a careless nature, but most institutions recognize that anyone can make an occasional error.

Students sometimes fear that they will be sued for malpractice if an error occurs. There is no way to guarantee that a nurse will not be sued. However, if an error occurs but steps are taken to assess the patient and reverse the effects of the error as soon as the error is discovered, it will be difficult to argue that the nurse had a pattern of irresponsible behavior. Nurses must remain vigilant in all nursing care activities to provide the best quality, careful nursing care.

How to Avoid Medication Errors

The basis of avoiding errors is using and acting on common sense. Read and adhere to institutional policies and procedures; do not try shortcuts. Read each order carefully, asking yourself whether this drug makes sense for this particular patient at this dosage. Look up any drug or dosage that seems questionable in a standard drug reference. Never assume that the physician was right, the pharmacist was right, or the previous nurse who administered the drug was right if there is any question in your mind. Be especially careful in taking verbal or telephone orders because it is easy to misunderstand what is said (see box, p. 43).

Double-check all dosage calculations. If you still feel uneasy about a drug amount, have a colleague or the pharmacy double-check it. If a dose seems unusually large or small, double-check it. For example, if the order was for 10 grains of aspirin, but, through an error in recording, it is noted as 100 grains, the dose would require 20 aspirin tablets, an unusually large amount for a patient. The other extreme also can happen. For example, the dose of ferrous sulfate (an iron preparation) for an adult may be listed as 30 mg. To administer that dose would require 1/10 tablet, an impossible task.

If possible, avoid distractions while preparing medications. Check each label 3 times: when taking the drug out of the drawer or cabinet, when checking the Kardex for the dose and time, and again at the bedside just before administering the drug. Leave medications in their labeled containers until you are at the bedside. Always check the patient's identity carefully. If the patient asks any questions that indicate a possible error, assume that the patient is right, and double-check. Examples include statements such as: "That doesn't look like my usual morning pill," "I already took that—the other nurse gave it to me earlier today," or "The doctor said I would have a different pill today."

Ask the patient about a history of allergies before administering any new drug. Finally, check each patient within a short period after administering medications. Administering medications is just one of many nursing responsibilities, but it can be one of the most dangerous if done carelessly.

NURSING PROCESS OVERVIEW

The Nursing Process With Drug Therapy

Assessment

Assessment includes gathering all the subjective and objective pertinent data about a patient, physically assessing the patient, and evaluating laboratory, radiographic, and other data. Throughout assessment the nurse analyzes the data and formulates nursing diagnoses.

Nursing Diagnoses

Nursing diagnoses are derived from the assessment data. With the possible exception of "Knowledge deficit," no single nursing diagnosis fits all situations related to drug therapy.

Patient Outcomes

Patient outcomes describe in measurable terms the goals of therapy in relation to the patient.

Planning/Implementation

The nurse develops the plan in response to the assessment of patient needs and the knowledge of the treatment plan. The plan should include goals and specific steps to reach the goals. The patient or family is included in the plan development. Implementation involves carrying out the plan. Planning and implementation should include individualizing the approach to fit the unique needs of the patient.

Evaluation

Evaluation involves determining the success of the plan and its implementation. The step includes determining whether the goals have been reached for the patient. It involves deciding whether the goals were appropriate for the patient. Finally, evaluation focuses on revising the overall plan.

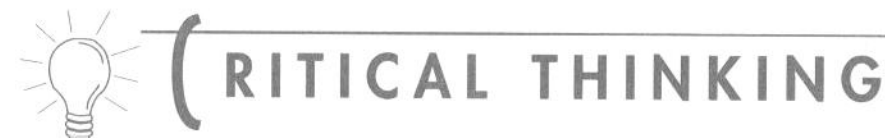

CRITICAL THINKING

APPLICATION

1. What are the steps of the nursing process?
2. Discuss how medication administration fits into the nursing process.
3. What are the five rights of drug administration?
4. List the basic teaching points about safe medication use that should be taught to all patients.
5. In the settings where you practice, who may prescribe drugs? Who prepares them? Who administers them?
6. What is the difference between the nurse practice act (or other legal statutes) and institutional policies and procedures?
7. What are some examples of medication errors?

CRITICAL THINKING

1. What kinds of information about drugs should be included in the patient teaching plan?
2. What are some factors that influence patient compliance?
3. When the nurse discovers that a medication error has occurred, what should be done?

SECTION II

Nursing Care Related to Drug Therapy

This section introduces the basic nursing activities involved in administering drugs to patients. Chapters 5 and 6 focus on the basic nursing activities involved in administering drugs.

CHAPTER 5 *Drug Administration* presents information and techniques that can assist the nurse in properly administering drugs to provide safe individualized patient care.

CHAPTER 6 *Calculating Drug Dosages* helps students achieve proficiency and develop confidence in this basic skill. Drug dosage calculations are presented as a guide to the level of proficiency expected of practicing nurses.

CHAPTER 7 *Over-the-Counter Drugs and Self-Medication* emphasizes the importance of these agents in nursing practice. The legal status of over-the-counter agents, their properties, and drug interactions are discussed. The material is a ready reference for the nurse in assessing the use of nonprescription medication.

CHAPTER 8 *Issues of Drug Abuse* guides the nurse in recognizing the impact of drug abuse on patient compliance and response. General principles and definitions are emphasized to aid the nurse in understanding the literature in this specialized area.

CHAPTER 9 *Care of the Poisoned Patient* introduces the study of adverse effects of chemicals, including drugs, on people.

CHAPTER 5

Drug Administration

OBJECTIVES

After studying this chapter, you should be able to do the following:

- *Explain differences between the unit-dose system and the stock drug system.*
- *Give examples of information about drug administration that must be recorded on the patient's record.*
- *Give examples of how administration of drugs to children or older adults may require more individualized planning.*
- *Describe how to administer drugs via a variety of routes.*

CHAPTER OVERVIEW

This chapter emphasizes drug administration. Drug therapy is only a part of total patient care, but for drug therapy to be successful it must be carried out properly. The patient has the right to receive the right drug, in the right dose, at the right time, via the right route.

The administration of drugs to patients is an opportunity for the nurse to continue to assess the patient's condition, to teach the patient in preparation for self-management of the health condition, to participate in discharge planning with the patient, and to evaluate the effectiveness of the care plan being implemented by the health care team. The reader should also study Chapter 3 carefully for information about the application of the nursing process to drug therapy.

KEY TERMS

buccal tablets
central venous catheters
deltoid muscle
dorsogluteal site
heparin lock
heparin well
implanted infusion port: OmegaPort or Port-A-Cath
intradermal injection
intramuscular injection
IV push
lingual spray
lozenges
nontunneled catheter
parenteral
peripherally inserted central catheter (PIC catheter or PICC)
rectus femoris muscle
stock drug system
subcutaneous injection
sublingual drugs
suppositories
suspension
troches
tunneled catheter: Broviac, Hickman, Groshong
unit dose system
vastus lateralis muscle
ventrogluteal muscle
Z-track technique

DRUG ADMINISTRATION SYSTEMS

The two major drug administration systems in common use today are the unit-dose system and the stock drug system. In the **unit-dose system** each dose of medication is individually wrapped, labeled, and supplied to the patient's unit in sufficient quantity to last 24 hours. On the patient unit each patient has a designated drawer, box, or container, and the exact number of ordered doses of medications for a 24-hour period is placed in that container by the pharmacy daily. When the nurse prepares to administer a drug, the patient's container is checked for the dose. The labeled medication is taken to the bedside. After the nurse verifies the patient's identity, the dose package is opened and the nurse administers the dose to the patient. This system has several advantages:

1. The medication remains in a labeled container until the nurse is at the bedside, thus reducing the chance of mixing up drugs.
2. Patients can be billed by exactly the number of medication doses that are taken.
3. Unauthorized use of medications is decreased.

Disadvantages include the increased cost for the pharmacy in setting up this system, the need for additional pharmacists or pharmacy technicians to resupply the patient units each 24 hours and to fill orders for stat and new orders, and the usual need for increased space in the pharmacy for storage of drugs in the unit-dose packages. The system builds in at least two opportunities to check the medication order, including when the physician's written order for drugs goes to the pharmacy to be filled and when the pharmacy stocks the patient's supply. The nurse then checks the drug when administering it.

In the **stock drug system** each patient unit is supplied with large-quantity stock containers of the drugs commonly used in that setting or institution. The nurse administering a drug takes the order sheet, Kardex, or medication card to the medication room and prepares the dose of the drug from the stock supply, usually putting the dose into a small medicine cup. The nurse then takes the drugs, now unlabeled, to the bedside, and, after checking the patient's identity, administers the prepared drugs. The advantages of this system are that the pharmacy need not restock the floor stock daily, calculation and preparation of doses require fewer pharmacy personnel since these duties are performed by the nurses, and stat and new orders can be filled immediately because the stock drugs are on the unit. Disadvantages are that the system is usually more time-consuming for the nursing staff, billing patients for exact drug use may be difficult, significant waste and inappropriate use of the stock drugs may occur (e.g., nurses and physicians using drugs for their own ailments), and medication errors are more common.

Most institutions combine the two systems. A hospital might supply all nonliquid oral forms in unit-dose packages but have the liquid forms in multiple-dose bottles, one bottle per patient. The nurse must learn as much as possible about the drug administration system so that valuable time is not lost in searching the patient unit for a drug that is available only in the pharmacy, or conversely, in calling the pharmacy for a drug already available on the patient unit.

RECORDING DRUG-RELATED INFORMATION

Recording drug administration is an important responsibility of the nurse. Forms for recording drug administration vary among agencies or institutions, but some general points usually do apply. The nurse should record that a dose was given as soon after administering the dose as possible. If a dose of medication is omitted, the reason must be noted, usually in the nurses' notes, on the form designated by the agency, or in the computer. Most institutions also require that doses given significantly early or late be accompanied by a notation explaining why. These records are legal documents, and information recorded on them should be legible and accurate.

Information related to the route of administration or to the drug itself may need to be recorded. Examples include the full-minute apical pulse, taken before a cardiotonic is administered; the blood glucose level, measured before a sliding-scale insulin dose is administered; the site of an injection; and the location of a topical nitroglycerin preparation. Such information is often noted in the same place the nurse recorded that the dose was administered.

Another important kind of information relates to individualized patient care; this includes the assessment, management, and evaluation of a specific patient. Assessment data might include the subjective and objective information that led the nurse to conclude that a prn drug was needed: for example, the oral temperature was 102°F, and the patient was shivering and complaining of generalized achiness. These data led the nurse to administer aspirin, an available prn option for that patient. Depending on the patient record system in use in that institution, such data might be recorded in the nurses' notes or patient progress notes, which may be paper forms or computer records. Information related to the management of a patient, such as the patient's tolerating physical therapy best when a prn analgesic is administered 1 hour before therapy, becomes part of the care plan. Another kind of drug management information relates to the actual techniques of administration. This information might be part of the care plan, or there might be adequate room on the medication record to include this information. An example of this kind of information is that the patient will take the drug more easily if it is crushed and mixed with applesauce.

Information related to the patient's response to the medication and the effectiveness of the drug (evaluation) should also be recorded. This information may include subjective or objective data; it is usually recorded in the nurses' notes or patient progress notes. Most of the forms in the patient's record are legal documents; therefore information recorded must be accurate, complete, and signed by the nurse.

ADMINISTERING DRUGS TO CHILDREN

Some drugs have been widely used in neonates and infants, and therefore dosage regimens are well documented; however, many drugs have not been studied in this population. Children are not simply "small adults." Because of the small size and immature organs of neonates and infants, doses must be carefully calculated. Administration of drugs must be monitored closely. Not only must the dose be correct, but also, since fluid overload can easily occur, the volume of medications being administered must be monitored closely.

Administering drugs to children presents unique challenges. Not only may the physiologic activity of the drug be altered (see Chapters 1 and 2), but the child may be unable or unwilling to take prescribed medications. For infants and toddlers, doses may be very small, requiring special care in calculation and preparation.

A developmental approach should be used in administering drugs to children. A tentative plan is prepared for drug administration based on knowledge of growth and development for different age groups. The plan is initially tentative because the child's chronologic age may not match his or her developmental age. As the nurse and the health care system get to know the child, effective individualized approaches can be noted in the care plan.

To understand the developmental approach, think about a 2-year-old who is to receive an injection and an oral medication. First, consider the available information about the child's general level of functioning, motor ability, interactions with other children, vocabulary, and ability to conceptualize. Then consider theories of child development such as those of Erikson, Freud, and Piaget for guidance. The 2-year-old, in Erikson's framework, is in the stage of autonomy vs. shame and doubt. Behaviors characteristic of this stage include negativism, difficulty making choices, separation anxiety, and ritual. The child shows pride in performing well, is able to feed self, and has a limited understanding of time.

A few nursing approaches for children include giving simple directions; describing honestly what will occur but not until shortly before administering the medications; and asking the child to administer the oral drug. Do not ask, "Do you want to take your medicine?" because the answer frequently is "No!" If possible, give the child a choice of beverage to accompany taking the oral drug, but limit the choice (e.g., milk or apple juice). Follow the same pattern each time drugs are administered. Use firmness and consistency. Be prepared with adequate but nonthreatening assistance to restrain the child for the injection. Give positive feedback when the child cooperates and assists, provide comfort as needed, and encourage family members to do the same. Children of this age often want to assist or cooperate but need guidance in how to do so.

Remember that children vary, and although a developmental approach provides guidance, it does not replace individualized assessment and planning. Children also differ from adults in their ability to understand and accept the intrusive nature of many of the routes of drug administration. The young child may be terrified of receiving eardrops because the child cannot see what the nurse is doing to the ears. Injections are painful, and young children may have unrealistic fears (e.g., that their insides will come out of the hole created by the needle). Simply applying a bandage over the injection site may eliminate this fear. These examples may be difficult for the adult caregiver to understand since adults have learned how to reason. Adults may also dislike injections, even fear them, but they understand that the injection is fast and for their overall benefit.

Children's level of comprehension is very concrete until the early teens. Thus children may have difficulty understanding why an injection in the thigh could help their earache. Children also have trouble understanding time relationships and thinking about long-term consequences. Thus long-term drug therapy for treating tuberculosis, seizures, or rheumatic fever may be difficult for the young child to understand.

A few additional guidelines related to techniques of administration include the following. Do not dilute medications in a large volume of liquid or food; if the child does not finish eating all of it, the nurse does not know how much medication has been consumed. Do not disguise medications in a favorite or essential food; the child may be unwilling to eat that food again. Do not try to trick the child into taking medications; be honest but caring in approaching children.

Use drawings, simple stories, coloring books, and toys dealing with medications and hospitalization. Explain the steps of administering the drug to preschool and young school-age children in a manner appropriate for their age. Allow children to play out their feelings. In a setting where children are frequently treated, have a toy box available containing items such as small dolls, medicine cups, and plastic syringes without needles to allow children to pretend, before or after medications are administered.

Do not underestimate the child's ability to understand or adjust to medication administration. At early ages many children can begin to accept responsibility for medication administration, especially for chronic health problems. For example, children 6 to 8 years old can be taught to self-administer insulin correctly.

There are other potential problems with medication administration and children. Some of these relate to the home environment. Problems that might place a child at risk include the following:

- Inappropriate use of medications originally prescribed for an adult in the household, without approval from a physician that the drug or dose is appropriate for the child
- Medications left within easy reach of young children, with the potential that a child will overdose
- Inaccurate dosage measurement, which might occur, for example, if spoons of different capacities are used to measure doses

- Using a medication prescribed for one child to treat others in the family when a definitive diagnosis on the other children has not been made
- Lack of knowledge of parents or caregivers that some medications should not be used in children in certain situations, for example, administering aspirin to treat fever in a child with chickenpox
- Referring to medications as "candy," which may cause children to not understand the serious nature of medications

The nurse who can visit the family in the home may be able to identify some of these problems, if they exist, and work with the family to correct them.

ADMINISTERING DRUGS TO OLDER ADULTS

Older adult patients can also present special care considerations for the nurse. As mentioned in Chapters 1 and 2, the physiologic changes that accompany aging influence the patient's response to medications. Medication use among the older adults is generally higher than among younger groups. As many as two thirds of Americans older than age 65 take at least one prescription drug; of these, at least one third take three or more drugs. Physiologic changes that may occur in older adults have been outlined earlier in this book. There is, however, great variability in the older adults. Some individuals at age 65 show marked physiologic changes, whereas others in their eighties or nineties show few physiologic changes. Some older adults take many medications, whereas others take few or none.

Individualized assessment and planning are important when working with older adults. An important role for the nurse is to make certain that all medications ordered for a particular patient are still necessary. Sometimes as side effects to one drug develop, an additional drug is prescribed to treat them. Side effects to the second drug develop, and these are treated with a third drug. It may be difficult for the physician, the nurse, and the patient to understand what the drug regimen is designed to do.

Another problem occasionally encountered with the older adults is the use of several health care providers, who may not be communicating with one another about the patient. Thus a patient may have an ophthalmologist, a cardiologist, a podiatrist, and a urologist, each prescribing treatments and drugs for various problems. This situation can result in too many drugs being taken, some of which may be antagonistic to each other or contraindicated with one of the drugs. Even intelligent, mentally alert patients can have difficulty managing a complicated medication regimen that may include drugs to be taken before and after meals, some once a day, others more often during the day, with the dose of other drugs changing based on the day of the week or the day of the month. If a complicated drug regimen is combined with the effects of chronic disease, possible poor nutrition, or other problems, it is not surprising that some older adult patients are at great risk from their medications.

Some older adults remain vigorous, physically active, and mentally alert. Many, however, have one or more physical problems that make medication usage difficult or potentially hazardous. For example, cataracts and glaucoma are both more prevalent in older adults, as are alterations in vision from strokes and other neurologic problems. Other patients have vision problems resulting from a general decline in visual acuity that has evolved over the years. Vision problems in older adults may make reading drug labels and package inserts and preparing the correct dose of a medication difficult. Alterations in vision may make it difficult for patients to read test results correctly or to monitor their weight (because they cannot read the scale). Hearing may decline in some patients. Alterations in hearing may place older adults at risk for misunderstanding verbal instructions about how to take medications correctly.

Physical dexterity may be altered in some patients. Arthritic changes, paralysis secondary to stroke, or other problems may make it difficult for older adults to manipulate items such as pill bottles, syringes, blood glucose testing equipment, and small pills or tablets.

Many older adults live on fixed low incomes. Medications are often expensive. Older adult patients who would like to take their medications as ordered may have difficulty because they cannot afford the medication or cannot physically get to the drugstore to pick up their prescription. Some patients may not be able to afford the drug in the dosing frequency prescribed; therefore they try to save money by taking doses only half as often as ordered (see boxes on p. 52).

Some older adults may also be poorly nourished. This situation may be due to lack of money, difficulty getting to the store, or difficulty eating certain foods (because of lacking teeth or having poorly fitting dentures). Still other reasons may be lack of knowledge about a well-rounded nutritious diet or lack of energy or interest in cooking regular meals (e.g., if the person lives alone). If the patient is poorly nourished, the serum albumin level may be low, causing a potential problem in the effects of protein-bound drugs. General poor nutrition may place the patient at risk for increased side effects from some drugs.

Another problem that older adults face is having family or health care team members assume that a decline in their condition represents a natural part of aging, without adequate patient assessment. Weakness, loss of balance, confusion, memory loss, slurred speech, fatigue, and loss of appetite are but a few symptoms that could be due to drug side effects and should not be attributed to aging.

Older adult patients must be approached as adults. Older adults who have taken many drugs over the years may have established elaborate rituals associated with taking drugs. The ritual may involve factors such as the time of day, the order in which the drugs are taken, or the fluid used to swallow the drugs. Ask patients about their usual practices before rush-

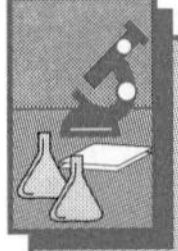

RESEARCH HIGHLIGHT

Too Many Medications, Too Little Money: How Do Patients Cope?

— SJ Chubon, RM Schulz, EW Lingle, MA Coster-Schulz: Public Health Nurs 11(6)4:412-415, 1994.

PURPOSE

In South Carolina, Medicaid pays for three prescriptions a month for Medicaid recipients. Many Medicaid recipients need more than three prescribed medications per month. The purpose of this study was to explore what patients who have multiple prescribed drugs do when the cost of only three of their prescriptions is provided.

METHOD

This was a qualitative pilot study with a convenience sample. Pharmacists in two small towns helped to identify Medicaid recipients taking more than three prescribed medications. Prospective participants were contacted in writing. Those willing to participate were paid $20. Subjects were interviewed in the participant's home by an experienced public health nurse. Subjects showed their medications to the nurse and discussed how they managed. Interview results were analyzed for common themes and unique experiences.

RESULTS

This study included 19 subjects: 17 women and 2 men. One subject was a child, but the others were adults. Of the subjects, 14 were over age 60. The mean age of the adults was 68.7 years. The mean number of drugs prescribed during the preceding year was 7.6. Medical diagnoses reported included diabetes, hypertension, heart disease, chronic lung disease, cancer, and asthma.

Subjects reported taking the following actions when they were faced with a prescription medication not paid for by Medicaid: (1) paid out of pocket (100%), (2) obtained medication in other ways (58%), (3) got money from someone else (42%), (4) did not get the medicine at all (42%), (5) changed the way medicine was taken (37%), and (6) took another person's medicine (11%). Those who obtained the medication in other ways reported receiving samples from the physician or obtaining medications from the pharmacist on credit until they could pay. Those who got money from someone else usually identified their children as a source of this additional money, although one person had taken out a loan to buy prescriptions. Prescriptions not filled included ones for digoxin, glyburide, furosemide, albuterol sulfate, metaproterenol sulfate, and sulindac.

IMPLICATIONS

Nurses working with patients on Medicaid or patients with limited resources for obtaining prescription medications should assess patients carefully to see if the drugs are being used as prescribed. Patient teaching may need to include guidelines about which medications can be omitted if necessary. Nurses should also use opportunities to advocate for their patients and to contact legislators and policymakers about the needs of patients.

GERIATRIC CONSIDERATION

Reducing Drug Costs

Prescription drugs can be costly. Possible ways to reduce costs for patients include the following:

- Ask the physician if the drug can be prescribed in the generic form.
- Shop around (via telephone) for the best buy. Pharmacies vary in their prices.
- If the prescription is for a new drug, ask the physician for a few samples, or ask the pharmacist to fill part of the prescription (e.g., to give you 10 tablets of the 100 ordered tablets) until you see whether this drug causes serious side effects.
- If a drug must be taken for an extended period, is there any organization through which drugs can be purchased at a reduced cost? For example, through the American Association of Retired Persons (AARP), members can buy large quantities of AARP medicines at reduced rates. However, these drugs must be ordered through the mail, so this service is most helpful with drugs that will be needed on a long-term, continuing basis.

ing in at 10 AM to administer a handful of drugs. When possible, allow patients to continue their usual routine.

Older adults may also be more sensitive to nausea as a side effect. This sensitivity combined with the potential interaction of a large quantity of drugs may compound the nausea. It may be necessary to readjust the dosage schedule to spread out the prescribed medications over the course of the day. Also, if the patient must drink 6 to 8 ounces of fluid or more to take all the medications, they should not be administered just before a meal. After drinking a full glass of liquid, the patient may not feel like eating a complete meal.

DRUG ADMINISTRATION SCHEDULES

In the hospital or nursing home the nurse determines the times to administer the medications. In the home the patient must do it. Scheduling may be difficult, and it may require incorporating many of the following adjustments (among others):

- Multiple daily doses of the same drug should be evenly spaced throughout the 24 hours to help maintain serum drug levels (see Chapter 1).

- Drugs with known interactions should not be administered at the same time (e.g., cholestyramine with digoxin).
- Drugs that interact with specific foods should not be given concurrently with those foods (e.g., tetracycline and milk).
- Drugs known to work best if given before or after a meal must be scheduled (e.g., sucralfate).
- Some drug doses must be scheduled early in the day for appropriate effect (e.g., insulin).
- The patient's sleep should not be interrupted any more than necessary. At home the patient may not get up to take any medications during the night.
- In the hospital some drugs are arbitrarily scheduled at a time during the day to allow for the return of laboratory results (e.g., warfarin).

When a patient is taking many medications, scheduling can be a challenge for the nurse and an even larger challenge for the patient.

Patients with multiple chronic health problems may need to take several drugs simultaneously. The combination of drugs or the total amount of fluid needed by the patient to swallow the drugs may be nauseating. If the patient refuses to take all the medications, tires before all the drugs are taken, or becomes too nauseated to take all the drugs, the nurse must ensure that the more necessary drugs are taken first and the less necessary ones are left until last. Consider a patient receiving a cardiotonic, an antihypertensive, a diuretic, a potassium replacement, a vitamin, and an iron supplement at 10 AM. It is presumed that all these drugs are necessary for management of the patient's condition. However, the nurse may decide that the cardiotonic, antihypertensive, diuretic, and potassium replacement are of greater priority. This is not to suggest that the nurse can simply decide not to administer certain medications but that the nurse is frequently required to exercise judgment and make decisions on short notice. A better long-term solution to this multiple drug problem might be to schedule the vitamin and the iron supplement at a time when the patient is taking fewer drugs and will then have less difficulty in taking all that are ordered. See Chapter 4 for additional discussion of medication scheduling.

TECHNIQUES FOR ADMINISTERING DRUGS

The box on p. 54 lists the steps to be followed in administering all drugs. For more detailed descriptions or additional illustrations, see textbooks of nursing fundamentals.

Stay informed about agency policies regarding infection control and guidelines from the Centers for Disease Control and Prevention. Wear gloves when administering medications if there is a chance of exposure to body fluids. Follow agency guidelines for disposing of contaminated needles and always be vigilant in working with needles. Keep up to date on immunizations (e.g., hepatitis B immunization) and follow agency guidelines if a needle stick occurs.

Oral Route

Drugs are most frequently administered via the oral route. This route is safe, convenient, and acceptable for most patients and medications.

After carefully checking and preparing the medications ordered, identify the patient, help the patient sit upright (if possible), and then hand the medications and a glass of water or other preferred liquid to the patient. The patient then puts the pills, tablets, or capsules in the mouth and swallows them with the offered fluid. The patient should drink enough fluid to ensure that the medication reaches the stomach. Drugs that lodge in the esophagus can cause irritation and burning and may result in poor absorption. Approximately 4 ounces of fluid is usually sufficient, but encourage the patient to drink more unless contraindicated. Patients who are not sitting upright may need additional fluid to ensure that the medication has reached the stomach.

Ensure that the medication was swallowed and is not being hidden in the patient's mouth. Although this situation is rare, it can occur with confused individuals or those with certain psychiatric problems. After the patient swallows the drug, record that the medication has been taken.

Many patients have difficulty swallowing whole tablets or capsules. Break scored tablets along the lines indicated. It may be possible to separate the halves of capsules and pour out the powdered drug into another liquid or soft food such as applesauce. Crush tablets and mix with water or food. Especially with children, use as little applesauce or other food as possible. Otherwise, the child may feel full or refuse the rest of the applesauce, and the nurse has no way of knowing how much of the prescribed dose was actually consumed. See the box on p. 55 for a list of drug forms that should not be crushed or chewed. If in doubt, consult the pharmacist before crushing tablets or breaking open capsules.

Children sometimes take medications wrapped in a jelly sandwich. Another way to encourage the child is to give the medication in a cup and follow it with a "chaser" of water, milk, or carbonated beverage in another medication cup. Children like the small cups and are not overwhelmed with a large volume of fluid. When choosing a food or fluid to give a child to help disguise or take medications, do not select items with high sugar content if the medication must be taken on a regular basis because the item may contribute to dental caries. For children with diabetes, use sugar-free vehicles.

Although in some institutions the pharmacy will send crushed dosage forms to the nursing unit, it is usually the nurse's responsibility to crush the medication. There are several ways to do this. Some agencies supply pill crushers in the nursing unit. A mortar and pestle may be used. Be sure that these implements are clean before use, and wash away any remaining drug residue and dry them after preparing the dose. It may be possible to place the tablet inside a plastic or paper medication cup and then place a second cup over the pill. Any handy blunt instrument can then be used to crush the tablet between the layers of the cups. Alternatively, place the pill be-

GENERAL STEPS IN DRUG ADMINISTRATION

1. At the start of the workday, review each patient's record, noting the medical and nursing diagnoses, current problems, relevant laboratory findings, and plan of health care.
2. Compare the physician's original order against the working tools (may be medication Kardex, medication cards, computer printout, or computer screen—whatever is used in that setting to guide the nurse in preparing drugs).
   a. Check for accuracy of transcription: Drug name? Drug dose? Route of administration? Frequency of administration?
   b. Check for appropriateness of the order. Does this drug make sense for this patient? Is this dose in the usual range for a patient of this age and weight?
   c. Other: Have any automatic expiration dates passed? Are there new laboratory values to be considered, such as serum electrolyte levels, serum drug levels, culture reports, or renal or liver function studies?
3. Look up any new drugs or check any drug information that is unclear.
4. Check the medication supply.
   a. Is stock bottle supply adequate for the shift? If not, reorder from the pharmacy.
   b. Check each patient's drawer or box of drugs. Are the drugs present?
   c. Are any missing drugs in the refrigerator, on the back of the medication cart, at the bedside? Where else?
   d. Are there sufficient supplies to prepare and administer the drugs (straws, water cups, medication cups, spoons, mortar and pestle, syringes)?
5. Review the specific drugs. Are there any special assessments to be made or data to check before any drug is administered? Examples might include measurement of apical pulse, blood pressure, temperature, weight, urine, or blood test.
   a. Organize equipment that might be needed.
   b. Make a list if necessary.
6. Check care plans (if not already done) to note personal preferences, previous problems, and nursing care approaches. Make a list of items to remember, such as applesauce, juices, coffee, crackers, yogurt, jelly sandwich, ice cream, or other foods to disguise flavors.
7. Just before preparing the drugs, wash hands.
8. Check the working tool and obtain the medication. Read the label carefully, checking the drug, the dose, and the route of administration.*
9. Pour or prepare the dose. If from a stock bottle, read the label again before replacing the bottle. If from a unit dose, check the label; do not remove the drug from the package.
10. Prepare all medications for that patient. If preparing medications in the medication room, prepare the medications for all the patients who are to receive them.
11. Go to the bedside, and identify the patient (if possible, use all three methods):
    a. Call the patient by name. (Be especially careful if there is more than one patient on the unit with the same last name.)
    b. Ask the patient to state his or her full name.
    c. Check the patient identification band. (This may be the only possible way to identify the infant, small child, or confused adult.)
12. Assess the patient.
    a. Note any changes since you last saw the patient.
    b. Obtain any objective data needed before administering the drugs such as apical pulse, blood pressure, or breath sounds.
    c. Obtain any appropriate subjective information.
    d. If you did not previously know the patient or if new drugs are being administered, check on history of allergy.
13. If the data obtained in step 12 were not acceptable, withhold the corresponding drugs. For example, if the apical pulse is 50 beats/min, do not administer the cardiotonic drug (use agency policies as guides). Other drugs may be given if the patient's condition is satisfactory.
14. Draw the curtain or otherwise ensure privacy, if needed.
15. Administer the medications, helping the patient as needed. If the medicines are in unit-dose packages, open the packages. Make certain the patient takes the medication. Do not leave any medications at the bedside unless authorized by a physician's order or written institutional policy.
16. Assist the patient to resume a comfortable position.
17. Wash hands.
18. If using a medication cart, and the medication record is kept with the cart, immediately record that the drugs were given. If using a different system, administer all medications, then return to the medication record and record that the drugs were given.
19. Depending on the drug, the patient, and the usual policies and procedures, notify appropriate individuals (e.g., nurse in charge, physician) about doses that were withheld.
20. Record other appropriate information such as data obtained during assessment, drugs withheld and why, or changes in the patient's condition.
21. Make appropriate additions to the care plan.
22. Check on the patient at appropriate intervals to evaluate the response to drug therapy.

*The next few steps vary slightly, depending on whether the drugs are prepared in the medication room, such as with a stock drug system, or in the patient's room, such as with a medication cart and unit-dose system.

DRUG FORMS THAT SHOULD NOT BE CRUSHED OR CHEWED

- Enteric-coated tablets.
- Sustained-release forms. These often have the following suffixes attached to the drug name:
  - Dur (*Duration*)
  - SR (*Sustained Release*)
  - CR (*Controlled or Continuous Release*)
  - SA (*Sustained Action*)
  - Contin (*Continuous*)
  - LA (*Long Acting*)
- Trade names that imply sustained release such as spansules, extentabs, extencaps.
- Trade names with the bid (twice a day) abbreviation in the name, such as Theobid, Lithobid, and Cardabid.
- Liquid-containing capsules, although occasionally it may be acceptable to puncture the capsule and squeeze out the contents; consult the pharmacist or manufacturer.

The name alone may not provide enough information. Consult the pharmacist if in doubt. Some forms that look like sustained forms are not, and vice versa. Some capsules containing small, slow-release pellets may be opened, and the pellets may be sprinkled on applesauce or gently mixed into liquid or food, but they should not be crushed or dissolved.

Scored tablets may be broken along the scored line but should not be chewed or crushed.

tween two metal spoons and crush it. Also, some unit-dose packages are sturdy enough to allow the pill or tablet to be crushed in the package. Regardless of how the drug is crushed, be careful to check that all the powdered drug is brushed into the cup that you give the patient.

As an alternative to crushing medications, obtain a liquid form of the drug. Many drugs are available in liquid forms as suspensions or solutions. Make substitutions carefully; be sure to consult the physician and pharmacist. For example, a sustained-release form of a drug might be available in tablet form, but the only liquid preparation available may not be a sustained-release form; therefore dosage frequency may require adjustment.

It is generally easy to measure the prescribed dose in a capsule or tablet form, but liquid preparations require more care. If the drug is in **suspension** form, shake the container thoroughly before pouring the dose. Inadequate shaking of suspensions can result in the patient receiving a weaker dose from the top of the bottle and a stronger dose near the bottom of the bottle, as the unsuspended particles of drug collect. In the institutional setting medication cups are usually provided for measuring the prescribed dose unless the drug is supplied in the unit dose from the pharmacy. Place the medication cup on a flat surface or hold it upright at eye level to check that the correct dose has been poured. The base of the meniscus should be at the level of the desired dose (Figure 5-1). For small amounts of liquids or odd quantities, measure the dose with a syringe. It is not acceptable to estimate 2 ml or 12.5 ml of a drug.

In the home patients usually use household tablespoons and teaspoons for measuring dosages. Encourage patients to use the same spoon each time since household spoons are not standardized and switching spoons may result in varying dosages. Tell patients to read the pharmacy label to see whether liquid forms must be stored in the refrigerator.

The availability of a liquid form of a drug does not necessarily ensure patient cooperation in taking the drug. Many liquid forms, especially tinctures and elixirs, may be very unpleasant tasting. Patients may be more willing to take a crushed tablet in food than to take the drug in the liquid form. Some patients may take liquid forms better through a straw placed near the back of the mouth. If the preparation can stain teeth, ensure that a straw is used so that the medication is delivered to the back of the throat, bypassing contact with the teeth. Cutting the straw in half may make it easier for children to manage.

A factor influencing the sequence of oral drug administration is the use or particular property of a drug. For example, Xylocaine Viscous, an oral preparation of lidocaine hydrochloride, is sometimes prescribed to produce relief of oral discomfort in stomatitis; it accomplishes this by producing local anesthesia. Administer this drug last if several drugs are being administered simultaneously because this drug may interfere with swallowing. Antitussives should usually be taken last because they generally should not be followed with water. Not all oral drugs are to be swallowed; sublingual or buccal tablets should dissolve in the mouth. Administer drugs to be taken via the sublingual or buccal route last, after drugs that are to be swallowed have been consumed.

Regardless of specific problems and their solutions, the quality of nursing care can be improved and much time saved if you record on the patient medication Kardex or care plan anything unique about the administration of medications to each patient.

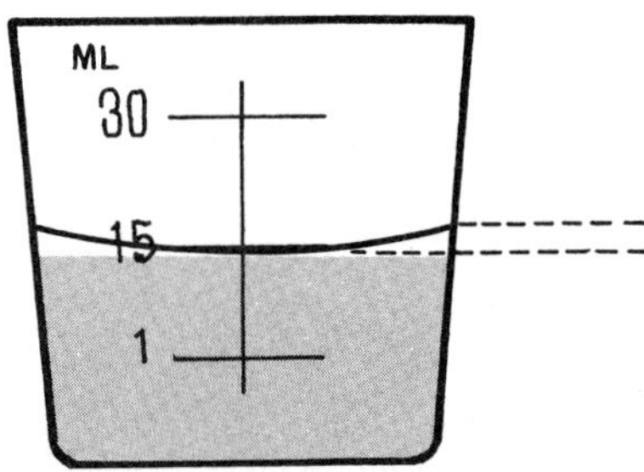

FIGURE 5-1

Reading meniscus. Meniscus is caused by surface tension of solution against container walls. Surface tension causes formation of concave or hollowed curvature on solution surface. Read level at lowest point of concave curve.

Sublingual, Buccal, Troche, Lozenge, and Lingual Spray Forms

Sublingual drugs are in tablet form but are placed under the tongue to dissolve. The most frequently prescribed sublingual drugs are the nitrates and nitrites for anginal heart pain. Instruct the patient to let the tablet dissolve under the tongue. Tell the patient not to drink any fluid, eat, or smoke while the drug is dissolving. This route of administration may be new to the patient, so make certain that the patient understands how to use drugs taken sublingually. Teach family members to administer drugs via this route when the patient is unable to do so, if appropriate for the patient's situation.

Teach patients to hold **buccal tablets** between the cheek and the gum and allow them to dissolve. Tell them to alternate cheeks with each dose of medication to minimize the chance for irritation of the mucosa. Report any oral irritation to the physician. Dissolve **troches** and **lozenges** in the mouth. These drug forms are usually designed to allow for slow release of the drug (i.e., over several minutes). Teach patients to avoid drinking, eating, or smoking until troches, lozenges, sublingual tablets, or buccal tablets have dissolved.

Another oral form is the **lingual spray.** Teach patients to spray one or two jets from a small canister into the mouth, under the tongue (as prescribed). The canister delivers a specific dose with each jet.

Feeding Tubes

Most medications that can be administered orally also can be administered via feeding tubes. Liquid preparations are preferred, but some medications can be finely crushed and mixed with sufficient water to ensure complete passage of the drug to the stomach (see the box on p. 55). Before administering any drug via a tube, verify that the tube is in the correct place. Refer to appropriate texts of nursing fundamentals for details about the care of patients with feeding tubes. If the drugs do not form a solid precipitate, mix them together and administer. Otherwise, administer the drugs one at a time, followed by a small amount of water (about 30 ml) to flush the drug through the tube, to help maintain the patency of the tube, and to ensure that subsequent drugs do not precipitate with residue remaining in the tube from an earlier drug. Do not mix the drugs for administration with the tube feeding itself. After the final drug is administered, clear the tube with water. Remember to include the amount of fluid used to flush the tubing in the totals for the patient's fluid intake.

Parenteral Medications: Injections

The word **parenteral** means outside the intestines, but in common usage it is usually limited to injections. There are many kinds of injections, which are named by indicating the site at which the medication is deposited. Intradermal, intramuscular, intravenous, and subcutaneous injections are all commonly used in everyday practice. Other injection sites, commonly used only by the physician, include intracardiac (usually reserved for resuscitation efforts), intrathecal (into the subarachnoid space via lumbar or ventricular puncture), and intraarticular (into a joint). The term *hypodermic* is being replaced gradually by *subcutaneous.*

There are advantages and disadvantages associated with parenteral administration. This route is used in patients who have difficulty swallowing, who are not alert, or who lack an adequate gag reflex. It can be used for a patient unwilling or unable to take other, usually oral, medications. (If multiple doses are required, intravenous administration is usually preferred in children because it is less intrusive). Insulin, heparin, and some other medications may be administered only parenterally. On the other hand, drugs administered via this route are generally considered irretrievable. A slight chance of infection exists because the integrity of the skin is broken. Inadvertent administration into the vascular space is also possible, although rare. Damage to muscles and nerves can also occur. Parenteral injections are also uncomfortable.

Carefully calculate and prepare the prescribed dose. Many injectable medications are dry powders and must be reconstituted before administration. Although the pharmacy can do this, sometimes the nurse must accomplish the task. Carefully read the manufacturer's information regarding reconstitution of dry medication. There may be restrictions on what fluids may be used for this purpose, or a specific diluent may be supplied by the manufacturer.

Not only must the appropriate diluent be obtained, but also the correct amount of diluent must be added to the dry powder. Beginning practitioners and students often find it difficult to understand the instructions related to reconstitution. For example, one form of penicillin states that certain amounts of diluent may be added to the 1,000,000-unit vial to provide the dilutions listed, stating, "Add 9.6 ml, 4.6 ml, or 3.6 ml to provide 100,000 units, 200,000 units, or 250,000 U/ml, respectively." Another vial used for some drugs combines the diluent and powder in a single glass vessel containing two compartments (Figure 5-2). Mix the diluent and powder in the closed vial before withdrawing the dose. Consult the pharmacist or a nursing supervisor if you have questions about reconstituting powder for injection (see box, p. 58).

Write the date, time of reconstitution, and concentration on the vial of reconstituted medication. Many institutions also require that the nurse initial the vial and put the patient's name on it. Reconstituted medications must often be stored in the refrigerator. Many vials are provided in single-dose concentrations; however, in pediatric settings, where the prescribed dose may be quite small, the nurse may use only a portion of the contents of a medication vial. Remember to read the label before using stored medications and observe expiration dates. Once reconstituted, many medications may be safely used for a short period.

Not all medications for injection are supplied in vials. Many come in small glass ampules, from which a single dose is withdrawn, and the ampule is discarded (Figure 5-3). A small metal saw may be supplied with the ampules. If supplied, use the saw and make two to three passes across the neck of the ampule. Do not saw through the glass, but make a scored line as a guide for breaking the ampule. To protect

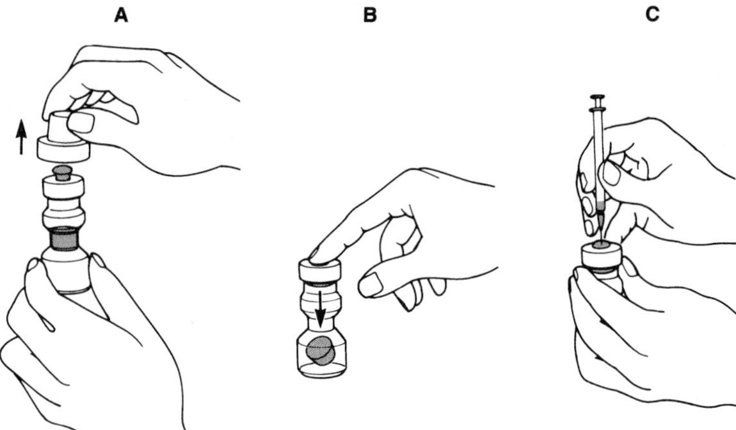

FIGURE 5-2
Drug mixing vial. **A,** Remove protective cap from vial. **B,** Push rubber plunger on top of vial. This action forces small rubber plug between upper and lower compartment into lower compartment, which allows powder and diluent to mix. Rotate vial between hands to speed mixing. Clean top of plunger with alcohol. **C,** Insert needle of syringe into plunger and withdraw dose. For best results needle must go straight into plunger.

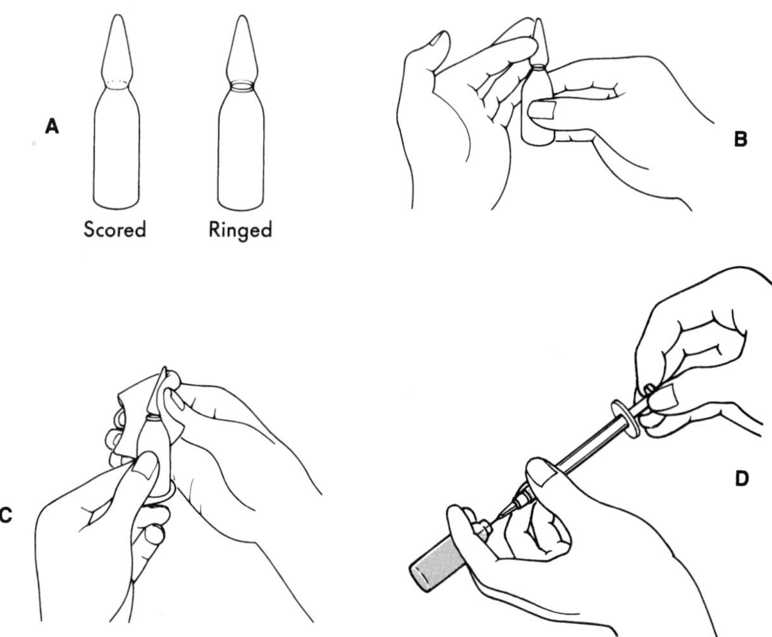

FIGURE 5-3
A, Examples of scored and ringed glass ampules. **B,** Hold ampule upright and gently flick top to shake medication into bottom of ampule. **C,** Hold vial with alcohol wipe or gauze and snap off top. **D,** Withdraw medication from bottom half of ampule.

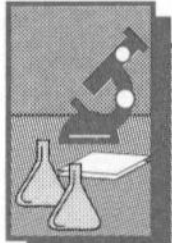

RESEARCH HIGHLIGHT

Defining Unnecessary Disinfection Procedures for Single-Dose and Multiple-Dose Vials

— T Buckley, SM Dudley, LG Donowitz: Am J Crit Care 3(6):448, 1994.

PURPOSE

Agency procedures describing techniques for drug preparation vary. This study was designed (1) to evaluate the need for cleansing the top of a single-dose medication vial and (2) to compare the effectiveness of cleaning the top of multiple-use vials with alcohol vs. povidone-iodine and alcohol.

SAMPLE AND METHODOLOGY

The rubber stoppers of five single-dose vials from each of 20 packages (N = 100) were cultured after the top of the vial was removed. The rubber stoppers of 87 previously used multiple-dose vials of antibiotics from the refrigerator of the neonatal intensive care unit were cultured. All these vials had been routinely cleaned using this technique: cleansing with a povidone-iodine pad, allowing the vial to sit for 3 minutes, and then wiping with 70% isopropyl alcohol to remove the povidone-iodine. After a change in institution practice to cleaning multiple-use vials with alcohol-only, 100 multiple-use vials that had been cleansed in this manner were cultured.

FINDINGS

Of the 100 single-dose vials cultured, 99% of the surfaces were sterile. One culture was positive for three colonies of *Staphylococcus epidermidis.* Of the multiple-dose vials cleaned with povidone-iodine followed by alcohol, 83 (95%) were sterile. Of the multiple-use vials cleaned with alcohol only, 100% of the surface cultures were sterile.

IMPLICATIONS

This study supports the view that the rubber stopper of single-use drug vials is sterile when the cap is removed and thus needs no further disinfection. With multiple-use vials, what seems like a more thorough procedure (cleaning with two agents instead of one) may not be more effective. The time involved in cleaning multiple-dose vials and the cost of two agents were not necessary in this institution. Cleaning multiple-dose vials with alcohol only was more effective than using two agents. Two limitations identified by the authors of this study were that all the multiple-use vials contained antibiotics and all were stored in the refrigerator.

CRITICAL THINKING: Are there procedures you have been taught that could be reevaluated? Are there measures in your agency that could be streamlined without compromising patient care? How could these be tested?

your fingers from getting cut, wrap the ampule in a piece of gauze or paper towel before opening it. Sharply snap the top off the ampule. Use a filter needle on the syringe, if one is available, to prevent small slivers of glass from entering the syringe. After withdrawing the dose, replace the filter needle with the needle for the injection.

Other medications are provided in prefilled syringes. The advantage of these syringes is fast and easy preparation. However, they are also more expensive. Most agencies stock prefilled syringes for narcotics and for selected other situations when drugs must be immediately available, such as the emergency drug box or resuscitation cart. Several manufacturers produce prefilled syringes, and techniques for activating and using the products vary. Consult the agency or institution for information about devices used in any individual setting. See Figure 5-4 for an illustration of one kind of holder for prefilled syringes.

The choice of syringe and needle to be used for any specific medication depends on the information obtained from assessment of the patient, the route of administration to be used, the characteristics of the fluid to be injected (e.g., aqueous or oil based), and the volume of medication to be delivered. Sample syringe sizes include 1 ml tuberculin and insulin syringes and 2.5, 5, and 10 ml syringes. Larger syringes are available but are rarely used for medication administration via the parenteral route. Use tuberculin syringes, marked in 0.01 ml gradations, when the volume to be administered is small. Insulin syringes are available in 0.5 or 1 ml volumes, although some institutions stock an insulin syringe with a maximum volume of 25 or 35 U. Do not substitute tuberculin and insulin syringes for each other.

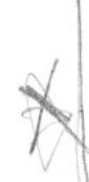

Needles vary in length and gauge, from 3/8 inch to 3 or more inches in length and from 14 gauge (large lumen) to 28 gauge (small lumen). Most institutions limit the variety of needles and syringes in stock, so the nurse may have a choice of five syringes and five needle sizes on the nursing unit. The smaller lumen (larger gauge) needles are usually used for intradermal injections. Subcutaneous injections are usually given with a ½- or ⅝-inch, 23- or 25-gauge needle. Intramuscular injections are usually given with a 19- or 21-gauge, 1½- to 2-inch needle; a 16- or 18-gauge needle may also be used (see box, p. 60).

After preparing the ordered dose and choosing the appropriate needle and syringe, go to the patient's bedside to administer the injection. Check the patient's name band to verify his or her identity, draw the curtain or otherwise ensure privacy, explain what is going to happen, and assist the patient to assume the necessary position. If the patient is unable or unwilling to assist in positioning, bring someone to assist you. Assess the injection site, locate the anatomic landmarks, and smoothly administer the injection. Help the patient return to a comfortable position. Dispose of the syringe and needle according to the procedures of the agency. Record that the medication has been given, noting the location so

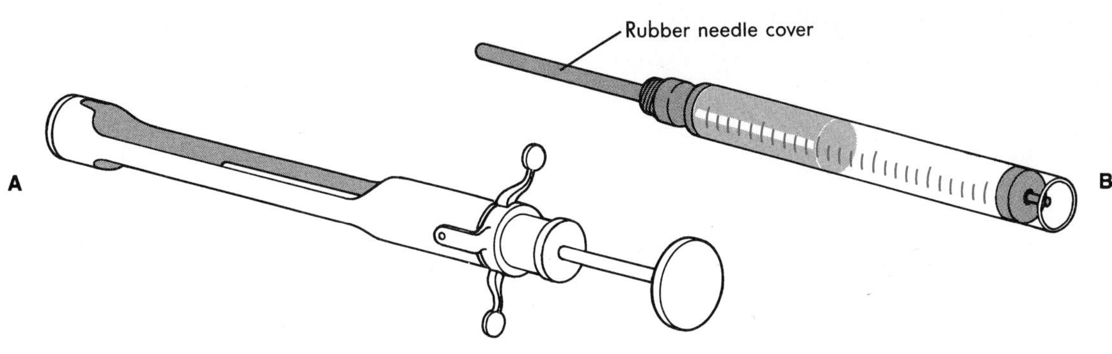

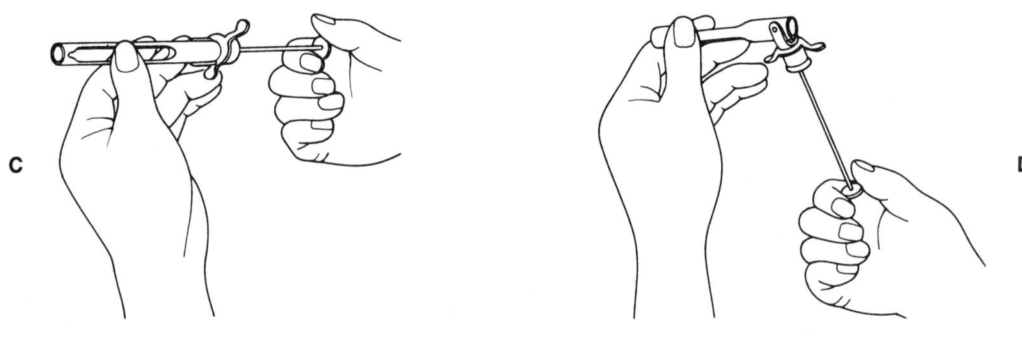

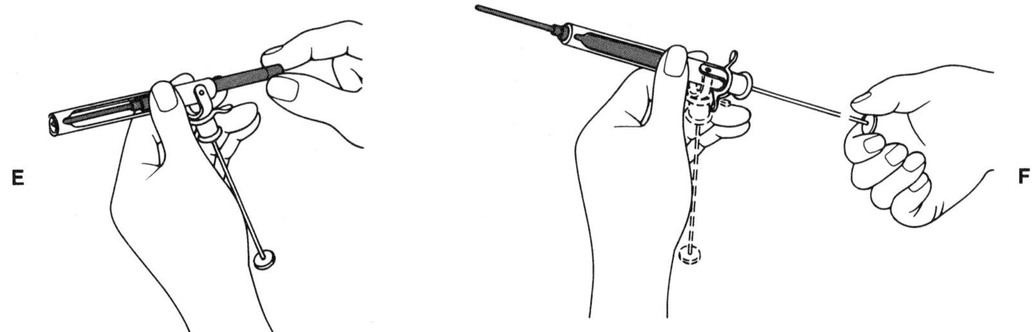

FIGURE 5-4
Prefilled medication cartridge and holder. **A,** Reusable stainless steel cartridge holder. **B,** Disposable prefilled medication cartridge. Note rubber needle cover. Also note threads just below needle and on rubber plug. **C,** Pull back on plunger. **D,** Open holder at hinge. **E,** Insert medication cartridge, and rotate it clockwise to screw cartridge into holder. **F,** Swing plunger back in place and turn plunger to secure it to small screw in rubber plug.

PREPARATION OF OIL-BASED MEDICINES FOR INTRAMUSCULAR ADMINISTRATION

Oil-based medicines are released more slowly because it takes the oil longer to be absorbed from the muscle than aqueous solutions. Administer oil-based medicines via the intramuscular route only, never intravenously.

Heat the unopened vial or ampule in warm water for several minutes to decrease oil viscosity.

Roll the vial vigorously between the hands to resuspend the medication, which is usually an inconspicuous film on the side of the ampule. Resuspension is adequate when no particles of medication remain on the bottom or sides of the vial. Failure to shake or roll the vial sufficiently results in inaccurate dosage and erratic absorption.

Draw up the correct dose into a syringe fitted with a large-bore (19- to 21-gauge), 1½-inch needle (for an adult), and administer the dose immediately, before the oil cools.

Inject the medicine, exerting slow, even pressure on the plunger. Attempting to inject too rapidly can cause pressure to increase within the syringe, and the needle and syringe may separate, causing loss of medication.

Use large muscle masses, such as the buttock, thigh, or ventrogluteal site. In infants and small children, use the vastus lateralis muscle.

The oil base can produce palpable lumps because it is absorbed slowly. Record injection sites, rotate them, and avoid the deltoid muscle.

that injection sites can be rotated. Check the patient again to make certain no untoward effects have occurred and to evaluate whether the drug is working as anticipated.

Record any aspects of the injection that are unique to the patient on the medication Kardex or patient care plan to assist other nurses in providing individualized care. More detailed information about drawing up medications, handling equipment, and administering injections can be found in a text of nursing fundamentals. Practice in giving injections is important in helping students become accurate, efficient, and confident.

Intradermal Injection

An **intradermal injection** is made just below the epidermis, or outer layer of skin (Figure 5-5). Such an injection is used for allergy testing and for administration of local anesthetics. Use a small-bore needle and a small-volume syringe, such as a 1 ml tuberculin syringe. The volume injected is usually small, less than 0.5 ml. The most frequently used sites for allergy testing are the medial surface of the forearm and the back.

When preparing for the injection, clean the chosen skin surface with alcohol. Allow the surface to dry or wipe off the alcohol with a sterile sponge. Hold the skin taut with one hand. With the other hand, hold the syringe at a 10- to 15-degree angle, with the needle bevel up, and gently but smoothly puncture the skin until the bevel is completely under the skin surface. Inject the prescribed amount or an amount that creates a raised wheal resembling a mosquito bite. If a wheal is not produced or if the site bleeds, you probably made too deep an injection and should repeat it. If several injections are given in the same site (e.g., on the same forearm), label them with a pen, especially if the reaction is to be checked at 48 hours.

Subcutaneous Injection

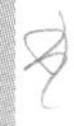

A **subcutaneous injection** is used to place medication below the skin into the subcutaneous layer (see Figure 5-5). The volume of a subcutaneous injection is usually <1 ml, and usually a ½- or ⅝-inch, 23- or 25-gauge needle is used. Insert the needle at a 45-degree angle, although it may be inserted at a 90-degree angle if the patient has heavy subcutaneous tissue or the nurse has pinched the subcutaneous tissue between thumb and fingers, holding the subcutaneous tissue up from the underlying muscle tissue. The usual injection technique is used. Choose the site, cleanse it with alcohol, let the alcohol dry or wipe it off with a sterile sponge, hold the skin taut, insert the needle, and aspirate for blood. If no blood is present, gently but smoothly inject the medication. Alternatively, cleanse the skin as described, then gently pinch the subcutaneous tissue between the thumb and the other fingers. Insert the needle, aiming it for the pocket created between the subcutaneous tissue being pinched and the tissue below.

The two medications most frequently administered via this route are heparin and insulin, and controversy continues about specific aspects of their administration. For additional discussion about the administration of these two drugs, consult Chapter 20 and Chapter 63. The usual sites for subcutaneous injection are illustrated in Figure 5-6.

Intramuscular Injection

Intramuscular injection is probably the method most familiar to students and patients. Most people have received medication via this route in the form of antibiotics or immunizations. Because the muscle layer is below the subcutaneous layer of skin, a long needle is used, usually 1½ inches, often of large lumen size, such as 19 or 21 gauge. Insert the needle at a 90-degree angle (see Figure 5-5). The choice of needle is influenced by the viscosity of the medication to be injected, the muscle to be used, and the size and age of the patient. A frequent error of beginning students is to choose too short a needle for administration of a medication to an overweight adult via a large muscle mass such as the vastus lateralis or dorsogluteal area.

The intramuscular technique is the same as other injection techniques previously outlined. Carefully prepare the ordered medication. Take the syringe to the bedside, and check the name band to verify the patient's identity. Draw the curtain or otherwise ensure privacy. Assist the patient to assume the necessary position. Identify appropriate anatomic land-

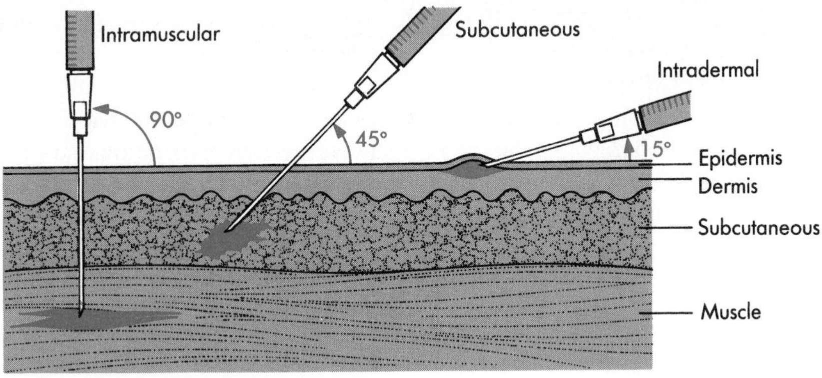

FIGURE 5-5
Comparison of angle of injection and location of deposition of medication for intramuscular, subcutaneous, and intradermal injections.

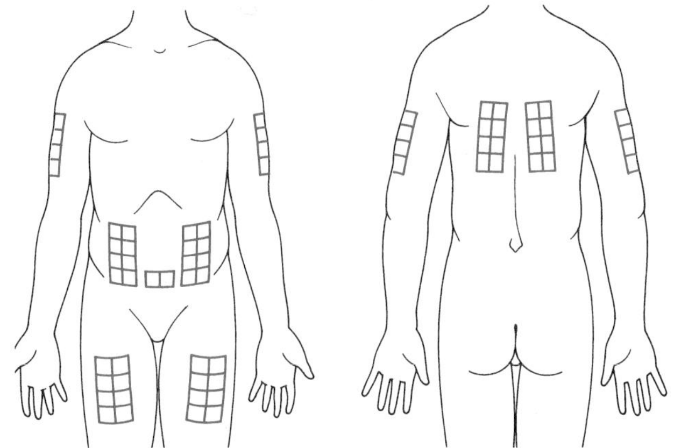

FIGURE 5-6
Commonly used subcutaneous injection sites.

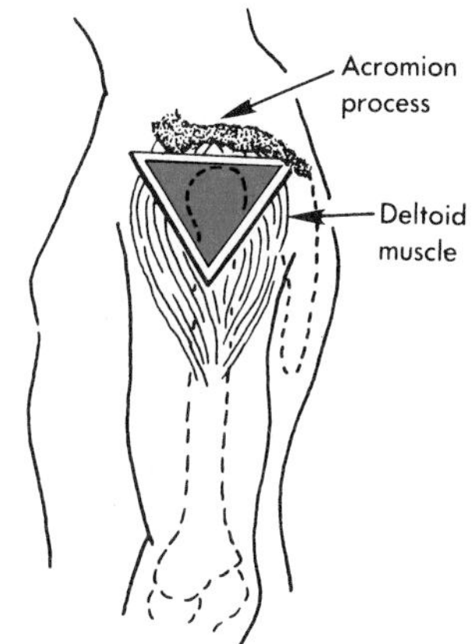

FIGURE 5-7
Deltoid muscle injection site roughly forms inverted triangle, with acromion process as base. Muscle may be visible in muscular patients.

marks to help define the injection site. Cleanse the skin, and let it dry. Hold the skin taut or gently pinch the skin. Swiftly insert the needle at a 90-degree angle, aspirate for blood, and if no blood is present, gently but smoothly inject the medication. If blood oozes after the needle is withdrawn, apply gentle pressure and a bandage if needed. Help the patient assume a comfortable position. Dispose of needle and syringe as directed by agency policy and then record that the medication has been given. Finally, check the patient again.

The **deltoid muscle,** located on the upper arm, is the site used for intramuscular injection of certain immunizations. It forms a triangular shape, with the base of the triangle along the acromion process and its peak ending about one third of the way down the upper arm (Figure 5-7). In muscular patients the deltoid muscle may be clearly visible. In other patients it may be necessary to palpate it. This muscle is small in children, many smaller-than-average patients, and older adults, so it can accommodate only small volumes of injected fluid (e.g., 1 ml). Depending on the patient's clothing, bruises or needle marks may be visible, which may be unacceptable to the patient. The radial nerve is nearby. The advantage of the deltoid muscle is that it is easily accessible.

The **dorsogluteal site** is made up of several gluteal muscles, although the gluteus medius is the muscle most often used for injections. As indicated in Figure 5-8, there are two ways to define this site. One way is to divide the buttocks on one side into imaginary quadrants and administer the injection in the upper outer quadrant. The second method is to locate the posterosuperior iliac spine and the greater trochanter of the femur and then draw an imaginary line between them. Give the injection up and to the side of this line. It is important to have a clear view of the area to help define the landmarks. Have the patient lie down, with the toes pointed inward, which helps foster muscle relaxation and thus decreases discomfort. Do not use this site for children younger than 3 years because the muscles are not yet well developed and because of the proximity of the sciatic nerve. In most ambulatory adults the dorsogluteal muscles are well developed and can accommodate an injection volume up to 5 ml if necessary, although any volume >3 ml may be uncomfortable to the patient.

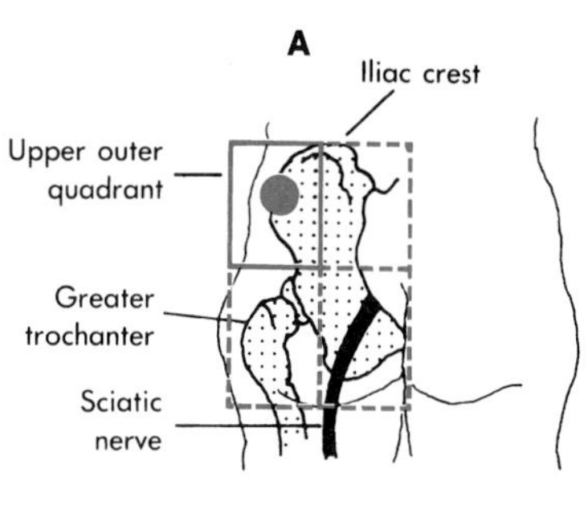

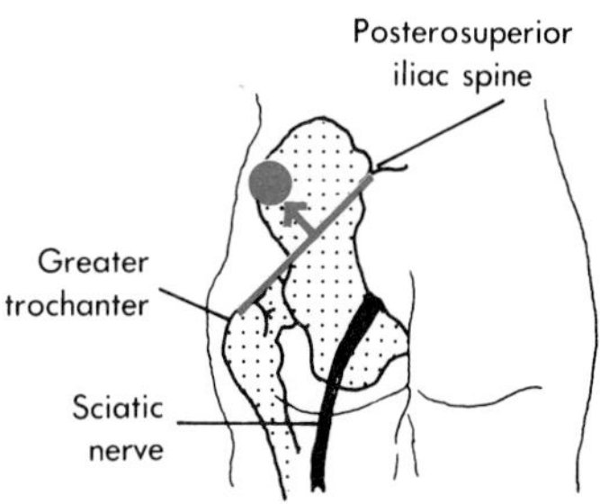

FIGURE 5-8
Two accepted methods for defining dorsogluteal injection site. **A,** Patient's buttocks can be divided on one side into imaginary quadrants. Center of upper outer quadrant should be used as injection site. **B,** Nurse locates site by palpation of posterosuperior iliac spine and greater trochanter, then draws imaginary line between them. Injection site up and out from that line should be used.

The **Z-track technique** can be used with any intramuscular injection, although it was first described for administration of an iron preparation that stains the skin if it leaks out. The dorsogluteal site is most frequently used for injections requiring the Z-track technique. When you prepare the drug to be administered, measure the ordered amount of drug into the syringe, then draw 0.1 to 0.3 ml of air into the syringe, and change the needle. When administering drugs via the Z-track method, pull the skin taut to one side, causing the layers of skin to slide sideways. While the skin is pulled laterally, insert the needle, then inject the medication and the small amount of air smoothly and slowly. Pause for 10 seconds before removing the needle. Withdraw the needle, then allow the skin to relax (Figure 5-9). This process disrupts the track created by the needle, preventing seepage, and possible skin discoloration caused by the medication. Do not massage or rub the site.

Both the **vastus lateralis muscle** and the **rectus femoris muscle** are found in the thigh. As shown in Figure 5-10, the two muscles lie side by side. Place one hand on the patient's upper thigh and one hand on the lower thigh. The area between your hands should represent the middle third of the thigh and the middle third of the underlying muscle. The vastus lateralis is lateral to midline, whereas the rectus femoris is in the midline. The vastus lateralis is the preferred injection site for children because it is well developed and has few major nerves that could be injured. This site is also satisfactory for adults. The rectus femoris is most often the site chosen by adults who self-administer intramuscular injections because it is easily accessible. The acceptable volume for injection in these sites varies with the age of the patient and the size of the muscle, but up to 5 ml may be administered in one injection to the well-developed adult.

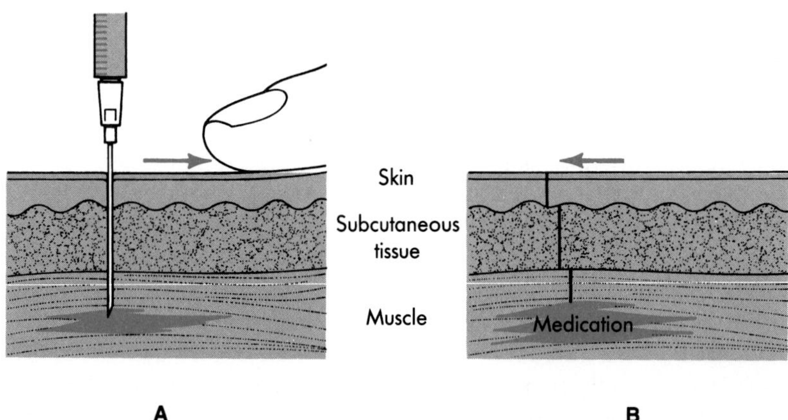

FIGURE 5-9
A, In Z-track intramuscular injection, skin is pulled laterally, then injection is administered. **B,** After needle is withdrawn, skin is released. This technique helps prevent medication from leaking.

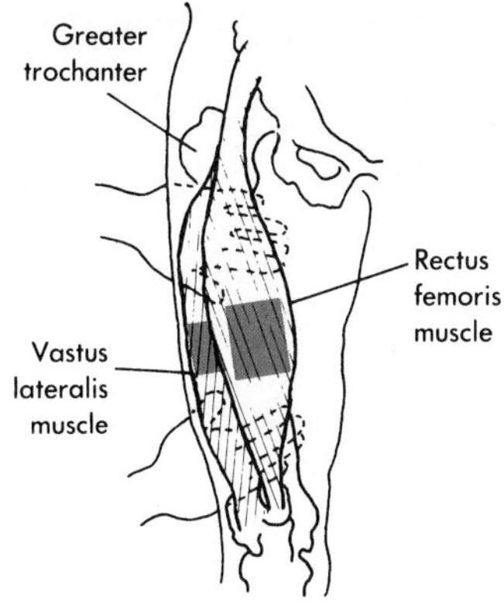

FIGURE 5-10
To define vastus lateralis and rectus femoris muscle sites, place one hand below patient's greater trochanter and one hand above patient's knee. Space between two hands defines middle third of underlying muscle. Rectus femoris muscle is on anterior thigh; vastus lateralis muscle is on lateral thigh.

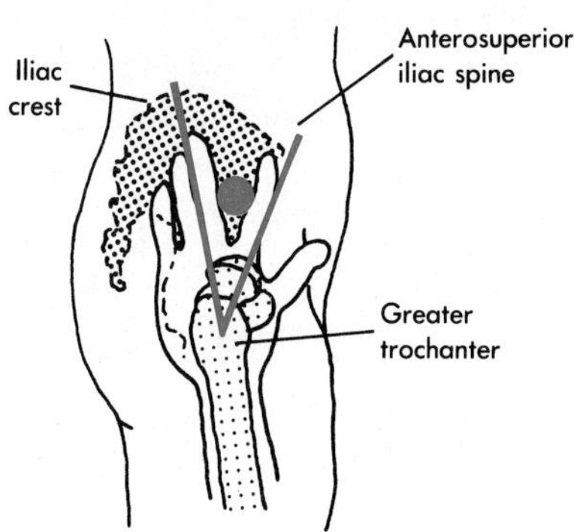

FIGURE 5-11
To locate ventrogluteal muscle injection site, place palm of hand on greater trochanter of femur. Make V with fingers, with one side running from greater trochanter to anterosuperior iliac spine and other side running from greater trochanter to iliac crest.

To define the **ventrogluteal muscle,** create a V between the index finger and the remaining three fingers. Place the palm on the greater trochanter of the femur, with one side of the V extending from the greater trochanter to the iliac crest and the other side running from the greater trochanter to the anterosuperior iliac spine (Figure 5-11). This muscle may accommodate up to 5 ml of drug in adults.

Intravenous Injection

The administration of drugs directly into the vascular system via the intravenous (IV) route is widely used today for a variety of reasons. If an IV infusion line is already in place, IV infusion is easy. Drugs begin to take immediate effect. IV injection avoids side effects caused by intramuscular injection. On the other hand, errors can be serious, even fatal, since medications administered via this route take effect quickly. The possibility of infection resulting from direct access to the vascular system is also present.

In many settings the venipuncture and establishment of the IV infusion is done only by members of the IV team or comparable group. If no designated team exists, many agencies or state nurse practice acts require special instruction, classes, and supervised practice in venipuncture techniques before nurses are permitted to perform this technique in their usual setting. Become familiar with the specific practices and policies of your agency or institution.

First, inspect the forearms and choose the venipuncture site. Figure 5-12 illustrates the location of veins commonly used in the forearm. Figure 5-13 illustrates the location of veins on the dorsal aspect of the hand. Other veins, such as those in the feet, are used only if absolutely necessary; some agencies may require a specific physician order if they are used. Problems associated with thrombophlebitis are more common with venipuncture of the lower extremities. Scalp veins are used in infants. If the patient is to have repeated venipunctures, choose a distal site rather than a proximal one. The rationale is that with each subsequent venipuncture the site should be moved more proximally (i.e., closer to the major vessels of the chest).

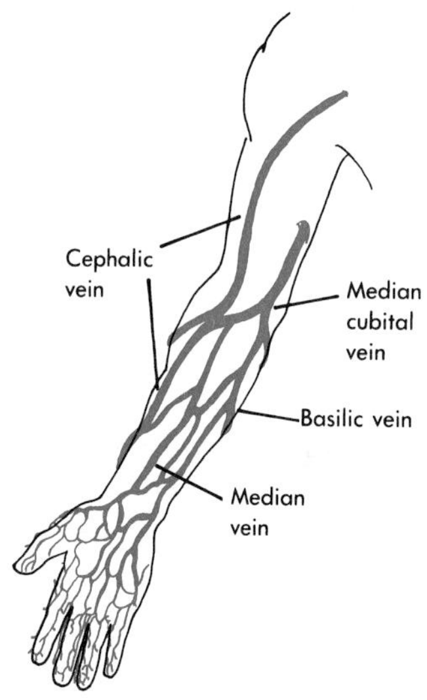

FIGURE 5-12
Veins of medial aspect of forearm commonly used for venipuncture.

After choosing a site and preparing the necessary equipment (needle, intracatheter, heparin well, tubing, blood collection devices, medication, and tape), apply a tourniquet several inches above the expected insertion site. Put on gloves, and palpate the vein to further define its location. Then cleanse the skin with alcohol, povidone-iodine solution, or other cleansing substance. Allow the area to dry or wipe it with a sterile sponge. With one hand, stabilize the extremity

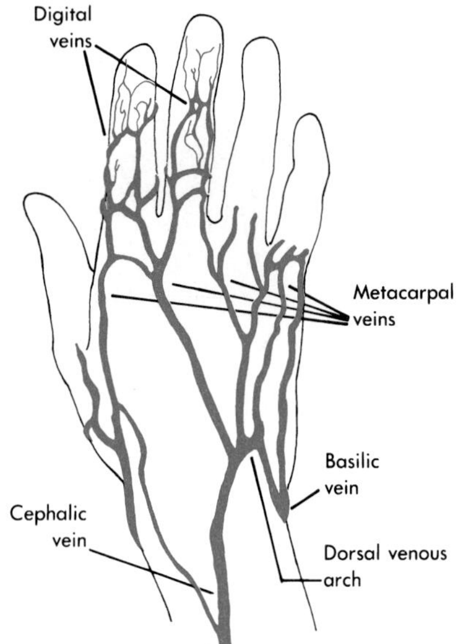

FIGURE 5-13
Major veins of dorsum of hand.

and the vein; with the other hand, hold the venipuncture needle bevel up. Approach the insertion site at a slight angle, about 10 degrees. Puncture the skin and then the vein. Experienced nurses can feel the vein wall being punctured. If blood appears in the tubing or syringe, release the tourniquet. Slowly inject the medication into the vein, draw the blood, or secure the infusion device to the forearm, depending on the reason for the venipuncture.

To remove any needle or tubing from a vein, put on gloves, carefully remove any securing tapes and dressing, place a sterile sponge over the insertion site, and apply gentle pressure. With the other hand, swiftly withdraw the needle or catheter, pulling straight back from the angle of insertion; then apply firm pressure for 2 to 5 minutes to prevent bleeding or bruising. Apply a bandage over the insertion site. Dispose of any needles and syringes according to agency procedures. Record any medication that has been administered, and check the patient again. Further elaboration of these techniques can be found in texts of nursing fundamentals and agency procedure manuals. In addition, the Centers for Disease Control and Prevention in Atlanta have established guidelines for preventing infections in venipuncture and IV infusions.

Heparin lock. Nurses may administer IV medications via a **heparin well** or **heparin lock.** This device consists of a needle attached to a short length of tubing capped by a piece of resealable rubber. The needle is placed in the vein; the device is then secured to the forearm. Its advantage is that medication can be administered via the IV route, but the patient does not need to be attached to continuous IV infusions or have repeated venipunctures for each dose of medication. Heparin wells are particularly helpful in children who require IV medications but not additional fluids. When not receiving a dose of medication, the patient can be up and around, not restricted by long IV tubing.

Heparin may be administered via heparin well, as described in Chapter 20. One method for administering other medications by intermittent infusion via heparin well is to insert and secure the heparin well and then prime it with 1 ml of a 10 U/ml heparin solution. Solutions of 10 U/ml are available in prepackaged syringes or multiple-dose vials, or the pharmacy or the nurse can mix the heparin with normal saline solution to achieve the desired concentration. Each time a drug is administered, cleanse the rubber insertion site with alcohol or another cleansing agent; flush the well with 1 to 2 ml of normal saline solution (this step may be omitted if the drug to be administered is compatible with heparin); administer the prescribed medication via push or infusion; flush the well with 1 to 2 ml of normal saline solution; then fill the well with 1 ml of the solution containing 10 U/ml heparin. The purpose of leaving the heparinized solution in the well is to prevent blood from clotting in the needle. Many agencies have found that normal saline solution left in a heparin well is as good as a dilute heparin solution in maintaining patency of the heparin well. Follow the institution's policies and procedures.

Intravenous tubing. Another way to administer IV medications is via tubing in place for the patient who is receiving constant IV fluids. At least two variations should be noted. The nurse must frequently administer a small amount, usually <5 ml, of drug. This is often called **IV push** drug. Prepare the drug, and verify the patient's identity. Then locate an injection site on the IV tubing. Cleanse the site with alcohol or another solution. Then inject 2 ml of normal saline solution (this step may be omitted if the IV push drug is compatible with the fluids infusing). Administer the ordered drug, and then administer another 2 ml of normal saline. Readjust the ongoing infusion to provide the ordered rate. Most commercially available IV tubings have check valves, or one-way valves, as part of the tubing (Figure 5-14). If a check valve is not present, however, clamp the tubing above the injection site before administering the drug and proceed as outlined above. If there is no check valve or if the tubing is not clamped, the injected medication will go in the direction of lower pressure, which may be up toward the bag or bottle of fluid instead of down toward the patient. Avoid this situation. When the medication goes toward the large bag or bottle of fluid the patient does not receive the complete dose until the bag is empty; drugs administered after that dose may not be compatible with the drug remaining in the fluid line.

The second method of giving IV drugs is to administer a bolus of medication. The drug is prepared and diluted in a larger volume of fluid, at least 50 to 100 ml in adults, which is usually administered for a period of 20 to 60 minutes. This volume can then be administered in several ways. One method is to add the drug to an in-line device such as a burette or volume-limiting device and then fill the device with 50 to 100 ml of the infusing IV fluid. The ongoing fluids are

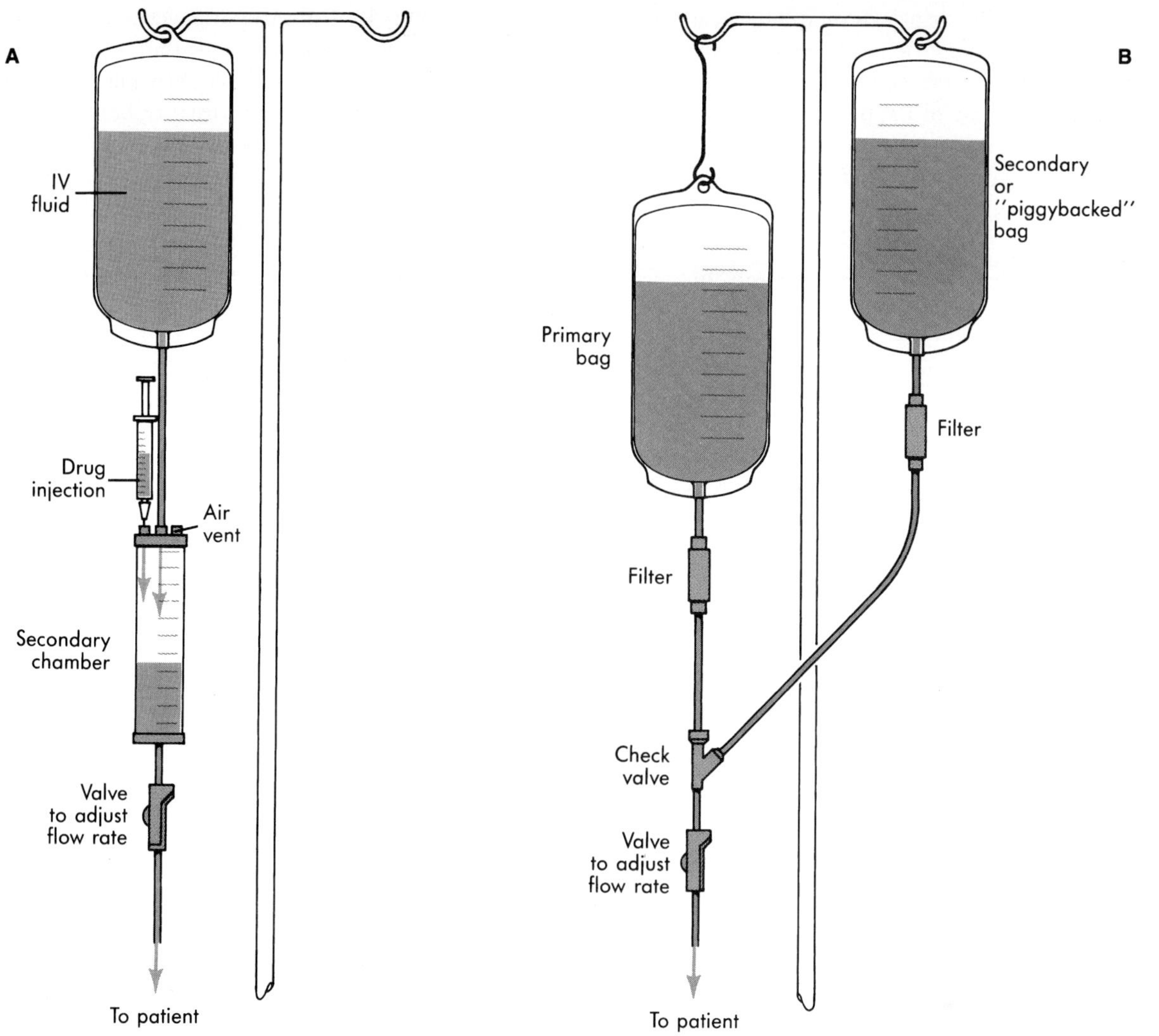

A
IV fluid
Drug injection
Air vent
Secondary chamber
Valve to adjust flow rate
To patient

B
Secondary or "piggybacked" bag
Primary bag
Filter
Filter
Check valve
Valve to adjust flow rate
To patient

FIGURE 5-14
Example setups for intermittent drug infusion. **A,** Drug is injected into secondary chamber, where it may be further diluted with IV fluid. Upper fluid reservoir may be temporarily closed while drug infuses. **B,** Secondary or "piggybacked" bag containing drug diluted in 50 to 100 ml of fluid is hung at level higher than primary bag. Contents of higher bag will infuse first, then contents of lower bag resume infusing. Check valve prevents medication from flowing into primary bag. Note that both lines have a filter.

temporarily stopped, the bolus is allowed to infuse, and then the ongoing fluids are continued. Commercially available infusion tubing that has two ports for hanging IV bags or bottles may also be used. These tubing systems have an identified port for attaching the primary fluids and a secondary port for attaching the intermittently administered bolus containing the drugs (see Figure 5-14).

The third method of administering IV drugs is to prepare the drug in a small volume of fluid and then attach IV tubing and a needle. Prime the tubing by running sufficient fluid through the tube to eliminate any air. Insert the needle into an identified insertion site on the tubing of the ongoing infusion after the site has been cleansed. The initial or primary infusion is clamped, the bolus containing the drug is allowed to infuse, then the continuous fluids are restarted. You may then discard the secondary infusion tubing and needle. To be effective and efficient, become familiar with the equipment and procedures used in your agency.

Central venous catheters and multilumen catheters. Central venous catheters are inserted for venous access in many patients. Central, in this case, refers to a large, more central vein, close to the heart, as opposed to a smaller, more peripheral vein. There are several kinds of venous access devices. Therefore, to provide correct nursing care, it is important to find out what kind of device is being used in each patient and for what purposes it is being used. One type of device is a nontunneled catheter, intended usually for 10 to

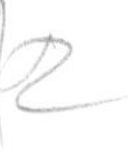

14 days of use. It may be a single or multilumen catheter, inserted into the subclavian or internal jugular vein, with the tip advanced into the superior vena cava, or further, depending on the intended use of the device (Figure 5-15). The catheter may be used for hemodynamic monitoring. Another type of device is a **tunneled catheter** such as the Broviac, Hickman, or Groshong catheter. The tip of the catheter is inserted into the internal or external jugular or cephalic vein, and the tip rests in the superior vena cava. The other end is tunneled through the subcutaneous tissue for 5 to 8 cm and exits through a small skin incision in the chest. With care these catheters can remain in place for months to years.

Another type of device is an **implanted infusion port** such as the OmegaPort or Port-A-Cath. With these devices a reservoir or port is implanted subcutaneously against a bony structure such as along the ribs of the chest wall. The port is attached to a catheter, typically a Hickman or Groshong catheter, which is tunneled subcutaneously to the selected vein. The implanted infusion port is designed to withstand 1000 to 2000 punctures by a needle. These devices can remain in place for months to years.

Recently, **peripherally inserted central catheters (PIC catheters or PICCs)** have been used more frequently. As the name implies, the catheter is inserted peripherally, usually in the basilic or cephalic vein in the antecubital space. The catheter is threaded through the vein so the tip rests in the superior vena cava. With care these devices can remain in place for months or longer.

Each of these catheters and ports, except the PIC catheter, must be inserted by the physician. Some states and some agencies will permit specially trained nurses to insert these. All these devices can be used to withdraw blood samples, as well as administer blood products, hyperalimentary products, and medications. Because the distal end of the catheter is in an area of high blood flow and volume, it permits infusion of large volumes of fluids. Also, central venous catheters allow administration of more irritating fluids and drugs than can be administered via peripheral IV lines. There is always the risk of infection or of introducing air with such catheters, especially when those with multiple ports are used.

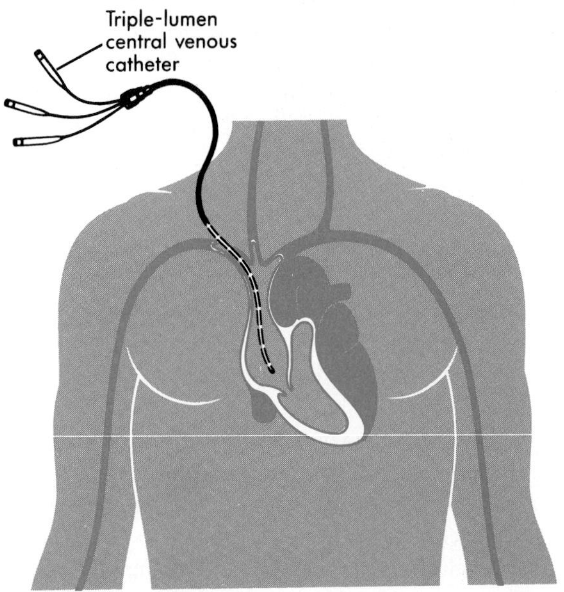

FIGURE 5-15
Triple-lumen central venous catheter in place.

Usually, care for the catheter and the insertion site is more rigorous for a centrally placed catheter than for a standard peripherally placed catheter. (A PIC catheter is a central line, even though it is inserted peripherally.) For example, cleansing of an injection port on a peripheral catheter may be done with an alcohol swab, whereas the port on a central line may require cleansing with a povidone-iodine solution. Also, there may be special dressing change procedures for the dressing covering the catheter insertion site. Follow agency procedures. Monitor the patient for signs of infection such as fever, redness at the insertion site, and increased white blood cell count.

For multilumen catheters, care of the ports not in use is important to keep the lumens patent. Follow agency procedure. Different types of catheters may require different protocols. One protocol is to change the cap on each port weekly or when it appears worn. Wear sterile gloves during cap changes, and discard contaminated caps carefully. Irrigate the ports not in use with 2.5 ml of heparinized solution (10 U/ml of heparin) every 12 to 24 hours. Irrigate a port after each intermittent infusion is given via that port. If blood is drawn via a port, irrigate the port after the sample is obtained. Cleanse the insertion site every 48 hours.

With an implanted infusion port, the skin must be punctured with a needle each time the patient must receive medication; however, there is no daily cleansing procedure as there is with the partially implanted catheters. To use an implanted device, put on sterile gloves and cleanse the site with a povidone-iodine solution (or as agency protocol directs). With one hand, palpate and locate the injection site. After the device is defined and stabilized with one hand, use the other hand to puncture the skin and septum with a Huber-type needle attached to a syringe containing sterile saline solution (Figure 5-16). The Huber-type needle is designed to prevent excessive damage to the rubber septum. The needle has a deflected point and a side opening to prevent coring of the septum. The needle may be bent 90 degrees to facilitate attaching infusions. Push the needle in far enough to feel it touch the back of the device. Aspirate blood to help determine patency, and then inject saline to flush the system. The device may be used to obtain blood samples, administer constant or intermittent infusions, or inject medications. After use, flush the device with a heparinized solution. Review the manufacturer's directions and request guidance in using these devices until comfortable with their use and operation.

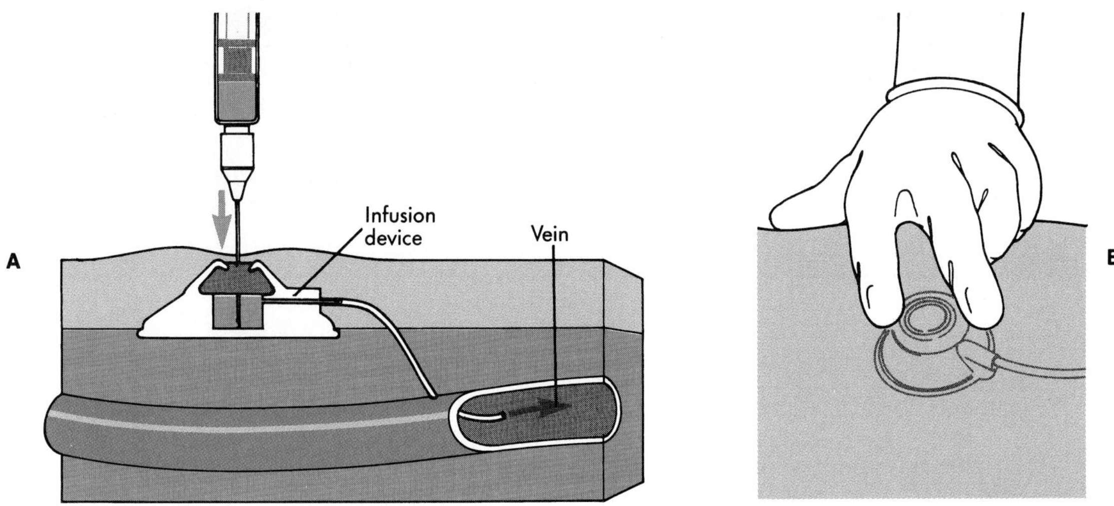

FIGURE 5-16
Implanted infusion device. **A,** Side view illustrating needle inserted through skin and top of infusion device. Distal end of device is in vein. **B,** Use one hand to secure device before inserting needle.

Drug Pumps

Several types of drug pumps for slowly injecting a medication are now available for patients' home use. Cancer chemotherapy, narcotic infusion for severe pain, or insulin therapy are the most common uses of drug pumps. One such device is the autosyringe pump, which consists of a syringe with a battery attachment for slow injection. This device injects the medication subcutaneously or attaches to an implanted infusion port such as the Port-A-Cath or a partially implanted catheter such as a Hickman catheter. Follow the manufacturer's instructions when preparing and using a drug pump, and have the patient give a return demonstration before discharge.

Information about calculation of infusion rates is included in Chapter 6. Additional general guidelines for care of the patient receiving an IV infusion are given in Chapter 17.

Rectal Medications

Administering medications via the rectal route is an alternative for patients who are nauseated or unable to swallow. Drugs administered via this route are usually in the form of a suppository or enema.

The procedure for administering medication by enema is the same as that for any enema. The goal is to have the patient retain the medication for as long as possible. Therefore a small-volume retention enema is administered. After preparing the medication and any other necessary equipment, go to the bedside, and verify the patient's identity. Explain briefly what will be done. Then draw the curtain or otherwise ensure privacy. Position the patient on the left side. Place adequate protective covering on the bed. Put on gloves, and lubricate the applicator or tubing tip with water-soluble jelly or lubricant (Figure 5-17). Separate the patient's buttocks with one hand, and ask the patient to take a deep breath. Use the other hand to insert the tubing or tip the desired distance. Administer the medication slowly to avoid stimulation and immediate expulsion. Withdraw the applicator, and gently hold the buttocks together until the patient's immediate urge to defecate has subsided. Wash the patient's buttocks, and assist the patient in returning to a comfortable position. Instruct the patient to try to hold the medication at least 30 minutes (or as indicated by the nature of the medication).

Suppositories are medications that have been mixed with cocoa butter, glycerin, or other substances that allow them to remain solid at room temperature but permit them to melt and release the medication when they contact the warm rectal mucosa. Suppositories are stored in the refrigerator to keep them firm. If a suppository is too soft to insert easily, run it under cold water (if foil wrapped) or place it in the refrigerator to help harden it before administering. The general procedure for administration is similar to that for the enema. Wear a finger cot or glove for inserting the suppository. Moisten the suppository with a water-soluble lubricant. Insert the suppository about a finger's distance into the rectum in adults, past the anal sphincter (Figure 5-18). If the suppository is not inserted far enough, it will be uncomfortable to the patient and will be quickly expelled. It may be necessary to place a small gauze pad over the anus to absorb oozing medication after the suppository has been inserted. If the suppository was intended to cause defecation, the patient may defecate as soon as the urge occurs. Unless the medication was prescribed to stimulate defecation, instruct the patient to retain the suppository as long as possible and to report when it is expelled.

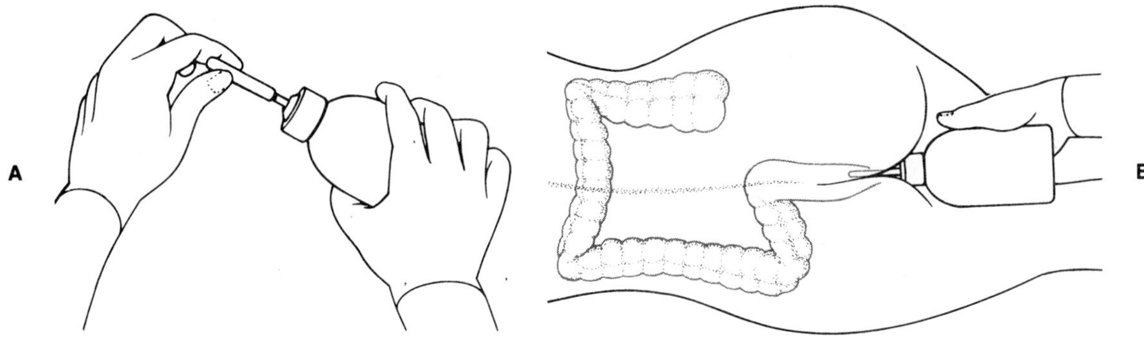

FIGURE 5-17
Administering single-dose enema. Position patient on left side, and place protective covering on bed. **A,** After donning gloves, remove cover from tip. Apply water-soluble lubricant if tip is not already lubricated. **B,** Gently insert applicator tip and squeeze bottle to propel medication into patient's rectum.

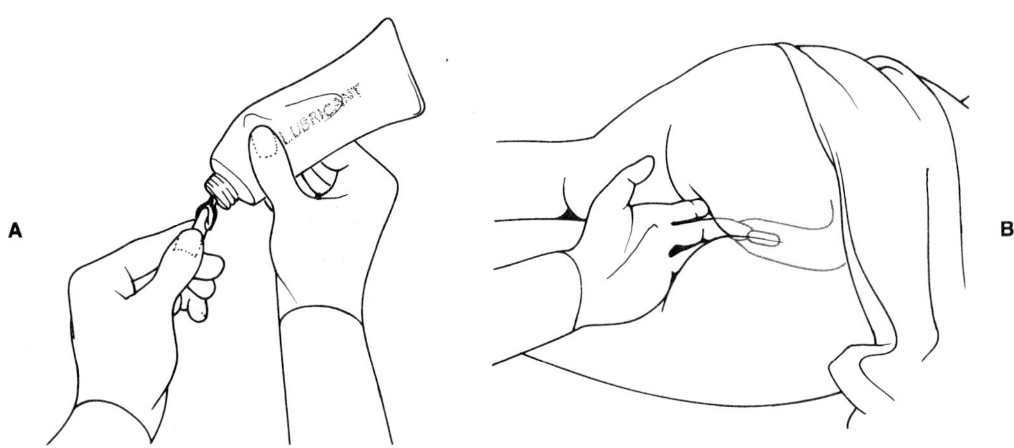

FIGURE 5-18
Inserting suppository. After positioning patient and removing suppository from package, don nonsterile gloves. **A,** Lubricate suppository with water-soluble lubricant. **B,** Insert suppository past anal sphincter.

Vaginal Medications

Vaginal medications can take the form of douches or irrigations, creams, or suppositories. The patient may be able to choose the form she prefers.

Many women are familiar with over-the-counter douche preparations and may feel comfortable with their use. For best effect, administer douches with the patient lying down. Moisten the tip of the tubing or applicator with water or a water-soluble lubricant. Insert the applicator or end of the tubing about 2 inches initially. Then advance it another 1 to 2 inches as the fluid is allowed to run in by gravity. A text on fundamentals of nursing offers more complete information about douching.

Insert vaginal suppositories by pushing them in with a gloved finger or with an applicator supplied by the manufacturer. The suppository may be lubricated with water or a water-soluble lubricant before being administered. It is important to place the suppository high in the vaginal vault, or the patient will expel it rapidly.

If the patient is taking a dose once daily, insert the vaginal suppository just before the patient goes to sleep so that it will remain in the vaginal vault all night and not drain out or be expelled. If the dose is given more than once daily, instruct the patient to remain lying down for a short period after administration so that the medication will not be quickly lost. Instruct the patient to continue the medication even during the menstrual period and to avoid the use of tampons while taking vaginal medications. It is usually necessary for the patient to wear a sanitary napkin during the course of therapy.

Insert vaginal creams with the applicator supplied by the manufacturer. The same guidelines outlined under vaginal suppositories apply. Creams are generally messier than suppositories, and patients may not accept them as well. If the applicator is reused for several doses, wash and dry it after each dose.

Skin Application

Many medications are applied to the skin, but it is such an easy and common route of administration that the nurse or patient may inadvertently become too casual about it. Some topical preparations, such as emollients for dry skin, may be applied liberally, as needed. Most skin medications, however, must be measured and applied as ordered to prevent the patient from receiving too large a dose. Avoid direct contact with the medication to prevent sensitization and to avoid the effects of the medication. Wear gloves and apply the medication with applicators, gauze, or cottonballs; or make certain that the medication is applied directly from the measuring guide, as is done with topical nitroglycerin preparations (see Chapter 15). Depending on the medication, rotate application sites, and avoid applying the medicine to abrasions, cuts, or other areas where the skin is no longer intact. Some topical preparations require dressings. If in doubt, ask the physician about the goals of therapy, and consult the pharmacist to determine the most effective method of administering the drug.

Nitroglycerin ointment is one type of skin application (Figure 5-19). The dose is ordered in inches, and the oint-

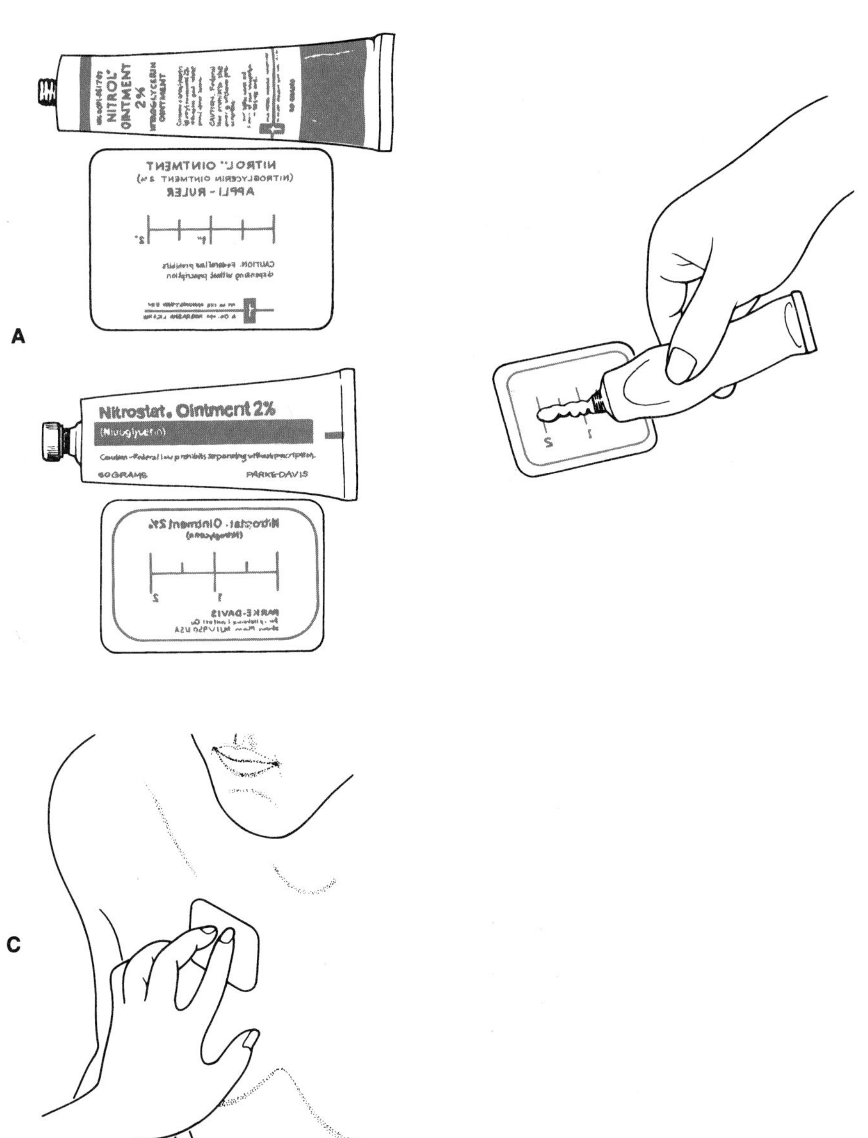

FIGURE 5-19

A, Nitroglycerin ointment and papers for measuring doses. **B,** Gently squeeze out a line of ointment along paper guide for prescribed length. **C,** Apply ointment to patient's skin. Clear plastic wrap may be applied over site to increase absorption and keep ointment from staining clothing.

ment is supplied with small papers printed with a 2-inch measuring guide. Squeeze out an even line of ointment of the prescribed length. Place the paper ointment-side down on the patient. Avoid rubbing in the ointment, although it is usually permissible to press the paper guide sufficiently to spread out the dose. Clear plastic wrap may be ordered to be placed over the paper and ointment to facilitate absorption and prevent staining of clothing.

A recent development in topical application is the single-dose, adhesive-backed delivery system, or transdermal patch (Figure 5-20). Examples include several types of nitroglycerin preparations, estrogen, and a scopolamine preparation. Refer to the manufacturer's literature for guidelines about the specific product. Review instruction sheets with the patient; these provide illustrations and additional information. Information includes the preferred location for application, frequency of changing, and the effect of contact with water on the delivery system while swimming or bathing.

Eye Medications

Eye medications are usually in the form of drops or ointments. Eyedrops are supplied in small volumes since each dose is contained in 1 or 2 drops. Avoid contaminating the dropper. Each patient in an institutional setting should have a separate bottle of eyedrops. Before administering eyedrops, be certain which eye is to be medicated (if not both). A frequent source of errors is confusion about the abbreviations for left eye (os), right eye (od), and both eyes (ou). Have the patient lie down or sit with the head tilted back. With your hand holding the dropper, place your hand on the patient's cheek or forehead to stabilize your hand and help prevent injury to the eye. Use the thumb (or fingers) of your other hand to gently pull down the lower lid; it may be necessary to use a small gauze sponge or cotton ball to help do this and avoid contaminating the eye. Drop the dose into the lower conjunctival sac, never onto the eyeball.

Nurses may find the following modification of technique helpful when administering eyedrops to patients who blink easily. Place the patient in the supine position, with the head turned to one side, about 45 degrees from midline. The eye to receive the eyedrops should be uppermost. With the eye closed, drop the prescribed dose on the inner canthus of the eye. Have the patient slowly turn from the side to midline, then toward the other side, while blinking. The eyedrops will move via gravity and surface tension into the conjunctival sac.

Eye ointments are applied much the same way as eyedrops. Squeeze a thin line of ointment onto the lower conjunctival sac, close the eye, and gently rub the eyelid to help distribute the dose (Figure 5-21).

A newer drug form available for eye medications is the sustained-release insert, such as the Ocusert Pilo-20 or Pilo-40 systems. This form of pilocarpine was designed for patients with a poor history of compliance or with conditions that make accurate instillation of eyedrops difficult, such as poor vision or arthritis. Place the insert into the upper or lower conjunctival sac. The medication is released slowly, over several days. Instruct patients to make sure that the insert is in place every morning since the unit may fall out at night. The unit is designed to be replaced weekly. Other drugs may become available in this form or in other new forms. Consult the manufacturer's literature and patient instruction sheet for specific guidelines about new drug forms, both to update your personal knowledge and to teach patients and their families.

Caution patients to read labels carefully, especially on refilled prescriptions. Only medications labeled for ophthalmic use should be put into the eye. Eyedrops should be kept in a

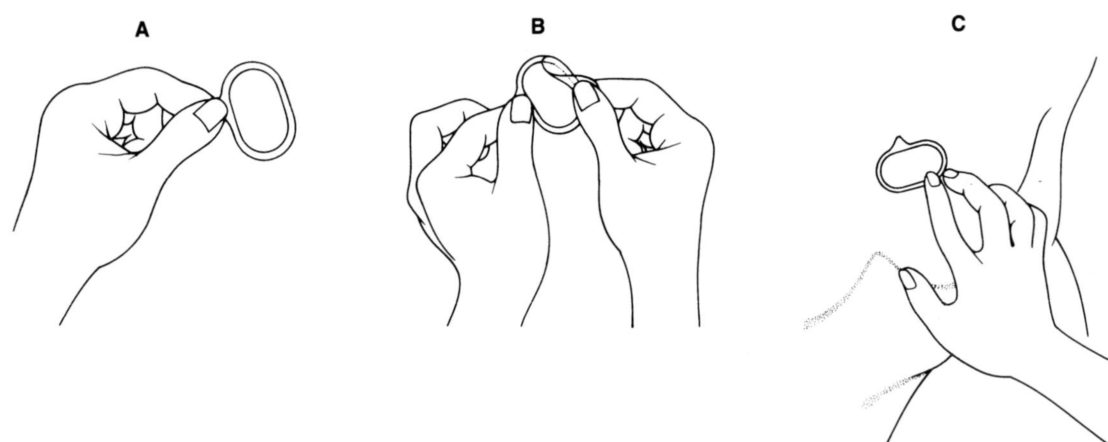

FIGURE 5-20
Transdermal patch. **A,** Hold patch by small wing. **B,** Remove protective backing. **C,** Place patch on chosen skin site and press into place. Sites should be changed or alternated with each successive dose.

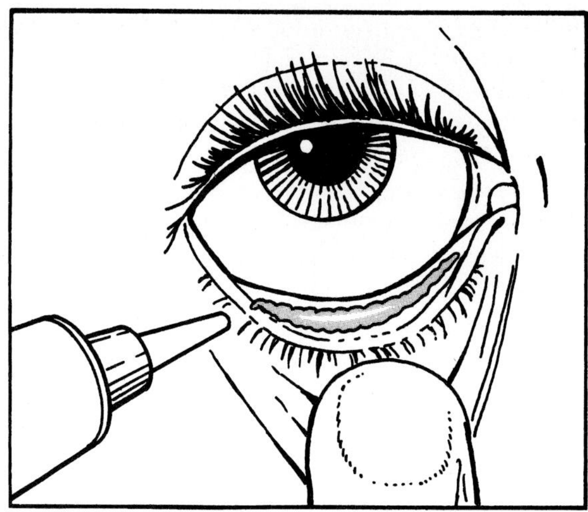

FIGURE 5-21
Administering ophthalmic ointment. To instill ointment, gently pull lower lid down as patient looks upward. Squeeze ophthalmic ointment into lower sac. Avoid touching tube to eyelid.

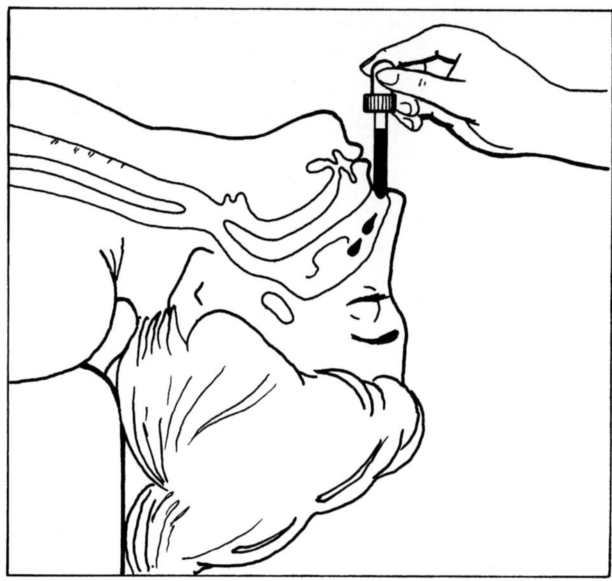

FIGURE 5-22
Administering nosedrops. Have patient gently blow nose. Open medication and draw liquid up to calibration on dropper. Instill medication. Have patient remain in position for 2 to 3 minutes. Repeat on other side if necessary.

safe place, away from other similarly shaped containers. Occasionally patients have inadvertently put glue or other toxic substances in their eyes because they did not read the label or depended on feel to select the bottle or tube of medication. Many medications cause patients to experience blurry vision briefly, so warn patients not to drive or engage in other dangerous activities immediately after using eye medications. Finally, instruct patients that the use and misuse of eye medications can have serious consequences, so eye medications should only be used as prescribed.

Nosedrops and Sprays

To instill nosedrops, have the patient lie down with the head over the edge of the bed (Figure 5-22). Support the patient's head with one hand while instilling the drops with the other. When the patient's head is in the midline, the nosedrops primarily reach the ethmoid and sphenoid sinuses; turning the patient's head toward the side will facilitate having the drops reach the maxillary and frontal sinuses. Have the patient remain in this position briefly, and then, if possible, bend over into a head-down position to help distribute the drug. Tell the patient to avoid blowing the nose for several minutes so that the medication will not be expelled.

Administering nose spray requires that the patient inhale via one nostril while occluding the other and squeezing a spray applicator. Remove the applicator from the nostril before releasing the pressure on the other nostril to avoid pulling sensitive nasal mucosa to the applicator opening. Have the patient keep the head upright or tilted slightly back. Many nose sprays are available over the counter, especially nasal decongestants (see Chapter 7). Caution the patient to use these sprays only as needed, for as short a period as possible, and only as directed.

Ear Medications

Most ear medications are in the form of drops. Have the patient lie down with the affected ear up. Keep the medication at body temperature. In adults or children older than 3 years, pull the top of the ear up and back to straighten the ear canal, then gently instill the prescribed number of drops. If the patient is a child younger than 3 years, pull the ear down and straight back (Figure 5-23). Have the patient remain with the affected ear up for 10 minutes to allow the medicine to disperse. A medication-soaked cottonball plug may be gently and loosely placed in the ear to prevent oozing; a dry cottonball will absorb the medication. If it is necessary to treat the other ear, repeat the procedure with the other ear after the 10-minute waiting period.

Endotracheal Tubes

Occasionally it is necessary to administer drugs via an endotracheal tube. Use this route only if necessary and only if specified by the physician. Drugs typically administered via this route include epinephrine, atropine, lidocaine, and surfactants. Dilute the prescribed dose in 5 to 10 ml of sterile water and saline solution. Attach a long needle or soft catheter to the syringe. Auscultate the lungs to verify placement of the endotracheal tube. The patient should remain in the supine position. Instruct the patient to hyperventilate for three to five breaths. Remove the ventilator or resuscitation bag, and inject the medication through the endotracheal tube as deeply as the catheter or needle permits. Do not puncture the tube with the needle. Reattach the resuscitation bag or venti-

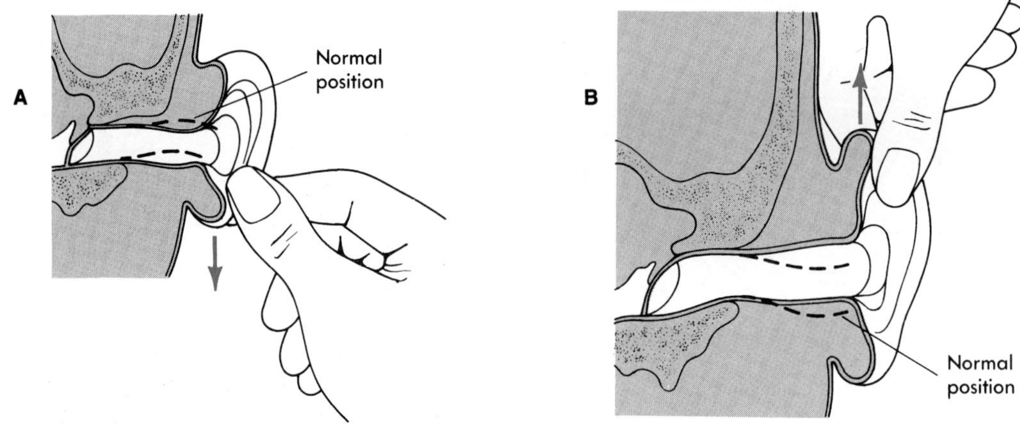

FIGURE 5-23
Straightening ear canal for administration of ear medication. Patient is lying on side with ear up. **A,** For child younger than 3 years, pull ear down and straight back. **B,** For all others, pull top of ear up and back.

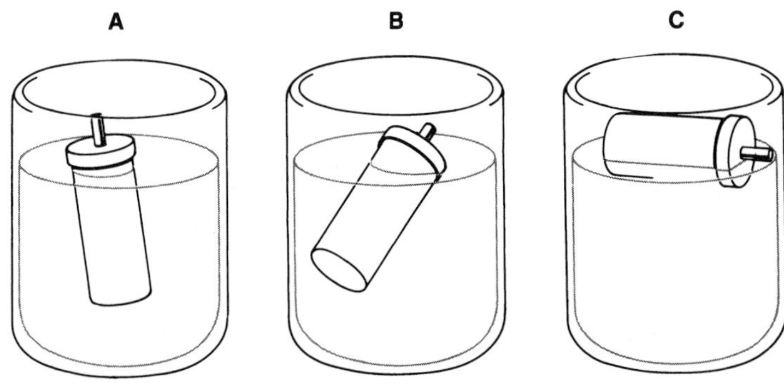

FIGURE 5-24
Checking canister for medication. This check could be done for metered-dose inhaler (see Chapter 27) or canister with nitroglycerin spray. **A,** Canister is full. **B,** Canister is partially full. **C,** Canister is nearly empty. This method of estimating how much medication remains is satisfactory for most drugs. Read manufacturer's instructions, however, because number of sprays used per canister must be counted for some drugs.

lator, and tell the patient again to hyperventilate for three to five breaths. Assess the patient's response to the medication.

Intraosseous Infusion

Intraosseous infusion may be used in emergency situations in children when an IV infusion cannot be started. In this technique a special needle is inserted into a large bone. Proper placement of the needle must be verified through aspiration of bone marrow. Drugs, fluids, or blood can then be infused. Although establishing an intraosseous infusion is easier than starting an IV infusion for small children and infants, several potential hazards, including infection, are associated with this technique. If this technique is used in your agency, request instruction in its use, and carefully review the protocol and procedure.

Implanted Dosage Forms

Some drugs may be delivered by subcutaneous implantation, a procedure usually performed by the physician. Some male hormones and a female contraceptive (levonorgestrel [Norplant]) are administered this way. See Figure 64-1 for an illustration of this form. The advantage is that the drug is slowly released over months to years, so the patient does not need to remember to take daily or more frequent doses. Disadvantages include the need for a minor surgical procedure to administer new doses, the possibility of small scar formation, and the possibility that the patient may forget to return for subsequent doses.

Inhalation

A few drugs are administered via inhalation, one of the most difficult routes of administration. For best results this method requires a cooperative patient who can inhale deeply and can manage the psychomotor tasks of using the equipment and preparing the medication. Often, however, the patient is a child or anxious or hypoxic because of the condition being treated, such as asthma.

In the hospital or institutional setting, inhalation therapy is fairly common, in the form of oxygen therapy via nasal cannula, nasal catheter, or some form of face mask. Other drugs may also be administered via intermittent positive pressure breathing (IPPB) machines. Trained respiratory therapists are often available to provide assistance. The nurse faces the greatest challenge in ensuring correct use of inhalation therapy in the outpatient setting.

Several inhalation drug delivery systems, such as metered-dose inhalers and turboinhalers, are available. Each system has advantages and disadvantages. Carefully review the literature supplied by the manufacturer, including the patient instruction sheet. Do not attempt to teach patients how to use the delivery system if they are short of breath or anxious. Make certain that patients show a satisfactory return demonstration before concluding that they can use the prescribed drug correctly. Remind patients to keep hand-held nebulizers and other equipment clean to prevent contamination and infection. Instruct patients to use the product only as ordered to prevent side effects, drug overdose, and drug dependency. See Chapter 27 for an illustration of a metered-dose inhaler. Figure 5-24 illustrates how the patient can estimate the amount of drug remaining in a canister. This method is helpful for patients using metered-dose inhalers or nitroglycerin lingual spray forms.

Other Drug Delivery Systems

New drug delivery systems are constantly being developed as a response to a problem in patient compliance, either an inability or an unwillingness of patients to comply. This might occur with limited vision, severe arthritis, or other medical conditions. The nurse faced with an unfamiliar delivery system should consult the manufacturer's literature and the patient instruction sheet that often accompanies the dosage form.

NURSING PROCESS OVERVIEW

Drug Administration

Assessment

When assessing a patient, ask why this patient might need a prescribed drug. Identifying the reason for each prescription helps the nurse detect inadvertent errors in which the wrong drug may be administered.

Obtain objective and subjective data from the patient to aid in determining the need and effectiveness of drug use. Determine any patient preferences regarding drug use and incorporate these if possible. Determine the developmental level of children to aid in planning nursing care approaches.

Nursing Diagnoses

Not all patients require the formulation of nursing diagnoses as a consequence of drug therapy. Most patients are not knowledgeable about a specific drug at the start of drug therapy. Other diagnoses may develop as the patient develops side effects, is unable to manage self-administration, or has collaborative problems as potential complications.

Patient Outcomes

The patient will improve as a result of the efforts of the health care team, and medications may be one part of therapy. The patient will experience no serious side effects of drug therapy, or the side effects will be diagnosed quickly and handled effectively.

Planning/Implementation

Implementing the therapeutic plan involves proper administration of the prescribed medications. The nurse should seek information about specific drugs from a variety of sources, including the physician, the pharmacist, and current printed materials. For a student nurse the prospect of learning about all the medications to be administered is likely to be overwhelming. After a nurse is in practice, however, repeated administration of medications facilitates development of a basic understanding of frequently used drug categories.

Not only must the nurse know about the prescribed medications, but the nurse must also exercise caution that the prescribed medication is what the patient actually receives. Thus medications should remain in labeled packages or containers until they are administered.

The patient has a right to receive the medication in the correct dose. Regardless of how drugs are supplied to the patient care unit, check labels carefully and double-check all dosage calculations. Some nurses have difficulty with the mathematic calculations necessary for determining correct doses; have a colleague verify dosage calculations rather than possibly subjecting the patient to an incorrect dose of medications. Consult the pharmacy for additional help. Successful drug therapy may depend on the proper timing of drug doses, as discussed in Chapter 1. To ensure that the patient receives each drug via the right route of administration, check that the route of administration ordered for each drug is appropriate for that drug. Learn how to develop medications via each route.

Develop a sense of suspicion whenever a medication order seems to be out of the ordinary. Double-check a dose of medication that seems unusually large or small. When at the bedside, if the patient seems hesitant to take the medication, stating that it is new or not what is usually taken, double-check the physician's orders before administering the medication. Record that a patient has received a medication as soon as possible after administration to avoid inadvertent duplicate administration by other members of the health care team.

Evaluation

The major question during evaluation is whether the medication is working as expected. The nurse must know what was expected of the medication, have initial baseline data about the patient, and know what parameters to assess to determine whether the drug is working as desired. Determine whether there were any problems associated with the route, time, or dose of medication, and make appropriate notation on the Kardex or care plan.

Critical Thinking

APPLICATION

1. Describe the differences between a unit-dose system and a stock drug system.
2. In your practice settings, where is information about medications recorded?
3. What are some problems you may encounter in administering drugs to older adult patients?
4. For each of the routes of medication administration listed below, answer the following questions:
   - What are advantages and disadvantages of this route?
   - Are there considerations unique to older adult patients or children with this route of administration?
   - How is a drug administered via this route?

   a. Oral route: Pills, capsules, tablets
   b. Oral route: Suspensions, tinctures, elixirs, syrups, and solutions
   c. Oral route: Sublingual tablet, buccal tablet, troche, lingual spray, and lozenge forms
   d. Oral drugs through feeding tubes
   e. Intradermal injections
   f. Subcutaneous injections
   g. Intramuscular injections
   h. Intravenous injections
   i. Z-track intramuscular injections
   j. Rectal enemas and suppositories
   k. Vaginal douches, creams, and suppositories
   l. Skin applications: Creams, ointments that must be measured, and transdermal patches
   m. Eyedrops and eye ointments
   n. Nosedrops and sprays
   o. Eardrops
   p. Drugs via inhalation

CRITICAL THINKING

1. Which is used in your practice setting: unit-dose system or stock drug system?
2. How can you use theories of Erikson, Freud, or Piaget as a guide in administering medications to children?
3. How can you, as a nurse, decide how to advise patients which drugs are "more important" and *must* be taken vs. those drugs that are "less important"?

CHAPTER 6

Calculating Drug Dosages

OBJECTIVES

After studying this chapter, you should be able to do the following:

- *Define common abbreviations used in drug orders, such as gtt, prn, and po.*
- *Perform calculations based on the strength of solutions of drugs.*
- *Calculate drug dosages based on the patient's body weight.*
- *Calculate infusion rates for drugs administered intravenously.*
- *Calculate pediatric drug dosages.*

KEY TERMS

body surface area
Clark's rule
gram
liter
stock or stock solution
Young's rule

CHAPTER OVERVIEW

Chapters 1 and 5 discussed the routes by which a drug may be given to a patient and the importance of careful control of drug levels in the body. Administering the proper drug dose by the appropriate route is the first step in ensuring that the desired drug concentration appears in the bloodstream. In this chapter the focus is on how to calculate drug dosages.

Students with good arithmetic skills can readily acquire the ability to solve problems of the level included in this chapter, but many students initially experience difficulty because they have forgotten the basic rules of arithmetic and algebra. Such students should review these rules before attempting the drug dosage calculations.

CALCULATING DRUG DOSAGES: ROLE OF THE NURSE

The nurse shares moral and legal responsibility with physicians and pharmacists in administering drugs. In many hospitals pharmacists calculate and prepare the drug for administration to the patient, according to the physician's order. This practice does not remove responsibility from the nurse who administers the drug to the patient. The nurse must verify that the correct drug at the proper dose has been prepared (see Chapter 5). For this reason the nurse should be familiar with the forms of drugs and be able to recognize common medications.

The nurse should also question a physician's order for a drug when that order seems inappropriate. For example, the nurse should question a drug dose that is outside the normal clinical dosage range. The nurse has access to several sources of information about specific drugs, including the pharmacist, the package insert supplied by the manufacturer, and references (see Chapter 3).

READING DRUG ORDERS

Physicians and pharmacists sometimes use a system of abbreviations in writing orders or prescriptions. These abbreviations are derived from Latin and Greek words and phrases. Although Latin and Greek are no longer used in medical writing, use of the phrases persists through custom. For this reason the nurse must be familiar with the common abbreviations listed in Table 6-1. Many of the abbreviations designate how to administer a drug. For example, a physician's order might read "penicillin G 100,000 U q3h, po." This order would be translated as "100,000 units (U) of penicillin G are to be given every 3 hours (q3h) by mouth (po)."

Pharmaceutical abbreviations can be confusing, and the nurse must be certain that the physician's intent is clearly understood. Among the most troublesome are the abbreviations *ad lib* and *prn*. A drug given prn is given at the prescribed interval if the patient requires the drug. For example, after surgery a patient might have the following order on the chart: "Morphine 10 mg q4h, prn." Every 4 hours the nurse should assess the patient; if the patient is comfortable, the nurse may postpone the dose. According to the drug order, morphine may be given less often than every 4 hours but not more often. In contrast, a medication prescribed ad lib is given whenever the patient needs it. Such abbreviations are used as medical shorthand to save time in communicating between medical personnel. If the use of an abbreviation creates any uncertainty, the physician or the pharmacist should be consulted for clarification.

TABLE 6-1 Pharmaceutical Abbreviations

ABBREVIATION/PHRASE	TRANSLATION
ad lib (ad libitum)	freely; as much or as often as wanted
aa (or $\overline{aa}$) (ana)	of each
ac (ante cibum)	before meals
bid (bis in die)	twice daily
$\bar{c}$ (cum)	with
gtt (guttae)	drops
hs (hora somni)	at bedtime
non rep (or non repetat) (non repetatur)	do not repeat
od (oculus dexter)	right eye
os (oculus sinister)	left eye
ou (oculus uterque)	both eyes
pc (post cibum)	after meals
po (per os)	by mouth
pr (per rectum)	by rectal route
prn (pro re nata)	according to circumstances
qs (quantum sufficit [satis])	as much as is necessary
qd (quaque die)	every day
qh (quaque hora)	every hr
q4h	every 4 hr
qid (quarter in die)	4 times daily
ss (or $\overline{ss}$) (semis)	one half
stat (statim)	immediately
tid (ter in die)	3 times daily

UNITS OF DRUG DOSAGE

In clinical practice, nurses encounter situations in which they must translate a physician's order for a certain drug dosage into the proper number of tablets or the proper volume of drug for an individual patient. This section is intended to prepare the student nurse to handle these problems with skill and confidence.

Before turning to the simple arithmetic required to solve dosage problems, the student must be familiar with the appropriate systems of units. The metric system (Table 6-2) is an international system that is most commonly used for drug dosage calculations. The primary units the student must be familiar with are units of mass and volume because most problems to be solved are expressed in units of drug mass and drug volume.

The primary unit of mass within the metric system is the **gram** (gm). With the use of prefixes, this unit can be adjusted to express thousands of grams (1 kilogram [kg] = 1000 gm) or thousandths of grams (1 milligram [mg] = 0.001 gm). The prefixes *deci-* and *centi-*, meaning ⅒ and 1/100, respectively, are used less often. The primary unit of volume within the metric system is the **liter** (L). With prefixes, the

TABLE 6-2 Common Systems of Units

SYSTEM	UNIT OF MASS	UNIT OF VOLUME
Metric	Gram (gm)	Liter (L)
Apothecary	Grain (gr)	Minim (m)
Household	Pound (lb)	Pint (pt)

liter is commonly divided into thousandths (1 L = 1000 milliliters [ml]) and less commonly into millionths (1 L = 1,000,000 microliters [μL]) or hundredths (1 L = 10 deciliters [dl]). The milliliter (ml) is the metric volume unit equivalent to the older unit commonly encountered in the clinic, the cubic centimeter (cc). These relationships are summarized in Table 6-3.

The metric system possesses many advantages in terms of ease of calculation and convenience of units. Nevertheless, other units of mass are occasionally encountered. For instance, body weight may be expressed in pounds rather than kilograms. Another instance is the grain (gr), the unit of mass in the apothecary system. This older system was retained for a few drugs, such as aspirin and morphine, that have been used medically for decades, but dosages of these drugs are now most commonly calculated in milligrams. Equivalents between the metric system and the other less commonly used systems are listed in Table 6-4.

Abbreviations for the various units are not entirely standardized in the medical literature. For example, gram may be abbreviated *Gm, gm,* or *g.* One set of abbreviations has been adopted for use throughout this book. Table 6-5 summarizes the abbreviations in use for various units.

The nurse in practice deals with solutions of drugs on a daily basis. A solution is a given mass of solid substance dissolved in a known volume of fluid (weight/volume or w/v) or a given volume of a liquid substance dissolved in a known volume of another fluid (volume/volume or v/v). The concentration of a w/v solution is always expressed as units of mass per units of volume. Common concentration units are gm/ml, gm/L, and mg/ml. Concentrations are also commonly expressed as percentages, based on the definition of a 1% solution as 1 gm of solid/100 ml of solution. Proportions are also used as expressions of concentrations. For example, *1:1000* designates a solution containing 1 gm/1000 ml of solution. Blood levels of certain metabolites are frequently expressed as mg% (mg/100 ml) of solution. *Mg/100* ml is equivalent to *mg/deciliter (dl);* that is, a 1 mg% solution is the same as a 1 mg/dl solution. The relationship between the various expressions of concentration is illustrated in Table 6-6.

TABLE 6-3 Equivalents Within Metric System

Units of mass	Units of volume
1 kg = 1000 gm	1 L = 1000 ml
1 gm = 1000 mg	1 ml = 1000 μL
1 mg = 1000 μg	

TABLE 6-4 Conversion Between Measurement Systems

APOTHECARY		METRIC
15 grains (gr)	=	1 gm*
1 dram (dr)	=	4 gm
15 minims (m)	=	1 ml
1 fluid dram (f dr)	=	4 ml
HOUSEHOLD		**METRIC**
1 teaspoon (t)	=	5 ml
1 tablespoon (T)	=	15 ml
1 fluid ounce (f oz)	=	32 ml (or 30 ml)†
1 pint (pt)	=	480 ml (or 500 ml)†
1 quart (qt)		960 ml (or 1000 ml)†
1 gallon (gal)		3.85 L (or 4 L)†
1 pound avoirdupois (lb)		0.46 kg

*Two factors have been used for converting grams to milligrams. Older conversion factor is 65 mg = 1 gr. This factor is basis for aspirin and acetaminophen formulations (i.e., a 5 gr aspirin tablet contains 325 mg of aspirin). More recently agreed on conversion factor is 60 mg = 1 gr. This new conversion factor is easier to use for drugs (e.g., morphine) that are frequently administered in small doses (fractions of grains). For example, ¼ gr of morphine equals 15 mg when new conversion factor is used. It is important to remember that these factors are simply estimates agreed on for ease of calculation. All problems presented in this book use conversion 15 gr = 1000 mg.

†Values in parentheses have been used because they are more easily measured in most clinical glassware.

TABLE 6-5 Abbreviations Summary

UNIT	ABBREVIATION USED IN THIS TEXT	OTHER ACCEPTABLE ABBREVIATIONS
Gram	gm	Gm, g
Milligram	mg	mgm
Microgram	μg	mcg
Liter	L	l
Milliliter	ml	cc*

*Used for gases only.

TABLE 6-6 Equivalents of Concentration Expressions

%	RATIO	gm/L	mg/ml	mg/dl	μg/ml
10	1:10	100	100	10,000	100,000
1	1:100	10	10	1,000	10,000
0.1	1:1000	1	1	100	1,000
0.01	1:10,000	0.1	0.1	10	100
0.001	1:100,000	0.01	0.01	1	10
0.0001	1:1,000,000	0.001	0.001	0.1	1

CALCULATIONS

Calculating the Strength of Drug Solutions

To calculate the concentration of a drug solution, use the following equation:

$$\text{Concentration} = \frac{\text{Mass of drug}}{\text{Volume of solution}}$$

If you know any two of these quantities, you can solve directly for the third, provided all the quantities are expressed in the same system of units. Therefore as a first step in the solution of any problem, it may be necessary to convert units from one system to another, as seen in Example 1.

Example 1

Prepare 1 L of a 5% solution.

You know:

1. Volume of solution (1 L)
2. Concentration (5%)

To solve:

1. Convert all quantities to the same system of units:

$$5\% = 5\text{ gm}/100\text{ ml};\ 1\text{ L} = 1000\text{ ml}$$

2. Substitute the known quantities into the equation:

$$5\text{ gm}/100\text{ ml} = \text{Mass of drug}/1000\text{ ml}$$

3. Solve for mass of drug:

$$\text{Mass} = \frac{1000 \times 5\text{ gm}}{100\text{ ml}} = 50\text{ gm}$$

In other words, if 50 gm of the drug is dissolved in enough diluent to make a final volume of 1 L, the result is a 5% solution.

Example 2

What is the strength of a 2 L solution containing 10 gm of drug?

You know:

1. Mass of drug (10 gm)
2. Volume of solution (2 L)

To solve, substitute the known quantities into the equation:

$$\text{Concentration} = \frac{110\text{ gm}}{2\text{ L}} = \frac{5\text{ gm}}{\text{L}}$$

The strength of this solution could be expressed equally well as 0.5% (0.5 gm/100 ml) or as a 1:200 solution (see Table 6-6).

Example 3

How much of a 2% solution can be prepared with 6 gm of drug?

You know:

1. Concentration (2%)
2. Mass of drug (6 gm)

To solve:

1. Convert all quantities to the same system of units:

$$2\% = 2\text{ gm}/100\text{ ml}$$

2. Substitute the known quantities into the equation:

$$2\text{ gm}/100\text{ ml} = 6\text{ gm}/\text{Volume of solution}$$

3. Solve for volume of solution:

$$\text{Volume} = \frac{6\text{ gm} \times 100\text{ ml}}{2\text{ gm}} = 300\text{ ml}$$

Self-Test for Proficiency in Drug Calculations

After thorough study of the previous section, you should be able to work the following problems. Check your answers and see the calculations worked out at the end of this chapter.

Set 1: Conversions of units and expressions of concentration

1. A solution is labeled 1:50. Express this concentration in the following units:
   a. gm/L
   b. mg/ml
   c. %
   d. mg%
   e. μg/ml
2. The body weight of a patient is given as 150 pounds. What is the body weight expressed in kilograms?

Calculating the Strength of Diluted Solutions

The preceding examples have all dealt with weight/volume problems. In examining volume/volume problems, the basic equation can be modified slightly and the problems can be solved in much the same way as before. The equation becomes:

$$(\text{Concentration of solution}) \times (\text{Volume of solution}) = (\text{Concentration of stock}) \times (\text{Volume of stock})$$

Stock or **stock solution** is a concentrated form of a drug that must ordinarily be diluted before use. With the use of this equation, calculations are performed as shown in the following examples.

Example 4

Prepare 500 ml of a 1% solution from a 1:25 stock.

You know:

1. Volume of solution (500 ml)
2. Concentration of solution (1%)
3. Concentration of stock (1:25)

To solve:

1. Convert all quantities to the same system of units:

$$1\% = 1\text{ gm}/100\text{ ml}$$
$$1{:}25 = 4\text{ gm}/100\text{ ml}$$

2. Substitute the known quantities in the equation:

$$\frac{500\text{ ml} \times \text{gm}}{100\text{ ml}} = \frac{4\text{ gm}}{100\text{ ml}} \times \text{Volume of stock}$$

3. Solve for the unknown:

$$\frac{500 \text{ ml} \times 1 \text{ gm}}{100 \text{ ml}} \times \frac{100 \text{ ml}}{4 \text{ gm}} = 125 \text{ ml}$$

Example 5

How much of a 0.5% solution can be prepared from 10 ml of a 20% solution?

You know:

1. Concentration of solution (0.5%)
2. Volume of stock (10 ml)
3. Concentration of stock (20%)

To solve:

1. Convert all quantities to the same system of units:

$$0.5\% = 0.5 \text{ gm/100 ml}$$
$$20\% = 20 \text{ gm/100 ml}$$

2. Substitute the known quantities in the equation:

$$\frac{0.5 \text{ gm}}{100 \text{ ml}} \times \text{Volume of solution} = \frac{20 \text{ gm}}{100 \text{ ml}} \times 10 \text{ ml}$$

3. Solve for the unknown:

$$\text{Volume of solution} = \frac{20 \text{ gm}}{100 \text{ ml}} \times 10 \text{ ml} \times \frac{100 \text{ ml}}{0.5 \text{ gm}} = 400 \text{ ml}$$

Self-Test for Proficiency in Drug Calculations

After thorough study of the previous section, you should be able to work the following problems. Check your answers and see the calculations worked out at the end of this chapter.

Set 2: Dilution of stock solutions

1. A stock solution of a drug contains 10,000 U/ml.
   a. Calculate the amount of stock that must be included in 500 ml of infusion fluid if a 150-pound patient is to receive 20,000 U of drug in this volume.
   b. Calculate the concentration of the diluted drug.
2. Prepare 1 quart of a 2% solution from a 1:10 stock.
3. How would you prepare 1 gallon of a 5% solution from a 50% solution?

Calculating Drug Dosages

All the examples thus far have dealt with the preparation of a drug for administration. The next step is the use of those materials to fulfill the physician's drug order for a patient. The equation is:

$$\text{Body weight} \times \text{Dosage} = \text{Volume of drug} \times \text{Drug concentration}$$

A drug dosage is expressed as units or mass of drug per body weight of patient. For example, 0.1 gm of drug/kg body weight is a drug dosage expression, but 0.1 gm of drug is not. Occasionally a physician may order a dose of, for example, 500 mg of an antibiotic to be taken every 4 hours. Technically this form does not constitute a drug dosage, but in practice it is understood that 500 mg is the appropriate dose for an average-size patient; that is, the intended dosage is 500 mg/70 kg body weight. More accurate dosages, of course, must be calculated for persons who deviate greatly from the normal weight range or when highly toxic drugs are involved. Common types of problems in drug dosage are presented in the following examples.

Example 6

A 100 kg patient is to receive a dose of 4 U/kg body weight. How many milliliters of the 100 U/ml stock solution are required?

You know:

1. Drug dosage (4 U/kg body weight)
2. Patient body weight (100 kg)
3. Concentration of the drug to be administered (100 U/ml)

To solve:

1. Substitute the known quantities in the equation:

$$100 \text{ kg} \times \frac{4 \text{ U}}{\text{kg}} = \text{Volume of drug} \times 100 \text{ U}$$

2. Solve for volume of drug:

$$\text{Volume of drug} = 100 \text{ kg} \times \frac{4 \text{ U}}{\text{kg}} \times \frac{1 \text{ ml}}{100 \text{ U}} = 4 \text{ ml}$$

Example 7

The attending physician has left orders for infusion with 25,000 U of a drug in 0.5 L of normal saline solution. The drug is supplied as 50,000 U/ml stock solution. What volume of the drug stock would you use to make up the 0.5 L drug solution for administration? What is the dosage if the patient weighs 100 kg?

To solve:

1. Set up the following proportion to calculate the volume of stock to be added to make the infusion mixture:

$$\frac{25{,}000 \text{ U}}{\text{ml of stock}} = \frac{50{,}000 \text{ U}}{1 \text{ ml}}$$

$$\text{ml of stock} = 0.5 \text{ ml}$$

2. Dosage is defined as the amount of drug per unit of body weight.

Therefore the dosage is:

$$\frac{25{,}000 \text{ U}}{100 \text{ kg}} = \frac{250 \text{ U}}{\text{kg}}$$

Self-Test for Proficiency in Drug Calculations

After thorough study of the previous section, you should be able to work the following problems. You can check your answers and see the calculations worked out at the end of this chapter.

Set 3: Drug dosages

1. A 70 kg patient is to receive 1.2 gm of a drug administered in a 3 ml volume. What is the concentration of the drug solution administered to the patient, and what is the drug dosage?
2. A 60 kg patient is to receive 600 mg of a drug administered in a 2 ml volume. What is the drug dosage?

3. A certain drug is dispensed in tablets marked 250 mg. The drug package insert says that the dose of the drug is not to exceed 10 mg/kg. If a 60 kg adult patient receives 2 tablets, will the dosage exceed what the manufacturer considers safe?
4. A certain patient is to receive a drug at a dose of 5 mg/kg. The drug is supplied in a vial marked 500 mg/ml. What volume of drug from the vial should be administered to a 70 kg patient?
5. A certain drug is known to cause thrombophlebitis when given intravenously at high concentrations. For this reason the package insert says the drug must be infused at a concentration of less than 10 mg/ml. A 50 kg patient is to receive 500 mg of the drug by intravenous (IV) infusion. What is the drug dosage, and what volume will need to be infused?

Calculating Infusion Rates

Many drugs must be administered intravenously by slow infusion rather than as a rapid bolus injection. Large volumes of fluids of various types are also given by IV infusion. Disposable infusion sets are available from several manufacturers. These sets are commonly calibrated to deliver 10, 12, 15, 20, 50, or 60 drops/ml (abbreviated gtt/ml) of fluid. The nurse in practice can find the calibration, or drop factor, for any particular infusion set by examining the package in which it is supplied. Usually a hospital has only two sizes available to minimize confusion: one regular, or macrodrip, set of 10, 12, or 15 gtt/ml and one pediatric, or microdrip, set of 50 or 60 gtt/ml.

Calculations of infusion rates can be carried out with the following equation:

$$\text{gtt/ml} = \frac{\text{gtt/ml calibration}}{\text{60 min/hr}} \times \frac{\text{Total ml to be administered}}{\text{Total hours of infusion}}$$

The use of this formula is illustrated in the following examples.

Example 8

A physician's order reads "3500 ml 5% dextrose in water IV in 24 hours." What is the correct infusion rate if the infusion set delivers 60 gtt/ml?

You know:

1. gtt/ml calibration (60 gtt/ml)
2. Total amount to be administered (3500 ml)
3. Total length of infusion (24 hr)

To solve, substitute the known quantities in the equation:

$$\text{gtt/min} = \frac{\text{60 gtt/ml}}{\text{60 min/hr}} \times \frac{\text{3500 ml}}{\text{24 hr}} = \text{145 to 146 gtt/min}$$

Example 9

To give 50 ml of antibiotic solution IV in 30 minutes, what should the infusion rate be in drops per minute? The infusion set is calibrated for 60 gtt/ml.

You know:

1. Total amount to be administered (50 ml)
2. Total length of infusion (0.5 hr)
3. gtt/ml calibration (60 gtt/ml)

To solve, substitute the known quantities in the formula:

$$\text{gtt/min} = \frac{\text{60 gtt/ml}}{\text{60 min/hr}} \times \frac{\text{50 ml}}{\text{0.5 hr}} = \text{100 gtt/min}$$

Example 10

If an infusion set calibrated for 15 gtt/ml is running at a rate of 45 gtt/min, how much time will be required to infuse 1 L of fluid?

You know:

1. gtt/ml calibration (15 gtt/ml)
2. Total volume to be administered (1000 ml = 1 L)
3. Flow rate (45 gtt/min)

To solve, substitute the known quantities in the equation:

$$\text{45 gtt/min} = \frac{\text{15 gtt/ml}}{\text{60 min/hr}} \times \frac{\text{1000 ml}}{\text{Hours of infusion}}$$

The formula can be rearranged to solve for the number of hours:

$$\text{Hours of infusion} = \frac{\text{15 gtt/ml}}{\text{60 min/hr}} \times \frac{\text{1000 ml}}{\text{45 gtt/min}} = \text{5.55 hr}$$

Self-Test for Proficiency in Drug Calculations

After thorough study of the previous section, you should be able to solve the following problems. You can check your answers and see the calculations worked out at the end of this chapter.

Set 4: Calculating IV infusion rates

1. The physician's order reads "1000 ml of D5W IV in 8 hours." What is the correct infusion rate if the administration set delivers 10 gtt/ml?
2. To give 50 ml of antibiotic solution intravenously in 30 minutes, what should the infusion rate be in drops per minute if the infusion set is calibrated to deliver 10 gtt/ml?
3. Half a liter of normal saline solution is to be infused over a 5-hour period. The infusion set delivers 20 gtt/ml. What should the rate of infusion be?
4. The physician's order reads "1000 ml D5W in 24 hours." If the infusion set calibration is 60 gtt/ml, how many drops per minute should be administered?
5. An infusion of 500 ml of IV fluid is to be carried out over 3 hours. What infusion rate must be used with an infusion set delivering 10 gtt/ml?

Calculating Pediatric Dosages

Calculation of pediatric dosages requires special knowledge of each drug and how it interacts with the unique metabolism of the infant (see Chapter 2). Some drugs may be given to children and infants in doses that are in the same proportion to body weight as the doses used in adults. Other drugs must be given in greatly reduced doses because the infant is more sensitive or is incapable of metabolizing the drug as rapidly as an adult. Physicians take these considerations into account when determining recommended pediatric doses. For many drugs the pediatric doses listed in various drug reference publications include a statement indicating that the dosage may be calculated for children according to their body weight, for example, but should not exceed a stated upper limit.

Several methods for calculating pediatric dosages exist. Three methods are presented here. The first method, called **Young's rule,** is based on the age of the child and applies to children between 1 and 12 years of age. The equation is:

$$\text{Child's dose} = \frac{\text{Age of child in years}}{\text{Age of child in years} + 12} \times \text{Adult dose}$$

The use of Young's rule is illustrated in the following example.

Example 11

What is the appropriate dose of aspirin for a 3-year-old child? A normal adult dose is 650 mg.

You know:

Adult dose (650 mg)

To solve, substitute the known quantities in the equation:

$$\text{Child's dose} = \frac{3 \text{ years}}{3 + 12} \times 650 \text{ mg} = \frac{1}{5} \times 650 \text{ mg} = 130 \text{ mg}$$

A second method for calculating pediatric dosages is based on a comparison of the child's weight to the average weight of an adult. This formula, which applies to all ages of children, is called **Clark's rule.** The equation is:

$$\text{Child's dose} = \frac{\text{Weight of child in pounds}}{150 \text{ pounds}} \times \text{Adult dose}$$

The use of Clark's rule is illustrated in the following example.

Example 12

What is the appropriate dose of aspirin for a 30-pound child if the normal adult dose is 650 mg?

You know:

1. Weight of the child (30 lb)
2. Adult dose (5 gr)

To solve, substitute the known quantities in the equation:

$$\text{Child's dose} = \frac{30 \text{ lb}}{150 \text{ lb}} \times 650 \text{ mg} = 130 \text{ mg}$$

Note that Clark's rule and Young's rule give the same answer when the child is not much lighter or heavier than the normal weight for age. The 30-pound 3-year-old child used in examples 11 and 12 is near the normal weight for that age. Clark's rule is considered the more accurate of the two rules since it will adjust dosage for a child who does deviate from normal weight.

The most accurate method of calculating pediatric dosage is based on the **body surface area** of the child's body relative to that of an adult. Surface area is obviously more difficult to measure than age or weight. Measurements under laboratory conditions yield 1.7 square meters (m^2) as the average body surface area for an adult. Measurements taken under similar conditions with children have allowed the construction of charts and nomograms that relate the child's body weight to surface area. An example of such a chart is shown in Table 6-7. The equation used for the drug dose calculation is:

$$\text{Child's dose} = \frac{\text{Surface area of child in m}^2}{1.7 \text{ m}^2} \times \text{Adult dose}$$

The use of the formula is illustrated in the following example.

Example 13

What dose of meperidine (Demerol) does a child weighing 10 kg require?

The adult dose of meperidine is 50 mg. To calculate the dosage on the basis of body surface area, determine from Table 6-7 the surface area that corresponds to a body weight of 10 kg. That value is 0.46 m^2. With that information you can solve the problem.

You know:

1. Suface area of child (0.46 m^2)
2. Adult dose (50 mg)

To solve, substitute these values in the equation:

$$\text{Child's dose} = \frac{0.46 \text{ m}^2}{1.7 \text{ m}^2} \times 50 \text{ mg} = 13.5 \text{ mg}$$

Self-Test for Proficiency in Drug Calculations

After thorough study of the previous section, you should be able to work the following problems. Check your answers and see the calculations worked out in at the end of this chapter.

TABLE 6-7 Body Surface Area as a Function of Weight

WEIGHT		SURFACE	APPROXIMATE	WEIGHT		SURFACE	APPROXIMATE
kg	lb	AREA (m^2)	AGE OF PATIENT	kg	lb	AREA (m^2)	AGE OF PATIENT
4	8.8	0.25	3 wk	19	41	0.73	5 yr
5.7	12.5	0.29	3 mo	21	47	0.82	6 yr
7.4	16	0.36	6 mo	24	53	0.90	7 yr
10	22	0.46	1 yr	27	59	0.97	8 yr
12	27	0.54	2 yr	32	71	1.12	10 yr
14	31	0.60	3 yr	39	86	1.28	12 yr
16	36	0.68	4 yr	70	150	1.7	Adult

Set 5: Calculating pediatric doses

1. A physician orders the antibiotic cephalexin for a 25-pound child. The normal adult dose for this drug is 250 mg qid. Use Clark's rule to calculate the dose for this child. Does the prescribed dose fall within the recommended dose of 6 to 12 mg/kg listed in the package insert?
2. You are to give a 5-year-old child phenobarbital. The adult dose is 60 mg. Use Young's rule to calculate the appropriate dose for the child.
3. A 10-year-old child requires codeine sulfate. The normal adult dose is 30 mg. Use body surface area to calculate the appropriate dose for this child.
4. You must give aspirin to a 4-year-old child. Adults take 325 or 650 mg of aspirin, depending on the severity of the pain to be relieved. Use Young's rule to calculate the appropriate dose for the child, based on the maximum adult dose.
5. A 12 kg infant is to receive atropine. The normal adult dose is 0.3 mg (300 μg). What is the appropriate dose for this infant, based on body surface area?
6. You are to give penicillin G to a 40-pound child. The adult dose is 300,000 U. Use Clark's rule to calculate the child's dose.

NURSING PROCESS OVERVIEW

Calculating Drug Doses

Assessment

The patient and ordered medications should be assessed individually. Is the drug appropriate? What is the usual dose, and is the dose ordered within the normal range? Is there anything about the patient that would indicate that an ordered dose is too large or too small?

Planning/Implementation

Calculate dosages systematically. Have a colleague check calculations if the dose seems unusual or if the mathematic calculations are difficult. Do a "common sense" check also: 2 tablets might make sense but 20 tablets? If an intramuscular (IM) dose is calculated at 7 ml, is there an error? Most IM doses do not exceed 2 ml. A dose can be too small; for example, should an IV dose of 0.02 ml be 2 ml?

Evaluation

Is the patient achieving the desired result? Are there side effects? Are they severe? What data indicate a prescribed dose is too high or too low? What should be recorded?

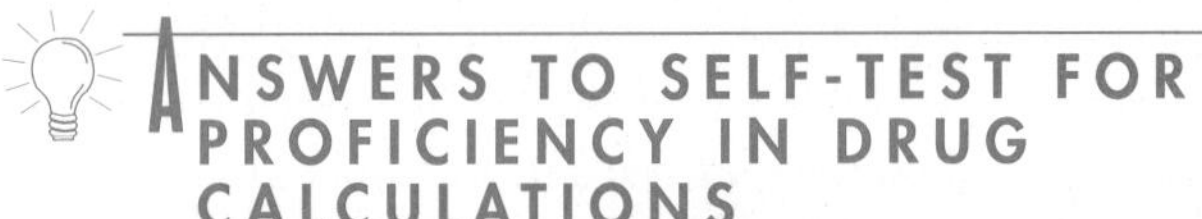

ANSWERS TO SELF-TEST FOR PROFICIENCY IN DRUG CALCULATIONS

At the end of each section in the text, there are questions designed to assist the student in developing proficiency. The correct answer for each self-test question is given below, followed by the calculation.

Solutions to set 1

1. The solution is labeled *1:50.* Ratio is defined as gm:ml, with both usually expressed as whole numbers. Therefore 1 gm/50 ml is the expression of concentration. You may now readily carry out the other conversions required. The answers are given first, followed by the calculation.
   a. *20 gm/L:* 1 gm/50 ml = ? gm/1000 ml. (Remember that 1 L = 1000 ml.) ? gm = (1000 ml × 1 gm)/50 ml = 20 gm/L.
   b. *20 mg/ml:* 1 gm = 1000 mg. Therefore: 1000 mg/50 ml = ? mg/1000 ml; ? mg = (1000 ml × 1 mg)/50 ml = 20 mg/ml.
   c. *2%:* Percentage is defined as gm/100 ml. Solving by proportion: 1 gm/50 ml = ? gm/100 ml. Therefore: ? gm = (1 gm × 100 ml)/50 ml = 2 gm. Thus the solution of 2 gm/100 ml is 2%.
   d. *2000 mg%:* Mg% is defined as mg/100 ml. Solving by proportion: 1 gm/50 ml = ? mg/100 ml. Therefore: ? mg = (1000 mg × 100 ml)/50 ml = 2000 mg. Thus the solution of 2000 mg/100 ml is 2000 mg%.
   e. *20,000 μg/ml:* 1 mg = 1000 μg. Therefore: 20 mg/ml = 20,000 μg/ml.
2. From Table 6-4, you find that 1 lb = 0.46 kg. Therefore, solving by proportion: 0.46 kg/1 lb = ? kg/150 lb. Thus: ? kg = (0.46 kg × 150 lb)/1 lb = 69 kg.

Solutions to set 2

1. a. *2 ml:* Calculate the *amount of stock* that contains 20,000 U. Solving by proportion:

$$\frac{10{,}000\ \text{U}}{1\ \text{ml}} = \frac{20{,}000\ \text{U}}{?\ \text{ml}}$$

$$?\ \text{ml} = \frac{(1\ \text{ml})\ (20{,}000\ \text{U})}{10{,}000\ \text{U}} = 2\ \text{ml}$$

   b. *40 U/ml:* Diluted drug is 20,000 U in 500 ml, so

$$\frac{20{,}000\ \text{U}}{500\ \text{ml}} = 40\ \text{U/ml}$$

2. Dilute 200 ml of 1:10 stock to 1 qt (1000 ml): 1:10 stock 4 1 gm/10 ml; 1 qt 4 1000 ml; 2% solution 4 2 gm/100 ml. To make 1 qt of 2% solution would require:

$$\frac{2\ \text{gm}}{100\ \text{ml}} = \frac{?\ \text{gm}}{1000\ \text{ml}}$$

? gm = (2 gm × 1000 ml)/100 ml = 20 gm. To get 20 gm from the 1:10 stock:

$$\frac{1\text{ gm}}{10\text{ ml}} = \frac{20\text{ gm}}{?\text{ ml}}$$

$$?\text{ ml} = (20\text{ gm} \times 10\text{ ml})/1\text{ gm} = 200\text{ ml}$$

3. *Add 400 ml of the 50% stock solution to 3600 ml of water:* 1 gal = 4000 ml, a 5% solution = 5 gm/100 ml, and a 50% solution = 50 gm/100 ml. Therefore the volume of stock solution to be added equals:

$$\frac{(5\text{ gm}/100\text{ ml}) \times 4000\text{ ml}}{(50\text{ gm}/100\text{ ml})} = 400\text{ ml}$$

Note that this volume is to be mixed with 3600 ml of water for the final volume of the solution to be 1 gallon.

Solutions to set 3

1. *The concentration is 0.4 gm/ml, and the dosage is 17 mg/kg:*

$$\text{Concentration} = 1.2\text{ gm}/3\text{ ml} = 0.4\text{ gm/ml}$$
$$\text{Dosage} = 1.2\text{ gm}/70\text{ kg} = 0.017\text{ gm/kg} = 17\text{ mg/kg}$$

2. Dosage is 10 mg/kg:

$$\text{Dosage} = 600\text{ mg}/60\text{ kg} = 10\text{ mg/kg}$$

3. *Dosage = 8.33 mg/kg. Therefore the dose as prescribed should be within the accepted safety limits:*

$$\frac{2\text{ tablets}}{\text{Dose}} \times \frac{250\text{ mg}}{\text{Tablet}} = \frac{500\text{ mg}}{\text{Dose}}$$

Therefore: 500 mg/60 kg = 8.33 mg/kg.

4. *0.7 ml:* (5 mg/kg) × 70 kg = 350 mg drug in each dose. Therefore:

$$\frac{350\text{ mg}}{500\text{ mg/ml}} = 0.7\text{ ml volume from the vial}$$

5. *Dosage = 10 mg/kg and the minimum infusion volume is 50 ml:*

$$\text{Dosage} = \frac{500\text{ mg}}{50\text{ kg}} = 10\text{ mg/kg}$$

$$\text{Minimum infusion volume} = \frac{500\text{ mg}}{10\text{ mg/ml}} = 50\text{ ml}$$

Solutions to set 4

1. *20 to 21 gtt/min:*

$$\text{gtt/min} = \frac{10\text{ gtt/ml}}{60\text{ min/hr}} \times \frac{1000\text{ ml}}{8\text{ hr}} = 20\text{ to }21\text{ gtt/min}$$

2. *16 to 17 gtt/min:*

$$\text{gtt/min} = \frac{10\text{ gtt/ml}}{60\text{ min/hr}} \times \frac{50\text{ ml}}{0.5\text{ hr}} = 16\text{ to }17\text{ gtt/min}$$

3. *33 to 34 gtt/min:*

$$\text{gtt/min} = \frac{20\text{ gtt/ml}}{60\text{ min/hr}} \times \frac{500\text{ ml}}{5\text{ hr}} = 33\text{ to }34\text{ gtt/min}$$

4. *41 to 42 gtt/min:*

$$\text{gtt/min} = \frac{60\text{ gtt/ml}}{60\text{ min/hr}} \times \frac{1000\text{ ml}}{24\text{ hr}} = 41\text{ to }42\text{ gtt/min}$$

5. *27 to 28 gtt/min:*

$$\text{gtt/min} = \frac{10\text{ gtt/ml}}{60\text{ min/hr}} \times \frac{500\text{ ml}}{3\text{ hr}} = 27\text{ to }28\text{ gtt/min}$$

Solutions to set 5

1. *Dosage prescribed = 3.8 mg/kg, which is less than the suggested lower limit of 6 mg/kg:*

$$\text{Child's dose} = (25\text{ lb} \times 250\text{ mg})/150\text{ mg} = 42\text{ mg}$$
$$25\text{ lb} = 11\text{ kg}$$
$$\text{Dosage} = 42\text{ mg}/11\text{ kg} = 3.8\text{ mg/kg}$$

2. *17.6 mg:*

$$\text{Child's dose} = \frac{5\text{ years}}{5 + 12} \times 60\text{ mg} = 17.6\text{ mg}$$

3. *19.8 mg:* According to Table 6-7, body surface area of 10-year-old child = 1.12 m^2.

$$\text{Child's dose} = (1.12\text{ m}^2/1.7\text{ m}^2) \times 30\text{ mg} = 19.8\text{ mg}$$

4. *2.5 gr:*

$$\text{Child's dose} = \frac{4\text{ years}}{4 + 12} \times 650\text{ mg} = 162\text{ mg}$$

5. *0.01 mg:* According to Table 6-7, body surface area of 12 kg infant = 0.54 m^2.

$$\text{Child's dose} = \frac{0.54\text{ m}^2}{1.7\text{ m}^2} \times 0.3\text{ mg} = 0.01\text{ mg}$$

6. *80,000 U:*

$$\text{Child's dose} = \frac{40\text{ lb}}{150\text{ lb}} \times 300{,}000\text{ U} = 80{,}000\text{ U}$$

CHAPTER 7

Over-the-Counter Drugs and Self-Medication

Lynn Roger Willis

OBJECTIVES

After studying this chapter, you should be able to do the following:

- *Explain the difference between over-the-counter medications and prescription drugs.*
- *Describe the advantages and disadvantages of fixed combinations of active ingredients.*
- *Explain the proper use of effective classes of over-the-counter agents.*
- *Discuss the dangers associated with continuous use of over-the-counter agents such as weight-loss products, laxatives, or sleeping medications.*

KEY TERMS

fixed combination products
nonsteroidal antiinflammatory drugs (NSAIDs)
over-the-counter (OTC) medications
placebos
sun protection factor (SPF)
teratogenicity

CHAPTER OVERVIEW

As health professionals, nurses focus on medications ordered for the patient by the physician. It is important to remember that patients also self-medicate, using a wide array of over-the-counter medications. In certain circumstances over-the-counter medications may significantly influence the effects of prescribed agents. This chapter summarizes the properties of most classes of over-the-counter agents. In later chapters how prescription drugs influence the same body systems will be discussed.

REGULATION OF OVER-THE-COUNTER DRUGS

Over-the-counter (OTC) **medications** are medicinal agents deemed safe enough for sale without a prescription. Products intended for the self-medication of a variety of illnesses have been sold in the United States since colonial times. Until the early twentieth century no restrictions governed the contents, potency, purity, safety, efficacy, sale, or advertising of these products, which came to be known as *nostrums* or *patent medicines.* Consequently, some were of marginal safety at best, and most provided no obvious therapeutic benefit. Most patent medicines were harmless and ineffective, but many contained alcohol, narcotics, or other dangerous drugs in unspecified quantities.

Some control of the patent medicine industry was achieved with passage of the first Pure Food and Drug Act of 1906 (see Chapter 3). This act required that package labels accurately list the ingredients of medicinal products. Any substance present but not listed on the label was deemed an adulterant. A later amendment to the act, the Sherley Amendment (1912), forbade false and fraudulent labeling claims. In 1938 a new Food and Drug Act was enacted. It required proof of safety for all medicinal products intended for sale. In 1952 the Durham-Humphrey Amendment to the 1938 act specified (1) drugs safe enough for sale without a prescription (over the counter) and (2) drugs deemed sufficiently dangerous or unsuitable for self-medication to require sale by prescription only.

Present control of OTC drugs stems from the Kefauver-Harris Amendment of 1962, which required proof of efficacy and safety and lack of **teratogenicity** (the ability to cause birth defects). This amendment affected all drugs introduced after 1962 and all drugs that had entered the market since 1938. To meet the conditions of this amendment, the Food and Drug Administration (FDA) convened several panels of experts to review the classes of OTC drugs and assign each to one of the following categories:

- Category I: Recognized as safe and effective for the claimed therapeutic indication
- Category II: Not recognized as safe and effective
- Category III: Additional data needed to decide safety or effectiveness

Drugs assigned to category I can be sold to the general public. Those in category II cannot. Drugs in category III, if generally recognized as safe, may be sold even though the evaluation of their safety and effectiveness has not been completed.

Since this review process began, many unsafe or ineffective OTC drugs and products have disappeared from the market. Others have undergone labeling changes or have been redesigned. However, since manufacturers are not required to indicate whether the drugs in their products are in category I or III, OTC products cannot be assumed to be effective simply because they are sold. Some consumer interest groups have objected to the sale of drugs in category III, apparently in the belief that a drug should be considered unsafe and ineffective unless proven otherwise. Such groups have also challenged the assignment of other drugs to category I. Until the FDA review panels have completed their work, the therapeutic benefit of some OTC drugs will remain questionable.

COMMON PROPERTIES OF OVER-THE-COUNTER DRUGS

Low Doses

Today's manufacturers of OTC products are concerned with safety. The toxicity of a drug varies in direct proportion to the dose administered; that is, the higher the dose, the greater the risk of toxicity. Thus most OTC products contain low, sometimes less-than-therapeutic, amounts of active ingredient. As such, they may serve as little more than **placebos** (inactive substances usually presented in the guise of an active medicine), especially for such subjective complaints as minor pain, itching, and sleeplessness. For such indications proof that a drug is effective may be difficult to establish, even when adequate dosage is provided.

Combination of Ingredients

Many OTC products contain several drugs. The drugs may be totally different, or they may be of the same or similar pharmacologic classification. When drugs are combined, adverse interactions may occur. Although the risk of interactions is low for the drugs in a given product, it is not so low when other drugs are taken simultaneously.

OTC products with several ingredients are termed **fixed combination products;** that is, the doses of the drugs in the product are fixed within the tablet or other dosage form and cannot be altered. For example, if a tablet contains 4 mg of antihistamine and 60 mg of decongestant, a patient who needed to increase the antihistamine dosage would also have to take more of the decongestant. Complete control of drug dosage is possible with readily available single-drug products, and such products can often be purchased less expensively than the heavily advertised combination products. By understanding the pharmacology of the drugs in OTC products and the specific needs of the patient, the nurse can advise a rational method of product selection.

MAJOR CLASSES OF OVER-THE-COUNTER DRUGS

The classes of OTC drugs chosen for discussion in this chapter include analgesic drugs, cold and cough remedies, weight-control products, and sleep aids; their component drugs are discussed in other chapters. Also discussed are ophthalmic products, acne treatments, sunscreens, topical antiinfectives, and hemorrhoidal products.

Analgesics

Aspirin, acetaminophen, ibuprofen, and naproxen are the most effective OTC analgesic drugs available. Nearly all OTC analgesic products intended for internal consumption contain one of these drugs. Aspirin, ibuprofen, and naproxen are

OTC members of a larger class of drugs known as **nonsteroidal antiinflammatory drugs (NSAIDs).** These drugs inhibit the synthesis of prostaglandins by inhibiting cyclooxygenase. This action may be related to the mechanism by which they produce analgesia. Acetaminophen is chemically unrelated to aspirin, naproxen, or ibuprofen. Its mechanism of action differs from that of NSAIDs, and it can be used by people who cannot tolerate NSAIDs. The complex pharmacology of these drugs is discussed in detail in Chapter 30.

Aspirin

Aspirin in doses of 650 mg relieves minor pain and reduces fever in most adults. Higher doses (as in "extra-strength" products) provide little additional relief for most people. Aspirin also relieves the pain and inflammation of arthritic disorders; however, this effect requires higher than usual doses, which must be used under medical supervision.

Aspirin produces numerous side effects. Although it normally presents no problem for individuals who take the drug only occasionally, it may be troublesome for those who take it regularly or are particularly sensitive to it. For example, aspirin inhibits platelet aggregation. As little as one 650 mg dose of aspirin may double the bleeding time for several days. Aspirin also irritates the stomach lining, sometimes causing pain, discomfort, and, on occasion, bleeding, which can cause the loss of 5 to 10 ml of blood in the stool each day. The bleeding is ordinarily of no consequence with occasional use of the drug, but those who take aspirin frequently may develop iron deficiency anemia resulting from long-term blood losses. Individuals with a history of peptic ulcer or intestinal bleeding or those who are taking anticoagulant drugs should not take aspirin.

Various dosage forms for aspirin are available, reflecting efforts by manufacturers to overcome some of the problems it causes. Aspirin is available in buffered, effervescent, and enteric-coated tablets to minimize gastric irritation. Timed-release tablets are available for persons who must take aspirin regularly. Since aspirin is unstable in aqueous solution, liquid forms are not available.

Acetaminophen

Acetaminophen is as effective as aspirin at relieving minor aches and pains and reducing fever. Maximum analgesic and antipyretic effectiveness are achieved in most adults with 650 mg of either drug. Higher doses (as in "extra-strength" products) provide little, if any, additional relief for most people, but they appear to be more effective than usual doses in some people. Unlike aspirin, acetaminophen does not relieve the pain and inflammation of arthritic disorders.

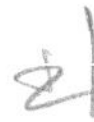

Acetaminophen (Datril, Tylenol, and other brands) is remarkably free of side effects. It does not affect blood-clotting mechanisms, nor does it irritate the stomach lining. Rarely, acetaminophen causes an allergic reaction, often a skin rash. It may also damage the liver but only in association with overdosage.

Acetaminophen is stable in solution and is available in a variety of pleasant-tasting syrups. Both aspirin and acetaminophen are available in inexpensive but reliable generic forms.

Ibuprofen and Naproxen

Ibuprofen (Advil, Nuprin) has been available OTC since 1984. Naproxen (Aleve) was granted OTC status in 1994. These drugs are members of a large family of NSAIDs (see Chapter 30) and were approved for OTC sale largely because they have a somewhat wider margin of safety than either aspirin or acetaminophen, especially in cases of overdose.

Ibuprofen and naproxen are recommended for people who cannot tolerate aspirin, but this recommendation requires rather narrow interpretation. People who are allergic to aspirin are also likely to be allergic to these drugs. Similarly, ibuprofen and naproxen irritate the gastric mucosa and may cause gastrointestinal (GI) tract bleeding. The drugs are often promoted as less likely than aspirin to cause gastric irritation, but some people may find them as troublesome as aspirin in this regard. For such people acetaminophen remains the preferred alternative. No therapeutic advantage is gained by taking any of these drugs together; indeed, doing so increases the risk of adverse effects.

Although ibuprofen and naproxen are usually superior to aspirin or acetaminophen for relieving certain types of pain, such as that associated with menstrual cramps, dental work, and severe muscle strains, they are no more effective than aspirin or acetaminophen against most other types of mild pain and generally are more expensive. Consequently, nurses should exercise discretion and judgment when recommending them.

Cold Remedies

Most of the available OTC cold remedies (e.g., Contac, Dristan, Novahistine) contain a sympathomimetic drug to relieve nasal and sinus congestion, an antihistamine to dry excessive nasal secretions, or an analgesic drug to relieve minor aches and pains. Some products also contain caffeine, vitamins, a laxative, or other substances. A few products contain only a single drug, usually a sympathomimetic or an antihistamine, but most cold remedies are combination products.

Sympathomimetic drugs relieve nasal stuffiness and congestion by constricting the blood vessels in swollen nasal membranes, decreasing local blood flow and swelling. When the swelling is relieved, the breathing passages open. The sympathomimetic drugs commonly included in OTC cold remedies as decongestants are phenylephrine, phenylpropanolamine, and pseudoephedrine. These drugs are available in many products, and their pharmacologic characteristics are discussed in Chapter 29. Phenylephrine is the least reliable of the three because stomach acid reduces its activity, and its absorption into the blood is often erratic.

Sympathomimetic drugs can cause stimulation of the central nervous system (CNS) and generalized vasoconstriction. As a result the side effects of irritability, nervousness, insomnia, headache, and hypertension can occur. Individuals with high blood pressure, thyroid disease, or heart disease are cautioned against taking these drugs unless directed to do so by their physician. The vasoconstrictive effects of sympathomimetics are intensified by monoamine oxidase inhibitors (e.g., Marplan, Nardil), which may be prescribed to treat depression (see Chapter 53) and may cause alarming and dangerous elevations of blood pressure and threat of stroke.

The rationale for including an antihistamine in a product intended to treat symptoms of the common cold is not based on antagonism of histamine receptors. Unless the cold is associated with conditions of increased histamine release, such as allergic rhinitis, antagonism of histamine receptors will be of no use (see Chapter 28). Instead, the justification for including antihistamines in OTC cold remedies rests largely on their anticholinergic action, which reduces secretion of mucus by the nasal and bronchial mucosa and produces a drying effect. This effect, however, is not impressive, especially at approved OTC doses.

The therapeutic index of antihistamines is high, and little risk of serious toxicity exists for adults. The most prominent side effects of antihistamines are drowsiness and sedation. These effects occur with all OTC antihistamines and doses. They pose a potentially serious threat to operators of motor vehicles or persons in hazardous occupations. Cold remedies that are promoted as "nondrowsiness formulas" generally do not contain an antihistamine.

The analgesic-antipyretic ingredients most often found in OTC cold remedies are aspirin or acetaminophen. Although aspirin and acetaminophen relieve the aches, pains, and feverishness associated with the common cold, it is never necessary to purchase a cold remedy that contains an analgesic. If analgesia is desired, aspirin or acetaminophen can be obtained separately at considerable savings and should be taken only as necessary.

No clear rationale exists for including caffeine, vitamins, laxatives, or other drugs in OTC cold remedies. The dose of caffeine provided in OTC cold remedies is generally far less than that contained in a cup of coffee. Vitamins are necessary only for correction of a vitamin deficiency and provide no therapeutic benefits for a cold sufferer. Laxatives, likewise, are of no known value for treatment of a cold.

Cough Remedies

If a cough accompanies a cold, it may be productive or nonproductive. A productive cough removes phlegm from the lower respiratory tract and generally should not be suppressed. A nonproductive cough is dry and, because of local irritation caused by the rapid movement of air, may be self-perpetuating. Nonproductive coughs can be safely suppressed and relieved with an OTC cough suppressant (antitussive) drug. Expectorants are also included in many OTC cough remedies. The detailed pharmacologic properties of expectorants and antitussives are discussed in Chapter 29.

Expectorants

The use of expectorants in clinical medicine is controversial. The controversy stems partly from a lack of objective evidence that expectorant drugs are effective and partly from confusion concerning the expected effect of an expectorant drug. By one definition, an expectorant should promote the expulsion of mucus, phlegm, and fluid from the lungs and bronchial passages; that is, it should enhance the productiveness of a cough. By another, it should relieve a dry, irritating cough by causing the secretion of soothing and protective mucus in the airway. There is little evidence to suggest that expectorant drugs are any better than placebo for promoting the expulsion of phlegm or relieving a cough.

Guaifenesin is the only expectorant approved for use in OTC cough remedies. It stimulates the reflex production of bronchial secretions by irritating the gastric mucosa. In higher dosage it causes nausea and vomiting.

Cough Suppressants

Three antitussive drugs have been approved for OTC status by the FDA. They are codeine, dextromethorphan, and diphenhydramine. Each one relieves coughs by suppressing the cough reflex center in the brain.

Codeine once was the most widely used antitussive agent, but because it is an opioid narcotic that can cause psychologic and physical dependence, its popularity has waned. In truth, the risk of dependence with codeine is less than that for morphine, and it is virtually nonexistent when the drug is used in recommended doses for short periods of time. Nevertheless, none of the other drugs in this class has a potential for dependence, and they have proved to be more popular among consumers.

The side effects most often associated with the use of codeine are nausea, constipation, and drowsiness. The drowsiness is caused by depression of the CNS and is intensified by other CNS-depressant drugs (e.g., barbiturates, alcohol, and antihistamines). Codeine should not be taken with any other CNS-depressant drug. Poisoning with codeine causes respiratory depression.

Abuse of OTC cough preparations that contain codeine has been a problem in the United States, and varying restrictions on their sale have been enacted by state legislatures. These restrictions range from a limit on the quantity that can be purchased by an individual to complete prohibition of sale without a prescription.

Dextromethorphan is a nonnarcotic cough suppressant with approximately the same antitussive potency and efficacy as codeine. As with codeine, dextromethorphan suppresses the cough reflex center in the brain, but it does not cause dependence or respiratory depression. Side effects are uncommon and generally mild, consisting largely of drowsiness and GI tract upset. Overall, dextromethorphan is the best choice for cough suppression, and the great majority of OTC antitussive products contain it.

Diphenhydramine, an antihistamine, is also an effective cough suppressant. It is nonnarcotic and therefore does not cause dependence. In adults the drug suppresses coughs at a dosage of 25 mg every 4 hours. Drowsiness commonly occurs at this dosage, however, and severely limits the usefulness of this drug for many people. Paradoxically, diphenhydramine may cause stimulation, not sedation, in small children. This effect and its high propensity to cause drowsiness in adults makes it the least useful of the approved antitussive drugs.

Decongestant Nosedrops and Nasal Sprays

Several sympathomimetic drugs are available without a prescription as nosedrops and nasal sprays for the symptomatic and temporary relief of nasal congestion. These drugs include phenylephrine, ephedrine, and naphazoline, which are short-acting decongestants that are used as frequently as every 3 or 4 hours, and xylometazoline and oxymetazoline, which are long-acting decongestants that are used only 2 or 3 times a day.

Topical decongestants have advantages over oral decongestants, but there are also some serious disadvantages. Since the drops and sprays apply the drugs directly to the congested nasal membranes, the onset of action and relief of congestion occur rapidly. In addition, only small amounts of the drugs need be administered since they are applied locally. Therefore the incidence and severity of systemic side effects (e.g., elevated blood pressure) are reduced. On the other hand, the intense localized vasoconstriction in the nasal mucosa can cause "rebound congestion," in which the congestion that returns when the effect of the drug has dissipated may be worse than the congestion that existed in the first place. A vicious cycle can then develop in which the drug that originally relieved congestion now becomes the cause of it. If unrecognized, this cycle of futile treatment can lead to chronic nasal stuffiness that will no longer respond to the decongestant drugs. Rebound congestion probably cannot be totally avoided when topical decongestants are used, but it can be minimized if the drugs are used only sparingly and strictly according to directions.

Nasal sprays are most convenient for adults and older children, and nosedrops are often preferable for use in young children. Topical decongestants should not be given to children younger than 2 years except as directed by a physician.

Weight-Control Products

Obesity is most frequently defined as a condition in which body weight is more than 20% greater than the ideal body weight. It is a complex problem that requires complex treatment. Drug treatment of obesity is of limited value at best. Amphetamines (see Chapter 54) have been prescribed for weight control. They, and related drugs, suppress appetite via a central mechanism, but the appetite remains suppressed only as long as sufficient levels of the drug are present in the brain. When the effect of the drug dissipates, hunger returns. Unless the patient willfully resists the temptation to overeat, drug treatment will be of no value. Moreover, tolerance to the appetite-suppressing action of these drugs develops quickly, and the drugs may produce dependence. Amphetamines are not available without a prescription.

Weight loss occurs if the rate at which calories are expended exceeds the rate at which they are obtained in the diet. No available OTC product enhances the rate at which calories are expended. They can aid only in reducing caloric intake. To that end, it matters little if a dietary aid possesses true pharmacologic activity. A placebo can be totally effective in some persons if they consume fewer calories while taking it. OTC drugs for promoting weight loss consist mainly of phenylpropranolamine, bulk-producing agents, and benzocaine.

When an OTC weight-control product is selected or recommended, the importance of a practical, balanced, and nutritious diet plan (preferably supervised by a family member, friend, nurse, registered dietitian, or physician) cannot be emphasized too strongly. By themselves, OTC products do not produce weight loss. The success of a weight-loss program depends on faithful maintenance of diminished caloric intake.

Phenylpropanolamine

Phenylpropanolamine is structurally related to ephedrine and amphetamine. Its pharmacologic characteristics are similar to those of amphetamine, but phenylpropanolamine is less potent. Phenylpropanolamine clearly suppresses appetite in experimental animals, but its effectiveness in humans is questionable. The drug has been assigned to category I because in controlled clinical trials human subjects who took the drug lost more weight by the end of the study than did untreated control subjects. The problem with these results is that the weight losses, and the differences between treated and untreated groups in these studies, were small. Often people who did not receive phenylpropanolamine lost nearly as much weight as did those who had received the drug.

Amphetamine-like side effects can occur with phenylpropanolamine. The most common of these are nervousness, insomnia, headache, nausea, and elevated blood pressure. Persons with diabetes mellitus, heart disease, hypertension, or thyroid disease should not take phenylpropanolamine, except on the advice of a physician.

Phenylpropanolamine may be unexpectedly dangerous in rare people. Since 1985, 11 cases of cerebral hemorrhage have been reported in persons taking this drug. Ten of the eleven cases involved women, and several apparently occurred after the recommended dosage had been taken.

When recommending a dietary aid containing phenylpropanolamine, the nurse should emphasize the questionable value of the drug if caloric intake is not also reduced, the development of tolerance after long-term use of the drug, and the side effects if the recommended daily dosage is exceeded.

Bulk-Producing Agents

A variety of bulk producers are sold as aids to weight reduction. When taken with 1 or 2 glasses of water, they tend to expand and swell in the stomach, thereby producing a feeling of fullness and a loss of appetite. Examples of OTC bulk producers are methylcellulose, carboxymethylcellulose, agar, psyllium hydrophilic mucilloid, and karaya gum. Unfortunately, the swollen bulk spends little time in the stomach, moving rapidly into the intestine, where it stimulates peristalsis and may exert a laxative effect. Some bulk producers are also marketed as laxatives and stool softeners (see Chapter 24). Bulk producers are probably no more effective at suppressing appetite and caloric intake than is drinking 2 or 3 glasses of water before meals, but the FDA has approved bulk-producing agents for dietary use.

Benzocaine

Several OTC weight-control products contain the local anesthetic drug benzocaine in tablets or in chewing gum. Presumably, benzocaine anesthetizes the gastric mucosa or the mucous membranes in the mouth, thereby reducing appetite or removing the pleasurable sensation of taste. There is no conclusive evidence that either effect promotes weight loss.

Sleeping Aids

Insomnia disrupts the restful nights of nearly everyone from time to time. Some people have difficulty falling asleep; others may awaken in the middle of the night and be unable to go back to sleep. The cause of sleep difficulties may be physiologic or psychologic. In most cases the difficulties are temporary.

A wide variety of common remedies for sleeplessness may be tried. They include warm baths, a dull book, and a glass of warm milk or wine. In severe cases of insomnia the assistance of a physician may be sought, and a powerful sedative-hypnotic drug may be prescribed (see Chapter 51). Many people fear the addictive properties of these drugs, but they find little or no relief from home remedies. Between these extremes lies the OTC sleeping aid.

The FDA severely restricts the number of drugs that can be sold as OTC sleeping aids. OTC sleeping aids may contain an antihistamine alone or an antihistamine with aspirin or acetaminophen. Diphenhydramine is the only antihistamine recognized by the FDA as safe and effective for use as an OTC sleeping aid. Doxylamine succinate, another antihistamine, may legally be sold in OTC sleeping remedies, but its safety and clinical effectiveness are still under investigation.

Antihistamines have utility as OTC sleeping aids because of their tendency to cause drowsiness. This tendency, plus a wide margin of safety, lends credence to marketing claims for the effectiveness of antihistamines in the treatment of occasional insomnia. An analgesic drug is included in some preparations on the assumption that mild nighttime pain may contribute to sleeplessness. Clinical comparisons of antihistamines with placebo in sleep laboratories tend to reinforce the claims of effectiveness, but some authorities remain doubtful.

The most common side effects produced by antihistamines are drowsiness or dizziness, although young children, older adults, and patients with CNS dysfunction may exhibit signs of stimulation at therapeutic doses. The sedating effects of these drugs are additive with ethanol and other CNS depressants, and the potential for poisoning exists when an acute overdose of the antihistamine is taken with another depressant drug. Other side effects of antihistamines include blurred vision, tinnitus, and dry mouth.

Product selection in this category of drugs is relatively simple because of the limited number of available active ingredients. It is very important for the nurse to assess the cause of sleeplessness and the need for a sleeping aid. If mild pain is keeping someone awake, relief of the pain with aspirin or acetaminophen will often be sufficient to allow sleep to occur. If anxiety is the cause, antihistamine-induced drowsiness may be helpful, but it may also be no more effective than a glass of warm milk or a warm bath, although more expensive. Wise nursing counsel may be the most effective remedy for patients with mild insomnia.

Ophthalmic Products

OTC ophthalmic products are intended only for the symptomatic, short-term relief of mild self-limiting conditions such as eye fatigue, tearing, redness, or the itching and stinging associated with allergic or chemical conjunctivitis. The products are sold as eyewashes, artificial tears, and decongestants. Conditions involving marked eye pain or blurred vision require attention by a physician.

All OTC ophthalmic products must be clear, odorless, colorless, and sterile solutions with a pH and tonicity approximating that of natural tears. They must also contain preservatives to maintain sterility. Sterility cannot be maintained indefinitely, however, and bacterial contamination may be transferred to the eye. Thus cloudy or discolored solutions should be discarded.

OTC ophthalmic products contain a variety of nonmedicinal ingredients. Tonicity adjusters (e.g., dextran, glycerin) prevent excessive tearing that can dilute and wash away active ingredients. Antioxidants and stabilizers (sodium bisulfite, metabisulfite) prevent the chemical alteration of the ingredients. Buffers (e.g., boric acid) maintain the pH of the solution within a range of 6 to 8. Solutions of higher or lower pH may irritate the eyes. Wetting agents (polysorbate 80) reduce surface tension. Preservatives (e.g., benzalkonium chloride) prevent bacterial growth. Viscosity-increasing agents (gelatin, polyethylene glycol) spread the solution over the eye.

Decongestant ophthalmic products contain a sympathomimetic drug (ephedrine hydrochloride, naphazoline hydrochloride, phenylephrine hydrochloride, or tetrahydrozoline hydrochloride). Local application of one of these drugs to the eye promptly relieves the symptoms of allergic conjunctivitis. By constricting dilated blood vessels in the white of the eye, they also relieve the bloodshot look and restore the normal white color to the eyes. Sympathomimetic drugs also stimulate the adrenergic receptors affecting pupillary size and may cause dilation of pupils (mydriasis). For this reason these products should not be used by persons with narrow-angle glaucoma.

Problems may occur with decongestant ophthalmic products. Rebound congestion can occur by the same mechanism as described for topical nasal decongestants. It can be minimized or avoided by using the medicine only occasionally and strictly according to directions. In addition, these products will be ineffective if the cause of the symptoms is within the eyeball. The medicine may mask a bacterial infection.

Acne Medications

Acne vulgaris frequently afflicts adolescents. For them, prevention and treatment of even mild attacks of the disease, with its unsightly pimples and scars, are given high priority. The pimples and skin eruptions of acne are called *comedones.* They consist of a mixture of sebum, produced by the sebaceous glands of the hair follicles, and epithelial cells shed by the infundibulum of the follicle. Acne is associated with excessive production of sebum, which impairs the normal washout of infundibular cells as they are shed. The cells become compacted and plug the follicle, which then becomes distended with accumulated sebum and cells. The condition is relieved by removal of the plug by lancing the comedo or by the natural growth of the hair, which brings the plug to the surface. This form of acne, termed *noninflammatory,* is not usually associated with scarring. Scarring is more likely to occur with the inflammatory form of the disease, which is characterized by pustule formation and local inflammation. In the inflammatory form comedones do not open at the skin surface to relieve the pressure within the hair follicle. An inflamed follicle may rupture beneath the skin surface and spread sebum, cells, and bacteria to surrounding tissues. Whereas noninflammatory acne can be treated with OTC products, cases of inflammatory acne should be referred to a physician.

External factors may contribute to the development of acne. These factors include personal hygiene, diet, and self-image. Personal hygiene combats excessive skin oiliness, but compulsive and vigorous cleansing of the skin has not proved to be more effective in preventing acne than normal washing. Since bacterial infection is not ordinarily associated with acne, the use of antibacterial soaps and antiseptic solutions is neither necessary nor recommended.

The role of diet in acne is controversial. Chocolate has long been condemned as a causative factor, but there is no evidence of a cause-and-effect relationship between chocolate and acne. Similarly, evidence does not support the need for dietary restrictions of sweets, nuts, and greasy foods. Until a clearer understanding of acne and its cause emerges, individual trial and error with diet, hygiene, and other factors should neither be excluded nor discouraged.

Desquamating Agents

Noninflammatory acne is treated symptomatically. Treatment consists of removing excess sebum from the skin by washing and promoting the production and turnover of new skin to prevent closure of the pilosebaceous orifices of the hair follicle. The skin should be washed with warm water, mild soap, and a soft washcloth, no more than 3 times daily. The washing and rubbing produce some drying and peeling of the skin. Closure of the pilosebaceous orifices can be prevented by the topical application of mildly irritating agents, which promote desquamation (peeling) and stimulate growth of new skin cells.

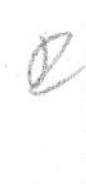

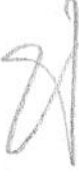

OTC desquamating agents include sulfur (2% to 10%), resorcinol (1% to 4%), and salicylic acid (0.5% to 2%). Resorcinol and salicylic acid often appear in alcoholic solutions that dry quickly and do not leave a visible film. Some products contain all three agents. Dosage forms of these drugs include creams, lotions, gels, and liquids. Ointment bases tend to be greasy and messy. Some soaps include desquamating agents, but this formulation is irrational because rinsing and drying remove the agents from the skin.

Benzoyl peroxide is a stronger irritant and desquamating agent than is sulfur, resorcinol, or salicylic acid. Used in concentrations of 5% to 10%, it generally produces mild stinging and warming of the skin. For most acne problems benzoyl peroxide is probably no more effective than the milder agents and should be used only after the milder irritants and faithful adherence to a regular skin-washing schedule have been unsuccessful. Benzoyl peroxide is highly irritating and should not contact the eyelids, neck, or lips. Its use should be discontinued if severe and prolonged stinging or irritation occurs.

More serious forms of acne require treatment with medications available only by prescription. Antibiotics may be used topically or orally in low doses. Isotretinoin may be effective in severe cases when the patient is unresponsive to other therapy.

Sunscreen Products

The sun emits principally two types of ultraviolet radiation, UVA and UVB. UVA radiation causes darkening, or tanning, of the skin. UVB radiation causes sunburn. Sunburn occurs when UVB radiation damages small blood vessels in the skin, causing them to become leaky and congested. Many people incorrectly consider sunburn a harmless, although painful, price to pay for a seasonal tan.

UVA radiation tans the skin by stimulating production of the dark pigment, *melanin.* The darkness of the tan depends on how much melanin is produced. People who do not tan easily do not produce enough melanin. Melanin absorbs UVA and UVB radiation and protects the skin from harmful effects of ultraviolet radiation. Naturally dark skin contains more melanin than pale skin and is correspondingly better protected.

The harmful effects of ultraviolet radiation can be serious, permanent, and potentially life threatening. These effects, including premature aging and wrinkling of the skin and skin cancer, occur after years of repeated exposure and may occur without significant episodes of sunburn. Sunscreens diminish the harmful consequences of ultraviolet radiation by absorbing or reflecting it. Used correctly, they prevent sunburn, premature aging of the skin, and reduce the risk of skin cancer. Chemical sunscreens selectively absorb and screen out most of the harmful burning radiation but permit tanning radiation to reach the skin. Physical sunscreens scatter and reflect all ultraviolet radiation. They prevent sunburn well, but they also prevent tanning.

Twenty-one chemical sunscreens have been approved by the FDA. Those most commonly available include aminobenzoic acid, cinoxate, homosalate, menthyl anthranilate, oxybenzone, and padimate O. Sunscreen products may contain one or several of these agents. Physical sunscreens include titanium oxide and zinc oxide in ointments and creams. They are intended for complete coverage of small areas of sunburn-prone skin such as the nose and lips.

Not all suntan products contain sunscreens. Some contain cosmetically appealing but otherwise inactive ingredients such as cocoa butter, mineral oil, and lanolin. None of these ingredients prevents sunburn or promotes tanning.

Some drugs, cosmetics, and soaps sensitize a person's skin to ultraviolet radiation and cause it to burn more easily than usual. Examples of such photosensitizing drugs include tetracycline antibiotics (see Chapter 42) and diuretics (see Chapter 14). Photosensitivity reactions are triggered by UVA radiation. Most sunscreens absorb little, if any, of this radiation and will not prevent it. Those that do block UVA radiation include menthyl anthranilate and oxybenzone.

The effectiveness of sunscreens is rated by the **sun protection factor (SPF)**, which is listed on the product label. The SPF relates the amount of time it takes a person to get a mild sunburn without sunscreen protection to the time required after a sunscreen has been applied to the exposed skin. For example, skin that ordinarily burns after 30 minutes of exposure to the sun will, if treated with a sunscreen with an SPF of 4, be able to stay in the sun for 2 hours (4 times as long) before it burns to the same degree. A sunscreen with an SPF of 8 protects 8 times as long (4 hours). Products with SPFs greater than 8 screen out tanning and burning radiation. Therefore persons who desire a tan should not use a sunscreen with an SPF higher than 8. Products with higher SPF values (some go as high as 50) screen out nearly all tanning and burning radiation. These products offer approximately equal protection from the radiation and differ only in the length of time that they allow a person to stay exposed to the sun. In some cases the higher SPF is of marginal value. For example, a sunscreen with an SPF of 15 would let someone who normally burns in 60 minutes stay in the sun for 15 hours. This would extend the time of protection into the night.

The choice of SPF depends on how easily a person burns or tans. The FDA recommends products with an SPF of 8 or more for people who always burn and never tan, 6 to 7 for people who always burn and minimally tan, 4 to 5 for people who burn moderately and tan gradually, 2 to 3 for people who burn minimally and always tan well, and 2 for people who rarely burn and tan profusely.

Sunscreens should be applied at least 30 minutes before each exposure to the sun to allow the chemicals time to penetrate the skin. Some products, such as aminobenzoic acid, should be applied 1 to 2 hours before exposure. No sunscreen or suntan product will promote a deeper tan than a person's skin can naturally produce. If skin does not readily produce melanin, it will never tan as well as skin that readily produces the pigment.

Topical Antiinfective Drugs

Serious infections of the skin require systemic antiinfective agents that are available by prescription. In certain situations more minor infections of the skin may respond to topical application of agents directly at the site of infection. Drugs used in this way tend to be too toxic for systemic use, but in the low doses used topically they are safe enough to be available without a prescription.

Antifungal Products

Several common tineal (fungal) infections of the skin generally respond to self-medication with OTC products, although responsiveness depends on the strain of fungus, the site of infection, and the severity and duration of the infection. Microorganisms most often responsible for superficial tineal infections in humans are *Trichophyton, Microsporum, Epidermophyton,* and *Candida* species. OTC products are effective only for acute superficial infections. Chronic and extensive infections respond slowly if at all and often require the attention of a physician. Fungal infections of the toenails or fingernails and those that have penetrated the hair shafts generally respond poorly to OTC antifungal products. The nurse should exercise care in selecting or recommending OTC antifungal medications. If the condition involves an apparent tineal infection of the foot (athlete's foot), groin, or scalp, reasonably rapid results can be expected from OTC products. Patients with suspected fungal infections of other body regions should be referred to a physician.

OTC antifungal preparations include keratolytic agents, fungistatic agents, and fungicides. Keratolytic preparations include selenium sulfide and Whitfield's ointment (containing benzoic acid [6%] and salicylic acid [3%]). These agents irritate the skin and cause peeling of the superficial layers to expose deeper sites of infection to other antifungal compounds. Selenium sulfide stops cellular growth when it is applied in concentrations of 1% to 2%. It is a common and effective ingredient in antidandruff preparations.

Fungistatic agents include fatty acids and salicylanilide. Sodium propionate and undecylenic acid are fungistatic fatty acids. Sodium propionate is effective in 1% solution and 5% ointment. Undecylenate is effective as the acid (5%) and as the zinc salt (20%). It is commonly used as an ointment, powder, or spray for the relief of athlete's foot.

The fungicidal drug tolnaftate is effective against the majority of superficial fungal infections except *Candida* species. Tolnaftate is sold as powder, liquid, cream, spray, or gel (all 1%). Relief of itching occurs within several days, but complete suppression of the infection generally requires 2 to 3 weeks of treatment. If the skin is rough and scaly, prior treatment with a keratolytic agent to remove the scale improves the effectiveness of tolnaftate.

Antibacterial Products

The antibiotic drugs available without a prescription include bacitracin, neomycin sulfate, polymyxin B sulfate, tetracycline hydrochloride, chlortetracycline hydrochloride, and oxytetracycline hydrochloride. The FDA OTC Panel on Antimicrobial Drugs recognizes skin-wound antibiotics and skin-wound protectants. The former includes products for the treatment of overt skin infections; the latter refers to products with antibiotics added to prevent the subsequent infection of a wound and the growth of organisms in the product. All OTC antibiotics sold as skin-wound antibiotics were classified in category III. All but neomycin sulfate were classified in category I for use as skin-wound protectants.

When used as directed, the OTC topical antibiotics are generally safe. However, their low concentration in the available products makes their effectiveness against skin-wound infections questionable. Bacitracin, neomycin sulfate, and polymyxin B sulfate are nephrotoxic if absorbed systemically. With ordinary topical use such toxicity is rare. In view of the questionable topical efficacy of the drugs and their potential toxicity, their use is not recommended.

Hemorrhoidal Products

Environment, heredity, and posture have contributed to the incidence of a number of painful anorectal disorders, the most prevalent of which is hemorrhoids. Hemorrhoids are varicosities produced by increased pressure in the hemorrhoidal veins. Upright posture, hypertension, coughing, pregnancy and labor, physical exertion, straining during defecation, and rectal carcinoma can contribute to hemorrhoids. These varicosities, which can occur within or outside the anorectal line, are associated with itching, burning, inflammation, and swelling. Mild pain and discomfort are common; however, bleeding, prolapse of an internal hemorrhoid, and severe chronic pain require the attention of a physician.

OTC products for the treatment of anorectal disorders are intended for the symptomatic relief of pain, itching, and burning. They contain a variety of pharmacologic agents, including local anesthetics, vasoconstrictors, antiseptics, astringents, emollients or lubricants, keratolytics, anticholinergics, and a variety of miscellaneous agents such as counterirritants and wound-healing agents.

The FDA OTC Panel on Hemorrhoidal Drug Products has ruled on the efficacy of these agents. Antiseptics, wound healers, and anticholinergics all have been classified as category II hemorrhoidal products. Local anesthetics have been judged effective for relief of the itching and burning of hemorrhoids. Of the many local anesthetics available, only two are safe and effective: benzocaine (5% to 20%) and pramoxine hydrochloride (1%). Ephedrine sulfate, epinephrine hydrochloride, and phenylephrine hydrochloride are vasoconstrictor drugs that have been judged effective for the symptomatic relief of hemorrhoidal itching and swelling, although conclusive evidence of effectiveness on swollen hemorrhoidal tissue itself is lacking. Presumably, the vasoconstrictor drugs directly constrict the vascular smooth muscle in the anorectal area.

A variety of emollients or lubricants (protectants) have been recommended for use in hemorrhoidal preparations. These include calamine, cocoa butter, cod liver oil, glycerin, mineral oil, petrolatum, shark liver oil, and zinc oxide. All can be administered to the rectum externally and internally except glycerin, which is intended for external use only. Petrolatum may be the most effective of these agents. To be effective, the total protectant concentration of an OTC hemorrhoidal product should be 50%.

Mildly keratolytic agents such as aluminum chlorhydroxy allantoinate relieve the itching and burning of hemorrhoids. Their usefulness is confined to the external anal tissues. Stronger agents, such as resorcinol and sulfur, are not recommended.

Astringents coagulate skin cell protein, thereby protecting underlying skin cells from dehydration and irritation. Calamine, zinc oxide, and hamamelis water (witch hazel) have been judged effective for the relief of hemorrhoidal itching, irritation, and pain. Calamine and zinc oxide may be applied externally and internally to anorectal tissue, whereas hamamelis water is intended for external use only. Antiseptics are no more effective than washing with soap and water for the prevention of anorectal infections. Antiseptics may adversely alter the normal bacterial flora in that region.

Anticholinergic drugs (e.g., atropine; see Chapter 11) are of dubious value in OTC hemorrhoidal preparations. These drugs are not absorbed through the skin and, if applied to the external anal tissues, do not relieve itching or pain. They can be absorbed across the rectal mucosa, however, and in sufficient dosage can interfere with autonomic nerve function throughout the body. There is no evidence that a local or systemic anticholinergic effect is of any value in treating hemorrhoids.

A counterirritant drug distracts from the discomfort of itching, irritation, and pain by stimulating local nerve endings to provide a sensation of warmth, tingling, or coolness. Counterirritation forms the therapeutic basis for the relief of minor muscle aches and pain by OTC remedies that provide deep-heating and penetrating warmth. These remedies do not directly affect muscles. Instead, their effects are localized to the skin, where they stimulate local sensory nerve endings. However, since no sensory nerves occur in the rectal mucosa, there is no rational basis for including a counterirritant in an internal hemorrhoidal preparation. A counterirritant may provide temporary relief of pain and itching if applied externally to the anorectal region. Menthol is the only recommended counterirritant for external hemorrhoidal preparations.

Wound-healing agents include an extract of brewer's yeast, skin respiratory factor (SRF), cod liver oil, and vitamins A and D. No convincing evidence of their effectiveness as wound healers has been found; until such evidence emerges, their value in the treatment of hemorrhoids is questionable.

OTC products for the treatment of hemorrhoids and other mild anorectal disorders are provided in a variety of dosage forms including ointments, creams, suppositories, pads, and foams. Ointments (oil base), creams (water soluble), and gels are equally effective in delivering active ingredients to the affected areas. Devices such as the *pile pipe,* a tube having lateral exit ports, are useful for applying the medication directly into the rectum. Suppositories are not particularly useful for the treatment of hemorrhoids. They may slip beyond the affected site, releasing their active ingredients in contact with healthy mucosa. In addition, with suppositories the degree of coverage of the affected area may be erratic and cannot be controlled. Finally, because suppositories must melt to release their active ingredients, relief of painful symptoms is delayed. Foams provide no advantages over ointments and creams; moreover, they are messy.

Personal hygiene and normal bowel habits are important in the successful treatment of hemorrhoids. Many physicians recommend taking sitz baths or soaking with astringent solutions as an adjunct to the use of OTC products for the relief of mild itching and burning sensations. In addition, the diet should be adjusted to avoid either excessively loose or compact stools.

NURSING PROCESS OVERVIEW

Over-the-Counter Drugs

OTC, or nonprescription, drugs do not form a major part of the clinical responsibilities of the practicing nurse. Nevertheless, the nurse is frequently sought as a source of information on these agents. The following presentation is one suggestion for a method of patient counseling about nonprescription medications.

Assessment

Since the patient is involved in self-care, assist the individual to clearly state what condition or symptoms are to be treated. For example, if the individual is seeking a medication to treat the symptoms of a cold, lead the person to consider exactly what symptoms require treatment. For some persons a cough might be the most outstanding symptom, whereas for others it might be nasal congestion or headache.

Nursing Diagnoses

- Knowledge deficit related to not knowing how to self-medicate for minor health problems

Patient Outcomes

The patient will have symptomatic relief of the problem being treated, with no side effects.

Planning/Implementation

After leading the patient to define exactly what symptoms are to be treated, teach the patient what types of medications are available to treat these symptoms. Suggest that fixed combinations of ingredients are more difficult to use because dosages are impossible to regulate for each component of the combination. More control may be gained by using single agents at appropriate doses as necessary for defined symptoms. Suggest other sources of information about nonprescription drugs, such as the pharmacist.

Evaluation

Effectiveness of the treatment is evaluated by the patient involved in self-care. If the patient seeks advice because therapy is unsuccessful, have the patient consider whether the proper medication was administered for the symptom to be controlled and if the right dose was used.

NURSING IMPLICATIONS SUMMARY

General Guidelines: OTC Drugs

- If asked about OTC remedies, first assess the patient. What symptoms or problems require treatment? What has the patient used successfully in the past?
- Remember that many patients do not consider drugs purchased without a prescription as true drugs; that is, if questioned about medications they are taking, they may not think to include OTC preparations.
- As a part of assessment, ask specifically about medicine purchased at the drugstore or health food store. It may be helpful to include some leading questions such as: "Do you take any cold medicines, cough syrups, vitamins, or other medicines that you can buy without a prescription?" It may also help to know of local health problems or habits. For example, in an area where there are frequent high pollen counts, causing frequent allergy problems, ask questions about allergies and what the patient uses to relieve allergy symptoms.
- In asking how a patient uses OTC drugs, try to frame questions in a nonjudgmental way to learn about actual use patterns. Most patients want to use medications correctly and will welcome instruction about drug use but not if they feel defensive about their current practices.

Patient and Family Education

- Point out to the patient that many OTC preparations contain multiple drugs. Encourage the patient to consider purchasing products that contain only the drug needed. This may be difficult since the ingredients for a product may be listed in generic names, which are not usually familiar to the patient.
- Ideally, the nurse would accompany the patient to the drugstore and review product labeling during the instruction. In the absence of this possibility, suggest that the patient talk over the medication needs with the pharmacist. In addition, the pharmacist can help the patient choose the least expensive but most effective product available at that store.
- Talking about OTC drug use may provide the ideal opportunity to review general safe practices regarding drug use (see box on p. 40).
- Suggest that the patient periodically look over all the medications in the house and discard those that look discolored or crumbled or that have passed the expiration date. Emphasize to patients the need to discard medications in a way that children or animals cannot find them and take them. Small amounts of liquids can be poured down the sink or toilet, and a few remaining tablets or capsules can be flushed also. If there is a large quantity of medication, consider checking with a local pharmacy or poison control center for guidance about proper disposal.
- Encourage patients who are not obtaining relief from appropriate OTC medications to seek medical care for the problem.

CRITICAL THINKING

APPLICATION

1. The present laws that regulate the OTC drug industry have evolved from which law?
2. What classes of drugs did the Durham-Humphrey Amendment to the 1938 law create?
3. What does the Kefauver-Harris amendment to the 1938 law require?
4. What are the categories used by FDA review panels on OTC drugs to classify drugs?
5. List the advantages and disadvantages of fixed-ratio combination drug products.
6. Which analgesics are available without a prescription?
7. Name the ingredients of OTC cold remedies.
8. What are the major side effects of antihistaminic drugs?
9. List the OTC expectorant drugs.
10. Name the available OTC cough suppressants.
11. Which drugs are used in OTC products for weight control and treating obesity?
12. Phenylpropanolamine is related to which drugs? What are its side effects?
13. What is the rationale for the use of a bulk-producing agent in a weight-control product? How might you counsel patients about these?
14. What drugs are available in OTC sleeping aids?
15. List the classes of ingredients in OTC ophthalmic products.
16. What precautions should be exercised in the use of OTC ophthalmic products? How might you teach patients about these precautions?
17. List the commonly available OTC drugs for treatment of acne.
18. Distinguish between chemical and physical sunscreens.
19. Define sun protection factor (SPF).
20. OTC antifungal products include which drugs?
21. Distinguish between keratolytic, fungistatic, and fungicidal drugs.
22. Which antibiotics are currently available in OTC preparations?
23. List the ingredients of OTC hemorrhoidal products and describe their actions.

CRITICAL THINKING

1. A friend twists her ankle playing tennis, and asks you what medication she should take for pain. What factors should you consider in advising her?
2. What factors should you consider in choosing a cold remedy?
3. You have a cold and bad cough. What factors should you consider in buying a cold remedy and cough suppressant?
4. What nonmedicinal measures should you teach patients who wish to control their weight?
5. How would you assess the side effects of phenylpropanolamine?
6. You become aware that your neighbor's teenage daughter may be abusing OTC weight-control products in an effort to lose weight. What should you do?
7. Give some examples of situations in which an analgesic should be used at bedtime.
8. Your roommate is distressed by her acne. She is willing to let you advise her. Develop a plan to treat her acne.
9. In addition to applying sunscreen, what other measures can be used to limit skin exposure to the sun?
10. Develop a plan of care that includes nonmedication measures to treat hemorrhoids in a pregnant woman.

CHAPTER 8

Issues of Drug Abuse

Eleanor J. Sullivan
Sandra M. Handley

OBJECTIVES

After studying this chapter, you should be able to do the following:

- *Define drug use, misuse, abuse, and dependence.*
- *Identify the characteristics of an individual that may increase the risk of drug abuse.*
- *Identify the characteristics of drugs that may increase the potential for drug abuse.*
- *Recognize why certain drugs are attractive to specific individuals.*
- *Describe current drug abuse treatment modalities.*
- *Describe medications that are used in withdrawal and treatment.*
- *Apply the nursing process to care of patients who abuse drugs.*

KEY TERMS

drug abuse
drug dependence
tolerance
withdrawal

CHAPTER OVERVIEW

This chapter defines drug use, misuse, abuse, and dependence. Drug abuse is described in terms of risk factors for the individual and the abuse potential of specific drugs. The most frequently used drugs are discussed, including prescription drugs and alcohol. Current concepts of treatment and medications used in treatment and withdrawal are described.

OVERVIEW OF DRUG ABUSE

This chapter focuses on substances that are commonly used and abused, including legal drugs, such as prescription medications, alcohol, and tobacco, and illegal or illicit drugs, such as marijuana and cocaine. All drugs have the potential for abuse.

Nurses encounter patients with a variety of conditions. Often the physical or mental condition is related, directly or indirectly, to drug abuse. It is important that nurses routinely assess drug use/abuse in an initial workup and continue to consider its possibility throughout their care of the client. When drug abuse is part of the health care problem and is not addressed, care is incomplete, increasing the likelihood of recurrence. Underlying drug abuse may be a factor in as many as 40% of hospital admissions.

Current Definitions: Drug Abuse and Drug Dependence

Differentiating between drug misuse, abuse, and dependence is not simple. It is based on patterns of use, such as amount and frequency. Defining these terms is complicated by legal definitions. By legal definition, any use of an illicit or illegal drug is considered abuse. In health care the effects of drugs on the body and on the behavior of the individual is the concern.

Drug use occurs on a continuum from experimentation, infrequent use, regular use, abuse with resulting health and social problems, and dependence characterized by loss of control. Both drug abuse and drug dependence are diagnostic terms defined by the American Psychiatric Association's Diagnostic and Statistical Manual (DSM). The current version, DSM-IV, identifies the abused drug of choice as part of the diagnosis.

Drug abuse occurs when the individual's drug use becomes problematic, causing social and personal difficulties that stem from the drug use.

Diagnostic criteria for drug abuse is evaluated during a 12-month period. The patient's impairment must involve one or more of the following: (1) failure to fulfill major role obligations at work, school, or home; (2) use in physically hazardous situations; (3) recurrent substance-related legal problems; or (4) use despite persistent or recurrent social or interpersonal problems as a result of use.

Drug dependence is diagnosed when physiologic effects appear and/or when loss of control over the drug and its use becomes increasingly apparent.

Diagnostic criteria for drug dependence include the presence of at least three of the following factors within a 12-month period: (1) tolerance; (2) withdrawal; (3) substance taken in larger amount or longer period than intended; (4) persistent, unsuccessful efforts to cut down; (5) an increased amount of time spent procuring, using, or recovering from the effects of the substance; (6) other previously important activities are avoided or reduced because of substance use; and/or (7) continued use despite knowledge of a problem.

Use and abuse are complicated by legal issues. Some drugs are legal, whereas others are illegal. Both legal and illegal drugs can be used to meet the criteria for abuse or dependence. Some drugs such as tobacco and alcohol are legal for persons who meet certain criteria, such as age. Legality is not a diagnosis, but legal difficulties are one criterion for a diagnosis. In addition, legal problems can be an external condition that encourages the individual to recognize the problem and seek treatment. For example, legal difficulties such as repeatedly driving under the influence of drugs, particularly alcohol, can result in a drunk-driving charge, and the individual may be given a choice between incarceration or treatment. A charge of possession of an illegal drug also can result in individuals recognizing how out of control their use is.

Risk Factors for Drug Abuse

Not everyone who experiments with a drug develops personal and social complications or loses control of drug use. Why this happens to some individuals and not to others is a question that is not fully understood and the topic of much research. When this question is better answered, both prevention and treatment of drug abuse will benefit.

Although no one knows exactly who will develop a drug abuse problem, some characteristics of those who are at higher risk for abuse have been identified. Individual risk factors for drug abuse can be categorized as genetic, environmental, or a combination of the two.

Genetic Risk Factors

Research has identified that one risk factor for drug abuse is a family history of abuse, particularly by a mother, father, or sibling. The genetic component of alcohol abuse in particular has been well documented with twin and adoption studies. For instance, either twin with alcoholism in the biologic family background is more likely to become alcohol dependent when adopted into a nondrinking environment than either twin with no alcoholism in the biologic family background adopted into a drinking environment. Genetic risk is greater than environmental risk.

Environmental Risk Factors

The family environment is a major risk factor for drug abuse. A child who grows up with a drug-abusing parent receives both role modeling and interpersonal experiences that may promote eventual drug abuse either during adolescence or adulthood. Family relationships are distorted to accommodate the drug-abusing parent.

Coping skills are another modifier of risk. These skills reflect how an individual adapts his or her behavior in response to demands. Ineffective coping, or coping strategies overwhelmed by stress, are a major risk factor for drug abuse. Drugs are often used as a temporary measure to decrease the psychologic discomfort caused by high stress or poor coping strategies. This situation is promoted in our society by advertising that features alcohol and nicotine as a means of coping with stress. Individuals who model this behavior put themselves at risk for abuse by managing stress indirectly through drugs rather than directly through constructive action to decrease stress and cope.

Personal crises are a risk factor. Coping skills are tested during situational or maturational crises. Situational crises are those that result from specific stressors such as job loss, divorce, or death. Maturational crises are a result of reaching new development stages such as adolescence or young adulthood. These situational crises increase the risk for drug use and abuse when used to decrease the pressure, stress, or emotional pain. Sometimes the health care system facilitates abuse. For example, stress may produce physiologic symptoms for which a health care provider prescribes a minor tranquilizer. This type of drug is subject to abuse when used over an extended time in place of learning new and more effective coping strategies.

Ready access to drugs is another risk factor. Drug abuse by health care professionals is a source of professional and societal concern. Licensed health care professions have become increasingly active in identifying and addressing substance abuse among their members in recent years. For nurses, in particular, some of the risk factors for substance abuse include a family history of substance abuse, a history of health problems, and a history of depression. The availability of drugs and a professional culture in which a drug is offered for every problem encourage nurses to self-medicate, thereby increasing their risk of abuse. Nurses recovering from drug dependence often say that their use began with prescription pain medications for an injury and progressed to abuse and dependence. Many professional organizations now sponsor peer assistance organizations that help to identify substance abuse and resources for treatment and monitor the professional on return to employment.

GENERAL CHARACTERISTICS OF ABUSED DRUGS

Drugs that produce a pleasurable effect, such as an elevated mood, euphoria, or a calming effect are most likely to be abused. Drugs that do not produce a mood-altering effect are rarely intentionally abused. One exception is anabolic steroids, which are abused because of their muscle-building effects.

The National Institute of Drug Abuse sponsors the National Household Survey of Drug Use, which contacts randomly selected households in the United States to provide comprehensive information on current drug use in the United States. The data in Table 8-1 describe drug use during the month before the 1990 survey. The table graphically indicates that the most widely used drugs in 1990 were alcohol and nicotine and the most widely used illegal drug was marijuana. Six percent of the subjects claimed illicit use of a drug in the previous month, and a little over 1% stated that they had used psychotherapeutic drugs in a nonmedical manner in the previous month. The survey did not include caffeine.

TABLE 8-1 Drug Use in United States in Month Preceding National Household Survey of Drug Use, 1990

DRUG USE	ALL AGES (%)
Any illicit use	6.4
Nonmedical use of any psychotherapeutic	1.4
Alcohol	51.2
Total nicotine	30.2
Cigarettes	26.7
Smokeless tobacco	3.5
Marijuana/hashish (1)	5.1
Total cocaine (1)	1
Cocaine (1)	0.8
Crack cocaine (1)	0.2
Analgesics (1, 2)	0.8
Inhalants (1)	0.6
Stimulants (1, 2)	0.5
Tranquilizers (1, 2)	0.5
Hallucinogens (1)	0.3
Sedatives (1, 2)	0.3
Phencyclidine (PCP) (1)	0.2
Heroin (ever used) (1)	0.8
Needle use in last year	0.4

Data from the National Institute of Drug Abuse: National household survey of drug use, DHHS Pub No 91-1732, Washington, 1991.
1, Any illicit use; *2*, Nonmedical use of any psychotherapeutic.

Route of Administration

In general, the more rapidly a route delivers the substance to the brain, the greater the effect and the higher the addictive potential of the drug. For example, cocaine powder is usually taken intranasally (snorted), and crack cocaine is smoked. Although the nasal mucosa is highly vascular and snorting allows rapid blood-brain transfer, inhalation is a faster route. This shorter time appears to be a factor in the highly addictive nature of nicotine in cigarettes.

The route of administration may be of particular concern in its own right. One example is intravenous (IV) drug use with its danger of spreading infection, particularly HIV/AIDS, when IV materials are shared. IV use also exposes the individual to cellulitis and scarred or sclerosed veins. Ingestion of alcohol often causes damage to the gastrointestinal tract. The intranasal use of cocaine can cause deterioration of the nasal septum. These pathologic signs provide external clues to drug use.

Tolerance

Tolerance concerns the effect of the drug on the body over time. Tolerance has occurred when it takes increasing amounts of the drug to achieve the same physiologic or psychologic effect. Although tolerance is particularly characteristic of opiates, prolonged use of alcohol, barbiturates, and benzodiazepines also leads to tolerance.

Cross-tolerance describes a physiologic characteristic in which developing a tolerance to one drug also increases the tolerance to a related category of drugs. Tolerance to alcohol, a central nervous system (CNS) depressant, results in cross-tolerance to other CNS depressants such as benzodiazepines and many anesthetic agents. The tolerant individual may require a higher dose of anesthesia to achieve the desired level of surgical anesthesia. This is one reason why it is important to have a thorough drug history before any care is given.

Withdrawal

Drugs that produce tolerance, a physiologic change caused by the presence of the drug, also produce symptoms when the drug is withdrawn, particularly when withdrawn abruptly. **Withdrawal** symptoms are characteristic of the drug class and are often the opposite of the drug's action. Alcohol, a CNS depressant, produces withdrawal symptoms characterized by hyperactivity. Conversely, when cocaine, a CNS stimulant is withdrawn, one of the effects is depression and a loss of feeling and pleasure. These withdrawal effects are neurologic rebound effects; since the neurons have adjusted their neurotransmitters to the presence of the drug, when the drug is withdrawn, the body overproduces neurotransmitters or lacks the balancing effect of the drug. The withdrawal symptoms characteristic of alcohol, benzodiazepines, and barbiturates are the most dangerous and require careful monitoring. Individuals vary greatly in their potential for and range of withdrawal symptoms.

Dependence

Physical dependence follows tolerance when the lack of the drug produces withdrawal symptoms. Physiologic dependence was at one time considered the essential factor in drug dependence; however, recent DSM criteria recognize both physical and psychologic characteristics in a diagnosis of drug dependence.

Psychologic dependence describes the psychologic need to continue drug use. Psychologic tolerance is the individual's psychologic attachment to the drug, including the behaviors surrounding acquiring and using the drug and the feeling state accompanying use. This complex set of feelings and behaviors is reinforced through use and experience with the drug, and these behaviors make giving up drug use more difficult. Psychologic dependence is often related to the use of the drug to reduce stress, which eventually becomes the only means of stress reduction. As an understanding of neurophysiology and neurotransmitters increases, the boundary between physical and psychologic dependence blurs.

CHARACTERISTICS OF SPECIFIC DRUGS

The major characteristics of commonly abused drugs are summarized in Table 8-2.

Caffeine

Caffeine may be the most widely abused drug in the United States, although the effects of this abuse are much less obvious and are usually less harmful than those produced by other abused drugs. Caffeine abuse often takes place unwittingly. Consider the following example:

> John has a cup of coffee while dressing in the morning and a second cup at breakfast. At work he consumes another cup of coffee at the 10:30 AM coffee break. At lunch John drinks two glasses of iced tea. On afternoon coffee break he has a chocolate bar and a cola. Before he leaves work, John takes two Excedrin for a headache. At dinner he drinks two cups of tea. Before bed John takes two more Excedrin.

Why is John unable to sleep? John cannot sleep because he ingested about 1 gm of caffeine during this typical day.

TABLE 8-2 Major Characteristics of Commonly Abused Drugs

DRUG	PRIMARY ROUTE(S)	DEPENDENCY		DESIRED EFFECT	WITHDRAWAL EFFECT	TREATMENT
		PHYSIOLOGIC	PSYCHOLOGIC			
Caffeine	Ingestion	Yes	Yes	Mild stimulation	Headaches	None
Alcohol	Ingestion	Yes	Yes	Euphoria	Tremors	Benzodiazepines
Nicotine	Inhalation, buccal	Yes	Yes	Relaxation	Irritability	None
Marijuana, hashish	Inhalation, ingestion	No	Yes	Relaxation	None	None
Opioids	Injection, ingestion	Yes	Yes	Euphoria	Yes	Methadone
Inhalants	Inhalation	No?	No?	Euphoria	None	None
Cocaine	Inhalation, smoking	No?	Yes	Euphoria	Depression	None
Amphetamines	Ingestion, injection	No	Yes	Euphoria	Depression	Tapering dose
Hallucinogens	Ingestion, smoking	No	No	Distorted perception	None	None
Phencyclidine (PCP)	Smoking, ingestion	No	No	Euphoria	None	None
Benzodiazepines	Ingestion, injection	Yes	Yes	Relaxation	Tremors, seizure	Tapering dose
Barbiturates	Ingestion, injection	Yes	Yes	Euphoria, relaxation	Yes	Phenobarbital

Most people are aware of the caffeine content of coffee, which ranges from 80 to 150 mg per cup. Less well known is the fact that tea, colas, chocolate, and some nonprescription medications (e.g., Excedrin) also contain caffeine. In the example given John took more than ½ gm of caffeine in these forms.

Ingestion of more than 500 mg (½ gm) of caffeine daily produces a variety of CNS effects and cardiovascular reactions. Irritability or nervousness is a common complaint, along with sleep disturbances. Patients may report heart palpitations or say that their heart is "racing." These descriptions may suggest premature ventricular contractions and tachycardia, common symptoms of chronic caffeine toxicity. Diarrhea and GI irritation frequently accompany chronic overdosage with caffeine. Patients complaining of symptoms such as these should be questioned about their caffeine intake. The person taking the history should ask specifically about individual beverages, foods, and medications that contain caffeine to make an accurate estimate of intake. The caffeine content of commonly ingested substances is presented in Table 8-3.

Whether true psychologic dependence on caffeine can occur is questionable, but many people have great difficulty in eliminating caffeine from their diet. Nevertheless, patients with peptic ulcer disease should avoid caffeine. Pregnant women may wish to avoid caffeine because it freely passes to the fetus. Any person who ingests more than 200 mg of caffeine daily should be encouraged to reduce his or her caffeine intake to avoid the subtle onset of chronic toxicity.

TABLE 8-3 Caffeine Content of Commonly Ingested Substances

SUBSTANCE	CAFFEINE CONTENT
Foods and Beverages	
Coffee	
Brewed	80-150 mg/5 oz cup
Instant	85-100 mg/5 oz cup
Decaffeinated	2-4 mg/5 oz cup
Tea, brewed	30-75 mg/5 oz cup
Cocoa	5-40 mg/5 oz cup
Cola soft drinks*	35-60 mg/12 oz bottle or can
Nonprescription Medications	
Analgesics (Anacin and Vanquish)	32 mg/tablet
Excedrin	65 mg/tablet
Cold Medications	
Dristan AF	16.2 mg/tablet
Korigesic	30 mg/tablet
Stimulants	
Nodoz	100 mg/tablet
Vivarin	200 mg/tablet

*Many soft drinks other than colas contain caffeine as an additive. The label reveals the presence of caffeine but not the amount.

Alcohol

Alcohol is a CNS depressant. It is widely available, relatively inexpensive, and comes in a variety of forms, such as beer, wine, wine coolers, and distilled spirits. In the United States alcohol is commonly served in social settings, where it is thought to promote conviviality. Heavy drinking over time can produce psychologic dependence, particularly in those genetically predisposed. Physical damage most commonly appears in the liver and brain. The alcohol withdrawal syndrome can be serious, characterized by tremors, changes in level of consciousness, with progression to seizures and delirium tremens, which are life-threatening conditions. These withdrawal symptoms are treated with a decreasing dose of benzodiazepines, most often chlordiazepoxide (Librium) or diazepam (Valium). The patient must be carefully observed, and supportive therapy must be given as necessary for respiratory, cardiovascular, and seizure complications. Alcohol use and abuse are discussed in detail in Chapter 51.

Nicotine

Nicotine is both a stimulant and a depressant. It may be the drug with the highest addiction potential; that is, there is a high risk that someone who begins to use a nicotine product will progress to becoming physically dependent on this drug. The initial effect of nicotine is physical stimulation, but this stage is then replaced by a relaxation effect. Nicotine is commonly used by smoking, although smokeless tobacco products, such as chewing tobacco, are also widely used.

Since nicotine produces tolerance, the user must keep increasing the amount of drug used to derive the same effect. Nicotine produces physiologic and psychologic dependence. Once dependent, an individual finds it extremely difficult to abstain. Withdrawal symptoms include craving, restlessness, decreased concentration, and hyperirritability. Nicotine has only recently come to be seen as a drug, which represents a change in thinking about tobacco and both its abuse potential and social acceptability. Nicotine use contributes to a variety of serious health problems, including lung cancer, hypertension, and cardiovascular disease.

Marijuana

Marijuana and its stronger version hashish are not easily classified. Both are derived from the marijuana plant, but hashish is more concentrated. The active ingredient is tetrahydrocannabinol, also known as THC. Marijuana is usually consumed by inhalation or ingestion. The primary effect is relaxation and a sense of well-being accompanied by a distortion in one's sense of time. Tolerance for some of the physiologic effects can develop over time, and physical dependence has been demonstrated in animals at high dosages. Physical dependence in humans has not been clearly demonstrated. Marijuana may produce a psychologic dependence that is manifested by daily usage. Long-term use can produce an amotivational syndrome characterized by apathy and loss of motivation. Marijuana is stored in the fat cells of the body and released gradually; therefore in heavy smokers such syndromes may be related to the presence and continuous slow release of the drug in the body. There are no known withdrawal symptoms.

Cocaine

Cocaine is a stimulant drug. It is available in a white powder that is used intranasally (snorted) or in a less expensive solid form, crack cocaine, that can be smoked or injected intravenously. Either form produces an intense, short-lived euphoric high. Physical dependence on cocaine is unclear. However, with high doses of crack cocaine, withdrawal is characterized by an initial dysphoric reaction followed by depression, craving, prolonged sleep, and anhedonia (the inability to experience pleasure).

Amphetamines

Amphetamines are stimulants often taken initially to increase alertness or to stay awake. Continued use can progress from pills to IV use, which is more potent and dangerous. Amphetamine users often switch to a depressant drug to "come down" from the stimulant effects of the amphetamines and to get needed rest. These dramatic, drug-controlled physiologic changes frequently cause the individual to become exhausted and physically debilitated. Such polydrug use can also lead to dependency on both types of drugs. Prolonged amphetamine use produces a physiologic withdrawal characterized by depression. Amphetamines are described in Chapter 54.

Inhalants

Inhalants are substances such as airplane glue, gasoline, and cleaning products with vapors that produce a "high." Inhalation produces rapid neurologic effects, and many of the inhalants are neurotoxic. In addition, inhalation allows little dose control. The substance is often kept in a plastic bag that is then placed over the face and the vapors inhaled, which creates a real potential for asphyxiation. Inhalant use is most common in children and adolescents. However, health care professionals such as dentists and anesthesia personnel may abuse nitrous oxide.

Hallucinogens

Hallucinogens alter perceptions and thought processes. Most hallucinogens are smoked or ingested. LSD (D-lysergic acid diethylamide) is a hallucinogen that was popular in the 1960s and is becoming available again. Other hallucinogens include mescaline (peyote) and psilocybin, which are derived from mushrooms, and synthetic drugs such as MDA (3,4 methylenedioxy amphetamine) and MDMA (3,4 methylenedioxy methamphetamine), which are amphetamine derivatives with hallucinogenic properties. Although physical and psychologic dependence are not characteristic of hallucinogens, behavior is unpredictable and may put the individual in danger.

PCP (phencyclidine) is an anesthetic agent that is used and abused for its hallucinogenic properties. It is smoked sometimes in conjunction with marijuana cigarettes. Individuals who use PCP may experience altered sensation and decreased sensitivity to pain and may exhibit violent behavior.

Opioids

Opioids include drugs derived from the opium poppy and their synthetic derivatives. Many opioids are excellent analgesics (see Chapter 32). Heroin is an opioid available in a fine white powder that can be dissolved and administered intravenously or subcutaneously (skin popping). The drug produces a euphoric response. Unlike other opioids, heroin is illegal in the United States. Its addiction potential is very high with regular use because the individual rapidly develops increasing tolerance to the drug and must use more to achieve the same effect. Both physical and psychologic dependence develop as the individual becomes dependent not only on the drug but on the whole lifestyle that goes with use of the drug. There is a predictable set of withdrawal symptoms that occurs with heroin and other opioids. The individual experiences rhinitis, nausea, and diarrhea, then muscle cramps, twitching and tremors. This syndrome lasts 3 to 5 days but may last longer. Although the withdrawal syndrome is very uncomfortable, it is not physiologically dangerous.

COMMONLY ABUSED PRESCRIPTION DRUGS

Prescription drugs are legally available only by prescription from a licensed health care provider. Patients often believe that any drug prescribed by a health care practitioner is unquestioningly safe. These patients are not aware of the addictive potential of some drugs. If they have a problem with use, they may not discuss it with their health care provider. Patients may not take the medication appropriately, using too much, taking it too often, or taking it at inappropriate times. Providers may not collect enough information about the other drugs the patient is using or past experiences with drugs. Special problems include adding new medications to treat the side effects of other drugs, lacking knowledge of usual side effects, and multiple caregivers prescribing drugs in isolation.

Drugs that produce physical or psychologic addiction are extensively regulated in the United States and Canada, as described in Chapter 3. Three categories of controlled prescription drugs were included in the Household Survey: opioids (see preceding discussion), benzodiazepines, and barbiturates.

Benzodiazepines

Benzodiazepines are categorized as minor tranquilizers or antianxiety agents and were initially developed to treat short-term anxiety. They were at one time widely prescribed, particularly for women. The drugs were overused for their relaxation effects. It was found that when benzodiazepines are used over time physical and psychologic dependence result. Withdrawal symptoms can occur after heavy, prolonged use that includes tremors, anxiety, and potential for seizures. To avoid withdrawal after prolonged use, the dosage must be tapered gradually. Benzodiazepines are discussed in Chapter 51.

Barbiturates and Sedatives

Barbiturates and other sedatives comprise another category of prescription drugs subject to abuse. These drugs are prescribed for sleeplessness but also produce relaxation and euphoria. They can be taken by ingestion or injection, rapidly produce tolerance, and result in both physical and psychologic dependence. Withdrawal is characterized by hypotension, fever, and delirium and can result in seizures. As with benzodiazepines, tapering the drug, especially by substituting a long-acting barbiturate such as phenobarbital, is recommended. Barbiturates and sedatives are covered in Chapter 51.

Polydrug Abuse

Many drugs are used in combination, either concurrently (together) or sequentially (first one, then the next). Alcohol is more likely to be used alone than any other drug, and it is also commonly used in combination with other drugs because of its easy availability. Polydrug use also may occur because an individual is unable to locate the drug of choice and uses an available substitute or because the individual likes the combination. Alcohol and other depressants are often used concurrently. Sometimes an individual may use a second drug to counteract the effects of the first; for example, a depressant drug is used to "come down" from a stimulant. This behavior is a pattern of alternating use.

When either of these patterns has occurred over a long time, withdrawal is more complicated because the individual needs to withdraw from two drugs that often produce opposite effects.

TREATMENT FOR DRUG ABUSE

Treatment Programs

Treatment for substance abuse is currently undergoing great change as the health care system itself changes. The predominant model for treatment developed experientially is based on the program at Hazelden, Minnesota (near Minneapolis). This program, a 28-day inpatient model, became known as the "Minnesota Model." The Minnesota Model is based on Alcoholics Anonymous (AA) and often uses recovering individuals as counselors. Twelve-step groups, of which AA is the prototype, are self-help groups in which members, who are all recovering from alcohol or drug dependence, join together to offer each other support and direction. Twelve-step groups are not considered treatment but are frequently adjuncts to treatment and in some cases are the only modality used by an individual.

Withdrawal Treatment

A thorough history of drug use and tests of body fluids for drugs at admission are essential measures to make sure that all abused drugs are identified so that a safe plan of withdrawal can be instituted.

Medications used to treat withdrawal symptoms are administered to reestablish physiologic homeostasis. The need for withdrawal treatment depends on the specific drug abused, how much and how long it was abused, and the physical and psychologic characteristics of the individual. Withdrawal effects vary greatly from individual to individual depending on these factors. This variation seems to reflect differences in neurologic response among individuals. A history of prior withdrawal experiences is extremely helpful because it can identify former problem areas that are likely to recur. This is particularly true with alcohol.

The most dangerous substances for withdrawal are the CNS depressants: alcohol, benzodiazepines, and barbiturates, all of which produce physiologic tolerance. Severe alcohol withdrawal syndrome is called delirium tremens (DTs). DTs begin as tremors and agitation, progress to hallucinations and delirium, and sometimes result in death. History is an important predictor of withdrawal symptoms; this information should be routinely collected on admission. Careful monitoring of vital signs and mental status is crucial because early withdrawal symptoms are reflected in the vital signs as increased blood pressure and pulse and in an altered mental status. Early intervention with medications can prevent initiation of DTs; the alcohol withdrawal syndrome is very difficult to stop once started. Benzodiazepines used for alcohol withdrawal vary, but diazepam (Valium) and chlordiazepoxide (Librium) are frequently used on a schedule of decreasing dosage over 3 to 5 days. However, increasingly benzodiazepines are used on an as needed basis for patients who experience symptoms or have a history of severe withdrawal.

Barbiturate withdrawal is managed through a decreasing dose of a long-acting barbiturate, usually phenobarbital, over several days, depending on the dose the patient was using before treatment. The potential for seizures is high during barbiturate withdrawal because the drugs themselves decrease seizure potential.

Benzodiazepine withdrawal is usually managed by decreasing the dosage of diazepam over several days or weeks.

Opioid withdrawal can be treated several ways. Methadone is a long-acting opiate that can be administered once daily to prevent withdrawal symptoms. The use of methadone as a replacement drug for opiates has long been the treatment of choice; however, recent data suggest that this approach may increase the likelihood of relapse to opioid use. Other alternatives are the use of clonidine to relieve symptoms or the use of buprenorphine over 5 to 8 days.

Treatment of withdrawal from stimulant dependence depends on the symptoms. Withdrawal from cocaine may result in a state of depression and loss of feeling and pleasure that requires treatment with antidepressants. Amphetamine withdrawal may result in either depression or an amphetamine-induced psychosis. These effects are treated with an antidepressant or antipsychotic medication, respectively, until the specific symptoms are under control.

Because many drugs interact, both in effect and tolerance, withdrawal from a combination of drugs, particularly combinations of CNS depressants, deserve particular caution in treatment. It may be necessary to manage withdrawal from each drug sequentially, particularly with alcohol and barbiturates or alcohol and benzodiazepines. Sequential withdrawal means to withdraw one drug while continuing the use of the other until the individual's condition is stabilized from the first withdrawal. Then withdrawal from the other drug is initiated.

Medications to Promote Abstinence

Medications used in treatment are oriented toward helping the individual achieve and maintain abstinence from drugs. None of the medications is meant as treatment alone but rather as an adjunct to an ongoing program of recovery.

Antabuse is used to promote abstinence in alcohol-dependent patients. When taken daily, Antabuse produces extreme nausea if the individual uses alcohol. Antabuse is used primarily to discourage impulse drinking and to help patients gain confidence in their ability to abstain.

Naltrexone is sometimes used with opiate users. It blocks the binding sites for opiates so that, if used, the opiate does not produce a euphoria or "high," which is the psychologic reinforcement for opiate use. Naltrexone is a long-acting medication that can be given in a daily dose. A new use of naltrexone is in the treatment of alcohol abuse. It appears that naltrexone may decrease craving for alcohol.

Methadone is used as part of a maintenance program. Patients who have been stabilized on a maintenance dose of methadone receive methadone daily, under clinic supervision, for an indefinite period. Methadone becomes a long-term substitute for the opioid, and the patient must attend the clinic daily for methadone and for periodic urine screening for other drugs. The use of methadone maintenance is controversial. Those who favor methadone maintenance for long-term use with opioid abusers believe that it allows the patient to lead a productive life, particularly one free of crime, until the individual is ready to achieve abstinence. Those who oppose methadone maintenance do so because the drug use continues, although under controlled conditions. Achieving full abstinence from opiates in methadone maintenance programs has been rare after long-term treatment.

NURSING PROCESS OVERVIEW

Drug Abuse

Assessment

An important aspect of any initial patient assessment needs to be questions about drug use or abuse. This approach is important to (1) avoid withdrawal symptoms, (2) identify underlying reasons for physiologic findings (particularly alcohol), (3) appropriately medicate or anesthetize an individual, and (4) determine appropriate referral and treatment for the patient.

A tool frequently used for screening that can be easily inserted into any assessment tool is the CAGE and the Cage adapted to Drug Abuse, CAGEAID. It consists of four questions that can identify alcohol or other drug abuse. Recognizing, however, that not all patients will be honest, the nurse should keep the potential for drug abuse in mind whenever there are physical or other factors that suggest drug involvement. Open-ended questions can help the assessment progress, and a nonjudgmental approach to both the patient and the topic of drug abuse is vital.

A thorough drug history is an important component of assessment for all patients, not just those suspected of substance abuse. All current medications, both prescribed and over-the-counter, should be identified. For patients who use drugs, particularly drugs that produce withdrawal symptoms, this history is imperative. A drug history should include the specific drug, dosage, how often it is taken, and for what period of time. When the information is unclear or inconsistent, the nurse can return to the questions later. Some patients may need to write down their usage or bring in their medication bottles. A particular red flag for prescription drug abuse is multiple prescriptions or multiple prescribers. This is common in older adults.

During the course of treatment, the nurse should continue to assess the patient's behavior and mental status. Some patients may use drugs to treat a mental health problem such as depression that may reappear or intensify when drug use is terminated.

Nursing Diagnoses

A variety of nursing diagnoses may be indicated for patients who are intentionally or unintentionally abusing drugs. Common nursing diagnoses for patients who experience withdrawal from drugs are (1) Sensory-perceptual alteration, (2) Alteration in comfort, and (3) Potential for injury.

Patient Outcomes

Outcomes for patients who abuse drugs are related to (1) safe withdrawal from drugs, (2) stabilization of physical conditions aggravated by drug abuse, and (3) appropriate referral for treatment for the drug abuse if appropriate.

Planning/Implementation

Nursing responses to patients who abuse drugs include developing an understanding of how drug abuse is part of the patient's lifestyle. This understanding from the patient's point of view helps the nurse to determine what treatment and other resources would be most acceptable to the patient.

Patients who abuse drugs often need basic information on their drug of abuse, its characteristics, and problems associated with the drug. Often this will be new information. Information about withdrawal symptoms and any treatment of the withdrawal should be clearly explained to the patient. The nurse should be familiar with withdrawal symptoms related to the specific drug and closely monitor the patient through vital signs and mental status for changes consistent with withdrawal. There are several assessment scales for withdrawal from alcohol that quantify withdrawal symptoms, one of which is the CIWA, Clinical Institute Withdrawal Assessment Scale.

Information about current drug abuse treatment programs and their rationale is necessary to help the patient decide on the type and format of treatment that will be most helpful. This information should include a discussion of the disease concept of drug abuse and the role of 12-step groups in treatment and follow-up.

Education of family and significant others is vital to provide support and to encourage the patient to seek further appropriate treatment.

Particularly for older adults for whom prescription drug abuse has been partly inadvertent, there are various books on prescription medications that are directed at the lay public and can be suggested. The nurse should discuss medication administration such as timing, missed doses, and side effects and be certain that the patient understands the information. It is also important to teach patients about the issues involved in multiple drug use and in combining drugs with alcohol.

Evaluation

The patient should be able to verbalize an understanding of how drug abuse was involved in this health care episode and plan for further treatment if indicated. The patient's family should also be able to verbalize this information. The patient should understand any withdrawal symptoms experienced and their relationship to the drug abuse. The patient should understand the use of any prescription medications.

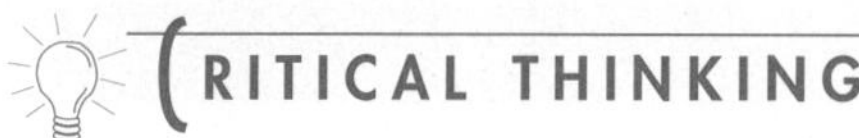

CRITICAL THINKING

APPLICATION

1. What are the criteria for diagnosing drug abuse? For drug dependence?
2. Describe some of the environmental risk factors for drug abuse.
3. Abused drugs tend to produce what kinds of mood changes?
4. What commonly abused drug has the highest addiction potential?
5. Which prescription drugs are most commonly abused?

CRITICAL THINKING

1. Describe the interrelationship between tolerance, withdrawal, and dependence.
2. Describe withdrawal treatment for CNS depressants.

CHAPTER 9

Care of the Poisoned Patient

OBJECTIVES

After studying this chapter, you should be able to do the following:

- *Discuss the importance of the field of clinical toxicology.*
- *Differentiate between toxicodynamics and toxicokinetics.*
- *Explain the rationale for nonspecific antidotes to poisons: decontamination, emesis and lavage, activated charcoal, and cathartics.*
- *Describe the basis for specific antidote categories: competitive antidotes, chelates, antibodies, and agents that produce metabolic alterations.*
- *Differentiate between diuresis and dialysis.*
- *Summarize nursing care implications for drugs discussed in this chapter.*

KEY TERMS

activated charcoal
cathartics
clinical toxicology
decontamination
diuresis
gastric lavage
ipecac syrup
specific antidote
toxicodynamics
toxicokinetics
toxicology

CHAPTER OVERVIEW

Toxicology is the study of poisons. A poison is a chemical substance that injures or kills when introduced into the body. There are literally thousands of potential poisons. Drugs, household and industrial chemicals, plants, pesticides, carbon monoxide, and heavy metals are the major agents of poisoning seen in clinical practice.

Poison control centers, located in communities throughout the United States, are usually identified in local telephone books. These centers provide the lay public and health professionals with information on the appropriate first aid and clinical management of suspected poisoning. Poisondex is a computerized database of more than 650,000 substances and includes information on most medicines and consumer products. Large poison control centers may also offer specialized poison treatment and consultation. Educational services such as professional training and poison prevention education for the public may also be offered.

Each year approximately 1.5 million cases are handled by poison control centers. More than 90% of all poisonings occur at home. Children younger than 3 years of age are the most frequent victims. These statistics highlight the tendency of young children to ingest pills, cleaning agents, and plants. Pills that are particularly attractive and troublesome to children include chocolate-flavored laxatives and vitamins (particularly those with iron given to pregnant women).

The U.S. mortality rate from poisoning of all types has recently been reported at approximately 12,000 deaths per year. Of these, about half are suicides and half are accidental. Less than 50 deaths per year are considered homicides.

Clinical toxicology is the study of care of the poisoned patient. Poisoning can be acute, subacute, or chronic, depending on the dose, length of exposure, and extent of tissue injury. In this chapter the primary emphasis is on the acutely poisoned patient. Acute poisoning is usually the immediate and direct result of a single excessive dose. Acute poisoning in children is most commonly caused by the ingestion of plants, drugs, or household products. In adults acute poisoning is often the result of a drug overdose. About 70% of adult drug overdose cases involve a central nervous system (CNS) depressant, commonly alcohol (23%) or a benzodiazepine (24%). Alcohol and benzodiazepines greatly potentiate the toxic effects of each other or other CNS depressants.

Therapeutic Rationale: Toxicodynamics and Toxicokinetics

The general principles of toxicology are those of pharmacology extended to excessive doses. (The principles relating drug dosage to drug action are discussed in Chapter 1.) The same factors that control pharmacokinetics and pharmacodynamics also apply to toxicology.

Toxicodynamics describes the harmful effects that a poison produces on the body. The graded dose-response curves described in Chapter 2 relate to both toxic effects and therapeutic effects. Therefore the symptoms of poisoning reflect the dosage of the poison. Treating the poisoned patient is frequently a complicated matter because the dose of the poison is seldom known with any accuracy and, further, because the identity of the poison itself may not be known. Therefore a thorough assessment of the patient is especially important in cases of poisoning. If the nature of the poison is known, the severity of the symptoms shown by the patient will be important in monitoring the course of treatment. If the nature of the poison is not known, the symptoms become vital in suggesting the nature of the poison. The application of toxicodynamics to the poisoned patient is demonstrated in Table 9-1, which lists symptoms and gives the common poisons that can cause them.

Toxicokinetics deals with the action of a poison in the patient as a function of time. It encompasses the absorption, distribution, localization, biotransformation, and elimination of the poison. The kinetics of a drug overdose, however, is not necessarily the same as that of the therapeutic dose. This is so because a large dose of drug may saturate and overwhelm one or more of the mechanisms controlling absorption, distribution, biotransformation, and elimination of therapeutic concentrations of the drug. Moreover, normal physiologic processes, such as heart rate, blood pressure, or respiration, may be compromised and thereby alter the disposition of the drug overdose. In this chapter toxicokinetics is presented as embodying the major steps in the care of the acutely poisoned patient. These steps include nonspecific antidotes to remove poison not yet absorbed, specific antidotes to counteract a few select poisons, and, occasionally, diuresis or dialysis.

Therapeutic Agents: Care of the Acutely Poisoned Patient

Nonspecific Antidotes

For a summary of information on nonspecific antidotes, refer to Table 9-2.

Decontamination

Decontamination is the removal or neutralization of a toxin. If the toxin is present on the clothing, skin, or eyes (e.g., insecticide spray), the clothing should be removed and the skin scrubbed well with soap and water. The eyes should be washed with a copious amount of warm water. If the patient has inhaled a noxious gas, that individual should be given fresh air or oxygen to breathe. When a poison or drug overdose has been swallowed, much of the substance usually remains unabsorbed for some time. In treating poisoned patients it is common to flush the poison from the gastrointestinal tract. Such techniques as induced vomiting (emesis), gastric lavage, administration of activated charcoal, and catharsis are appropriate to help eliminate a drug overdose that has been swallowed. The dosages for these nonspecific antidotes are listed in Table 9-2.

Emesis and Lavage

The stomach is emptied either by emesis or gastric lavage. There are three major points that determine whether vomiting or gastric lavage should be used. First, induction of vomiting is not appropriate when the patient might aspirate the vomitus. Therefore this method is contraindicated when the patient is lacking normal reflex control of gagging and vomiting, is unconscious, or is having seizures. Second, vomiting

TABLE 9-1 Physical Symptoms Produced by Common Poisons

SYMPTOMS	POISONING AGENT
Mental and Motor Symptoms	
Drowsiness, coma	Acetaminophen Alcohols Antihistamines Carbon monoxide Insulin Opioids (codeine, others) Salicylates Scopolamine Sedative-hypnotic drugs Tranquilizers Tricyclic antidepressants
Excitation, twitching, convulsions	Aminophylline Atropine CNS stimulants Carbon monoxide Cyanide Local anesthetics Organophosphate insecticides Phenothiazines
Agitation, delirium	Alcohols Aminophylline Atropine Lysergic acid diethylamide (LSD) Lead Marijuana Phencyclidine (PCP) Physostigmine
Paralysis	Foods containing *Clostridium botulinum* (botulism) Heavy metals
Ataxia (motor incoordination)	Alcohols Anticonvulsants Carbon monoxide Hallucinogens Heavy metals Hydrocarbons Sedative-hypnotics Tranquilizers
Cardiovascular and Renal Symptoms	
Increased pulse rate	Alcohols Amphetamine Aspirin Atropine Cocaine Parasympatholytics Sympathomimetics
Decreased pulse rate	Digitalis Opioids Parasympathomimetics
Hypertension	Amphetamine Sympathomimetics
Hypotension	Alcohols Aminophylline Aspirin Muscarine Nitrates, nitrites Opioids Sedative-hypnotics Tranquilizers
Oliguria, anuria	Carbon tetrachloride Ethylene glycol Heavy metals Methanol Mushrooms Petroleum distillates
Oral and Gastrointestinal Symptoms	
Acetone odor	Acetone Alcohol Salicylates
Almond odor	Cyanide
Garlic odor	Arsenic Dimethyl sulfoxide Phosphorus Organophosphate insecticides
Dry mouth	Amphetamine Antihistamines Atropine Opioids Phenothiazines
Excessive salivation	Arsenic Corrosives Mercury Mushrooms Organophosphate insecticides
Heavy vomiting	Aminophylline Corrosives Food poisoning Heavy metals Salicylates
Pupillary Symptoms	
Dilated pupils	Alcohols Anticholinergics Antihistamines CNS depressants CNS stimulants
Constricted pupils	Mushrooms Organophosphate insecticides Opioids
Nystagmus	Sedative-hypnotics

TABLE 9-1 Physical Symptoms Produced by Common Poisons—cont'd

SYMPTOMS	POISONING AGENT	SYMPTOMS	POISONING AGENT
Dermatologic Symptoms		**Pulmonary Symptoms**	
Jaundiced skin	Arsenic Carbon tetrachloride Mushrooms Naphthalene	Rapid breathing	Amphetamine Carbon monoxide Methanol Petroleum distillates Salicylates
Flushed skin	Alcohol Antihistamines Anticholinergics	Depressed respiration	Alcohol Opioids Sedative-hypnotics Tranquilizers
Cherry-red skin	Carbon monoxide Cyanide Nitrites	Wheezing	Mushrooms Opioids Organophosphate insecticides Petroleum distillates

TABLE 9-2 Nonspecific Antidotes

ANTIDOTE	TRADE NAME	ADMINISTRATION/DOSAGE	COMMENTS
Emetics			
✚ Ipecac	Ipecac syrup*	ORAL (in 8 oz water): *Children 6 mo-1 yr*—5-10 ml; *children 1-12 yr*—15 ml. *Adults*—30 ml. Vomiting within 30 min in 90% of patients. May repeat dose after 20-30 min if no vomiting has occurred.	Give only to conscious patient who has gag reflex and is not likely to aspirate vomitus. Do not give when vomitus will itself be injurious (acids, bases, hydrocarbons). Encourage patient to drink water. Water distends stomach and makes it more susceptible to action of ipecac syrup. Walking also helps to induce vomiting. Average return of stomach contents is 20%-60%. Keep vomitus for analysis.
Gastric Lavage			
Water 0.45% saline 0.9% saline		BY GASTRIC TUBE: *Young children*—10 ml/kg. *Adults*—300 ml.	If patient is in deteriorating condition, unconscious, prone to seizures, or lacking a gag reflex, nasotracheal intubation is necessary before lavage to protect airway. Use large-bore (28-40 Fr Ewald or Burke orogastric lavacutor) tubing to allow aspiration of tablets. Keep first wash for analysis. Continue washings until return is clear (2-20 L). Administering more than recommended volume distends stomach and may induce vomiting.
Activated charcoal	Acta-Char Charcoaid Charcodate† Insta-Char* Liqui-Char	ORAL OR BY GASTRIC TUBE: *Children*—15-30 gm in 4-8 oz water. *Adults*—25-50 gm in 8-16 oz water.	Administer as slurry within first hours of poisoning, after induced vomiting (charcoal will inactivate ipecac) or gastric lavage. Do not use with acetylcysteine in management of acetaminophen poisoning. Do not use magnesium sulfate as cathartic.
Cathartics			
Magnesium sulfate (Epsom salts), 10% solution		ORAL: *Children*—1-2 ml/kg. *Adults*—150-250 ml.	Do not use magnesium salts if patient has renal failure.
Magnesium citrate, 10% solution		ORAL: *Children*—1-2 ml/kg. *Adults*—150-250 ml.	Do not use citrate if activated charcoal has been given.

*Available in Canada and United States.
†Available in Canada only.

is not indicated when the regurgitated material can be damaging to the esophagus or lungs. Such material includes acids, bases, and nonaromatic or nonhalogenated hydrocarbons (oils and solvents). Third, induction of vomiting can take 20 to 30 minutes and therefore should not be used when time is critical.

The emetic of choice is **ipecac syrup,** which induces vomiting within 30 minutes in 90% of treated patients. With this agent 20% to 60% of the stomach contents can be emptied. Emetics such as salt water (sodium chloride), mustard water, and copper sulfate are considered dangerous and ineffective. When vomiting is induced, the vomitus should be saved for analysis. See the accompanying box for information on ipecac syrup abuse.

Gastric lavage is the preferred method of emptying the stomach in adults. The airway is first protected by an endotracheal tube. Use of a large-bore tube such as an Ewald or Burke tube allows tablets to be retrieved. Gastric lavage is less successful in children because a small-bore tube must be used. Tablets from some drug formulations partially deteriorate and then coalesce in the stomach to form a mass of undissolved drug that is too large to be washed out and yet is poorly soluble. Lavage is continued until the return is clear. It is important to note that the first wash is saved for analysis.

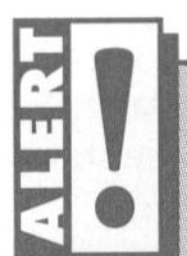

DRUG ABUSE ALERT

Ipecac Syrup

BACKGROUND

Normally ipecac syrup is administered to induce vomiting in an acute poisoning. Ipecac syrup is readily obtained at a drugstore. Chronic administration of ipecac is abuse. Such abuse occurs in some child abuse cases and in some cases of eating disorders. In eating disorders ipecac syrup may be taken to purge ingested food.

PHARMACOLOGY

Emetine HCl (ipecac alkaloid) is a safe drug for inducing vomiting in emergency home use. Administered chronically, however, it can produce many chronic symptoms. These may not be readily associated with abuse. Most of these symptoms relate to distorted electrolyte imbalances that arise from continual vomiting and loss of gastric fluids. The active alkaloid of ipecac also has a direct depressive action on heart and skeletal muscle.

HEALTH HAZARDS

Symptoms of continued ipecac administration include chronic diarrhea and vomiting, muscle weakness, colitis, cardiomyopathy, fever, edema, and electrolyte disturbances. Therapy for ipecac abuse is supportive while ipecac is discontinued.

Activated Charcoal

After emesis or lavage a slurry of activated charcoal may be administered through the lavage tube or a nasogastric tube, or it may be given orally. Because activated charcoal will absorb and inactivate ipecac, it should not be given until after vomiting has occurred. **Activated charcoal** absorbs a number of drugs and chemicals and thereby prevents their absorption into the body. The charcoal itself, with absorbed chemicals, is eliminated in the feces. Administration of activated charcoal is most effective if given within the first few hours of poisoning. If the poisoning is known to be caused by acetaminophen, activated charcoal should not be given. The antidote for acetaminophen is acetylcysteine, which is absorbed by activated charcoal.

Cathartics

Cathartics are the final common treatment to reduce absorption of poisons from the gastrointestinal tract by hastening their elimination. The preferred cathartics are sodium sulfate, magnesium sulfate, or magnesium citrate. However, magnesium citrate should not be used after charcoal administration because the citrate can displace poisons from charcoal. Oil-based cathartics such as mineral oil and castor oil are not used in treating poisoned patients because these oils can speed systemic absorption of some poisons. Cathartics are especially indicated under these circumstances: when enteric-coated tablets have been ingested, when poisoning occurred 1 hour or more previously, or when hydrocarbons have been ingested.

Specific Antidotes

A **specific antidote** is one that directly reverses the toxic action of the poison. In only 5% of poisoning cases is there a specific antidote (Table 9-3). Two specific antidotes, naloxone and flumazenil, are especially important in emergency department situations. They can be both diagnostic tools and potential treatments. Administration of naloxone (Narcan) to a patient who is comatose from an overdose of an opioid (heroin, morphine, pentazocine, propoxyphene) reverses the sedation within 2 minutes. Administration of flumazenil (Mazicon) to a patient who is comatose from an overdose of a benzodiazepine (e.g., chlordiazepoxide or diazepam) reverses the sedation within 1 minute.

Competitive Antidotes

At the receptor a specific antidote may compete for the toxin. Naloxone displaces narcotics (opioids) at the opioid receptor. Unlike other opioids, naloxone does not depress the respiratory center; therefore the occupation of the opioid receptor by naloxone protects against respiratory depression. Flumazenil is an antagonist of benzodiazepines, reversing the cognitive, psychomotor, hypnogenic, and electroencephalographic effects of benzodiazepines. Oxygen in high concentration competes with carbon monoxide in binding to hemoglobin to restore oxygenation. Atropine blocks the muscarinic receptor from the acetylcholine accumulated in anticholinesterase poisoning.

TABLE 9-3 Specific Antidotes

ANTIDOTE	POISON	ADMINISTRATION/DOSAGE	COMMENTS
Cholinergic Poisoning			
✣ Atropine	Anticholinesterase Organophosphates Physostigmine	INTRAVENOUS: *Children*—0.02 mg/kg. *Adults*—1-2 mg. This is initial dose. Repeat every 20 min until copious secretions are controlled.	Blocks muscarinic receptors to prevent peripheral actions of excessive concentrations of neurotransmitter, acetylcholine. See Chapter 11 for more information on actions of acetylcholine and how atropine blocks actions of acetylcholine. Muscarinic symptoms for which atropine is given include nausea, vomiting, diarrhea, sweat, increased bronchial and salivary secretions, and slow heart rate (bradycardia).
Pralidoxime chloride (PAM)	Anticholinesterase Organophosphates	*Organophosphate poisoning:* BY INFUSION in 100 ml saline over 15-30 min: *Children*—20-40 mg/kg. *Adults*—1-2 gm. A second dose can be given in 1 hr. *Carbamate (neostigmine, pyridostigmine) poisoning:* INTRAVENOUS: *Adults*—1-2 gm initially, followed by 250 mg every 5 min as necessary to reverse cholinergic crisis.	Reactivates enzyme acetylcholinesterase after inactivation by irreversible anticholinesterases or organophosphates. This allows acetylcholine to be degraded and relieves paralysis (overstimulation) caused by accumulated acetylcholine. Pralidoxime acts mainly outside CNS. In organophosphate poisoning, pralidoxime is given to restore neuromuscular function, especially to relieve paralysis of respiratory muscles. Atropine is given concurrently (see above) to relieve depression of respiratory center and to reverse muscarinic stimulation. In overdose by carbamate anticholinesterases (neostigmine, pyridostigmine and ambenonium, drugs for myasthenia gravis), pralidoxime antagonizes effects of these drugs on neuromuscular junction.
Physostigmine salicylate (Antilirium)	Antimuscarinic anticholinergic	INTRAVENOUS OR INTRAMUSCULAR: *Adults*—0.5-2 mg. INTRAVENOUS: *Children*—0.5 mg by slow (1 min) infusion: Repeat if needed at 5-10 min intervals until desired effect, or 2 mg total dose, is reached.	Reversible anticholinesterase that increases concentration of acetylcholine at its receptor sites. Reverses both CNS and peripheral anticholinergic effects. Useful for reversing toxic anticholinergic effects due to overdose of atropine and other belladonna alkaloids, tricyclic antidepressants, phenothiazines, and antihistamines. Central anticholinergic effects include anxiety, delirium, disorientation, hallucinations, hyperactivity, seizures, and—in extreme—coma, medullary paralysis, and death. Peripheral anticholinergic toxic effects include fast heart rate (tachycardia), fever, mydriasis (dilated pupils), vasodilation, urinary retention, decreased secretions, and decreased gastrointestinal motility.
Sedative Hypnotic/Opioid Poisoning			
Ethanol	Methanol Ethylene glycol	INTRAVENOUS: *Adults*—0.6 gm/kg + 7-10 gm over 1 hr; then 10 gm/hr maintenance. *Children*—0.6 gm/kg + 4-5 gm over 1 hr; 5 gm/hr maintenance.	All three alcohols are metabolized by aldehyde dehydrogenase. Ethanol is preferred substrate and thereby blocks metabolism of methanol and ethylene glycol to toxins formaldehyde and formic acid (both alcohols) and oxylate (ethylene glycol). Ethanol is given in additional loading dose to achieve blood level of 100 mg/dl.

Continued.

TABLE 9-3 Specific Antidotes—cont'd

ANTIDOTE	POISON	ADMINISTRATION/DOSAGE	COMMENTS
Sedative Hypnotic/Opioid Poisoning—cont'd			
Flumazenil (Mazicon)	Benzodiazepines	INTRAVENOUS: *Adults*—initially 0.2 mg administered over 30 sec; if desired level of consciousness is not obtained, a further dose of 0.3 mg may be administered over another 30 sec. Further doses of 0.5 mg may be administered over 30 sec at 1 min intervals to a cumulative dose of 3 mg. If patient relapses, repeat doses at 20 min intervals as needed, but no more than 1 mg at a time and no more than 3 mg per hour.	Reversible antagonist of benzodiazepine receptor. Reverses cognitive, psychomotor, hypnogenic, and electroencephalographic effects of benzodiazepines. Because flumazenil increases level of consciousness in cases of benzodiazepine overdose even in presence of alcohol intoxication, flumazenil helps in diagnosis. Symptoms of poisoning with barbiturates, alcohol, and phenothiazines are not affected. However, flumazenil may worsen toxicity of tricyclic antidepressants. Flumazenil is also used to improve recovery from surgical sedation with benzodiazepines.
Naloxone (Narcan)	Narcotics (opioids), including pentazocine, propoxyphene, diphenoxylate	INTRAVENOUS (May also give intramuscularly or subcutaneously): *Adults*—0.4-2 mg. Additional doses are repeated at 2-3 min intervals until patient responds or until 10 mg is given. *Children*—0.01 mg/kg with 0.1 mg/kg as subsequent dose.	Reversible antagonist of opioid receptor. Useful for reversing narcotic depression, including respiratory depression. Naloxone is preferred because it is pure opioid antagonist and causes no respiratory depression of its own. Naloxone is effective within 2 min and has duration of action of 1-4 hr. Because most opioids have a longer duration of action, effects of naloxone may wear off and patient may relapse, requiring additional naloxone.
Specific Metabolic Poisons			
Acetylcysteine (Mucomyst)	Acetaminophen	ORAL: 140 mg/kg as 5% solution mixed with soda, water, or grapefruit juice. Follow with 17 maintenance doses of 70 mg/kg every 4 hr.	Acetylcysteine restores sulfhydryl groups depleted by acetaminophen metabolism. This prevents toxicity to liver produced by metabolites of acetaminophen. Acetylcysteine should not be given with activated charcoal because charcoal absorbs it.
Amyl nitrite Sodium nitrite Sodium thiosulfate (Cyanide Antidote Package)	Cyanide	*Amyl nitrite:* Crush ampule on gauze and have patient inhale vapor. *Sodium nitrite:* Inject 10 ml of 3% solution after IV line is established. *Sodium thiosulfate:* Inject 50 ml of 25% solution after administration of sodium nitrite.	Cyanide has almond odor. Toxicity of cyanide is caused by its blockage of enzymes using oxygen in mitochondria (cytochrome oxidase), thereby depressing cellular respiration. Inhibition of cytochrome oxidase depends on binding of cyanide to ferric iron in cytochrome oxidase. Nitrite converts ferrous iron in hemoglobin to ferric iron, producing methemoglobin. This large pool of ferric iron in blood competes with cytochrome oxidase for cyanide, thereby restoring cellular respiration. Thiosulfate accelerates conversion of cyanide to relatively nontoxic thiocyanate, which is readily excreted in urine.

TABLE 9-3 Specific Antidotes—cont'd

ANTIDOTE	POISON	ADMINISTRATION/DOSAGE	COMMENTS
Metal Poisoning			
Deferoxamine mesylate (Desferal)	Iron	INTRAMUSCULAR, CONTINUOUS SUBCUTANEOUS, OR SLOW INTRAVENOUS: *Adults*—1 gm initially, 0.5 gm at 4 and 8 hr. Further doses if needed, up to 6 gm daily. For IV, do not give at rate greater than 15 mg/kg/hr. Administer IM if possible. *Children*—50 mg/kg/ IM or IV every 6 hr up to 15 mg/kg/hr by continuous IV. Maximum dosage: 6 gm/24 hr or 2 gm/dose.	Chelates iron and thereby prevents iron from entering cells and inhibiting chemical reactions. Chelate of iron and deferoxamine is rapidly excreted in urine, removing iron from body.
Dimercaprol (BAL)	Arsenic Gold Mercury Lead	INTRAMUSCULAR: Because dimercaprol is oil, give deep intramuscularly only. *Mild arsenic or gold poisoning:* 2.5 mg/kg 4 times daily, 2 days; 2 times, day 3; once daily, 10 days. *Severe arsenic or gold poisoning:* 3 mg/kg every 4 hr for 2 days, 4 times day 3; twice daily 10 days. *Mercury poisoning:* 5 mg/kg initially; 2.5 mg/kg 1.2 times daily for 10 days. *Acute lead poisoning:* 4 mg/kg alone initially, then at 4 hr intervals with calcium disodium edetate (administered at separate site). Maintain for 2-7 days.	Dimercaprol is a sulfhydryl compound that chelates arsenic, gold, and mercury and promotes their excretion in urine. Dimercaprol also reactivates affected sulfhydryl enzymes. Peak plasma concentrations occur 30-60 min after administration. Excretion is complete in 4 hr. Dimercaprol is not very effective for poisoning caused by antimony and bismuth. It is contraindicated in iron, cadmium, and selenium poisoning because chelates are more toxic, especially to kidney, than metal alone. Alkalinization of urine protects kidney from breakdown of dimercaprol-metal complex in acid urine. Common side effects of dimercaprol are rise in blood pressure with tachycardia (fast heart rate) and burning sensation of lips, mouth, and throat.
Edetate calcium disodium (calcium disodium versenate)	Lead	INTRAVENOUS: 50-75 mg/kg/day in 3-6 doses, each dose administered over at least 1 hr. Can continue for up to 5 days. Wait 2 days before resuming therapy for additional 5 days. INTRAMUSCULAR: Preferred route for children. Give 35 mg/kg twice daily. After 3-5 days, discontinue for 4 or more days.	Calcium-bound to EDTA is displaced by lead and resulting chelate is excreted in urine (50% in 1 hr: 95% in 24 hr). EDTA can produce toxic effects, including renal damage and irregularities in cardiac rhythm. Doses must be carefully monitored.
Penicillamine (Cuprimine, Depen)	Copper Lead Zinc Mercury	ORAL: *Adults*—1-1.5 gm daily in 4 divided doses on empty stomach for 1-2 mo. *Children*—30-40 mg/kg daily or 600-750 mg/m2 daily for 1-6 mo.	Penicillamine chelates copper, lead, zinc, or mercury, promoting their excretion in urine. Side effects include allergic reactions (principally rashes) and loss of sweet and salt tastes. Severe side effects include bone marrow depression and renal toxicity.

Chelates

Another category of action of specific antidotes is chelates, compounds that form a nontoxic complex with the toxin. Poisoning by heavy metals in particular is treated with chelates, which form a nontoxic complex with the metal; this complex is quickly eliminated, usually in the urine. Accumulation of the heavy metal is thereby reversed. Dimercaprol complexes arsenic, copper, lead, and mercury. Penicillamine, a drug used to treat rheumatoid arthritis and lupus (see Chapter 37) also complexes copper, lead, and mercury. Deferoxamine is a specific chelate for iron (see Chapter 22). Ethylenediaminetetraacetic acid (EDTA) is the chelate used for lead or cadmium intoxication.

Antibodies

In a few instances treatment with specific antibodies to the poison is possible. Antibodies to digoxin are available to counteract toxic levels of this important cardiac drug. These antibodies reverse the cardiac toxicity by complexing the digoxin and lowering the large pool of digoxin that is bound to plasma albumin. The digoxin then is not free to act. Antivenoms are antibodies for certain snake and spider venoms.

Metabolic Alterations

Specific antidotes may alter the metabolism of a toxin. Ethanol inhibits the biotransformation of methanol and ethylene glycol to toxic metabolites, particularly formic acid. Thiosulfate enhances the transformation of cyanide to the relatively nontoxic thiocyanate. Acetylcysteine restores the sulfhydryl groups of the liver after depletion by acetaminophen metabolism. Sulfhydryl groups protect the liver from toxic metabolites of acetaminophen. Physostigmine inhibits acetylcholinesterase, the enzyme that normally degrades acetylcholine. This action allows acetylcholine concentrations to rise at the synapses and compete with anticholinergic drugs blocking these receptors. This reversal by acetylcholine restores function in anticholinergic poisoning by drugs that are either anticholinergic, such as atropine or scopolamine, or have anticholinergic actions, such as antihistamines, tricyclic antidepressants, and antipsychotic drugs. Used as an antidote, pralidoxime reactivates acetylcholinesterase after it has been inactivated by an anticholinesterase poison. The poison is freed in an inactive form to be eliminated.

Diuresis and Dialysis

Diuresis

Diuresis can be used to hasten elimination of poisons excreted primarily by the kidneys. It is used when the level of poison in the blood is at a potentially fatal concentration, when the patient is in a coma, and when the patient otherwise has stable cardiovascular, respiratory, and renal function. Fluid diuresis, achieved with a potent loop diuretic such as furosemide, increases the glomerular filtration rate and thereby decreases the renal tubular reabsorption of the poison. Osmotic diuresis with mannitol or urea prevents reabsorption of the poison in the kidney by creating an osmotic load that effectively flushes the kidney tubule.

Alkalinization of the urine with sodium bicarbonate enhances the excretion of weak acids such as aspirin and phenobarbital by maintaining them in their ionized form, which is not reabsorbed readily. Similarly, acidification of the urine with ammonium chloride or ascorbic acid aids the excretion of weak bases such as amphetamine or phencyclidine by maintaining them in their ionized form, which is not reabsorbed. Diuretics are discussed fully in Chapter 14.

Dialysis

Dialysis is indicated in cases of extreme poisoning or renal failure when the poison is dialyzable. For instance, the anticoagulant warfarin and the cardiac glycoside digitoxin are tightly protein bound in the blood and therefore are not successfully removed by dialysis.

Hemodialysis is a highly technical and complex procedure in which the blood is shunted from the body and through tubing immersed in a physiologic buffer. Any chemical present in the blood but not in the buffer diffuses into the buffer because of the concentration gradient. The blood so dialyzed, or "washed," is continuously returned to the body. Salicylate, methanol, and ethylene glycol are especially effectively removed by hemodialysis.

Hemoperfusion is a relatively new technique in which the blood is pumped from a venous catheter through a column of absorbent material and returned to the patient. Anticoagulation with heparin is necessary to prevent the patient's blood from clotting in the cartridge. Hemoperfusion is effective for high-molecular-weight poisons with poor water solubility because the cartridge has a large surface area for absorption.

Peritoneal dialysis is the simplest dialysis technique, but, unfortunately, it is the most inefficient in removing the majority of drugs. In peritoneal dialysis physiologic buffer is introduced into the abdomen and left there for several hours before being drained and replaced. Because the gastrointestinal tract has a rich blood supply, the blood is dialyzed as it flows through the normal gastrointestinal network.

NURSING PROCESS OVERVIEW

Treatment of Poisoning

Assessment

Patients who have been exposed to poisons or who have ingested poisons may enter the health care system in any condition, from the child who is alert, oriented, and feeling fine after ingesting a handful of children's vitamins to the patient who requires resuscitation or is comatose and unable to provide any information about the toxic substances. Obtain a complete baseline assessment, including vital signs, mental status, blood pressure, weight, serum electrolyte levels, liver and renal function studies, blood gases, and electrocardiogram. The health history should include information about the poison(s) ingested (how much, when, what efforts have been tried as treatment) and preexisting health problems.

Nursing Diagnoses

- Anxiety related to treatment and/or possible outcome of treatment
- Altered comfort: nausea and vomiting from use of ipecac
- Ineffective airway clearance related to drug overdose with potential for aspiration

Patient Outcomes

The patient will recover from the poisoning episode with no ill effects. The nonspecific or specific antidote will successfully treat the poisoning, vomiting will end, and the patient will not aspirate and will be alert enough to clear airway. Suicidal patients will begin psychiatric care.

Planning/Implementation

Establish and maintain a patent airway with adequate ventilation. Other measures might include supportive care of the unconscious patient, administration of nonspecific or specific antidotes, and hospitalization for further observation or treatment. Monitor vital signs, blood pressure, and electrocardiogram as needed. Initiate and maintain intravenous therapy, monitor intake and output, monitor laboratory work (blood gases, liver and renal function studies, serum levels of suspected toxin[s] and/or antidotes), insert a nasogastric or orogastric tube for gastric lavage, or induce vomiting as ordered. Monitor mental status. Keep the patient and the family informed of actions being taken and their effect.

Evaluation

Effective treatment for overdose or exposure to toxins occurs when the poisonous substance is eliminated and the patient returns to normal without experiencing side effects associated with the poison or treatment. Most antidotes will not be administered on an outpatient basis. Before discharge, instruct the patient and the family about continuing care or observations required. If appropriate, give instructions about removing toxic substances from the home or workplace. Refer the patient to social services or a community-based nursing care agency if appropriate. Provide positive reinforcement about psychiatric care if recommended for the patient.

NURSING IMPLICATIONS SUMMARY

General Guidelines: Care of the Poisoned Patient

- Thoroughly assess any patient suspected of having ingested a toxic substance or a toxic amount of a generally nontoxic substance. If the patient's condition obviously requires emergency treatment, the initial assessment may be abbreviated until the patient is stabilized, then further assessment should be performed. Assess the following: blood pressure and vital signs, neurologic examination, level of respiratory effort, presence of cyanosis, breath sounds, electrocardiogram, complete visual inspection including nose and mouth, blood gases, serum electrolytes, renal and liver function tests, and weight. Obtain a detailed history from the patient and family about the suspected toxic agents, including the amount, how long ago the substance was ingested, efforts made to induce vomiting or dilute the substance, the age of the patient, and any coexisting medical problems. Save any samples of the toxic substance, vomitus, or stool; label carefully and send to the laboratory for analysis.
- Work quickly and efficiently to administer prescribed antagonists or other treatments, but remain calm. Reassure the patient and family that everything possible is being done. Families of children may be especially upset. Nurses who work in settings where overdoses or toxic ingestions are commonly seen (e.g., emergency departments, some occupational health settings) should know the following: location of emergency equipment for intubation, assisted ventilation, and resuscitation; telephone number of the nearest poison control center; location of reference guides to emergency treatment of overdoses; location of antidotes, antagonists, and equipment (e.g., lavage tubes) used in that setting; and general procedures to be followed in treating overdoses.
- Prevention of overdose is preferable to treatment for overdose; however, preventive health teaching is usually not appropriate during treatment of acute overdose. Nurses who work with patients or families in situations that involve drugs or toxic chemicals should review general safety measures on a regular schedule. Teaching points to review with patients and families to help prevent accidental ingestion of medicines or toxic household chemicals include: keep medications out of the reach of children, the incompetent, or the confused; keep medications in a locked cabinet; keep household products out of reach of children; keep drugs and chemicals in clearly and correctly labeled containers; use safety latches on cabinets and drawers; never refer to medicines as candy; treat all medicines with respect; use childproof caps when children are in the environment; use

Continued.

Nursing Implications Summary—cont'd

drugs only as prescribed; never double or increase the dose of any drug unless specifically directed to do so by the physician. Teach patients never to borrow medications prescribed for another person.

- Ipecac is available in small quantities without a prescription and should be kept in the home (out of the reach of children) for emergency treatment of overdose. However, teach families to call the poison control center before administering ipecac to ascertain that inducing vomiting is appropriate for the ingested substance. Teach patients to keep the number of the poison control center handy near the telephone.
- Instruct patients or families calling for emergency help to bring a sample of the drug or toxic substance and any vomitus to the emergency department when they bring the patient.

Ipecac

Drug Administration/Patient and Family Education

- Ipecac may be purchased without prescription and may be kept in the home. Do not administer ipecac until directed to do so by the physician or poison control center. Any ipecac remaining after a dose has been administered should be discarded. Check expiration dates.
- Have the patient drink a full glass of water (8 oz) after taking the ordered dose (½ to 1 full glass for a child). A frightened child may do better if the water is administered before the ipecac. Avoid milk products. Generally, if vomiting does not occur after the first dose, the dose is repeated in about 20 minutes. If vomiting does not occur after the second dose, take the patient to the emergency department. Do not give this drug to infants younger than 6 months of age. Children 6 months to 1 year of age should be treated in the emergency department.
- If the physician has also prescribed activated charcoal, give ipecac syrup first and administer the activated charcoal after vomiting has ceased. Do not induce vomiting in anyone who is drowsy because this may predispose to aspiration. Save vomitus and send it to the laboratory for analysis.

Activated Charcoal

Drug Administration

- Activated charcoal is most effective when administered within 30 minutes of ingestion of the poison. The mixture is unattractive. Put it into an empty soft-drink can to administer it to children. Mix charcoal with water or a small amount of fruit juice. Do not mix with ice cream, milk, sherbet, or chocolate syrup because these foods will decrease the ability of the charcoal to absorb the toxin. Activated charcoal adsorbs ipecac; do not administer these simultaneously. If multiple doses of activated charcoal are ordered, preparations that contain sorbitol should not be used for each dose because the total amount of sorbitol may cause diarrhea; alternate sorbitol-containing preparations with activated charcoal that does not contain sorbitol. Caution patients that activated charcoal may cause feces to turn black.

Cathartics

Drug Administration

- See Chapter 24 for additional information about saline cathartics. Do not use sodium salts if the patient has a history of heart disease. Do not use magnesium salts if the patient has a history of renal failure. Do not use magnesium sulfate if activated charcoal has been administered.

Atropine

- See Chapter 11 for additional information about atropine.

Pralidoxime Chloride

Drug Administration

- Review the information presented in Table 9-3. Keep a suction machine and intubation equipment readily available when using this drug. See Chapter 37 for a discussion of myasthenia gravis. Keep edrophonium, atropine, syringes, and a tourniquet handy when working with patients with myasthenia gravis. Monitor patients carefully. Side effects of pralidoxime may mimic effects of ingested substances: dizziness, blurred vision, diplopia, drowsiness, nausea, tachycardia, hyperventilation, and muscle weakness.

Physostigmine Salicylate

Drug Administration

- Review the information presented in Table 9-3. Monitor vital signs and blood pressure. Treat overdose of physostigmine with atropine, which should be kept at the bedside. Because the drug has a short duration of action (30 to 60 minutes), it may be necessary to repeat doses. Monitor the patient carefully. Physostigmine may be administered intravenously undiluted. Administer at a rate of 1 mg or less over 1 to 3 minutes (adults) or 0.5 mg per minute (children). Too rapid intravenous (IV) administration may cause convulsions, difficulty breathing, and bradycardia.

Ethanol

Drug Administration

- Ethanol can be administered intravenously or via orogastric or nasogastric tube. Orally, a 20% solution is preferred to reduce the risk of gastritis, but, if needed, any blended whiskey can be used. If the patient's condition warrants it, oral administration is preferred because the IV route is limited to 5% and 10% solutions. Monitor blood ethanol

NURSING IMPLICATIONS SUMMARY—cont'd

levels during therapy. Monitor vital signs, blood pressure, and electrocardiogram. When using ethanol for treatment of overdose, keep a suction machine and equipment for intubation and resuscitation at the bedside.

Flumazenil

Drug Administration

- Flumazenil may be administered via direct IV push at a rate of 200 µg over 15 seconds. It may also be diluted in D5W, normal saline, or 0.45% sodium chloride and 2.5% dextrose. See the manufacturer's literature for information about admixing with other drugs. Monitor level of consciousness and vital signs, especially respirations. Have a suction machine at the bedside. Anticipate the possibility of needing an artificial airway and ventilatory and circulatory support. Have drugs readily available to treat seizures. Monitor electrocardiogram and oxygenation via pulse oximetry. If resedation occurs, it may be necessary to repeat doses. Flumazenil is also discussed in Chapter 51.

Patient and Family Education

- Flumazenil is used in an acute care setting. If flumazenil has been used as part of outpatient surgery or procedures, warn the patient not to resume regular activities for at least 18 to 24 hours after discharge because psychomotor and memory deficits may persist that long. Give postdischarge instructions in writing to the patient and a responsible caretaker.

Naloxone

Drug Administration

- Monitor respirations. Naloxone should promptly increase the respiratory rate and volume. If it does not, the respiratory depression is probably not the result of narcotic overdose, or multiple agents were consumed or injected. Keep intubation and resuscitation equipment and drugs readily available if the patient manifests respiratory depression.
- Monitor vital signs and blood pressure. Naloxone has a relatively short half-life, and the dose may need to be repeated. Remember that in narcotic addicts this drug may precipitate withdrawal symptoms. Monitor neonates carefully. Naloxone may be used to treat neonatal respiratory depression, which may be present if narcotic analgesics were administered in large doses during labor and delivery or if the mother is a narcotic addict. If the mother is an addict, naloxone will precipitate withdrawal symptoms in the infant. Naloxone is also discussed in Chapter 31.

Acetylcysteine

Drug Administration

- Review Table 9-3 and see Chapter 29. Monitor vital signs and blood pressure. Side effects from acetylcysteine are rare; they include nausea, vomiting, and increase in blood pressure. Acetylcysteine has a bad odor; doses must be diluted before administration. The manufacturer's insert provides information about volumes of diluent to use per dose. Try chilling doses and have the patient take doses through a straw placed in a cup or container that is tightly capped. Doses vomited within 1 hour of administration must be repeated; check with the physician.

Cyanide Antidote Package

Drug Administration

- This combination of drugs (amyl nitrite, sodium nitrite, sodium thiosulfate) is recommended for cyanide poisoning and also for treatment of overdose with sodium nitroprusside (see Table 9-3 and Chapter 13). Side effects are rare. Monitor vital signs and blood pressure.

Deferoxamine Mesylate

Drug Administration

- Monitor blood pressure, vital signs, fluid intake and output, and serum iron levels. Rapid intravenous administration may cause hypotension, tachycardia, erythema, and urticaria. Anaphylactic reactions are rare, but keep epinephrine and intubation and resuscitation equipment handy. In acute iron poisoning, treat with deferoxamine in addition to lavage and/or induction of emesis, maintain a patent airway, control shock (IV fluids, vasopressors), and correct acidosis (administer sodium bicarbonate or other drugs).
- Intramuscular injection is the preferred parenteral route. Reconstitute powder with 2 ml of sterile water for injection for each 500 mg vial; use 8 ml for each 2 gm vial. Dissolve all powder before injecting dose. After subcutaneous injection some patients experience a local histamine-like reaction.
- Reserve IV injection for patients who exhibit signs of shock. Reconstitute powder as above, then further dilute with normal saline solution, dextrose injection, or lactated Ringer's injection. Administer at a rate not exceeding 15 mg/kg/hr.

Patient and Family Education

- Advise patients on long-term therapy to have regular ophthalmic examinations.
- Usually discontinue chelation therapy during pregnancy. Advise women considering pregnancy to consult the physician.
- Warn patients that deferoxamine may turn urine red.

Dimercaprol

Drug Administration

- Review Table 9-3. Monitor vital signs, blood pressure, and fluid intake and output. Monitor the blood urea nitrogen (BUN), and serum creatinine, serum electrolytes. Do not administer medicinal iron to patients receiving dimercaprol.

Continued.

NURSING IMPLICATIONS SUMMARY—cont'd

- To avoid skin contact with the drug when preparing doses, wear gloves. Keep the urine alkaline to facilitate chelation, and monitor the urine pH. For detailed instructions in preparing oil-based suspensions, see Chapter 5.

Patient and Family Education

- Inform patients that the drug may produce a garliclike odor to the breath. Inform parents that some children have a fever during therapy.

Edetate Calcium Disodium

Drug Administration

- Read the physician's orders carefully. Do not confuse edetate calcium disodium (used to treat lead poisoning) with edetate disodium (used to treat hypercalcemia). Assess urine output before administering. Because the chelate is excreted in the urine, patients with oliguria or renal disease may be unable to tolerate this drug. Monitor vital signs, blood pressure, BUN, urinalysis, serum electrolytes, serum creatinine, fluid intake and output, and electrocardiogram. Edetate calcium disodium interferes with the duration of action of zinc insulin preparations. Patients with diabetes who are receiving zinc insulin may need a change in dosage or drug while they are receiving edetate calcium disodium.
- IV injection is the preferred route of administration in children and in individuals with lead encephalopathy, although patients in the latter group must be monitored carefully for increased intracranial pressure.
- For intramuscular use, lidocaine or procaine may be added to the reconstituted solution to help prevent pain at the injection site (check with the physician or pharmacy). Assess the mouth and gums for development of sores. These sores should subside after drug therapy. Zinc replacement may be necessary between courses of therapy with edetate calcium disodium.

Penicillamine

- Review Table 9-3. Penicillamine is also used to treat rheumatoid arthritis, as discussed in Chapter 37.

CRITICAL THINKING

APPLICATION

1. What do the terms *toxicology* and *clinical toxicology* mean?
2. What is toxicodynamics, and why is it important clinically?
3. What is toxicokinetics, and why is it important clinically? How does toxicokinetics differ from pharmacokinetics?
4. How does the health professional use nonspecific antidotes in treatment of acute poisoning?
5. What is the role of cathartics in treating acute poisoning? Which drugs are recommended? Why?
6. Describe specific antidotes the health professional would consider for each of the following categories: competitive antidotes, chelates, antibodies, metabolic alterations.
7. When is diuresis indicated in treating acute poisoning? Describe fluid and osmotic diuresis and alkalinization and acidification of the urine. Explain when these processes may be helpful.
8. When is dialysis indicated in treating acute poisoning?

CRITICAL THINKING

1. Determine if your community has a poison control center. What services are offered by this center? Where is the number in the telephone directory?
2. Why is patient assessment so important in treating poisoning?
3. Contrast the uses of emesis and gastric lavage in emptying the stomach. What is the drug of choice for inducing vomiting? Why?
4. It is recommended that households with children have on hand a small quantity of ipecac. What are important teaching points about this drug?
5. When is the administration of activated charcoal indicated? When is it not indicated?
6. Differentiate between hemodialysis, hemoperfusion, and peritoneal dialysis.
7. What are important teaching points for promoting safety and decreasing the possibility of poisoning in the household?

SECTION III

How the Nervous System Controls Body Functions

A separate introductory section on neuropharmacology has been a feature of this textbook from its beginning. This format introduces the student to key concepts in neuropharmacology and asks the student to concentrate first on mechanisms and effects before proceeding to drugs and therapeutics. The autonomic and motor nervous systems provide the prototypes for our knowledge of neuropharmacology.

CHAPTER 10 *Introduction to Neuropharmacology* reviews these systems and the function and regulation of the neurotransmitters acetylcholine and norepinephrine.

CHAPTER 11 *Mechanisms of Cholinergic Control* reviews mechanisms of cholinergic drugs.

CHAPTER 12 *Mechanisms of Adrenergic Control* reviews mechanisms of adrenergic drugs.

The purpose of Chapters 11 and 12 is to introduce the student to the spectrum of mechanisms and therapeutic uses for drugs that affect these two neurotransmitters. The student is cautioned not to be concerned initially with actual drugs listed because these drugs, their therapeutic uses, and the implications for nursing are all discussed in detail in the following chapters. However, the student will find the detailed classification of drugs by mechanism useful as a review later in the course of study.

CHAPTER 10

Introduction to Neuropharmacology

OBJECTIVES

After studying this chapter, you should be able to do the following:

- *Differentiate between the motor nervous system and the autonomic nervous system.*
- *Distinguish between acetylcholine, norepinephrine, and epinephrine.*
- *Describe the divisions of the autonomic nervous system: sympathetic and parasympathetic.*
- *List the effects on tissues of sympathetic (adrenergic) stimulation and parasympathetic (cholinergic or muscarinic) stimulation.*
- *Describe the "fight or flight" response.*

KEY TERMS

autonomic nervous system
central nervous system
efferent neurons
neurotransmitter
parasympathetic (cholinergic) nervous system
reuptake
sympathetic (adrenergic) nervous system

CHAPTER OVERVIEW

Many different classes of drugs, used for a variety of therapeutic purposes, affect the nervous system at some level. Some of these drugs are designed to alter the function of some portion of the nervous system, whereas others alter functions of the nervous system as a side effect. A review of the anatomy and biochemical function of the nervous system is necessary to understand the mechanisms of these drugs and the array of side effects they produce. This chapter presents that review.

The **central nervous system** includes the brain and spinal cord. The functions of these structures are twofold: first, to monitor, convey, and process signals from sensory receptors throughout the body by way of ascending neuronal pathways and, second, to sequence information and convey signals to initiate or to modify body actions.

The neurons that relay information from the central nervous system to the rest of the body are called **efferent neurons.** The ascending sensory neurons and the efferent neurons form the peripheral nervous system. The peripheral nervous system is subdivided into the motor nervous system and the autonomic nervous system.

NEUROTRANSMITTERS

Neurotransmitters and Receptors

All neurons use neurotransmitters to contact neurons and other cells. A **neurotransmitter** is a chemical that is synthesized in the nerve cell and stored inside vesicles (sacs) in the terminal. Most neurons appear to make only one kind of neurotransmitter. When the neuron is stimulated, some of the vesicles merge with the nerve terminal membrane and quantities of neurotransmitter are released. There is a space between the neuron and the cell with which the neuron is communicating. This space is the synaptic cleft or synapse. The neurotransmitter molecules diffuse across the synapse and occupy specific receptors on the next cell. The function of the receptor is to recognize only one specific neurotransmitter and to initiate a cellular response to that neurotransmitter. The binding of the neurotransmitter to its receptor is reversible. When the neurotransmitter diffuses away from the receptor, the stimulation of the cell is terminated.

Two neurotransmitters, acetylcholine and norepinephrine, are the neurotransmitters of the peripheral nervous system. A given class of neurons, however, will use only one of these neurotransmitters. The synthesis and degradation of each neurotransmitter are discussed first. A description of where each neurotransmitter is found in the peripheral nervous system and the responses produced follows.

Acetylcholine

Acetylcholine is synthesized in the nerve terminal by the enzyme choline acetylase from choline and an acetate molecule activated by coenzyme A (Figure 10-1). This acetylcholine is packaged in vesicles. On stimulation of the nerve, some of the vesicles release acetylcholine into the synapse, where the acetylcholine diffuses to the opposing membrane and binds at the specific receptors for acetylcholine. In addition, the membrane contains the enzyme acetylcholinesterase, which degrades acetylcholine to acetate and choline. The acetylcholinesterase is very active, and the half-life of the acetylcholine released is only a few milliseconds. Any acetylcholine that diffuses from the synapse into the blood is degraded by nonspecific cholinesterases in the blood or tissues. Thus, when released, acetylcholine produces a response in the next cell by way of the acetylcholine receptor and/or is rapidly degraded by the membrane-bound enzyme acetylcholinesterase or by nonspecific cholinesterases in the blood plasma.

Norepinephrine and the Neurohormone Epinephrine

Norepinephrine is synthesized in the nerve terminal from the amino acid tyrosine (see Figure 10-1). Norepinephrine is a neurotransmitter because it is released from a neuron to act on an adjacent cell. The chromaffin cells of the adrenal medulla also synthesize norepinephrine but convert 80% to 85% of the norepinephrine to epinephrine. These adrenal stores of epinephrine and norepinephrine are released into the blood on stimulation of the adrenal medulla in response

to stress. Epinephrine is called a neurohormone because it is released into the blood to produce effects at distant sites.

Most norepinephrine is *not* degraded after release. Instead, it is taken back up into the neuron from which it was released and stored again in granules. This process is called **reuptake.** There are two enzymes that can degrade norepinephrine and epinephrine. Monoamine oxidase (MAO) is located in the mitochondria of most cells, including nerve terminals that release norepinephrine. Catechol *O*-methyltransferase (COMT) is found in the cytoplasm of most cells. Both MAO and COMT are found in large concentrations in the liver and kidney. Any norepinephrine that diffuses into the blood or any epinephrine in the blood is quickly degraded by the liver and/or kidney. No drugs are used that interfere with COMT, but in later chapters we shall see that drugs that inhibit MAO are used for treating depression, hypertension, and parkinsonism. Epinephrine and norepinephrine are metabolized to the common product vanillylmandelic acid (VMA). Because VMA is excreted in the urine, the measurement of VMA in collected urine is used as an index of sympathetic activity.

The main features of the peripheral nervous system and its neurotransmitters acetylcholine and norepinephrine are reviewed as a preparation for discussing drugs that act by modifying neurotransmitter action within the peripheral nervous system. The motor nervous system is discussed first and then the more complex autonomic nervous system.

MOTOR NERVOUS SYSTEM

The motor (somatic) nervous system is under both conscious and unconscious control to initiate muscle contraction (Figure 10-2). A motor neuron has a cell body in the spinal cord and contacts a striated muscle at a specialized region, the neuromuscular junction. Motor neurons are found in several cranial nerves and in all spinal nerves. Stimulation of a motor neuron releases acetylcholine at the neuromuscular junction, and the muscle cell reacts to acetylcholine by contracting. Stimulation of a motor neuron may arise as a result of a willed impulse originating in the brain and transmitted to the appropriate neuron in the spinal cord or, unconsciously, as a reflex. A reflex is initiated by sensory input (i.e., heat, touch, pressure, pain) that is transmitted to the spinal cord and then out to the motor neurons without processing by the brain.

AUTONOMIC NERVOUS SYSTEM

Divisions of the System

The role of the **autonomic nervous system** is to monitor and control internal body functions such as cardiac output, blood volume, blood composition, blood pressure, and digestive processes, primarily by modifying the tone of tissue smooth muscle and the quantity of tissue secretions (see Figure 10-2). The autonomic nervous system has two distinct efferent divisions, the **parasympathetic (cholinergic) nervous system** and the **sympathetic (adrenergic) nervous system.** Both divisions commonly act on a given organ but produce oppo-

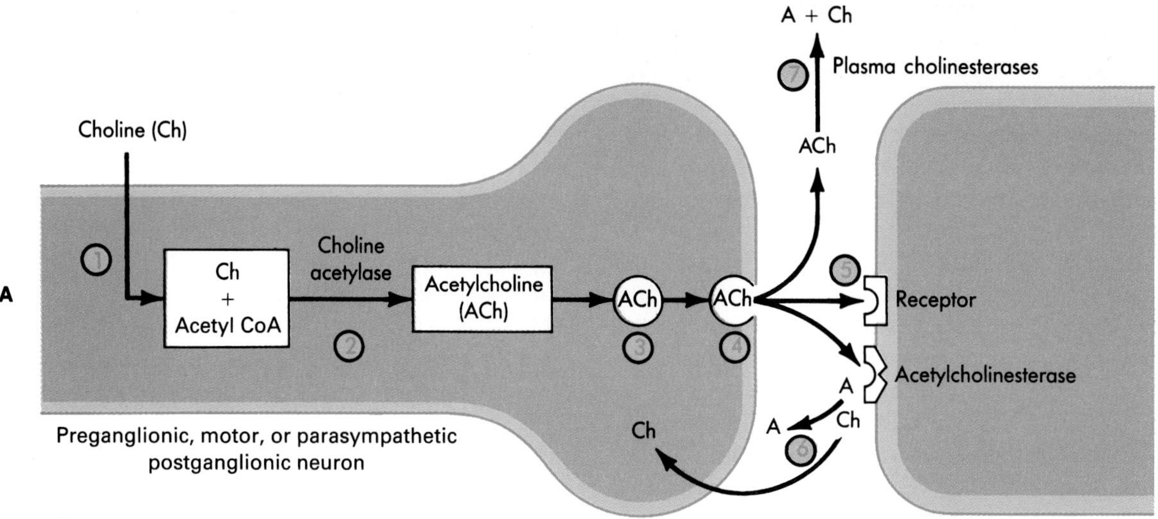

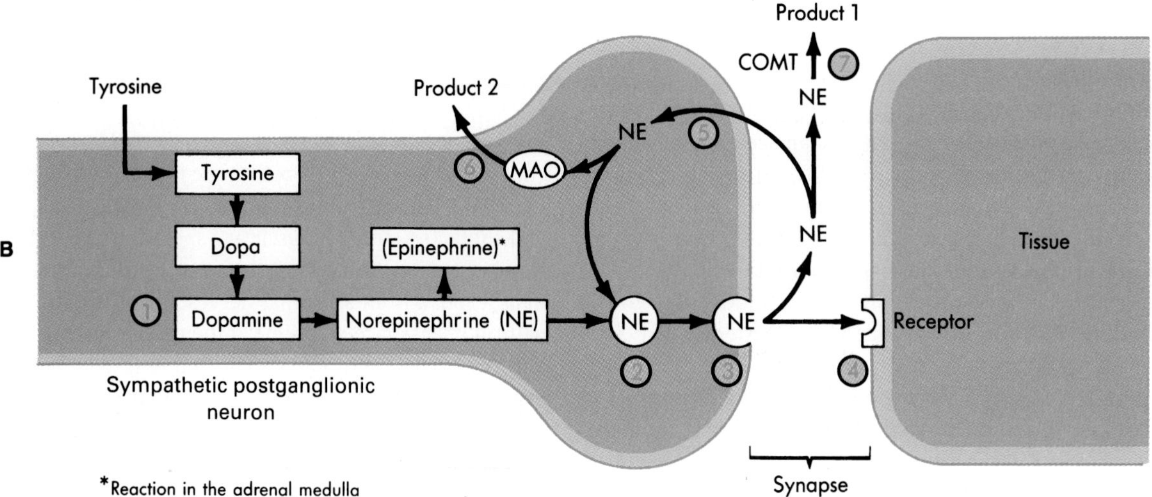

FIGURE 10-1

A, Acetylcholine. *(1)* Choline is taken up by neuron and *(2)* used to synthesize acetylcholine, which *(3)* is stored in vesicles. On stimulation of neuron *(4)*, some vesicles merge with membrane to discharge acetylcholine into synapse, where acetylcholine diffuses to *(5)* its receptor to activate cell, or to *(6)* acetylcholinesterase, enzyme that degrades acetylcholine. Plasma cholinesterases can also degrade acetylcholine. **B,** Norepinephrine. *(1)* Tyrosine is taken into neuron and in three reactions is converted to norepinephrine, which is *(2)* stored in vesicles. On stimulation of neuron *(3)*, some vesicles merge with membrane to discharge norepinephrine into synapse, where it diffuses to *(4)* its receptor to activate cell. Most of norepinephrine is *(5)* taken up by neuron and reused. Some norepinephrine is degraded by *(6)* mitochondrial enzyme monoamine oxidase (MAO) or *(7)* enzyme catechol-O-methyl transferase (COMT) found in most body tissues.

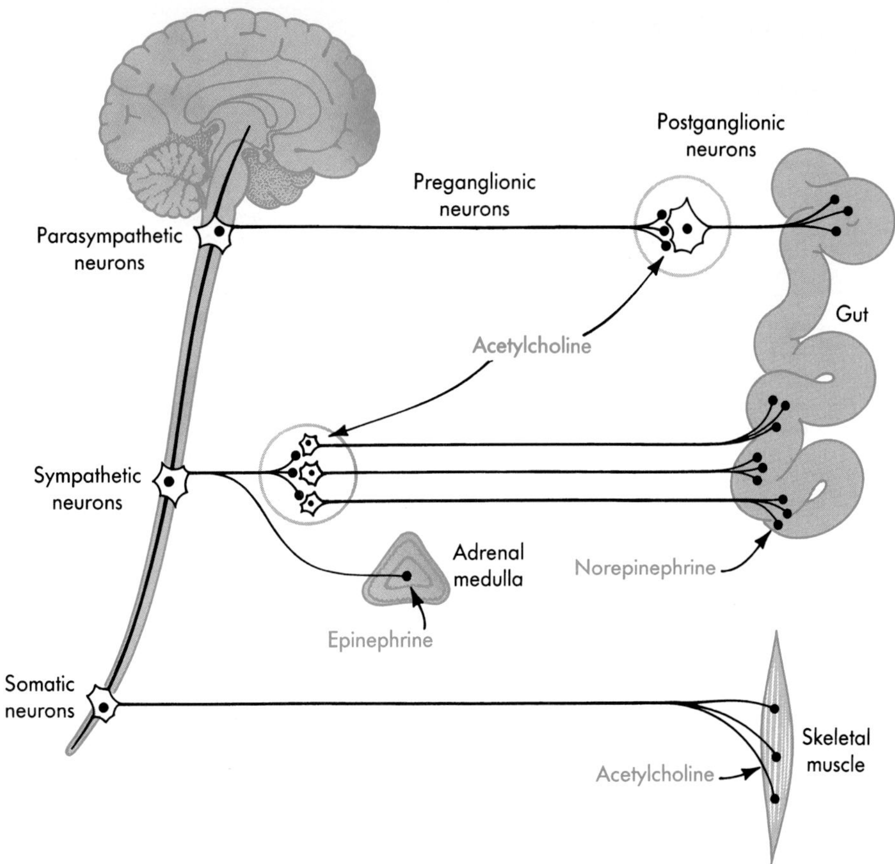

FIGURE 10-2
Neurotransmitters of autonomic nervous system. Acetylcholine and norepinephrine are released from neurons as indicated on adjacent cells. Epinephrine is released from adrenal medulla into blood to act throughout body.

site responses. This activity is highlighted in Table 10-1, in which the prominent effects of the two divisions on key tissues are summarized. For example, the parasympathetic division slows the heart rate, whereas the sympathetic division increases the heart rate. This dual antagonistic innervation is a hallmark of the autonomic nervous system; it allows full control of organ function according to bodily requirements. This antagonism is a result of two distinct kinds of receptors, adrenergic receptors and cholinergic receptors, coexisting on the same organ. In general, activation of the cholinergic receptor produces the opposite cellular response from activation of the adrenergic receptor.

Autonomic Tone

The concept of autonomic tone is also important. Although a minimal but constant release of each neurotransmitter affects each tissue, one branch of the autonomic nervous system is dominant and sets the tone of that tissue to coordinate with other tissues. The sympathetic nervous system provides the dominant tone for the cardiovascular system; therefore the magnitude of cardiac and blood pressure responses reflects predominantly the degree of sympathetic tone, which is itself determined and coordinated within the central nervous system. Parasympathetic control of the cardiovascular system is primarily that of a reflex decelerator system to protect against rapid rises in cardiovascular function. On the other hand, parasympathetic tone is coordinated within certain brain centers to dominate visual, digestive, and eliminatory functions and to determine the intensity of these responses. The role of the sympathetic nervous system is primarily that of an override mechanism to depress these functions in times of stress.

Preganglionic and Postganglionic Neurons

Each efferent division of the autonomic nervous system is a two-neuron system. The first neuron (preganglionic neuron) has its cell body in the brainstem or spinal cord and terminates outside the spinal cord in a special nervous tissue, a ganglion (see Figure 10-2). The first neuron sends a projection out of the spinal cord (preganglionic fiber) that contacts a second neuron (postganglionic neuron) within the ganglion. The neurotransmitter for the synapse in the ganglion is acetylcholine. The second neuron has its cell body in a gan-

TABLE 10-1 Autonomic Nervous System Actions

TISSUE	PARASYMPATHETIC (CHOLINERGIC OR MUSCARINIC) RESPONSE	SYMPATHETIC (ADRENERGIC) RESPONSE
Eye	Constriction (miosis) Accommodation (focus on near objects)	Dilation (mydriasis)
Glands	Increased salivation (copious, watery) Increased tears and secretions of respiratory and gastrointestinal tract	Increased sweating* Increased salivation (thick, contains proteins)
Heart	Decreased rate (negative chronotropy) Decreased strength of contraction (negative inotropy) Decreased conduction velocity through the atrioventricular node (negative dromotropy)	Increased rate (positive chronotropy) Increased strength of contraction (increased contractility or positive inotropy) Increased conduction velocity through atrioventricular node (positive dromotropy)
Bronchioles	Smooth muscle constriction (restricts airways)	Smooth muscle relaxation (opens airways)
Blood vessels	Constriction of vessels in heart (not a prominent effect in humans) Dilation of vessels in salivary gland and erectile tissues	Dilation of vessels in heart and skeletal muscle Constriction of vessels in skin, viscera, salivary gland, erectile tissues, kidney
Gastrointestinal tract		
Smooth muscle	Contraction	Relaxation
Sphincters	Relaxation	Contraction
Urinary bladder		
Fundus	Contraction	Relaxation
Trigone and sphincter	Relaxation	Contraction
Uterus		Contraction
Liver		Glycogenolysis

*Acetylcholine is the neurotransmitter for this sympathetic response. This is the exception to the rule that norepinephrine is the postganglionic neurotransmitter.

glion and by means of a postganglionic fiber innervates an internal organ, usually modifying the action of involuntary muscle such as smooth muscle or cardiac muscle.

Role of Acetylcholine, Norepinephrine, and Epinephrine

The most important pharmacologic difference between the parasympathetic and the sympathetic nervous systems is that the final postganglionic transmitter is different for the two divisions. The preganglionic neurotransmitter at the synapses within the ganglia for both divisions is acetylcholine. However, the parasympathetic nervous system also uses acetylcholine as a postganglionic neurotransmitter. Therefore the parasympathetic nervous system is often called the *cholinergic nervous system.* The sympathetic nervous system uses norepinephrine as the postganglionic transmitter. The sympathetic nervous system has another component, the neurohormone epinephrine. Epinephrine is released from the adrenal medulla as a reaction to stress. The adrenal medulla acts like a postganglionic neuron because it is innervated by a preganglionic fiber and on stimulation releases epinephrine. Epinephrine is carried by the blood throughout the body, where epinephrine not only activates tissue receptors for norepinephrine but also activates additional receptors more specific for epinephrine itself. The synonym for the sympathetic nervous system is the *adrenergic nervous system.* The term *adrenergic* comes from the British word for epinephrine, *adrenaline.* (Norepinephrine is also called *noradrenaline.*) The identity of the neurotransmitter at the various sites of the peripheral nervous system is diagrammed in Figure 10-2.

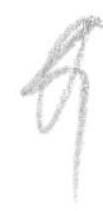

Characteristics of the Autonomic Nervous System

Functional Characteristics

Certain characteristics readily distinguish the parasympathetic and the sympathetic nervous systems functionally. These characteristic functions are listed in Table 10-1. The parasympathetic nervous system has dominant control over "regulatory" processes of the body, whereas the sympathetic nervous system provides immediate adaptation for "fight or flight." Indeed, the easiest way to remember the actions of the sympathetic nervous system (and by contrast the parasympathetic nervous system) is to review the "fight or flight" adaptations: the eyes dilate so that vision is improved even in dim light, the bronchioles dilate to let air flow to and from the lungs more readily, the heart beats faster and with greater strength to supply blood to muscle, the visceral blood vessels are constricted but muscle blood vessels are dilated so that the increased blood flow can meet the demands of cardiac and skeletal muscle for oxygen and nutrients, digestive and excretory processes are slowed, and the liver breaks down stored glycogen to provide glucose for fuel. All these responses represent actions of the sympathetic nervous system.

Anatomic Characteristics

The parasympathetic and the sympathetic nervous systems also differ in their anatomy. The postganglionic neurons of the two systems derive from distinct areas of the spinal cord. The efferent neurons for part of the parasympathetic nervous system arise in the lower area of the brain. These parasympathetic cell bodies include the respiratory and circulatory centers of the medulla, which control cardiovascular and gastrointestinal processes. The remainder of the preganglionic neurons of the parasympathetic nervous system arise from the sacral portion of the spinal cord and allow parasympathetic control of digestive, excretory, and reproductive processes. In contrast, the preganglionic neurons of the sympathetic nervous system all arise in the thoracic and lumbar regions of the spinal cord. Also, the number of postganglionic to preganglionic neurons is highly characteristic of each division. In the parasympathetic nervous system each preganglionic neuron contacts one or two postganglionic neurons so that there is discrete neuronal control over organ function. In contrast, the sympathetic nervous system may have 20 or more postganglionic neurons in contact with each preganglionic neuron so that the action on stimulation of preganglionic neurons is diffuse, in keeping with the "alarm" nature of the sympathetic nervous system.

CENTRAL NERVOUS SYSTEM: COMMENTS

The brain and spinal cord are more complex in their neuronal organization than is the peripheral nervous system. This complexity is necessary because information must be processed rather than just transmitted. This processing is accomplished in two ways. First, a given neuron may send out many axonal projections and thereby form synaptic junctions with many different neurons. This arrangement serves to send a flow of information to several areas for further processing. Second, a given neuron can receive information from more than one neuron. Thus dendrites from a given neuron may have synaptic junctions with axons from many neurons. This arrangement serves to collect information from different sources.

Neurotransmitters

An important difference between the central nervous system and the peripheral nervous system is the number of neurotransmitters believed to exist. In addition to acetylcholine and norepinephrine, the central neurotransmitters that will be encountered in discussing central nervous system pharmacology in later chapters include dopamine, serotonin, epinephrine, histamine, gamma aminobutyric acid (GABA), glycine, and enkephalins. Some neurotransmitters, in particular GABA and glycine, are inhibitory rather than excitatory. The neuronal response to these neurotransmitters is to develop a more negative resting potential with a decreased likelihood of firing rather than to depolarize more readily and fire.

Correlation of Function With Neurotransmitters

In the past few years nerve tracts have been described in the brain and characterized by their neurotransmitter content. These nerve tracts have cell bodies in different areas of the brain to collect information, but the neurons then converge and form synaptic junctions with many neurons in other regions of the brain. Through surgery or chemical destruction of specific nerve tracts it has been possible to associate control of mental and motor behavior with some of the nerve tracts and their neurotransmitters. Examples include a role for acetylcholine and dopamine in the central coordination of muscle movement (see Chapters 56 and 57), a role for dopamine in psychosis (see Chapter 52), a role for dopamine and serotonin in depression (see Chapter 53), and the role of enkephalins in analgesia (see Chapter 31). A current goal in neuropharmacology is to identify how drugs modify behavior through their modification of neurotransmitter synthesis, storage, release, action, and inactivation.

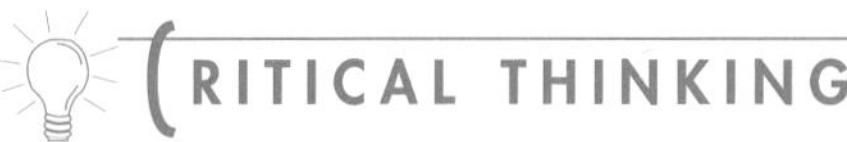

CRITICAL THINKING

APPLICATION

1. What are neurotransmitters?
2. Describe the synthesis, storage, release, and termination of action of acetylcholine and norepinephrine.
3. What are the two divisions of the autonomic nervous system? How are they involved in dual antagonistic innervation and in determining autonomic tone?
4. Describe the neurons of the autonomic nervous system and those of the motor nervous system with respect to anatomy and identity of the neurotransmitter used.

CRITICAL THINKING

1. Describe the "flight or fight" adaptations of the sympathetic nervous system. What objective data would you expect to find?
2. What would be the objective change in heart rate that you might see if you administer a drug that blocks the adrenergic stimulation?
3. What would be the effect on secretions (glands) of administering a drug that blocks the cholinergic stimulation?

CHAPTER 11

Mechanisms of Cholinergic Control

OBJECTIVES

After studying this chapter, you should be able to do the following:

- *Differentiate between muscarinic and nicotinic receptors.*
- *Describe the difference between direct- and indirect-acting cholinomimetic drugs.*
- *Explain the difference between reversible and irreversible acetylcholinesterase inhibitors.*
- *List three therapeutic uses of cholinomimetic drugs.*
- *Describe three kinds of cholinergic antagonists.*
- *Describe six therapeutic uses of muscarinic receptor antagonists (atropine).*

KEY TERMS

extrapyramidal motor effects
irreversible inhibitors
muscarine
reversible inhibitors

CHAPTER OVERVIEW

This chapter is intended to be read twice during a course in pharmacology. The beginner should read the chapter for the mechanisms and therapeutic applications but should not be overly concerned with the drugs given as examples. Later, in a course in pharmacology, the student can return to this chapter to review the mechanism of action of these drugs. The exception is the drug atropine, which is presented in detail in this chapter but not elsewhere.

In this chapter the basis of selective action of cholinergic drugs is explained. The emphasis is on how the therapeutic activities of these drugs arise from their selective action on classes of receptors for acetylcholine. Cholinergic drugs achieve their effects through stimulation and inhibition of receptors. The organ systems most prominently affected include the eye, gastrointestinal system, and muscle.

POPULATIONS OF CHOLINERGIC RECEPTORS AS DEFINED BY DRUG ACTION

In Chapter 10 three distinct populations of receptors for acetylcholine in the peripheral nervous system were presented: receptors on striated muscle at the neuromuscular junction, receptors on postganglionic neurons within the ganglia, and receptors on other innervated tissues.

Muscarinic Receptors

The distinction between acetylcholine receptors is not just anatomic. Chemical differentiation is made with **muscarine,** a chemical found in certain mushrooms, which mimics the effects of acetylcholine by slowing the heart rate or stimulating smooth muscle when applied to those tissues. Muscarine produces no effect when applied to skeletal muscles or to ganglia. Muscarine mimics acetylcholine only at the postganglionic receptors. The parasympathetic postganglionic receptors are therefore called *muscarinic receptors.*

As a cholinergic agonist, muscarine is a laboratory tool. It is encountered clinically only as a toxin responsible for acute mushroom poisoning. (Another kind of mushroom poisoning exists in which symptoms take several hours to appear.) The symptoms of acute mushroom poisoning appear within an hour or so of ingestion and consist of generalized parasympathetic overstimulation that includes glandular stimulation (sweating, tearing, salivation), an overactive gastrointestinal system (nausea, cramps, diarrhea), cardiovascular symptoms (flushed skin and slow heart rate), constricted pupils, and excessive urination.

Nicotinic Receptors

Nicotine, found in tobacco, is another cholinergic agonist. Nicotine is the laboratory agent that mimics the effects of acetylcholine at the skeletal muscle and ganglionic receptors. Therefore the "nicotinic" receptors are the ganglionic and neuromuscular receptors for acetylcholine. Nicotine is not an effective agonist for acetylcholine at the muscarinic receptors.

DIRECT- AND INDIRECT-ACTING CHOLINOMIMETIC DRUGS

Drugs that mimic the action of acetylcholine act by one of two mechanisms: directly, by mimicking acetylcholine (these drugs are chemically related to acetylcholine) or indirectly, by inhibiting acetylcholinesterase (these drugs allow acetylcholine to remain intact longer because its degradation is inhibited).

Acetylcholine itself is not commonly used as a therapeutic agent because it produces too many responses and because it is too rapidly degraded in the blood. Rarely, acetylcholine is used topically in eye surgery. Carbachol (Carbacel) and pilocarpine (Pilocar) are examples of direct-acting cholinomimetic drugs used principally in ophthalmology. Bethanechol (Urecholine) is the only direct-acting cholinomimetic drug used systemically.

Reversible and Irreversible Acetylcholinesterase Inhibitors

The acetylcholinesterase inhibitors can be subdivided into the reversible inhibitors and the irreversible inhibitors. The **reversible inhibitors,** as the name implies, bind to the enzyme reversibly, and therefore the drug effect wears off as the drug is eliminated from the body, usually in a few hours. Examples of reversible inhibitors of acetylcholinesterase include physostigmine (Eserine), pyridostigmine (Mestinon), and neostigmine (Prostigmin).

The **irreversible inhibitors** form a permanent covalent bond with acetylcholinesterase, and the enzyme must be completely replaced before the drug effect wears off, a process requiring days to weeks. The most common examples of irreversible acetylcholinesterase inhibitors are the organophosphate compounds, which include potent drugs for constricting the pupil (miotics): demecarium (Humorsol), echothiophate (Phospholine), and isoflurophate (Floropryl); the insecticides parathion and malathion; and several agents developed for chemical warfare. It is interesting to note that the antidote for poisoning by an irreversible acetylcholinesterase inhibitor is pralidoxime (PAM), which is itself an acetylcholinesterase inhibitor. PAM, however, is able to compete with the enzyme for the phosphate group of the inhibitor, thereby eliminating itself and the inhibitor from the enzyme, reversing the "irreversible" inhibition.

Therapeutic Uses of Cholinomimetic Drugs

Cholinomimetic drugs are used clinically for three effects in the peripheral nervous system:

1. To restore muscle tone in patients with myasthenia gravis or in surgical patients treated with tubocurarine. This is a nicotinic effect at the neuromuscular junction. The drugs used to increase muscle strength are all acetylcholinesterase inhibitors. Cholinomimetic drugs acting at the neuromuscular junction are discussed in Chapters 37 and 69.
2. To constrict the pupil (miosis), a muscarinic effect that is used in ophthalmology. Cholinomimetic drugs administered to act in the eye are described in Chapters 70 and 71.
3. To stimulate an atonic bladder or intestine. This is a muscarinic effect. Cholinomimetic drugs affecting the gastrointestinal system are discussed in Chapter 23.

Table 11-1 reviews the receptor selectivity of cholinomimetic drugs discussed in detail in other chapters. No clinical use is made of drugs stimulating nicotinic receptors of the ganglia. Ganglia are involved in so many responses that their stimulation by drugs is clinically useless.

TABLE 11-1 Receptor Selectivity of Cholinomimetic Drugs at Therapeutic Doses

GENERIC AND TRADE NAMES	MUSCARINIC RECEPTOR*	NICOTINIC† (NEUROMUSCULAR) RECEPTOR	THERAPEUTIC USES
Direct-Acting			
Bethanechol (Urecholine)	+	0	To stimulate atonic bladder or intestine
Carbachol (Carbacel and others)	+ [topical]		To cause miotic reaction (constriction of pupil)
Pilocarpine (Pilocar and others)	+ [topical]		To cause miotic reaction (constriction of pupil)
Indirect-Acting: Reversible Inhibitors of Acetylcholinesterase			
Ambenonium (Mytelase)	(+)	+	To restore muscle strength in myasthenia gravis
Edrophonium (Tensilon)	(+)	+	To diagnose myasthenia gravis; to differentiate myasthenic crisis from cholinergic crisis
Neostigmine (Prostigmin)	+	+	To restore muscle strength in myasthenia gravis To stimulate atonic bladder or intestine
Physostigmine (Eserine)	+ [topical]		To cause miotic reaction (constriction of pupil)
Pyridostigmine (Mestinon)	(+)	+	To restore muscle strength in myasthenia gravis
Indirect-Acting: Irreversible Inhibitors of Acetylcholinesterase			
Demecarium (Humorsol)	+ [topical]	(+) near eye	To cause miotic reaction (constriction of pupil)
Echothiophate (Phospholine)	+ [topical]	(+) near eye	To cause miotic reaction (constriction of pupil)
Isoflurophate (Floropryl)	+ [topical]	(+) near eye	To cause miotic reaction (constriction of pupil)
Pralidoxime (Protopam)	+	+	To reactivate acetylcholinesterase

*+, Stimulation; *(+)*, stimulation, at high concentrations, of muscles near eye; *0*, no stimulation.
†No drugs are used therapeutically that primarily stimulate nicotinic-ganglionic receptors. Stimulation of nicotinic-ganglionic receptors is a toxic effect of cholinomimetic drugs.

CHOLINERGIC ANTAGONISTS

Anticholinergic Drugs

As illustrated in Figure 11-1, each group of receptors for acetylcholine is characterized by a drug that blocks the action of acetylcholine at that type of receptor by occupying the receptor and preventing cholinergic action. Because each class of acetylcholine antagonist acts on a discrete receptor population, clinical use of each class of antagonist differs greatly. Table 11-2 reviews receptor selectivity of cholinergic receptor antagonists discussed in detail in other chapters.

Neuromuscular Receptor Antagonists

Tubocurarine primarily blocks the receptors for acetylcholine at the neuromuscular junction and thereby causes muscular relaxation or paralysis. Antagonists of the neuromuscular cholinergic receptor are used chiefly as an adjunct to anesthetics and will be discussed in Chapter 69.

Ganglionic Receptor Antagonists

The receptors for acetylcholine in the ganglia are blocked by hexamethonium, thus blocking transmission for both parasympathetic and sympathetic impulses. Antagonists like hexamethonium lack much specificity in the response produced. Limited use of drugs antagonizing the action of acetylcholine in the ganglia is made in treating severe cases of hypertension. One such drug, trimethaphan, is discussed in Chapter 13 along with the other antihypertensive drugs.

Muscarinic Receptor Antagonists

Atropine and scopolamine are the prototypes of drugs that block acetylcholine at the muscarinic receptors. These are the parasympathetic postganglionic receptors for acetylcholine on the heart, smooth muscle, and exocrine glands.

Atropine is an alkaloid originally derived from the leaves of the deadly nightshade, or *Atropa belladonna,* which belongs to the potato family. Several other plants also contain atropine and a related drug, scopolamine. These two drugs are often referred to as *belladonna alkaloids.* Many references to the use of these plants as medicinal agents are found in ancient medical literature. To this day, atropine remains the most useful and widely versatile of the antimuscarinic drugs.

Therapeutic Uses

1. Muscarinic receptor antagonists block secretions. Salivation is readily blocked by atropine. Indeed, one classic side effect of atropine is a dry mouth (xerostomia). Secretions in the respiratory tract are also inhibited by atropine. This inhibition of bronchial and salivary secretions is the desired effect when atropine is administered as a preanesthetic agent before surgery. The drying effect of atropine reduces secretions that may be involuntarily aspirated when the patient is drowsy or unconscious. Atropine and related drugs are moderately effective in depressing gastric acid secretion in patients with peptic ulcers. The role of cholinergic antagonists in treating gastrointestinal disorders is discussed in Chapter 23. Large doses of atropine and scopolamine dilate the blood vessels in the skin, especially around the face and particularly in children, thus producing a pronounced blushing. The mechanism for this vasodilation is not clear, but because sweating is inhibited by atropine, this flush may represent a mechanism to dissipate heat and a fever may be noted.

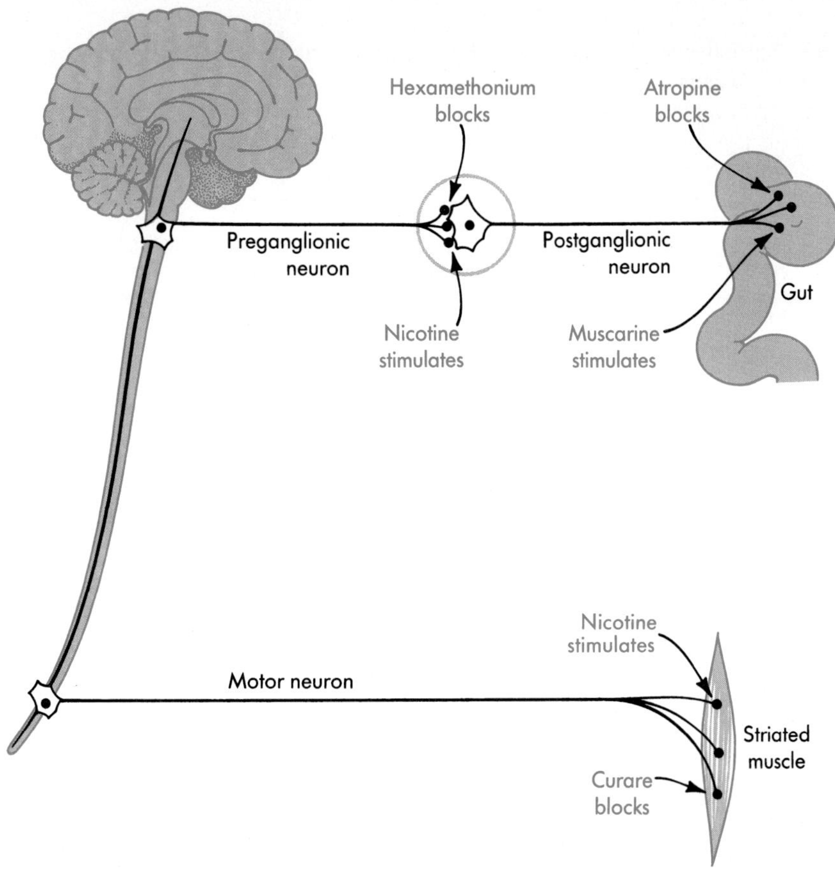

FIGURE 11-1

Acetylcholine is peripheral neurotransmitter at three receptor populations. Each receptor population is characterized by an agonist and an antagonist. Muscarine is agonist and atropine is antagonist of parasympathetic postganglionic (muscarinic) receptors. Nicotine is agonist and hexamethonium is antagonist of parasympathetic preganglionic (nicotinic) receptors. Nicotine is agonist and tubocurarine is antagonist of neuromuscular junction (nicotinic) receptors.

2. These agents depress an overactive gastrointestinal tract. A prominent antimuscarinic effect of atropine is to inhibit the tone and motility of smooth muscle. The gastrointestinal smooth muscle is very sensitive to atropine. Drugs affecting gastrointestinal motility are discussed in Chapter 23.
3. Muscarinic receptor antagonists dilate the eye (mydriasis) and paralyze accommodation (cycloplegia). Atropine is applied by drops to the eye to block the actions of acetylcholine. The result of this antagonism is dilation of the pupil, caused by relaxation of the circular muscles of the iris, and blurred vision, associated with paralysis of accommodation. This mydriasis and cycloplegia allow measurements of lens refraction, examination of the retina, and aid in the healing of some infections. Drugs affecting the eye are discussed further in Chapter 71. Atropine taken orally will also reach the eye. Photophobia (sensitivity to light) as a result of the dilation and blurring of vision (caused by the cycloplegia) are frequent side effects of oral administration of atropine.
4. These agents increase the heart rate. Atropine is administered to increase the heart rate by antagonizing the acetylcholine released by the vagus nerve at the atrioventricular node of the heart (Chapter 19).

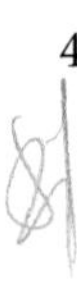

5. These agents relax bronchial smooth muscle. Ipratroprium alleviates bronchospasm, which is common in many pulmonary diseases.
6. These agents treat toxicity of cholinergic agents. The most frequent cause of cholinergic toxicity is overexposure to insecticides such as malathion and parathion, which are organic phosphate acetylcholinesterase inhibitors. Atropine will reverse the muscarinic effects (i.e., salivation, tearing, diarrhea, bradycardia) but will not reverse the neuromuscular paralysis. PAM, which regenerates acetylcholinesterase at all sites, is therefore the drug of choice.

Side effects may occur in addition to therapeutic effects. The side effects of atropine are extensions of the actions just described. The expected cardiovascular effect is an increase in the heart rate (tachycardia), although a slowing of the heart rate (bradycardia) may be noted with low doses administered intravenously. Dilated pupils and blurred vision are accompanied by an intolerance of the eye to light (photophobia) and, sometimes, eye pain. In addition to dry mouth and constipation, patients may experience nausea and vomiting. Urinary hesitancy or retention is common. The skin is dry and flushed, and some patients may develop a fever from the inability to dissipate heat through sweating.

TABLE 11-2 Receptor Selectivity of Cholinergic Receptor Antagonists (Anticholinergics) at Therapeutic Doses*

GENERIC AND TRADE NAMES	MUSCARINIC RECEPTOR	NICOTINIC (GANGLIONIC) RECEPTOR	NICOTINIC (NEUROMUSCULAR) RECEPTOR	THERAPEUTIC USES
Anisotropine	—	0	0	Same as homatropine
Atracurium (Tracrium)	0	0	—	Same as tubocurarine
✣ Atropine	—	0	0	To produce mydriasis (dilated pupil) and cycloplegia (paralysis of accommodation): eye topical; to reduce gastric acid secretion and gastrointestinal motility and tone of bladder and ureter: systemic use
Cyclopentolate (Cyclogyl)	— [topical]			To produce mydriasis and cycloplegia
Gallamine (Flaxedil)	(—)	0	—	Same as tubocurarine
Glycopyrrolate (Robinul)	—	0	0	Same as homatropine
Homatropine methylbromide (Homapin)	—	0	0	To reduce gastrointestinal hypermotility and gastric acidity
Ipratropium (Atrovert)	—	0	0	To relax bronchial smooth muscle
Methantheline (Banthine)	—	0	0	Same as homatropine methylbromide
Methscopolamine (Pamine)	—	0	0	Same as homatropine methylbromide
Metocurine (Metubine)	0	0	—	Same as tubocurarine
Oxyphencyclimine (Daricon)	—	0	0	To control gastrointestinal hypermotility, gastric acidity, and hypermotility of genitourinary and biliary tracts
Pancuronium (Pavulon)	0	0	—	Same as tubocurarine
Propantheline (Pro-Banthine)	—	0	0	Same as oxyphencyclimine
Scopolamine	—	0	0	Same as atropine
Succinylcholine (Anectine)	0	0	—	To depolarize skeletal muscle relaxant
Trimethaphan (Arfonad)	0	—	0	To lower blood pressure in selected cases of hypertensive crisis
Tropicamide (Mydriacyl)	— [topical]			Mydriasis and cycloplegia
✣ Tubocurarine (Tubarine)	0	(—)	—	To relax nondepolarizing skeletal muscle
Vecuronium (Nocuron)	0	0	—	Same as tubocurarine

*—, Inhibition; (—), inhibition at high concentrations; 0, no inhibition.

Other Uses

Drugs that are muscarinic receptor antagonists have other uses unrelated to peripheral muscarinic receptors. Many anticholinergic drugs also have effects in the central nervous system. Some drugs have antitremor activity and are used to relieve certain tremors called **extrapyramidal motor effects** caused by Parkinson's disease, other diseases, and some drugs. Anticholinergic drugs used in the treatment of parkinsonism are discussed in Chapter 56.

Differences in Central Nervous System Effects of Atropine and Scopolamine

Atropine, particularly in an overdose, produces generalized excitement, which in the toxic state may result in hallucinations. In contrast, although scopolamine can produce hallucinations, scopolamine also produces sleepiness, sedation, and amnesia. Scopolamine, unlike atropine, is effective in preventing motion sickness.

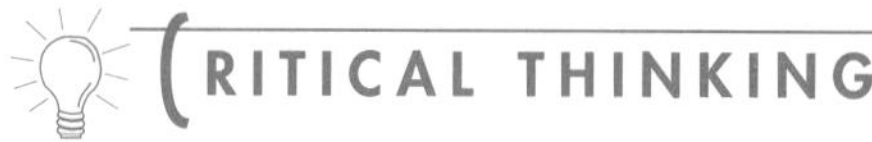

APPLICATION

1. What are muscarine and nicotine, and how do they relate to receptors for acetylcholine?
2. What are the three prototype antagonists, and with which receptor population is each associated?
3. List the five actions of atropine that the nurse would see as useful therapeutically.

CRITICAL THINKING

1. Contrast the mechanisms of a direct- and an indirect-acting cholinomimetic drug. How might this knowledge about a drug influence the frequency of patient assessment?
2. Compare and contrast the three therapeutic uses of cholinomimetic drugs with regard to the receptor stimulated.
3. What atropine-like (anticholinergic) side effects might the nurse anticipate that a patient would experience? How would you assess each effect you have listed?
4. Develop an argument for and against classifying nicotine, as found in cigarettes, as a drug.

CHAPTER 12

Mechanisms of Adrenergic Control

OBJECTIVES

After studying this chapter, you should be able to do the following:

- *Define catecholamine.*
- *Discuss alpha-1, alpha-2, beta-1, and beta-2 adrenergic receptors and the effect of stimulation of these receptors.*
- *Relate the activity of the beta-adrenergic receptors to the "fight or flight" concept mentioned in Chapter 10.*
- *Describe the role of cyclic adenosine monophosphate (AMP) in stimulation of the beta receptors.*
- *Define directly mimicking and indirect-acting adrenergic drugs.*
- *Explain the four mechanisms by which drugs interfere with adrenergic activity.*

KEY TERMS

adrenergic drug
alpha receptors
alpha-1 receptors
alpha-2 receptors
beta receptors
beta-1 receptors
beta-2 receptors
catecholamines
cyclic AMP
signal transduction

CHAPTER OVERVIEW

Like Chapter 11, this chapter is intended to be read as an introduction at the beginning of a course in pharmacology and again later as a review. When reading this chapter as an introduction, pay attention to the mechanisms and their associated effects. The drugs given as examples and their classification by mechanism of action will be of interest when the chapter is reviewed later.

This chapter explains the basis of selective action of adrenergic drugs. Emphasis is given to showing how the therapeutic activities of these drugs arise from their selective action on classes of receptors for norepinephrine and epinephrine. These drugs achieve their effects through stimulation or inhibition of receptors. The organ systems most prominently affected include the eye, bronchial smooth muscle, blood vessel smooth muscle, and the heart.

CATECHOLAMINES AND THEIR RECEPTORS

Naturally Occurring Catecholamines

Dopamine, norepinephrine, and epinephrine are naturally occurring **catecholamines** that function as neurotransmitters and neurohormones. Dopamine is derived from the amino acid tyrosine and is the chemical precursor of norepinephrine:

Tyrosine → Dopamine → Norepinephrine → Epinephrine

All three catecholamines are important neurotransmitters in the central nervous system (CNS). In the autonomic nervous system norepinephrine is the sympathetic postganglionic neurotransmitter, and epinephrine is the neurohormone released from the adrenal medulla in reaction to stress. Dopamine's role in the autonomic nervous system is not completely understood at present.

Classes of Adrenergic Receptors and Responses

Isoproterenol was the first synthetic catecholamine to be studied. The existence of two classes of adrenergic receptors was proposed in the late 1940s to explain the different physiologic effects elicited by norepinephrine, epinephrine, and isoproterenol. **Alpha receptors** are those receptors for which norepinephrine and epinephrine are equally potent, but isoproterenol is less potent. **Beta receptors** are those receptors for which isoproterenol is more potent than or as potent as epinephrine or norepinephrine. Subsequent studies over the years have expanded this classification to include two subtypes in each class: alpha-1, alpha-2, beta-1, and beta-2 receptors.

Alpha-1 Adrenergic Receptors

Alpha-1 receptors account for the primary responses elicited by norepinephrine released from sympathetic postganglionic neurons. Epinephrine is as potent as norepinephrine in stimulating alpha-1 receptors. Physiologic effects resulting from stimulation of alpha-1 receptors include the following:

1. Contraction of the radial muscles of the iris. The radial muscles are arranged like the spokes of a wheel so that contraction causes dilation of the pupil (mydriasis). Adrenergic drugs used therapeutically for this effect are discussed in Chapter 71.
2. Constriction of arterioles and veins, which causes an increase in blood pressure. Adrenergic drugs that are used to raise the blood pressure are discussed in Chapter 16.
3. Contraction of smooth muscle sphincters in the stomach, intestine, and bladder.
4. Contraction of the uterus (in women) and stimulation of ejaculation (in men).
5. Decreased secretions from the pancreas.
6. Breakdown of glycogen in the liver (glycogenolysis) and synthesis of glucose (gluconeogenesis).

Drugs mimicking the adrenergic effects listed in items 3 through 6 are not used therapeutically.

Systemic Effects of Activation of Alpha-1 Adrenergic Receptor

The general role of the alpha-1 receptor is to stimulate contraction of smooth muscle. The most prominent systemic effect is an increase in blood pressure resulting from the constriction of blood vessels, mainly arterioles. The blood vessels controlled by alpha-1 receptors are those that service the internal organs, mucosal surfaces, and skin. Blood pressure is in part a reflection of the degree of constriction of these blood vessels since blood pressure is determined by cardiac output and peripheral resistance to blood flow in blood vessels.

Local Vasoconstriction

Therapeutic use is made of local vasoconstriction by epinephrine and some other alpha-1 adrenergic receptor agonists (stimulants). Nasal decongestion may be achieved by local application of a vasoconstrictive drug (Chapter 29). Drug absorption from parenteral sites is slowed when a drug is injected along with a vasoconstricting agent. Local anesthetics in particular will have a longer duration of action when injected with epinephrine to slow systemic absorption.

Alpha-2 Adrenergic Receptors

The existence of a second class of alpha receptors, the alpha-2 receptors, was experimentally proved in the 1970s. Alpha-2 receptors were found presynaptically on sympathetic neuronal terminals. These presynaptic **alpha-2 receptors** inhibit further release of norepinephrine when they are stimulated. Presynaptic alpha-2 receptors therefore function as a negative feedback system to limit the amount of norepinephrine released from the neuron. Alpha-2 receptors are found on platelets where their activation results in platelet aggregation.

Alpha-2 receptors have also been found on the smooth muscle of the blood vessels that determine blood pressure—the resistance vessels. Like alpha-1 receptors, alpha-2 receptors mediate vasoconstriction to increase resistance and thereby increase blood pressure. Current thought is that the alpha-1 receptors are physically located primarily where sympathetic neurons innervate the blood vessel. Norepinephrine released from the sympathetic postganglionic nerve terminal performs two functions: (1) activation of the alpha-1 receptors on the tissue (usually to elicit smooth muscle contraction) and (2) activation of alpha-2 receptors on the nerve terminal, which inhibits further release of norepinephrine. The alpha-2 receptors on the blood vessel are believed to mediate vasoconstriction to blood-borne dopamine and catecholamine.

Alpha-2 receptors also control blood flow in the skin. Activation of alpha-2 receptors results in vasoconstriction. The fact that cold potentiates activation of alpha-2 receptors may explain the etiology of Raynaud's disease. This condition is characterized by intense cutaneous vasoconstriction leading to pain and, in the extreme, loss of digits. The therapeutic potential of drugs acting at alpha-2 receptors remains to be developed. The antihypertensive drugs clonidine and methyldopa have been found to stimulate the alpha-2 receptor. This action does not account for the antihypertensive effect of these drugs, which has been shown to be a result of their activity in the CNS.

Beta-1 Adrenergic Receptors

The **beta-1 receptors** are stimulated by norepinephrine and by epinephrine, but isoproterenol is a more potent stimulant than either of these drugs. Physiologic responses to activation of beta-1 receptors include the following:

1. Stimulation of the heart. There are three cardiac effects. Activation of the beta-1 receptor in the conducting tissue of the heart speeds the repolarization of the cells. An increase in heart rate (positive chronotropic effect) and an increase in impulse conduction speed (positive dromotropic effect) are the two consequences. Stimulation of the beta-1 receptors in the ventricular muscle increases the force of contraction (positive inotropic response). Drugs acting on beta-1 receptors that are used for stimulating the heart under certain restricted conditions are presented in Chapter 16.
2. Stimulation of the beta-1 receptor of fat tissue induces lipolysis, the breakdown of stored fat. The fatty acids that are released can then be used as energy sources by the heart and liver. No therapeutic use is made of drugs mimicking this adrenergic effect.

Beta-2 Adrenergic Receptors

In contrast to their relative activities on the beta-1 receptors, epinephrine and isoproterenol are equipotent in stimulating **beta-2 receptors,** whereas norepinephrine is a weak stimulant. Physiologic responses to activation of beta-2 receptors include:

1. Dilation of the bronchioles. The relaxation of bronchial smooth muscle decreases airway resistance and makes it easier to breathe. Drugs acting through activation of beta-2 receptors are used to treat patients with restricted airways, primarily caused by asthma or chronic obstructive lung disease. These drugs are discussed in Chapter 27.
2. Relaxation of uterine smooth muscle. Drugs acting through activation of beta-2 receptors, such as ritodrine and terbutaline, are used to stop premature labor by relaxing the pregnant uterus (see Chapter 65).
3. Dilation of the blood vessels in the skeletal muscle, brain, and heart. Activation of these beta-2 receptors causes vasodilation and shunts blood to the skeletal muscle, brain, and heart.
4. Breakdown of glycogen in the liver (glycogenolysis) and synthesis of glucose (gluconeogenesis). Note that these also are alpha-1 adrenergic effects. No therapeutic use is made of these actions.

Systemic Effects of Activation of Beta-Adrenergic Receptor

The value of the responses to two classes of beta receptors can be appreciated by recalling the "fight or flight" nature of the sympathetic nervous system discussed in Chapter 10. The heart rate and cardiac output increase because epinephrine reinforces the action of norepinephrine on the beta-1 receptors. Blood is shunted to muscle, brain, and heart, where stimulation of beta-2 receptors results in vasodilation, and from the skin and abdominal organs, where stimulation of alpha-1 receptors causes vasoconstriction. Epinephrine also stimulates the liver to break down glycogen to glucose, and it stimulates the fat cells to break down lipid to fatty acids to provide readily available energy sources for the body.

Table 12-1 reviews the receptor selectivity of these sympathomimetic drugs, discussed in detail in other chapters.

Signal Transduction: Second-Messenger Concept and Beta Receptor

The identification of hormones and neurotransmitters as molecules released to act at other, sometimes distal sites, raises the question of how the agents effect change once they are bound to their specific receptors. This is the problem of **signal transduction.** The first system to be well characterized was that of the beta receptor.

In the 1950s Earl Sutherland began the work of elucidating how epinephrine causes glycogenolysis (breakdown of glycogen to glucose) in the dog liver. He and his colleagues subsequently showed that epinephrine acts by binding to what we now recognize as the beta-2 receptor on the liver cell membrane. When the beta-2 receptor is occupied, there is a structural change that activates the membrane-bound enzyme adenylate cyclase.

As illustrated in Figure 12-1, this structural change is complex. When occupied, the beta receptor activates a transducer protein called G_s (s = stimulatory protein). G_s then activates adenylate cyclase. The active portion of adenylate cyclase is inside the cell. The enzyme catalyzes the conversion of adenosine triphosphate (ATP) to pyrophosphate (PP) and cyclic adenosine 3′, 5′-monophosphate (**cyclic AMP**). Cyclic AMP is the key to the intracellular action of epinephrine. Epinephrine is the hormone released to signal the cell to act. Cyclic AMP is the "second messenger" that translates the presence of epinephrine at the cell surface to the internal machinery of the cell. Many cyclic AMP molecules are formed as a result of each receptor occupation, amplifying the epinephrine signal. Cyclic AMP produces cellular effects by stimulating other enzymes. The enzymes present in the cell that can be stimulated by cyclic AMP determine the cellular response. In the liver the response is the breakdown of glycogen. In the heart the response is an increase in heart rate, force of contraction, and conduction speed. In smooth muscle the response is relaxation.

Recently it has been shown that the alpha-2 receptor is also linked to the adenylate cyclase. When occupied, the alpha-2 receptor activates a transducer protein called G_i (i = inhibitory protein). G_i then inhibits adenylate cyclase activity. Therefore the beta receptors (beta-1 and beta-2) and the alpha-2 receptor have opposite effects.

Activation of the alpha-1 receptor uses a different second messenger. This activation also initiates interaction

TABLE 12-1 Receptor Selectivity of Adrenergic Drugs

GENERIC AND TRADE NAMES	ALPHA RECEPTOR	BETA-1 RECEPTOR	BETA-2 RECEPTOR	CNS	MAIN THERAPEUTIC USES
Catecholamines					
✣ Dobutamine (Dobutrex)	0	+D	0	0	Increases cardiac contractility with little increase in heart rate or conductivity
Dopamine (Intropin)	(+)I	(+)I	0	0	Dilates renal arteries at low doses by activating dopamine receptors and preventing kidney shutdown in shock
Epinephrine	+D	+D	+	(+)	Treats anaphylactic shock Treats acute asthma attacks Limits systemic absorption of drugs applied for local action
Isoproterenol (Isuprel)	0	+D	+	(+)	Improves bronchodilation for asthma
Norepinephrine, levarterenol (Levophed)	+D	+D	0	(+)	Counteracts hypotension of spinal anesthesia
Noncatecholamines					
✣ Albuterol (Ventolin, Proventil)	0	0	+	0	Improves bronchodilation
Amphetamine	+I	+I	0	+	Depresses appetite Stimulates respiration Counteracts narcolepsy
Bitolterol (Tornalate)	0	0	+	0	Improves bronchodilation
Ephedrine	+I,D	+I,D	+	+	Improves bronchodilation for asthma Reduces congestion (nasal decongestant) Dilates pupil (mydriasis)
Fenoterol (Berotec)	0	0	+	0	Improves bronchodilation
Hydroxyamphetamine (Paredrine)	+I	+I	0	0	Dilates pupil (mydriasis)
Isoetharine (Bronkosol)	0	0	+	0	Improves bronchodilation
Mephentermine (Wyamine)	+I,D	+I,D	0	+	Counteracts hypotension of spinal anesthesia Depresses appetite
Metaproterenol (Alupent, Metaprel)	0	(+)	+	0	Improves bronchodilation
Metaraminol (Aramine)	+I,D	+I,D	0	0	Counteracts hypotension of spinal anesthesia
Methoxamine (Vasoxyl)	+D	0	0	0	Counteracts hypotension of spinal anesthesia Terminates paroxysmal atrial tachycardia
Naphazoline (Privine)	+	0	0	0	Reduces congestion (nasal decongestant)
Oxymetazoline (Afrin)	+	0	0	0	Reduces congestion (nasal decongestant)
Phenylephrine	+D	0	0	0	Reduces congestion (nasal decongestant) Terminates paroxysmal atrial tachycardia
Phenylpropanolamine	+I,D	+I,D	+	(+)	Reduces congestion (nasal decongestant)
Pirbuterol (Maxair)	0	0	+	0	Improves bronchodilation
Procaterol (Pro-Air)	0	0	+	0	Improves bronchodilation
Propylhexedrine (Benzedrex)	+	0	0	0	Reduces congestion (nasal decongestant)
Pseudoephedrine	+I,D	+I,D	+	(+)	Reduces congestion (nasal decongestant)
Ritodrine (Yutopar)	0	0	+	0	Stops premature labor
Terbutaline (Brethine, Bricanyl)	0	0	+	0	Improves bronchodilation
Tetrahydrozoline (Tyzine)	+	0	0	0	Reduces congestion (nasal decongestant)
Xylometazoline (Otrivin)	+	0	0	0	Reduces congestion (nasal decongestant)

+I, Indirectly acting (releases norepinephrine); *+D,* directly acts on receptor; *(+),* effect is modest except at high concentration; *0,* no effect.

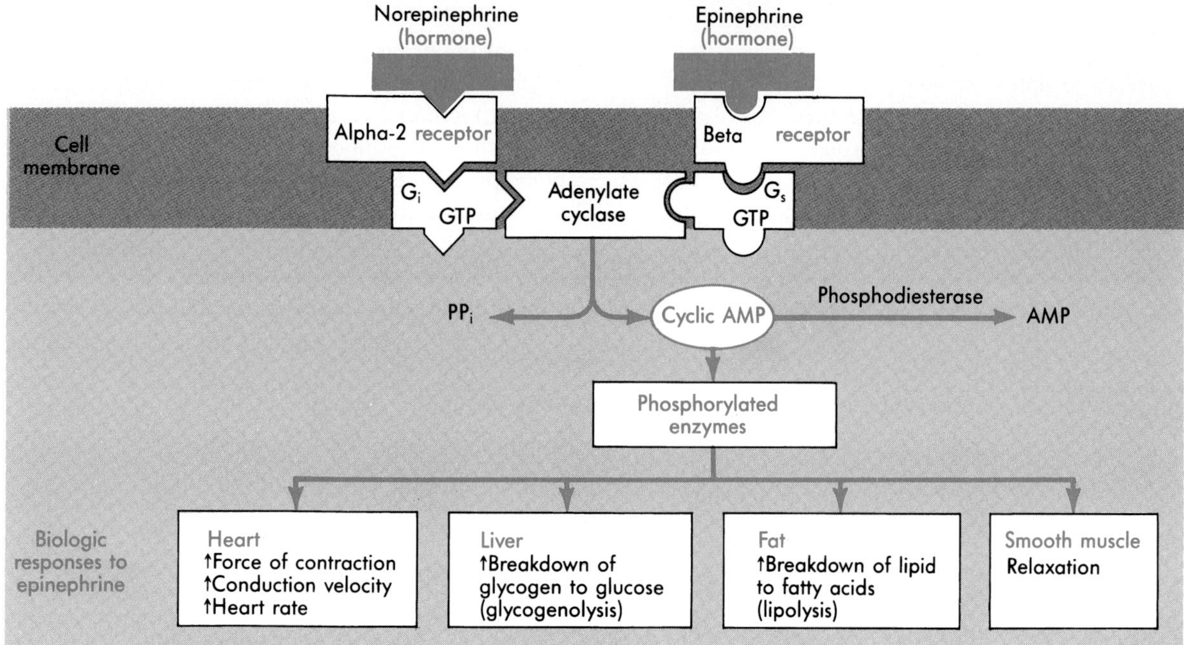

FIGURE 12-1

Second-messenger concept. Binding of hormone at cell surface initiates a series of reactions that modify activity through phosphorylation of key enzymes and thereby modify cellular responses. Cyclic AMP is second messenger because it carries message that hormone is at cell surface and translates this message into action by stimulating a phosphorylating enzyme (cyclic AMP–dependent protein kinase). Cellular responses to epinephrine characteristic for a given organ are given as examples of biologic responses mediated through cyclic AMP. Note that while beta-adrenergic receptor acts through a stimulatory G protein *(G_s)* to promote production of cyclic AMP, alpha-2 adrenergic receptor acts through an inhibitory G protein *(G_i)* to suppress production of cyclic AMP. ATP is substrate for adenylate cyclase, with cyclic AMP and pyrophosphate *(PPi)* being products. G proteins are regulated by binding and hydrolysis of guanosine triphosphate (GTP).

with a G-protein, but the result is activation of mechanisms that elevate intracellular calcium. The increased cytosolic concentration of calcium changes the activity of certain enzymes. The changes in enzymatic activities account for the actions produced by the activation of the alpha-1 receptor.

Two more features of the cyclic AMP system need to be highlighted. First, epinephrine is not the only hormone that stimulates the formation of cyclic AMP. Most polypeptide hormones, discussed in Chapter 58, are known to work through cyclic AMP. The exceptions are insulin, growth hormone, and prolactin. Each hormone has its specific receptor on its target tissues. This is why each hormone can have tissue-specific actions while using the same second-messenger system. Second, cyclic AMP is rapidly degraded by the enzyme phosphodiesterase to 5′-adenosine monophosphate (AMP). A few drugs have been identified that inhibit phosphodiesterase and thereby produce elevated cyclic AMP concentrations. The main drug of this type is theophylline and its dimer, aminophylline. Such drugs are used to produce vasodilation in cerebral ischemia and, more important, to treat asthma by promoting bronchial dilation (Chapter 27).

Therapeutic Uses and Features of Adrenergic Drugs

The therapeutic use of an **adrenergic drug** depends on whether it acts on alpha-1, beta-1, or beta-2 receptors. A variety of drugs have been synthesized that are relatively specific for activating a given receptor type and thereby directly mimic some portion of norepinephrine or epinephrine action. Other adrenergic drugs act by a second mechanism of action. These are indirect-acting adrenergic drugs, which act by causing the sympathetic postganglionic neurons to release norepinephrine. This increased amount of norepinephrine activates alpha-1, alpha-2, and beta-1 receptors. Drugs such as amphetamine, ephedrine, and mephentermine also act in the CNS, which both determines and limits their use. The catecholamines are relatively or completely ineffective when taken orally because they are rapidly destroyed in the gastrointestinal tract or by the liver, whereas many noncatecholamines can be taken orally.

DRUGS INHIBITING ADRENERGIC ACTIVITY

Table 12-2 lists the drugs that interfere with peripheral adrenergic activity and the therapeutic use of these drugs. Several different drug mechanisms interfere with adrenergic activity. These mechanisms include:

1. Blockade of alpha-adrenergic receptors
2. Blockade of beta-adrenergic receptors
3. Depletion of peripheral neuronal stores of norepinephrine
4. Inhibition of peripheral sympathetic activity through an action in the CNS

Each of these mechanisms will be discussed further in regard to the spectrum of physiologic effects produced.

Blockade of Alpha-Adrenergic Receptors

Each of the drugs phenoxybenzamine, phentolamine, and prazosin acts selectively to antagonize norepinephrine at the alpha-1 receptors. Infusion of one of these drugs into a person with normal blood pressure produces little change in blood pressure as long as the person is lying down. However, any sudden shift to the upright position causes orthostatic (postural) hypotension because the blockade of the alpha-1 receptors prevents the vasoconstriction necessary to redistribute blood flow. Therefore in orthostatic hypotension the

TABLE 12-2 Drugs Inhibiting Adrenergic Receptor Activity

GENERIC AND TRADE NAMES	ALPHA RECEPTOR	BETA-1 RECEPTOR	BETA-2 RECEPTOR	CNS	MAIN THERAPEUTIC USES
Alpha-Adrenergic Receptor Antagonists					
Phenoxybenzamine (Dibenzyline)	—	0	0	0	Treats hypertension related to pheochromocytoma Treats vasospastic disorders of digits (Raynaud's syndrome)
Phentolamine (Regitine)	—	0	0	0	Treats hypertension related to pheochromocytoma
Prazosin (Minipress)	—	0	0	0	Treats chronic hypertension
Terazosin (Hytrin)	—	0	0	0	Treats chronic hypertension
Beta-Adrenergic Receptor Antagonists					
Acebutolol (Sectral)	0	—	0	0	Treats chronic hypertension
Atenolol (Tenormin)	0	—	0	0	Treats chronic hypertension Treats angina prophylactically
Betaxolol (Betoptic)	0	—	0	0	Treats glaucoma (ophthalmic use)
Carteolol (Cartrol)	0	—	—	0	Treats chronic hypertension
Esmolol (Brevibloc)	0	—	0	0	Controls supraventricular tachycardia
Labetalol (Trandate, Vescal)	—	—	—	0	Treats chronic hypertension Treats angina prophylactically
Levobunolol (Betagan)	0	—	—	0	Treats glaucoma (ophthalmic use)
✤ Metoprolol (Lopressor)	0	—	0	—	Treats chronic hypertension Treats angina prophylactically
Nadolol (Corgard)	0	—	—	—	Treats chronic hypertension Treats angina prophylactically
Oxprenolol (Trasicor)	0	—	—	0	Treats chronic hypertension
Penbutolol (Levatol)	0	—	—	0	Treats chronic hypertension Treats angina prophylactically
Pindolol (Visken)	0	—	—	—	Treats chronic hypertension Treats angina prophylactically
Propranolol (Inderal)	0	—	—	—	Treats chronic hypertension Treats angina prophylactically Treats cardiac arrhythmias Treats migraine prophylactically
Sotalol (Sotacor)	0	—	—	0	Treats chronic hypertension
Timolol (Blocadren, Timoptic)	0	—	—	0	Treats chronic hypertension Treats glaucoma (ophthalmic use)
Drugs Depleting Neuronal Stores of Norepinephrine					
Guanadrel (Hylorel)	I	I	I	0	Treats severe chronic hypertension
Guanethidine (Ismelin)	I	I	I	0	Treats severe chronic hypertension
Reserpine (Serpasil)	I	I	I	—	Treats chronic hypertension
Drugs Inhibiting Sympathetic Activity Through CNS Action					
Methyldopa (Aldomet)	−CNS	0	0	—	Treats chronic hypertension
✤ Clonidine (Catapres)	−CNS	0	0	—	Treats chronic hypertension
Guanabenz (Wytensin)	−CNS	0	0	—	Treats chronic hypertension
Guanfacine (Tenex)	−CNS	0	0	—	Treats chronic hypertension

—, Inhibition; *0*, no effect; *I*, indirect inhibition resulting from depletion of norepinephrine stores; *−CNS*, decrease in peripheral sympathetic tone through action in central nervous system.

blood pools in the legs and drains from the head, causing fainting.

Other effects characteristic of blockade of the alpha-1 receptors include a pinpoint pupil (miosis), nasal stuffiness, or inhibition of ejaculation (in men).

The uses and pharmacokinetics of the alpha-1 receptor antagonists in the treatment of hypertension are discussed in Chapter 13.

Blockade of Beta-Adrenergic Receptors

Nonselective Antagonists

The physiologic effects of beta-receptor antagonists can be anticipated by considering the functions of the beta receptors. In the healthy person blockade of the beta-1 receptors in the heart causes little change at rest but limits the increase in cardiac functions normally elicited by exercise and hypertension. Conditions improved by beta-1 receptor blockade include angina, hypertension, and some cardiac arrhythmias. Recently, propranolol, metoprolol, and timolol have been found to be effective treatment for patients with angina to prevent recurrent heart attacks.

Beta-receptor antagonists are also effective in treating hypertension. However, when a beta-receptor antagonist is given with a vasodilator drug, the beta-receptor antagonist inhibits the reflex activation of the heart caused by the drop in blood pressure. For this reason a beta-receptor antagonist combined with a vasodilator is especially effective in treating hypertension. The use of beta-receptor antagonists in the therapy of hypertension is discussed in Chapter 13.

Blockade of beta-2 receptors limits bronchiole dilation and therefore can severely compromise pulmonary function in patients with asthma. This effect has led to the development of beta-1 selective antagonists (cardioselective antagonists) such as atenolol (Tenormin) and metoprolol (Lopressor).

Propranolol (Inderal) was the first beta-receptor antagonist approved for clinical use in the United States. It blocks both beta-1 and beta-2 receptors and is used to treat hypertension, angina, and cardiac arrhythmias. In addition, propranolol is an effective prophylactic in the treatment of migraine headaches, although the mechanisms involved are not clear.

Nadolol (Corgard) was introduced in 1980 as a nonselective beta-receptor antagonist for use in treating angina and hypertension. Additional nonselective beta-receptor antagonists that have been released for clinical use in the United States include labetalol (Trandate, Vescal), penbutolol (Levatol), and pindolol (Visken). Labetolol has alpha- and beta-antagonist action.

Timolol (Timoptic), betaxolol (Betoptic), levobunolol (Betagan), and metipranolol (OptiPranolol) are beta-receptor antagonists that are effective in treating glaucoma by reducing the production of aqueous humor in the eye. They are discussed with other ophthalmic drugs in Chapter 71. Timolol is also used as an antianginal agent.

Depletion of Peripheral Neuronal Stores of Norepinephrine

Guanethidine (Ismelin) and reserpine (Serpasil) are antihypertensive drugs that deplete norepinephrine from peripheral neurons.

Guanethidine is taken up into the postganglionic sympathetic nerve terminals, where it then prevents the release of norepinephrine. After several days the neuronal content of norepinephrine is depleted. Guanadrel is a more recent drug that has the same mechanism of action.

Reserpine also causes a depletion of norepinephrine stores not only in the periphery but also in the brain. The central action of reserpine is believed to contribute in a major way to the depression of sympathetic tone with this agent.

Reserpine and guanethidine are useful in treating chronic hypertension (Chapter 13) and Raynaud's disease (Chapter 15).

Inhibition of Peripheral Sympathetic Activity Through Central Nervous System Action

The CNS controls sympathetic activity, although the mechanism of this control is not understood. The preceding section indicated that part of the effect of reserpine is believed to be mediated through an action in the CNS. It is now recognized that two other antihypertensive drugs, clonidine (Catapres) and methyldopa (Aldomet), decrease sympathetic tone mainly through an action in the CNS. Guanabenz (Wytensin) and guanfacine (Tenex) are more recent antihypertensive drugs that have the same mechanism. The role of these drugs in the treatment of hypertension is described in Chapter 13.

CRITICAL THINKING

APPLICATION

1. Which are the three naturally occurring catecholamines, and where are they found?
2. What does the "second messenger" (cyclic AMP) do?
3. What are the four major drug mechanisms that inhibit adrenergic activity? What therapeutic use is made of each of these actions?

CRITICAL THINKING

1. What physiologic actions does the nurse associate with stimulation of the alpha-1 adrenergic receptor? Of the alpha-2 adrenergic receptor? Of the beta-1 adrenergic receptor? Of the beta-2 adrenergic receptor? What changes in objective data would you expect to see with each of these?
2. Compare and contrast the mechanism of action of direct-acting and indirect-acting sympathomimetic drugs.

SECTION IV

Drugs Affecting the Cardiovascular and Renal Systems

This section is divided into two groups: drugs that affect circulation and blood pressure, Chapters 13 through 17, and drugs that affect the heart, Chapters 18 and 19.

CHAPTER 13 *Antihypertensive Drugs* presents antihypertensive drugs according to their mechanism of action. The latest guidance in the use of antihypertensive agents is thoroughly discussed and integrated into the presentation.

CHAPTER 14 *Diuretics* covers diuretics, which are frequently used to help control blood pressure and treat conditions marked by fluid retention.

CHAPTER 15 *Antianginals and Other Vasodilators* focuses on the drugs used to treat angina and those used chiefly to treat impaired peripheral vascular circulation.

CHAPTER 16 *Drugs to Treat Shock* details the drugs used to reverse the condition of shock. Together Chapters 15 and 16 cover the pharmacologic aspects of circulation.

CHAPTERS 17—*Fluids and Electrolytes,* 18—*Cardiac Glycosides and Other Drugs for Congestive Heart Failure,* and 19—*Drugs to Control Cardiac Arrhythmias* are each devoted to a given area of therapeutics for which the pharmacologic factors are distinctly focused on a physiologic process: fluids and electrolytes, cardiac glycosides and the treatment of congestive heart failure, and antiarrhythmic drugs.

CHAPTER 13

Antihypertensive Drugs

OBJECTIVES

After studying this chapter, you should be able to do the following:

- *Discuss the factors that control blood pressure.*
- *List lifestyle modifications that may be used to help reduce blood pressure.*
- *Discuss the drug classes that may be used for initial drug therapy for hypertension.*
- *Describe modifications in antihypertensive therapy that may be needed for special populations: African-Americans, older adults, pregnant women, and patients with coexisting cardiovascular disease.*
- *Develop a plan of nursing care for patients who receive one or more of the following drug groups: beta-blockers, alpha-1 blockers, sympatholytics, centrally acting antihypertensives, angiotensin converting enzyme inhibitors, calcium channel blockers, other vasodilators, and alpha-1 and alpha-2 blockers.*
- *Develop a plan of nursing care for a patient with a hypertensive emergency being treated with diazoxide, sodium nitroprusside, or trimethaphan.*
- *Develop a teaching plan for a patient who has orthostatic hypotension or who needs to reduce sodium intake.*

KEY TERMS

angiotensin converting enzyme (ACE) inhibitors
beta-blockers
calcium channel blockers
essential hypertension
hypertensive emergency
vasodilator

CHAPTER OVERVIEW

Hypertension is generally defined as a resting systolic blood pressure >140 mm Hg or a diastolic blood pressure >90 mm Hg, or both, in an adult. In the United States it is estimated that this condition may apply to 50 million persons. High blood pressure reflects an increased tone of the arteries and arterioles. Renal, endocrine, or neurogenic diseases are found to be the cause of hypertension in 10% of patients with hypertension. The hypertension in these patients is treated by focusing on its cause. No primary cause of the hypertension can be found in the remaining 90% of patients with hypertension; this condition of unknown origin is called **essential hypertension.**

The patient with hypertension may have no symptoms of this disease but will have an increased risk of stroke, blindness, and heart and renal disease after 10 or more years of sustained high blood pressure that produces vascular and organ damage. The prevalence of hypertension is higher in older adults than in younger adults, higher in men than in women during the young adult and early middle-age range, but higher in women than men from middle age onward. Hypertension is more common in African-Americans, in those from the southeastern United States, and in poor and less educated individuals.

Effective drug therapy for hypertension has been available for two decades. Throughout this period, for patients controlling their hypertension with therapy, mortality from coronary heart disease has decreased by 50% and that from stroke by 57%. Also during this time, evidence from epidemiologic studies has accumulated to show that a systolic blood pressure >120 mm and/or a diastolic blood pressure >80 mm is associated with increased risks or morbidity, disability, and mortality. This chapter presents the drugs used to control hypertension and the rationale for their use.

Therapeutic Rationale: Hypertension

Physiology of Hypertension

The major factors that regulate blood pressure are diagrammed in Figure 13-1. These factors center around those that influence the circulating volume through adjustments of body salt and water (renal mechanisms) and those that influence the activity of the heart and blood vessels (cardiovascular mechanisms).

Renal Mechanisms

The kidney plays an important role in maintaining blood pressure through control of the salt and water content of the body (Chapter 14). A decrease in blood pressure stimulates the release of renin from the kidney. Renin release is partly controlled by beta-adrenergic receptors. Renin is a proteolytic enzyme that acts on a protein in the blood to produce the peptide angiotensin I. Angiotensin I is rapidly converted to angiotensin II, a small peptide that is a potent vasoconstrictor and therefore increases blood pressure. Angiotensin II also acts on the adrenal cortex to stimulate the secretion of aldosterone.

Aldosterone is the mineralocorticoid hormone that acts on the kidney to decrease the excretion of sodium and to increase potassium excretion. The resulting sodium retention expands the plasma and extracellular fluid volumes, which contribute to the elevation of blood pressure.

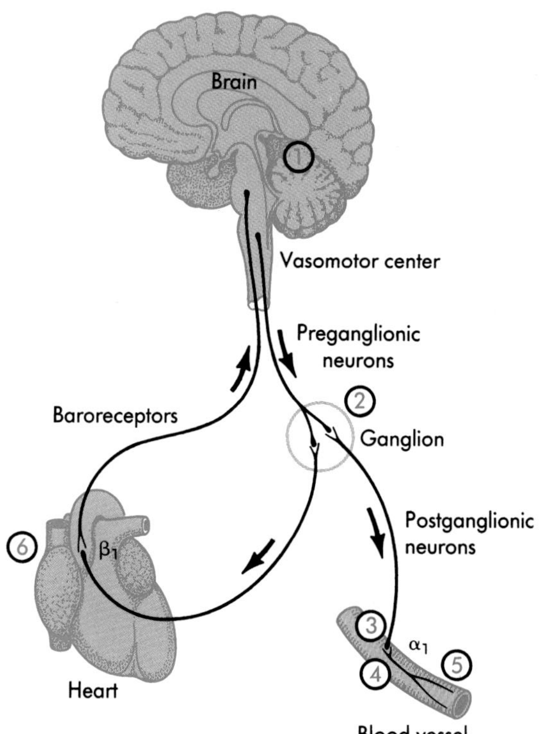

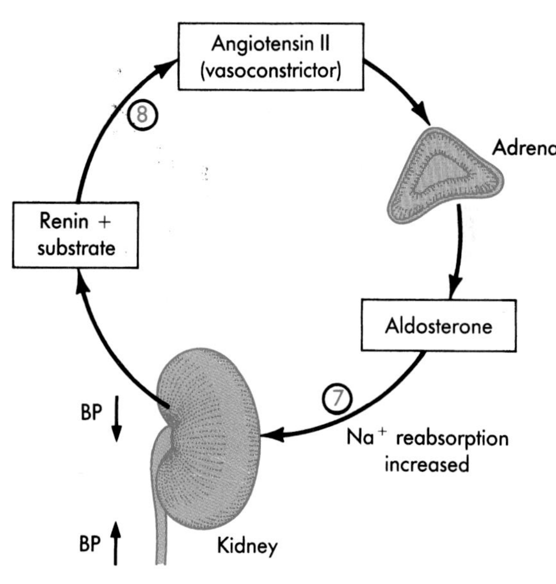

FIGURE 13-1
Numbers in diagram refer to mechanisms by which various antihypertensive drugs appear to act. *1*, Drugs acting centrally to depress sympathetic tone: clonidine, methyldopa, guanabenz, reserpine. *2*, Drug blocking ganglionic receptor for acetylcholine: trimethaphan. *3*, Drugs interfering with norepinephrine synthesis, storage, or release: guanethidine, guanadrel, reserpine. *4*, Drugs (a) blocking alpha-adrenergic receptor: prazosin, phenoxybenzamine, phentolamine, labetalol or (b) blocking angiotensin II receptor: losartan. *5*, Drugs directly dilating smooth muscle: hydralazine, minoxidil, sodium nitroprusside, diazoxide, calcium channel blockers. *6*, Drugs decreasing cardiac output: beta-blockers, calcium channel blockers. *7*, Drugs blocking sodium reabsorption: diuretics. *8*, Drugs inhibiting angiotensin II formation: ACE inhibitors.

Cardiovascular Mechanisms

Within the blood vessels, the blood pressure depends on the cardiac output and the resistance to blood flow in the blood vessels. Baroreceptors in the aorta and carotid sinus monitor the blood pressure and send the information to the brain. The brain integrates this information and adjusts the heart rate and resistance of the blood vessels, largely through the sympathetic nervous system, to fine-tune the blood pressure. The vasomotor center in the medulla is a major center in the brain that controls blood pressure. As the neurotransmitter of the sympathetic nervous system, norepinephrine raises blood pressure by stimulating the beta-1 receptors of the heart to increase cardiac output and by stimulating the alpha-1 receptors of the blood vessels, causing constriction and increasing resistance to blood flow. By contrast, in the central nervous system (CNS), norepinephrine is the neurotransmitter for nerve tracts that ultimately decrease blood pressure.

Atrial natriuretic factor (ANF) is a group of peptides released from the atrial tissue of the heart in response to stretch of the tissue. The primary effect of ANF is to increase diuresis and sodium excretion. Secondarily, ANF decreases renin release and thereby the level of angiotensin II and aldosterone. ANF also inhibits the release of vasopressin from the hypothalamus. The study of ANF is relatively new, and no current drug therapy is based on the actions of ANF.

Therapeutic Options for Hypertension

Lifestyle Modifications

Habits and lifestyle affect blood pressure. Counseling the hypertensive individual to control weight and sodium intake, to give up smoking and excessive alcohol consumption, and to exercise regularly is important in blood pressure management. Altering these habits and lifestyle risk factors can reduce blood pressure. For the mildly hypertensive individual, these changes may be the only treatment needed. Even if drug therapy is required, modification of these lifestyle factors will be additive and reduce the level of drug intervention required.

Antihypertensive Therapy

There has been an explosion of new drugs for the treatment of hypertension. Table 13-1 outlines those drugs that have a role in the treatment of hypertension. Agents that depress sympathetic tone encompass several adrenergic mechanisms because adrenergic drugs can lower blood pressure by decreasing the activity of the sympathetic nervous system peripherally or centrally. (Drug mechanisms that modify the activity of the sympathetic nervous system are reviewed in Chapter 12.) A variety of agents also alter vascular tone. Figure 13-1 shows the sites of action of antihypertensive drugs.

Choices for Drug Therapy

The Joint National Committee on Detection, Evaluation, and Treatment of High Blood Pressure updated and published its recommendations in 1993. Classification of hypertension has been changed from mild, moderate, and severe to four stages:

CLASSIFICATION OF BLOOD PRESSURE FOR ADULTS (>18 YR)

Category	Systolic	Diastolic
Normal	<130	<85
High normal	130-139	85-89
Stage 1	140-159	90-99
Stage 2	160-179	100-109
Stage 3	180-209	110-119
Stage 4	≥210	≥120

Treatment of hypertension has become more aggressive. Accumulated evidence shows that even what was formally labeled "mild" hypertension is associated with an increased incidence of cardiovascular disease and stroke, especially when other cardiovascular risk factors are present. For instance, a greater incidence of sudden death, usually caused by electrical dysfunction of the heart associated with poor coronary circulation or by myocardial infarction is seen among patients having both "mild" hypertension and atherosclerosis. Other risk factors include smoking, high cholesterol values (above 185 mg/dl), high lipid levels, abnormal glucose tolerance test, electrocardiographic abnormalities, and a family history of atherosclerosis. For individuals with these risk factors, even hypertension in the high normal range with a systolic blood pressure of 130 to 139 mm Hg and a diastolic blood pressure of 85 to 89 mm Hg should be carefully monitored, with emphasis on lifestyle modifications to control blood pressure.

Initial Drug Therapy

Drug therapy is generally advised for patients who fall in stage 1 or stage 2 hypertension, especially those with risk factors and with a blood pressure remaining at or above 140/90 mm Hg for 6 months despite attempts to change lifestyle factors. In general, drug therapy for hypertension is standard. Yet therapy is changing as more is being learned about hypertension and as new drugs become available. Current drug therapy is based on a treatment algorithm in which drug classes are substituted or added until blood pressure is brought under control.

Initial drug therapy begins with the administration of a single drug from one of several drug classes. Diuretics and beta-blockers are the preferred classes because these have been proven effective in many clinical trials. Other drug classes may be used, especially when beta-blockers and diuretics are ineffective. These drug classes include angiotensin converting enzyme, or ACE, inhibitors, calcium antagonists, alpha-1 receptor blockers and the alpha beta-blocker.

The most common choice is an oral diuretic, usually a thiazide or thiazide-like diuretic. Hydrochlorothiazide and chlorthalidone have been found effective in clinical trials. Diuretics are especially effective as single agents for African-American patients with hypertension. Diuretics inhibit renal tubular reabsorption, causing diuresis that leads to reduction of body salt and water (extracellular fluid). The loss of extracellular fluid is associated with reduction of arterial blood pressure, but the mechanism of this hypotensive action re-

TABLE 13-1 Categories of Antihypertensive Drugs

TYPE	DRUGS	ANTIHYPERTENSIVE ACTION
Drugs for Initial Therapy		
Diuretics		
Thiazide-type	Chlorthalidone Hydrochlorothiazide See also Table 14-1.	Reduces body salt and water; decreases arterial blood pressure; may reduce plasma volume. Often a diuretic alone is effective as antihypertensive agent. Diuretics counteract fluid retention caused by other antihypertensive drugs and/or enhance action of most antihypertensive drugs.
Loop	Bumetanide Ethacrynic acid ✤ Furosemide	More potent than thiazide-type. May need higher doses for patients with renal impairment or congestive heart failure.
Potassium-sparing	Amiloride Spironolactone Triamterene	Used mainly in combination with other diuretics to reverse or avoid hypokalemia; may cause hyperkalemia when combined with potassium supplements or ACE inhibitors.
Adrenergic inhibitors		
Beta-blocker	Atenolol Betaxolol Bisoprolol Metoprolol Nadolol ✤ Propranolol Timolol	Decreases cardiac output; decreases plasma renin activity. Preferred for patients with angina or after a heart attack. Atenolol, betaxolol, bisoprolol, and metoprolol are cardioselective and at low doses will not aggravate asthma.
Beta-blocker with intrinsic sympathetic activity	Acebutolol Carteolol Penbutolol Pindolol	Mechanism is same as other beta-blockers. Intrinsic sympathetic activity is advantage for patients with bradycardia and those with diabetes mellitus because they have fewer metabolic side effects.
Alpha beta-blocker	Labetalol	Acts like beta-blocker with alpha-1 blockade for vasodilation. May cause postural effects.
Alpha-1 blocker	Doxazosin Prazosin Terazosin	Blocks postsynaptic alpha-1 receptors on arterioles to cause vasodilation. Orthostatic hypotension is common. Used less commonly alone; more often combined with diuretic.
Angiotensin converting enzyme (ACE) inhibitors	Benazepril ✤ Captopril Enalapril Fosinopril Lisinopril Quinapril Ramipril	Blocks formation of angiotensin II, a potent vasoconstrictor, and prevents degradation of vasodilator bradykinin and certain prostaglandins. Especially useful in treating congestive heart failure and renovascular hypertension associated with diabetes and scleroderma.
Calcium antagonists (calcium channel blockers)	Amlodipine Diltiazem Felodipine Isradipine Nicardipine Nifedipine ✤ Verapamil	Blocks inward movement of calcium ion across cell membranes, resulting in smooth muscle relaxation (vasodilation). Diltiazem and verapamil also block slow calcium channels in heart.
Supplemental Antihypertensive Agents		
Centrally acting alpha-2 agonist	✤ Clonidine Guanabenz Guanfacine Methyldopa	Stimulates alpha-2 receptors in brain that inhibit peripheral sympathetic pathways.
Drugs interfering with storage and/or release of norepinephrine	Guanadrel Guanethidine Reserpine and related drugs	Guanadrel and guanethidine inhibit catecholamine release from peripheral neurons; reserpine depletes tissue stores of catecholamines.
Direct vasodilators	Hydralazine Minoxidil	Acts directly on vascular smooth muscle; not recommended in presence of other cardiovascular disease.

mains obscure. This hypotensive effect is not seen in normotensive patients. The volume depletion also produces a reduction in plasma volume, although it is not clear that this reduction persists after the first month of therapy. In addition, many antihypertensive drugs cause fluid retention, an action that limits their antihypertensive effect. Diuretics are therefore commonly given with other antihypertensive drugs. Diuretics are discussed in Chapter 14.

Instead of a diuretic, a beta-blocker may be given as the first drug. Hypertensive individuals with high plasma renin levels are especially responsive to beta-blockers and generally unresponsive to diuretics. This situation is so because beta-blockers inhibit the release of renin from the kidney. Unfortunately, renin levels cannot be reliably or readily determined at present. In general, however, Caucasian hypertensive patients in the younger age groups have high renin levels, whereas African-American hypertensive patients in the older age groups have low renin levels. A beta-blocker is also indicated for patients who have coronary artery disease. Beta-blockers have been shown to have a protective effect against sudden death in individuals who have had a heart attack, whereas diuretics may, through a lowering of potassium levels, increase the vulnerability of the compromised heart to sudden failure.

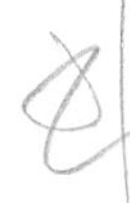

Calcium channel blockers are another choice as initial therapy. These agents act by preventing the entry of calcium into the smooth muscle layer of blood vessels. This action diminishes the contraction of the blood vessels and results in vasodilation. Calcium channel blockers decrease hypertension without causing reflex sympathetic stimulation or fluid retention. These drugs are especially effective as single agents for older adult patients, for those with angina, and for those with low plasma renin activity. Calcium channel blockers are tolerated by all age groups.

ACE inhibitors are effective in treating most forms of hypertension and for treating congestive heart failure. The ACE inhibitors are another choice for initial therapy suitable for all age groups, but they are more effective in Caucasian than African-American patients. ACE inhibitors block the formation of the potent vasoconstrictor, angiotensin II. The antihypertensive response is not associated with an increase in heart rate or cardiac output. ACE inhibitors are especially indicated for the hypertensive patient with heart failure.

Alpha-1 blocking agents are occasionally used as the initial antihypertensive agent. This drug class has a beneficial effect on hyperlipidemia. A limitation is the orthostatic hypotension characteristic of these agents. The alpha beta-blocker is also occasionally used as the initial drug.

After 3 to 6 months, the response of the patient is evaluated. If the response is inadequate, the drug dosage may be increased, another drug may be substituted, or a second drug from a different class may be added. The most common two-drug regimen involves the addition of an adrenergic inhibitor to diuretic therapy. The adrenergic inhibitor is commonly a beta-blocker. The choice of therapy will depend on how the patient tolerates the various side effects of the drug classes. A patient with stage 3 and stage 4 hypertension frequently requires a combination of two or three drugs to achieve control of blood pressure. The centrally acting alpha-1 agonists, the peripheral-acting adrenergic antagonists, and the direct-acting vasodilators are other choices for combination therapy.

Drug therapy can rarely be discontinued after the blood pressure is brought into a normal range. Frequently the drug dosage can be reduced with time. This reduction is important because antihypertensive drugs can produce uncomfortable side effects, whereas the hypertension itself may not produce uncomfortable symptoms, a situation that can make patient compliance with drug therapy difficult. Obesity and high salt intake are factors that aggravate hypertension. If a patient reduces weight and salt intake, drug requirements frequently may also be reduced.

Antihypertensive Therapy for Special Patient Populations

African-American Patients

Hypertension is more prevalent in African-Americans; it develops at an earlier age and is more severe than in Caucasians. In general, African-American hypertensive patients respond best to diuretics as monotherapy. ACE inhibitors and beta-blockers are generally less effective as single agents for African-American patients than for Caucasian patients. However, in combination with diuretics, ACE inhibitors and beta-blockers are equally effective in Caucasian and African-American hypertensive patients. Other antihypertensive drug classes, the calcium antagonists, alpha-1 blockers, and the alpha beta-blocker, are equally effective in both racial groups. African-Americans have a higher prevalence of salt sensitivity, obesity, and smoking—risk factors that can be modified with lifestyle changes.

Older Adult Patients

Approximately two thirds of the U.S. population aged 65 years or older has hypertension. A recent study examined the effect of treating older adult patients with an elevated systolic pressure but normal diastolic pressure. The incidence of both stroke and heart attack was reduced. Older patients are more sensitive to diuretics, beta-blockers, and the orthostatic hypotensive effects of other antihypertensive drugs. All classes of antihypertensive agents are effective in older adult patients, but only diuretics and beta-blockers have been used in clinical trials and have been shown to reduce cardiovascular disease and death.

Pregnant Patients

Hypertension during pregnancy imposes risk for both the mother and the fetus. Four diagnostic categories are recognized: chronic hypertension, preeclampsia-eclampsia, chronic hypertension with superimposed preeclampsia, and transient hypertension. Preeclampsia is a pregnancy-specific condition that develops primarily in first pregnancies after the twentieth week of gestation. It is characterized by increased blood pressure and is accompanied by proteinuria, edema, and occasionally by abnormalities of coagulation and liver function.

Eclampsia is the convulsive phase. Diet and bed rest are the first line of treatment for preeclampsia, but if high blood pressure persists, methyldopa, hydralazine, and beta-blockers have each proved effective in controlling blood pressure and improving fetal survival. If hypertension is unrelated to pregnancy, treatment should continue, although aggressive antihypertensive therapy is discouraged. However, ACE inhibitors are contraindicated during pregnancy because serious neonatal problems, including renal failure and death, have been reported when women have taken these drugs during pregnancy. Methyldopa, the most extensively evaluated antihypertensive agent used during pregnancy, has few adverse effects. Beta-blockers also appear safe when used during the latter part of the pregnancy. They may be associated with growth retardation of the fetus if used early in the pregnancy.

Patients With Coexisting Cardiovascular Disease

Cerebrovascular disease. Hypertension should be treated in a patient with cerebrovascular disease, but treatment may be suspended immediately after a stroke. Orthostatic hypotension should be avoided as a side effect of antihypertensive therapy.

Coronary artery disease. Beta-blockers or calcium antagonists, especially those that reduce the heart rate, are useful for patients with angina. Beta-blockers without intrinsic sympathomimetic activity are drugs of choice for patients who have had a myocardial infarction because these agents have been shown to reduce the risk of a subsequent attack and death.

Cardiac failure. ACE inhibitors, alone or in combination with digitalis or diuretics, are effective in reducing mortality caused by progressive congestive heart failure.

Left ventricular hypertrophy. Hypertrophy results from cardiac adaptation to the increased afterload imposed by elevated blood pressure. Beta-blockers and the calcium blockers diltiazem and verapamil are the preferred agents for treating hypertension because of their beneficial effect of decreasing afterload. Direct-acting vasodilators and ACE inhibitors may worsen the condition. Weight loss and salt restriction are beneficial.

Peripheral vascular disease. Hypertension is a major risk factor for atherosclerosis and aneurysms. However, there have been no studies to show whether controlling blood pressure alters the course of these diseases.

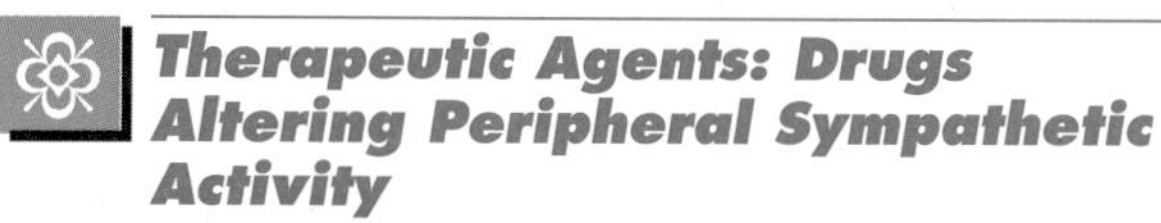

Therapeutic Agents: Drugs Altering Peripheral Sympathetic Activity

Antihypertensive drug that alter peripheral sympathetic activity include antagonists (blockers) of both the alpha- and beta-adrenergic receptors and drugs that interfere with the storage and/or release of norepinephrine, the adrenergic neurotransmitter. Each of these drug classes is discussed separately, and they are summarized in Table 13-2.

BETA-BLOCKERS

General Characteristics

Mechanism of Action

Beta-blockers are more precisely the beta-adrenergic receptor antagonists. Beta-1 adrenergic receptors are found principally in heart and fat tissue, stimulating heart function and lipolysis, respectively. Beta-2 adrenergic receptors mediate bronchodilation and peripheral vasodilation. The antihypertensive action of beta-blockers is not entirely clear, but it appears to result from the decreased cardiac output and from the inhibition of renin production by the kidney. The decreased cardiac output is a result of the inhibition of the beta-1 adrenergic receptors to decrease heart rate, contractility, and automaticity.

One goal in the development of new beta-blockers has been to develop cardioselective agents, drugs specific for the beta-1 receptor. The adverse side effects associated with blockade of beta-2 receptors include bronchospasm, prolongation of insulin-induced hypoglycemia, and aggravation of peripheral vascular insufficiency. However, the superiority of the cardioselective beta-blockers for avoiding these complications is marginal.

Another goal in the development of new beta-blockers has been to find drugs with some intrinsic sympathetic activity (partial agonists), as seen in acebutolol, carteolol, oxprenolol, and pindolol. These drugs should produce less cardiac depression and should be safer for patients with compromised cardiac function. The issue of improved safety remains to be proved.

Pharmacokinetics

The available beta-blockers do not differ in their antihypertensive effect. However, they do differ in their physiologic distribution and metabolism. Dosages of each of the drugs must be individualized for the patient. Some of the drugs must be given two or more times a day, whereas others require only once-a-day administration. Beta-blockers are metabolized by the liver and excreted in the urine.

Uses

Beta-blockers have been proven effective as antihypertensive agents when used alone or with a diuretic. They are most effective when given as a sole drug to hypertensive patients with high plasma renin levels. These patients are principally young white patients. Older African-American hypertensive patients tend to have low plasma renin concentrations and respond better to a diuretic alone or to a diuretic given with another type of sympathetic depressant.

A beta-blocker is needed when a direct-acting vasodilator, such as hydralazine or minoxidil, must be added to the therapy. These vasodilators alone cause a reflex increase in cardiac output because of their marked hypotensive effect. This reflex cardiac stimulation is blocked by the beta-blocker.

Text continued on p. 149.

TABLE 13-2 Drugs for Treatment of Chronic Hypertension

GENERIC NAME	TRADE NAME	ADMINISTRATION/ DOSAGE	COMMENTS
Beta-Adrenergic Receptor Antagonists (Beta-Blockers)			
Acebutolol hydrochloride	Monitan† Sectral*	ORAL: *Adults*—100 mg 2 times/day initially. Adjust weekly to control hypertension. Maintenance: 400-800 mg daily to control hypertension. Reduce dose by 50%-75% for patients with renal failure. Do not exceed 800 mg daily in older adults. FDA pregnancy category B.	Cardioselective drug. Indication: hypertension. Nonlabeled indications: angina, supraventricular arrhythmia, ventricular tachycardia, hypertrophic cardiomyopathy, myocardial infarction, mitral valve prolapse, thyrotoxicosis, anxiety.
Atenolol	Apo-Atenolol† Novo-Atenol† Tenormin*	ORAL: *Adults*—25-50 mg daily initially; increase gradually to 50-100 mg after 2 wk if necessary. Dosage reduced for patients with impaired renal function: 50 mg/day when creatinine clearance is 15-35 ml/min; 50 mg every 2 days when creatinine clearance is <15 ml/min. FDA pregnancy category D.	Cardioselective drug. Indications: hypertension, angina, myocardial infarction. Nonlabeled indications: supraventricular arrhythmia, ventricular tachycardia, hypertrophic cardiomyopathy, mitral valve prolapse, thyrotoxicosis.
Betaxolol	Kerlone	ORAL: *Adults*—10 mg daily initially; double after 1-2 wk if needed. Older adults may require less or more than usual adult dose. Reduce dose in half for patients with renal function impairment undergoing hemodialysis. FDA pregnancy category C.	Cardioselective drug. Indications: hypertension, glaucoma.
Bisoprolol fumarate	Zebeta	ORAL: *Adults*—5 mg daily initially; double after 1-2 wk if needed. Older adults may require less or more than usual adult dose. Reduce dose in half for patients with bronchospastic disease. FDA pregnancy category C.	Cardioselective drug. Indication: hypertension.
Carteolol hydrochloride	Cartrol	ORAL: *Adults*—2.5 mg daily initially; adjust to 10 mg if needed. Older adults may require less or more than usual adult dose. Dosage intervals are increased for patients with impaired renal function: 48 hr if creatinine clearance is 20-60 ml/min; 72 hr if creatinine clearance is <20 ml/min. FDA pregnancy category C.	Nonselective drug. Indication: hypertension. Nonlabeled indication: angina.
Metoprolol tartrate	Apo-Metoprolol† Betaloc† Lopressor Novometoprol† Toprol-XL	ORAL: *Adults*—50 mg every 12 hr initially; increase if necessary to no more than 120 mg every 8 hr. Extended-release: 100-400 mg once a day. Older adults may require less or more than usual adult dose. FDA pregnancy category C.	Cardioselective drug. Indications: hypertension, angina, myocardial infarction. Nonlabeled indications: supraventricular arrhythmia, ventricular tachycardia, hypertrophic cardiomyopathy, mitral valve prolapse, thyrotoxicosis, vascular headache, anxiety.

*Available in Canada and United States.
†Available in Canada only.

TABLE 13-2 Drugs for Treatment of Chronic Hypertension—cont'd

GENERIC NAME	TRADE NAME	ADMINISTRATION/ DOSAGE	COMMENTS
Beta-Adrenergic Receptor Antagonists (Beta-Blockers)—cont'd			
Nadolol	Corgard* Syn-Nadolol†	ORAL: *Adults*—40 mg daily initially; increase if necessary by 40-80 mg each week to maintenance daily dose of 80-320 mg. Older adults may require less or more than usual adult dose. Dosage intervals are increased for patients with impaired renal function: 24-36 hr if creatinine clearance is 31-50 ml/min; 24-48 hr if creatinine clearance is 10-30 ml/min; 40-60 hr if creatinine clearance is <10 ml/min. FDA pregnancy category C.	Nonselective drug. Indications: hypertension, angina. Nonlabeled indications: supraventricular arrhythmia, ventricular tachycardia, hypertrophic cardiomyopathy, myocardial infarction, mitral valve prolapse, thyrotoxicosis, vascular headache.
Oxprenolol hydrochloride†	Trasicor†	ORAL: *Adults*—20 mg 3 times/day initially; may increase by 60 mg daily every 1-2 wk if necessary. Total usual daily dose: 120-320 mg. Extended-release (for maintenance): 120-320 mg daily in morning.	Nonselective drug. Indication: hypertension. Nonlabeled indications: angina, hypertrophic cardiomyopathy, myocardial infarction, tremors, mitral valve prolapse.
Penbutolol sulfate	Levatol	ORAL: *Adults*—20 mg once a day. FDA pregnancy category C.	Nonselective drug. Indication: hypertension. Nonlabeled indication: angina.
Pindolol	Novo-Pindol† Syn-Pindolol† Visken*	ORAL: *Adults*—5 mg 2 times/day; may increase by 10 mg daily every 2-3 wk if necessary; usual daily dose: 45-60 mg. FDA pregnancy category B.	Nonselective drug. Indication: hypertension. Nonlabeled indications: angina, hypertrophic cardiomyopathy, mitral valve prolapse.
Propranolol hydrochloride	Apo-Propranolol† Detensol† Inderal Novopranolol†	ORAL: *Adults*—40 mg 2 times/day; increase gradually if needed to 120-240 mg daily. FDA pregnancy category C. *Children*—0.5-1 mg/kg daily in 2-4 divided doses. *Pheochromocytoma:* ORAL: *Adults*—20 mg 3 times/day to 40 mg 3 or 4 times/day for 3 days before surgery; given with alpha-adrenergic blocking medication.	Nonselective drug. Indications: hypertension, arrhythmias, hypertrophic cardiomyopathy, myocardial infarction, pheochromocytoma, vascular headache, tremors. Nonlabeled indications: anxiety, thyrotoxicosis, mitral valve prolapse, neuroleptic-induced akathisia.
Sotalol hydrochloride	Betapace Sotacor†	ORAL: *Adults*—80 mg 2 times/day; increase by 80 mg 2 times/day at weekly intervals as needed. Maintenance: 160 mg 2 times/day.	Nonselective drug. Indications: hypertension‡, angina‡, arrhythmias. Nonlabeled indications: hypertrophic cardiomyopathy, myocardial infarction, thyrotoxicosis, anxiety, mitral valve prolapse.
Timolol maleate	Apo-Timol† Blocadren	ORAL: *Adults*—10 mg 2 times/day initially; may increase weekly as needed. Maintenance: 20-40 mg daily. FDA pregnancy category C.	Nonselective drug. Indications: hypertension, myocardial infarction, vascular headache. Nonlabeled indications: angina, hypertrophic cardiomyopathy, pheochromocytoma, tremors, anxiety, thyrotoxicosis, mitral valve prolapse.
Alpha-1 Blockers (Alpha-1 Adrenergic Receptor Antagonists)			
Doxazosin mesylate	Cardura*	ORAL: 1 mg daily at bedtime. Maintenance: may increase every 2 wk, doubling dose to 16 mg/day if needed. FDA pregnancy category C.	Indication: hypertension. Nonlabeled indication: benign prostatic hypertrophy. Favorable side effect is lowering of cholesterol and triglyceride levels.

‡Use approved in Canada but not in United States.

Continued.

TABLE 13-2 Drugs for Treatment of Chronic Hypertension—cont'd

GENERIC NAME	TRADE NAME	ADMINISTRATION/ DOSAGE	COMMENTS
Alpha-1 Blockers (Alpha-1 Adrenergic Receptor Antagonists)—cont'd			
Prazosin hydrochloride	Minipress*	ORAL: *Adults*—initial dose 0.5 mg 2 or 3 times/day for 3 days. Maintenance: adjust gradually to 6-15 mg daily divided in 2 or 3 doses. FDA pregnancy category C.	Indication: hypertension. Nonlabeled indications: Raynaud's phenomenon (vasospasticity in digits), benign prostatic hyperplasia, toxicity of ergot alkaloids. Favorable side effect is lowering of cholesterol and triglyceride levels.
Terazosin hydrochloride	Hytrin*	ORAL: *Adults*—initially 1 mg at bedtime. Maintenance: adjust gradually to 1-5 mg daily. FDA pregnancy category C.	Indications: hypertension, benign prostatic hyperplasia. Favorable side effect is lowering of cholesterol and triglyceride levels.
Alpha-1, Alpha-2 Blockers (Nonspecific Alpha-Adrenergic Receptor Antagonists)			
Phentolamine hydrochloride Phentolamine mesylate	Regitine Rogitine†	*Prevention of dermal necrosis:* INTRAVENOUS: *Adults*—add 10 mg to each 1 of norepinephrine IV solution. In event of extravasation of IV norepinephrine, infiltrate 5-10 mg in 10 ml normal saline. *Before surgery for pheochromocytoma:* ORAL: *Adults*—50 mg every 4-6 hr. *Children*—25 mg every 4-6 hr. INTRAMUSCULAR, INTRAVENOUS: *Adults*—5 mg. *Children*—1 mg.	Indications: prevention or control of hypertension from pheochromocytoma before and during surgery; reversal of ischemia and prevention of necrosis of skin after IV administration or extravasation of norepinephrine.
Phenoxybenzamine hydrochloride	Dibenzyline	ORAL: *Adults*—10 mg daily. May be increased by 10 mg/day to maximum dose of 60 mg daily. *Children*—0.2 mg/kg body weight up to 10 mg once a day.	Irreversible inhibitor. Indication: control of hypertension and sweating from pheochromocytoma before surgery. Nonlabeled indication: treatment of urinary symptoms associated with benign prostatic hypertrophy.
Alpha- and Beta-Adrenergic Receptor Antagonist			
Labetalol hydrochloride	Trandate* Normodyne	ORAL: *Adults*—100 mg twice a day; adjust in 100 mg increments every 2 or 3 days as needed. Maintenance: 200-400 mg twice daily. INTRAVENOUS: *Adults*—20 mg injected slowly over 2 min with additional 40 mg or 80 mg injections at 10 min intervals until desired blood pressure is achieved or total equals 300 mg; alternatively, infuse at 2 mg/min for desired effect of 50-300 mg.	Nonselective beta-blocker, selective alpha-1 beta-blocker. Indication: control of hypertension.
Sympatholytic Drugs			
Deserpidine	Harmonyl	ORAL: *Adults*—250-500 mg in single or divided dose daily.	Rauwolfia alkaloid. Indication: hypertension. Nonlabeled indication: Raynaud's phenomenon.
Guanadrel	Hylorel	ORAL: *Adults*—5 mg twice daily initially; may increase to 20-75 mg daily divided into 2-4 doses.	Depletes norepinephrine in sympathetic neuron. Indication: severe hypertension.
Guanethidine monosulfate	Apo-Guanethidine† Ismelin*	ORAL: *Adults*—10-12.5 mg daily initially; may increase to 25-50 mg daily. *Children*—200 μg/kg body weight or 6 μg/m^2 body surface area daily.	Depletes norepinephrine in sympathetic neuron. Indications: severe hypertension, renal hypertension.

TABLE 13-2 Drugs for Treatment of Chronic Hypertension—cont'd

GENERIC NAME	TRADE NAME	ADMINISTRATION/ DOSAGE	COMMENTS
Sympatholytic Drugs—cont'd			
Rauwolfia serpentina	Raudixin Rauval Rauverid	ORAL: *Adults*—50-200 mg in single or divided dose daily.	Rauwolfia alkaloid. Indication: hypertension. Nonlabeled indication: Raynaud's phenomenon.
Reserpine	Novoreserpine† Reserfia† Serpasil† Serpalan	ORAL: *Adults*—100-250 mg daily. *Children*—5-20 μg/kg/body weight 150-600 μg/m^2 body surface area daily.	Rauwolfia alkaloid. Indication: hypertension. Nonlabeled indication: Raynaud's phenomenon.
Centrally Acting Antihypertensive Drugs			
✣ Clonidine hydrochloride	Catapres* Dixarit	ORAL: *Adults*—100 μg 2 times/day initially; may increase to 600 μg daily in divided doses. TRANSDERMAL: *Adults*—begin with system delivering 100 μg daily for 1 week; may increase dosage delivered weekly to 300 μg daily.	Decreases central sympathetic outflow. Indication: hypertension. Nonlabeled indications: diagnosis of pheochromocytoma; prophylaxis for vascular headaches; treatment of vasomotor symptoms of dysmenorrhea or menopause; aid in opioid withdrawal, nicotine withdrawal; treatment of Gilles de la Tourette's syndrome.
Guanabenz acetate	Wytensin	ORAL: *Adults*—4 mg 2 times daily initially; may increase every 1-2 wk by 4-8 mg daily. Maximum: 32 mg daily.	Alpha-2 agonist. Acts centrally to decrease sympathetic outflow. Indication: hypertension.
Guanfacine hydrochloride	Tenex	ORAL: *Adults*—1 mg daily at bedtime initially; may increase in 3-4 wk to 2 mg daily. Maximum: 3 mg daily.	Decreases central sympathetic outflow. Indication: hypertension.
Methyldopa	Aldomet* Apo-Methyldopa† Dopamet† Novomedopa†	ORAL: *Adults*—250 mg 2-3 times daily initially; may adjust after 2-day intervals. Usual maintenance dose: 500 mg daily. Maximum dose: 3 gm daily. *Children*—10 mg/kg body weight or 300 mg/m^2 body surface area daily divided into 2-4 doses. Maximum daily dose: 65 mg/kg body weight or 3 gm, whichever is less. INTRAVENOUS: *Adults*—250-500 mg in 100 ml 5% dextrose over 30-60 min; may repeat in 6 hr. *Children*—5-10 mg/kg body weight in 5% dextrose over 30-60 min; may repeat in 6 hr.	Decreases central sympathetic outflow. Indications: hypertension, hypertensive crises (IV).
Angiotensin Converting Enzymes (ACE) Inhibitors			
Benazepril	Lotensin	ORAL: *Adults*—10 mg daily; may increase to 20-40 mg daily in single or divided dose.	Inhibits production of angiotensin II, a potent vasoconstrictor. Indication: hypertension. Nonlabeled indications: congestive heart failure, hypertension of scleroderma.
✣ Captopril	Capoten*	ORAL: *Adults*—*Antihypertension:* 12.5 mg 2 or 3 times daily; may double dose after 1-2 wk. *Left ventricular dysfunction* (post–myocardial infarction): Initial dose of 6.25 mg; then 12.5 mg 3 times/day; may increase gradually to 25 mg 3 times/day. *Diabetic nephropathy:* 25 mg 2 times/day.	Inhibits production of angiotensin II, a potent vasoconstrictor. Indications: hypertension, congestive heart failure, left ventricular dysfunction after myocardial infarction, diabetic nephropathy. Nonlabeled indication: hypertension of scleroderma.

Continued.

TABLE 13-2 Drugs for Treatment of Chronic Hypertension—cont'd

GENERIC NAME	TRADE NAME	ADMINISTRATION/ DOSAGE	COMMENTS
Angiotensin Converting Enzymes (ACE) Inhibitors—cont'd			
		Congestive heart failure: 12.5 mg 2 or 3 times/day; may increase gradually to 50 mg daily. ORAL: *Children*—300 μg/kg body weight 3 times/day. *Newborns*—10 μg/kg body weight 2 or 3 times daily.	
Enalapril maleate	Vasotec*	ORAL: *Adults—Hypertension:* 5 mg daily initially; may increase after 1-2 wk. Maintenance: 10-40 mg daily divided into 1 or 2 doses. *Congestive heart failure; left ventricular dysfunction: Adults*—2.5 mg 1 or 2 times daily; may increase to 5-20 mg daily as 1 or 2 doses. INTRAVENOUS (Enalaprilat): *Adults*—1.25 mg over 5 min; may repeat in 6 hr.	Inhibits production of angiotensin II, a potent vasoconstrictor. Indications: hypertension, congestive heart failure, left ventricular dysfunction. Nonlabeled indication: hypertension of scleroderma.
Fosinopril	Monopril	ORAL: *Adults*—10 mg once a day; may increase to 20-40 mg.	Inhibits production of angiotensin II, a potent vasoconstrictor. Indication: hypertension. Nonlabeled indication: hypertension of scleroderma.
Lisinopril	Prinivil* Zestril*	ORAL: *Adults—Hypertension:* 10 mg once a day; may increase to 20-40 mg. *Congestive heart failure: Adults*—2.5-5 mg daily; may increase to 10-20 mg daily.	Inhibits production of angiotensin II, a potent vasoconstrictor. Indications: hypertension, congestive heart failure. Nonlabeled indication: hypertension of scleroderma.
Quinapril hydrochloride	Accupril	ORAL: *Adults*—10 mg once a day; may increase to 20-80 mg.	Inhibits production of angiotensin II, a potent vasoconstrictor. Indication: hypertension. Nonlabeled indications: congestive heart failure, hypertension of scleroderma.
Ramipril	Altace	ORAL: *Adults*—2.5 mg once a day; may increase to 20 mg.	Inhibits production of angiotensin II, a potent vasoconstrictor. Indication: hypertension. Nonlabeled indications: congestive heart failure, hypertension of scleroderma.
Calcium Channel Blockers			
✣ Diltiazem	Cardizem*	ORAL: *Adults*—30 mg 3 or 4 times a day initially; may increase gradually. Maximum: 360 mg daily. Also available in extended-release forms.	Vasodilation from blocking of calcium ion flow in smooth muscle membranes. Indications: hypertension, angina, supraventricular tachycardia.
Felodipine	Plendil Renedil†	ORAL: *Adults*—5 mg once daily, may increase after 2 wk to 10 mg daily.	Vasodilation from blocking of calcium ion flow in smooth muscle membranes. Indications: hypertension, angina.
Isradipine	DynaCirc	ORAL: *Adults*—2.5 mg 2 times/day; may increase gradually to 20 mg daily.	Vasodilation from blocking of calcium ion flow in smooth muscle membranes. Indication: hypertension.
Nicardipine	Cardene	ORAL: *Adults*—20 mg 3 times/day.	Vasodilation from blocking of calcium ion flow in smooth muscle membranes. Indications: hypertension, angina.

TABLE 13-2 Drugs for Treatment of Chronic Hypertension—cont'd

GENERIC NAME	TRADE NAME	ADMINISTRATION/ DOSAGE	COMMENTS
Calcium Channel Blockers—cont'd			
Nifedipine	Adalat* Apo-Nifed† Novo-Nifed† Nu-Nifed† Procardia	ORAL: *Adults*—10 mg 3 times/day. Maximum: 120-180 mg daily.	Vasodilation from blocking of calcium ion flow in smooth muscle membranes. Indications: hypertension, angina.
Verapamil	Calan Isoptin* Novo-Veramil† Nu-Verap† Verelan	ORAL: *Adults*—80-120 mg 3 times/day. Maximum daily dose: 480 mg. Extended-release: 240 mg once a day; may increase weekly to 240-480 mg daily. *Older adults*—40 mg 3 times/day initially. *Children*—4-8 mg/kg body weight daily in divided doses.	Vasodilation from blocking of calcium ion flow in smooth muscle membranes. Indications: hypertension, angina, supraventricular tachycardia. Nonlabeled indications: hypertrophic cardiomyopathy, vascular headache.
Other Vasodilators			
Hydralazine	Apresoline* Novo-Hylazin†	ORAL: *Adults*—10 mg 4 times/day for 2-4 days, then 25 mg 4 times/day; may increase to 50 mg 4 times/day after 1 week. *Children*—750 μg/kg body weight or 25 mg/m² body surface daily, divided into 2-4 doses. INTRAVENOUS, INTRAMUSCULAR: *Adults*—10-40 mg, repeated as needed. *Children*—1.7-3.5 mg/kg body weight or 50-100 mg/m² body surface daily, divided into 4-6 doses.	Direct-acting vasodilator. Indications: severe hypertension, hypertensive crisis. Nonlabeled indication: congestive heart failure.
Minoxidil	Loniten*	ORAL: *Adults*—5 mg daily as one or divided dose. Maintenance: 10-40 mg daily. *Children:* 200 μg/kg body weight daily as 1 or 2 doses, up to 50 mg daily.	Direct-acting vasodilator. Indication: severe hypertension.

Beta-blockers are also used in the treatment of angina (Chapter 15) and certain arrhythmias (Chapter 19) and after myocardial infarction. The use of these drugs after myocardial infarction is intended to prevent sudden death resulting from electrical abnormalities in the recovering heart. Specifically, atenolol, metoprolol, oxprenolol, propranolol, and timolol have been approved for use in reducing the incidence of sudden death after a heart attack.

Adverse Reactions and Contraindications

Clinical trials have shown beta-blockers to be well tolerated and effective in the treatment of hypertension. Adverse effects are reported in 10% of patients and are usually mild. The most common side effects are sleep disturbances, fatigue, cool extremities, reduced exercise tolerance, tingling in the fingers or toes, gastrointestinal (GI) upset, bronchospasm, depressed mood, and sexual dysfunction (impotence in men).

Patients with abnormal cardiovascular function are the most likely to encounter more serious side effects, such as pulmonary edema, hypotension, cardiac failure, and an atrioventricular nodal block.

Beta-blockers should not be discontinued abruptly because such an action may exacerbate angina, myocardial infarction, or ventricular arrhythmias. Instead, the dosage should be reduced gradually over 1 to 2 weeks with careful monitoring of the patient for these possible complications.

Beta-blockers are used with caution in patients whose health status could be worsened by this class of drugs; specific conditions include poor cardiac function, asthma, peripheral vascular disease, and diabetes. Blockade of beta-receptors can compromise cardiac function, induce bronchospasm, and inhibit peripheral vasodilation. Hypoglycemia normally elicits the discharge of epinephrine. The effects of this released epinephrine will not be noticed easily in a patient who is taking a beta-receptor–blocking drug. This is an important point for those patients with diabetes mellitus who are taking insulin or an oral hypoglycemic drug.

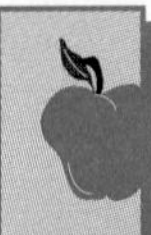

DIETARY CONSIDERATION

Sodium and Hypertension

Excessive intake of sodium is associated with fluid retention and hypertension in some individuals. The first step in decreasing sodium intake is to stop adding salt to food while cooking or to cooked food during meals. The next step is to eliminate processed foods that contain a large amount of added sodium, including:

- Relishes and pickles
- Salted popcorn, nuts
- Sauerkraut
- Bouillon cubes
- Salted crackers
- Potato chips, pretzels
- Canned, frozen, or dehydrated soup
- Bread, rolls, bran, bran flakes
- Processed cheese, cheese spreads
- Canned meat such as tuna and Vienna sausages
- Salt-cured meat such as bacon, ham, corned beef, salt pork, luncheon meats, frankfurters, and sausage
- Seasonings such as garlic or onion salts, or prepared mustard; meat extracts and tenderizers such as monosodium glutamate, soy sauce, and Worcestershire sauce; catsup; steak sauce; and cooking with salt pork or bacon grease

Instruct patients to read food ingredient lists and to limit or avoid foods containing salt, baking soda, monosodium glutamate, baking powder, and sodium compounds such as sodium benzoate, sodium citrate, sodium propionate, sodium alginate, sodium sulfite, sodium hydroxide, disodium phosphate, and sodium saccharin. Finally, instruct patients to limit or avoid foods naturally high in sodium such as milk, eggs, meat (including fish and poultry), cheese, beets and greens, carrots, celery, chard, spinach, kale, and white turnip roots.

Toxicity

Symptoms of overdose include severe dizziness or fainting, hypotension, irregular or slow heartbeat, difficulty in breathing, bluish-colored fingernails or palms of the hands, or seizures. These symptoms require treatment that includes gastric lavage and administration of activated charcoal followed by supportive therapy for specific symptoms.

Interactions

The therapeutic effects of beta-blockers are inhibited by cocaine, by sympathomimetic agents such as the bronchodilators, by xanthines such as theophylline, and by the centrally acting antihypertensive drugs clonidine and guanabenz. The hypotensive actions of beta-blockers are potentiated by most other antihypertensive agents. The calcium channel blockers diltiazem and verapamil are more likely than other drugs of their class to cause significant bradycardia when given with beta-blockers.

Allergen immunotherapy or the use of allergenic extracts for skin testing is not recommended for patients taking beta-blockers. The beta-blockers increase the potential for serious systemic reactions or anaphylaxis. They also impair glycemic control in diabetic patients taking insulin or oral hypoglycemic agents.

Specific Beta-Blockers

Acebutolol

Acebutolol (Sectral) is an intermediate-acting cardioselective beta-blocker with moderate intrinsic sympathomimetic activity (ISA). It is moderately well absorbed when taken orally. Acebutolol is metabolized by the liver, but the drug is mostly excreted unchanged, both in the urine and in the feces through enterohepatic circulation. The dosage is reduced for patients with renal function impairment.

Atenolol

Atenolol (Tenormin) is a long-acting cardioselective beta-blocker. Poorly absorbed from the GI tract, the drug is poorly metabolized by the liver and excreted in the urine. The time between doses must be increased in patients with impaired renal function.

Betaxolol

Betaxolol (Kerlone) is a long-acting cardioselective beta-blocker structurally related to metoprolol. It is well absorbed after oral administration and metabolized by the liver. Doses should be decreased in patients with renal impairment and for older adults. Betaxolol is also available for ophthalmic administration to treat glaucoma.

Carteolol

Carteolol (Cartrol) is a long-acting nonselective beta-blocker with moderate ISA. The drug undergoes minimal hepatic metabolism and is largely excreted unchanged in the urine. The dosage interval must be increased for patients with impaired renal function. Carteolol is available in an ophthalmic preparation for the treatment of glaucoma.

Labetalol

Labetalol (Normodyne, Trandate) has both alpha and beta receptor antagonist activities. The decrease in heart rate is not as pronounced with labetalol as with other beta-blockers. The alpha antagonist effect is more prominent with labetalol than the beta-antagonist effects, and a decrease in peripheral resistance is probably the major therapeutic effect. Labetalol is especially useful for treating hypertensive patients who also have angina. Orthostatic hypotension may be experienced early in therapy.

An intravenous (IV) preparation of labetalol is available for hypertensive emergencies, especially hypertensive encephalopathy, hypertension associated with extensive burns, and hypertension in patients with coronary artery disease or recent heart attack.

Metoprolol

Metoprolol (Lopressor, Betaloc) is a short-acting cardioselective beta-blocker. It is well absorbed from the GI tract and readily metabolized by the liver. Dosages do not need to be modified with hepatic or renal function impairment. Extended-release forms are available.

Nadolol

Nadolol (Corgard) is a long-acting nonselective beta-blocker. It is not well absorbed from the GI tract, and up to one fourth of the dose may be excreted in the feces. Absorbed drug is excreted unchanged in the urine. The time between doses must be increased in patients with impaired renal function.

Oxprenolol

Oxprenolol (Trasicor) is a short-acting nonselective beta-blocker with ISA. It is well absorbed and metabolized by the liver. Oxprenolol is available in Canada but not in the United States. An extended-release form is available.

Penbutolol

Penbutolol (Levatol) is a long-acting nonselective beta-blocker with ISA. It is well absorbed and metabolized by the liver; the metabolites are excreted in the urine.

Pindolol

Pindolol (Visken) is a short-acting nonselective beta-blocker with significant ISA. It is well absorbed when taken orally. Pindolol is metabolized by the liver, but about half the dose is excreted unchanged in the urine.

Propranolol

Propranolol (Inderal), a nonselective beta-blocker, is the oldest of the clinically used beta-blocking drugs. It is well absorbed orally and readily metabolized by the liver. Propranolol is short acting but is available in extended-release forms. It is also available as an oral solution and in an injectable form. Propranolol has several approved indications in addition to those as an antianginal, antiarrhythmic, and antihypertensive agent. These indications include prophylactic treatment against sudden death after a myocardial infarction; adjunct to the treatment of the adrenal tumor pheochromocytoma; treatment of tremors; and prophylaxis for vascular headache.

Sotalol

Sotalol (Sotacor) is a very long-acting nonselective beta-blocker. It is moderately well absorbed and poorly metabolized by the liver. Most of the drug is excreted unchanged in the urine. Patients with renal failure should be given the drug less frequently. In the United States sotalol is approved for the treatment of cardiac arrhythmias but not approved for the treatment of hypertension. However, sotalol is approved as an antianginal and antihypertensive agent in Canada.

Timolol

Timolol (Blocadren, Apo-Timol) is a short-acting nonselective beta-blocker. It is well absorbed from the GI tract and metabolized by the liver. Timolol is also approved for use as prophylactic treatment for vascular headache and against sudden death after a myocardial infarction. An ophthalmic formulation is available for the treatment of glaucoma.

ALPHA-1 BLOCKERS

General Characteristics

Mechanism of Action

Alpha-1 adrenergic receptors are found on vascular smooth muscle, where they mediate vasoconstriction in response to sympathetic nerve stimulation. Blockade of these receptors therefore results in vasodilation. Both arterioles and veins dilate, reducing the total peripheral resistance.

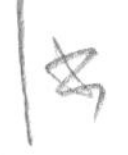

Pharmacokinetics

Alpha-1 blockers are taken orally one or more times a day, depending on the drug. The major pharmacologic difference between the alpha-1 blockers is their duration of action. They are metabolized by the liver, and metabolites are excreted in the urine.

Uses

Alpha-1 blockers are largely used as second or third drugs in the treatment of hypertension. A favorable side effect is a reduction in cholesterol and triglyceride levels. Moreover, reflex tachycardia is not common, in contrast with other classes of direct vasodilators. A diuretic is usually necessary because the alpha-1 adrenergic blockers tend to cause fluid retention.

Alpha-1 blockers are also useful in treating benign prostatic hyperplasia. These drugs reduce the tone of the prostatic smooth muscle, thereby decreasing pressure on the urethra and allowing urine to pass more freely.

Adverse Reactions and Contraindications

The most common side effects are dizziness, light-headedness, palpitations, and fainting caused by orthostatic hypotension. For this reason the dosage is often started low and raised gradually to allow patients to develop some tolerance to the orthostatic hypotension. Other complaints may include weakness, fatigue, drowsiness, blurred vision, nasal congestion, nausea, edema, and weight gain.

Because blood pressure is lowered to a degree that can interfere with the perfusion of blood in the heart, attacks of angina may be precipitated by alpha-1 adrenergic blockers.

Interactions

Antiinflammatory drugs tend to cause fluid retention, and this effect may be worsened with alpha-1 adrenergic blockers. Alcohol has a vasodilator effect that increases the risk for dizziness and fainting.

Specific Alpha-1 Blockers

Doxazosin

Doxazosin (Cardura) can be taken just once a day. This drug is well absorbed orally.

Prazosin

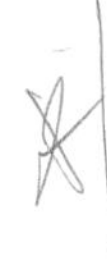

Prazosin (Minipress) has a shorter duration of action than the other alpha-1 blockers. It is commonly given with a diuretic. Since marked orthostatic hypotension may occur when the drug is first administered, the dosage is started low or given at bedtime.

Terazosin

Terazosin (Hytrin) is effective alone or with a diuretic in treating hypertension. The drug is long acting. It is the only alpha-1 blocker specifically approved for treating benign prostatic hyperplasia.

SYMPATHOLYTIC DRUGS

Sympatholytic drugs are those drugs that interfere with the storage and/or release of norepinephrine. The drugs in longest use are the rauwolfia alkaloids. Because these drugs cause a variety of side effects, they are no longer in wide use but may prove effective in cases refractory to the newer drugs.

Guanethidine

Mechanism of Action

Guanethidine (Ismelin) enters peripheral sympathetic neurons; it is taken into the cell by the same mechanism as for the reuptake of norepinephrine. Inside the neuron guanethidine blocks norepinephrine release. Guanethidine does not cross the blood-brain barrier and therefore produces no central effects. Because norepinephrine is not available for release from peripheral sympathetic neurons, both peripheral vascular resistance and cardiac output are decreased.

Pharmacokinetics

The effects of guanethidine may take 1 to 2 weeks to reach the maximum therapeutic response to a given dosage regimen. Moreover, the effects of guanethidine persist for 7 to 10 days after therapy is discontinued.

Uses

Guanethidine is a very potent antihypertensive drug that is restricted for use in controlling severe hypertension.

Adverse Reactions and Contraindications

A number of uncomfortable side effects arise from the depletion of peripheral norepinephrine stores. Orthostatic (postural) hypotension is a special problem with guanethidine therapy. The tone of blood vessels is diminished by guanethidine, and, if the patient moves suddenly from a reclining to a standing position, the appropriate vascular changes cannot take place quickly enough for proper blood redistribution to occur. The blood stays in the periphery and drains from the head on standing, resulting in fainting. Patients taking guanethidine must be instructed to change body positions slowly. Other side effects resulting from the depletion of norepinephrine include a slow heart rate (bradycardia) and diarrhea. This diarrhea, which occurs after meals, can be severe and of an explosive nature. In men failure of erection or ejaculation may arise as a result of the loss of vascular tone. Guanethidine also causes sodium retention; therefore a diuretic is administered concurrently.

Contraindications for guanethidine therapy include the presence of angina, cerebral insufficiency, or coronary artery disease–conditions that are further compromised by the loss of vascular tone.

Interactions

A number of drug interactions have been noted for guanethidine. Patients taking guanethidine are supersensitive to administered catecholamines. Patients become less responsive to guanethidine when an indirect-acting adrenergic drug (e.g., amphetamine or ephedrine) or a tricyclic antidepressant drug is taken. The indirect-acting adrenergic drugs release stored norepinephrine from neurons, an action that overcomes the effect of guanethidine to block release of norepinephrine. Tricyclic antidepressants block the uptake of guanethidine into the neuron so that guanethidine cannot reach its site of action.

Guanadrel

Guanadrel (Hylorel) has actions similar to those of guanethidine but with more rapid onset of action and shorter duration of action. The side affects of guanadrel are similar to those of guanethidine but less severe.

Reserpine and Related Drugs

Reserpine (Serpasil), Deserpidine (Harmonyl), and rauwolfia serpentina (Raudixin and others) and related drugs are often called rauwolfia alkaloids because reserpine was originally isolated from the *Rauwolfia serpentina* bush of India. Reserpine was originally used as an antipsychotic drug but has been replaced by the phenothiazine tranquilizers for this use. Reserpine is effective in lowering blood pressure because it depletes stores of norepinephrine from neurons both in the CNS and the peripheral nervous system. The central action produces sedation and tranquilization. The reported incidence of depression with reserpine has varied from 27% to 40%. Occasionally, patients who take reserpine will become severely depressed to the point of attempting suicide. More commonly, patients complain of a lethargic feeling, an increased appetite, and increased dreaming. Nightmares are sometimes a complaint.

Other side effects of reserpine can be related to the decreased sympathetic tone, such as, vasodilation that results in a flushed, warm feeling and nasal congestion. Some side effects of reserpine can be related to the predominant parasympathetic tone when sympathetic tone is depressed: salivation, stomach cramps, and diarrhea. Because reserpine augments gastric acid secretion through the increased parasympathetic tone, it should not be used in patients with a peptic ulcer.

Therapeutic Agents: Centrally Acting Antihypertensive Drugs

Clonidine, guanabenz, guanfacine, and methyldopa exert their antihypertensive activity through actions in the CNS.

SPECIFIC DRUGS

Clonidine

Mechanism of Action

Clonidine (Catapres) has an antihypertensive effect that results from its action in the CNS. It activates alpha-2 receptors in the vasomotor center of the medulla, an action that inhibits activity of the sympathetic nervous system. Heart rate and cardiac output are decreased and account for the reduction in blood pressure.

Pharmacokinetics

Clonidine is well absorbed and becomes effective within 1 hour when taken orally. A transdermal system is also available for administering clonidine that requires 2 to 3 days before an effect is seen. Over half the drug is excreted unchanged in the urine.

Patients with impaired renal function may require lower doses or less frequent administration.

Uses

Clonidine is commonly used with a diuretic in antihypertensive therapy. New therapeutic uses for clonidine have been developed. Clonidine is used in the prophylaxis of vascular headaches and to treat the vasomotor symptoms of menopause. The symptoms of opioid withdrawal and nicotine withdrawal can often be controlled by clonidine. Gilles de la Tourette's syndrome, a condition of severe and multiple tics, is alleviated by clonidine therapy.

Adverse Reactions and Contraindications

Common side effects of clonidine therapy include drowsiness, dry mouth, and constipation. Sudden discontinuance can be dangerous. After discontinuing therapeutic doses for 12 to 48 hours, many patients experience symptoms of a sympathetic rebound: restlessness, insomnia, tremors, increased salivation, and increased heart rate (tachycardia). If clonidine is not reinstated, further symptoms follow: headaches, abdominal pain, and nausea. The most severe reaction is a hypertensive crisis that is best treated in the hospital with a combination of alpha-blocking and beta-blocking drugs: phentolamine and propranolol. To avoid these withdrawal problems, clonidine doses are gradually reduced over a week or more.

Interactions

The hypotensive action of clonidine may be decreased by antidepressants or appetite suppressants. If beta-blockers are taken concurrently, they should be discontinued gradually before clonidine is discontinued. If clonidine is discontinued while the patient is still taking a beta-blocker, this situation increases the risk of a clonidine-withdrawal hypertensive crisis.

Guanabenz

Guanabenz (Wytensin) has a mechanism of action similar to that of clonidine; it inhibits sympathetic activity by activating alpha receptors in the CNS. Guanabenz has a long duration of action, 12 to 24 hours, and may require only once-a-day dosage. It is metabolized and excreted in the urine.

The most common side effects are drowsiness, dry mouth, dizziness, weakness, and headache. Withdrawal rebound hypertension can occur if guanabenz is discontinued abruptly.

Guanfacine

Guanfacine (Tenex), like clonidine and guanabenz, appears to act in the CNS. By stimulating central alpha-adrenergic receptors, there is a decreased sympathetic outflow and a lowering of blood pressure. Guanfacine has a long duration of action, about 24 hours, and can be taken once a day. It is well absorbed and is metabolized in the liver. The most common side effects are drowsiness, dry mouth, depression, and confusion.

Methyldopa

Mechanism of Action

Methyldopa (Aldomet) is taken into sympathetic neurons and metabolized to methylnorepinephrine. Methylnorepinephrine is stored in granules and released on stimulation of the neuron. Methylnorepinephrine is called a *false transmitter* because it takes the place of norepinephrine.

Until recently the antihypertensive effect of methylnorepinephrine was believed to result from the ineffectiveness of methylnorepinephrine as a vasoconstrictor. Recently it has been shown that methylnorepinephrine is a potent vasoconstrictor, so the action of methylnorepinephrine as a false transmitter for peripheral sympathetic neurons does not account for the antihypertensive effects of methyldopa. The effect of methyldopa in the CNS to decrease the activity of the sympathetic nervous system is now believed to account for the antihypertensive effect of the drug. Methyldopa decreases sympathetic tone and has a tranquilizing effect on behavior.

Pharmacokinetics

Methyldopa is administered orally two to four times daily. An injectable form of methyldopate is available for IV administration in a hypertensive crisis. However, methyldopate is relatively slow acting and does not act immediately to lower blood pressure. Methyldopa and its sulfated metabolite are excreted in the urine.

Uses

Methyldopa is used to treat moderate-to-severe hypertension, including that complicated by renal diseases. Methyldopa appears to be safe for the fetus when taken in the last trimester. An injectable form, methyldopate, is used in the treatment of hypertensive crisis. Because methyldopate has a slow onset of action, it is not the sole initial therapy for a hypertensive crisis.

Adverse Reactions and Contraindications

Side effects common to methyldopa are related largely to the decrease in central sympathetic activity. Drowsiness is common at the beginning of treatment. Unpleasant sedation, depressed mood, and nightmares are occasional complaints. Tiredness and fatigue may be noted. Peripheral effects include a slow heart rate (bradycardia), diarrhea, dry mouth, and occasional ejaculatory failure in men.

Interactions

Occasionally, methyldopa causes a false-positive Coombs' test. A positive Coombs' test indicates hemolytic anemia, but it is rare for the patient taking methyldopa to have hemolytic anemia in spite of the positive test. Methyldopa may also cause a mild alteration of liver function tests. Methyldopa is therefore not a drug to use for patients who already have impaired liver function, because the drug will interfere with evaluating the course of the disease. This alteration of liver tests ordinarily occurs during the first 6 weeks of therapy, and it is reversed by discontinuing methyldopa.

Sympathomimetic drugs decrease the hypotensive effect of methyldopa and may themselves give exaggerated vasopressor responses. Methyldopa may cause hyperexcitability in patients receiving monoamine oxidase inhibitors.

Therapeutic Agents: Vasodilators for Treating Chronic Hypertension

Vasodilators that are used to treat chronic hypertension are presented in the following three sections: angiotensin converting enzyme inhibitors, calcium channel blockers, and other vasodilators.

ANGIOTENSIN CONVERTING ENZYME INHIBITORS

General Characteristics

Mechanism of Action

Angiotensin II is a potent vasoconstrictor. As seen in Figure 13-1, angiotensin II is formed from angiotensin I by angiotensin converting enzyme. When this enzyme is inhibited, the amount of angiotensin II formed decreases. **Angiotensin converting enzyme (ACE) inhibitors** therefore decrease the amount of the potent vasoconstrictor, angiotensin II. The ACE inhibitors also block the degradation of bradykinin and thus increase the amounts of this important vasodilator peptide. The net effect of ACE inhibitors is to decrease peripheral vascular resistance. This action makes the ACE inhibitors useful in treating congestive heart failure and hypertension.

Pharmacokinetics

ACE inhibitors are effective orally. They differ primarily in whether they are transformed to active metabolites. Benazepril, enalapril, fosinopril, and quinapril all give rise to active metabolites. Excretion tends to be predominantly renal.

Uses

ACE inhibitors have rapidly found a role in the treatment of chronic hypertension. These drugs are used alone or with a diuretic or other drug in the treatment of mild to severe hypertension. ACE inhibitors are also useful in treating renovascular hypertension by altering renal blood flow for patients with diabetic nephropathy or renal scleroderma.

ACE inhibitors are combined with diuretics and digitalis therapy for the treatment of congestive heart failure that is not responsive to other measures.

Adverse Reactions and Contraindications

ACE inhibitors are well tolerated and have little if any adverse effects on the CNS function or on carbohydrate or lipid metabolism. Dizziness, a skin rash, swelling, and an increase in serum potassium levels (hyperkalemia) have been reported. Some patients develop a cough during therapy that begins as a tickling sensation and progresses to a dry, nonproductive persistent cough that becomes worse at night. The cough disappears when the drug is withdrawn.

Patients with a history of angioedema, impaired renal function, a renal transplant, on renal dialysis or with renal artery stenosis should not be given ACE inhibitors. ACE inhibitors can cause fetal and neonatal problems and should not be administered to pregnant women. There is evidence for some ACE inhibitors that they are excreted in breast milk, so these drugs should not be taken by nursing mothers.

Interactions

Drug interactions have been reported for the ACE inhibitors. Foods or drugs high in potassium may contribute to hyperkalemia. The hypotensive effect of ACE inhibitors is enhanced by diuretics, alcohol, and beta-blockers. Patients who are sodium or water depleted through diuretic therapy should begin taking ACE inhibitors at about half the regular dose. Nonsteroidal antiinflammatory drugs (NSAIDs), especially indomethacin, may antagonize the antihypertensive effect of the ACE inhibitors and cause sodium retention leading to edema.

Specific ACE Inhibitors

Benazepril

Benazepril (Lotensin) is rapidly absorbed and metabolized by the liver. However, benazepril is also highly protein bound, and the main metabolite, benazeprilat, is also active, so the duration of action is 24 hours.

Captopril

Captopril (Capoten) is rapidly absorbed after oral administration and is effective within 1 hour. About half of the drug is excreted unchanged in the urine, and there is no active metabolite.

Enalapril

Enalapril (Vasotec) is a prodrug designed to be absorbed orally. On absorption, enalapril is deesterified to the active drug, enalaprilat, which is an inhibitor of angiotensin converting enzyme like captopril. However, patients with liver disease may be unable to activate enalapril.

Enalaprilat injection (Vasotec injection) is the active form of enalapril in a dosage form suitable for treatment in a hypertensive emergency.

Fosinopril
Fosinopril (Monopril) is slowly absorbed orally and metabolized by the liver and gastric mucosa to an active metabolite, fosinoprilat. Since the metabolite has a long duration of action, the drug's duration of action is about 24 hours.

Lisinopril
Lisinopril (Prinivil, Zestril) is poorly absorbed, is not protein bound, and is not metabolized by the liver. Lisinopril is excreted in the urine unchanged. The duration of action is about 24 hours. The dosage must be greatly reduced for patients with impaired renal function.

Quinapril
Quinapril (Accupril) is well absorbed and metabolized by the liver and gastric mucosa to an active metabolite, quinaprilat, which is highly protein bound. The duration of action is about 24 hours.

Ramipril
Ramipril (Altace) is rapidly absorbed and metabolized by the liver to ramiprilat, which has about six times the activity of ramipril itself. The duration of action is about 24 hours.

CALCIUM CHANNEL BLOCKERS

General Characteristics

Mechanism of Action
Calcium channel blockers decrease the entry of calcium into smooth muscle and thereby lower vascular tone, an action that reduces peripheral resistance and blood pressure. This reduction in blood pressure can produce a reflex increase in heart rate. Cardiac function is also depressed because of reduced intracellular calcium. Each of the various calcium channel blockers differs in its relative effect on vascular and cardiac tissue. In general, calcium channel blockers are useful for patients with coexisting angina (see Chapter 15).

Pharmacokinetics
Calcium channel blockers are generally well absorbed, and most have reduced bioavailability because the drug is extensively metabolized by the liver on absorption. Most of these agents are protein bound in the blood. Excretion of the drug or its metabolites is in the urine and feces.

Uses
Calcium channel blockers have rapidly become important in the treatment of various cardiovascular diseases. These drugs are effective in the treatment of angina, arrhythmias, and hypertension. In the treatment of hypertension, calcium channel blockers may be used alone or in combination with one or more other drugs, most commonly a diuretic.

Adverse Reactions and Contraindications
Calcium channel blockers are well tolerated by various age and ethnic groups, and side effects are generally mild. Older adults may be more sensitive to the effects of these drugs than younger groups are. Headaches, dizziness, and edema are complaints in 20% or less of patients. Calcium channel blockers have not been tested in pregnant women. Adverse fetal effects have been found in animal studies when very large doses were given. Some of the calcium channel blockers have been found in breast milk.

Concern has been raised that calcium channel blockers may increase the rate of heart attacks or death. The fast-acting form of nifedipine at high dosage has been specifically implicated by recent studies as increasing mortality. Studies are underway to determine how safe calcium channel blockers are in general.

Interactions
Calcium channel blockers depress the atrioventricular (AV) nodal conduction that may lead to heart block. Beta-adrenergic blockers act synergistically with calcium channel blockers to depress both AV conduction and cardiac contractility. The digitalis glycosides act in an additive manner with the calcium channel blockers to depress AV conduction. These drugs should be used with caution in patients with congestive heart failure.

Specific Calcium Channel Blockers

✣ *Diltiazem*
Diltiazem (Cardizem) depresses both the sinoatrial (SA) and AV nodes but produces little negative inotropic effect (decrease in the strength of the heartbeat). It is effective in dilating coronary vessels, making it a good antianginal agent. Diltiazem is well absorbed orally and extensively metabolized. The onset of action is 30 to 60 minutes for the tablet form and 2 to 3 hours for the extended-release capsule form. The duration of action is 4 to 8 hours for the tablet form, 12 hours for the sustained-release capsule form, and 24 hours for the controlled-dose capsule form. Diltiazem is extensively metabolized, and metabolites are excreted in the urine and feces.

Felodipine
Felodipine (Plendil) is a potent peripheral vasodilator that does not depress the SA or AV node. The drug is well absorbed but extensively metabolized by the liver after absorption. Felodipine is effective in 2 to 5 hours and has a duration of action of 24 hours. Metabolites are excreted in the urine.

Isradipine
Isradipine (DynaCirc) is a potent vasodilator that does not depress the SA or AV node. With its use there tends to be a

reflex increase in heart rate in response to the vasodilation. Isradipine is used primarily as an antihypertensive agent. It is effective in 2 to 3 hours and has a duration of action over 12 hours. Isradipine is extensively metabolized, and metabolites are excreted in the urine and feces.

Nicardipine

Nicardipine (Cardene) is more selective for vascular smooth muscle than for cardiac muscle. This means that nicardipine is a potent vasodilator and also dilates the coronary vessels with little or no depression of conductivity. It is used both as an antihypertensive agent and an antianginal agent. Nicardipine is well absorbed and rapid acting; it has duration of action of about 8 hours. It is extensively metabolized, and metabolites are excreted in the urine and feces.

Nifedipine

Nifedipine (Procardia, Adalat) is similar to nicardipine in being more selective for smooth muscle than for cardiac muscle. It has no real effect on the AV node and so does not directly depress the heart rate. It is used both as an antihypertensive agent and an antianginal agent. Nifedipine is rapidly absorbed with an onset of action of 20 minutes and a duration of action of 4 to 8 hours. Extended-release forms are available with longer durations. The drug is readily metabolized, and metabolites are excreted in the urine and feces.

Verapamil

Verapamil (Calan, Isoptin) depresses the SA and AV nodes, an action that makes it a useful antiarrhythmic drug (Chapter 19). A slowing of the heart rate (bradycardia) is common. Verapamil is used as both an antihypertensive agent and an antianginal agent. It is well absorbed. The onset of action is 4 to 12 hours, and the duration of action is 8 to 10 hours. Extended-release forms have a 24-hour duration of action. Verapamil is readily metabolized, and metabolites are excreted in the urine and feces.

Other Vasodilators

Hydralazine

Hydralazine (Apresoline) acts directly on arteriolar smooth muscle to cause relaxation. The mechanism is not known. The drop in arterial blood pressure is great enough to activate the baroreceptors of the aorta. This activation causes a reflex stimulation of the heart that increases cardiac output and partially compensates for the fall in blood pressure (reflex tachycardia). Hydralazine also causes sodium retention. Because hydralazine causes reflex stimulation of the heart and increases sodium retention, it is most effective in reducing hypertension when added to a diuretic to counteract the sodium retention and a beta-blocker (propranolol, nadolol, or metoprolol) to block the reflex stimulation of the heart.

Side effects common to hydralazine include headache, palpitation, loss of appetite, nausea, vomiting, and diarrhea. In the absence of a beta antagonist, hydralazine can cause angina in susceptible individuals as a result of the reflex stimulation of the heart. Hydralazine is not a good drug for a patient with angina, coronary artery disease, or congestive heart failure because of the indirect cardiac effects.

An occasional effect of long-term therapy at high doses of hydralazine is the appearance of a "lupuslike" syndrome. Lupus erythematosus is an autoimmune disease with symptoms of fever, joint pain, chest pain, edema, and circulating antibodies to DNA. The syndrome induced by hydralazine is similar, but it is reversed when the drug is discontinued. The appearance of lupuslike symptoms is infrequent when smaller doses of hydralazine are used in combination with diuretic and sympathetic blocking drug. Patients on hydralazine therapy are monitored for the appearance of the anti-DNA antibodies.

Minoxidil

Minoxidil (Loniten) is a direct-acting vasodilator like hydralazine, but it is more potent. This drug must be given with a diuretic to control fluid retention and a beta-receptor blocker to prevent reflex tachycardia. A side effect of minoxidil is excessive hairiness, which may develop after a few weeks of treatment. Some patients experience transient nausea, headaches, or fatigue when treatment is started.

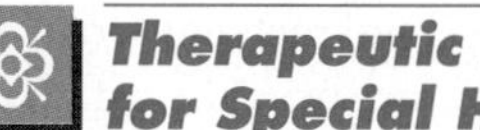

Therapeutic Agents: Drugs Used for Special Hypertensive Situations

Alpha-1, Alpha-2 Blockers

Phentolamine

Mechanism of Action

Phentolamine (Regitine, Rogitine) is a short-acting and reversible alpha-adrenergic receptor antagonist. The major effects of phentolamine are vasodilation resulting from blockade of alpha-1 adrenergic receptors and cardiac stimulation believed to be associated with blockade of the presynaptic alpha-2 adrenergic receptors. (The presynaptic alpha-2 adrenergic receptors are associated with uptake of norepinephrine; see Chapter 12.)

Pharmacokinetics

This drug is not well absorbed orally, and IV or intramuscular administration is more common.

Uses

Phentolamine has specific clinical uses as a vasodilator. One use is to lower blood pressure in patients with a tumor of the adrenal medulla that secretes large amounts of epinephrine (the tumor is called a pheochromocytoma). Another use is to lower blood pressure in patients who are being treated with a monoamine oxidase inhibitor and are suffering from the "cheese reaction," a hypertensive crisis that can be reversed with phentolamine. (See Chapter 53

PATIENT PROBLEM

Orthostatic Hypotension

THE PROBLEM

The blood pressure drops markedly as the individual moves from lying to sitting or sitting to standing position.

SIGNS AND SYMPTOMS

Dizziness, lightheadedness, weakness, and syncope (fainting)

ASSOCIATED OR CONTRIBUTING FACTORS

Long periods of standing; hot weather; hot showers or baths; ingestion of alcohol; exercise, especially when followed by immobility; and dehydration

PATIENT AND FAMILY EDUCATION

- Tighten calf muscles regularly while standing, or take a break to walk around frequently.
- If possible, sit instead of standing at work.
- Reduce the temperature of baths and showers.
- Wear support stockings. In severe cases tailor-made waist-high stockings may be needed.
- Avoid the use of alcohol.
- Move slowly from lying to sitting position. Hold on to something to provide support while moving from lying to sitting or standing position.
- Maintain adequate fluid intake to avoid dehydration, especially in the summer or if perspiring profusely.
- If the problem is severe, consult the physician. A change in drug or dose may be needed.

ADDITIONAL NURSING CARE MEASURES

- Monitor the blood pressure with patient lying, sitting, and standing. To document hypotension, check both arms.
- Supervise ambulation. Instruct patients with marked hypotension to call for assistance when moving from a reclining to a standing position.

for a discussion of the "cheese reaction.") A third use is to treat patients who are being withdrawn from the antihypertensive drug clonidine and may suffer a temporary hypertensive crisis.

A major use of phentolamine is to infiltrate a site where levarterenol (norepinephrine) or metaraminol has leaked into the tissue surrounding the infusion site. Phentolamine reverses the profound vasoconstriction that can otherwise cause tissue death.

Phentolamine, usually with papaverine, may be used in the treatment of impotence. The drugs are administered intracavernosally within 2 hours of intercourse.

Adverse Reactions and Contraindications

Side effects of the systemic use of phentolamine include hypotension, a rapid heart rate (tachycardia) as a reflex response of the body to the hypotension, nasal congestion associated with the vasodilation, and general GI upset. Caution should be used in administering phentolamine to patients with angina, coronary insufficiency, or a history of heart attacks.

Interactions

Phentolamine antagonizes the vasopressor action of sympathomimetic drugs such as dopamine, epinephrine, and phenylephrine.

Phenoxybenzamine

Mechanism of Action

Phenoxybenzamine (Dibenzyline) is an irreversible and nonselective blocker of alpha-adrenergic receptors.

Pharmacokinetics

Phenoxybenzamine is given orally. The onset of action takes several hours. Because the drug combines irreversibly with alpha-adrenergic receptors, the effect is cumulative over a week with daily dosing. The duration of action is prolonged, 3 to 4 days after a single dose. Phenoxybenzamine is metabolized by the liver with renal and biliary excretion of metabolites.

Uses

Phenoxybenzamine is used to control the high blood pressure caused by the elevated plasma levels of epinephrine in patients with the adrenal tumor pheochromocytoma when they are not yet ready for surgical removal of the tumor. Phenoxybenzamine is also used to dilate blood vessels in the skin, as in the treatment of Raynaud's phenomenon, in which there is a prominent neurogenic vasoconstriction of the blood vessels of the skin, particularly in the hands and feet (Chapter 15).

Adverse Reactions and Contraindications

The prominent side effect of phenoxybenzamine is orthostatic hypotension (see box). Reflex tachycardia, nasal congestion, and GI upset are other common side effects of phenoxybenzamine resulting from its alpha-adrenergic antagonist activity.

Interactions

A major source of drug interactions with phenoxybenzamine is overstimulation of beta-adrenergic receptors by drugs such as epinephrine, which have both alpha- and beta-adrenergic receptor agonist activity. The blockade of alpha receptors allows beta-receptor activation to go unopposed. Tachycardia is exaggerated. The vasodilator activity of drugs (as of the opioids) is exaggerated in the presence of phenoxybenzamine.

Therapeutic Agents: Drugs Used in Hypertensive Emergencies

A **hypertensive emergency** cannot be simply defined. The blood pressure may be severely elevated or only moderately elevated. The important feature is that there is impending end-organ damage, usually of the brain, heart, or eyes. Unstable neurologic symptoms that suggest damage to the brain include headache, restlessness, confusion, and even convulsions. Hemorrhaging may be apparent in the eye. Drugs currently used to treat hypertensive emergencies by rapidly lowering blood pressure are listed in Table 13-3.

Vasodilators

Diazoxide

As a **vasodilator,** diazoxide (Hyperstat) acts directly to relax arteriolar smooth muscle. This action lowers blood pressure but does not affect the venous side of circulation. Diazoxide is therefore not useful for those conditions requiring the decreased venous return produced by trimethaphan.

The advantage of diazoxide treatment is that a bolus of the drug can be given intravenously over 30 seconds and will usually be effective in 5 minutes and remain effective for 2 to 12 hours. Blood pressure does not need to be continuously monitored as with trimethaphan treatment. The patient rarely be-

TABLE 13-3 Drugs Used in Hypertensive Emergencies

GENERIC NAME	TRADE NAME	ADMINISTRATION/ DOSAGE	COMMENTS
Diazoxide	Hyperstat*	INTRAVENOUS: *Adults*—150 mg or 5 mg/kg body weight. *Children*—5 mg/kg body weight. Administered over 30 sec. May be repeated after 30 min.	Direct-acting vasodilator. Acts rapidly (2-5 min) and lasts 2-12 hr. Increases venous return and cardiac output. Blood pressure fall is rarely excessive, so blood pressure monitoring is not critical.
Enalaprilat	Vasotec	INTRAVENOUS: *Adults*—1.25 mg administered over 5 min every 6 hr. Use 0.625 mg for patients undergoing diuretic therapy or in renal failure.	An ACE inhibitor, drug is in active form for IV administration. Clinical response should be seen in 1 hr.
Labetalol	Normodyne Trandate*	INTRAVENOUS: *Adults*—20 mg or 0.25 mg/kg injected over 2 min. Additional injections of 40-80 mg may be given at 10 min intervals until blood pressure control is achieved or total dose of 300 mg has been given. Alternatively, may be infused at rate of 2 mg/min.	Mixed alpha and beta blocker. Clinical response is seen in about 5 min.
Methyldopate hydrochloride	Aldomet*	INTRAVENOUS: *Adults*—250-500 mg in 100 ml 5% dextrose, administered slowly over 30-60 min. Maximum dose is 1 gm in 6 hr. INTRAVENOUS: *Children*—5-10 mg/kg in 5% dextrose, administered over 30-60 min. Maximum dose is 65 mg/kg body weight or 3 gm daily.	Centrally acting antihypertensive. Clinical response may take several hours. Duration of action is 10-16 hr.
✤ Nitroglycerin	Nitro-Bid* Nitrol Nitrostat* Tridil*	INTRAVENOUS: *Adults*—initially 5 μg/min; increase in 5 μg increments every 3-5 min until clinical response or 20 μg/min is reached.	Direct-acting vasodilator. Doses are stated for non-PVC infusion sets. PVC may absorb nitroglycerin. IV nitroglycerin is also used to reduce cardiac load or as antianginal agent in emergency situation. Effective immediately.
Sodium nitroprusside	Nipride* Nitropress	INTRAVENOUS: *Adults*—dissolve 50 mg in 500-1000 ml of 5% dextrose. Infuse 0.5 to 10 μg/kg/min. Solution must be protected from light and discarded after 4 hr. *Children*—1.4 μg/kg/min.	Direct-acting vasodilator. Acts rapidly (1-2 min). Continuous infusion is necessary to maintain hypotensive effect. Decreased venous return occurs with no change in heart rate. Blood pressure must be carefully monitored and infusion rate adjusted to maintain desired level.
Trimethaphan camsylate	Arfonad*	INTRAVENOUS: *Adults*—0.1% (1 mg/ml) infusion in 5% dextrose. Rate of infusion is begun at 0.5-1 mg/min and increased gradually until blood pressure falls by 20 mm Hg. After several minutes, rate is again increased until blood pressure reaches desired level.	Rapidly acting drug blocks acetylcholine receptors in ganglia. Inhibits sympathetic and parasympathetic nervous systems and decreases venous return and cardiac output. Blood pressure must be carefully monitored because hypotensive effect is variable and unpredictable.

*Available in Canada and United States.

comes excessively hypotensive. Diazoxide causes retention of sodium and water, which must be treated with a diuretic. Diazoxide also causes hyperglycemia.

Nitroglycerin

Nitroglycerin (Nitro-Bid IV, Nitrostat IV, Tridil) acts directly to relax smooth muscle with a greater effect on the venous than the arterial circulation. The advantage of nitroglycerin is its immediate action; it must be continuously infused. Since nitroglycerin is absorbed by PVC plastic, special non-PVC infusion sets are used.

Sodium Nitroprusside

Sodium nitroprusside (Nipride) acts directly on the smooth muscle of both arterioles and venous vessels. The result is an immediate decrease in blood pressure with no increase in venous return. There are no notable side effects with short-term use of nitroprusside. Blood pressure must be constantly monitored, and the drug is administered by intravenous (IV) drip. Nitroprusside is unstable in light, so it should not be used more than 4 hours after it is dissolved. Side effects arise from the use of nitroprusside for several days. Some of it is metabolized to thiocyanate, which can produce ringing in the ears (tinnitus), blurred vision, and hypothyroidism.

Ganglionic Blocking Drug: Trimethaphan

Trimethaphan (Arfonad) blocks the receptors for acetylcholine in the ganglia and is a ganglionic blocking drug. Ganglionic blocking drugs inhibit both sympathetic and parasympathetic activity and therefore have limited clinical use. Trimethaphan is used in treating some hypertensive emergencies. Because this drug has a short duration of action, it is administered by continuous IV drip; during this time blood pressure must be constantly monitored. Side effects result from the inhibition of both sympathetic and parasympathetic tone. Severe hypotension can result from the inhibition of sympathetic tone. IV drip is then discontinued until the blood pressure begins to rise again. Side effects from loss of parasympathetic tone include pupillary dilation, loss of accommodation, drying of mucous surfaces, constipation, and urinary retention.

The disadvantages of trimethaphan therapy are that blood pressure must be carefully monitored and that the loss of pupillary reflexes makes it difficult to monitor ongoing neurologic damage to the brain (when neurologic damage was the presenting set of symptoms). In addition, trimethaphan can be unpredictable in its effects; patients already taking antihypertensive medication or those with a reduced blood volume may be unusually sensitive to trimethaphan. Some patients do not respond readily to trimethaphan; others are initially responsive but become unresponsive later.

Trimethaphan does decrease venous return of blood and lower cardiac output. These actions are helpful when the patient has a condition such as a dissecting aortic aneurysm, hypertensive encephalopathy, acute left ventricular failure, or cerebral hemorrhage, because the pressure is removed from the weakened tissue.

NURSING PROCESS OVERVIEW

Antihypertensive Drugs

Assessment

Assess the blood pressure with the patient at rest. Check both arms. Some physicians order lying, sitting, and standing blood pressure measurements. Monitor weight, serum electrolytes, blood urea nitrogen, and measures of renal and cardiovascular function. Obtain a dietary history that focuses on sodium intake. Assess patterns of smoking and alcohol consumption.

Nursing Diagnoses

- Sexual dysfunction related to drug's side effect: impotence
- Noncompliance related to intolerable side effects
- Risk for orthostatic hypotension

Patient Outcomes

The patient will maintain blood pressure within normal range. The patient will not discontinue antihypertensive medication without consulting the health care provider. The patient will not experience intolerable side effects.

Planning/Implementation

Patients in hypertensive crisis may be admitted to the acute care setting for cardiac monitoring and intravenous drug therapy. Otherwise, therapy may be started in the hospitalized or ambulatory patient. Monitor the blood pressure and other vital signs, intake and output, weight, serum electrolyte levels, blood glucose levels, and other laboratory data specific to the side effects of individual drugs. In preparation for discharge, teach the patient about prescribed drugs and other prescribed therapies: sodium restriction, weight loss, smoking cessation, limited alcohol intake, and regular exercise.

Evaluation

Ideally, therapy will lower the blood pressure to below 140/90 mm Hg without serious side effects. Ascertain that the patient can explain the hazards of untreated hypertension, how to take the prescribed medications safely, why additional drugs such as diuretics or potassium may be needed, what to do about anticipated side effects, how to follow any dietary restrictions, and when to call the physician. If necessary, teach the patient to record weight or blood pressure on a regular basis. If the patient is interested, refer him or her to local smoking-cessation clinics.

NURSING IMPLICATIONS SUMMARY

General Guidelines: Antihypertensives

Drug Administration/Patient Education

- Encourage the patient to lose weight to reach a desirable body weight and to restrict dietary intake of sodium because these changes may reduce the need for antihypertensive drug therapy. Other lifestyle changes that may lessen the need for antihypertensive medication include stopping smoking, cutting back on caffeine intake, and exercising regularly.
- Assess the patient thoroughly and thoughtfully on a regular basis. Poor compliance with drug therapy may result if the patient feels worse, not better, while taking antihypertensives. The patient may feel reluctant to discuss side effects such as impotence and may discontinue a drug if this or other side effects occur. In addition, the cost of drug therapy, especially when two or more drugs are required, may be prohibitive.
- Reinforce the need to take these medications as directed and not to discontinue therapy abruptly or without consulting the physician.
- Work with the patient to develop a system for remembering to take medicines. Activities such as marking off a calendar when doses are taken or preparing a week of doses at one time may keep the patient more involved and help to serve as a reminder.
- Instruct the patient about orthostatic hypotension, a common side effect of antihypertensive therapy (see box on p. 157).
- Monitor blood pressure and pulse at least every 4 hours when a patient begins antihypertensive therapy, during periods of dosage adjustment, or when orthostatic hypotension is a problem. Assess the blood pressure with the patient lying, then sitting, then standing; check both arms. For selected patients, it may be necessary to instruct a family member to measure and record the blood pressure in the home setting.
- Supervise the ambulation of the hospitalized patient undergoing antihypertensive therapy to guard against injury in case the patient becomes dizzy or faint. Be especially alert with older adult patients, who are more sensitive to drug effects.
- Teach the patient to keep all health care providers informed of all drugs being used and to avoid over-the-counter medications unless approved by the physician. The incidence of hypotensive episodes is increased if the patient taking antihypertensives takes other drugs that also cause hypotension, including diuretics, CNS depressants, barbiturates, antihistamines, or alcohol.
- Monitor the daily weight of the hospitalized patient. Weigh the patient under standard conditions (same time, same scales, same amount of clothing). Observe for signs of fluid retention such as pitting edema (edema characterized by indentations that remain in the skin for seconds to minutes after pressure has been applied by the examiner's finger); dependent edema; and tight rings, shoes, and clothing. Auscultate the lungs to detect pulmonary rales. If possible, instruct the patient to monitor and record his or her weight at home. Report to the physician a weight gain in excess of 2 lb/day or 5 lb/wk. Record intake and output in the hospitalized patient. Refer the patient to a dietitian or teach the patient about dietary sodium (see box on p. 150).
- When a patient is taking a combination product containing two or more drugs, teach about each drug in the product and assess for side effects for each drug. For example, Apresoline contains hydralazine and hydrochlorothiazide; the drug Ser-Ap-Es contains hydralazine, hydrochlorothiazide, and reserpine.
- If a dose is missed, instruct the patient to take the dose as soon as it is remembered, unless within 2 hours of the next dose, and then to resume the usual dosing schedule. Emphasize that the patient should not double up for missed doses.
- Caution the patient to avoid driving or operating hazardous equipment if sedation or sleepiness occurs. Review the box on p. 300 for measures to help patients with dry mouth.

Intravenous Antihypertensive Therapy

- Monitor the patient's blood pressure and pulse every 3 to 5 minutes until stable, then every 15 to 30 minutes. Use an electronic infusion monitor and/or a microdrip infusion set to titrate the drug dose more accurately. Monitor the electrocardiogram. Ensure that the patient remains in bed for up to 3 hours after drug administration. Keep the call bell within reach and the siderails up.

Beta-Blockers

Drug Administration

- See general guidelines for antihypertensives.
- Take the apical pulse for a full minute before administering a dose. If the pulse is <60 beats/min in an adult or <90 to 110 beats/min in a child, withhold the dose and notify the physician. Specific guidelines may vary with an individual patient or by physician preference. Be especially alert to bradycardia if the patient is also taking a cardiac glycoside. Monitor the blood pressure. Review the general guidelines. Monitor the general parameters of cardiovascular function, including intake, output, daily weight, and serum electrolyte. Because beta-blockers accumulate in the presence of renal failure, monitor the blood urea nitrogen levels. Treatment of overdose with beta-blockers is symptomatic.

NURSING IMPLICATIONS SUMMARY—cont'd

- Bronchospasm occurs occasionally. Assess for signs of respiratory distress, auscultate lung sounds, and monitor respiratory rate.
- Assess the patient for signs of depression, including withdrawal, insomnia, anorexia, and lack of interest in personal appearance.
- If beta-blockers are being used for treatment of angina pectoris, see the Nursing Implications Summary in Chapter 15 (p. 194).

Intravenous Atenolol

- May be given by direct IV push at a rate of 5 mg injected evenly over 5 minutes. Monitor blood pressure, pulse, and electrocardiogram.

Intravenous Labetalol

- May be given by direct IV push at a rate of 20 mg or less over at least 2 minutes. May be further diluted to provide a constant infusion. For example, dilute 200 mg (40 ml) in 160 ml of diluent to form a concentration of 1 mg/ml. Compatible with most IV fluids, including D5W, NS, D5NS, D5 in 0.2%, 0.33%, or 0.45% NS, Ringer's injection, or lactated Ringer's injection. Use microdrip tubing and/or a volume- or rate-controlling device to titrate dose precisely. Monitor blood pressure every 2 to 5 minutes until stable. During IV administration, keep the patient supine. After administration, monitor blood pressure every 15 to 30 minutes until stable; this may take up to 3 hours. There is Y-site incompatibility with cefoperazone, nafcillin, and sodium bicarbonate. Mixing labetalol with other drugs in syringe or solution is not recommended.

Intravenous Metoprolol

- May be given by direct IV push. Administer dose over at least 1 minute. Monitor blood pressure, pulse, and electrocardiogram.

Intravenous Propranolol

- Check dose carefully; IV dose is much smaller than oral dose. May be given undiluted or diluted in 5% dextrose solution. Administer at a rate of 1 mg/min or more slowly. Monitor blood pressure, pulse, and electrocardiogram.

Patient and Family Education

- Emphasize the importance of taking these drugs as prescribed for optimal benefit. Caution the patient not to discontinue these drugs without consulting the physician and not to let prescriptions run out. Stress that several weeks of therapy may be needed to gain maximum effects. Orthostatic hypotension may be a problem (review the box on p. 157).
- Instruct the patient to take oral doses with meals or snacks to reduce gastric irritation. Instruct the patient to swallow extended-release forms whole without chewing, crushing, or breaking (unless the tablet is scored). Instruct the patient taking concentrated oral propranolol to measure the dose with the calibrated dropper provided, then to mix the dose with a small amount of liquid or food such as water, juice, soda, applesauce, or pudding. Tell the patient to take the dose immediately after preparing it and to eat all the mixture to ensure that the whole dose is consumed.
- Emphasize the following points to the patient. For missed doses of atenolol, betaxolol, carteolol, labetalol, nadolol, penbutolol, sotalol, or extended-release oxprenolol or propranolol: Take when remembered—unless within 8 hours of next scheduled dose, then omit. For missed doses of other beta-blockers: Take when remembered—unless within 4 hours of next scheduled dose, then omit. Do not double up for missed doses. Wear a medical identification tag or bracelet.
- Many side effects can occur with beta-blockers. Tell the patient to report any unexpected sign or symptom to the physician. Teach the patient to report signs of thrombocytopenia (unexplained bruising or bleeding) or of agranulocytosis (unexplained fever or sore throat). Teach patients with diabetes that beta-blockers may mask the symptoms of hypoglycemia; these patients should monitor blood glucose levels carefully during periods of dosage adjustment or when starting or stopping the drug. Tell the patient that if drowsiness occurs, driving or operating hazardous equipment should be avoided until this effect wears off. Instruct the patient to notify the physician if drowsiness is severe or persistent.

Alpha-1 Blockers: Doxazosin, Prazosin, and Terazosin

Drug Administration/Patient and Family Education

- See general guidelines for antihypertensives.
- A "first-dose" reaction may occur within 30 to 90 minutes after the initial dose has been administered. Monitor blood pressure; anticipate that orthostatic hypotension and/or fainting may occur. Supervise the patient closely during the first 2 hours after the first dose. A first-dose reaction is more common in older adults. It also may occur if the dosage is increased. To help minimize this reaction, the first dose is often limited to 1 mg; also the first dose can be given at bedtime, if possible.
- Nasal congestion or runny nose may be a problem. Inform the patient that this side effect may decrease with continued use of the prescribed drug. Caution the patient to avoid the use of over-the-counter medications to self-treat this annoying side effect.

Continued.

NURSING IMPLICATIONS SUMMARY—cont'd

- Caution the patient to avoid driving or operating hazardous equipment until the effects of these medications are known. Blurred vision, dizziness, and lethargy may be common.
- Before discharge, teach the patient how to monitor for fluid retention. If diuretics are also prescribed, explain the importance of taking all drugs as ordered for maximum effects.
- These drugs are especially prone to cause orthostatic hypotension, particularly when therapy is started and during periods of increasing dosage. See box on p. 157 for a discussion of orthostatic hypotension. Instruct the patient to take the first dose and any increased doses at bedtime and to be especially careful when getting up at night during the first few days of therapy. Warn the family members about this side effect so that they will not be frightened and will know that they should make the patient lie down until he or she is no longer dizzy.
- When terazosin is being used to treat benign prostatic hypertrophy, teach the patient that 2 to 6 weeks of therapy may be needed before symptoms improve.

Sympatholytic Drugs: Guanethidine and Guanadrel

Drug Administration/Patient and Family Education

- See general guidelines for antihypertensives.
- Diarrhea may be severe (see Chapter 24). The drugs may cause hypoglycemia. Instruct the patient with diabetes to monitor blood glucose levels closely during the start of therapy and periods of dosage adjustment. Dry mouth may occur (see box on p. 300). Nasal congestion may be a problem. Caution the patient to avoid treatment with over-the-counter products without consulting the physician.

Reserpine and Related Drugs

Drug Administration/Patient and Family Education

- See general guidelines for antihypertensives.
- Serious mental depression is a side effect. Assess the patient carefully for changes in mood or affect; assess for anorexia, insomnia, impotence, withdrawal, and mood swings. Instruct the family to report the development of any change in the patient's personality.
- Take doses with meals or snack to reduce gastric irritation.
- Monitor the patient's pulse. Tell the patient to notify the physician if noticeable changes in heart rate occur. Explain that several weeks of therapy may be necessary to see the full drug benefit.

Centrally Acting Antihypertensive Drugs: Clonidine, Guanabenz, and Guanfacine

Drug Administration/Patient and Family Education

- See general guidelines for antihypertensives.
- Dry mouth may occur (see box on p. 300). Constipation may occur (see box on p. 304). Caution the patient to avoid driving or operating hazardous equipment if drowsiness occurs.
- Emphasize to the patient the importance of not discontinuing these drugs abruptly. Teach the patient to have prescriptions refilled before the supply on hand runs out. Patients who may not comply with dosage schedules should not take these drugs. See discussion of withdrawal symptoms (p. 153). If an oral dose is missed, instruct the patient to take it as soon as it is remembered, unless within 2 hours of the next dose. Teach the patient not to double up for missed doses. If two or more doses are missed, the patient should notify the physician.
- Clonidine is available in a transdermal form. Review the instruction leaflet provided by manufacturer with the patient. Emphasize the following points. Do not cut or trim the patch. Remove the old patch. Apply the new patch to clean hairless area, but avoid areas of skin irritation or scars. Rotate sites. If the patch becomes loose or falls off, replace it with a fresh one; if it is only slightly loose, cover it with an adhesive overlay provided by the manufacturer. Replace the patch weekly. If a patch is overdue for replacement by 3 days or more, notify the physician; do not apply two patches at once. To discard the patch, fold it in half, sticky sides together. Discard the patch out of reach of children.

Methyldopa

Drug Administration/Patient and Family Education

- See general guidelines for antihypertensives.
- Dry mouth may occur (see box on p. 300). Depression is a side effect. Assess the patient carefully for changes in mood or affect; assess for anorexia, insomnia, impotence, withdrawal, and mood swings. Instruct the family to report the development of any change in the patient's personality. Diarrhea may occur.
- Nasal congestion may be a problem. Caution the patient to avoid treatment with over-the-counter products without consulting the physician.
- Methyldopa may alter liver function tests. Teach the patient to report the development of malaise, fever, right upper quadrant abdominal pain, or any change in the color or consistency of stools. Monitor liver function tests. Tell the patient that urine may darken if exposed to the air.

NURSING IMPLICATIONS SUMMARY—cont'd

- The IV form is methyldopate hydrochloride. Dilute the dose in 100 to 200 ml of 5% dextrose in water. Administer dose as an infusion over 30 to 60 minutes. Avoid intramuscular or subcutaneous administration.

Vasodilators for Treating Chronic Hypertension: ACE Inhibitors

Drug Administration

- Monitor serum potassium levels.

Intravenous Enalapril

- Check the dose; a single IV dose is much smaller than the oral dose. May be given undiluted; or dilute with up to 50 ml of a compatible IV solution (see manufacturer's guidelines). Administer the dose over at least 5 minutes. Monitor blood pressure and pulse. Keep the patient supine until the blood pressure is stable.

Patient and Family Education

- See general guidelines for antihypertensives.
- Caution the patient to avoid excessive amounts of foods high in potassium (see the dietary consideration box on potassium, p. 170). Teach the patient to avoid salt substitutes unless approved by the physician, because these often contain large amounts of potassium.
- Tell the patient to take captopril on an empty stomach, 1 hour before meals, unless instructed otherwise by the physician. Other ACE inhibitors may be taken on a full or empty stomach. If a dose is missed, it should be taken as soon as remembered, unless close to the time for the next dose. Tell the patient not to double up for missed doses. Instruct the patient to report the development of fever, sore throat, or signs of infection. Caution the patient to avoid driving or operating hazardous equipment if dizziness develops; if dizziness is severe, consult physician.

Calcium Channel Blockers

- See Nursing Implications Summary in Chapter 15 (p. 194).

Hydralazine

Drug Administration

- Hydralazine may be administered intramuscularly or intravenously (direct IV). It is recommended that it not be mixed with infusion fluids. Administer intravenously at a rate of 10 mg over 1 minute.

Patient and Family Education

- See general guidelines for antihypertensives.
- Diarrhea may occur (see Chapter 24). Teach the patient to monitor weight and to assess for fluid retention. Tell the patient to notify the physician if lupuslike symptoms develop (see p. 156).
- Instruct the patient to report the development of tingling of fingers or numbness because this sensation may signal peripheral neuropathy; pyridoxine may be prescribed. Instruct the patient to take oral doses with food or a snack to reduce gastric irritation. Tell the patient to avoid driving or operating hazardous equipment if dizziness develops.

Minoxidil

Patient and Family Education

- See general guidelines for antihypertensives.
- This drug may cause hypertrichosis (excessive hairiness) after several weeks of therapy. Instruct the patient to report this side effect. The hair can be shaved, bleached, or removed, depending on the location and severity. Caution the patient not to discontinue the medication without contacting the physician. The excessive hair growth may slowly disappear after several months of therapy.
- The side effect of hypertrichosis led to the development of topical minoxidil (Rogaine), used to stimulate hair growth in men who are balding. Instruct the patient to follow the instructions supplied by the manufacturer. Wash hair daily before applying solution, and dry scalp and hair thoroughly. Apply the prescribed amount, with the applicator supplied. Wash hands to remove any solution left on the hands. Do not use a hair dryer to dry the scalp after drug application. If topical minoxidil is used at night, wait at least 30 minutes after applying solution before going to bed. If a dose is missed, the patient should apply it as soon as it is remembered, unless it is close to the time for the next dose; the patient should not double up for missed doses. Tell the patient to report local side effects (e.g., itching, scalp burning, skin irritation) or systemic effects (e.g., dizziness, flushing, headache, tingling of hands or feet, or weight gain).
- Instruct the patient to report the development of shortness of breath, increased heart rate, or changes in heart rhythm. Teach the patient to monitor resting pulse and to report increases of 20 or more beats per minute above normal to the physician. Assess for distended jugular veins and pulmonary rales.

Alpha-1, Alpha-2 Blockers: Phenoxybenzamine and Phentolamine

Drug Administration

Intravenous Phentolamine

- Dilute 5 mg with 1 ml of sterile water; may be further diluted. Administer at a rate of 5 mg or less over 1 minute. Monitor blood pressure and pulse every 30 seconds, and monitor electrocardiogram. Do not leave the patient unattended until stable. Treat overdose with dopamine; do *not* use epinephrine.

Continued.

NURSING IMPLICATIONS SUMMARY—cont'd

- When the drug is used to treat extravasation, 5 to 10 mg of phentolamine is diluted in 10 ml of sodium chloride injection, and the area of extravasation is infiltrated with this solution with a small-bore needle. There may be other protocols in different agencies. Phentolamine may also be added to infusions of norepinephrine to prevent damage from extravasation.

Patient and Family Education

- See general guidelines for antihypertensives.
- Nasal congestion may be a problem. Inform the patient that this side effect may decrease with continued use of the prescribed drug. Caution the patient to avoid the use of over-the-counter medications to self-treat this annoying side effect.
- Tachycardia may be a problem. Teach the patient to take and record his or her resting pulse; increases of 20 or more beats per minute above normal should be reported to the physician. Orthostatic hypotension may develop (see box on p. 157).
- Phenoxybenzamine may cause dry mouth (see the box on p. 300). Caution the patient to avoid driving or operating hazardous equipment if drowsiness, confusion, or unusual tiredness develop. Phenoxybenzamine may also cause sexual dysfunction. Question the patient tactfully about sexual problems; many patients are reluctant to discuss sexual difficulties. Sexual problems may prompt the patient to discontinue the medication. Provide emotional support as needed. Remind the patient not to discontinue the medication without notifying the physician.
- (Intracavernosal injection of phentolamine and/or papaverine is discussed in the Nursing Implications Summary of Chapter 15, p. 194.)

Drugs Used in Hypertensive Emergencies

Drug Administration

- Drug dose may be titrated to the patient's blood pressure. Use microdrip tubing or an infusion monitor to regulate infusion. Do not leave the patient unattended until stable. Keep siderails up. Ideally the patient should be in an intensive care unit. Monitor electrocardiogram, blood pressure, pulse, respirations, acid-base balance, oxygenation via pulse oximetry, level of consciousness, intake, output; insertion of a Foley catheter may be necessary. These drugs should not be mixed with other drugs in an infusion or a syringe. Keep the patient and family informed of the patient's condition.

Intravenous Diazoxide

- Administer dose quickly, undiluted (e.g., 150 mg over 10 to 30 seconds). Because diazoxide is highly alkaline, avoid intramuscular or subcutaneous injection. Make certain that the IV line is patent before administering, and inspect the insertion site for irritation or redness. If extravasation occurs, apply ice packs. Treat drug overdose or severe hypotension with dopamine. Monitor the patient's blood glucose level because the diazoxide may cause hyperglycemia; insulin may be necessary.

Intravenous Nitroglycerin

- Before administration nitroglycerin injection must be diluted in D5W or 0.9% sodium chloride injection. Mix well. Use glass solution bottles and non-PVC infusion sets. See manufacturer's instructions regarding dilution instructions. Use microdrip tubing or an infusion monitor to help regulate the dosage precisely.

Intravenous Sodium Nitroprusside

- Dilute as directed by the manufacturer. Do not use an IV filter. Do not use if highly discolored; may be used if faintly brownish in color. Cover prepared infusion with sleeve provided by manufacturer or aluminum foil to protect from light. It is not necessary to cover the drip chamber or the tubing. Titrate dose based on physician guidelines and patient response; a typical dose is 3 μg/kg of body weight/min (adults) or 1.4 μg/kg/min (small children). Use microdrip tubing and an infusion control device. Monitor serum cyanide and thiocyanate concentrations with prolonged use.
- To treat overdose, discontinue nitroprusside and administer amyl nitrate (Chapter 15 and Chapter 9) for 15 to 30 seconds every minute until a sodium nitrite solution for IV administration can be prepared. Administer a 3% sodium nitrite solution in a dose of 4 to 6 mg/kg over 2 to 4 minutes. After this solution has been administered, inject sodium thiosulfate intravenously, 150 to 200 mg/kg. Monitor the patient carefully. Signs of overdose can reappear for up to several hours, and sodium nitrite and sodium thiosulfate can be repeated at half the dose listed. Monitor thiocyanate levels if the drug is used longer than 72 hours. Use dopamine to correct hypotension.

Intravenous Trimethaphan

- Dilute a 500 mg ampul in 500 ml D5W to produce a concentration of 1 mg trimethaphan per milliliter. Titrate the dose based on physician guidelines and patient response; a typical initial dose is 0.5 to 1.0 mg/min. Use microdrip tubing and an infusion control device. Monitor the patient's response closely. If blood pressure does not drop with the patient in the supine position, try raising the head of the bed. Monitor the patient closely for signs of cerebral anoxia; note that the drug produces pupillary dilation so this objective sign may be of little significance. To treat severe hypotension, use phenylephrine or try dopamine.

CRITICAL THINKING

APPLICATION

1. Describe the renal mechanisms that control blood pressure.
2. Describe the cardiovascular mechanisms that control blood pressure.
3. Name the beta-blockers that the nurse might see used as antihypertensive drugs. How does blockade of the beta-receptors lower blood pressure? What are the side effects of these drugs? What are cardioselective beta-blockers? List three cardioselective beta-blockers.
4. How does the action of phenoxybenzamine differ from that of phentolamine?
5. How does the use of prazosin differ from that of phentolamine?
6. List which antihypertensives act by interfering with storage and/or release of norepinephrine.
7. List which antihypertensives act centrally to inhibit sympathetic activity.
8. How do ACE inhibitors work? What are their limiting side effects?
9. How do calcium channel blockers decrease hypertension?
10. List those antihypertensives used in the chronic treatment of hypertension that are direct-acting vasodilators.
11. Which drug is both an alpha- and a beta-adrenergic antagonist?
12. List three drugs used to control a hypertensive emergency. Specify the mechanism of action for each drug.
13. What is orthostatic hypotension? Which antihypertensive drugs are commonly associated with orthostatic hypotension as a side effect?
14. Which antihypertensive is associated with the synthesis of a false transmitter?
15. Describe reflex tachycardia. Which antihypertensive drugs does the nurse anticipate to cause reflex tachycardia?

CRITICAL THINKING

1. Lifestyle modifications that may help lower blood pressure are described in this chapter. Describe at least five specific interventions a patient can use to help stop smoking.
2. For what situations might the nurse see phentolamine used as an antihypertensive drug? What is the mechanism of action?
3. Develop a teaching plan for a patient taking an ACE inhibitor.
4. Develop a teaching plan for a patient taking a calcium channel blocker.
5. What is a limiting side effect of reserpine? How can the nurse assess the patient for this side effect?
6. What education can the nurse provide about orthostatic hypotension as a side effect of antihypertensive drugs?
7. What reaction may occur with the sudden discontinuation of clonidine? What counsel can the nurse give?
8. Why is patient compliance with antihypertensive therapy frequently poor? What actions can the nurse take to increase compliance?
9. Hypertension is a major health problem that requires chronic drug therapy. The drugs may be costly and may cause annoying or embarrassing side effects. Treatment of hypertension may also necessitate lifestyle changes (e.g, sodium restriction, weight loss). Try some role-playing activities in which one student practices asking another student ("the patient") about how well the patient is complying with drug therapy. Try to develop questions that are nonjudgmental (to avoid putting the patient on the defensive) and yet not superficial.

CHAPTER 14

Diuretics

OBJECTIVES

After studying this chapter, you should be able to do the following:

- *Explain why increasing sodium excretion is a desirable action of diuretics.*
- *Name the loop diuretics.*
- *Identify the class of diuretics with the highest potency.*
- *Name conditions for which loop diuretics or thiazide diuretics are used.*
- *Develop a nursing care plan for a patient receiving a loop diuretic, thiazide diuretic, potassium-sparing diuretic, carbonic anhydrase inhibitor, or osmotic diuretic or a combination of two diuretics.*

KEY TERMS

carbonic anhydrase inhibitors
diuretics
homeostasis
loop diuretics
nephron
osmotic diuretics
potassium-sparing diuretics
thiazide diuretics

CHAPTER OVERVIEW

Diuretics are drugs that increase urine flow. There are several mechanisms by which drugs can produce this effect, but the clinically important drugs of this class act on the kidney. This chapter reviews pertinent renal physiology and discusses the mechanism of action and clinical properties of diuretic drugs.

Therapeutic Rationale: Diuretics

The kidneys regulate water and electrolyte balance in the body. Diuretics act at various sites within the kidney to modify salt and water excretion. The mechanisms by which these drugs act can be understood by first considering normal renal function and then considering how diuretics alter the normal processes.

Function of the Nephron

The functional unit of the kidney is the **nephron** (Figure 14-1). Glomerular filtration is the first step in the production of urine. Blood contacts a filtering surface in the glomerulus, where water and small molecules pass into the tubule, leaving behind most proteins and protein-bound small molecules. The remainder of the nephron adjusts the salt and water content of the tubular fluid to achieve **homeostasis,** a balanced condition in which the body retains the salt and water required for proper function and eliminates the excess. For the purpose of understanding diuretic drugs, this discussion is limited to six ions or molecules: sodium (Na^+), chloride (Cl^-), potassium (K^+), water (H_2O), bicarbonate (HCO_3^-), and organic ions.

Sodium Ion Sites

Sodium ion freely enters tubular fluid from the glomerulus so that fluid entering the proximal convoluted tubule has the same sodium ion content as blood. The proximal convoluted tubule actively removes sodium ion from the tubule. No further sodium ion is removed in the descending limb of Henle's loop, but in the ascending limb sodium ion follows chloride ion out of the tubule. In the distal convoluted tubule sodium ion is removed by an active pump like that in the proximal convoluted tubule or by a pump that exchanges sodium ion for potassium ion. With the latter pump sodium ion is reabsorbed, whereas potassium ion is excreted.

Chloride Ion Sites

Chloride ion is primarily removed from tubular fluid in the ascending limb of Henle's loop. This active removal of chloride ion draws sodium ion along with it and effectively dilutes tubular fluid.

Potassium Ion Sites

Potassium ion is not the primary ion involved in the action of any diuretic drug; diuretics are designed to alter sodium ion excretion patterns. Nevertheless, potassium excretion is altered by some of these agents, and the effects on some patients may be detrimental. Potassium ion may be reabsorbed in the ascending limb of Henle's loop. Secretion of potassium occurs in the distal convoluted tubule, where the ion is exchanged for sodium ion (see Figure 14-1).

Water Sites

Water may be recovered from the tubule by diffusion in the proximal convoluted tubule and in the descending limb of Henle's loop. The ascending limb of Henle's loop and the dis-

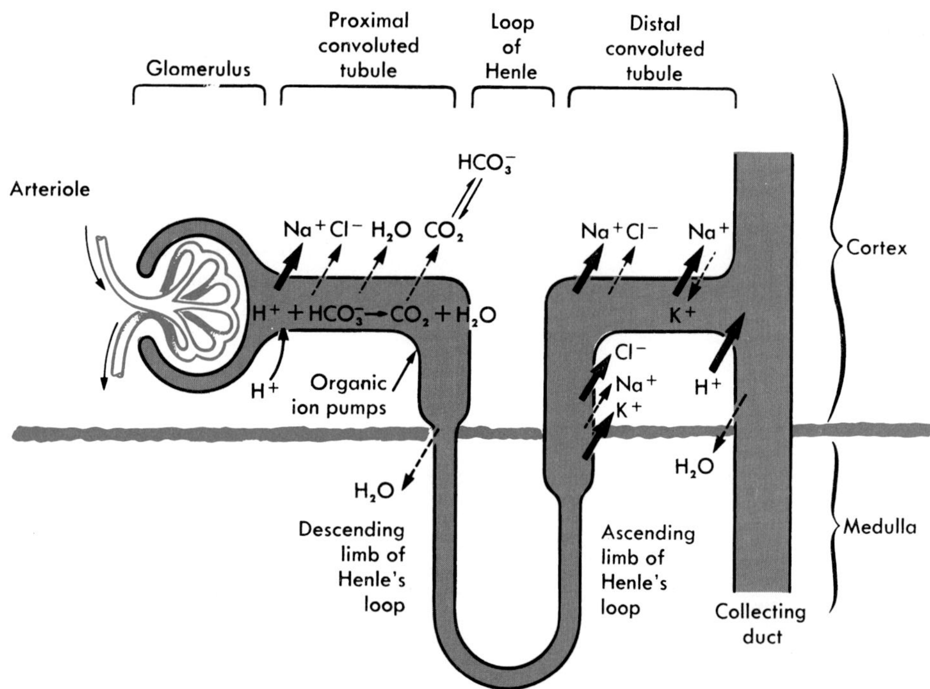

FIGURE 14-1
Sites of secretion and reabsorption of salt and water in nephron. Active (energy-requiring) processes are designated by *bold arrows;* passive diffusion is designated by *broken arrows.*

tal convoluted tubule are relatively impermeable to water. Final urine concentration is achieved in the collecting duct. Removal of water at this site is regulated by antidiuretic hormone (ADH), which increases permeability of the tissue to water and thereby increases water retention.

Bicarbonate Sites

Bicarbonate, which is the main buffer for the blood, freely enters tubular fluid from the glomerulus and must be recovered for the body to maintain proper acid-base balance. Reabsorption of bicarbonate occurs in the proximal convoluted tubule and depends on the enzyme carbonic anhydrase. Carbonic anhydrase converts hydrogen ion and bicarbonate ion in the tubular fluid to carbon dioxide and water. Carbon dioxide can freely pass into the tubular epithelial cell and is reabsorbed, whereas bicarbonate ion stays in the tubule. The reabsorbed carbon dioxide is quickly reconverted to bicarbonate within the kidney cell and may reenter the bloodstream.

Organic Ion Pumps

The kidney can rapidly secrete complex ions such as amino acids and other natural compounds. This secretion occurs near the proximal convoluted tubule in the cortical portion of the descending limb of Henle's loop. Many drugs, including several diuretics, enter tubular fluid by this mechanism, which is referred to as an *organic anion pump.* Since some diuretics work only from within the tubule, the action of the drug depends at least in part on the proper function of the organic ion pump.

Mechanism of Diuretic Action

The diuretics considered in this chapter achieve their effects mainly by increasing sodium ion excretion. Since water tends to follow sodium ion in the kidney, it is excreted when sodium ion is excreted. Several distinct mechanisms for increasing sodium ion excretion exist, and all may be understood in terms of the renal physiology just discussed. Specific patterns of ion excretion produced by the classes of drugs are summarized in Table 14-1, and mechanisms are discussed in detail in the following sections.

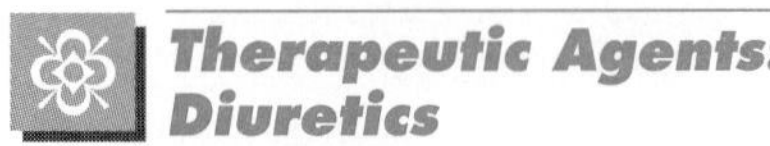

Therapeutic Agents: Diuretics

Loop Diuretics

Bumetanide, ethacrynic acid, furosemide, torsemide

Mechanism of Action

Bumetanide, ethacrynic acid, furosemide, and torsemide (Table 14-2) are called **loop diuretics** because the primary site of their diuretic action is in Henle's loop. These drugs inhibit active reabsorption of chloride ion in the ascending limb of Henle's loop. Since chloride ion reabsorption is prevented, passive reabsorption of sodium ion is also blocked. Therefore sodium chloride is retained in the tubule and excreted in urine, carrying water with it. Although 99.4% of the sodium ion entering tubular fluid is usually reabsorbed, under the influence of loop diuretics only 70% to 80% of the sodium ion is reabsorbed, along with an equivalent amount of chloride ion. Potassium ions and calcium ions are also excreted in higher than normal amounts in response to these drugs (see Table 14-1). At high doses, furosemide may occasionally increase bicarbonate excretion, whereas other loop diuretics have little direct effect on such excretion.

Although all loop diuretics are similar in their mechanism of action, bumetanide is much more potent than other loop diuretics. For example, 1 mg of bumetanide given orally is as effective as approximately 40 mg of furosemide.

Pharmacokinetics

Loop diuretics are well absorbed from the gastrointestinal (GI) tract, producing a diuretic effect within 1 hour of administration. With intravenous (IV) doses, diuresis occurs within 5 to 10 minutes (see Table 14-2).

Ethacrynic acid should not be given by intramuscular (IM) or subcutaneous injection since the drug can cause severe pain and irritation at the injection site. Torsemide also is used parenterally only intravenously. Other loop diuretics can be given intramuscularly, but the IV route is preferred for parenteral administration.

Loop diuretics are bound to proteins in the bloodstream and in the protein-bound form are not available for glomeru-

TABLE 14-1 Diuretic Effects on Tubular Transport

DRUG	EXCRETION INCREASED					EXCRETION BLOCKED		
Loop diuretics	Na^+	H_2O	K^+	Cl^-	—	Uric acid	Li^+	—
Thiazides and related drugs	Na^+	H_2O	K^-	Cl^-	HCO_3^-	Uric acid	Li^+	—
Potassium-sparing diuretics	Na^+	H_2O	—	—	HCO_3^-	—	—	K^+, H^+
Carbonic anhydrase inhibitors	Na^+	H_2O	K^-	—	HCO_3^-	Uric acid	—	—
Osmotic diuretics	(Na^+)*	H_2O	(K^+)*	(Cl^-)*	—	—	—	—

Li^+, Lithium ion; *H^+*, hydrogen ion.
*Large doses.
NOTE: The effects on ion transport shown are those commonly observed in humans during chronic therapy with normal clinical doses. With prolonged therapy, ions whose excretion is increased may become depleted from the body, whereas those whose excretion is blocked may accumulate. Lithium ion accumulation is clinically important only for those patients receiving lithium carbonate therapy for bipolar disorder. Uric acid accumulation is usually important only for those patients predisposed to gout.

TABLE 14-2 Loop Diuretics

GENERIC NAME	TRADE NAME	ADMINISTRATION/DOSAGE	DIURETIC EFFECT ONSET	PEAK	DURATION
Bumetanide	Bumex	ORAL: *Adults*—0.5-2 mg each morning; if needed, a second dose may be given 4-5 hr later. Usual daily doses are <10 mg. FDA pregnancy category C.	30 min	1-2 hr	4-6 hr
		INTRAVENOUS: *Adults*—initially 0.5-1 mg to relieve pulmonary edema; repeat dose in 2 hr if needed.	5-10 min	15-20 min	3-4 hr
Ethacrynic acid	Edecrin*	ORAL: *Adults*—50-100 mg initially; thereafter 50-200 mg daily. FDA pregnancy category B. *Children*—25 mg initially, increasing by 25 mg to maintain.	30 min	1-2 hr	6-8 hr
		INTRAVENOUS: *Adults*—50 mg. *Children*—1 mg/kg.	5-10 min	15-20 min	1-3 hr
Furosemide	Lasix* Myrosemide Novosemide† Uritol†	ORAL: *Adults*—20-80 mg once or twice daily. FDA pregnancy category C. *Children*—2 mg/kg initially, increasing by 1 or 2 mg/kg after 6-8 hr; maximum dose, 6 mg/kg.	30-60 min	1-2 hr	6-8 hr
		INTRAVENOUS: *Adults*—20-40 mg once or twice daily. *Children*—1 mg/kg initially, increasing by 1 mg/kg after 2 hr; maximum dose 6 mg/kg.	5-10 min	15-20 min	1-3 hr
Torsemide	Demadex	ORAL: *Adults*—5-20 mg once daily, adjusted as needed for therapeutic effect. Maximum daily dose: 200 mg. FDA pregnancy category B.	60 min	1-2 hr	6-8 hr
		INTRAVENOUS: *Adults*—5-20 mg once daily, adjusted as needed for therapeutic effect. Maximum daily dose: 200 mg.	5-10 min	1 hr	6-8 hr

*Available in Canada and United States.
†Available in Canada only.

lar filtration. These diuretics are secreted into the tubule by the organic anion pump in the cortical portion of the descending limb of Henle's loop. The effectiveness of loop diuretics depends on their ability to enter tubules, since diuresis is produced from within the tubule. In the kidney, ethacrynic acid exists primarily as the free drug and as a complex with cysteine. The cysteine-ethacrynic acid complex is much more effective than the free drug.

Excretion of loop diuretics is primarily renal, but some biotransformation to active and inactive products occurs. In renal failure the half-life of bumetanide and torsemide are unchanged, which suggests that biotransformation may be a highly effective route of elimination for these drugs.

Uses

Since loop diuretics promote the loss of excess salt and body water, they can control edematous states, such as those occurring in congestive heart failure, renal disease, cirrhosis of the liver, lymphedema, nephrotic syndrome, and ascites associated with cirrhosis or malignancies. The loop diuretics furosemide and torsemide are also used as second-line drugs for hypertension. Because loop diuretics cause rapid diuresis, rapid weight loss may occur as large volumes of fluid are lost (see box, p. 170).

Adverse Reactions and Contraindications

Electrolyte depletion, marked by weakness or lethargy, dizziness, leg cramps, anorexia, vomiting, and possibly mental confusion, may occur gradually. GI tract disturbances are also common with loop diuretics. Symptoms may include diarrhea, loss of appetite, and stomach pain or cramping. Ethacrynic acid causes GI tract disturbances more often than other loop diuretics, especially in patients receiving the drug continually for several months. A sudden, severe, watery diarrhea indicates the drug should be withdrawn. The physician may discontinue ethacrynic acid permanently if these symptoms arise.

Orthostatic hypotension is common with these powerful diuretics. Patients who tend to rise quickly from a sitting or

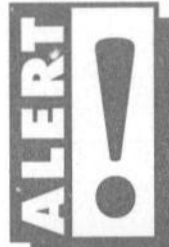

Drug Abuse Alert

Diuretics

BACKGROUND

Diuretics may be abused by patients obsessed with weight loss. The acute weight loss produced by diuretics has been exploited by some diet clinics that may initiate the program with a diuretic so that dramatic weight loss will occur early; however, this weight loss is short-lived, and the earlier weight recurs with rehydration. Such acute weight loss is occasionally exploited in high school and college wrestling programs; the diuretics allow a wrestler to meet a weight limit at weigh-in, and the athlete usually attempts to rehydrate before wrestling. Diuretics may also be abused by patients, obsessed with excretory functions, who use the drugs to achieve large volumes of urine. Such patients, who may also abuse cathartics, often view this ritualistic drug-taking as purification of the body.

PHARMACOLOGY

Diuretics promote an acute loss of body water and therefore cause an immediate drop in body weight. The amount of diuresis is related to the dose and strength of the drug used and also to the patient's water balance.

HEALTH HAZARDS

Long-term use of diuretics can cause severe electrolyte imbalances, especially if patients are not receiving careful counseling on dietary practices. If patients are receiving drugs from more than one physician or from unauthorized sources, follow-up care to monitor for the development of side effects may be lacking. The use of these drugs in weight control is unjustified, especially in healthy young athletes with no preexisting edema.

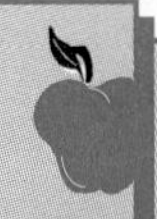

Dietary Consideration

Potassium Sources

Some drugs, especially the loop and thiazide diuretics, steroids, and amphotericin B, cause excessive loss of potassium, resulting in hypokalemia (low blood potassium levels). In mild cases hypokalemia may go unnoticed, but in severe cases it may contribute to toxicity from other drugs, as well as cardiac toxicity. Good dietary sources of potassium include:

- Citrus fruits and juices
- Bananas
- Grape, cranberry, apple, pear, and apricot juices
- Cereals
- Leafy vegetables
- Meat, fish, and fowl
- Salt substitutes (read label)
- Coffee, tea, and cola beverages
- Nuts and peanut butter

Some sources of potassium may be contraindicated in persons who must also limit sodium intake. Licorice can cause potassium excretion and should be avoided by patients experiencing hypokalemia.

lying position must learn to move slowly to allow accommodation of blood pressure (see box, p. 157). The most serious danger is risk of injury from falls.

Loop diuretics increase the loss of potassium and calcium ions, as well as sodium and chloride ions (see Table 14-1). Excessive potassium loss impairs proper functioning of the heart, skeletal muscle, kidneys, and other organs. Many physicians routinely prescribe a potassium replacement for their patients receiving loop diuretics for prolonged periods (see box above). Loss of calcium may rarely be sufficient to produce tetany. Most patients do not require calcium replacement, but serum calcium levels should be observed periodically. Uric acid excretion is partially blocked by loop diuretics. In susceptible patients gout may develop, but for most patients the increase in serum uric acid produces no symptoms. Loop diuretics affect ion transport in several body organs other than the kidneys. Altered sodium and potassium transport may be associated with toxicity to certain cells in the inner ear. Transient or permanent deafness has been observed in patients receiving loop diuretics, especially those who receive high doses or those who have reduced renal function in whom the drugs accumulate. Ototoxicity is more likely with ethacrynic acid than with other loop diuretics.

Loop diuretics impair glucose tolerance in some patients and rarely precipitate diabetes mellitus. Some patients experience sensitivity to sunlight while taking furosemide. Lupus erythematosus may be activated by ethacrynic acid and furosemide. Large doses of bumetanide may cause severe muscle pain (myalgia), chest pain, and premature ejaculation.

Loop diuretics should be used sparingly, if at all, in severe renal impairment. These drugs are less effective in these patients because the drugs fail to reach their site of action in the tubule. Loop diuretics also tend to accumulate in these patients, creating a greater risk of drug toxicity.

Toxicity

The loop diuretics are the most potent diuretics known. Their rapid, powerful action must be carefully monitored to avoid profound dehydration and salt depletion. Dehydration with reduction in blood volume can precipitate circulatory collapse. Vascular thromboses and emboli may be generated, especially in older adult patients (see box, p. 171).

Interactions

The potassium-depleting effect of loop diuretics makes these drugs dangerous for patients receiving digitalis. Lowered potassium content in tissues predisposes the heart to toxicity from cardiac glycosides, which may include fatal arrhythmias. Corticosteroids are also potassium-depleting agents and may add to the danger of electrolyte imbalance when given with loop diuretics.

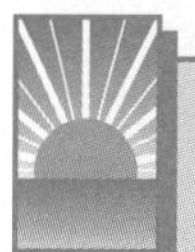

GERIATRIC CONSIDERATION

Diuretics

THE PROBLEM

Older adult patients are often more sensitive to the effects of diuretic drugs than are other adult patients. For example, loop diuretics and thiazides can cause excessive hypotension and severe electrolyte imbalances. Potassium-sparing diuretics more often cause hyperkalemia in older adults than in others.

SOLUTIONS

- Dosages of these drugs for older adults may be lower than for other adults.
- Blood pressure should be carefully monitored.
- Precautions should be taken against orthostatic hypotension.
- Electrolyte balance should be carefully monitored.
- Dietary counseling may be required to maintain potassium balance.

Loop diuretics lower the renal clearance of lithium, a drug used to control manic cycles in manic-depressive psychosis. Under these conditions, lithium may accumulate and severe toxicity may occur. These drugs are ordinarily not given together.

Loop diuretics have an antihypertensive action that may be additive with that of other antihypertensive agents. Care is required to prevent excessive hypotension when these drugs are used with antihypertensives.

The ototoxic effect of loop diuretics may be potentiated by aminoglycoside antibiotics (see Chapter 43), which are also ototoxic. This combination should be avoided because permanent deafness may result.

When given with loop diuretics, amphotericin B has the potential for increasing the risk of nephrotoxicity, ototoxicity, and hypokalemia.

Loop diuretics are strongly bound to serum proteins and may therefore displace other drugs from protein-binding sites. This action increases the concentration of the free, active form of the displaced drug. The anticoagulant warfarin is displaced in this way by loop diuretics. Higher concentrations of unbound warfarin produce greater anticoagulant effects and may produce toxicity.

Thiazide Diuretics

Mechanism of Action

Thiazide diuretics have multiple effects on the nephron. These diuretics block sodium and chloride ion reabsorption in the distal convoluted tubule. This action leads to increased excretion of sodium chloride and body water and establishes a new state of salt and water balance in which there is a lower level of body sodium than before the drug was given. Thiazide diuretics also inhibit carbonic anhydrase in the proximal convoluted tubule, thereby elevating the excretion of bicarbonate ion and an additional increment of sodium ion. This effect is lost after a few days. Potassium excretion is also enhanced by the thiazide diuretics, but this effect is not required for diuresis and is usually considered a toxic side effect.

Pharmacokinetics

Thiazide diuretics are well absorbed from the GI tract and may take action in the kidney within 1 hour of ingestion. Peak diuretic action can occur from 2 to 6 hours after an oral dose, depending on which thiazide preparation is used. Various preparations differ in timing and duration of diuretic effects (Table 14-3). In general, the longer acting thiazide diuretics are highly bound to serum proteins. Their long duration of action is related to their slow elimination from these protein-binding sites.

Thiazide diuretics remain primarily in the extracellular water in the body except for the drug concentrated in the kidneys. Thiazides are secreted into the renal tubule by the organic anion pump. Most of the dose leaves the body by this route. Some drug is eliminated by the liver, which secretes these drugs into the bile. Chlorothiazide sodium may be administered intravenously. The onset of action is somewhat more rapid by this route, but the duration of effect is not greatly altered from that of oral doses. This preparation must never be administered intramuscularly or subcutaneously. Great care should be taken to prevent leakage of the drug into the tissues when it is given intravenously.

Uses

Thiazide diuretics are less potent than loop diuretics and are more suitable for use by outpatients. The drugs can control edema associated with heart or kidney disease, as well as that caused by corticosteroid or estrogen therapy. The use of thiazide diuretics in controlling hypertension is discussed in Chapter 13.

Adverse Reactions and Contraindications

Long-term use of thiazide diuretics can cause fluid and electrolyte imbalance, which may produce thirst, weakness, lethargy, restlessness, muscle cramps, and fatigue. The electrolyte imbalance most likely to occur is excessive potassium and chloride ion loss. The loss of these ions leads to metabolic alkalosis. Potassium supplements may be required to remedy this situation. Chloride loss alone is usually mild and does not require treatment.

Calcium excretion is blocked by thiazide diuretics, and increased serum calcium levels may result. The parathyroid glands may also be affected by long-term therapy with these diuretics. Uric acid excretion is also blocked, and the increased blood levels may precipitate an attack of gout in susceptible individuals.

Thiazide diuretics irritate the GI tract and may cause side effects ranging from simple nausea and vomiting to constipation, jaundice, and pancreatitis.

TABLE 14-3 Thiazide Diuretics and Agents With Similar Mechanisms

GENERIC NAME	TRADE NAME	ADMINISTRATION/DOSAGE	DIURETIC EFFECT ONSET	PEAK	DURATION
Thiazide Diuretics					
Bendroflumethiazide	Naturetin*	ORAL: *Adults*—initially, 5 mg once daily; maintenance, 2.5-5 mg once daily or less frequently. FDA pregnancy category C. *Children*—maximum dosage 0.4 mg/kg daily in 1 or 2 doses; reduce dose for maintenance.	1-2 hr	4 hr	6-12 hr
Benzthiazide	Exna Hydrex	ORAL: *Adults*—50-100 mg once daily. FDA pregnancy category C. *Children*—1-4 mg/kg daily in 3 doses initially; dose reduced for maintenance.	2 hr	4-6 hr	12-18 hr
Chlorothiazide	Diuril	ORAL: *Adults*—0.25 to 1 gm once daily. FDA pregnancy category B. *Children*—22 mg/kg daily in 2 doses. *Infants <6 mo*—10-20 mg/kg daily in 2 doses.	2 hr	4 hr	6-12 hr
Chlorothiazide sodium	Diuril (sodium)	INTRAVENOUS: *Adults*—500 mg twice daily.	15 min	30 min	6-12 hr
Cyclothiazide	Anhydron	ORAL: *Adults*—1-2 mg once daily; maintenance, 1 mg 2-4 times weekly. FDA pregnancy category C. *Children*—initially, 0.02-0.04 mg/kg daily; reduce dose for maintenance.	2-4 hr	7-12 hr	18-24 hr
Hydrochlorothiazide	Diuchlor-H† Esidrix HydroDiuril* Oretic Urozide†	ORAL: *Adults*—initially, 25-100 mg once or twice daily; maintenance, 25-100 mg daily or less frequently. FDA pregnancy category B. *Children*—1-2 mg/kg daily in 2 doses. *Infants <6 mo*—up to 3 mg/kg daily.	2 hr	4 hr	6-12 hr
Hydroflumethiazide	Diucardin Saluron	ORAL: *Adults*—50-100 mg; once daily for low doses; divided doses over 100 mg daily. FDA pregnancy category C. *Children*—1 mg/kg daily; adjust as needed for maintenance.	1-2 hr	3-4 hr	18-24 hr
Methyclothiazide	Aquatensen Duretic† Enduron	ORAL: *Adults*—2.5-10 mg once daily. FDA pregnancy category B. *Children*—0.05-0.2 mg/kg daily.	2 hr	6 hr	24 hr
Polythiazide	Renese	ORAL: *Adults*—1-4 mg once daily; maintenance, 0.5-8 mg daily, according to response. *Children*—0.02-0.08 mg/kg daily.	2 hr	6 hr	36 hr
Trichlormethiazide	Metahydrin Naqua Trichlorex	ORAL: *Adults*—1-4 mg once daily. FDA pregnancy category C. *Children*—0.07 mg/kg daily in single or divided dose.	2 hr	6 hr	24 hr
Nonthiazide Diuretics With Thiazide-like Mechanisms					
Chlorthalidone	Hygroton* Thalitone Uridon†	ORAL: *Adults*—25-100 mg after breakfast daily or less frequently. FDA pregnancy category B. *Children*—2 mg/kg once daily for 3 days/wk.	2 hr	2 hr	48-72 hr
Indapamide	Lozide† Lozol	ORAL: *Adults*—2.5 mg/day taken in morning; may be increased after few days to 5 mg/day. FDA pregnancy category B.	1-2 hr	2.3-3.5 hr	24-72 hr
Metolazone	Diulo Mykrox Zaroxolyn*	ORAL: *Adults*—5-20 mg once daily for extended-release tablets. For prompt metolazone tablets, dose is 0.5 mg once daily. FDA pregnancy category B.	1 hr	2 hr	12-24 hr
Quinethazone	Hydromox	ORAL: *Adults*—50-100 mg once daily, or 150-200 mg alternate days or 3 times weekly.	2 hr	6 hr	18-24 hr

*Available in Canada and United States.
†Available in Canada only.

Thiazides may cause orthostatic hypotension. Chlorothiazide sodium may lower glomerular filtration rate when given intravenously. This does not affect most patients, although a patient with already reduced renal function may be adversely affected.

Thiazides are usually avoided in patients with severe impairment of renal function or anuria. Thiazides are less effective in these patients and may worsen renal function. Thiazides are also avoided in jaundiced infants because they may displace bilirubin from protein-binding sites, thereby increasing the risk of hyperbilirubinemia or kernicterus.

Toxicity

Thiazides affect the central nervous system (CNS). Mild symptoms include dizziness, headache, and paresthesia. At high concentrations such as those found in drug overdose, mental lethargy may progress to coma, although heart function and respiration are not markedly depressed. Overdose requires stomach evacuation, with monitoring of electrolyte balance and renal function.

Interactions

Since thiazide diuretics have hypotensive activity, they may potentiate the action of other antihypertensive agents, especially those that act at ganglionic or peripheral adrenergic sites (see Chapter 13). Thiazide diuretics are often included in fixed combinations that are marketed primarily as antihypertensives. Examples of these fixed combinations are shown in Table 14-4.

Thiazides cause loss of potassium, producing hypokalemia. Potassium loss is enhanced when thiazide diuretics are given with corticosteroids or adrenocorticotropic hormone (ACTH). Hypokalemia may make patients more sensitive to digitalis toxicity.

Thiazide diuretics frequently alter the requirement for insulin or other hypoglycemic agents. A diabetic patient who must receive one of the thiazides should be carefully observed during the first few days of thiazide therapy to prevent loss of diabetes control.

Lithium excretion is blocked by thiazides and other diuretics. The increased danger of lithium toxicity prevents the safe concurrent use of these drugs.

Cholestyramine and colestipol are solid resins used orally to treat hyperlipidemias (see Chapter 21). These agents can lower absorption of thiazide diuretics.

Potassium-Sparing Diuretics

Amiloride, spironolactone, triamterene

Mechanism of Action

Potassium-sparing diuretics (Table 14-5) inhibit the pump mechanism that normally exchanges potassium for sodium in the distal convoluted tubule (see Figure 14-1). This pump is controlled by mineralocorticoid hormones, such as aldosterone, which increase sodium retention and promote potassium loss. Aldosterone is present in greater than normal amounts in edematous states resulting from congestive heart failure, nephrotic syndrome, and hepatic cirrhosis.

Spironolactone competitively blocks the action of aldosterone in the sodium-potassium exchange pump, thereby causing sodium to remain in the tubule and to be excreted. Potassium is not pumped into the tubule, so it is not excreted. Triamterene produces the same effects as spironolactone but by a direct mechanism that does not depend on aldosterone. Spironolactone is most effective when the aldosterone level is elevated, whereas the more rapidly and directly acting triamterene and amiloride are effective at any level of aldosterone.

Since the sodium-potassium pump in the distal convoluted tubule is ordinarily responsible for reabsorbing only a small fraction of the sodium from the tubule, blockage of this pump increases sodium excretion only slightly. This limits the effectiveness of the potassium-sparing agents as diuretics.

Pharmacokinetics

Spironolactone, a steroid derivative, is not highly water soluble but is formulated using very fine particles to improve absorption from the GI tract. Peak therapeutic effects with spironolactone are observed several days after treatment begins (see Table 14-5). This delay is related to the mechanism of action of the drug and is not a result of delay in absorption or other pharmacokinetic properties of the drug.

Spironolactone is extensively metabolized much the same as the natural mineralocorticoids it chemically resembles. Metabolites of spironolactone appear in urine and in lesser quantities in bile. Triamterene, although not a steroid like spironolactone, is also relatively insoluble in water. Intestinal absorption is somewhat variable but usually satisfactory. Most of the orally administered dose appears in the urine within 24 hours. The drug enters the renal tubule by glomerular filtration and tubular secretion. Unlike spironolactone, the peak effect of this drug is observed within a day.

Amiloride is more water soluble than triamterene or spironolactone and is excreted primarily renally. About 60% of an oral dose is recovered unchanged in urine within 48 hours of administration. Absorption of the drug is impaired if it is taken with food.

Spironolactone is highly protein-bound in the blood, whereas triamterene is only moderately bound, and amiloride exists primarily as free drug.

Uses

Amiloride, spironolactone, and triamterene can be used to control edema in congestive heart failure, cirrhosis of the liver, and nephrotic syndrome. Spironolactone may ameliorate the effects of excessive aldosterone levels in patients with the endocrine disorder hyperaldosteronism. It may also be useful in treating hypertension and reversing potassium loss. Amiloride is also used for adjunctive therapy of hypertension.

Adverse Reactions and Contraindications

Spironolactone, triamterene, and amiloride may cause dangerous increases in serum potassium levels. Patients with

TABLE 14-4 Fixed Combinations Including a Thiazide

COMPONENTS	TRADE NAMES	USE/ORAL ADULT DOSE
Thiazide With ACE Inhibitor		
Hydrochlorothiazide + captopril	Capozide	Antihypertensive; 1 tablet 2 or 3 times daily
Hydrochlorothiazide + enalapril	Vaseretic	Antihypertensive; 1 tablet daily
Hydrochlorothiazide + lisinopril	Prinzide, Zestoretic	Antihypertensive; 1 to 2 tablets once daily
Thiazide With Alpha-Blocker		
Polythiazide + prazosin	Minizide	Antihypertensive; 1 capsule 2 or 3 times daily
Thiazide With Beta-Blocker		
Bendroflumethiazide + nadolol	Corzide*	Antihypertensive; 1 tablet daily
Chlorthalidone + atenolol	Tenoretic*	Antihypertensive; 1 or 2 tablets once daily
Hydrochlorothiazide + bisoprolol	Ziac	Antihypertensive; 1 or 2 tablets once daily
Hydrochlorothiazide + metoprolol	Lopressor HCT	Antihypertensive; 1 or 2 tablets daily
Hydrochlorothiazide + pindolol	Viskazide†	Antihypertensive; 1 or 2 tablets once daily
Hydrochlorothiazide + propranolol	Inderide LA	Antihypertensive; 1 capsule daily
Hydrochlorothiazide + timolol	Timolide*	Antihypertensive; 1 tablet twice daily
Thiazide With Centrally Acting Antihypertensive		
Chlorthalidone + clonidine	Combipres*	Antihypertensive; 1 to 2 tablets 2 to 4 times daily
Chlorothiazide + methyldopa	Aldoclor, Supres†	Antihypertensive; 2 to 4 tablets daily
Hydrochlorothiazide + methyldopa	Aldoril,* Dopazide†	Antihypertensive; 2 to 4 tablets daily
Thiazide With Potassium-Sparing Diuretics		
Hydrochlorothiazide + amiloride	Moduretic,* Moduret	Diuretic or antihypertensive; 1 or 2 tablets daily
Hydrochlorothiazide + spironolactone	Aldactazide,* Spirozide	Antihypertensive; 2 to 4 tablets daily Diuretic; 1 to 4 tablets daily
Hydrochlorothiazide + triamterene	Dyazide,* Maxzide	Diuretic or antihypertensive; 1 or 2 capsules daily
Thiazide With Rauwolfia		
Chlorothiazide + reserpine	Diupres	Antihypertensive; 1 or 2 tablets 1 or 2 times daily
Hydrochlorothiazide + reserpine	Hydropres,* Mallopres	Antihypertensive; 1 tablet 1 to 4 times daily
Methyclothiazide + deserpidine	Enduronyl, Dureticyl†	Antihypertensive; ½ to 1 tablet daily
Polythiazide + reserpine	Renese-R	Antihypertensive; ½ to 2 tablets daily
Trichlormethiazide + reserpine	Metatensin	Antihypertensive; 1 to 2 tablets daily
Thiazide With Vasodilator		
Hydrochlorothiazide + hydralazine	Apresazide, Aprozide	Antihypertensive; 1 capsule or tablet twice daily
Thiazide With Rauwolfia and Vasodilator		
Hydrochlorothiazide + reserpine + hydralazine	Ser-Ap-Es,* Unipres	Antihypertensive; 1 to 2 tablets 3 times daily

ACE, Angiotensin converting enzyme.
*Available in Canada and United States.
†Available in Canada only.

TABLE 14-5 Potassium-Sparing Diuretics

GENERIC NAME	TRADE NAME	ADMINISTRATION/DOSAGE	DIURETIC EFFECT		
			ONSET	PEAK	DURATION
Amiloride	Midamor*	ORAL: *Adults*—5-10 mg daily as a single dose. FDA pregnancy category B.	2 hr	6-10 hr	24 hr
Spironolactone	Aldactone* Novospiroton†	ORAL: *Adults*—25-200 mg daily in divided doses. *Children*—1-3 mg/kg daily in divided doses.	Effects build over period of days		
Triamterene	Dyrenium*	ORAL: *Adults*—25-100 mg daily with meals; do not exceed 300 mg daily. FDA pregnancy category B. *Children*—2-4 mg/kg daily in divided doses.	2-4 hr (Maximal effect not seen for several days)		

*Available in Canada and United States.
†Available in Canada only.

impaired renal function or excessively high potassium intake are especially at risk. The earliest sign of hyperkalemia may be an irregular heartbeat. Fatal cardiac arrhythmias can occur.

Spironolactone can cause various endocrine alterations, since the drug chemically resembles not only mineralocorticoids but also androgens and progestins. Women may observe menstrual irregularities, hirsutism, and deepening of the voice. Men may observe gynecomastia (breast development) and have difficulty in achieving or maintaining erection. Symptoms in both sexes are usually reversed when the drug is discontinued.

Spironolactone produces tumors in rats exposed to the drug for long periods. It should be restricted to cases in which the benefit clearly outweighs this risk. Spironolactone should not be used to control edema in pregnancy. If the drug is used by lactating women, breastfeeding should be discontinued because metabolites appear in breast milk.

Triamterene and amiloride may produce a reversible azotemia revealed by an increased blood urea nitrogen (BUN) level. Triamterene has also been linked to blood dyscrasias and to photosensitivity. Skin rashes, GI tract disturbances (especially with spironolactone), dizziness, and fever have been observed in patients receiving potassium-sparing diuretics.

All potassium-sparing diuretics are contraindicated in patients with hyperkalemia.

Toxicity

Patients who overdose on potassium-sparing diuretics should have their stomachs evacuated. Electrolyte balance and renal function should be carefully monitored.

Interactions

Two potassium-sparing diuretics should not be administered concurrently, nor should these drugs be administered to a patient receiving potassium supplements or ingesting a diet high in potassium.

Use of the potassium-sparing diuretics with antihypertensive agents may require reduction in doses of the latter drugs, since spironolactone, triamterene, and amiloride may have additive antihypertensive effects with these agents. When spironolactone is combined with other diuretics, dosages may require reduction. Spironolactone can prevent distal tubular reabsorption of sodium, making diuretics that act upstream of this site in the nephron even more effective. Amiloride given in fixed combination with hydrochlorothiazide is not as effective in preventing hypokalemia as are spironolactone and triamterene.

Spironolactone reduces vascular responsiveness to norepinephrine. This effect may impair maintenance of normal blood pressure in patients receiving local or general anesthesia.

Anticoagulant drugs are more potent when given with potassium-sparing diuretics, which may result in excessive anticoagulation and the risk of bleeding.

Lithium toxicity is increased by potassium-sparing diuretics, as lithium excretion is blocked. Spironolactone increases the half-life of digoxin, leading to digoxin accumulation. Careful monitoring and dosage adjustment is required to keep digoxin blood levels in a safe range.

Carbonic Anhydrase Inhibitors

✣ Acetazolamide, dichlorphenamide, methazolamide

Mechanism of Action

Diuretics that inhibit carbonic anhydrase in the kidney prevent secretion of hydrogen ion into the renal tubule and prevent reabsorption of carbon dioxide from the renal tubule (Table 14-6). As a result, excretion of bicarbonate is rapidly increased and urine becomes alkaline. **Carbonic anhydrase inhibitors** have diuretic action because sodium ion accompanies the excreted bicarbonate. Bicarbonate excretion is much greater than sodium ion excretion, and these drugs are classified as weak diuretics. Moderate amounts of

TABLE 14-6 Carbonic Anhydrase Inhibitors

GENERIC NAME	TRADE NAME	ADMINISTRATION/DOSAGE	CLINICAL EFFECT		
			ONSET	PEAK	DURATION
Acetazolamide	Acetazolam† Diamox*	ORAL, INTRAVENOUS: *Adults*—250-375 mg once daily; alternate-day therapy may be used. FDA pregnancy category C.	About 1 hr (oral) IV: 2 min	2-4 hr (oral) IV: 15 min	6-12 hr (oral) IV: 4-5 hr
Dichlorphenamide	Daranide	ORAL: *Adults*—initially 100-200 mg, then 100 mg every 12 hr until desired effect achieved; maintenance, 25-50 mg 1-3 times daily. FDA pregnancy category C.	0.5-1 hr	2-4 hr	6-12 hr
Methazolamide	Neptazane*	ORAL: *Adults*—25-100 mg 2 or 3 times daily. FDA pregnancy category C.	2-4 hr	6-8 hr	10-18 hr

*Available in Canada and United States.
†Available in Canada only.

potassium, phosphate, and chloride ion are also lost in urine. When carbonic anhydrase inhibitors are given for long periods, metabolic acidosis may occur. Since metabolic acidosis prevents the diuretic action of these drugs, they are not suitable for long-term continuous administration as diuretics.

Pharmacokinetics

Carbonic anhydrase inhibitors are well absorbed from the GI tract. The most widely used drug of this class, acetazolamide, is concentrated in the kidneys, where tissue levels may be 2 to 3 times the plasma concentration within 30 minutes to 2 hours of an oral dose. Acetazolamide enters the tubule by the organic anion pump. The drug also inhibits carbonic anhydrase in other tissues.

Acetazolamide is sometimes given on alternate days rather than continuously (see Table 14-6). This therapy is designed to prevent the kidney from becoming resistant to the action of the drug (e.g., to prevent metabolic acidosis). During the day without the drug, acetazolamide is cleared from the body and kidney function returns to its predrug condition. When the drug is readministered on the following day, it is as effective as when first given.

Uses

Carbonic anhydrase inhibitors are primarily used to treat glaucoma. In addition, acetazolamide is used for convulsive disorders, altitude sickness, and familial periodic paralysis. Because acetazolamide alkalinizes the urine, it may be used to dissolve uric acid or cystine stones in the urinary tract.

Adverse Reactions and Contraindications

Reactions to these drugs are uncommon, especially when they are used in intermittent or short-term therapy. Drug precipitation in urine has occurred, causing the formation of stones.

Carbonic anhydrase inhibitors act directly on the CNS, causing paresthesia, nervousness, sedation, lassitude, depression, headaches, vertigo, and other symptoms. Patients may complain of unusual tiredness or weakness. The conditions of patients already experiencing respiratory acidosis may worsen from these drugs, which tend to produce metabolic acidosis.

Carbonic anhydrase inhibitors cause a range of GI tract symptoms including diarrhea, loss of appetite, nausea, vomiting, metallic taste, and weight loss.

Carbonic anhydrase inhibitors are usually not given to patients at risk for electrolyte disturbances, e.g., adrenocortical insufficiency, hypokalemia, acidosis, hepatic disease, or renal failure.

Toxicity

Renal function and acid-base balance must be carefully monitored in patients who have excessively high blood levels of carbonic anhydrase inhibitors.

Interactions

Carbonic anhydrase inhibitors produce more marked potassium excretion than sodium excretion. Potassium depletion is therefore likely to occur. This possibility is made even more likely by corticosteroids or ACTH given concomitantly. Digitalis toxicity is increased in the presence of low serum potassium levels.

Excretion of amphetamines, anticholinergics, mecamylamine, and quinidine is slowed because carbonic anhydrase inhibitors alkalinize the urine. Alkaline urine also blocks the effects of methenamine, which requires an acidic environment to be converted to formaldehyde, the active metabolite.

Osmotic Diuretics

Osmotic diuretics are nonelectrolytes that are filtered by the glomerulus but not significantly reabsorbed or metabolized. Therefore osmotic diuretics enter renal tubules and are highly concentrated in renal tubular fluid.

The high osmolality in tubules reduces reabsorption of water, which increases the production of urine. At high doses, some increase in sodium excretion is produced, but this effect is not observed in most clinical circumstances. These drugs are therefore exceptions to the generalization that sodium excretion precedes water excretion during diuretic therapy.

Osmotic diuresis may be used clinically to prevent permanent damage during acute renal failure. The usefulness of osmotic diuresis in these cases frequently depends on maintaining adequate urine volume without altering electrolyte balance. Osmotic diuretics also increase the osmolality of plasma, which allows reduction of osmotic pressure inside the eye and in cerebrospinal fluid.

The agents currently used as osmotic diuretics, mannitol and urea, are usually administered intravenously. Mannitol is the preferred agent.

Toxicity produced by these agents depends on how much drug is administered and how much the drug affects fluid balance. These drugs are retained within the extracellular space and can cause an acute expansion of extracellular fluid volume during IV administration. This volume expansion may be hazardous to a patient with reduced cardiac reserve.

Fluid and electrolyte imbalances may develop, especially if a degree of renal impairment exists. Under these circumstances the diuretics tend to accumulate in the blood and may cause dangerous shifts in salt and water balance.

Pulmonary congestion, acidosis, thirst, blurred vision, convulsion, nausea and vomiting, diarrhea, tachycardia, fever, and angina-like pain may be noted occasionally. Local irritation with thrombophlebitis can also occur. Urea should not be used in a patient with liver failure because the high levels of urea may place additional demands on liver function.

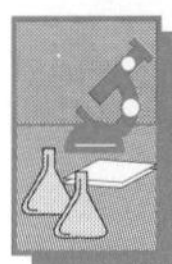

RESEARCH HIGHLIGHT

Mannitol Injections: With or Without Filter Needles? A Cost-Effectiveness Analysis

—AS Zbrozek, E Agbara, M Head: Nurs Econ 12(4):196, 1994.

PURPOSE

Mannitol is an osmotic diuretic available in several concentrations. At room temperature, solutions with a concentration >20% may crystallize. It is possible to dissolve the crystals by heating the solution. Nevertheless, the manufacturer recommends using an administration set with a filter. While reviewing hospital practice, a large Texas hospital learned that the use of filters in administering mannitol was not consistent throughout the hospital. The hospital wanted to investigate whether using a filter was actually cost-effective.

SAMPLE AND METHODOLOGY

Rather than using a prospective study, which could take many months and possibly place patients at risk, the authors chose to use an economic analysis. A decision tree was developed, and values were placed on each of the branches of the tree. Factors in the formulation included the cost of a filter needle ($0.33), the mortality rate given a crystallization complication (10%), the patient age (40 years with a mean life expectancy of 77 years), and the estimated average medical cost of caring for a patient with morbidity attributable to failure to filter crystallized mannitol ($500), which assumed a mean of 1 day additional length of stay of $400. The formula was used with a worst-case scenario (an incidence of crystallization complications elevated to 5%), and a best-case scenario (a level of crystallization complications lowered to 0.5%).

FINDINGS

In all scenarios created with the formula used, the use of filter needles is a cost-effective nursing care measure. Variables included patient age (20, 40, and 60 years); morbidity ($100 and $500), and incidence of crystallization.

IMPLICATIONS

The cost-effectiveness of many nursing care activities needs to be determined. Many research methods can be used to evaluate the effectiveness of various aspects of patient care. Using a mathematical model may take less time than other methods; it certainly prevents patients from inadvertent risk while the study is being completed. It is important to develop a decision tree and a mathematical model that reflects a realistic situation. In this case a practice recommended by the manufacturer appears to be a cost-effective measure that takes little nursing time.

CRITICAL THINKING: Are there nursing care procedures you have been taught that could be evaluated with this approach? What are the pitfalls of using mathematical analysis and not other methods, such as chart review or prospective patient care studies?

NURSING PROCESS OVERVIEW

Diuretics

Assessment

Perform a total patient assessment, focusing on the presenting signs and symptoms and appropriate laboratory and other objective data that would help further define the nature of the patient's condition. Assess the patient's intake, output, weight, and blood pressure and observe for signs of electrolyte imbalance, fluid retention, or dehydration.

Nursing Diagnoses

- Fluid volume deficit related to furosemide therapy as manifested by excessive urine output, decreased skin turgor, and orthostatic hypotension
- Potential complication: Hypokalemia, or with potassium-sparing diuretics, hyperkalemia
- Risk for sleep pattern disturbance related to nocturia secondary to diuretic therapy

Patient Outcomes

The patient will have diuresis without drug-related side effects. The nurse will manage and minimize episodes of electrolyte imbalances. The patient will have drug dosage and dosing schedule adjusted to minimize sleep disturbance.

Planning/Implementation

Determine what actions are required to aid drug therapy. For example, dietary and fluid restrictions may be required to speed fluid removal and to prevent reaccumulation. Monitor fluid intake and output, serum electrolyte levels, BUN level, uric acid level, body weight, and blood pressure and observe for the appearance of new signs or symptoms. Watch for side effects such as ototoxicity with ethacrynic acid.

Evaluation

Diuretic therapy is effective if excess fluid is lost and blood pressure is maintained and if abnormalities in electrolyte status or side effects do not result. For some patients, it is necessary to tolerate minor side effects to achieve required diuresis. Potassium depletion may be treated with potassium supplements. Teach the patient why the medication is necessary, what the major possible side effects are, and what symptoms should be reported to the physician. Discuss why additional medications such as potassium supplements may be needed. Teach selected patients to record daily weight, fluid intake and output, and blood pressure. If the physician has prescribed a restricted diet, verify that the patient understands how to choose menus within the limits of the diet plan. Be aware of the potential for abuse with these compounds (see box on p. 170).

Nursing Implications Summary

General Guidelines: Diuretics

- Carefully measure and record fluid intake and output. Report unexpected findings to the physician. For example, oliguria (scanty urine output) or anuria (no urine output) are unexpected after an increase in a diuretic dose. Patients who are at home are not usually required to measure intake and output, except in the case of severe kidney or heart disease, but encourage the patient to report abnormal output.
- Weigh the patient in the short-term care setting daily. Weigh the patient under standard conditions (e.g., at the same time [usually in the morning], after the patient has voided or the catheter bag has been emptied, but before breakfast). Use the same scale each day, and have the patient wear the same amount of clothing. If appropriate to their ability and resources, teach patients who are at home how to keep daily or weekly weight records. Instruct patients to report to the physician weight gains or losses greater than 2 lb/day or 5 lb/wk unless otherwise instructed by the physician.
- Monitor the blood pressure regularly. Although all patients receiving diuretic therapy would be expected to experience an initial drop in blood pressure, older adults, those receiving IV diuretics, and those also taking antihypertensives may experience a precipitous fall in blood pressure and in rare instances may go into shock. Other drugs that can cause hypotension, and can thus potentiate hypotension in patients receiving diuretics, include CNS depressants, barbiturates, narcotics, and antihypertensives. Initially, monitor the blood pressure with the patient in the standing, sitting, and lying positions and compare the measurements from each arm.
- Review with the patient the symptoms of orthostatic hypotension (see box on p. 157). Caution the patient to avoid the use of alcohol because it enhances hypotension.
- To monitor for fluid retention, measure the patient's abdominal girth or the circumference of one or both legs. To ensure accurate measurement, mark the patient's skin with small ink marks to indicate the correct placement of the tape measure from day to day.
- Check dependent areas daily for the presence of or change in the amount of pitting edema. In pitting edema an indentation or depressed area made by the examiner's finger remains visible in the skin for seconds to minutes after the pressure has been released. Dependent areas where this is more likely to occur include the sacral area and the feet and legs.
- Observe the patient for symptoms of dehydration, including thirst, decreased skin turgor, nausea, light-headedness, weakness, increased pulse, oliguria, decreased blood pressure, and elevated hemoglobin, hematocrit, and BUN levels.
- Assess the patient for electrolyte abnormalities, and monitor the serum levels of potassium, sodium, calcium, magnesium, and bicarbonate. The signs and symptoms of common electrolyte abnormalities are summarized in Table 17-1.
- Teach patients the importance of taking potassium supplements, if prescribed, and work with them to find a preparation they are willing to take (see Chapter 17). Many effervescent preparations are unpalatable. Enteric-coated tablets have been implicated in small bowel ulceration. Oral solutions are the preferred form of therapy, but they are often unpleasant tasting. Dilute these solutions in juice or milk to reduce the risk of gastric irritation and to make the taste tolerable. Instruct patients to take potassium with meals to reduce gastric irritation. Encourage hypokalemic patients to increase dietary intake of potassium-rich foods (see box on p. 170).
- Caution the patient taking diuretics not to switch to salt substitutes without first consulting the physician. Salt substitutes contain a variety of electrolyte salts, and the exact proportions vary from product to product. A patient may inadvertently contribute to electrolyte abnormalities by using a salt substitute. For example, a patient taking a potassium-sparing diuretic may develop hyperkalemia if a salt substitute containing a high portion of potassium salts is used.
- Refer the patient as needed to the dietitian for instruction about special dietary restrictions, which may include sodium, calories, cholesterol, and other factors.
- Teach patients about their need for diuretic therapy, and review the anticipated side effects of the prescribed drugs. Poor compliance may stem from patient annoyance caused by frequent and excessive urination. Instruct patients to take once-daily diuretics in the morning and to take twice-daily diuretics in the morning and the last dose by 6 PM to avoid interrupting sleep to urinate.
- If diuretics are prescribed for hypertension, emphasize the importance of taking all drugs prescribed, even if the patient has no symptoms of hypertension. Teach patients that drug therapy for hypertension may be required for the rest of their lives.
- Dehydration and hypovolemia can contribute to thromboembolic disorders. Assess the patient for pain in the chest, calves, and pelvis that might indicate thromboembolism.
- For some patients intermittent therapy (every other day or M-W-F) will achieve the desired effects with fewer side effects.
- Teach the patient to take diuretics as ordered. If a dose is missed, it should be taken as soon as remembered, unless within a few hours of the next dose (this varies with the frequency of the dosing schedule), in which case it should be omitted and the regular dosing schedule resumed. Tell the patient not to double up for missed doses.
- Thirst is often a frequent side effect (see patient problem box on dry mouth, p. 300).

NURSING IMPLICATIONS SUMMARY—cont'd

- Remind the patient to keep all health care providers informed of all drugs being taken.

Loop Diuretics

Drug Administration

- Review the general guidelines for patients receiving diuretics. Assess the patient for development of hyponatremia, hypocalcemia, hypokalemia, and hypochloremic alkalosis (see Table 17-1).
- Monitor serum electrolyte levels. Monitor blood glucose levels because these drugs may cause hyperglycemia.
- Review drug interactions, and counsel the patient as appropriate.
- Assess patients receiving warfarin and loop diuretics for signs of excessive anticoagulation (see Chapter 20).
- Monitor serum uric acid levels, and assess the patient for signs of gout.
- Assess the patient for signs of ototoxicity, which include tinnitus (ringing in the ears), reduced hearing acuity, and vertigo.
- Question the patient about allergy to sulfonamides, thiazide diuretics, or any other loop diuretics before administering first doses. Observe for allergic response, including development of rashes.
- Teach patients taking the oral liquid form to measure doses with the calibrated dropper provided with the drug or to use a specially marked measuring spoon or medication cup to measure doses.

Intravenous Bumetanide

- Bumetanide is usually given undiluted but may be mixed with 5% dextrose in water (D5W), normal saline, and lactated Ringer's solution.
- Administer dose evenly for a 2-minute period. After IV administration, monitor blood pressure every 15 to 30 minutes until stable, keep siderails up, and supervise ambulation.

Intravenous Ethacrynic Acid

- Ethacrynic acid may be given undiluted, or 50 mg may be diluted in 50 ml of D5W or 0.9% normal saline. Do not mix with other drugs. Do not administer if solution is discolored or contains particulate matter. Administer at a rate of 10 mg or less over a 1-minute period, or infuse total dose over 30 minutes. Check the infusion site carefully; thrombophlebitis is common, and extravasation causes pain and tissue irritation. After IV administration, monitor blood pressure every 15 to 30 minutes until stable, keep siderails up, and supervise ambulation.

Furosemide

- Furosemide may be given undiluted or added to D5W, normal saline, or lactated Ringer's injection. Inspect the solution before administering, and do not use it if it is yellow. Do not mix furosemide with other drugs.
- Administer at a rate of 40 mg evenly administered for a 1- to 2-minute period. If administered as an infusion, use an infusion control device and administer no faster than 4 mg/min. After IV administration, monitor blood pressure every 15 to 30 minutes until stable, keep siderails up, and supervise ambulation.

Intramuscular Furosemide

- IM injection of furosemide may cause transient pain at the injection site.

Intravenous Torsemide

- Torsemide may be given undiluted, at a rate of 1 dose evenly administered for a 2-minute period.

Patient and Family Education

- See the general guidelines for patients receiving diuretics.
- Potassium supplements are often prescribed concomitantly with loop diuretics. Emphasize the importance of taking potassium supplements as prescribed, refer to the dietitian as needed, and review good dietary sources of potassium. Instruct the patient that diarrhea, vomiting, and anorexia (loss of appetite), if prolonged or severe, may also cause hypokalemia and should be reported to the physician. Caution patients also taking a cardiac glycoside to be especially careful to avoid hypokalemia. Review other drug interactions with the patient, as appropriate.
- Caution patients with diabetes to monitor blood glucose levels carefully because hyperglycemia may occur, requiring an adjustment in diet or dose of insulin.
- Instruct the patient to report signs of agranulocytosis (depressed production of white blood cells [leukopenia]), including unexplained fever, chills, sore throat, or enlarged lymph nodes. This is a rare but serious side effect of drug therapy (see patient problem box on p. 268).
- Instruct the patient to take oral preparations with meals or just after eating to reduce gastric irritation. Warn the patient in renal failure that bumetanide may cause myalgia. Tell the patient to report skin changes, rashes, photosensitivity (see box on p. 649), nausea, vomiting, or any unexpected sign or symptom.

Thiazide Diuretics

Drug Administration

- See the general guidelines for diuretic therapy. Thiazides may cause hypokalemia, hypochloremia, alkalosis, hyponatremia, and hypomagnesemia. Monitor the patient for these electrolyte abnormalities and monitor serum electrolyte levels (see Table 17-1).
- Monitor the patient's blood glucose levels because thiazide diuretics may cause hyperglycemia.

Continued.

NURSING IMPLICATIONS SUMMARY—cont'd

- Review drug interactions, and counsel the patient as appropriate.
- Monitor serum uric acid levels, and assess for signs of gout.
- Monitor the serum BUN levels and lipid levels.

Parenteral Chlorothiazide

- Dilute each vial (0.5 gm) with at least 18 ml of sterile water. Dilute further if desired with D5W or sodium chloride injection. Do not mix with other drugs or blood products. Administer at a rate of 0.5 gm or less over a 5-minute period.
- Check the insertion site for signs of extravasation since the drug is extremely alkaline. Do not administer intramuscularly or subcutaneously. Thiazides can cause a paradoxical antidiuretic effect in patients who have diabetes insipidus (see Chapter 59).

Patient and Family Education

- See the general guidelines for diuretic therapy.
- Potassium supplements may be prescribed, but patients may be able to prevent hypokalemia by increasing their daily dietary intake of potassium-rich foods (see box on p. 170). If potassium supplements are prescribed, emphasize the importance of taking these as ordered. Instruct patients that diarrhea, vomiting, and anorexia, if prolonged or severe, can also cause hypokalemia and should be reported to the physician. Concomitant administration of adrenal corticosteroids may also predispose the patient to hypokalemia.
- Caution patients with diabetes to monitor blood glucose levels carefully because hyperglycemia may occur, requiring an adjustment in diet or insulin dosage. Instruct patients to take oral doses with meals to reduce gastric irritation.
- Review the problem of photosensitivity (see box on p. 649).

Potassium-Sparing Diuretics

Drug Administration

- See the general guidelines for diuretic therapy.
- Potassium-sparing diuretics may cause hyperkalemia or hyponatremia. Assess the patient for these electrolyte imbalances and monitor serum electrolyte levels (see Table 17-1).
- Many combination products are available containing both a potassium-depleting diuretic and a potassium-sparing diuretic. The combination is designed to promote diuresis while maintaining normal serum potassium levels. Patients receiving combination drugs are potentially at risk for side effects caused by any of the component drugs (see Table 14-4). Instruct the patient to report the development of any unexpected sign or symptom.
- Monitor BUN levels.

Patient and Family Education

- Patients should take doses with meals or a snack to reduce gastric irritation. Spironolactone tablets may be crushed and mixed in syrup or fluid of the patient's choice. The triamterene capsule may be opened and the contents mixed with food or fluid for patients who have difficulty swallowing.
- If a potassium-sparing diuretic has been newly prescribed or if a potassium-sparing diuretic is prescribed in addition to a potassium-depleting diuretic, emphasize the need to omit previous potassium supplements that may have been ordered; consult the physician. In addition, instruct the patient to limit intake of potassium-rich foods (see box on p. 170).
- Instruct the patient to avoid salt substitutes that contain potassium while taking potassium-sparing diuretics.
- Caution patients taking triamterene that photosensitivity may develop (see box on p. 649).

Carbonic Anhydrase Inhibitors

Drug Administration

- Review the general guidelines for diuretic therapy.
- Monitor serum electrolyte levels, and assess the patient for electrolyte abnormalities, especially metabolic acidosis (see Table 17-1). Intermittent therapy may be used to limit the development of acidosis.
- Read the physician's orders carefully. Tablets and extended-release capsules are available. Review drug interactions, and counsel the patient as appropriate.
- Monitor serum uric acid and blood glucose levels.
- Monitor the patient for signs of kidney stone formation, such as renal colic (severe flank pain), hematuria (blood in the urine), and oliguria.

Intravenous Acetazolamide

- Dilute each 500 mg of acetazolamide with at least 5 ml of sterile water for injection, and administer at a rate of 500 mg over at least a 1-minute period. The drug may be further diluted with standard IV fluids and administered over 4 to 8 hours. Avoid IM injection, which is very painful.

Patient and Family Education

- Review the guidelines for diuretic therapy.
- Instruct patients with diabetes to monitor blood glucose levels; a change in diet or insulin dose may be required. Review expected effects and possible side effects. Instruct the patient to report any unexpected sign or symptom. Instruct the patient to avoid driving or operating hazardous equipment if drowsiness, dizziness, light-headedness, or visual changes occur and to notify the physician.
- A metallic taste in the mouth may occur. Sucking sugarless hard candy, chewing sugarless gum, brushing the teeth, or rinsing the mouth frequently may help.
- Photosensitivity may occur (see box on p. 649)

NURSING IMPLICATIONS SUMMARY—cont'd

Osmotic Diuretics

Drug Administration/Patient and Family Education

- See the general guidelines for diuretic therapy.
- Monitor serum electrolyte levels and assess for electrolyte abnormalities (see Table 17-1). Assess the patient for signs of circulatory overload. Monitor vital signs for blood pressure, intake and output, and daily weight. Assess breath and heart sounds. Monitor the patient for signs of pulmonary congestion or congestive heart failure, including dyspnea, labored respiration, tachypnea, tachycardia, distended neck veins, rales, agitation, fluid retention, and weight gain.
- Osmotic diuretics are often given to patients with increased intracranial pressure. Assess level of consciousness and monitor indicators of cerebral function, including blood pressure, pulse, intracranial pressure, and Glasgow Coma Scale or institutional equivalent.
- Determine the desired daily fluid balance with the physician. The infusion rate may be titrated to output. Diuresis may be copious, especially initially; a urinary catheter may be needed. If the urine output falls below 30 to 50 ml/hour, notify the physician.
- Oral fluids may not be permitted. Occasional ice chips may be permitted to help relieve thirst.
- If extravasation occurs, osmotic diuretics cause local skin and tissue damage. Before starting infusion, check that the IV line is secure and patent, with no signs of redness or infiltration, and that the rate of flow is not sluggish. Inspect infusion site regularly. If infiltration is suspected, discontinue infusion and restart in another site.

Intravenous Mannitol

- Read the physician's order carefully. Mannitol is available in several concentrations. Do not confuse mannitol with mannitol hexanitrate, an antianginal drug. It is not necessary to dilute mannitol. Check ampule or bottle for crystallization, a common problem. If crystals are present, warm the container under running water until crystals dissolve. Cool to body temperature before administering. Use an in-line IV filter for 15%, 20%, and 25% solutions. Do not add to other IV solutions, medications, or blood products. The rate of administration is usually 1 to 2 gm/kg for a 30- to 90-minute period but may vary. (See also box on p. 177.)

Intravenous Urea

- Urea must be diluted to make a 30% solution (30% solution equals 30 gm of urea/100 ml or 300 mg/ml). Dilute with D5W or D10W or with 10% invert sugar in water; some manufacturers supply the diluent. Patients with hereditary fructose intolerance (aldolase deficiency) may have a severe reaction to the invert sugar solution if it is used as a diluent. Symptoms include hypoglycemia, nausea, vomiting, tremors, coma, and convulsions. Infuse at a rate of 4 ml/min (1200 mg/min) or slower. Use only fresh solutions, and discard any unused portions. Do not mix with blood or other drugs in the same syringe.
- These drugs are rarely used outside of the short-term care setting. Keep the patient and family informed of the patient's condition.

CRITICAL THINKING

APPLICATION

1. What is the nephron?
2. What is the function of the glomerulus?
3. Where is sodium reabsorbed from the renal tubule?
4. How is bicarbonate ion recovered from tubular fluid? Where does this occur?
5. What is the general mechanism by which all diuretics except osmotic diuretics act?
6. What is the specific mechanism of action of loop diuretics?
7. What side effects are characteristic of loop diuretics?
8. How does bumetanide differ from the other loop diuretics?
9. What is the specific mechanism of action of thiazide diuretics?
10. What side effects are characteristic of thiazide diuretics?
11. What is the specific mechanism of action of potassium-sparing diuretics?
12. What side effects are associated with potassium-sparing diuretics?
13. How are carbonic anhydrase inhibitors used clinically?
14. What side effects are characteristic of carbonic anhydrase inhibitors?
15. What reactions occur with osmotic diuretics?

CRITICAL THINKING

1. Develop a nursing care plan for a patient receiving one of the diuretics discussed in this chapter. How can you assess the drug's effectiveness? About what drug interactions should you instruct the patient?
2. Your older adult patient tells you the physician just began diuretic therapy, but the patient cannot remember the name of the drug. What should you warn the patient about?

CHAPTER 15

Antianginals and Other Vasodilators

OBJECTIVES

After studying this chapter, you should be able to do the following:

- *Describe drug therapy for angina pectoris, including differentiating among the nitrates, the beta-adrenergic blocking drugs, and the calcium channel–blocking drugs.*
- *Discuss the rationale for drug treatment of vasospastic disorders.*
- *Develop nursing care plans for patients receiving drugs from the following groups: nitrates, beta-adrenergic blocking drugs, calcium channel–blocking drugs, vasodilating drugs for vascular disease, and pentoxyfylline.*

KEY TERMS

angina pectoris
classic angina
coronary atherosclerosis
Raynaud's disease
unstable angina
variant angina (Prinzmetal's angina)
vasodilators

CHAPTER OVERVIEW

This chapter covers drugs used primarily to improve circulation: sympathomimetic drugs and selected vasodilators. Because beta-blockers and calcium channel blockers have gained widespread use in the treatment of angina, these drug classes are also discussed.

Vasodilators improve blood flow by increasing the size of the blood vessels. Vasodilation has been used in treating angina and peripheral vascular disease. Although some of the activity of vasodilators may be related to alpha- or beta-adrenergic receptors, most vasodilators work by a mechanism that was not understood until recently. As an understanding of these diseases progresses, the role of vasodilators is being reevaluated. Vasodilators used primarily as antihypertensive agents are discussed in Chapter 13.

Therapeutic Rationale: Angina

Blood Circulation to the Heart

The heart has a very high requirement for oxygen and nutrients. These needs are met by the coronary circulation (Figure 15-1) because the heart muscle cannot use the blood pumped through its chambers. The right and left coronary arteries originate at the aorta as it leaves the heart. The left coronary artery divides into the circumflex branch and the anterior descending branch. The three major vessels of the heart are thus the right coronary artery, circumflex coronary branch of the left coronary artery, and the anterior descending branch of the left coronary artery. These vessels divide and subdivide to the capillaries that finally service the individual cardiac cells. Ordinarily, the heart receives an adequate supply of blood through these coronary vessels.

Angina Pectoris

Angina pectoris, which literally means a choking of the chest, is the result of a temporary insufficiency of oxygen to the heart. The heart has a large requirement for oxygen and normally extracts maximum amounts of oxygen from the coronary circulation. The increased oxygen demands of the heart associated with increased work are normally met by increased coronary blood flow.

In about 1 of 50 American adults the coronary arteries become narrowed by fatty deposits that develop just underneath the inner lining of the vessel. This condition is called **coronary atherosclerosis.** The flow of blood in affected vessels is reduced, and the dependent heart muscle no longer receives an adequate blood supply. As the atherosclerosis worsens, the vascular system in the heart compensates by developing additional blood vessels (collateral circulation) to bypass the affected vessel. If a large enough area of the heart muscle does not receive sufficient oxygen, pain results.

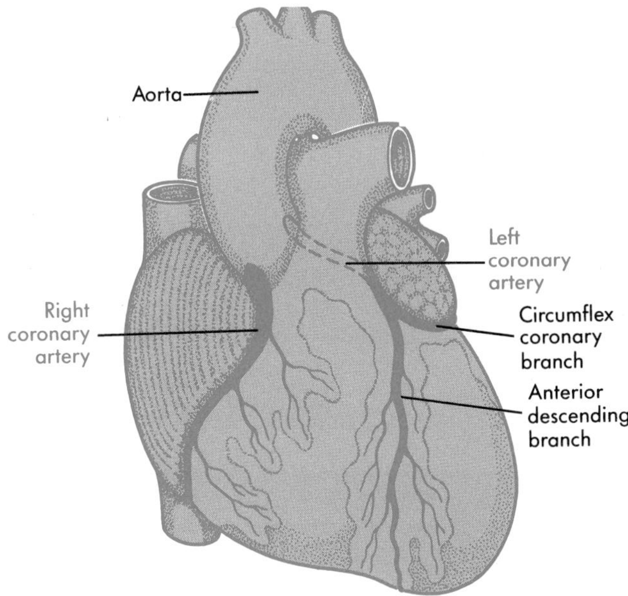

FIGURE 15-1
Coronary arteries. The three major coronary arteries are right coronary artery and two branches of left coronary artery; circumflex coronary branch and anterior descending branch. These arteries supply blood for heart muscle. Occlusion of one or more of these arteries can cause angina.

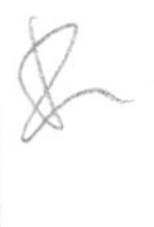

Anginal pain is a sudden, severe, and pressing pain that begins behind the breast bone and radiates up to the left shoulder and arm. Often this pain initially may be a feeling of acute chest discomfort; it also may be felt in the neck, jaw, teeth, arms, or elbows, areas to which cardiac pain is physiologically referred. The pain gradually wears off when the person stops and rests. Drugs that increase the heart rate, decrease blood flow to the heart, or cause fluid retention may precipitate anginal episodes. Drugs shown to increase anginal attacks include bromocriptine, diazoxide, digitalis, dobutamine, dopamine, ergotamine, fluorouracil, hydralazine, indomethacin, minoxidil, nifedipine, prazosin, propranolol, and thyroid hormone.

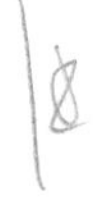

Classic angina is often called *stable angina* or *exertional angina.* In classic angina the large coronary arteries are obstructed by atherosclerosis to the point that blood flow cannot increase to supply more oxygen required by increased work. Coronary atherosclerosis is the most common cause of angina.

Variant angina (Prinzmetal's angina) has a different origin than classic angina. Variant angina is caused by spasms of the large coronary arteries that result in obstruction of blood flow. These coronary spasms have no relationship to exercise and may occur at rest. Variant angina frequently has a daily rhythm, with episodes being more common in the morning. However, most patients with variant angina also have coronary atherosclerosis; in these patients anginal pain may also occur with exertion.

Unstable angina refers to angina that has a changing intensity. Pain comes at decreasing levels of exertion and often at rest. Patients who progress to unstable angina are the most likely to have a heart attack and should be medically reviewed immediately.

The treatment of angina depends on the recognition that the supply of oxygen to the heart does not meet the demand. On a long-term basis the demand for oxygen can be decreased by altering secondary factors that are known to adversely affect the heart. These factors include smoking, excess weight, hypertension, arrhythmias, anxiety, anemia, and lack of regular exercise. The major risk factors for the progression of atherosclerosis are cigarette smoking, hypertension, and high serum cholesterol levels. Evidence affirms that alteration of these risk factors in patients with angina related to coronary atherosclerosis does prolong life.

Coronary artery bypass surgery may be indicated when angina is severe because of coronary atherosclerosis. In this type of surgery one or more of the main coronary vessels is bypassed with a graft from the aorta to the lower end of the vessel. Replacement of vessels severely narrowed by atherosclerosis greatly improves coronary blood flow. About 70%

of patients have no further angina, and another 20% have markedly reduced angina.

Percutaneous transluminal coronary angioplasty (PTCA) is a nonsurgical procedure for opening a coronary artery narrowed by atherosclerosis. A balloon catheter is inserted into the narrowed area. The balloon is inflated, and the vessel is widened. The PTCA procedure is most effective in patients with severe angina who have only one severely narrowed coronary artery. This is usually the left coronary artery servicing the more worked left ventricle.

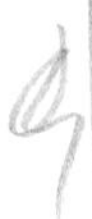

Therapeutic Agents: Angina

Drug therapy for angina pectoris rests with three classes of drugs. The nitrates primarily offer acute relief of angina. The beta-blockers offer long-term relief in classic angina. The calcium channel blockers are especially effective in relieving the coronary spasms of variant angina. These three drug classes are discussed in detail in the following sections.

NITRATES

General Characteristics

Mechanism of Action

Nitric oxide is now recognized to be the *endothelium-derived relaxing factor (EDRF)* responsible for relaxation of vascular smooth muscle resulting in vasodilation (Figure 15-2). Nitrates are broken down to nitric oxide. However, within cells, the endogenous source of nitric oxide is the amino acid arginine.

The nitrates were originally believed to dilate the coronary blood vessels, thereby increasing blood flow in the heart. It is now understood that most patients with angina have atherosclerosis of the coronary vessels and that atherosclerotic vessels cannot dilate. Furthermore, insufficient oxygen (ischemia) is itself a potent vasodilator; thus the coronary vessels are already dilated during an anginal attack. The nitrates act to dilate arterioles and veins in the periphery, thereby lowering blood pressure. The reduced blood pressure means that the work of the heart is greatly reduced. This reduced workload lowers the oxygen demand of the heart.

Pharmacokinetics

The organic nitrates, nitroglycerin, erythrityl tetranitrate, and isosorbide dinitrate, relieve anginal attacks within a few minutes when administered sublingually. The organic nitrates are rapidly degraded by the liver, and therefore large doses are required for prophylactic use. Moreover, tolerance rapidly develops, reducing the duration of relief.

Uses

The nitrates, particularly nitroglycerin, are the mainstay of antianginal medication. The nitrates are most effectively used as needed to relieve an acute anginal attack. Patients who understand the factors that precipitate their own anginal attacks can take these medications prophylactically just before those activities.

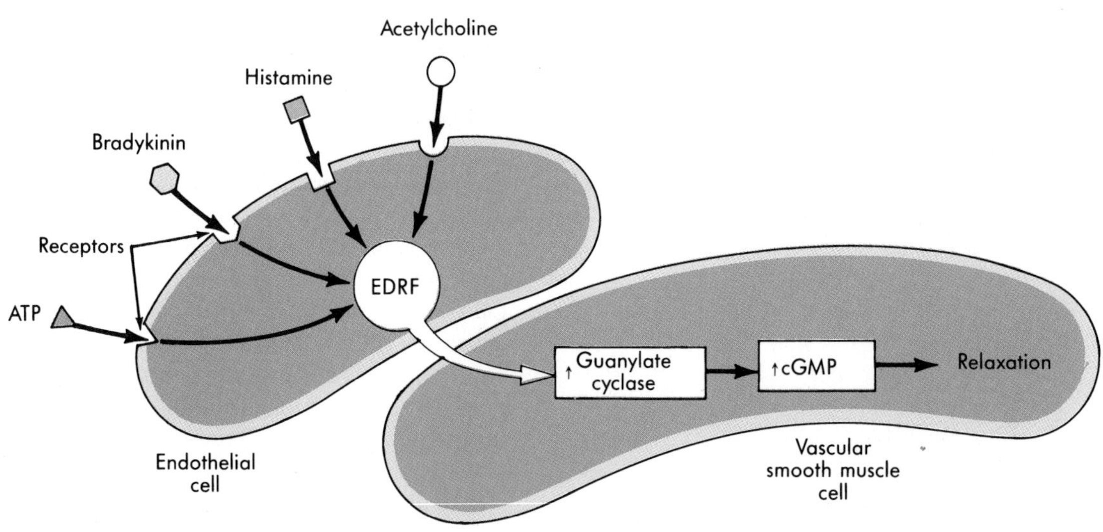

FIGURE 15-2
Endothelium-derived relaxing factor (EDRF) is nitric oxide. Nitric oxide is a very potent vasodilator. Endothelial cell produces nitric oxide from arginine, an amino acid, in response to various substances such as acetylcholine, histamine, bradykinin, and adenosine triphosphate (ATP). However, nitrates are also broken down to nitric oxide. Nitric oxide diffuses into vascular smooth muscle cells and stimulates enzyme, guanylate cyclase, which produces second-messenger cyclic guanosine monophosphate (GMP). Cyclic GMP activates intracellular events that result in vasodilation.

The organic nitrates are administered orally in large doses to provide prophylactic treatment for angina.

Adverse Reactions and Contraindications

The side effects of sublingual nitrates result from the generalized vasodilation they produce. These side effects include flushing, headache, and dizziness. The flushing is a result of the vasodilation in the "blush" area of the neck and face. The headache is a result of the pressure imposed by dilated blood vessels in the brain. The incidence of headaches decreases 2 to 3 weeks after initial therapy. The dizziness is the result of the generalized hypotension. The patient should sit or lie down to avoid fainting after taking one of these drugs.

Nitrates should not be taken by patients with recent head trauma because of the increase in cerebrospinal fluid pressure. Patients for whom hypotension is a risk, especially after a myocardial infarction, should not take these drugs.

Toxicity

Severe hypotension is usually transitory. The legs should be elevated to aid venous return. Severe hypotension is accompanied by a reflex increase in heart rate, which increases the workload for the heart and makes the pain worse.

Interactions

The hypotensive effects of nitrates are enhanced by alcohol, beta-blockers, calcium channel blockers, and antidepressants. Patients taking drugs with anticholinergic action may have a dry mouth that delays dissolution of sublingual and buccal preparations.

Specific Nitrates

For summary information on specific nitrates, refer to Table 15-1.

Nitroglycerin

Nitroglycerin is considered the drug of choice for angina. When nitroglycerin is taken sublingually, its effect begins in 30 seconds, is maximal in 3 minutes, and lasts for about 10 minutes. A drawback to nitroglycerin is that it decomposes when exposed to light or heat. Nitroglycerin can also volatilize from the tablets, which therefore must be kept in airtight containers.

Several dosage forms for nitroglycerin are available. A variation of the sublingual form is nitroglycerin lingual aerosol, which allows the drug to be sprayed, in a metered form, on or under the tongue. The aerosol is a substitute for the sublingual tablets in the short-term relief of an anginal attack. Extended-release buccal forms are intended for prophylactic use. Extended-release capsules and tablets have up to 10 times the sublingual dose. These are swallowed and are effective for 8 to 12 hours. Nitroglycerin is very lipid soluble and probably enters the body from the gastrointestinal tract through the lymphatics rather than the portal blood.

Nitroglycerin may also be administered through the skin. A measured amount of nitroglycerin ointment is spread on a nonhairy part of the body and held in place with plastic wrap taped over the area. This route of administration is said to produce relief for up to 3 hours. Nitroglycerin is also available impregnated in a polymer bonded to an adhesive bandage (Figure 15-3). This disk is applied to the skin, and nitroglycerin is absorbed through the skin (transdermally) for a period of 24 hours. The unit should be applied to a site free of hair, and the bandage should be placed at a new site each time to avoid irritation.

Nitroglycerin is administered intravenously in acute heart failure. Nitroglycerin can reduce the myocardial ischemia that results when the left side of the heart is failing. Because blood is not being pumped out effectively, pressure builds in the left ventricle. Pulmonary edema results, since blood backs up in the lungs. Nitroglycerin is an effective dilator of the coronary arteries and therefore allows more oxygenated blood to reach the troubled heart muscle. The heart is able to perform better, and the symptoms of acute heart failure are relieved.

Erythrityl Tetranitrate

Erythrityl tetranitrate is the longest acting of the sublingual or chewable organic nitrates. This drug becomes effective in 5 minutes, and its effects last for 4 hours. This is a long duration compared to nitroglycerin or even isosorbide dinitrate, and therefore erythrityl tetranitrate is better for prophylactic use than for relief of acute attacks. Erythrityl tetranitrate is also available for oral administration.

Isosorbide Dinitrate

Isosorbide dinitrate is another organic nitrate that can be taken sublingually or chewed. It is effective in 2 to 5 minutes and can act for 1 to 2 hours.

Pentaerythritol Tetranitrate

Pentaerythritol tetranitrate has not been proved effective for the prophylactic treatment of angina.

BETA-BLOCKERS

General Characteristics

Mechanism of Action

Beta-blockers decrease the oxygen requirements of the heart by reducing its workload. Blocking the beta-1 adrenergic receptors of the heart decreases the heart rate and the force of contraction, and a decrease in blood pressure follows. These actions also benefit coronary circulation by decreasing the resistance in the coronary circulation. However, beta-blockers are not vasodilators.

There are two subclasses of beta-receptors: beta-1 and beta-2. (For further discussion of beta-receptors, see Chapter 12.) The cardioselective beta-blockers are relatively selective for the beta-1 receptors. However, this selectivity is di-

TABLE 15-1 Drugs Prescribed for Relief of Angina Pectoris

GENERIC NAME	TRADE NAME	ADMINISTRATION/DOSAGE	COMMENTS
Nitrates and Nitrites			
Erythrityl tetranitrate	Cardilate*	SUBLINGUAL, ORAL, OR BUCCAL: *Adults*—5-10 mg 3 times/day. If required, dose may be increased every 2-3 days up to 30 mg 3 times/day. Onset: 5 min for sublingual; 30 min for oral. Duration: 4 hr.	Prophylactic treatment prevents anginal attacks. Hypotension, headaches, and tolerance to nitrates are possible side effects.
Isosorbide dinitrate	Iso-Bid Isordil* Isotrate Sorbitrate Others	SUBLINGUAL: *Adults*—2.5-5 mg. Chewable: 5-10 mg. Onset: 2-5 min. Duration: 1-2 hr. ORAL: *Adults*—5-30 mg 4 times daily. Timed-release forms, 40 mg 2-4 times/day. Onset: 15-30 min. Duration: 4-6 hr.	Drug relieves acute angina attacks. It is possibly effective prophylactically, especially if taken in anticipation of stressful situation. Hypotension is side effect limiting dose. It is possibly effective as prophylactic treatment to prevent anginal attacks. Headache can be severe. Tolerance to nitrates may develop.
Isosorbide mononitrate	Monoket IMDUR	ORAL (tablets): *Adults*—20 mg 2 times/day, 7 hr apart. ORAL (extended-release): *Adults*—30 or 60 mg once daily. May increase to 120 mg if needed. FDA pregnancy category C.	Drug is for prophylaxis and long-term treatment of angina due to coronary artery disease.
✣ Nitroglycerin	Nitroglycerin Nitrostat	SUBLINGUAL: *Adults*—Tablets of 0.15-0.3 mg initially, up to 0.6 mg as required in individual. Individual dosages may be repeated at 5-minute intervals, up to 3 tablets in 15 min. Peak action: 3 min. Duration: 10 min.	Drug is direct-acting vasodilator. It is drug of choice for angina pectoris. Patient takes at onset of acute anginal episodes or in anticipation of an episode, as before exercise or sex. Storage containers should be kept cool to prevent disintegration and airtight to prevent volatilization.
	Nitrolingual*	SUBLINGUAL: *Adults*—1 or 2 metered doses (400 μg/dose) on or under tongue. Repeat at 5-minute intervals for relief of anginal attack.	Sublingual spray should afford relief after total of 3 doses in 15 min.
	Niong Nitrong* Nitronet Klavikordal	ORAL (sustained-release): *Adults*—2.5-6.5 mg every 8-12 hr. Onset: slow variable. Duration: 8-12 hr.	Drug provides prophylactic administration of nitroglycerin. Effectiveness of this mode of therapy is not established. Tolerance to nitrates may develop.
	Nitrogard* Nitrogard SR*	BUCCAL: *Adults*—1 mg 3 times/day. May increase to 2 mg. Kept in mouth for several hours. May increase to 4 times/day or add extra for acute prophylaxis, but no more than every 2 hr.	Nitroglycerin is released from polymer base over several hours to achieve long duration of action.
✣ Nitroglycerin ointment, 2%	Nitro-Bid* Nitrol* Nitrong*	TOPICAL: *Adults*—Initially 1 inch is spread over area of skin. This is increased by ½-inch increments as required. Absorption is improved by covering area with plastic. Onset: 30-60 min. Duration: up to 3 hr.	Drug provides prophylactic administration of nitroglycerin. Effectiveness of this mode of therapy is not established. Excessive dose may cause violent headache. Area of administration will be irritated and should be rotated. On termination of treatment, area and frequency of administration should be reduced gradually over 4-6 weeks to prevent withdrawal reactions.
	Nitrodisc, Nitro-Dur Transderm-Nitro	TOPICAL: Apply to site free of hair. Do not apply to hands or feet. Change daily to new site.	Nitroglycerin is impregnated into polymer bound to adhesive bandages. Drug is absorbed through skin over 24 hr.
Pentaerythritol tetranitrate	Peritrate* Pentylan	ORAL: *Adults*—Initially 10-20 mg 4 times/day. If required, dosage may be adjusted up to 40 mg 4 times/day. Onset: 30 min. Duration: 4-5 hr.	Drug is possibly effective as prophylactic treatment for angina pectoris. Hypotension, headaches, and tolerance to nitrates are possible side effects. Tablets are taken 30 min before or 1 hr after meals and at bedtime. Drug is taken on empty stomach.

*Available in Canada and United States.
†Available in Canada only.

TABLE 15-1 Drugs Prescribed for Relief of Angina Pectoris—cont'd

GENERIC NAME	TRADE NAME	ADMINISTRATION/DOSAGE	COMMENTS
Nitrates and Nitrites—cont'd			
	Duotrate Peritrate SA*	ORAL (sustained-release): *Adults*—30-80 mg twice day. Onset: 30-60 min. Duration: 12 hr.	Drug is possibly effective as prophylactic treatment for angina pectoris. Hypotension, headaches, and tolerance to nitrates are possible side effects. Tablets are taken 30 min before or 1 hr after meals and at bedtime. Drug is taken on empty stomach.
Beta-Adrenergic Blocking for Angina			
Acebutolol	Monitan† Sectral*	ORAL: *Adults*—200 mg 2 times/day initially, then adjusted according to response.	Drug is cardioselective. Dosage should be reduced for patients with reduced liver or kidney function.
Atenolol	Apo-Atenolol† Novo-Atenol† Tenormin*	ORAL: *Adults*—50-200 mg once daily.	Drug is cardioselective. Dose is given every other day to patients with severely impaired renal function.
Carteolol	Cartrol	ORAL: *Adults*—Up to 10 mg daily.	Drug is nonselective. Dosage interval is increased for patients with severely impaired renal function.
Labetalol	Normodyne Trandate*	ORAL: *Adults*—150-300 mg 2 times/day.	Drug is nonselective. It also has alpha-1 adrenergic blocking effects.
Metoprolol	Apo-Metoprolol† Betaloc† Lopressor* Novometoprol†	ORAL: *Adults*—50 mg 3 or 4 times/day. For prophylaxis after myocardial infarction: 100 mg 2 times/day.	Drug is cardioselective. It is readily metabolized by liver. Bioavailability is increased by food.
Nadolol	Corgard	ORAL: *Adults*—40-80 mg daily.	Drug is nonselective. It is excreted unchanged in urine. Dosage interval is increased in patients with renal impairment.
Penbutolol	Levatol	ORAL: *Adults*—20-40 mg once daily.	Drug is nonselective. It is excreted unchanged in urine.
Pindolol	Syn-Pindolol† Visken*	ORAL: *Adults*—10 mg 4 times/day.	Drug is nonselective. It is well metabolized.
✣ Propranolol	Inderal*	ORAL: *Adults*—10-20 mg 3 or 4 times/day. Increase as required. Maintenance dose is usually 160-240 mg/day, in 4 doses.	Drug is nonselective. It is well absorbed and extensively metabolized by liver.
Sotalol	Betapace Sotacor	ORAL: *Adults*—Initially 80 mg 2 times/day. Increase at weekly intervals as needed.	Drug is nonselective. It is excreted unchanged in the urine. Dosage interval is increased in patients with renal impairment.
Timolol	Apo-Timolol† Blocadren*	ORAL: *Adults*—10-30 mg 2 times/day. Prophylaxis for myocardial infarction is 10 mg 2 times/day.	Drug is nonselective. It is well absorbed and extensively metabolized by liver.
Calcium Channel Blockers			
Amlodipine	Norvasc	ORAL: *Adults*—5-10 mg once daily.	Drug is a potent peripheral arteriolar vasodilator.
Bepridil	Bepadin Vascor	ORAL: *Adults*—Initially 200 mg once daily. Increase after 10 days, if necessary, to 300 mg once daily. Maximum dose is 400 mg/day.	Drug also has significant cardiac effects: negative inotopy and bradycardia.
Diltiazem	Cardizem	ORAL: *Adults*—60 mg every 6 hr.	Drug is best taken before meals.
Felodipine	Plendil Renedil†	ORAL: *Adults*—10 mg once a day.	Geriatric patients may be more sensitive.
Nicardipine	Cardene	ORAL: *Adults*—20 mg 3 times daily, adjusted for need and tolerance.	Drug is a potent peripheral vasodilator. Reflex increase in heart rate masks negative inotropy.

Continued.

TABLE 15-1 Drugs Prescribed for Relief of Angina Pectoris—cont'd

GENERIC NAME	TRADE NAME	ADMINISTRATION/DOSAGE	COMMENTS
Calcium Channel Blockers—cont'd			
Nifedipine	Adalat Apo-Nifed† Novo-Nifedin† Nu-Nifed† Procardia	ORAL: *Adults*—Initially 10 mg 3 times/day. If required, increase dose every 3-7 days. Maximum dose is 180 mg daily.	Drug is a potent peripheral vasodilator. Reflex increase in heart rate masks negative inotropy.
✣ Verapamil	Apo-Verap† Calan Isoptin* Novo-Veramil†	ORAL: *Adults*—240-480 mg daily in 3 or 4 divided doses.	Drug depresses sinoatrial and atrioventricular nodes and causes extensive first-pass metabolism. Half-life is increased in patients with cirrhosis, and dose should be lowered by 70%.

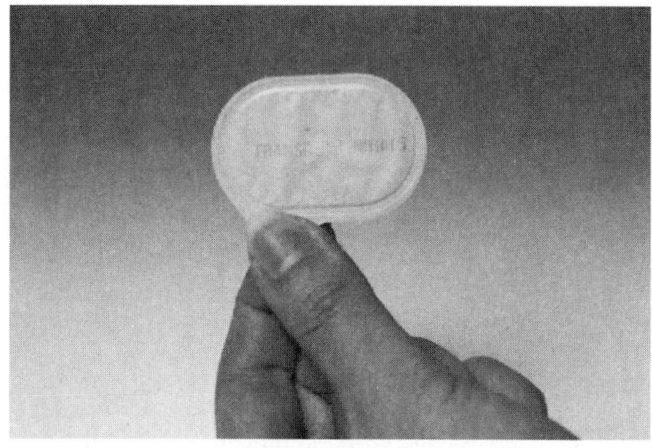

FIGURE 15-3
Transderm-Nitro delivery system for controlled release of nitroglycerin for prevention of angina. *(Courtesy Summit Pharmaceuticals, Division of Ciba-Geigy.)*

minished at higher doses. There is no evidence that any particular beta-blocker is better than another in the management of angina. Patients with asthma, diabetes, or peripheral vascular disease are better able to tolerate the selective beta-1 blockers. Beta-1 selective drugs include acebutolol, atenolol, and metoprolol. Nonselective drugs include nadolol, oxprenolol, pindolol, propranolol, sotalol, and timolol.

Pharmacokinetics

Beta-blockers are administered orally. The frequency of administration depends on the given drug. They are generally well absorbed and metabolized by the liver. Metabolites are generally excreted in the urine, although some metabolites are excreted in the feces through the biliary system.

Uses

Beta-blockers have become widely used in the management of classic angina. A beta-blocker is commonly prescribed as prophylactic therapy, and nitroglycerin is prescribed for acute anginal attacks. Long-term therapy reduces the frequency of anginal pain and decreases the requirements for nitroglycerin. The effective dose is highly individual for each patient. One index of dosage is the decrease in resting heart rate. In patients who have severe angina, enough medication may be given to lower the resting pulse to 50 to 60 beats per minute. If gastrointestinal side effects such as nausea, cramping, or diarrhea occur, taking the drug with meals may lessen these symptoms.

Beta-blockers are widely used as antihypertensive agents. This use is discussed extensively in Chapter 13.

Another prophylactic use of beta-blockers is to prevent sudden death following a heart attack. Several studies have shown that administration of a beta-blocker after a heart attack reduces the incidence of sudden death by as much as 40%. In addition to reducing the workload of the heart, other actions of beta-blockers such as the antiarrhythmic and antiplatelet functions may be important.

Adverse Reactions and Contraindications

The most common side effects of beta-blockers are fatigue and mental lassitude. Depression, nightmares, and psychosis are more severe central nervous system (CNS) side effects sometimes seen. Peripheral vasoconstriction may cause cold hands or feet. Sexual dysfunction, including impotence, is a side effect, especially of propranolol and timolol. Beta-blockers are contraindicated for patients with severely impaired heart or circulatory function (e.g., congestive heart failure, heart block, severe sinus bradycardia, and Raynaud's phenomenon). It is important to note that withdrawal of beta-blockers should be gradual. Sudden withdrawal can lead to unstable angina, a myocardial infarction, or even sudden death.

Adverse effects of beta-blockers include bronchospasm, hypoglycemia, and impairment of peripheral circulation. The bronchospasm arises from blockade of the beta-2 receptors of the bronchi. Beta-blockers mask symptoms of hypoglycemia such as an increase in heart rate and blood pressure. This makes it more difficult for patients with diabetes to monitor their blood glucose. Dilation of peripheral blood vessels is mediated by beta-2 receptors. These adverse effects are less common with the beta-1 selective blockers.

Interactions

Beta-blockers inhibit glycogen breakdown, a process normally stimulated by epinephrine and norepinephrine. This interferes with the action of insulin and oral antidiabetic agents. Beta-blockers may exaggerate the hypotensive effects of other drugs such as calcium channel blockers, clonidine, diazoxide, guanabenz, and reserpine.

Specific Beta-Blockers

There are now many beta-blockers on the market. Those that have been specifically approved for use in the United States as antianginal agents are atenolol, metoprolol, nadolol, and propranolol. Acebutolol, carteolol, labetalol, penbutolol, pindolol, sotalol, and timolol are additional beta-blockers used in the United States unofficially as antianginal drugs. Atenolol, metoprolol, propranolol, and timolol have been approved for prophylaxis against myocardial reinfarction. Specific beta-blockers are listed in Table 15-1.

Acebutolol

Acebutolol (Monitan, Sectral) is an intermediate-acting, cardioselective beta-blocker. The drug is metabolized by the liver and excreted both through the kidney and feces. Dosage should be reduced for patients with reduced liver or kidney function.

Atenolol

Atenolol (Tenormin) is a long-acting, cardioselective beta-blocker. Poorly absorbed from the gastrointestinal tract, the drug is not metabolized but excreted unchanged in the urine. The time between doses must be increased in patients with impaired renal function.

Carteolol

Carteolol (Cartrol) is a long-acting, nonselective beta-blocker. It is well absorbed and excreted largely unchanged in the urine. The dosage interval is increased for patients with impaired renal function.

Labetalol

Labetalol (Normodyne, Trandate) is a long-acting, nonspecific beta-blocker that also has selective alpha-1 adrenergic blocking effects. It is well absorbed, metabolized by the liver, and excreted in the urine.

Metoprolol

Metoprolol (Betaloc, Lopressor) is a short-acting, cardioselective beta-blocker. It is well absorbed from the gastrointestinal tract and readily metabolized by the liver.

Nadolol

Nadolol (Corgard) is a long-acting, nonselective beta-blocker. It is not well absorbed from the gastrointestinal tract, and up to one fourth of the dose may be excreted in the feces. Absorbed drug is excreted unchanged in the urine. The dosage interval is increased for patients with renal failure.

Penbutolol

Penbutolol (Levatol) is a short-acting, nonselective beta-blocker. It is well absorbed and highly protein bound. The drug is excreted unchanged in the urine.

Pindolol

Pindolol (Visken) is a short-acting, nonselective beta-blocker. It is well absorbed and metabolized by the liver.

Propranolol

Propranolol (Inderal), a nonselective beta-blocker, is the oldest of the clinically used beta-blocking drugs. It is well absorbed orally, but it is readily metabolized by the liver.

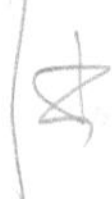

Sotalol

Sotalol (Betapace, Sotacor) is a nonselective beta-blocker. It is well absorbed and excreted primarily unchanged in the urine. The interval between doses must be increased for patients with impaired renal function.

Timolol

Timolol (Apo-Timolol, Blocadren) is a short-acting nonselective beta-blocker. It is well absorbed from the gastrointestinal tract and metabolized by the liver.

CALCIUM CHANNEL BLOCKERS

General Characteristics

Calcium channel blockers, also called calcium antagonists or calcium entry blockers, are a class of drugs currently used in the treatment of angina, certain arrhythmias (Chapter 19), and hypertension (Chapter 13).

Mechanism of Action

Skeletal muscle has extensive stores of calcium in the sarcoplasmic reticulum, but both cardiac muscle and vascular smooth muscle lack these stores and must depend on the influx of extracellular calcium for the maintenance of contraction, or tone. The calcium channel blockers interfere with the initial influx of calcium through specific calcium channels on the cell surface.

Pharmacokinetics

Calcium channel blockers are administered orally for prophylactic treatment of angina. They are generally metabolized by the liver, with metabolites being excreted in the urine and sometimes the feces through biliary excretion.

Uses

Prophylactic treatment of angina. The calcium channel blockers decrease the oxygen requirements of the heart through several actions. They reduce peripheral vascular resistance by a systemic vasodilation. This means that the workload of the heart is decreased. Calcium channel blockers dilate the coronary vessels by inhibiting contractility of coronary smooth muscle. This action is especially important for relief from variant angina, in which coronary spasm prevents blood flow. However, it is becoming clear that there is a varying degree of coronary spasm even in classic angina. Patients with asthma, diabetes, and peripheral vascular disease, who cannot tolerate beta-blockers, can benefit from calcium channel blockers. The calcium

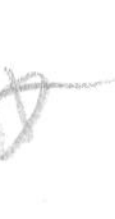

channel blockers also reduce the cardiac contractility (negative inotropy), which decreases the oxygen requirement of the heart. These agents increase coronary blood flow through coronary vasodilation more selectively than they inhibit cardiac contractility. Without this selective preference, the calcium channel blockers would not be clinically useful because they would overly compromise cardiac function. The various drugs of this class differ in the degree of selectivity in coronary vasodilation vs. decreased cardiac contractility.

Antihypertensive therapy. The vasodilator effect of calcium channel blockers makes them useful antihypertensive agents. (See Chapter 13 for a complete discussion.)

Antiarrhythmic therapy. Verapamil and diltiazem are used to treat supraventricular tachyarrhythmias.

Adverse Reactions and Contraindications

In general, the side effects of calcium channel blockers are mild. Headaches, light-headedness, and constipation are the most common ones. Some patients may feel unusually tired or weak. Side effects that require medical attention include difficulty in breathing, skin rash, heart rate less that 50 beats per minute or an irregular or pounding heartbeat, or edema in the lower limbs.

Interactions

There are several important interactions of calcium channel blockers with other drugs. Beta-blockers and calcium channel blockers, if given concurrently, may cause cardiac problems. These problems include a conduction block or arrhythmias and hypotension. Diltiazem and verapamil may inhibit the liver metabolism of several drugs, including carbamazepine, cyclosporine, quinidine, theophylline, and valproate. This may allow these drugs to reach toxic levels in the body. Digitalis glycosides may also accumulate in the presence of calcium channel blockers, resulting in excessive slowing of the heart or a heart block. Disopyramide depresses the force of the heartbeat (negative inotropic effect) and should not be administered within 48 hours of a calcium channel blocker.

Specific Calcium Channel Blockers

Five calcium channel blockers are currently approved in the United States for use in the treatment of angina: bepridil (Vascor), diltiazem (Cardizem), nicardipine (Cardene), nifedipine (Aldalat, Procardia), and verapamil (Calan, Isoptin). Felodipine (Plendil, Renedil) and isradipine (DynaCirc) are also used as antianginals. Calcium channel blockers used in the treatment of hypertension are covered in Chapter 13.

Bepridil

Bepridil (Vascor) is a nonselective calcium channel blocker that affects both cardiac and smooth muscle. It is used for the management of angina. It is rapidly absorbed. The 24-hour duration of action allows once a day dosage.

Diltiazem

Diltiazem (Cardizem) produces cardiac effects similar to those produced by verapamil. The incidence of dizziness, headache, and hypotension is less with diltiazem than with nifedipine and verapamil.

Diltiazem is well absorbed orally and has a duration of action of 4 to 8 hours. Extended-release capsules are available. Diltiazem is extensively metabolized; metabolites are excreted in the urine (35%) and in the feces (65%).

Felodipine, Isradipine, Nicardipine, Nifedipine

Felodipine (Plendil), isradipine (DynaCirc), nicardipine (Cardene), and nifedipine (Adalat, Procardia) are calcium channel blockers chemically related as dihydopyridines. Dihydopyridines are selective for vascular smooth muscle and are potent coronary and peripheral vasodilators. The cardiodepressant effect of dihydopyridines is minor because they do not depress the sinoatrial or atrioventricular nodes and because reflex sympathetic activity caused by hypotension counteracts the negative inotropic effect. The hypotensive effect can be accompanied by a reflex tachycardia. If combined with a beta-blocker, these calcium channel blockers may produce excessive hypotension and rarely heart failure.

Dihydopyridines are well absorbed orally. Felodipine has a 24-hour duration of action and isradipine more than 12 hours. Nicardipine and nifedipine have a 4- to 8-hour duration of action, but nifedipine is available in extended-release forms.

The side effects most frequently reported are related to peripheral vasodilation: headaches, hypotension, flushing, tingling in the extremities, and edema.

✣ Verapamil

Verapamil (Calan, Isoptin) depresses the atrioventricular node (negative chronotropism and negative dromotropism), an action that makes it a useful antiarrhythmic drug (Chapter 19). A slowing of the heart rate (bradycardia) is common. Verapamil does not cause a pronounced decrease in blood pressure, and therefore reflex sympathetic activity to stimulate the heart is minimal. The slowing of the heart rate and the decrease in blood pressure reduce the oxygen requirements of the heart. Verapamil increases coronary blood flow, which increases the oxygen available to the heart.

Although verapamil is readily absorbed, it is rapidly metabolized by the liver. The tablet form must be taken three or four times a day, but extended-release tablets and capsules are available. Verapamil is generally well tolerated, with constipation being the most common side effect. Verapamil is contraindicated for patients with atrioventricular conduction disturbances or congestive heart failure.

NURSING PROCESS OVERVIEW

Antianginal Drugs

Assessment

Patients with angina pectoris have a primary single complaint: chest pain. Obtain a thorough patient assessment, focusing on the subjective and objective signs. Determine the pulse, respiration, blood pressure, and level of consciousness. Question about the onset and duration of the pain, and ask about previous similar episodes and treatments. Obtain an electrocardiogram and appropriate laboratory work, including serum enzyme concentrations. When there is doubt as to the cause of chest pain, the usual practice is to treat the patient as if a myocardial infarction has occurred.

Nursing Diagnoses

- Potential altered health maintenance related to insufficient knowledge about prescribed antianginal drugs
- Potential for injury related to orthostatic hypotension secondary to vasodilator therapy

Patient Outcomes

The patient will be able to use antianginal drugs as prescribed to treat or prevent attacks of angina. The patient will not experience side effects related to vasodilation or will demonstrate actions to lessen the problems with side effects, such as sitting down before using sublingual nitroglycerin. The patient will be able to explain any lifestyle changes prescribed.

Planning/Implementation

Administer drugs as ordered. Assess for further chest pain, monitor for drug side effects, and begin teaching the patient about the drugs in anticipation of the patient's discharge from the hospital. Work with the patient and family to identify stresses that may precipitate angina attacks and plan possible ways to decrease these stresses. Instruct the patient about other prescribed therapies: losing weight, stopping smoking, controlling blood pressure, and exercising regularly. Refer the patient as needed to the dietitian, the local heart association, or the visiting nurse association.

Evaluation

The drugs used to treat angina are successful if the pain is relieved and the patient experiences no side effects resulting from drug therapy. The drugs do not halt the progression of disease. Before the patient's discharge from the hospital, determine that the patient can explain when and how to take the medications prescribed, can describe the drug side effects and how to treat them, and can explain what to do if drug therapy does not relieve the symptoms, how to correctly store the medication, and how to test for its continued effectiveness.

Therapeutic Rationale: Peripheral Vascular Disease

Vasospastic Disorders

Blood flow to the arms and legs, particularly the hands and feet, can be limited by peripheral vascular disease. Basically, the blood vessels may be narrowed by arteriosclerosis or by spasm of the vessels (vasospasm). If the vessel narrowing is a result of arteriosclerosis, vasodilator drugs are of little value. Vasodilator drugs may worsen the condition because vessels narrowed by arteriosclerosis do not dilate; adjacent vessels dilate and shunt the blood away from the occluded area. Blood flow in the occluded vessel therefore is reduced, not increased, by vasodilator drugs. On the other hand, if the narrowing of the vessel is a result of vasospasm, drugs are of benefit.

Raynaud's disease is the classic vasospastic disease in which primarily the fingers and toes are affected. In Raynaud's disease the blood vessels of the digits are readily thrown into spasm by cold or emotion and turn blue or white. Warming restores blood flow. Currently, the most successful drug treatment of Raynaud's disease is reported with two drugs that have been used to treat hypertension: reserpine and guanethidine. These drugs interfere with sympathetic innervation. Reserpine depresses sympathetic tone by depleting stored norepinephrine in the neurons. Guanethidine acts at the sympathetic neuron by blocking the release of norepinephrine and depleting norepinephrine stores. These drugs and their side effects are discussed fully in Chapter 13.

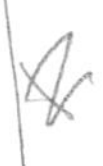

Impaired Cerebral Blood Flow

Vasodilators are sometimes prescribed to improve blood flow in the brain, particularly in older adult patients with arteriosclerosis of cerebral vessels who have suffered strokes or show signs of mental impairment. The problem is cerebral ischemia (insufficient oxygen to areas of the brain). Controlled medical trials are showing that this drug therapy is of little value. There is some medical opinion that vasodilator drugs may make the situation worse by shunting blood away from the unreactive, damaged vessels to areas with adequate blood flow already, as described for peripheral vascular insufficiency resulting from arteriosclerosis. Cyclandelate, ergoloid mesylates, and papaverine are sometimes prescribed to improve cerebral blood flow. There is no evidence that these drugs alter the progression of cerebral arteriosclerosis. They may improve some symptoms on a short-term basis.

Therapeutic Agents: Peripheral Vasodilators

Unfortunately, a large number of "vasodilator" drugs advertised for treating peripheral vascular spasm are of doubtful clinical value. These drugs include cyclandelate, isoxsuprine, nicotinyl alcohol, nylidrin, and papaverine.

Specific Vasodilators

For summary information on specific vasodilators, refer to Table 15-2.

Cyclandelate

Cyclandelate (Cyclospasmol) acts directly on vascular smooth muscle to cause relaxation. In the laboratory cyclandelate is a more effective vasodilator than papaverine, but the clinical effectiveness of cyclandelate is considered doubtful. Side effects include belching and heartburn, flushing, headache, weakness, and an increased heart rate.

Ergoloid Mesylates

Ergoloid mesylates (Hydergine) produce vasodilation in contrast to the ergot alkaloids, which produce vasoconstriction (Chapter 65). Ergoloid mesylates are of definite value in treating brain disease secondary to hypertension, but the benefit is related to the fall in blood pressure. These alkaloids act centrally to reduce vascular tone and slow heart rate. They act peripherally to block alpha-adrenergic receptors. These alkaloids are available in a sublingual dosage form. Sublingual irritation, nausea, and gastrointestinal tract upset are the side effects. The dihydrogenated ergot alkaloids can markedly reduce heart rate through their central effect of lowering sympathetic tone.

Flunarizine

Flunarizine (Sibelium) is a calcium channel blocker available in Canada to treat cerebral vascular disorders. The drug relieves symptoms of dizziness, vertigo, and tinnitus.

Isoxsuprine

Isoxsuprine (Vasodilan, Vasoprine) was originally thought to stimulate beta-receptors, but its vasodilating action is not blocked by drugs that are antagonists of the beta-receptors.

TABLE 15-2 Vasodilator Drugs

GENERIC NAME	TRADE NAME	ADMINISTRATION/DOSAGE	COMMENTS
Cyclandelate	Cyclospasmol*	ORAL: *Adults*—300-400 mg 4 times/day. Can be decreased gradually to 100-200 mg 4 times/day.	Direct vasodilator for use in vasospastic disorders may cause gastrointestinal tract disturbances.
Ergoloid mesylates	Hydergine*	SUBLINGUAL, ORAL: *Adults*—1 mg 3 times/day.	Drug can cause marked bradycardia. It relieves symptoms in hypertensive brain disease by lowering blood pressure.
Flunarizine†	Sibelium†	ORAL: *Adults*—10 mg once daily in evening.	Calcium channel blocker is indicated for prophylaxis of migraine.
Isoxsuprine	Vasodilan* Vasoprine	ORAL: *Adults*—10-20 mg 3-4 times/day. INTRAMUSCULAR: *Adults*—5-10 mg 2-3 times daily.	Drug is a direct-acting vasodilator with no proven use.
Nicotinyl alcohol	Roniacol† Ronigen Rycotin	ORAL: *Adults*—50-100 mg 3 times/day. ORAL (timed-release): *Adults*—300-400 mg every 12 hr.	Drug is a direct vasodilator that causes pronounced blushing. Gastrointestinal tract disturbances, tingling sensation, and rashes are side effects. Use has not been proved effective for any vasospastic disorders.
Nimodipine	Nimotop	ORAL: *Adults*—60 mg every 4 hr, beginning within 4 days after subarachnoid hemorrhage and continuing for 21 days.	Calcium channel blocker treats cerebral vasospasm after subarachnoid hemorrhage.
Nylidrin hydrochloride	Arlidin* PMS Nylidrin†	ORAL: *Adults*—3-12 mg 3-4 times/day.	Drug stimulates beta-adrenergic receptors and directly dilates vessels. It may cause dizziness, tachycardia, and hypotension.
Papaverine hydrochloride	Many trade names	ORAL: *Adults*—100-300 mg, 3-5 times/day. ORAL (timed-release): *Adults*—150 mg every 12 hr. Can give up to 150 mg every 8 hr or 300 mg every 12 hr. INTRAVENOUS: *Adults*—30-120 mg, over 1-2 min. INTRAMUSCULAR: *Adults*—30-120 mg.	Drug depresses heart. It directly relaxes smooth muscle, particularly of large blood vessels. Use is to relieve smooth muscle spasm in vascular disease or colic. Its effectiveness has not been proved.
Pentoxifylline	Trental*	ORAL: *Adults*—400 mg 3 times daily, with meals.	Drug is not vasodilator. It reduces blood viscosity and improves red blood cell flexibility to improve blood flow.

*Available in Canada and United States.
†Available in Canada only.

Clinical tests have not demonstrated any usefulness for isoxsuprine. Side effects include flushing, hypotension, dizziness, an increased heart rate, and occasionally a rash.

Nicotinyl Alcohol

Nicotinyl alcohol (Ronigen, Rycotin) has been used as a vasodilator but without good evidence of clinical effectiveness. This drug causes a pronounced flushing, postural (orthostatic) hypotension, and gastrointestinal tract upset. It can also cause a rash.

Nimodipine

Nimodipine (Nimotop) is a calcium channel blocker approved to treat cerebral vasospasm following subarachnoid hemorrhage. This action alleviates the cerebral ischemia that can follow a stroke and, by maintaining blood flow, protects the brain from deterioration. This use of a calcium channel blocker is seen as the beginning of a new therapeutic approach for the treatment of various neurologic disorders. Calcium channel blockers for neurologic use cross the blood-brain barrier.

Nylidrin

Nylidrin (Arlidin) is the classic example of a drug that stimulates blood flow in muscle. The rationale is to stimulate the beta-receptors of the blood vessels to produce vasodilation. However, blood vessels of the muscle, not the skin, have beta-receptors, so the approach is of little value in vasospastic disorders of the digits. The beta-blocker propranolol does not entirely reverse this stimulation, so nylidrin is believed to also act directly on smooth muscle. Side effects attributed to nylidrin include trembling, nervousness, weakness, dizziness, palpitations, and nausea and vomiting.

Papaverine

Papaverine (various trade names) relaxes smooth muscle. In large doses papaverine also depresses cardiac muscle, slowing conduction and prolonging the refractory period. Papaverine has long been used as a smooth muscle relaxant for ischemia of the brain, periphery, or heart. As with the other vasodilator drugs, there is little good evidence that papaverine improves peripheral vascular circulation. Side effects of papaverine can include flushing of the face, malaise, gastrointestinal tract upset, and headache. Other reported side effects include excess perspiration, loss of appetite, increased heart rate, and increased depth of respiration. Rarely, a hypersensitivity reaction involving the liver is seen. Symptoms of the liver damage may include jaundice, eosinophilia, and altered results of liver function tests.

Blood Viscosity-Reducing Drug: Pentoxifylline

Pentoxifylline (Trental) is a different type of drug for the treatment of peripheral vascular disease. Pentoxifylline increases the flexibility of red blood cells and reduces blood viscosity. These actions improve blood flow through narrowed vessels.

Pentoxifylline is administered as an adjunct to surgery for the treatment of intermittent claudication. Side effects are rare, but include dizziness, headache, nausea, or vomiting. Drug interactions include the potentiation of antihypertensive drugs. Smoking may interfere with the therapeutic action of pentoxifylline because nicotine constricts blood vessels. Toxic symptoms of pentoxifylline include excitement and seizures.

NURSING PROCESS OVERVIEW

Vasodilator Therapy in Peripheral Vascular Disease

Assessment

Assess the patient and obtain a history about onset and course of vascular disease. Assess the blood pressure and pulses, including peripheral pulses. Assess for altered sensation, poor healing of injuries on the feet, cool extremities, or symptoms of altered cerebral blood flow. Perform a mental status examination.

Nursing Diagnoses

- Potential for injury related to orthostatic hypotension associated with drug therapy
- Alteration in comfort: headache related to vasodilator therapy
- Alteration in comfort: nausea related to drug therapy

Patient Outcomes

The patient will be able to explain how to take prescribed medications correctly. The patient will demonstrate actions to minimize injury from side effects, such as sitting down when dizziness develops. The patient will be able to describe drug side effects and explain that some side effects will diminish with continued drug use. The patient will not discontinue medications without consulting the physician.

Planning/Implementation

Monitor the presenting signs and symptoms, especially blood pressure and pulses, and look for drug side effects. Instruct the patient about prescribed medications and begin teaching the patient about prevention of trauma to areas with decreased perfusion. Instruct the patient about other prescribed therapies: an exercise program, weight loss, and restriction of certain activities.

Evaluation

It is difficult to measure the effectiveness of these drugs. Before the patient's discharge from the hospital, determine that the patient can explain when and how to take the ordered medications, the side effects that might occur, and the situations that would require notification of the physician.

Nursing Implications Summary

Antianginal Drugs

Drug Administration

- In patients with chest pain, assess blood pressure and pulse; auscultate lungs and heart; assess intensity, duration, location, and quality of pain; assess response to medication; check for presence of diaphoresis, precipitating factors, electrocardiographic changes, or subjective and objective degree of patient distress; and obtain patient history. Chest pain in the person with a history of angina pectoris may have other causes.
- In the hospital it is often customary to keep a small supply of sublingual nitroglycerin tablets at the bedside of patients with a history of angina pectoris. Instruct patients to use as needed but to notify the nurse when tablets are used. Record the frequency of use, as well as a patient assessment, in the nurses' notes. Count and replenish the tablets each shift.

Patient and Family Education

- Encourage the patient to make all recommended lifestyle changes, including losing weight to reach desirable body weight, lowering cholesterol levels, ceasing smoking, and engaging in a regular exercise program after approval by the physician. Assist the patient and family in identifying activities that trigger anginal attacks such as eating a heavy meal, engaging in strenuous physical activities, lifting heavy objects, being exposed to cold weather, and having sex. Work with the patient to develop ways to decrease the frequency of attacks or to decrease the likelihood that activities will cause anginal pain to develop.
- Encourage the patient to notify the physician if the frequency, intensity, duration, location of pain, or response to antianginal drugs changes. Instruct the patient to avoid the use of alcohol, as it potentiates the hypotensive effects of the nitrates and nitrites. Remind the patient to keep all health care providers informed of all drugs being used because diuretics, antihypertensives, CNS depressants, narcotics, and sedatives may potentiate the hypotensive effects of the antianginal drugs. Encourage the patient to maintain regular contact with the primary health care provider and not to stop drug therapy without medical consultation.
- If a headache regularly occurs when antianginal drugs are taken, it may indicate too high a dosage. For some patients it may be necessary to use mild analgesics with antianginal therapy; consult the physician.

Nitrates and Nitrites

Drug Administration

Intravenous Nitroglycerin

- Consult the manufacturer's literature for specific instructions about dilution, dosage, and administration. Use a microdrip infusion set and a volume control or rate-controlling device to prevent overdosage and to accurately titrate the dose. Nitroglycerin migrates into plastic tubing. Dilutions should be prepared and kept in glass bottles. Use nonpolyvinyl chloride tubing. Monitor the blood pressure, heart rate, electrocardiographic changes, and pulmonary capillary wedge pressure (PCWP). Use intravenous nitroglycerin only in settings where drugs and experienced personnel to treat cardiovascular emergencies are available.

Patient and Family Education

- If syncope (fainting), dizziness, or hypotension occurs with nitrate or nitrite use, instruct the patient to lie down before taking the prescribed dose of medication. Ascertain that the patient can correctly use sublingual drug forms before the patient's discharge. This may be a new dosage form for the patient. In addition, teach the family how to place a dose under the patient's tongue in the event the patient cannot do it. Tell the patient not to eat, drink, chew tobacco, or smoke while the dose is dissolving.
- Review the standard instructions with the patient and family for antianginal agents used to relieve an attack of angina. When chest pain develops, the patient should sit down, then use one tablet, letting it dissolve under the tongue or in the cheek, or chew a chewable tablet. If relief is not obtained, the patient should repeat the dose in 5 minutes and again in another 5 minutes if needed, for a total of 3 tablets. If the pain persists after 3 tablets, the patient should notify the physician or seek medical help. These guidelines may be individualized based on the patient, the patient's condition, and the physician's preference.
- Instruct the patient to take oral nitrates with meals or a snack to reduce gastric irritation. Review the ordered drugs carefully with the patient, as well as exactly how and when to take the prescribed drugs, since there are many dosages and drug forms available for these drugs.
- Storage instructions for these drugs include keeping drugs out of the reach of children and not storing in the bathroom or near the kitchen sink or other damp areas. Check expiration dates and replace drugs as needed. For sublingual nitroglycerin, follow the previous instructions and keep tablets in the original glass container. Once the bottle is opened, remove the cotton and do not replace it. Replace the cap tightly and quickly each time the bottle is opened. Do not put other medicines in the same bottle with the nitroglycerin. When pouring a dose (a tablet), pour one or more tablets into the lid of the bottle, take the dose out, and return remaining tablets to the bottle. Avoid replacing tablets from the palm of the hand into the bottle. Instruct the patient to obtain a small glass bottle from the pharmacist for carrying a small number of pills. Do not carry the small bottle too close to the body, because body warmth may cause the pills to lose their strength.
- To prevent an attack of angina, instruct patients to take the prescribed drug before engaging in the activity ex-

NURSING IMPLICATIONS SUMMARY—cont'd

pected to produce anginal pain. For sublingual or chewable forms, this may be 5 to 10 minutes before engaging in such activities; for extended-release forms, patients may need to take the antianginal drug several hours before the activity. For specific patient needs, consult the physician.

- If doses are missed, instruct patients to take the dose as soon as remembered, unless within 2 hours of the next dose (extended-release forms or isosorbide dinitrate). Do not double up for missed doses.

Buccal Extended-Release Forms

- For buccal extended-release tablets, place the dose between the cheek and upper gum or between the upper lip and gum and allow it to dissolve over 5 hours. When eating or drinking, place the dose between the upper lip and gum. If the patient wears dentures, place the tablet between the cheek and gum. Tell the patient not to use chewing tobacco while using this form. Replace the tablet if it is accidentally swallowed. Tell the patient not to go to sleep with a tablet still in the mouth. Sublingual erythrityl tetranitrate, isosorbide dinitrate, and nitroglycerin tablets may also be administered buccally.

Chewable Tablets

- For chewable tablets, instruct the patient to chew it well, then hold it in the mouth for at least 2 minutes before swallowing. Instruct the patient not to drink, smoke, eat, or chew tobacco while using this form.

Extended-Release Capsules and Tablets

- Instruct the patient to swallow extended-release capsules whole, without chewing, crushing, or breaking.

Lingual Aerosol Forms

- Review the patient instruction leaflet supplied by the manufacturer. To use, remove the cover. Do not shake the container. Hold the container upright, close to the patient's mouth. Spray 1 or 2 sprays (as prescribed by the physician) under the tongue. Close the mouth. Avoid swallowing for 1 or 2 minutes. This drug may be used like nitroglycerin tablets: when an attack of angina occurs, the patient should administer a dose as prescribed. If no relief is obtained in 5 minutes, the patient should repeat the dose. If there is no relief in another 5 minutes, the patient should repeat the dose. If no relief occurs after a total of 3 doses in 15 minutes, the patient should seek medical attention or notify the physician. The prescription may be modified for individual patient needs and by physician preference.

Topical Transdermal Forms

- Review the patient instruction leaflet supplied by the manufacturer. Do not trim or cut the adhesive patch. Remove the previous patch before applying a new patch. Rotate sites to avoid skin irritation. Apply the patch to an area that is clean and dry, with little or no hair. Avoid scratches, scars, or existing skin irritation. If the patch loosens or falls off, replace it with a new one. Side effects are the same as for other antianginal drugs in this group. Transdermal forms should not be used to treat an acute attack of angina. Tolerance to this therapy may be lessened if the patches are not used continuously; some physicians may prescribe a patch-free period each day (e.g., during the night).

Topical Ointments

- Review the patient instruction leaflet supplied by the manufacturer. Remove the ointment from a previous dose before applying a fresh dose. Measure the prescribed amount of ointment, using the measuring paper supplied by the manufacturer. Gently spread the ointment over a small area of about the same size each time with the measuring paper or small applicator (not the fingertips). Do not massage the ointment into the skin. Apply to areas with little or no hair. Avoid scratches and scars. Rotate sites to avoid skin irritation. Cover the area with plastic kitchen wrap or other dressing only if ordered by the physician. If a dressing is prescribed, it should be used each time the drug is used. If a dose is missed, apply it as soon as remembered, unless it is within 2 hours of the next dose, then follow the usual dosing schedule. Do not use more ointment than ordered and do not double up for missed doses.

Amyl Nitrite

- Amyl nitrite is rarely used for treatment of angina. Instruct the patient and family to wrap the ampule in a cloth or handkerchief, break the glass ampule within its protective covering, then have the patient inhale several deep breaths.

Beta-Blockers

- See Nursing Implications Summary in Chapter 13 (p. 160).

Calcium Channel Blockers

Drug Administration

- Assess the patient with complaints of chest pain for intensity, duration, location, and quality of pain; response to medications; presence of diaphoresis; vital signs, blood pressure, and electrocardiographic changes; precipitating factors; patient history; auscultation of heart and lung sounds; and other subjective complaints. Chest pain in the patient with a history of angina pectoris may be due to other causes also.
- In patients taking calcium channel blockers, monitor the blood pressure, pulse, intake and output, and weight. Signs of fluid retention are peripheral edema and subjective complaints of tight shoes and rings. Signs of heart failure

Continued.

NURSING IMPLICATIONS SUMMARY—cont'd

include dyspnea on exertion, distended jugular veins, orthopnea, or moist rales on pulmonary auscultation.

- If calcium channel blockers are prescribed for hypertension, see the general guidelines for patients receiving antihypertensives in Chapter 13 (p. 160).

Nifedipine

- To administer sublingually or intrabuccally, puncture the fluid-filled capsule and squeeze the drug into the mouth. The patient may chew the capsule to break it and direct the contents to the cheek or under the tongue.

Diltiazem

- Administer intravenous (IV) doses undiluted for a period of at least 2 minutes in the adult. Monitor the electrocardiographic changes and the blood pressure. Diltiazem may also be diluted and administered as an infusion. See the manufacturer's literature for various dilutions. Use microdrip tubing or an infusion control device to help maintain an even infusion. Monitor blood pressure, pulse, and electrocardiographic changes.

Verapamil

- Administer IV doses undiluted over at least 2 minutes in the adult and 3 minutes in the older adult patient. Monitor the electrocardiographic changes and the blood pressure.

Patient and Family Education

- See the box on p. 157 for a discussion of orthostatic hypotension and the box on p. 304 for a discussion of constipation.
- If appropriate, teach the patient to take and record the pulse daily at home. Instruct the patient to report a change of 10 beats per minute in the resting pulse or a pulse rate less than 50 beats per minute. Appropriate candidates for such instruction may be those on multiple-drug regimens or those in whom control of side effects has been difficult. If appropriate, instruct the patient to monitor and record weight on a regular basis. Instruct patients to report a weight gain of greater than 2 lb/day or 5 lb/wk. Instruct the patient to report the development of tight rings, shoes, or clothing or signs of peripheral edema.
- Because of potential drug interactions with other medication, instruct the patient to keep all health care providers informed of all drugs being used. Instruct the patient to avoid the use of any over-the-counter preparations unless first cleared by the physician. In addition to using these drugs as prescribed, the patient may find additional relief by losing weight, stopping smoking, limiting caffeine intake, avoiding extremes of temperature, and becoming involved in a regular exercise program. The patient should consult the physician.
- Emphasize to the patient the importance of taking these drugs as prescribed and not discontinuing them without consultation with the physician. If a dose is missed, instruct the patient to take the missed dose as soon as remembered, but not within 2 hours of the next scheduled dose. Instruct the patient not to double up for missed doses.
- Headache may develop after a dose of medication is taken but will last only a short time. This side effect should gradually diminish with continued use of the drug. Instruct the patient to report any signs of liver problems such as right upper quadrant abdominal pain, jaundice, change in color or consistency of stools, fever, or malaise.
- The calcium channel blockers may cause tender gums or swelling or bleeding gums. Encourage the patient to have regular dental examinations. Review oral hygiene practices; encourage regular flossing and brushing. If gum problems develop, the patient should check with the physician or dentist.
- Instruct the patient to swallow extended-release capsules or tablets whole, without crushing or chewing. Instruct the patient using extended-release diltiazem capsules to check with the physician before changing brands of medication; the different brands should be given on different dosing schedules. Instruct the patient to take extended-release verapamil tablets whole, without chewing or crushing, unless the physician has authorized breaking extended-release verapamil tablets in half.

Bepridil

- Encourage the patient to take doses with meals or at bedtime if nausea is a problem.

Peripheral Vasodilators

Drug Administration

- Monitor the blood pressure and pulse when beginning therapy or when changing doses.

Isoxsuprine

- Intramuscular (IM) doses of isoxsuprine may cause hypotension and tachycardia. Monitor the blood pressure and pulse.
- If isoxsuprine is used to prevent labor, monitor intensity, frequency, and duration of uterine contractions. Monitor fetal heart rate at regular intervals.

Nimodipine

- See nursing interventions for calcium channel blockers discussed earlier in this chapter. For patients who cannot swallow, withdraw the fluid from within the capsule and administer via a feeding tube, followed by 30 ml of 0.9% sodium chloride. To withdraw dose, puncture both ends

NURSING IMPLICATIONS SUMMARY—cont'd

of the capsule with an 18-gauge needle and withdraw fluid into a syringe.

Papaverine

- Administer IV doses of papaverine undiluted at a rate of 30 mg or less over 2 minutes. IM injection is preferred. Monitor the electrocardiographic changes, pulse, respiration, and blood pressure during IV administration and for 1 hour afterward.

Patient and Family Education

- Instruct the patient to take doses with meals or antacids to diminish gastrointestinal tract symptoms. Review information about orthostatic hypotension with the patient (see box on p. 157). Hypotension may be potentiated in patients receiving vasodilators who are also receiving other drugs that can cause hypotension such as diuretics, antihypertensives, CNS depressants, narcotics, and sedatives. Instruct the patient to keep all health care providers informed of all medications being taken.
- Instruct the patient to avoid the use of alcohol because it potentiates the hypotensive effects of vasodilators. Instruct the patient to avoid smoking, which reduces peripheral blood flow.
- Instruct the patient to swallow timed-release formulations whole, without chewing or crushing. Encourage the patient to maintain desirable body weight to help decrease symptoms from peripheral vascular disease. Warn the patient that nicotinyl alcohol, pentoxifylline, or papaverine may produce pronounced flushing, which is not harmful. Caution the patient to avoid driving or operating hazardous equipment if side effects such as dizziness, weakness, drowsiness, or double vision occur.
- Encourage the patient to take peripheral vasodilators as prescribed. Regular long-term use may be necessary for full benefit to occur. Instruct the patient to take missed doses as soon as remembered, unless within 2 hours of the next dose. Do not double up for missed doses.
- Nylidrin may cause palpitations, especially if taken at bedtime. Work with the patient to develop a dosage schedule that avoids taking the last dose at bedtime.
- Papaverine or phentolamine may be used to produce erections in some impotent men. The patient should clean off the base of the penis with alcohol and inject the prescribed dose into the base of the penis as instructed by the physician. After injection, the patient should massage the penis and attempt intercourse within 2 hours. Teach the patient to consult the physician if the erection lasts more than 4 hours, the erection is painful, there is bleeding at the injection site that does not stop after pressure is applied, a lump develops where the medication was injected, or the penis is becoming curved.
- Instruct patients taking pentoxifylline to avoid the use of aspirin or aspirin-containing products while taking this drug. Assess patients for hypersensitivity or intolerance to methylxanthines before administering pentoxifylline. Methylxanthines include caffeine, theophylline, and theobromine (the active ingredients in coffee, tea, and chocolate). Pentoxifylline is contraindicated in persons with intolerance to methylxanthines.

CRITICAL THINKING

APPLICATION

1. What is the origin of angina? Describe the differences between classic (exertional) angina, variant angina, and unstable angina.
2. How do the nitrates relieve angina?
3. How do the beta-blockers relieve angina? What are their side effects?
4. How do the calcium channel blockers relieve angina?
5. What are two causes of insufficient blood flow to the digits? Which cause is amenable to drug therapy? What role do vasodilators play?
6. List the seven drugs used as vasodilators for improving peripheral circulation. What are some of their common side effects?

CRITICAL THINKING

1. How might the type of angina influence a teaching plan for a patient?
2. Outline the main teaching points for patients taking nitrates.
3. For which patients are the cardioselective beta-blockers especially indicated?
4. What would you include in the teaching plan for a patient taking a beta-blocker?
5. Why are calcium channel blockers especially effective for variant angina?
6. What would you teach a patient about the calcium-channel blockers?

CHAPTER 16

Drugs to Treat Shock

OBJECTIVES

After studying this chapter, you should be able to do the following:

- *Discuss the use of sympathomimetic amines in the treatment of shock.*
- *Develop nursing care plans for patients receiving sympathomimetic amines.*

KEY TERMS

anaphylactic shock
reflex bradycardia
shock
sympathomimetic drugs

CHAPTER OVERVIEW

Sympathomimetic drugs restore functions mediated through adrenergic receptors. These drugs are used primarily in the treatment of shock, a condition of poor tissue perfusion in which selective adjustment of cardiac or vascular function may prevent shock from becoming irreversible and progressing to death.

Therapeutic Rationale: Shock

Shock is a disruption of circulation. Frequently, the blood pressure is too low to force blood through vital tissues. Poor perfusion of the brain results in confusion or coma; poor perfusion of the kidney results in low urine output (<30 ml/hr); and poor perfusion of the skin makes the skin cold and clammy. In shock, the body has already activated the sympathetic nervous system to increase blood pressure. Fluid replacement or fluid addition is often the first choice in treating shock to overcome the decrease in the circulating volume caused by the constriction of the peripheral blood vessels. Selected use of direct-acting sympathomimetic amines is made in treating certain types of shock, raising blood pressure by increasing peripheral resistance (activation of alpha-1 adrenergic receptors) or by increasing cardiac output (activation of beta-1 adrenergic receptors).

Therapeutic Agents: Direct-Acting Sympathomimetic Drugs

As discussed in Chapter 12, the sympathetic nervous system plays a major role in controlling cardiovascular function. Stimulation of the alpha-adrenergic receptors of blood vessels causes vasoconstriction. On a systemic level, this vasoconstriction shows up as a higher blood pressure. Stimulation of the cardiac beta-1 receptors increases heart rate and force of contraction, resulting in an increased cardiac output. Stimulation of the beta-2 receptors, found primarily in the blood vessels of the skeletal muscle, causes vasodilation. Only in unusual circumstances, however, does systemic stimulation of the beta-2 receptors decrease blood pressure. The net change in cardiovascular function produced by direct-acting **sympathomimetic drugs** depends on the degree of activity at the three adrenergic receptor subtypes.

✣ DOPAMINE

Mechanism of Action

Dopamine (Dopastat, Intropin) is a naturally occurring catecholamine capable of acting at alpha- and beta-adrenergic receptors, as well as at its own specific dopaminergic receptors. Appropriate doses of this catecholamine can be selected such that cardiac output is increased while heart rate and mean blood pressure remain unchanged. The unusual and highly desirable property of dopamine is that renal blood flow is directly stimulated at these same doses. Renal function may therefore be maintained in patients being treated for shock as long as supportive therapy maintains adequate blood volume.

Pharmacokinetics

Dopamine must be administered by constant intravenous (IV) infusion. Dopamine is rapidly taken up and stored or destroyed by tissues. The infusion rate must be meticulously adjusted to achieve the desired therapeutic results.

Uses

Dopamine is the most widely used sympathomimetic amine for treating shock. The action of dopamine may be controlled by the rate of infusion. Dopamine is used primarily as a renal vasodilator to prevent renal failure in shock and secondarily to increase cardiac output. At low doses (0.5 to 2 μg/kg/min), dopamine acts exclusively on dopamine receptors in the renal arterioles to cause vasodilation. At higher doses (1 to 10 μg/kg/min), dopamine acts at cardiac beta-1 receptors to stimulate cardiac contractility. The beta-1 receptors controlling heart rate and the alpha-receptors controlling blood pressure are not activated. At doses above these, dopamine causes the release of norepinephrine, thereby increasing heart rate and blood pressure.

Adverse Reactions and Contraindications

Dopamine can cause tachycardia (fast heart rate), palpitation, nausea and vomiting, angina, headache, hypertension, and vasoconstriction. A reduction or discontinuance of dopamine infusion is usually sufficient to reverse side effects because dopamine has such a short plasma half-life. Leakage of dopamine around the infusion site must be avoided, but if extravasation does occur, the alpha-adrenergic receptor antagonist phentolamine should be infused into the area to reverse vasoconstriction. Untreated extravasation can cause tissue death and sloughing.

Like the other sympathomimetic amines, dopamine is contraindicated for patients predisposed to cardiac arrhythmias.

Interactions

Dopamine is not stable in alkaline solutions and should not be made up in a sodium bicarbonate solution. Patients medicated with a monoamine oxidase inhibitor require only 10% of the usual dose of dopamine. Tricyclic antidepressants potentiate the hypertensive action of dopamine. Dopamine should not be administered to women in labor receiving an oxytocic drug because a severe persistent hypertension may be produced. Patients receiving one of the general anesthetics that sensitize the heart to catecholamines may develop arrhythmias if dopamine is administered. Since dopamine dilates renal arteries, the action of diuretic drugs is potentiated.

DOBUTAMINE

Mechanisms of Action

Dobutamine (Dobutrex), like dopamine, at low doses will selectively increase the contractility of the heart without increasing the heart rate. Dobutamine neither stimulates the dopamine receptors of the kidney blood vessels nor releases norepinephrine. At high doses, dobutamine does increase heart rate and conduction velocity (beta-1 adrenergic receptor) and stimulates beta-2 adrenergic receptors.

Pharmacokinetics

Dobutamine has a plasma half-life of about 2 minutes and must be administered by continuous IV infusion. Dobutamine is rapidly metabolized to inactive compounds in the liver.

Uses

Dobutamine improves cardiac output in patients with congestive heart failure with little effect on heart rate or systolic blood pressure.

Adverse Reactions and Contraindications

Increased heart rate and blood pressure are the most frequent side effects and can be reversed by lowering the infusion rate. Palpitations, shortness of breath, angina, nausea, and headache are infrequent side effects of dobutamine. Dobutamine is contraindicated for patients in whom the increased force of contraction would be dangerous, as in idiopathic hypertrophic subaortic stenosis.

Interactions

Drugs that may sensitize the heart to the inotropic effects of dobutamine include hydrocarbon inhalation anesthetics and the reserpine antihypertensives. Dobutamine may block the effectiveness of the beta-blockers and several other antihypertensive agents: guanadrel, guanethidine, and nitroprusside.

EPINEPHRINE

Mechanism of Action

Epinephrine is a potent agonist of the beta-1 receptors of the heart, increasing heart rate and force of contraction. This cardiac stimulation is achieved with an increase in the oxygen demand of the heart, which may not be tolerable in cardiac disease. Epinephrine also stimulates alpha-receptors to cause vasoconstriction, particularly of the vessels in the skin, mucosa, kidney, and visceral organs. Epinephrine also stimulates beta-2 receptors, which alter blood flow because the receptors mediate vasodilation in the blood vessels in skeletal muscle. The overall response to IV administration of epinephrine is a marked increase in heart rate and force of contraction with little or no increase in blood pressure.

Pharmacokinetics

Epinephrine is not active when given orally because it is rapidly inactivated by the gastric mucosa. Epinephrine is administered intramuscularly or subcutaneously. Epinephrine may be inhaled from a nebulizer for relief of bronchospasm. IV administration of epinephrine must be done very slowly and cannot be done using one of the epinephrine suspensions. Intracardiac injection of epinephrine is a last step in attempting cardiac resuscitation when other measures have failed.

Epinephrine is rapidly degraded by monoamine oxidase and catechol *O*-methyltransferase of the liver and kidney. Epinephrine is unstable in alkaline solutions and when exposed to light or air. Pink or brown solutions should not be used.

Uses

Epinephrine, administered as soon as possible, is the drug of choice for treating **anaphylactic shock.** Anaphylactic shock is the result of massive histamine release caused by an allergic reaction and must be promptly treated. Histamine causes profound vasodilation and bronchial constriction. Epinephrine opposes the actions of histamine: epinephrine produces vasoconstriction, raising the blood pressure, and relaxes the bronchioles, restoring breathing. Epinephrine quickly reverses the edema of the larynx and the bronchospasm of anaphylactic shock.

Epinephrine may be administered systemically or by inhalation for relief of bronchospasm resulting from asthma or allergic reactions. Because epinephrine causes vasoconstriction, it is applied topically as a hemostatic agent. Epinephrine injection prolongs the action of local anesthetics by slowing their systemic absorption.

Adverse Reactions and Contraindications

Fear and anxiety are side effects of epinephrine arising from stimulation of the central nervous system. Other side effects include a throbbing headache, dizziness, and pallor caused by vasoconstriction. Stimulation of skeletal muscle causes tremor and weakness, and stimulation of the heart causes palpitation. These effects are usually transient. Hyperthyroid and hypertensive patients are prone to an exaggerated hypertensive response to epinephrine. Cerebral hemorrhage and cardiac arrhythmias are serious reactions to epinephrine.

Epinephrine is contraindicated for patients receiving a general anesthetic that sensitizes the heart to catecholamines. Neither patients with narrow-angle glaucoma nor women in labor should receive epinephrine. Epinephrine must be used with extreme care in patients with cardiac arrhythmias, cardiovascular disease, hypertension, or hyperthyroidism. The hyperglycemic, hypoinsulinemic effects of epinephrine will interrupt control of diabetes mellitus.

Interactions

Epinephrine should not be administered simultaneously with isoproterenol because the combination can cause cardiac arrhythmias. Cardiac effects of epinephrine are also potentiated by tricyclic antidepressants, antihistamines, thyroxine, digitalis, and mercurial diuretics. A hypertensive response to epinephrine may be seen in patients receiving a monoamine oxidase inhibitor or oxytocin.

ISOPROTERENOL

Mechanism of Action

Isoproterenol (Isuprel) is a synthetic catecholamine that stimulates beta-1 and beta-2 adrenergic receptors but has little activity on alpha-adrenergic receptors. Isoproterenol will therefore stimulate heart rate and cardiac output. At sufficient doses of isoproterenol, blood pressure will fall because activation of the beta-2 receptors of the blood vessels in skeletal muscle will shunt blood to the muscles and lower peripheral resistance. Smooth muscle, particularly the bronchial and gastrointestinal tract smooth muscle, is relaxed by isoproterenol. Isoproterenol is effective in treating bronchospasm when administered by inhalation.

Pharmacokinetics

Isoproterenol is not very effective orally. Absorption from a sublingual site is unreliable. Isoproterenol may be given effectively subcutaneously, intramuscularly, or intravenously. The catechol *O*-methyltransferase of the liver and other tissues is the major enzyme for degrading isoproterenol.

Uses

The principal use of isoproterenol is as a bronchodilator (see Chapter 27). Isoproterenol is infrequently used as a cardiac stimulant in heart block and in cardiogenic shock secondary to a myocardial infarction or septicemia.

Adverse Reactions and Contraindications

Side effects of isoproterenol include palpitation, tachycardia (fast heart rate), headache, and flushing of the face. Sweating and mild tremors, nervousness, dizziness, and nausea may be experienced. Patients taking digitalis or otherwise disposed toward cardiac arrhythmias should not receive isoproterenol.

Interactions

Isoproterenol should not be administered with epinephrine because together they can induce severe cardiac arrhythmias.

LEVARTERENOL [NOREPINEPHRINE]

Mechanism of Action

Levarterenol (Levophed), or norepinephrine, the neurotransmitter of the sympathetic nervous system, is a potent agonist of the alpha-1 and beta-1 adrenergic receptors when administered as the drug levarterenol. Levarterenol has relatively little effect on the beta-2 adrenergic receptors.

Levarterenol produces a potent peripheral vasoconstriction and inotropic response. Blood flow is shifted from the skin and visceral and renal vessels (where blood vessels are constricted) to the heart and brain (where blood vessels do not have alpha-receptors). On administration, levarterenol initially raises blood pressure dramatically. The increase is quickly great enough to stimulate the baroreceptors in the aorta, thereby triggering reflex stimulation of the vagus nerve, a physiologic process called **reflex bradycardia** (slow heart rate), which results because stimulation of the vagus nerve releases acetylcholine. Acetylcholine, however, slows the heart, and vagal stimulation from administration of acetylcholine counteracts the direct stimulation of the heart by levarterenol. The net result of administering levarterenol is therefore an increase in blood pressure with a modest and variable change in heart rate but very strong contractions of the heart.

Pharmacokinetics

Levarterenol is ineffective when taken orally, being rapidly degraded in the stomach. This drug is administered intravenously, and if it does infiltrate the infusion site, the alpha-adrenergic receptor antagonist phentolamine must be infiltrated in the area to counteract the profound vasoconstriction that may lead to tissue ischemia.

Levarterenol is rapidly inactivated by the liver. Like native norepinephrine, levarterenol is taken up and stored in sympathetic neurons identical to the native norepinephrine.

Uses

Levarterenol is used to restore blood pressure in acute hypotensive states but only after blood volume has been restored. In the absence of adequate blood volume, tissue perfusion is inadequate after vasoconstriction by levarterenol in spite of increased blood pressure. Kidney perfusion in particular is poor. Levarterenol provides a temporary treatment when the brain or heart is compromised in shock. Levarterenol may be used immediately after cardiac arrest has been terminated to restore and maintain blood pressure.

Adverse Reactions and Contraindications

Anxiety and a slow, forceful heartbeat are common side effects from administration of levarterenol. Some patients may develop a transient hypertension that is evidenced by a severe headache.

Levarterenol is contraindicated for patients who have vascular thrombosis because the resulting vasoconstriction could cause tissue death. Levarterenol should not be used to raise blood pressure in patients anesthetized with a drug that sensitizes the heart to catecholamine-induced arrhythmias (see Chapter 68).

Interactions

Administration of levarterenol to a patient taking an antidepressant drug (either a monoamine oxidase inhibitor or a tricyclic antidepressant) may cause a severe hypertensive response, since antidepressant drugs interfere with the degradation and reuptake, respectively, of norepinephrine. A persistent hypertensive response may be elicited if levarterenol is administered after an oxytocic drug during labor.

METHOXAMINE

Methoxamine (Vasoxyl) acts selectively to stimulate alpha-adrenergic receptors. Methoxamine, which is administered intravenously or intramuscularly, increases blood pressure for a period of 60 to 90 minutes. This vasopressor action is used to treat the hypotension of anesthesia during surgery, primarily for spinal anesthesia when the patient is conscious and aware of the unpleasant effects of hypotension. The increased blood pressure in a patient with normal blood pressure will cause a reflex slowing of the heart rate (reflex bradycardia). Use of this action is made in terminating episodes of paroxysmal supraventricular tachycardia.

Side effects of methoxamine include sustained hypertension with a severe headache. Goose flesh (pilomotor erection), desire to urinate, and vomiting are occasional side effects.

Like the other sympathomimetic vasopressors, methoxamine should be used with caution in patients with heart disease or hypertension and is potentiated in patients receiving oxytocic drugs, monoamine oxidase inhibitors, tricyclic antidepressants, or general anesthetics of the type that sensitizes the heart to catecholamines.

PHENYLEPHRINE

Phenylephrine (Isophrin, Neo-Synephrine) acts selectively to stimulate alpha-adrenergic receptors. Phenylephrine's effect is shorter in duration (20 to 50 minutes) than methoxamine's, but otherwise the description of methoxamine and its uses, side effects, and drug interactions can be applied to phenylephrine.

Phenylephrine is used mainly as a nasal decongestant (see Chapter 29); it is also used to dilate the pupil (see Chapter 71). These actions result from stimulation of alpha-adrenergic receptors.

Therapeutic Agents: Indirect-Acting Sympathomimetic Drugs

Indirect-acting sympathomimetic drugs cause the release of norepinephrine from sympathetic neurons. The norepinephrine so released accounts for the activity of the drug. Like methoxamine, the selective alpha-adrenergic receptor agonist, the indirect-acting sympathomimetic amines are used primarily in treating the hypotension of spinal anesthesia. During spinal anesthesia, the sympathetic ganglia lying near the spinal cord may be affected, thereby disrupting sympathetic control of blood pressure. This is usually not to a degree that is life threatening, but the sensation is unpleasant to the conscious patient. The indirect-acting sympathomimetic amines act directly on the postganglionic nerve terminals to release norepinephrine and restore blood pressure.

EPHEDRINE

Mechanism of Action

Ephedrine is the prototype of the indirect-acting sympathomimetic amines, although ephedrine can be shown to have direct sympathomimetic actions at alpha- and beta-adrenergic receptors. Ephedrine, which has been isolated from several plants, has been used in Chinese medicine for 2000 years.

Pharmacokinetics

Ephedrine is active for 4 to 6 hours when administered orally, subcutaneously, intramuscularly, or intravenously.

Uses

The major use of ephedrine is as a bronchodilator (see Chapter 27). Ephedrine, seldom used as a vasopressor, is not included in Table 16-1. The vasopressor response to ephedrine is primarily a result of cardiac stimulation, increasing blood pressure through an increase in cardiac output.

Adverse Reactions and Contraindications

Ephedrine is a potent stimulant of the central nervous system, and this stimulation is the major side effect. Insomnia, agitation, euphoria, and confusion may be noted. Delirium and hallucinations can occur at high doses. As with other sympathomimetic drugs, headache, palpitation, nausea and vomiting, and difficulty in voiding may be side effects. Repeated administration of ephedrine decreases the effectiveness of the drug. This rapidly developing tolerance (tachyphylaxis) results from the depletion of stored norepinephrine.

Ephedrine should be used cautiously in patients with hypertension, hyperthyroidism, diabetes mellitus, or (in males) prostate obstruction.

Interactions

The vasopressor response to ephedrine is potentiated by monoamine oxidase inhibitors, tricyclic antidepressants, and oxytocic drugs. Cardiac arrhythmias may be precipitated by ephedrine in the presence of digitalis or one of the general anesthetics that sensitize the heart to catecholamines.

METARAMINOL

Mechanism of Action

Metaraminol (Aramine) has both direct alpha-adrenergic agonist activity and an indirect sympathomimetic activity. Metaraminol can deplete norepinephrine stores on repeated administration to cause tachyphylaxis.

Pharmacokinetics

Metaraminol is administered intravenously, intramuscularly, or subcutaneously, with the onset of action being 1 to 2 minutes, 10 minutes, and 15 to 20 minutes, respectively. The activity persists for 20 to 60 minutes. Larger doses are administered by IV infusion, and care must be taken to avoid leakage of the drug at the infusion site. Metaraminol produces a rise in diastolic and systolic blood pressure, but heart rate is usually decreased as a result of reflex bradycardia. The force of contraction of the heart is increased.

Uses

Metaraminol is used clinically only to treat certain acute hypotensive states, as in spinal anesthesia.

Adverse Reactions and Contraindications

Metaraminol does not have any pronounced central nervous system effects. Otherwise side effects, contraindications, and drug interactions are identical to those described for ephedrine.

MEPHENTERMINE

Mechanism of Action

Mephentermine (Wyamine) is an indirect-acting sympathomimetic drug. The major effect of mephentermine is an in-

TABLE 16-1 Sympathomimetic Drugs Used to Treat Hypotension and Shock

GENERIC NAME	TRADE NAME	ADMINISTRATION/DOSAGE	COMMENTS
Dobutamine hydrochloride	Dobutrex*	INTRAVENOUS: *Adults*—2.5-10 μg/kg/min. A 12.5-25 mg/ml solution is made and used.	To stimulate cardiac contractility in cardiogenic shock.
✣ Dopamine hydrochloride	Intropin* Revimine†	INTRAVENOUS: *Adults*—1 ampule (40 mg of chloride salt in 5 ml) is diluted in 250 ml (800 μg/ml) or 500 ml (400 μg/ml) of solution. Initial intravenous infusion is 2-5 μg/kg/min. Onset: 5 min. Duration: 10 min.	To maintain renal blood flow in shock with mild cardiac stimulation.
✣ Epinephrine hydrochloride	Adrenalin chloride* EpiPen Sus-Phrine	INTRAMUSCULAR, SUBCUTANEOUS, INTRAVENOUS: *Adults*—0.5 ml of 1:1000 solution intramuscularly or subcutaneously followed by 0.25-0.5 ml of 1:10,000 solution intravenously every 5-15 min. *Children*—0.3 ml of 1:1000 solution intramuscularly. May be repeated every 15 min for 1 hr if necessary. Onset: minutes. Duration: 1-4 hr.	To treat anaphylactic shock.
Isoproterenol hydrochloride	Isuprel hydrochloride*	INTRAVENOUS: *Adults*—1-2 mg (5-10 ml) diluted in D5W and infused at rate of 1-10 μg/min. Onset: minutes. Duration: 1-2 hr.	To stimulate cardiac contractility.
Levarterenol (norepinephrine) bitartrate	Levophed bitartrate*	INTRAVENOUS: *Adults*—2-8 ml of 0.2% solution in 500 ml D5W and given by continuous infusion for desired response. Onset: immediate. Duration: minutes.	To maintain blood pressure in life-threatening situations.
Mephentermine sulfate	Wyamine sulfate	INTRAVENOUS: *Adults*—1 gm is diluted in 1 L D5W and given by continuous infusion to maintain pressure. Onset: immediate. Duration: 30-45 min.	To maintain arterial blood pressure during spinal, epidural, or general anesthesia.
Metaraminol bitartrate	Aramine	INTRAMUSCULAR, INTRAVENOUS: *Adults*—2-5 mg as a single intravenous injection or 200-500 mg diluted in 1 L D5W given by continuous infusion to maintain pressure. Alternatively, 5-10 mg given intramuscularly. Onset: 1-2 min. Duration: 20-60 min.	To maintain blood pressure during spinal, epidural, or general anesthesia.
Methoxamine hydrochloride	Vasoxyl*	INTRAMUSCULAR, INTRAVENOUS: *Adults*—5-20 mg in a single intramuscular dose or 2-5 mg intravenously (slow IV). Onset: immediate. Duration: 60 min.	To maintain blood pressure during spinal and general anesthesia. To control hypotension after ganglionic blockade.
Phenylephrine hydrochloride	Neo-Synephrine hydrochloride*	ORAL, INTRAMUSCULAR, SUBCUTANEOUS, INTRAVENOUS: *Adults*—1-10 mg intramuscularly or subcutaneously; 0.25-0.5 mg given intravenously or 10 mg in 500 ml D5W infused slowly; 20 mg 3 times/day orally for orthostatic hypotension. Onset: minutes. Duration: 1-2 hr.	To maintain blood pressure during general and spinal anesthesia. To treat orthostatic hypotension and paroxysmal atrial tachycardia.

*Available in Canada and United States.
†Available in Canada only.

creased blood pressure resulting from increased cardiac output and peripheral vasoconstriction.

Pharmacokinetics

The effects of mephentermine persist for 30 to 60 minutes after subcutaneous administration and continue for up to 4 hours after intramuscular administration. Mephentermine can also be administered as a single IV dose. Mephentermine does not cause the tissue irritation characteristic of most vasopressor drugs.

Adverse Reactions and Contraindications

Side effects of mephentermine are minimal and include drowsiness, weeping, incoherence, and, occasionally, convulsions. Contraindications and drug interactions are those described for other vasopressor drugs.

NURSING PROCESS OVERVIEW

Sympathomimetic Drugs

Assessment

Sympathomimetics treat shock, which can be caused by trauma, blood loss, burns, sepsis, cardiac failure (cardiogenic shock), anaphylaxis, and extreme reactions to some drugs. The patient in shock appears pale, with clammy skin. The blood pressure is usually low or may even be absent; the pulse rate may be increased and thready. If alert, the patient may complain of fear of impending doom and may be anxious. The respiratory rate may be increased. Perform a rapid assessment, including the pulse, respirations, blood pressure, and level of consciousness. Examine for obvious causes of the shock. Monitor appropriate laboratory work: arterial blood gas concentrations, serum electrolyte concentrations, hematocrit and hemoglobin values, and serum glucose.

Nursing Diagnoses

Nursing diagnoses include the following:
- Risk for decreased cardiac output
- Risk for arrhythmias
- Risk for hypovolemic shock
- Risk for electrolyte imbalances
- Risk for septicemia
- Risk for renal insufficiency

Depending on the clinical picture of the patient, one or more of these risks may exist.

Patient Outcomes

The nurse will manage and minimize the complications associated with the potential complications identified for the patient. The patient will achieve and maintain a satisfactory blood pressure without experiencing permanent effects caused by the potential complication.

Planning/Implementation

Administer ordered vasopressors to increase and maintain the blood pressure; use an infusion control device and/or a microdrip infusion set. Monitor the vital signs frequently, as often as every 5 minutes. Administer ordered replacement fluids and blood. Monitor intake and output; a Foley catheter may be inserted. Monitor the level of consciousness. Use a cardiac monitor to assess the patient's condition. Have available emergency care equipment, such as a suction machine and resuscitation equipment. Remain with the patient and stay calm. Continue to assess for changes in patient status and drug side effects. Keep the patient and family informed of what is being done.

Evaluation

Drugs to treat shock are successful if the blood pressure is maintained to provide adequate tissue perfusion. Few vasopressors are used in self-management situations; most are used only in the short-term care setting for the patient in shock. Epinephrine may be prescribed for patients with a history of previous serious allergic response. Before discharge, the patient should be able to explain when epinephrine should be used and how to use it, to demonstrate the correct administration technique, and to explain the side effects that result from the medication; the patient also should know when to seek emergency assistance.

NURSING IMPLICATIONS SUMMARY

General Guidelines: Sympathomimetic Drugs

Drug Administration

- For safe care of the patient requiring IV sympathomimetic drugs for the treatment of shock or hypotension, use a microdrip IV administration and/or an electronic IV monitor or regulator to accurately control the rate of fluid and drug administration. Monitor the blood pressure and pulse every 2 to 5 minutes until the blood pressure and rate of drug administration are stable, then every 15 minutes. Do not leave the patient unattended. Monitor the cardiac output, pulmonary artery pressure, pulmonary capillary wedge pressure (PCWP), central venous pressure (CVP), or other available indicators of hemodynamic response. Monitor the electrocardiographic changes. Monitor intake and output; monitor urinary output every 30 to 60 minutes. Monitor serum electrolytes.
- Read drug labels carefully because some drug forms are not indicated for IV administration. Do not administer any drug intravenously if sediment or discoloration is visible. Do not mix sympathomimetic drugs with other drugs in a syringe or in IV solutions. If in doubt, consult the pharmacist. Observe the patient for development of hypertensive crisis. If it does occur, slow or stop vasopressor drugs, notify physician, and administer specific drug antidotes or phentolamine, an adrenergic blocking drug, as ordered.
- Avoid extravasation of these drugs. All sympathomimetic drugs cause vasoconstriction, which can lead to tissue necrosis or sloughing. Administer these drugs through a central venous catheter if possible. In the event of extravasation, the physician may order the site of injury infiltrated with a solution of 5 to 10 mg of phentolamine diluted in 10 to 15 ml of normal saline solution.

NURSING IMPLICATIONS SUMMARY—cont'd

- Many of these preparations contain bisulfites, which can cause an allergic reaction in susceptible individuals. Although uncommon in the general population, this reaction may be seen more often in persons with a history of asthma. Symptoms include dizziness; feeling faint; bluish discoloration of the skin; skin rash or hives; swelling of the face, eyelids, or lips; and difficulty breathing. If possible, obtain a history of allergy or previous health problems preceding drug administration. Observe all patients for unexpected drug reactions. Keep the patient and family informed of the patient's condition. Provide calm reassurance. Note that shock produces a sense of impending doom and a feeling of anxiety. Administration of adrenergic medication may also produce a tachycardia and palpitations, which contribute to a sense of anxiety.
- In many agencies, standard dilutions for these drugs are available in the short-term care units. The manufacturer's insert provides detailed instructions about various dilutions and compatible IV fluids. Some of these drugs are available premixed (prediluted) and ready for infusion. Read labels carefully. Calculate dosages and dilutions carefully.

Dopamine

Drug Administration

- Dilute the concentrate for injection before infusion. Follow dilution guidelines for the agency. One protocol states "add 5 ml of concentrate containing 40 mg dopamine per ml (total of 200 mg of dopamine) to 500 ml of compatible IV solution to obtain a final concentration of 400 μg/ml."

Dobutamine

Drug Administration

- Dilute the concentrate for injection to a volume of at least 50 ml with a compatible IV solution before administration. The final concentration should be no greater than 5000 μg/ml (5 mg/ml). Solutions that are slightly pink in color may still be used. After mixing with IV solution, use within 24 hours.

Ephedrine

Drug Administration

- Ephedrine may be given undiluted. Administer at a rate of 10 mg or less over 1 minute.

Epinephrine

Drug Administration

- The usual dose of epinephrine in anaphylactic shock is 0.1 to 1 ml (0.1 to 1 mg) of 1:1000 solution given subcutaneously.
- For direct IV administration, epinephrine is available prediluted in syringes in a concentration of 1:10,000, or this concentration can be made by diluting 1 ml of 1:1000 solution to at least 10 ml with normal saline. For direct IV administration, use at a rate of 1 mg or less over 1 minute or longer. For infusion, the solution may be further diluted in 250 to 500 ml of 5% dextrose in water (D5W) and titrated to patient response.
- Epinephrine may be administered via the endotracheal route. Avoid administering epinephrine and isoproterenol simultaneously because they are both cardiac stimulants.
- Monitor the blood glucose in patients receiving epinephrine, since this drug causes hyperglycemia.

Isoproterenol

Drug Administration

- For direct IV administration, administer each 1 ml of a 1:50,000 solution over 1 minute (1 ml of 20 μg/ml or 1 ml of 0.02 mg/ml). For infusion, dilute 1 mg (5 ml of 200 μg/ml or 0.2 mg/ml) of a 1:5000 solution in 250 ml of D5W. Titrate dose to patient response.

Levarterenol [Norepinephrine]

Drug Administration

- Dilute with D5W injection, with or without normal saline, before use. In the usual dilution, add 4 mg of drug to 1000 ml of D5W injection for a concentration of 4 μg/ml, or add 4 mg of drug to 250 ml of D5W injection for a concentration of 16 μg/ml.

Mephentermine

Drug Administration

- Mephentermine may be given undiluted at a rate of 30 mg or less over 1 minute. It may also be diluted by adding 600 mg to 500 ml of diluent to make a dilution of 1 mg/ml, and infusion may be titrated to patient response.

Metaraminol

Drug Administration

- A single dose up to 5 mg may be given undiluted, at a rate of 5 mg over 1 minute. Metaraminol may also be diluted with D5W for injection or normal saline for injection. See manufacturer's directions for further guidelines. Titrate to patient response.

Methoxamine

Drug Administration

- Methoxamine may be given undiluted at a rate of 5 mg or less over at least 1 minute. The solution may also be diluted by adding 40 mg of methoxamine to 250 ml of D5W and titrating the rate to patient response.

Phenylephrine

Drug Administration

- For direct IV administration, dilute 10 mg (1 ml) with 9 ml of sterile water for injection; administer over 20 to 30 seconds for paroxysmal supraventricular tachycardia or over at least 1 minute for other conditions. For infusion, dilute 10 mg in 500 ml of diluent, and titrate to patient response.

CRITICAL THINKING

APPLICATION

1. List the direct-acting sympathomimetic drugs. What is their receptor selectivity and what physiologic actions result?
2. List the indirect-acting sympathomimetic drugs. What is their receptor selectivity and what physiologic actions result?
3. What are symptoms of anaphylactic shock?
4. Which drug would the nurse expect to see used as a renal vasodilator?
5. Which drug is used as a selective stimulant of cardiac contractility?

CRITICAL THINKING

1. Which drug would the nurse expect to see used to treat anaphylactic shock? What is the usual dosage range and how is it administered?
2. Develop a teaching plan for the patient discharged to home with a "bee sting" kit containing epinephrine.
3. Why are sympathomimetic drugs sometimes administered during spinal anesthesia?
4. Develop a table that compares and contrasts the drugs listed on Table 16-1. Some factors to compare include site of action, side effects, and advantages and disadvantages.

CHAPTER 17

Fluids and Electrolytes

OBJECTIVES

After studying this chapter, you should be able to do the following:

- *Explain what forces control the movement of water between body compartments.*
- *Describe the causes and signs of dehydration, and suggest fluids to reverse dehydration.*
- *Describe the causes and signs of fluid excess, and suggest ways to control it.*
- *Describe appropriate nursing actions in response to common problems encountered with intravenous fluids.*

KEY TERMS

diffusion
hydrostatic pressure
hyperkalemia
hypernatremia
hypokalemia
hyponatremia
interstitial fluid
intracellular fluid
isotonic
metabolic acidosis
metabolic alkalosis
oncotic pressure
osmosis
respiratory acidosis
respiratory alkalosis

CHAPTER OVERVIEW

Fluids and electrolyte solutions are used to reestablish proper salt and water balance. Since these solutions are used to return the body to homeostasis, they may be thought of as drugs. This chapter reviews the general classes of fluids and solutions that are commonly used in clinical practice. Although a full discussion of the clinical indications for these solutions is outside the scope of a pharmacology text, the most important physiologic and clinical factors in the use of these solutions are covered.

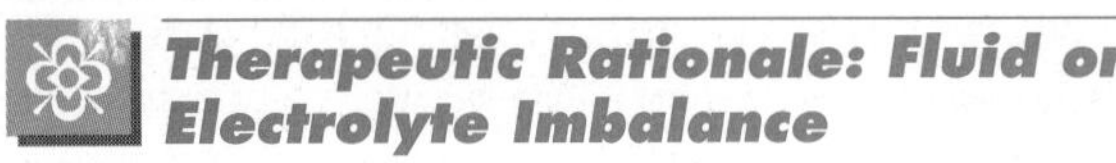

Therapeutic Rationale: Fluid or Electrolyte Imbalance

Regulation of Salt and Water Balance

Fluid Compartments

Water comprises 60% of the weight of an average person. Although water passes easily through most tissues, certain physical and permeability barriers allow the body to be divided into compartments in which water content may be independently regulated. For example, a 70 kg person would contain 42 L of water, of which 28 L are inside cells (Figure 17-1). This water, along with its dissolved solutes, is called **intracellular fluid.** The **interstitial fluid** bathes the outside of cells and allows them to excrete waste products and receive nutrients. Plasma constitutes an important separate fluid compartment similar to interstitial fluid, but it is more accessible to manipulation and testing. Extracellular fluid primarily includes interstitial fluid and plasma but also other fluids such as lymph and cerebrospinal fluid.

Composition of Body Fluids

The fluid compartments in the body differ in the concentration of important ions and other solutes. In plasma the major solute is sodium chloride (Figure 17-2). The primary buffers maintaining the pH of blood at 7.4 are bicarbonate (HCO_3^-, 27 mEq/L) and protein (16 mEq/L). Interstitial fluid is similar to plasma except that the protein content is much reduced.

Inside the cell, high concentrations of protein and potassium are found, but the sodium ion concentration is much lower. Phosphate is the major buffer for intracellular fluid. Phosphate is shown in Figure 17-2 as PO_4^{-3} but is actually present as a mixture of HPO_3^{-2} and $H_2PO_3^{-1}$. Magnesium ion, an important component of critical enzyme systems, is also a significant constituent of intracellular fluid.

Movement of Fluid and Electrolytes Between Compartments

Water moves freely through the vascular walls separating plasma from interstitial fluid and through the cell membranes separating intracellular fluid from interstitial fluid. Movement of ions and other solutes is rigidly controlled so that optimum concentration differences are maintained between compartments. The concentrations of these solutes influence the disposition of water among the compartments. To understand the distribution of water and the various solutes, certain concepts from chemistry and physiology must be recalled.

Osmosis describes the movement of water across a semipermeable membrane (a membrane that selectively limits passage of some chemicals). For example, a cell membrane is semipermeable. The direction of movement is determined by the concentration of solutes in the water on either side of the membrane. Water moves toward the solution having the higher concentration. Osmosis reduces the difference in concentration of the solutions on either side of a semipermeable membrane.

The movement of water by osmosis across semipermeable membranes creates osmotic pressure. For example, if a glucose solution is enclosed in a synthetic membrane that allows water but not glucose to pass through the membrane and the sealed sac is submerged in pure water, two things will happen. Water will enter the sac at a greater rate than it leaves the sac. As water enters the solution-filled sac, pressure inside the sac increases and opposes the entry of more water. The pressure required to completely prevent the net movement of water into the sac is a measure of the osmotic pressure of the solution.

The osmotic properties of a solution relate to the concentration of solute, but the number of particles (ions, atoms, or

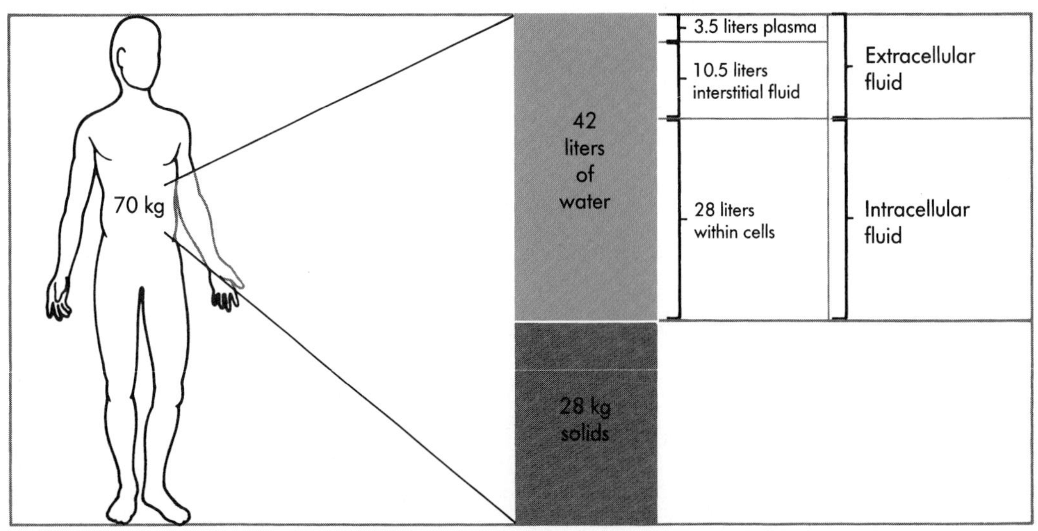

FIGURE 17-1
Distribution of water in men. In women, about 50% of body weight is found as water, but proportion of intracellular to extracellular fluid is same as for men.

molecules) is important, not the mass of the solute. For example, a 0.5 molar solution of glucose contains 90 gm/L of glucose and has a potential osmotic pressure of 9650 mm Hg. In contrast, a 0.5 molar solution of sodium chloride contains 29 gm/L of sodium chloride and has a potential osmotic pressure of 19,300 mm Hg. The greater potential osmotic pressure of the sodium chloride solution results from the ionization of sodium chloride to release two particles for every molecule of salt, a sodium ion and a chloride ion. Glucose does not ionize, and each molecule of the glucose remains a single particle.

Osmolarity of the extracellular fluid is determined mainly by the concentration of sodium chloride. Solutions that have the same osmolarity as plasma are called **isotonic.** Isotonic solutions include 5% dextrose and 0.9% sodium chloride solutions. Hypertonic solutions have an osmolarity above that of plasma (>310 mOsm/L); hypotonic solutions have lower osmolarity than plasma.

Oncotic pressure regulates the movement of water between plasma and interstitial fluid. This pressure is generated by the difference in protein concentration between plasma and interstitial fluid. Although most solutes in plasma pass freely through pores of the vascular walls that separate plasma from interstitial fluid, proteins cannot leave plasma by that route. Since proteins act like any other solute to cause the movement of water, movement of water from interstitial fluid toward plasma is promoted.

Without a balancing force, oncotic pressure tends to dilute the protein in plasma and increase pressure in the plasma compartment. Oncotic pressure is balanced by **hydrostatic pressure** generated by the force of contraction of the heart. In the arteriolar vasculature where blood pressure is highest, hydrostatic pressure predominates over oncotic pressure. In the arteriolar side of capillaries, water, along with dissolved nutrients and other solutes, moves from plasma into the interstitial fluid, where it is available to cells. Pressure on the venous side of the capillaries is lower. This lower venous pressure is not sufficient to fully block the movement of water. Therefore oncotic pressure is the predominant regulator on the venous side of capillaries and allows water and solutes, including waste products, to move back into the plasma compartment.

Diffusion describes the movement of solutes across semipermeable membranes. The direction of movement is toward the less concentrated solution. As with osmosis the process lowers the difference in concentration between the two solutions. Free diffusion of most ions and solutes takes place between plasma and interstitial fluid, but the cell membrane is not normally permeable to most solutes found in extracellular fluid. Sensitive control of uptake and release of solutes is maintained by active transport systems on the cell membrane. For example, the high intracellular concentration of potassium is maintained by the action of Na^+, K^+-ATPase, an active transport system that hydrolyzes a molecule of adenosine triphosphate (ATP) to exchange three sodium ions for two potassium ions. Other active transport systems maintain the high intracellular concentrations of phosphate and magnesium ion.

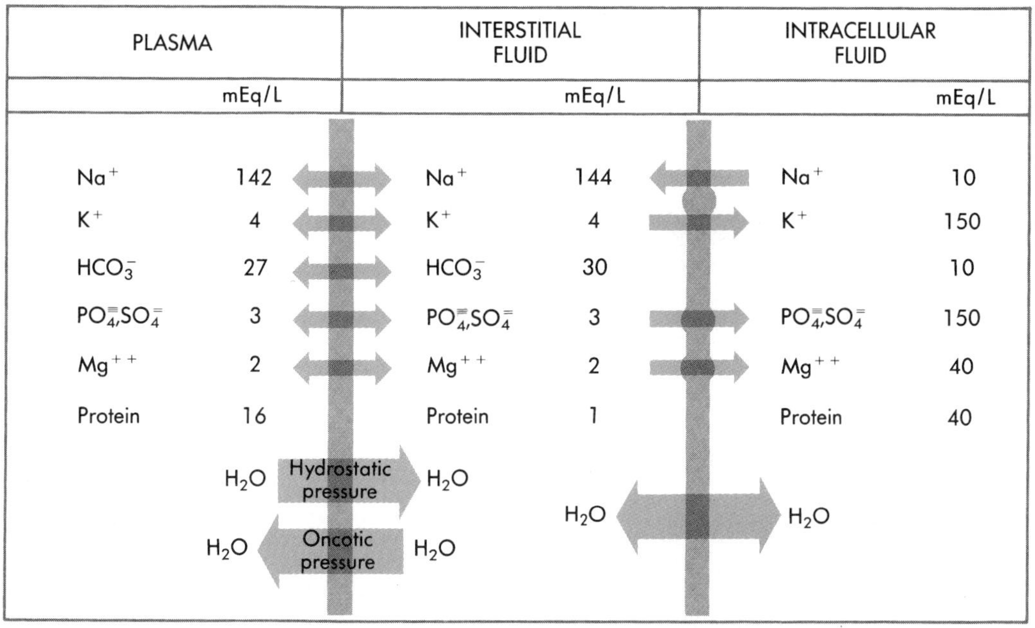

PLASMA	mEq/L	INTERSTITIAL FLUID	mEq/L	INTRACELLULAR FLUID	mEq/L
Na^+	142	Na^+	144	Na^+	10
K^+	4	K^+	4	K^+	150
HCO_3^-	27	HCO_3^-	30		10
$PO_4^=, SO_4^=$	3	$PO_4^=, SO_4^=$	3	$PO_4^=, SO_4^=$	150
Mg^{++}	2	Mg^{++}	2	Mg^{++}	40
Protein	16	Protein	1	Protein	40

H_2O Hydrostatic pressure H_2O

H_2O Oncotic pressure H_2O

H_2O H_2O

FIGURE 17-2
Movement of water and solutes between body compartments. *Double-headed arrows* represent simple diffusion; *straight arrows* indicate pressure-regulated processes. *Arrows passing through or in contact with circles* represent active transport of solutes.

Clinical Indications for Fluid Therapy

Loss of Extracellular Fluid Volume

Several clinical conditions can cause water and solutes to be lost from the extracellular fluid compartment. For example, sudden hemorrhage, prolonged vomiting, excessive diarrhea, or plasma loss through large areas of burned skin may cause fluid and salt loss, but the fluid remaining in the extracellular compartment may for a time stay essentially normal in composition. If the fluid loss is excessive and uncompensated, the patient may enter hypovolemic shock, in which the blood volume becomes so depleted that organ perfusion is compromised. The symptoms of this condition include lowered blood pressure, increased heart rate, rapid respiration, restlessness, pale and clammy skin, and decreased urine output. Without adequate perfusion the kidneys may fail completely. Hypovolemic shock is potentially life threatening and requires rapid replacement of fluid and electrolytes to restore the proper distribution of volume throughout the body.

In certain conditions, extracellular fluid volume may be decreased primarily by water loss. For example, patients who fail to take in adequate water may suffer dehydration. This condition is common in older adults who may have inefficient thirst centers in the brain. Unconscious patients lose between 1000 and 1700 ml of water in insensible perspiration, breath, and urine each day; this water must be replaced daily to avoid dehydration. In certain circumstances watery diarrhea and high-volume renal failure may cause loss of water in excess of salt loss (see box). All these circumstances may require replacement of lost volume and restoration of the proper proportion of solutes in the extracellular fluid.

Fluid deficiency requiring therapy is associated with weight loss in excess of 5% of normal body weight, dry lips and eyes, decreased blood pressure, and depressed central nervous system (CNS) activity. Skin turgor is also diminished.

Fluid Excess

In certain conditions extracellular fluid volume is expanded to a degree that may impair cardiovascular functioning, in part by increasing venous pressure. Fluid excess may arise from conditions impairing the body's ability to eliminate fluid such as heart failure or renal impairment. Alternatively, fluid excess can arise from the improper administration of intravenous (IV) fluids. The main route for elimination of excess fluid is through the kidneys. Treatment aims to prevent further overload and, if necessary, to assist the kidneys by pharmacologic means. For example, digitalis given to strengthen contraction of the heart in heart failure improves perfusion of the kidneys and assists in mobilizing and eliminating excess fluid. Diuretics also enhance urine production.

Signs of fluid excess include swelling and edema, bounding pulse, distension of the jugular vein, difficult or noisy breathing, and warm, moist skin.

Electrolyte Imbalances

The proper concentrations of ions and solutes in the extracellular compartment can be disrupted by diseases or medical interventions (Table 17-1).

Sodium ion. Sodium is the major ion determining the osmolarity of plasma and interstitial fluid. **Hypernatremia** (excessive sodium ion concentration in plasma) can arise when a patient loses water but retains salt. Alternatively, hypernatremia may arise when excessive sodium has been administered with fluids or medications. In hypernatremia, water moves from cells into the extracellular fluid in an attempt to reduce the sodium ion concentration and restore equal osmolarity between the fluid compartments. **Hyponatremia** (plasma sodium concentrations less than 130 mEq/L) arises most commonly in patients who are losing water and elec-

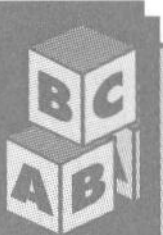

PEDIATRIC CONSIDERATION

Diarrhea in Infants

THE PROBLEM

In most cases diarrhea is mild and self-limiting, but infants and young children may be thrown into dangerous states of dehydration and electrolyte imbalance if diarrhea is severe or prolonged. Hypotension and coma can arise when fluid losses equal 5% of body weight; losses of 10% can cause shock, and death ensues at higher losses.

ASSOCIATED OR CONTRIBUTING FACTORS

In underdeveloped nations diarrhea is a significant cause of mortality in infants and children, with death resulting from dehydration and electrolyte imbalance. Poor sanitation may expose children and adults to infectious agents that cause diarrhea. Even if the diarrhea is caused by bacterial contamination of food or water, treatment is often successful if salt and water balance are maintained. Intravenous replacement of fluids is expensive, unavailable to many people, and unnecessary in the majority of cases. Aggressive oral replacement with properly balanced solutions is first-line treatment.

SOLUTIONS

- Oral rehydration therapy (ORT) should begin early in the course of the disease.
- In the United States preparations are available under the trade names Lytren, Pedialyte, Rehydralyte, and Resol.
- In Canada, Lytren and Pedialyte are available.
- In other countries the World Health Organization (WHO) Diarrheal Disease Control Program supplies ORS-bicarbonate or ORS-citrate in premeasured packets that are mixed with 1 L of potable water before use.

trolytes but are receiving water without adequate electrolyte replacement. In an extreme case this condition is called *water intoxication.* The low sodium ion concentration of the extracellular fluid causes water to move into cells in an attempt to restore equal osmolarity between the two compartments.

Potassium ion. Hyperkalemia (excessive potassium ion concentration in plasma) causes less osmotic disturbance than a sodium ion imbalance, but potassium ion imbalances can be life threatening because cardiac function may be impaired. Potassium-induced cardiac dysfunction appears in the electrocardiogram (ECG) as depressed ST segments, widened QRS complexes, and peaked T waves. Hyperkalemia may result from massive tissue injury when large numbers of cells die, releasing their high intracellular concentrations of potassium into the extracellular fluid. Renal failure may also cause retention of potassium, as may the potassium-sparing diuretics discussed in Chapter 14.

Hypokalemia (low potassium ion concentration in the plasma) can result from the use of diuretics such as furosemide, ethacrynic acid, or the thiazides. Poor nutrition or poor gastrointestinal (GI) tract absorption may also result in hypokalemia. Vomiting depletes the body of potassium, along with fluid and other salts. Replacement of potassium is necessary to restore normal function, but the replacement should be spread out over several days to avoid excessive cardiac stress.

Hydrogen ion and bicarbonate ion. The balance of these ions regulates the pH of plasma and interstitial fluid. An increase of hydrogen ion over bicarbonate ion lowers the pH of extracellular fluid, causing acidosis. An increase of bicarbonate ion over hydrogen ion causes a rise in pH of the extracellular fluid, or alkalosis. Acid-base imbalances arise from respiratory or metabolic causes. **Respiratory acidosis** arises when pulmonary ventilation is impaired. Without adequate ventilation the carbon dioxide concentration in blood rises. In the blood, carbon dioxide becomes carbonic acid, which lowers blood pH. Pneumonia, pulmonary obstructive disease, and depressed respiration can produce respiratory acidosis. Therapy is aimed at the underlying disease. **Metabolic acidosis** arises when excess acid is produced, as in diabetic acidosis, lactic acidosis, starvation, or certain types of poisoning.

Respiratory alkalosis can be induced by hyperventilation, through which excessive amounts of carbon dioxide are lost. **Metabolic alkalosis** arises when excess hydrogen ion is lost, as in prolonged vomiting or nasogastric suctioning. Respiratory alkalosis seldom requires IV therapy, but metabolic alkalosis is often treated with isotonic saline. During metabolic alkalosis, bicarbonate excretion becomes limited by the progressive depletion of sodium. Administering isotonic saline allows the kidneys to sacrifice the sodium required to accompany excreted bicarbonate. With this assistance the kidneys usually reestablish acid-base balance.

Therapeutic Agents: Fluid and Electrolyte Solutions

Hydrating Solutions

Conditions such as hemorrhage or shock, in which plasma volume is suddenly reduced, require replacement of fluid as initial therapy. Replacement of lost fluid volume allows maintenance of kidney function, preventing further development of dangerous electrolyte imbalances. Perfusion of other vital organs is also maintained by this strategy.

Sodium Chloride in Water

Isotonic saline (Table 17-2) replaces extracellular fluid volume and treats sodium depletion and metabolic alkalosis. Dangers associated with its use include circulatory overload and hypernatremia. Metabolic acidosis may arise when ex-

TABLE 17-1 Common Electrolyte Imbalances

SOLUTE	NORMAL CONCENTRATION IN PLASMA	SIGNS OF DEFICIENCY	SIGNS OF EXCESS
Sodium ion	136-145 mEq/L	Anorexia, nausea, vomiting; increased intracranial pressure; oliguria leading to anuria	Dry, sticky membranes; fever; weakness and disorientation; oliguria
Potassium ion	3.5-5 mEq/L	Muscle weakness; diminished tendon reflexes; paralytic ileus; cardiac arrhythmia	Nausea and vomiting; muscle weakness; electrocardiographic changes
Bicarbonate ion	24-31 mEq/L (pH 7.35-7.45)	Metabolic acidosis (pH <7.35); weakness; deep, rapid breathing (Kussmaul); stupor or unconsciousness	Metabolic alkalosis (pH >7.45); hypertonicity of muscles; depressed respirations; tetany
Calcium ion	4.7-5.6 mEq/L	Tetany; prolonged QT interval on electrocardiogram	Weakness, fatigue, thirst; nausea, anorexia; muscle cramping
Magnesium ion	1.3-2.3 mEq/L	Flushing, hypertension; neuromuscular irritability	Nausea, vomiting; diarrhea, colic

TABLE 17-2 Parenteral Therapy Solutions

SOLUTION	IV DOSAGE	COMMENTS
Calcium gluceptate (22%, or 0.9 mEq Ca^{++}/ml) or Calcium gluconate (10%, or 0.47 mEq Ca^{++}/ml)	Doses are individualized.	Calcium solutions may be used to resuscitate the heart, to treat hyperkalemia, to treat magnesium intoxication, or to replace calcium in patients receiving large volumes of citrated blood.
✣ Dextrose in water (2.5%, 5%, 10%, 20%, 25%, 38%, 40%, 50%, 60%, 70%)	Isotonic (5%) 90 to 125 ml/hr is usual but may range much higher; doses of hypertonic solutions are individualized for specific purposes.	Isotonic dextrose (D5W) maintains or replaces fluid without altering electrolytes. Hypertonic dextrose is used to prevent brain damage caused by hypoglycemic shock or to supply extra calories (see Table 17-4).
✣ Dextrose in saline (2.5%, 5%, or 10% dextrose in various combinations with 0.11%, 0.2%, 0.225%, 0.3%, 0.45%, or 0.9% [NaCl])	Doses are adjusted as needed for specific fluid and electrolyte needs of patient.	Hypotonic solution (2.5% dextrose, 0.45% NaCl) drives fluid from plasma into interstitial space. Isotonic solutions supply calories and replenish salt and water.
✣ Dextrose in saline (5% dextrose with 0.2%, 0.225%, 0.33%, 0.45% or 0.9% NaCl and 0.075%, 0.15%, 0.224%, or 0.3% KCl)	Doses are adjusted as needed for specific fluid and electrolyte needs of patient.	Mixture replenishes salt and water when potassium replacement is also required. Dosage must be carefully monitored to avoid potassium overload, especially when renal function is compromised.
✣ Dextrose with electrolytes (5% with Electrolyte No. 48, No. 75, Ionosol, Isolyte, Normosol, Plasma-lyte; 50% with Electrolytes pattern A, B, or 1)	Refer to specific information supplied with individual preparation.	Complex mixtures are used in special circumstances to correct massive electrolyte imbalances.
KCl in water (0.1, 0.2, 0.3, 0.4, 1.5, 2, or 3 mEq/ml)	Solution must be diluted before use and administered at rates <10-15 mEq/hr for minimally depleted patients or up to 40 mEq/hr for severely depleted patients.	Solutions are strongly hypertonic (15% = 2000 mEq/L) as supplied and must be diluted before administration. Concentrations are commonly 40-60 mEq/L.
Lactated Ringer's solution (0.6% NaCl, 0.03% KCl, 0.02% $CaCl_2$, 0.31% Na lactate)	90-125 ml/hr is commonly used.	Balanced salt solution supplies, in mEq/L, the following ions: Na^+ 130, K^+ 4, Ca^{++} 3, Cl^- 109. It is used to maintain or restore fluid and electrolyte balance, especially when mild acidosis is also present. A portion of the lactate present is converted to bicarbonate, which elevates blood pH.
Magnesium sulfate (10%, 12.5%, 20%, 50%)	A 10% solution should be infused at rates <1.5 ml/min. More concentrated solution is for intramuscular administration.	Nearly isotonic solution (10%) is used to reverse severe magnesium deficiencies such as maintenance during total parenteral nutrition and to control convulsions of eclampsia.
✣ NaCl in water (0.45%, 0.9%, 3.0%, 5.0%)	Isotonic (0.9%) and hypotonic (0.45%) solutions are infused at 90-125 ml/hr but may range much higher for initial therapy; 3% solution is infused up to 80 ml/hr and 5% solution up to 50 ml/hr.	Isotonic saline supplies 154 mEq/L of Na^+ and 154 mEq/L of Cl^-. It is used to replace sodium and water loss.
Ringer's solution (0.86% NaCl, 0.03% KCl, and 0.033% $CaCl_2$)	Dosage of 90-125 ml/hr is commonly used.	Balanced salt solution supplies, in mEq/L, the following ions: Na^+ 147, K^+ 4, Ca^{++} 4.5, Cl^- 156. It is used to maintain or restore fluid and electrolyte balance. Additional K^+ is required to correct severe potassium depletion.
Sodium bicarbonate in water (4.2%, 5%, 7.5%, 8.4%)	Doses are calculated to reverse acidosis (individualized for each patient).	Commercially available solutions are hypertonic and must be diluted before use. One liter of 1.4% $NaHCO_3$ contains 167 mEq/L of Na^+. This nearly isotonic solution reverses metabolic acidosis.

cess chloride ion promotes bicarbonate ion loss in the kidneys. Hypokalemia may arise as excess sodium ion forces potassium ion excretion by the kidneys. Hypertonic saline solutions should be used in small volumes and administered carefully to correct severe hyponatremia. Use of sodium chloride that contains preservative requires special precautions (see box).

Ringer's Solution and Lactated Ringer's Solution

Ringer's solution and lactated Ringer's solution are used to replace fluid, sodium, and other electrolytes (see Table 17-2). Often called *balanced* or *maintenance solutions,* these preparations are appropriate to replace volume if renal function is not seriously compromised. The potassium found in these solutions cannot be eliminated by the body and may accumulate to dangerous levels unless the kidneys are functioning. For this reason renal function must be established before these fluids are administered.

Ringer's solution is appropriate replacement therapy for patients who have lost fluid and electrolytes through the alimentary tract, for burn patients, for postoperative patients, and for patients with dehydration or sodium depletion. Lactated Ringer's solution is most appropriate for patients who, along with other electrolyte imbalances, have acidosis. The lactate in this solution, converted to bicarbonate by the liver, provides stronger basic cations in the blood than the simple inorganic salt solutions.

Dextrose in Water

Dextrose, or glucose, in an isotonic solution (5%) is appropriate for most situations in which rehydration is needed. In addition to fluid, the solution supplies about 170 cal/L or 560 kJ/L. Electrolytes are not supplied in this solution. Hypertonic glucose solutions are given slowly to avoid tissue damage. These hypertonic solutions may be used to shift fluid from the interstitial space into the plasma. Isotonic dextrose solutions may be infused through peripheral veins, but hypertonic dextrose solutions should be infused through a central vein to avoid excessive irritation.

Dextrose solutions may have other components added for infusion, but not all additives are compatible. For example, dextrose solutions are never used in the same IV line with whole blood because the glucose causes hemolysis (rupture of red blood cells). The pharmacist can provide information about compatibilities of IV fluids.

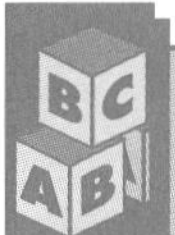

PEDIATRIC CONSIDERATION

Benzyl Alcohol

THE PROBLEM

Benzyl alcohol is a bacteriostatic agent commonly used in solutions of sodium chloride and other drugs. Neonates are especially sensitive to this agent, and deaths have occurred when solutions containing benzyl alcohol were used in this age group.

SOLUTIONS

- Avoid administration of bacteriostatic saline (with benzyl alcohol) to newborns.
- Do not dilute drug with bacteriostatic saline if the drug is to be used in newborns.
- With newborns, do not flush IV lines with bacteriostatic saline.

Solutions to Correct Specific Electrolyte Imbalances

Dextrose in saline may be used to hydrate patients and to replace sodium loss. Five percent dextrose in 0.9% saline has about the same properties as normal saline.

Five percent dextrose in 0.45% saline may be used to shift fluid from plasma into the interstitial space, which may cause difficulty for patients with cardiac, renal, or liver disease who also have edema and poor venous return.

Potassium chloride is often added to IV fluids to replace potassium lost from the GI tract or through the kidneys. Replacement must be undertaken carefully to avoid causing hyperkalemia and its dangerous side effects. Dosage is calculated from a knowledge of approximate loss for the individual patient.

Magnesium sulfate is used to correct severe magnesium deficiencies. The 10% solution is nearly isotonic and may be used intravenously, but the 50% solution is strongly hypertonic and is used intramuscularly.

Plasma Expanders

In hemorrhage or hypovolemic shock, rapid filling of the plasma compartment may be a lifesaving measure. This volume replacement may be accomplished in several ways (Table 17-3), depending on the patient's needs.

Whole blood can be used in patients who have lost more than 20% of their blood volume. Crossmatching to test for blood group compatibility is required, although O-negative blood can be used until crossmatched blood is available. Whole blood replaces fluid, electrolytes, and oxygen-carrying capacity lost through hemorrhage. Before use, whole blood must be tested for evidence of viruses, including hepatitis and human immunodeficiency virus (HIV).

Plasma is a natural cell-free fluid that performs all the functions of whole blood except for oxygen transport. Crossmatching is not required.

Human albumin and *plasma protein fractions* expand plasma volume by increasing the plasma protein concentration. The resulting increase in plasma oncotic pressure causes water to move from the interstitial space into the plasma compartment. The albumin preparation contains appreciable amounts of sodium that may cause problems for certain patients with cardiovascular disease.

Dextran and *hetastarch* are complex carbohydrate molecules too large to pass out of the capillaries or vascular

TABLE 17-3 Blood, Blood Components, and Blood Substitutes

PREPARATION	DOSAGE/ADMINISTRATION	COMMENTS
Whole blood	One unit = 450 ± 45 ml blood + 63 ml CPD (citrate-phosphate-dextrose) or CPDA-1 (citrate-phosphate-dextrose-adenine), administered intravenously through a 170 µm filter.	Whole blood is used to treat patients who have lost more than 20% of blood volume. Whole blood acts as volume expander and maintains oxygen transport.
Plasma	Monitored by clinical response to IV infusion.	Plasma is used as volume expander when oxygen transport is not seriously impaired.
Albumin, human (5%, 25%) (Albuminar, Albutein, Buminate, Plasbumin)	Adjusted according to patient's need, but should be <250 gm/48 hr.	Albumin is used to expand plasma volume. Normal human serum albumin preparations contain significant amounts of Na^+, which may be dangerous for patients on sodium-restricted diets.
Plasma protein fraction (5%) (Plasmanate, Plasma-Plex, Plasmatein, Protenate)	*Adults*—1-1.5 L of 5% solution infused at 5-8 ml/min, adjusted as necessary. *Children*—33 ml/kg infused at 5-10 ml/min to correct dehydration.	Plasma protein fraction is used to correct hypovolemic shock in adults, to correct dehydration in children, and to supply protein to patients with deficiencies. Human plasma protein fraction is 83% albumin, <17% globulin, and <1% gamma globulin.
Dextrans (Dextran 40, Dextran 70, Dextran 75)	Infusion rates may be rapid initially, but total daily dose should not exceed 20 ml/kg.	Dextran 40 (molecular weight 40,000) has effects that last 2-4 hr. Dextran 70 (molecular weight 70,000) and Dextran 75 (molecular weight 75,000) are cleared by kidney more slowly than Dextran 40; duration of action of these preparations is about 12 hr. They are used for shock.
Hetastarch (6% in 0.9% NaCl) (Hespan)	Rates of infusion for acute hemorrhagic shock are 20 ml/kg/hr or less.	Hetastarch is used as plasma volume expander in shock or hypovolemia.

TABLE 17-4 Fluids Used for Total Parenteral Nutrition

SOLUTION	IV DOSAGE	COMMENTS
Hypertonic dextrose (50% or 70%)	Solution is diluted with water or amino acid solutions to about 12.5% before use. Longer term therapy may require 25% to 30% solutions. Minimum adult requirement for dextrose is about 150 gm daily. Initial infusion of 1000-1200 ml of 12.5% dextrose approximates that requirement; dosage can be gradually increased as needed to meet caloric requirements.	Solutions must be administered into central vein with sufficient blood flow to dilute glucose. Special care is taken to maintain aseptic conditions because these catheters remain in use for prolonged periods. Infusion should be terminated gradually to avoid rebound hypoglycemia.
Crystalline amino acids (Aminosyn, BranchAmin, FreAmine, HepatAmine, NephrAmine, Novamine, ProcalAmine, RenAmin, Travasol, TrophAmine)	Solution may be given at about 1 gm/kg body weight per day, as needed to prevent protein breakdown and negative nitrogen balance. Solutions contain mixtures of essential and nonessential amino acids. TrophAmine and Aminosyn contain taurine, an amino acid required by neonates.	A 3.5% solution is nearly isotonic, supplies 140 cal/L, and may be administered via peripheral vein. Various commercial amino acid solutions include appreciable amounts of sodium and other electrolytes.
Intralipid, Nutrilipid (10% or 20%)	Solution may be given by peripheral vein 1 ml/min for 10% or 0.5 ml/min for 20% over 30 min initially as needed to supply calories (20% contains 2000 cal/L) or to replace essential fatty acids. Children and infants require lower infusion rates. Lipids should supply no more than 60% of total calories. Dosage should not exceed 2.5 gm fat/kg body weight daily.	Soybean oil 10% or 20% is stabilized with egg yolk phospholipids with glycerol to adjust to isotonicity. Major fatty acids contained in these preparations are linoleic and oleic.
Liposyn (10% or 20%)	Same as Intralipid.	Safflower oil 10% or 20% is stabilized with egg phospholipids. This preparation contains more linoleic acid but much less linolenic acid than Intralipid.

walls. Therefore these compounds are restricted to the vascular space. They generate osmotic forces that cause water to enter the blood vessels, thereby expanding plasma volume.

Intravenous Hyperalimentation

Patients unable to take oral foods and fluids require maintenance with IV nutrients. Dextrose solutions supply some calories. However, only about 3 L of fluid can be administered daily without overloading the circulatory system. Therefore about 500 calories can be supplied each day from isotonic dextrose solutions. For longer term therapy, more calories from different sources are required. Total parenteral nutrition (TPN) is now possible using synthetic amino acids, dextrose, and fat emulsions (Table 17-4).

Hypertonic dextrose is required for TPN. Solutions for administration are prepared from 50% or 60% dextrose stock solutions, but as they are administered the concentration of dextrose is only 25% to 30%. This hypertonic solution must be administered via a large central vein in which blood flow is sufficient to dilute the strong glucose solution and prevent tissue damage. A 10% dextrose solution is hypertonic but can be given peripherally without damage to veins.

Amino acids are used in TPN to prevent negative nitrogen balance and breakdown of protein in the body. Pure amino acid solutions, rather than protein hydrolysates, are preferred. At 3.5% concentrations the amino acid solutions offer about 140 cal/L and a variety of electrolytes. Extra potassium is often required by patients receiving amino acid solutions, since potassium is depleted by amino acid metabolism.

Fat emulsions may be administered intravenously during TPN to prevent essential fatty acid deficiency. Since fats have a high caloric content, these preparations may supply a significant proportion (up to 60%) of the daily caloric requirement.

Vitamin and mineral supplements may need to be added to the TPN fluids. A variety of these preparations exist, allowing individual design of the nutrition program.

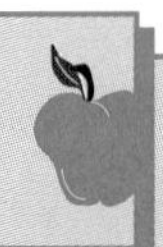

DIETARY CONSIDERATION

Vitamins

Vitamins are among the essential nutrients. If the patient's diet is varied and plentiful, vitamin deficiencies are rare. Digestive disorders and certain drugs can interfere with vitamin absorption. Good sources of major vitamins are listed in the following examples.

Vitamin A (Retinol)
Liver, kidney, fish liver oils, cream, butter, whole milk, whole-milk cheese, fortified margarine, skim milk, skim-milk products, and dark green and deep yellow fruits and vegetables (all contain a precursor of vitamin A)

Vitamin D
Exposure to sunlight, fortified milk, liver, egg yolk, butter, cream, fish, and liver oils

Vitamin E
Widely distributed in foods, especially wheat germ and vegetable oils

Vitamin K
Fruits and leafy vegetables, cereals, dairy products, meat, and tomatoes

Vitamin C (Ascorbic Acid)
Citrus fruits, other fruits, and vegetables

B-COMPLEX VITAMINS

Thiamine
Organ meats, legumes, nuts, whole or enriched grain products, wheat germ, and brewer's yeast

Riboflavin
Milk and milk products, organ meats, eggs, leafy green vegetables, and whole or enriched grain products

Niacin
Meats, legumes, nuts, peanut butter, and whole-grain and enriched-grain products. Tryptophan, a niacin precursor, is also found in protein foods of animal origin.

Pantothenic Acid
Liver, kidney, salmon, eggs, legumes and peanuts, whole grains, milk, fruits, vegetables, molasses, and yeast

Biotin
Organ meats, egg yolk, legumes, nuts, and mushrooms

Folic Acid
Leafy green vegetables, orange juice, liver peanuts, legumes, whole-grain products, and wheat germ

Vitamin B_{12}
Animal protein products only (meat, milk, fish and shellfish, eggs, and cheeses)

Pyridoxine
Meat, fish, egg yolks, legumes and nuts, potatoes, whole grains, wheat germ, yeast, prunes and raisins, and bananas

TABLE 17-5 Intravenous Infusion: Problems, Signs and Symptoms, and Suggested Nursing Actions

PROBLEM	SIGNS AND SYMPTOMS	NURSING ACTIONS
Pain during infusion	Patient discomfort	Slow rate of infusion because some drugs are irritating to veins. Warm IV fluids to room temperature before hanging. Rule out phlebitis (below).
Occluded infusion	Decreased rate of infusion or no infusion Backup of blood into tubing Possible discomfort	Check to see that clamp is open or electronic device is turned on. Inspect tubing for kinks. Remove dressing over insertion site (using aseptic technique); check for kinks, remove old dressing, and retape insertion site. If fluid level in bag or bottle is low, raise level of bag or bottle or replace it with full bag or bottle. With some infusion devices (e.g., Port-A-Cath) or with multilumen central catheters, use thrombolytics such as urokinase to dissolve clots occluding IV flow; follow agency policies. If all else fails, restart IV.
Extravasation (leaking of fluid or drug into tissue surrounding vein, caused by tear in vein)	Decreased rate of infusion or no infusion Patient discomfort Puffiness, edema of extremity or insertion site Coolness distal to insertion site No blood return when bag or bottle is lowered below level of insertion site	Discontinue IV and restart line at another site. Apply warm soaks (follow agency procedure). If drug is known to be caustic (e.g., mechlorethamine), carry out any specific measures, including infiltration of area with steroids or drug antidote; consult physician or agency policies.
Phlebitis (irritation or inflammation of the vein)	Patient discomfort Red streak coursing arm Site is warm to touch Possible edema	Slow rate of infusion, while doing further assessment. If phlebitis is confirmed, discontinue IV and restart line at another site. Apply warm soaks (follow agency procedure).
Septicemia	Fever, chills, symptoms of shock, malaise, hypotension Normal appearance of IV insertion site Headache, nausea, vomiting	Notify physician. Rule out other causes (respiratory tract infection, urinary tract infection, wound infection). Discontinue IV line, culture catheter tip and fluid (or as agency procedure directs), and restart IV line at another site.
Fluid overload	Noisy, rapid respiration, rales Distended neck veins Increased pulse rate or blood pressure Distress Puffiness, edema of dependent areas Weight gain	Slow infusion rate to keep line open. Notify physician.
Embolism	Shortness of breath Chest and shoulder pain Cyanosis Hypotension, weak pulse Loss of consciousness	Place patient on left side, in Trendelenburg's position. Notify physician. Remain with patient, taking vital signs.

NURSING PROCESS OVERVIEW

Fluids and Electrolytes

Assessment

Observe the patient for edema, especially in dependent areas; check skin turgor; auscultate breath and heart sounds; and monitor the vital signs, weight, and fluid intake and output. Observe the patient for specific electrolyte level imbalances. Observe for signs of nutritional deficiency, remembering that weight and intake measures alone are poor indicators. Monitor appropriate laboratory values, including serum electrolyte, blood urea nitrogen (BUN), and blood gas levels. If the patient is receiving IV fluids or nutrition, observe the administration setup, starting at the level of the patient. Check the insertion site; observe for signs of infiltration or infection; and check the placement and patency of the tubing, the rate of flow, and the amount of fluid remaining.

Nursing Diagnoses

- Risk for electrolyte imbalances
- Risk for negative nitrogen balance
- Risk for septicemia
- Risk for fluid volume excess related to excessive IV fluid intake

Patient Outcomes

The nurse will manage and minimize problems related to the potential complications listed above. The patient will exhibit no edema from excessive fluid intake.

Planning/Implementation

The decision to initiate, terminate, or change the fluid and electrolyte therapy depends on the ongoing and cumulative database gathered during assessment. Keep the patient informed about the goals of therapy. Enlist the help of the patient and family in monitoring the IV line, and encourage them to report any unexpected subjective or objective finding. Continue to monitor the parameters identified above. Observe patients for the desired and undesired effects of therapy. Label all IV fluids and medications carefully, monitor their rate of flow and their effects, and record carefully.

Evaluation

Therapy with fluids and electrolytes is effective if desired goals have been achieved without harmful consequences to the patient. If an oral electrolyte replacement is prescribed, review with the patient and family how the medication is administered, work with the patient to find an acceptable dosage form, review the need to continue the medication as desired, review side effects, and discuss situations that should cause the patient to call the physician or nurse (e.g., signs of electrolyte overload). Instruct the patient to measure fluid intake and output or weight at home. If the patient is to continue hyperalimentation at home, instruct the patient and family about the desired goals of therapy and review the technical tasks associated with the therapy (how to care for the insertion site, how to change the bottle, and what to do if the infusion line fails to function). Refer patients to social service and a visiting nurse agency as needed.

NURSING IMPLICATIONS SUMMARY

General Guidelines: Care of Patient Receiving IV Fluids

- Maintain vigilance whenever working with IV fluids or drugs because the administration of any substance directly into the vascular system can cause serious and rapid consequences.
- Inspect the patient receiving IV fluids at least hourly. Assess for correct infusion rate; and inspect the bag or bottle, tubing, monitoring devices, and area surrounding the insertion site. Assess for signs of fluid overload and observe for any of the common problems associated with IV fluid therapy. See Table 17-5 for a summary of common IV problems and suggested nursing actions.
- Monitor skin turgor, intake and output, and weight; inspect dependent areas for edema; monitor vital signs; auscultate heart and lung sounds; and monitor central venous pressure and pulmonary capillary wedge pressure if available.
- Be familiar with agency or institutional policies and procedures regarding IV administration. Policies may specify who may start IV administrations, who may add electrolyte solutions or drugs to infusions, and what the procedures are for routinely changing the tubing or insertion site or for redressing central line insertion sites.
- Use measures to prevent complications of IV administration, in addition to assessing for their development and subsequent treatment. For example, cleanse insertion sites thoroughly before initiating IV therapy, and wear sterile gloves when starting the IV line. Cleanse injection ports well with an alcohol or povidone-iodine solution before puncturing them. Use a Luer-Lok type of connection to prevent accidental pulling apart of IV tubing. Choose insertion sites where catheters are less likely to be dislodged by patient movement, and tape catheters securely. Wear gloves when discontinuing IV catheterization.

Continued.

Nursing Implications Summary—cont'd

- Become familiar with the IV equipment used in the agency. Read the package inserts and attend in-service programs about new equipment.
- Check infusion rates carefully. If you have difficulty calculating IV drip rates, check calculations with another nurse. If a drip rate seems excessively fast or slow, discuss this with another nurse. Some agencies require that two nurses check the infusion rate for infants and small children. See Chapter 6 for information about calculating IV rates of infusion.
- Inspect IV solutions carefully before using. Do not use solutions that are discolored, are leaking, or contain particulate matter.
- Choose a needle or catheter, administration set, and tubing length appropriate for the patient and the drug. For example, the larger the diameter of the needle or catheter, the faster the fluid will infuse, but the larger the diameter, the more difficult it is to insert the needle or catheter into the chosen vein. The higher the fluid reservoir (bag or bottle) is above the patient, the faster the rate of infusion; generally, the reservoir should be about 36 inches above the insertion site. The viscosity of the fluid influences the rate of flow; for example, blood infuses more slowly than normal saline or 5% dextrose solutions. The greater the length of tubing from the fluid reservoir to the patient, the slower the rate of flow. Choose a tubing long enough to allow safe movement by the patient but short enough to ensure that the tubing will not get tangled in the siderails or significantly restrict flow. Finally, choose an administration set appropriate to the ordered rate of flow. For example, if the rate of flow is 150 ml/hr, the drip rate on a minidrip set that delivers 60 gtt/ml would be 150 gtt/min, almost too fast to count. That same rate of administration with a set that delivers 10 gtt/ml would be 25 gtt/ml, an easy rate to count. Use a minidrip set for infants or small children, when a keep open or slow rate is in use, or when drug dose is measured according to patient response such as when an IV drug (e.g., dopamine) is adjusted based on the patient's blood pressure.
- Use volume control devices to limit the volume a patient could receive in a specified time period; an example is Buretrol, a volume control device attached to the IV tubing between the fluid reservoir and the patient. The nurse fills the volume control device with a specified volume of fluid and adjusts the flow rate. The patient can receive only the volume contained in the device, until it is refilled. For example, consider an infant requiring IV fluids. Even if a 500 ml reservoir bag were hung instead of a 1000 ml bag, the danger of fluid overload would be significant if all 500 ml were to infuse rapidly. The nurse could fill the volume control device with the amount ordered for 1 hour (e.g., 30 ml for this patient) and adjust the flow rate. Even if all of the fluid in the device would infuse rapidly, the danger of fluid overload would be much less than with 500 ml. Volume control devices permit the addition of medications to the fluid in the chamber.
- IV pumps and controllers are widely used today. These electronic devices help maintain a constant rate of flow. Because they contain alarms, they warn the nurse when a problem has occurred. The IV pump delivers the IV fluid with pressure, whereas the IV controller adjusts the rate of fluids infusing via gravity. Become familiar with devices used in the agency. Electronic devices do not replace careful patient assessment and nursing care but can assist in managing IV therapy.
- The use of in-line IV filters for all medications and solutions is not universally accepted. Nevertheless, many agencies require them. Familiarize yourself with the advantages of the filters in use in your agency. For example, some filters remove only particulate matter, and some do not have air eliminating capability. The 0.22 μm filter can remove particulate matter, fungi, bacteria, and air but cannot filter TPN solutions because it is too small. Tubing for blood administration is equipped with a filter. Fat emulsions cannot be filtered.
- Label all fluid reservoirs as directed by agency procedure. A common way is to place a length of adhesive tape along the side of the bag or bottle next to the volume markers on the container. The correct fluid level per hour is marked on the tape. For example, if 1000 ml of fluid is started at 8 AM and the fluid is to infuse at 100 ml/hr, there should be 900 ml remaining at 9 AM and 800 ml at 10 AM. Thus any nurse on duty can determine at a glance whether the infusion is running at the correct rate. If the infusion is not correctly timed, do not try to catch up by doubling or increasing the rate for the next hour or two. Assess the situation and, if necessary, restart the infusion at another site. If the solution is infusing too rapidly, slow the rate and assess the patient for signs of fluid overload (see Table 17-5). If the extra volume infused was minimal and the patient's condition is satisfactory, resume the prescribed rate. If the volume is excessive or signs of fluid overload are present, maintain the IV at the keep open rate and notify the physician.
- Label all IV solutions carefully, especially when additives such as potassium, vitamins, heparin, insulin, and other drugs have been included. Record the administration of all IV solutions carefully. See Chapter 5 for additional information about IV administration.

Oral and Intravenous Potassium

Drug Administration

- Potassium chloride (KCl) is the most frequently administered electrolyte added to IV fluids. (Most sodium chloride administered is supplied by manufacturers in commonly used concentrations; potassium chloride is more often added by the nurse or pharmacy.) Ascertain that the patient has adequate kidney function before administering IV potassium. Always dilute potassium chloride before administering it intravenously. Carefully check the dose before adding it. Carefully label containers to which potassium has been added.

NURSING IMPLICATIONS SUMMARY—cont'd

- Monitor the patient's ECG changes and serum potassium level. See Table 17-1 for signs of common electrolyte imbalances. The classic ECG changes seen with low potassium (hypokalemia) include ST segment depression, flattened T waves, presence of U waves, and ventricular arrhythmias. The classic ECG changes with high potassium (hyperkalemia) include tall thin T waves, prolonged PR interval, ST depression, widened QRS complex, and loss of P waves.
- Carefully check the rate of administration of IV potassium. The usual dosage is 20 to 60 mEq/24 hr. If needed, IV potassium may be given at a rate of 10 to 15 mEq/hr of a solution containing 40 mEq/L unless the patient is severely potassium depleted.
- To treat hyperkalemia, discontinue potassium replacements (IV or oral) and limit potassium-rich foods (see box on p. 170). Emergency treatment includes IV sodium bicarbonate, calcium gluconate (if not contraindicated by existing cardiac conditions), and IV glucose and insulin (which help shift potassium into the cell). Dialysis may also be used.
- Subacute hyperkalemia is treated with cation exchange resins such as sodium polystyrene sulfonate (Kayexalate, SPS suspension, others), which exchanges sodium for potassium in the intestine. The effect is not evident for several hours to 1 day after administration. The resin is given orally, via nasogastric tube, or as a retention enema. Adverse effects include hypokalemia, hypocalcemia, anorexia, nausea, vomiting, and constipation. Monitor electrolyte levels. When the resin is given orally or via nasogastric tube, constipation is common, so a mild laxative may be administered concurrently. For oral administration, dilute the drug in water, syrup, fruit juice, or soft drink.
- Monitor potassium levels carefully in patients with cardiac conditions because hypokalemia potentiates the effects of cardiac glycosides. Do not administer potassium to patients receiving potassium-sparing diuretics (see Chapter 14).

Patient and Family Education

- Review with patients the importance of taking potassium preparations as ordered. Some patients will be able to maintain potassium levels through dietary intake of potassium-rich foods (see box on p. 170).
- Work with patients to find an acceptable form of potassium. Oral preparations are often unpalatable or difficult to swallow. Enteric-coated tablets have been implicated in small bowel ulceration. Effervescent preparations are often unpalatable, and patients soon stop taking them. Oral solutions work well but often have a bitter, salty taste.
- Dilute oral solutions in juice or milk if acceptable to the patient. Avoid tomato juice if the patient is on a low-sodium diet.
- Dissolve the soluble powders, granules, or tablets in at least 4 ounces of juice or water; avoid tomato juice if the patient is following a low-sodium diet. Allow fizzing to stop before the patient drinks the dose.
- Extended-release tablets and capsules should be swallowed whole without being chewed or crushed. A few tablets may be crushed or broken and a few capsules may be opened, but most should not be; check with the pharmacist.
- Instruct patients to take potassium with meals to reduce gastric irritation.
- Instruct patients to take missed doses if remembered within 2 hours of when scheduled, otherwise omit missed dose, and resume regular dosing schedule. Do not double up for missed doses.

Magnesium Sulfate

Drug Administration/Patient and Family Education

- Magnesium sulfate is administered orally to promote defecation (see Chapter 24) and parenterally to treat or prevent hypomagnesemia. It is also available as an anticonvulsant, especially in pregnancy-induced hypertension (PIH).
- See Table 17-1 for signs of magnesium imbalances. If magnesium imbalance is suspected, monitor the serum magnesium level.
- Intramuscular (IM) administration of magnesium is painful. Use large muscle masses and rotate sites. Inject the drug slowly.
- The goal in treating PIH is to obtain a serum level that inhibits seizures but does not cause respiratory or cardiac paralysis. Several dosage regimens are followed for this purpose; most are initiated with a loading dose, followed by a maintenance dose. Assess the deep tendon reflexes, respiratory rate, ECG changes, and urinary output. If reflexes diminish or cease, if the respiratory rate decreases, or if the urinary output falls below 30 to 100 ml/hr, the dose of magnesium sulfate may require reduction. ECG changes due to increasing magnesium levels include prolonged PQ interval and widened QRS complex. Monitor vital signs, intake and output, and serum magnesium levels. Monitor fetal heart sounds. In severe cases, monitor maternal ECG changes and attach a fetal monitor to assess infant status. Newborns of mothers who received magnesium sulfate should be monitored for several hours after delivery for signs of hypermagnesemia (see Table 17-1).
- Administer the 10% solution (1 g/10 ml or 8 mEq/10 ml) at a rate of 1.5 ml/min. Dilute the 50% solution to a 20% solution or less before IV administration.
- Have available equipment for resuscitation in settings where parenteral magnesium sulfate is administered. Have available calcium gluconate and calcium gluceptate as specific antidotes for magnesium overdose.

Sodium Bicarbonate

Drug Administration/Patient and Family Education

- Sodium bicarbonate is given orally to neutralize gastric acid (see Chapter 26) and to alkalinize the urine.
- During resuscitation efforts, administer sodium bicarbonate via direct IV push to help correct metabolic acido-

Continued.

sis. It is usually included in the emergency drug box or on the resuscitation cart, packaged in labeled, filled syringes.

- For general IV administration the drug is diluted and administered at a rate of 2 to 5 mEq/kg over 4 to 8 hours. Signs of overdose are metabolic alkalosis and hypernatremia (see Table 17-1). Monitor serum electrolyte and arterial blood gas levels.

Calcium

Drug Administration/Patient and Family Education

- Oral calcium compounds are used as antacids (see Chapter 26). Read the physician's orders carefully.
- IV calcium compounds include calcium gluconate, calcium chloride, and calcium gluceptate. When possible, warm drug to body temperature before administering. The IV route is preferred in infants, but scalp veins should be avoided because extravasation may cause tissue necrosis. Monitor ECG changes during IV administration. Keep patient recumbent for 30 minutes after IV administration; monitor blood pressure and serum calcium levels.
- If IV administration is not possible, calcium gluceptate, calcium gluconate, or a combination of calcium glycerophosphate and calcium lactate may be administered intramuscularly. (Do not give calcium chloride intramuscularly.) Use large muscle masses and rotate injection sites. If >5 ml is to be administered intramuscularly to an adult, divide the dose in half and administer via two injections. With children, determine whether the dose should be divided.
- Severe hypocalcemia may manifest as tetany. Chvostek's sign and Trousseau's sign may be positive (see a text on physical assessment). Pad the siderails. Have resuscitation equipment readily available.
- Review with patients taking oral calcium supplements foods that are rich in calcium (see box on p. 751). Hypercalcemia is discussed in Chapter 62.

Blood, Plasma, Albumin, and Plasma Protein Fraction

Drug Administration

- Review the general guidelines for care of patients receiving IV fluids and other replacement solutions (p. 217).
- Whole blood is administered via a blood infusion tubing set, which usually contains an in-line filter. The infusion is established, usually with normal saline in the primary line; solutions with dextrose may hemolyze the blood, and solutions containing calcium, as in lactated Ringer's solution, may clot the blood. The blood is then piggybacked to the primary solution via the second port in the set. This method helps prevent the blood from clotting; it also helps maintain a patent IV access line, even if infusion of the blood must be stopped, as might happen with an allergic reaction.
- Monitor hematocrit and hemoglobin levels, intake and output, and vital signs.
- Before beginning the transfusion, carefully check the patient's identification bracelet and the label on the container of blood. Blood type incompatibility is potentially fatal; death can occur after infusion of as little as 50 to 100 ml of an incorrect blood type. Most institutions provide specific, detailed procedures to ensure that blood is carefully checked beforehand. Signs and symptoms of a transfusion reaction include flushing, nausea, hypotension, increased pulse rate, difficulty breathing, tightness in the chest, chills, fever, headache, substernal chest pain, vomiting, and sense of impending doom. In addition, hematologic changes may occur, including disseminated intravascular coagulation (DIC), thrombocytopenia, and spontaneous bleeding. If the patient is anesthetized or unconscious, this reaction may be difficult to recognize.
- After initiating the transfusion, remain with the patient for 10 to 15 minutes, monitoring and recording the vital signs. Thoroughly investigate any unanticipated occurrence; stop the infusion, but maintain a patent IV access line by restarting the priming solution, and notify the physician. Hypersensitivity reactions include rashes, itching, and the symptoms of a transfusion reaction noted above. Minor reactions can frequently be treated with antihistamines or corticosteroids, but occasionally emergency life support measures, including epinephrine, are required. Know beforehand where emergency drugs and equipment are kept.
- Febrile reactions usually begin within the first 15 minutes of infusion but may not begin until 1 to 2 hours later. They are characterized by fever (39.4° to 40°C [103° to 104°F]), chills, headache, and malaise. Stop the infusion, notify the physician, and investigate the cause.
- Do not mix any medications with blood. If it is necessary to administer an IV medication via the same IV access line, stop the blood infusion, flush the line with saline, inject the medication, flush the line again with saline, and resume the blood infusion. Blood cells are large, so a large diameter needle or catheter should be used.
- Circulatory overload is more common when whole blood is administered, when the patient is an older adult or an infant, or when the patient has cardiac disease. Monitor vital signs and cardiac and lung sounds, and observe for respiratory difficulty and cough.
- When fluid overload is a concern or large volumes must be transfused, whole blood components may be prescribed, such as packed red cells, platelets, cryoprecipitated factor VIII (for patients with hemophilia), and fibrinogen. These products are smaller in volume than whole blood but are generally administered the same way.
- Complete administration of whole blood within 2 to 4 hours; after this time, the blood may clot. (In extreme emergencies, pressure applied to the bag will afford delivery within 10 minutes or less.)
- Blood products deteriorate rapidly if not stored properly and used promptly. Do not thaw frozen products until they are to be used. Do not procure blood from the blood bank until the patient is ready for the infusion. Do not

leave blood products in the patient care unit. Check and observe expiration dates of all blood products. Plasma, albumin, and plasma protein fraction are derived from blood, and the same general guidelines apply.

Dextran

Drug Administration

- Monitor weight, blood pressure, pulse, and intake and output. Assess for signs of fluid overload (see p. 216). Monitor hematocrit, hemoglobin, serum electrolytes, serum protein, and serum protein electrophoresis levels. Assess patients for bleeding.
- Notify physician if urine output falls below 30 ml/hr.
- Monitor patients for signs of allergic reaction. If blood must also be administered, flush tubing thoroughly between blood and dextran infusion because dextran causes blood to coagulate in tubing.
- Use only clear solutions. If crystallization has occurred, heat bottle in warm water until crystals dissolve before administering. If drawing blood for laboratory tests, note on the requisition that dextran is being administered, because it may cause false high serum glucose levels and alterations in other blood tests.

Hetastarch

Drug Administration

- Monitor for allergic reactions. Monitor vital signs. Monitor hematocrit, hemoglobin, plasma proteins, and platelet levels. Assess patients for signs of bleeding.
- Flush tubing with saline or change tubing before administering blood.

Total Parenteral Nutrition (TPN)

Drug Administration/Patient and Family Education

- Review the general guidelines for care of patients receiving IV fluids (p. 217).
- TPN, or hyperalimentation, must be administered via a central infusion line for solutions more concentrated than 10% dextrose. The central line is placed by the physician using aseptic technique, as described in Chapter 5.
- Follow aseptic technique when manipulating the TPN infusion. These fluids provide favorable conditions for the growth of harmful bacteria. It is essential to prevent infection. Follow agency procedures for maintenance of TPN. Procedures usually specify how often to dress the insertion site, what method to use for dressing, what agent to use to clean injection sites (e.g., povidone-iodine or alcohol), and how often to change tubing.
- Monitor vital signs and assess for fluid overload (see p. 216). Monitor the patient's temperature every 4 hours in the hospital. Instruct the patient at home to notify the physician if fever develops.
- Hypertonic dextrose, amino acids, and fat emulsions are the mainstay of TPN therapy. The rate of flow, additives (vitamins, minerals, and electrolytes), and their concentrations must be ordered specifically by the physician. Most agencies have devised a protocol for monitoring the patient, including the frequency of blood work such as serum electrolyte levels, albumin levels, BUN levels, liver function studies, and blood glucose levels; the frequency of vitamin and mineral infusions; the procedures for culturing the catheter tip and fluid if infection develops; and the frequency of weighing the patient.
- Do not add medications to the solution or administer medications via the TPN line unless specifically permitted by agency protocol or the pharmacist. Usually, if other IV medications are needed, a separate peripheral IV line must be started and maintained.
- Maintain the infusion at a steady rate; usually an electronic monitoring device is used. Erratic infusion rates may cause fluctuations in blood glucose levels, which induces hyperglycemia and hypoglycemia. If the infusion stops or must be discontinued abruptly, standing orders are (at most facilities) to begin a peripheral infusion of 10% dextrose to prevent hypoglycemia. When the need for TPN therapy has resolved, gradually slow the rate of infusion to prevent hypoglycemia.
- Assess the patient for appearance of dry, flaky skin; hair loss; and rashes. These signs may indicate essential fatty acid or zinc deficiency.
- Prepare TPN solutions in a laminar flow hood, where risk of contamination is low.
- Some patients are suitable candidates for TPN administration at home. Assess learning needs with the patient and family. Provide reassurance. Ascertain that the patient and family are able to manipulate the equipment. Refer the patient to a social services agency and to a community-based nursing care service.

Amino Acid Infusions

Drug Administration

- Review the general guidelines for TPN. Assess for common side effects (nausea, vomiting, flushing, and a sensation of warmth). Less common are chills, headache, abdominal pain, dizziness, rashes, hyperglycemia, and glycosuria.
- Monitor intake and output; serum electrolyte, magnesium, blood ammonia, phosphate, serum protein, cholesterol, and BUN levels; liver function studies; and blood glucose levels. Observe for signs of essential fatty acid deficiency (hair loss and dry, flaky skin).
- Vitamins, electrolytes, trace elements, heparin, and insulin may be administered via the same IV line, but other medications should not be. Do not premix these drugs with amino acid infusions; administer via a Y-connector.
- Use an IV filter. Infuse at a rate not exceeding 4 mg/kg/hr of nitrogen. Infuse at a steady rate; use an electronic infusion monitor if available.

Fat Emulsions

Drug Administration/Patient and Family Education

- Assess for history of allergy to eggs, legumes, soybeans, or previous fat emulsion before use.

Continued.

NURSING IMPLICATIONS SUMMARY—cont'd

- See the general guidelines for IV therapy. Administer fat emulsions via a central or peripheral IV line. Read the manufacturer's information supplied with the bottle of fat emulsion. Fat emulsion should comprise no more than 60% of the total daily caloric intake. Inspect before using. If the emulsion has cracked (the oil separated from the other products), it should not be used. Do not shake the emulsion.
- Assess for side effects including thrombophlebitis, vomiting, chest pain, back pain, and allergic reactions. Begin the infusion slowly (e.g., 1 ml/min) and observe the patient. If no untoward effect has occurred after 15 to 30 minutes, increase the rate of infusion to the desired rate. Monitor serum triglyceride levels. Fat emulsions can cause hyperlipidemia, which should clear between infusions; if not, withhold the next dose and notify the physician.
- Do not filter a fat emulsion. If it is piggybacked into a line incorporating a filter, the fat emulsion must be inserted below the level of the filter (closer to the patient).

Vitamins

Drug Administration/Patient and Family Education

- Water-soluble vitamins may be given intravenously, whereas fat-soluble vitamins are administered via IM injection. Vitamins should be given parenterally when oral intake and digestion are compromised. Patients with vitamin deficiencies who are able to eat and digest food should be counseled to increase their dietary intake of vitamin-rich foods (see box on p. 215).

CRITICAL THINKING

APPLICATION

1. What are the three main fluid compartments of the body?
2. What are the major buffers of plasma?
3. What is the major difference in composition between plasma and interstitial fluid?
4. What is osmosis?
5. What solute primarily determines the osmotic strength of plasma?
6. What is oncotic pressure?
7. Does the protein content of plasma cause water to move into or out of blood vessels?
8. What is hydrostatic pressure?
9. Does hydrostatic pressure cause water to move into or out of blood vessels?
10. What are signs of fluid overload?
11. What are the uses of isotonic saline?
12. What dangers are associated with saline administration?
13. What is the primary use for isotonic dextrose?
14. Dextrose solutions must not be mixed with whole blood for administration. Why?
15. What organ system must be functioning before potassium replacement is begun?

CRITICAL THINKING

1. How are cells able to maintain high intracellular concentrations of potassium, phosphate, and magnesium?
2. What are signs of dehydration or fluid deficit? Give examples of patients who are at high risk for dehydration.
3. What can cause fluid excess or overload? Give examples of patients who are at high risk for fluid overload.
4. What is hypernatremia? Hyponatremia? How would you assess for these?
5. What is hyperkalemia? Hypokalemia? How would you assess for these?
6. What is respiratory acidosis? How does it differ from metabolic acidosis? How would you assess for these?
7. What is respiratory alkalosis? How does it differ from metabolic alkalosis? How would you assess for these?
8. Compare and contrast isotonic saline, Ringer's solution, and lactated Ringer's solution.
9. Why are solutions of large molecular weight proteins or carbohydrates able to expand plasma volume?
10. What special precautions for administration are necessary with hypertonic dextrose for parenteral nutrition?
11. What additional supplement may be required by patients receiving amino acid solutions for parenteral nutrition?
12. What is the primary advantage of fat emulsions in parenteral nutrition? What are some nursing care precautions in administering fat emulsions?
13. What teaching points are necessary for patients and families administering TPN in the home?

CHAPTER 18

Cardiac Glycosides and Other Drugs for Congestive Heart Failure

OBJECTIVES

After studying this chapter, you should be able to do the following:

- *Explain where the signal to beat originates in the heart and how it is transmitted throughout the heart.*
- *Explain what the mechanism of action of cardiac glycosides is and why these drugs are used in the treatment of congestive heart failure.*
- *Discuss the toxicity expected with cardiac glycosides.*
- *Discuss why dopamine or dobutamine may be useful in the treatment of congestive heart failure.*
- *Explain how diuretics may be useful in the treatment of congestive heart failure.*
- *Develop a nursing care plan for a patient receiving a cardiac glycoside.*

CHAPTER OVERVIEW

Congestive heart failure leads to symptoms that may be traced back to the failure of the heart muscle to adequately pump the blood delivered to it. Although the condition cannot be cured, many medications can improve the situation by acting directly on the heart or by acting at other sites to relieve symptoms and indirectly aid the heart.

KEY TERMS

action potential
atrioventricular (AV) node
automaticity
cardiac glycosides
chronotropic
conduction velocity
congestive heart failure
contractility
depolarization
dromotropic
excitability
Frank-Starling law
hypertrophy
rate
sinoatrial (SA) node

Therapeutic Rationale: Congestive Heart Failure

Cardiac Structure and Function

Electrical Activity of the Heart

To understand the action of drugs on the heart, it is important to understand how the cells and tissues of the heart communicate with each other to produce the integrated function of the whole organ.

Action potential is a burst of electrical activity in a cell. Frequently described as cell firing, the process is similar to the conduction of impulses along a nerve fiber. The first event in the process is rapid **depolarization** in which sodium rushes into the cell. This event stimulates adjacent cells to depolarize. Repolarization occurs more slowly than depolarization and involves movements of several ions. The ionic changes generated by an action potential cause myocardial fibers to contract.

Automaticity is the ability of certain heart cells to depolarize spontaneously to initiate a beat (contraction of the whole heart). Normally a heartbeat is initiated in the **sinoatrial (SA) node,** and all other cells of the heart follow in response to the signal from the SA node. When other cells in the heart spontaneously depolarize and initiate competing beats, serious arrhythmias result. This tendency to spontaneously depolarize is referred to as **excitability.** Certain drugs increase the excitability of cells by reducing the energy necessary to depolarize the cell, and some drugs can decrease cell excitability.

Conduction velocity is the rate at which an electrical impulse passes through the **atrioventricular (AV) node.** There is a delay in transmission of the impulse to beat from the atrium to the ventricle produced by the AV node. This delay regulates the temporal separation in atrial and ventricular contractions.

Dromotropic refers to factors affecting conduction velocity. A positive dromotropic response is an increase in conduction velocity, whereas a negative dromotropic response is a decrease in that velocity.

Rate is the number of beats or ventricular contractions per minute. In normal hearts, this is the rate of SA node firing. *Bradycardia* means a slow heart rate. *Tachycardia* means a fast heart rate. **Chronotropic** refers to changes in heart rate. Positive chronotropic effects are increases in heart rate; negative chronotropic effects are decreases in heart rate.

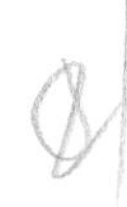

Contractility is measured as the strength of the muscular contraction of the heart. *Inotropic* refers to factors affecting the strength of cardiac contraction. A positive inotropic response is an increase in cardiac contractility. A negative inotropic response is a decrease in cardiac contractility.

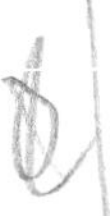

Conductive Tissues of the Heart

The heart is formed of muscle similar in many respects to skeletal muscle but different in that many of the fibers conduct and contract. This property facilitates rapid conduction of action potentials. Action potentials do not pass directly between the atria and ventricles because they are insulated from each other by a ring of nonconductive tissue. The independence of the atria and ventricles as contractile units is important in regulating the heartbeat.

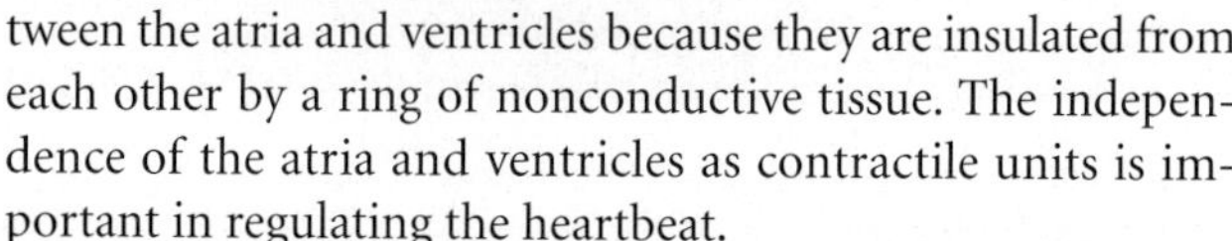

Within the heart the impulse to beat normally originates at the SA node, a specialized group of automatic cells in the right atrium (Figure 18-1). Another group of specialized fibers, the AV node, transmits this impulse to the ventricles after an important delay. The heart is innervated by the sympathetic and parasympathetic branches of the autonomic nervous system (Figure 18-2). The vagus nerve is part of the parasympathetic nervous system; its action is localized in the nodes. Stimulation of the vagus nerve releases acetylcholine, which slows the rate of depolarization and makes the cells less excitable. In the SA node, these actions decrease the rate of firing, which reduces heart rate. Stimulation of the vagus nerve also decreases conduction velocity through the AV node. This slowing of conduction velocity increases the temporal separation between contraction of atria and ventricles and therefore slows heart rate.

Sympathetic nerve fibers innervate the atria and ventricles. Stimulation of the sympathetic nerves releases norepinephrine, which activates the beta-1 adrenergic receptors of the heart. Activation of the beta-1 receptors in the conducting tissue of the heart speeds repolarization of the cells. The results are an increase in heart rate (positive chronotropic effect) and an increase in conduction velocity (positive dromotropic effect). Stimulation of the beta-1 adrenergic receptors in the ventricular muscle increases the force of contraction (positive inotropic response).

Alterations of Myocardial Output

Frank-Starling Law

The volume of blood that the heart delivers per second to the arteries varies with stress, exertion, and other factors. How the heart regulates its output to meet these variable demands is described by the **Frank-Starling law.** This principle of physiology states that the force of muscular contraction is directly related to the stretch of the muscle; the more a muscle is stretched, within mechanical limits, the stronger is its subsequent contraction. With respect to the heart, this principle means that, when the ventricles are filled with larger than normal volumes of blood, they contract with greater than normal force to deliver their entire contents to the arteries. Normally, blood does not accumulate in the veins, and all the blood coming to the heart is pumped into the arteries.

When the healthy heart responds to acute exercise, the Frank-Starling law applies. The heart increases its force of contraction and hence its output. If cardiac muscle fibers are stretched beyond their mechanical limits, the strength of contraction decreases and cardiac output falls.

Sympathetic Nervous System Stimulation

Stimulation of the sympathetic nervous system also increases the rate of contraction of the heart, which is a second mechanism for increasing output. The peak efficiency of the heart

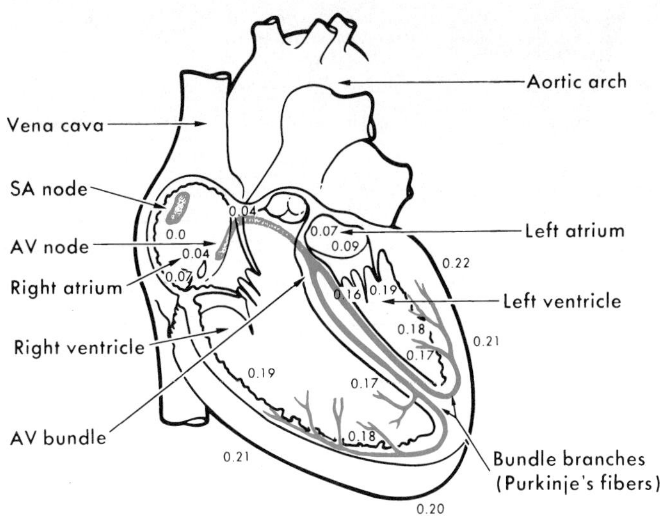

FIGURE 18-1
Transmission of action potentials through heart. Initiation of heartbeat occurs at sinoatrial (SA) node, and action potential is transmitted throughout atria before passing through atrioventricular (AV) node to ventricles. Numerals designate seconds it takes for impulse to travel from SA node to anatomic site designated by numeral. All parts of atria have received impulse with 0.09 seconds, but transmission to ventricles is delayed during its passage through AV node so that ventricles do not begin to contract until 0.16 seconds after SA node firing. Delay allows atria to contract and fill ventricles before ventricles begin to contract to force blood from heart.

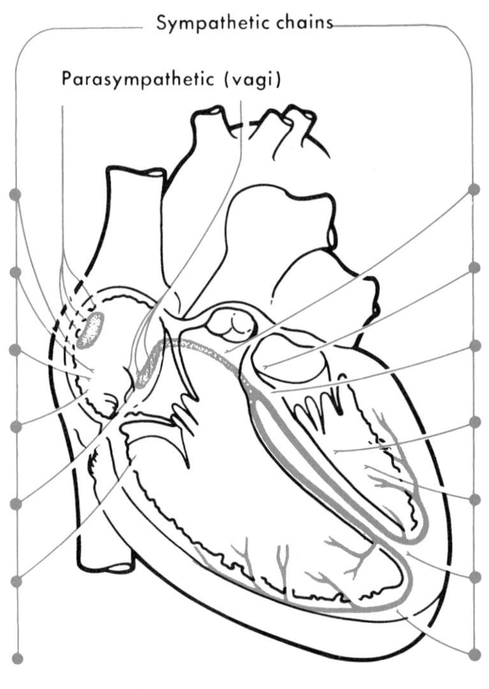

FIGURE 18-2
Autonomic innervation of heart.

under these conditions is reached at about 150 to 175 beats per minute. Faster rates result in incomplete filling of the ventricles and reduce the overall efficiency of the pump.

Cardiac Hypertrophy

If the heart is subjected to chronic demands for increased output, it may enlarge. This condition is called **hypertrophy** of the myocardium and may be a normal response to chronic stress. For example, long-distance runners and tennis players may have enlarged hearts. In other cases the enlargement of the heart may signal a pathologic process. For example, in chronic heart failure the myocardial output gradually falls below the required level, resulting from the failure of the myocardium as a pump. As the output falls, the normal regulatory mechanisms come into effect. Hypertrophy of the heart may occur as the body seeks to increase the efficiency of the pump. Sympathetic stimulation may also be increased to increase the heart rate and hence the output. In many cases, in the absence of acute demands on the heart, these mechanisms enable a weakened heart to maintain sufficient output. Patients may not complain of symptoms but on examination may have an enlarged heart and high heart rate.

Congestive Heart Failure

If the regulatory mechanisms fail and cardiac output falls below venous return, **congestive heart failure** results. The symptoms arise directly from insufficient cardiac output. The blood pooled in the veins produces increased venous pressure. The excessive venous pressure stretches cardiac muscle fibers beyond their limit, and as predicted by the Frank-Starling law, the strength of contraction falls further. The kidneys do not receive sufficient blood flow to maintain salt and water balance. Edema of the lungs and periphery develops as fluid leaks into tissues from the capillaries. The typical patient in congestive heart failure is therefore short of breath and has a rapid pulse resulting from sympathetic stimulation of the heart, obvious swelling of the hands and feet, and an enlarged heart. All these acute symptoms may be relieved by increasing cardiac output. The drugs discussed in the next section are used primarily for this purpose.

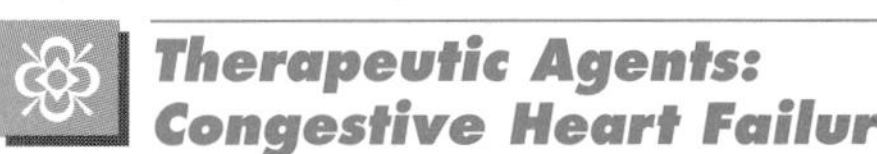

Therapeutic Agents: Congestive Heart Failure

Cardiac Glycosides

Glycosides are complex steroidlike structures linked to glucose molecules. The drugs discussed in this section are referred to as **cardiac glycosides** because of their potent action on the heart. *Digitalis* has been used as a generic term to refer to digoxin and digitoxin; these drugs originally derived from extracts of the plant *Digitalis purpurea* and related species.

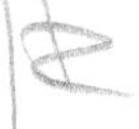

Digoxin and Digitoxin

Mechanism of Action

Biochemically, cardiac glycosides inhibit Na^+, K^+-ATPase and promote accumulation within heart cells of the calcium necessary for contraction. These actions increase contractility, which increases cardiac output, improves blood flow to the kidneys and periphery, reduces venous pressure, and allows excess fluid to be excreted as edema clears. The diuretic effect of cardiac glycosides results from these actions on the heart.

Pharmacokinetics

The available cardiac glycosides are similar in intrinsic potencies, but they differ markedly in pharmacokinetic properties (Table 18-1). These properties largely determine the dosage and dosing schedule for the individual preparations (Table 18-2).

TABLE 18-1 Pharmacokinetics of Cardiac Glycosides

	DIGOXIN	DIGITOXIN
Oral absorption	60%-100%	90%-100%
Plasma protein binding	23%	97%
Plasma half-life	32-48 hr	5-7 days
Route of excretion	Renal	Hepatic
Oral administration		
Onset of action	1-2 hr	1-4 hr
Peak effect	2-6 hr	8-14 hr
Duration of action	2-6 days	14 days
Intravenous administration		
Onset of action	5-30 min	—
Peak effect	1-4 hr	—
Duration of action	2-6 days	—

TABLE 18-2 Summary of Inotropic Agents

GENERIC NAME	TRADE NAME	ADMINISTRATION/DOSAGE	COMMENTS
Digitoxin	Crystodigin Digitaline†	ORAL: *Adults*—initially 0.6 mg, then 0.4 mg in 4-6 hr, followed by 0.2 mg 4-6 hr later (for rapid loading) or 0.2 mg twice daily for 4 days (for slow loading). Maintenance doses range from 0.05-0.3 mg daily. FDA pregnancy category C.	Dosage forms are inconvenient for children. Digoxin is more conveniently administered.
Digoxin	Lanoxin*	ORAL (Tablets): *Adults*—initially 0.75-1.25 mg divided into 2 or more doses given at 6-8 hr intervals (for rapid loading). Maintenance dose, also used for slow loading, is 0.125-0.5 mg daily. FDA pregnancy category C. *Children* (elixir)—loading doses that follow should be divided and administered every 6-8 hr. Premature infants: 0.02-0.035 mg/kg. Newborns: 0.025-0.035 mg/kg. Infants-2 yr: 0.035-0.06 mg/kg. 2-5 yr: 0.03-0.04 mg/kg. 5-10 yr: 0.02-0.035 mg/kg. Older than 10 yr: usual adult dose (tablets). Maintenance dose for premature infants is 20%-30% of loading dose; for all other children, 25%-35% of loading dose.	Bioavailability of digoxin from tablet is variable and may be as low as 60%.
	Lanoxicaps Lanoxin†	ORAL (capsules) and INTRAVENOUS: *Adults*—loading dose of 0.4-0.6 mg followed by 0.1-0.3 mg 2 or 3 more times at 4 to 6 hr intervals. Maintenance dose ranges from 0.05 to 0.35 mg daily. *Children*—loading doses that follow are divided and administered every 6 hr. Premature infants: 0.015-0.025 mg/kg. Newborns: 0.02-0.03 mg/kg. Infants-2 yr: 0.03-0.05 mg/kg. 2-5 yr: 0.025-0.035 mg/kg. 5-10 yr: 0.015-0.03 mg/kg. Older than 10 yr: 0.008-0.012 mg/kg. Maintenance dose for premature infants is 20%-30% of oral loading dose; for all other children, 25%-30% of oral loading dose.	Oral absorption from solution in soft gelatin capsule is nearly 100%.
Amrinone	Inocor	INTRAVENOUS: *Adults*—initially, 0.75 mg/kg body weight given slowly over 2 or 3 min. Repeat after 30 min if needed. Maintenance, 0.005-0.01 mg/kg/min, according to clinical response. FDA pregnancy category C.	Patients with atrial flutter may require pretreatment with digitalis to prevent ventricular arrhythmia. Patients require adequate fluid intake to maintain adequate cardiac fluid filling so that response to amrinone is optimal.

*Available in Canada and United States.
†Available in Canada only.

Half-lives of cardiac glycosides may extend to 7 days (see Table 18-1). With repeated equal doses of a drug, the plateau of drug concentration in the blood is not achieved for about four elimination half-times (see Chapter 1). Therefore these long half-lives for cardiac glycosides mean that the final desired therapeutic concentration of drug in blood would not be achieved for weeks after the start of therapy. To avoid a long delay in achieving therapeutic concentrations, cardiac glycosides are administered first in a loading dose. The loading dose is designed to rapidly raise the concentration in blood to the therapeutic range. After the loading dose or doses, a smaller dose is administered on a regular schedule. This smaller dose, called the *maintenance dose,* maintains the concentration of drug in the therapeutic range. This dose is continued indefinitely or until some change in the patient's condition requires adjustment.

Digitoxin is given orally in a dose to produce and to maintain the therapeutic level in plasma of 14 to 26 ng/ml. The dose required to produce the maximum therapeutic effect varies considerably from patient to patient and must be individualized. Digitalizing, or loading, doses range from 0.4 to 1.2 mg/day. Since 97% of this drug is reversibly bound to protein in blood and is inactive, the dose must reflect that only 3% of the dose in the bloodstream is active. Since the half-life of digitoxin is about 6 days, about 10% of the total body store of the drug is excreted each day. The routine daily dose of the drug must compensate for this loss. Maintenance doses should be expected to range from 0.05 to 0.3 mg/day. Consideration of the half-life of the drug is also important when toxicity occurs; toxicity may persist for long periods because the drug is slowly removed from the system.

Digoxin is usually given orally in a dose that produces and maintains the therapeutic plasma level of 0.8 to 1.6 ng/ml. Dosage regimens must be individualized. Digitalizing doses range from 0.75 to 1.25 mg/day. This drug is less highly bound to plasma protein than digitoxin and has a shorter half-life. The maintenance dose must replace the 37% of the total body store of the drug that is lost every day. Maintenance doses commonly range from 0.05 to 0.5 mg/day, depending on the drug form used.

Uses

Cardiac glycosides are used to treat congestive heart failure because they directly improve the strength of the heart muscle, elevating cardiac output. Cardiac glycosides are also widely used to control cardiac arrhythmias (see Chapter 19).

Adverse Reactions and Contraindications

There is such a small difference between the therapeutic dose and doses that cause side effects that most patients taking cardiac glycosides experience drug-related difficulties. The symptoms may be neurologic, visual, cardiac, or even psychiatric. They often tend to be vague and easily confused with those of congestive heart failure.

The neurologic or central nervous system (CNS) effects of cardiac glycosides are now recognized as significant sources of many side effects observed with these drugs. Anorexia, nausea, and vomiting result from stimulation of the chemoreceptor trigger zone in the CNS. Weakness, fatigue, fainting, and other neurologic symptoms also may originate in the CNS. Visual disturbances such as dimness of vision, double vision, blind spots, flashing lights, or altered color vision also occur. Psychiatric disturbances range from mood alterations to psychoses or hallucinations.

Patients receiving cardiac glycosides must be checked frequently for the appearance of extra heartbeats or other arrhythmias. It is routine practice in many hospitals to omit the dose if the heart rate is less than 60 beats per minute. Although bradycardia is the most common sign of digitalis-induced arrhythmias, other changes in heart rate are possible. For this reason, any change in heart rate or rhythm should be noted and reported.

Cardiac glycosides are contraindicated in patients with any sign of prior toxicity with one of the drugs. The drugs are also routinely avoided in ventricular fibrillation. Risk of arrhythmias may be increased by hyperkalemia, myxedema, pulmonary disease, or cardiac disease. (See the accompanying box for a selected geriatric consideration.)

Toxicity

Because the toxic reactions caused by cardiac glycosides are dose related, they are somewhat predictable (see Chapter 2). For example, bradycardia may be an early sign of rising blood concentrations of cardiac glycosides, but as concentrations continue to rise, the arrhythmias appear; tachycardia and ultimately ventricular fibrillation and death may occur. Blood

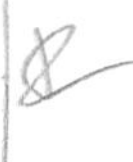

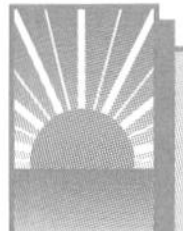

GERIATRIC CONSIDERATION

Cardiac Glycosides

THE PROBLEM

Older adult patients receiving cardiac glycosides may have diminished renal or hepatic function and a decreased volume of distribution for cardiac glycosides. They are also more prone to electrolyte imbalances, including hypokalemia, which can increase drug toxicity. Appetite suppression caused by digoxin can aggravate the problem of poor nutrition in frail older adult patients.

SOLUTIONS

- Adjust doses carefully to avoid toxicity. Maintenance doses may be lower in older adult patients than in younger adults.
- Watch carefully for signs of electrolyte imbalance.
- Instruct the patient about appropriate dietary practices that minimize risk of electrolyte imbalances.
- Do not assume that complaints of fatigue, weakness, mood alterations, or other signs of toxicity are a normal part of aging or of heart disease, and observe patients carefully.

levels of cardiac glycosides are routinely monitored to aid in establishing safe doses and in diagnosing drug toxicity.

Accidental poisoning of children with preparations of cardiac glycosides is not uncommon. Patients who are around small children should be warned of the potential danger their medicine poses to curious toddlers.

With digoxin or digitoxin overdose, patients may continue to be at risk during the lengthy period required to eliminate these long-acting agents. If arrhythmias or hyperkalemia becomes life threatening, digoxin immune FAB (Table 18-3) can be administered to rapidly neutralize free drug. Arrhythmias and electrolyte imbalance can be reversed within 30 minutes. The inotropic effect of the cardiac glycosides persists for several hours longer.

Interactions

Toxicity of the cardiac glycosides may be increased by the presence of other drugs. For example, potassium-depleting diuretics such as thiazides or loop diuretics (see Chapter 14) may predispose a patient to cardiac toxicity, because a low intracellular potassium level increases the likelihood of arrhythmias.

Adrenergic Drugs

Stimulation of the beta-1 class of adrenergic receptors in the heart directly increases cardiac contractility by increasing cyclic adenosine monophosphate (cyclic AMP) in heart muscle. An increase in cyclic AMP can also be achieved by blocking phosphodiesterase, the enzyme that degrades cyclic AMP. Drugs with these actions may be of value in treating symptoms of acute or chronic congestive heart failure.

Dobutamine

Dobutamine directly stimulates myocardial beta-1 receptors, but it has little effect on beta-2 receptors and alpha-receptors, which predominate in blood vessels. Dobutamine does not activate dopamine receptors in renal vasculature. The drug has little tendency to increase heart rate or to elevate blood pressure. These properties make it an attractive agent for increasing cardiac output in severely ill patients. A disadvantage of dobutamine is that it must be given intravenously and has a short duration of action. This drug is therefore appropriate only for acute cardiac decompensation. See Chapter 16 for a more detailed discussion of this drug.

TABLE 18-3 Treatment of Cardiac Glycoside Overdose

GENERIC NAME	TRADE NAME	ADMINISTRATION/DOSING
Digoxin immune Fab	Digibind	INTRADERMAL: *Adults*—0.1 ml of 0.1 mg/ml solution. Inspect for redness and wheal 20 min later. Do not administer full dose if reaction is positive. FDA pregnancy category C. INTRAVENOUS: *Adults*—give amount equimolar to total amount of digoxin or digitoxin in body. Digoxin immune Fab in a dose of 40 mg binds approximately 0.6 mg of drug. Consult package insert for aid in calculating dosage.

Dopamine

Dopamine directly stimulates myocardial beta-1 receptors but also causes indirect stimulation at this site by releasing norepinephrine from nerve terminals in the heart. Dopamine also stimulates alpha receptors in blood vessels and dopamine receptors in renal vasculature. Low doses increase renal blood flow, thus promoting diuresis. Higher doses directly stimulate the heart. Vasoconstriction caused by alpha-receptor stimulation appears with the highest doses. Since dopamine can limit cardiac output by these actions in peripheral vessels, it is usually selected only for patients in congestive heart failure complicated by hypotension. Like dobutamine, dopamine must be administered intravenously and has a very short duration of action. See Chapter 16 for a more detailed discussion of this drug.

Amrinone

Amrinone is intended for short-term intravenous (IV) use in congestive heart failure when response to other agents has been poor. The drug rapidly increases cardiac output and is additive in its effects with digitalis. The exact mechanism of action of amrinone is not yet completely understood, although the drug inhibits phosphodiesterase. In addition, it has some activity as a vasodilator in the periphery.

Diuretics

Diuretics control the pulmonary edema that accompanies severe congestive heart failure. The agent most commonly selected is furosemide, although other diuretics may also be effective (see Chapter 14).

In addition to relieving pulmonary edema, a side effect of congestive heart failure, diuretics may directly improve cardiac function in some patients. In end-stage congestive heart failure, venous pressure is elevated sufficiently to cause heart muscle fibers to stretch excessively during filling of the chambers. Diuretics lower the pressure forcing blood into the heart chambers. As a result, the muscle fibers are not so abnormally stretched; they are then able to contract with greater power. Therefore contractility of the heart muscle is improved. The major consideration limiting the use of diuretics in congestive heart failure is the risk of causing electrolyte or fluid imbalances, which may be especially dangerous to patients in heart failure. Volume depletion or excessive dehydration must be avoided. Patients receiving digitalis should be carefully observed to prevent complications because diuretics tend to alter potassium concentration in the blood (see Chapter 14).

Vasodilators

Vasodilators reverse the persistent vasoconstriction in late chronic congestive heart failure resulting from long-term compensatory sympathetic nervous system stimulation. Sympathetic nervous system stimulation may drive a failing heart, but it constricts peripheral blood vessels, thereby reducing cardiac output and increasing the workload of the heart. Vasodilators reduce the resistance against which the left ventricle must force blood. Cardiac output is thus increased, and workload is reduced.

Several classes of vasodilators are used in congestive heart failure. Nitroprusside (see Chapter 15) can be used for short-term IV therapy in severely ill patients. This agent is often given with an adrenergic agent such as dobutamine or dopamine.

Angiotensin converting enzyme (ACE) inhibitors captopril, enalapril, and lisinopril (see Chapter 15) may also produce vasodilation that is useful in controlling congestive heart failure. These oral agents are used with diuretics and cardiac glycosides for therapy for chronic congestive heart failure.

NURSING PROCESS OVERVIEW

Cardiotonic Therapy

Assessment

Obtain baseline assessment data, including the vital signs and blood pressure, weight, fluid intake and output, serum electrolyte and blood urea nitrogen (BUN) levels, electrocardiographic (ECG) changes, and other laboratory data. Auscultate heart and lungs and assess for the presence and location of edema. Obtain any subjective history of recent dysfunction such as dyspnea on exertion, shortness of breath, inability to perform activities of daily living, and orthopnea (needing to sleep with the head supported or elevated on several pillows).

Nursing Diagnoses

- Risk for health maintenance related to insufficient knowledge of cardiac glycoside therapy
- Risk for electrolyte imbalance or hypokalemia

Patient Outcomes

The patient will be able to manage adding cardiac glycosides to the daily routine, that is, will take the drug regularly at approximately the same time, with few if any side effects. The nurse will manage and miminize episodes of electrolyte imbalance.

Planning/Implementation

Monitor the weight, fluid intake and output, ECG changes, serum electrolyte levels, blood pressure, and other parameters of cardiovascular function. Auscultate the heart and lungs.

Evaluation

Before discharge, make sure patients can explain why and how to take all prescribed medication, what interrelations may exist (e.g., the need to take potassium supplements if certain diuretics and cardiac glycosides are prescribed together), how to plan meals within prescribed dietary limitations, what side effects are anticipated, and what situations require consultation with a physician. If appropriate, patients should be able to measure pulse, correctly record weight or pulse, and state what decisions should be made based on assessment of these data.

NURSING IMPLICATIONS SUMMARY

Cardiac Glycosides

Drug Administration

- Observe the patient carefully. Desired effects of therapy include a decrease in pulse rate; slower, less labored respirations; diuresis with accompanying weight reduction; less coughing; less distended neck veins; and better tolerance of exertion. At the same time observe for signs of toxicity. Many of the symptoms are seen in older or chronically ill persons and may not be recognized as drug toxicity. Symptoms include abdominal discomfort, fatigue, confusion, restlessness, anorexia, nausea, and vomiting.
- Take the apical pulse for a full minute before administering a cardiac glycoside. Withhold the dose if the pulse is below 60 beats per minute in an adult or below 90 to 110 beats per minute in an infant or small child; notify the physician. Guidelines may vary according to institution or physician.
- Monitor the serum potassium and other electrolyte levels. Digitalis toxicity is aggravated in hypokalemia. If the potassium level is below normal range, notify the physician. Signs of hypokalemia are noted in Table 17-1. Recall that vomiting, chronic diarrhea, nasogastric suctioning, and alkalosis contribute to hypokalemia, as can administration of potassium-depleting diuretics, long-term steroid therapy, amphotericin B, and long-term glucose therapy.
- Monitor serum drug levels when available. Withhold the drug and notify the physician if the serum drug level is higher than the therapeutic range.
- Monitor intake and output, daily weight, vital signs, and heart and lung sounds. Assess for dependent edema in the sacral area and feet and ankles. Assess for jugular venous distention. Use data from central venous or arterial lines if available. Monitor ECG changes; the cardiac glycosides can

Continued.

NURSING IMPLICATIONS SUMMARY—cont'd

cause PR interval prolongation, ST segment sagging, AV blockage, and other arrhythmias.

- Read the physician's orders and drug labels carefully; do not confuse digoxin with digitoxin.

Intravenous Digoxin

- Monitor the apical pulse and check serum electrolyte and drug levels before administering intravenous digoxin. It may be administered undiluted or diluted in 4 ml of sterile water, normal saline, or 5% dextrose in water (D5W); use diluted solution as soon as prepared. Administer each dose evenly over at least 5 minutes. If possible, monitor ECG changes during IV administration.

Patient and Family Education

- Review with the patient the expected benefits and possible side effects of drug therapy. Review in detail the signs of drug toxicity, especially if the patient is an older adult because older adults are more sensitive to the effects of cardiac glycosides.
- Discuss the importance of maintaining an adequate potassium level. Review sources of dietary potassium (see box on p. 170). Patients with heart disease may need instruction about sodium-restricted, weight-reduction, and low-cholesterol diets; refer such patients to a dietitian as needed.
- Review all medications the patient is taking, and emphasize the importance of taking them as prescribed. These may include diuretics, potassium replacements, and antihypertensives.
- If appropriate for their abilities, resources, and medical conditions, instruct patients to monitor and record the apical pulse on a regular basis. It may also be appropriate to instruct patients to measure and record weight on a regular basis. Instruct patients to report weight gain greater than 2 lb/day (1 kg/day) or 5 lb/wk (2 kg/wk) to the physician.
- Instruct the patient to take cardiac glycosides with meals or snacks to lessen gastric irritation. The liquid form may be dispensed with a calibrated dropper; instruct the patient to measure doses with this dropper.
- For maintenance therapy, cardiac glycosides are usually taken once a day. For missed doses, instruct the patient to take the dose as soon as remembered on the day it was missed if within 12 hours of the usual time the dose is taken. Instruct the patient not to double up for missed doses and to take only one dose a day unless otherwise directed by the physician. Refer the patient as needed to community-based nursing care services.
- Remind the patient to keep cardiac glycosides out of the reach of children, to keep all health care providers informed of all drugs being taken, and not to self-medicate with over-the-counter drugs without consulting the physician.
- Suggest that patients wear a medical identification tag or bracelet indicating that they are taking cardiac glycosides.

Amrinone

Drug Administration

- Review the information about cardiac glycosides.
- Monitor the platelet count and other parameters noted above.
- Follow the dosage charts supplied by the manufacturer. Amrinone may be given as a bolus; administer dose over 2 to 3 minutes. It may be administered into fluids containing dextrose but should not be diluted with solutions containing dextrose. If given as an infusion, use microdrip tubing and an electronic infusion monitor.
- Monitor the ECG changes and other data available from central venous or arterial lines.
- Amrinone is incompatible with furosemide. A precipitate will form of the two drugs mix in the same tubing.
- Amrinone is used only in the short-term care setting. Keep the patient and family informed of the patient's condition.

Digoxin Immune FAB

Drug Administration

- Review the manufacturer's insert for the latest guidelines.
- Skin testing may be prescribed before the full dose is given (see manufacturer's guidelines). Be prepared to treat an anaphylactic reaction. Patients who are allergic to digoxin immune FAB should not be given the full dose unless absolutely necessary. Have personnel, equipment, and drugs for resuscitation available.
- Prepare ordered dose and administer over 30 minutes, using IV tubing with a 0.22-micron filter unless cardiac arrest is imminent. Digoxin immune FAB may be given as a bolus in that situation. Monitor the ECG changes and data from central venous and arterial lines as available.
- Monitor serum level of cardiac glycosides and serum electrolyte levels.
- Keep the patient and family informed of the patient's condition.

CRITICAL THINKING

APPLICATION

1. How does heart muscle differ from skeletal muscle?
2. What is the purpose of the ring of nonconductive tissue that separates the atria from the ventricles?
3. Where does the impulse to beat originate in the healthy heart?
4. What structure transmits the impulse to beat from the atria to the ventricles?
5. What is the physiologic effect of cardiac glycosides on the heart?
6. What is the mechanism of action of cardiac glycosides?
7. What is the mechanism by which cardiac glycosides produce diuresis in a patient with congestive heart failure?
8. How do digitoxin and digoxin differ in plasma protein binding and route of excretion?
9. Which cardiac glycoside has the longest elimination half-time?
10. What is the purpose of the loading dose at the beginning of therapy with cardiac glycosides?
11. Do cardiac glycosides have a high or a low therapeutic index?
12. What drugs increase the likelihood of cardiac glycoside toxicity?
13. How may diuretics improve function in a failing heart?
14. How do vasodilators relieve symptoms of congestive heart failure?

CRITICAL THINKING

1. What is the effect of parasympathetic stimulation on the heart?
2. What is the effect of sympathetic stimulation on the heart?
3. How does the Frank-Starling law apply to the heart?
4. What symptoms are typical of congestive heart failure? How would you assess for these?
5. What toxicity is common with cardiac glycoside therapy? What should you assess while monitoring for this toxicity?
6. Why are pulse rates measured before administering each prescribed dose of cardiac glycosides? What parameters should you use in assessing pulse rate data?
7. What inotropic drugs other than cardiac glycosides are used in congestive heart failure? What is the basis for their action in congestive heart failure?
8. How do diuretics relieve pulmonary congestion in congestive heart failure? How should you assess for this?

CHAPTER 19

Drugs to Control Cardiac Arrhythmias

OBJECTIVES

After studying this chapter, you should be able to do the following:

- *Explain how normal heart rhythm is maintained.*
- *Describe the four classes of antiarrhythmic agents.*
- *Explain how each class of antiarrhythmics suppresses arrhythmias.*
- *Discuss the cardiotoxicity of antiarrhythmic drugs.*
- *Develop a nursing care plan for a patient receiving an antiarrhythmic.*

KEY TERMS

arrhythmias
atrial flutter
automaticity
bradycardia
ectopic foci
fibrillation
premature ventricular contractions (PVCs)
refractory period
tachycardia

CHAPTER OVERVIEW

Cardiac **arrhythmias** are defined as any deviation from the normal rate or pattern of heartbeat. Heart rates that are too slow (**bradycardia**), too fast (**tachycardia**), or irregular are included in this classification. Arrhythmias are also referred to as *dysrhythmias.*

To understand the pharmacologic control of arrhythmias, recall the physiologic control mechanisms of the heart. The impulse to beat originates in the sinoatrial (SA) node; it spreads through the atria, causing them to contract, then passes through the artioventricular (AV) node and enters the ventricles, causing contraction of that tissue (see Chapter 18). The electrical activity that allows this communication is discussed first in this chapter, followed by a description of classes of antiarrhythmic agents and individual drugs.

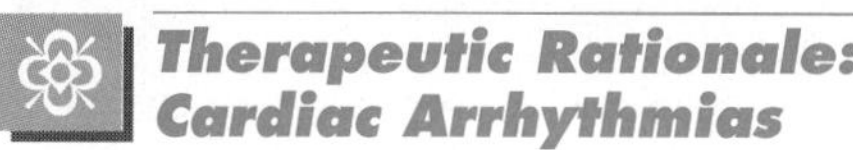

Therapeutic Rationale: Cardiac Arrhythmias

Electrophysiology of the Heart

Action Potentials

An action potential describes changes in electrical potential between a cell and its environment over time. Typical action potentials for three types of cardiac tissue are illustrated in Figure 19-1. Atrial and ventricular patterns are quite similar. Both begin with a rapid depolarization, marked by 0 on the curves, which is caused by a rapid rush of sodium ion (Na^+) into the cell. The inside of the cell therefore becomes more positive as the electrical potential shifts from about −90 mV to about +20 mV. Shortly thereafter, chloride ion (Cl^-) enters the cardiac cell, so the electrical potential becomes more negative. This phase is marked by 1 on the curve. During the relatively long plateau period, marked phase 2 on the curve, sodium ion and calcium ion (Ca^{++}) slowly enter the cell, while potassium ion leaves the cell. As time progresses, the sodium and calcium ions stop flowing in, but potassium ion continues to flow out (phase 3). During this phase the electrical potential continues to become more negative. In the final phase of the action potential, sodium ion flows out of the cell in exchange for potassium ion, which enters the cell. At the end of this cycle, the cell has returned to the resting potential of about −90 mV and has regained the ability to generate another normal action potential. From the beginning of phase 0 until sometime during the middle of phase 3, atrial or ventricular cells cannot be stimulated to beat again. This span of time is referred to as the **refractory period.** In nodal tissue the refractory period lasts well beyond phase 3 of the action potential.

Automaticity of Normal Sinoatrial Nodal Cells

The action potential for the SA nodal tissue differs from that of atrial and ventricular cells. Most important in terms of cardiac physiology is the gradual depolarization that occurs during phase 4 (see Figure 19-1). This ability to gradually shift from a potential of about −70 mV to −50 or −40 mV triggers the start of the action potential (phase 0) in SA nodal cells. This process is called **automaticity:** the cells need no externally applied stimulus to initiate an action potential.

Electrocardiogram

In the clinical setting, information about the function of a patient's heart must be gained from electrocardiographic (ECG) tracings (Figure 19-2). These ECG tracings may be related to action potentials in various parts of the heart. The change in potential marked in Figure 19-2 as P (the P wave) is produced by the initial depolarization of atrial cells (phase 0 on the action potential). Very shortly after this wave of depolarization, the atrium contracts to complete filling of the ventricles. The waves marked Q, R, and S (QRS complex) result from depolarization of the ventricles. Repolarization of the atria occurs at this time but is masked by large changes produced by the ventricles. Ventricular contraction occurs between the QRS complex and the midpoint of the T wave. The T wave is generated by repolarization (phase 1 through 3 of the action potential) of the ventricles.

Mechanisms Producing Arrhythmias

Arrhythmias occur because of disorders in pacing of the heartbeat and/or disorders in conducting the impulse to beat through cardiac tissues. Disorders in cardiac pacing are frequently related to changes in automaticity of the heart. For example, the normal pacemaker of the heart, the SA node, may become overstimulated by the sympathetic nervous system. Catecholamine neurotransmitters for this branch of the nervous system increase automaticity of the SA node. As a result, phase 4 on the action potential curve is steepened and shortened, phase 0 is triggered more frequently, and the heart beats more rapidly. In contrast, if the vagus nerve is predom-

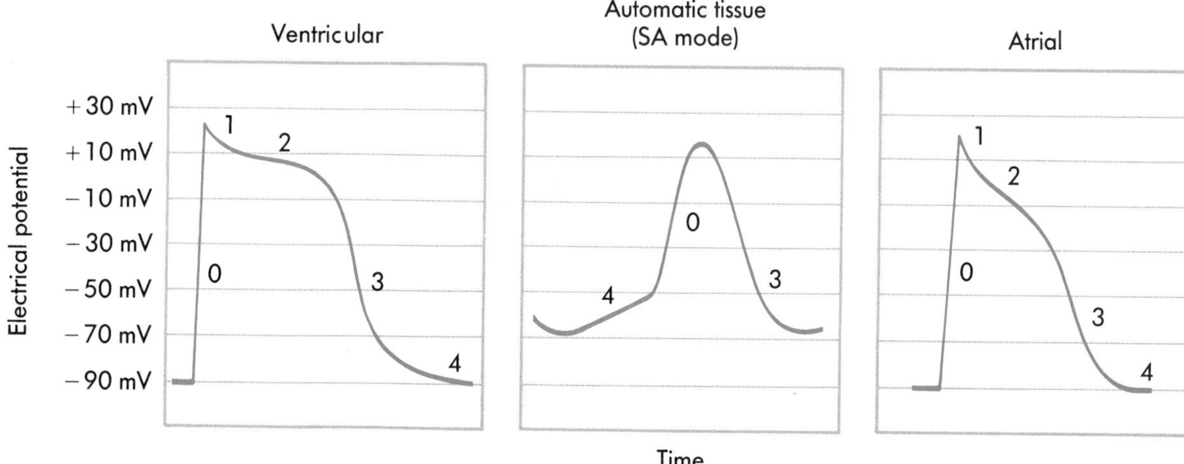

FIGURE 19-1
Typical action potential for three types of cardiac tissues. Action potentials are determined in laboratory in tissues from experimental animals.

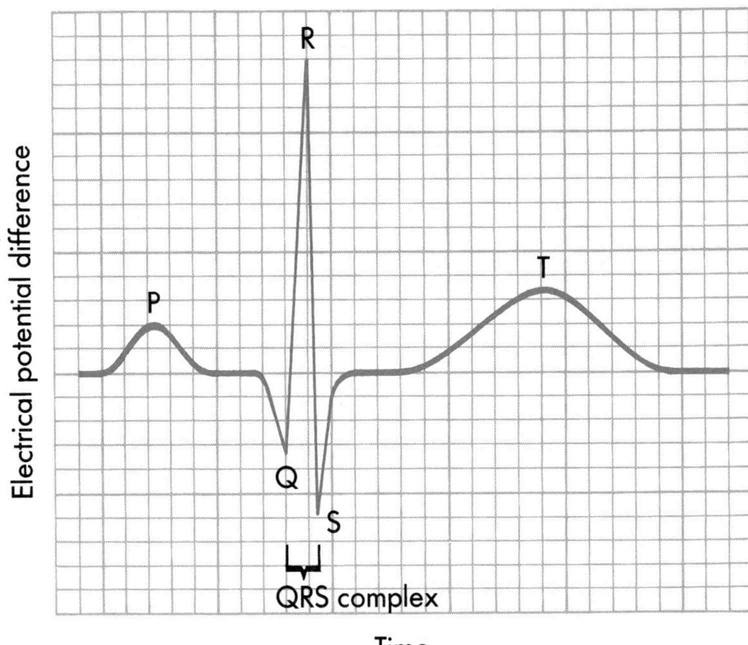

FIGURE 19-2
ECG tracing showing pattern typical of normal heart function.

inant and sympathetic stimulation is removed, heart rate decreases. This action occurs because acetylcholine from the vagus nerve decreases the automaticity of the SA node.

Sinus tachycardia, a rapid atrial rate, may not be harmful unless the ventricular rate is also abnormally increased. Many physicians do not give antiarrhythmic drugs to patients with rapid atrial rates and no other symptoms. Sinus tachycardia may be produced in healthy persons by anxiety; ingestion of coffee, tea, or other caffeinated products; alcoholic beverages; or smoking. Sympathomimetics, anticholinergics, or phenothiazines may also induce transient sinus tachycardia.

Sinus bradycardia is usually of minor importance and not treated. If bradycardia is associated with reduced cardiac output, atropine may be prescribed. Atropine increases the heart rate by blocking the effects of vagal nerve stimulation.

In addition to disorders in pacing at the SA node, the heart may suffer altered rates resulting from **ectopic foci** of automatic cells. Ectopic foci are groups of cells in the atria or the ventricles that spontaneously beat independently of the SA node. These groups of automatic cells may replace the SA node as the primary pacer for the heart, work in combination with the SA node so that the heart responds to both pacemakers, or interfere with SA nodal pacing so that neither pacing system is effective.

Premature ventricular contractions (PVCs) occur when the ventricles beat in response to both the SA node and an abnormal pacemaker. The ECG pattern shows a normal QRS complex following a P wave (see Figure 19-2), plus an abnormal QRS complex that is isolated from a P wave. These arrhythmias are found even among healthy persons. If PVCs are rare, they are ordinarily not treated unless the patient is recuperating from a myocardial infarction (MI). If the patient complains of palpitations with the PVCs, mild sedatives may be prescribed. Abstaining from coffee, tea, other caffeinated products and cigarettes may also control the condition.

When PVCs occur frequently or in rapid succession or with other signs of cardiac disease, treatment may be instituted with any one of several antiarrhythmic agents (Table 19-1). If these contractions are caused by a previous MI, lidocaine is the drug of choice in the hospital. *Ventricular tachycardia* usually relates to ectopic foci that are stimulating PVCs. Lidocaine is again the drug of choice, but many other drugs may also be effective.

Conduction disorders are primarily of two types. One involves an alteration in conduction time across the AV node. The AV node prevents the ventricles from receiving the impulse to beat until the atria have contracted and filled the ventricles (see Chapter 18). If the ventricles contract prematurely, ineffective pumping occurs, because the chambers will be only partially filled. If the delay in transmission through the AV node becomes too long, skipped heartbeats may occur, since the AV node may still be in the refractory period from the last beat when the next impulse arrives from the SA node.

The second type of conduction disorder involves conduction through contracting tissue. If an area of heart muscle becomes oxygen starved (ischemic) or damaged, it may not only fail to contract, but it may also fail to conduct an action potential properly. Ordinarily an action potential spreads across the tissue in a pattern that allows all parts of the tissue to contract at the proper time so that the heart pumps efficiently. This damaged region alters the pattern of stimulation, and the subsequent contraction may not be rhythmic or effective. Occasionally the damaged area may alter conduction so that a phenomenon called *reentry* occurs. In reentry, the action

TABLE 19-1 Classification of Antiarrhythmics With Indications for Use

CLASS	DRUGS	EFFECT ON ACTION POTENTIAL	INDICATIONS FOR USE
I	Disopyramide Moricizine Procainamide Quinidine	Depress phase 0; may prolong action potential duration	Ventricular arrhythmias; supraventricular arrhythmias (quinidine only)
I-B	Lidocaine Mexiletine Tocainide	Depress phase 0 without involving autonomic nervous system	Ventricular arrhythmias
I-C	Flecainide Propafenone	Depress phase 0 markedly; profound slowing of conduction	Ventricular arrhythmias, life-threatening
II	Esmolol	Depress phase 4 depolarization	Supraventricular and other tachyarrhythmias; acebutolol for premature ventricular contractions
III	Amiodarone Bretylium	Prolong phase 3 repolarization	Ventricular arrhythmias
IV	Diltiazem Verapamil	Depress phase 4 depolarization; lengthen phase 1 and 2	Supraventricular tachyarrhythmias

potential from a single impulse to beat passes more than once through the same group of cells. In the extreme case, reentry may produce a continuous cycle or loop of electrical activity through part of the tissue that prevents the heart from contracting properly.

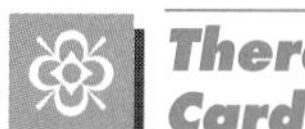

Therapeutic Agents: Cardiac Arrhythmias

The classification system described in Table 19-1 is based on effects of the drugs on the action potential (see Figure 19-1). The classification system demonstrates the mechanistic relatedness of drugs that might otherwise seem unrelated. Even within groups, however, effects of the drugs may differ somewhat. Table 19-2 lists the specific actions and reactions generated by each drug.

Antiarrhythmics may have other applications. For example, propranolol, esmolol, sotalol, and oxprenolol block beta-adrenergic receptors (see Chapters 12 and 13); in the heart this action slows the rate at the SA node and slows conduction through the AV node. The effect at both sites is to slow heart rate. Anticholinergic drugs, such as atropine, may produce the opposite effect by blocking the muscarinic receptors by which the heart responds to vagal nerve stimulation. Calcium channel blocking drugs such as verapamil and diltiazem primarily change the responses of cells highly dependent on the so-called slow calcium current (e.g., AV nodal cells or cells in ischemic regions of muscle). Local anesthetics, such as lidocaine and related drugs, alter cardiac cell membranes and thus change the sodium ion influx that causes phase 0 of the action potential.

Table 19-3 gives an alphabetic listing of drugs used to control arrhythmias. In the following presentation the drugs are grouped according to mechanistic class.

CLASS I ANTIARRHYTHMIC DRUGS

Class I antiarrhythmic drugs depress phase 0 of the action potential (see Figure 19-1) and prolong action potential duration. The effective refractory period is therefore prolonged in atria and ventricles, making the tissue less electrically responsive. Class I antiarrhythmics are indicated for prophylaxis and treatment of ventricular arrhythmias (premature contractions and tachycardia); quinidine and procainamide may also be used to treat atrial tachycardia or fibrillation.

Disopyramide

Mechanism of Action

Disopyramide slows conduction and prolongs the effective refractory period in atrial and ventricular tissues, but has little effect on the AV node or the His-Purkinje system.

Pharmacokinetics

Disopyramide is rapidly and almost completely absorbed orally. Biotransformation in liver produces metabolites with antimuscarinic and antiarrhythmic activities. About half of each dose is eliminated unchanged in urine. Dosage adjustment may be required, based on assessment of renal function.

Serum concentrations of disopyramide are not a reliable guide for adjusting dosage because of the large patient-to-patient variation in protein binding.

Adverse Reactions and Contraindications

Difficulty in urination, which is an antimuscarinic effect, may be experienced by 10% to 20% of treated patients. Up to 10% of patients suffer hypotension (dizziness or fainting), altered heart function (change in rhythm or heart failure), or fluid retention (congestive heart failure). Dry mouth, another antimuscarinic effect, is very common but not dangerous.

TABLE 19-2 Mechanism of Action of Antiarrhythmics

DRUG	PREDOMINANT MECHANISM OF ANTIARRHYTHMIC ACTION	SUMMARY OF CARDIAC ACTIONS			ADVERSE REACTIONS
		CONDUCTION VELOCITY	AUTOMATICITY	CONTRACTILITY	
Adenosine	Slows conduction through AV and SA nodes.	Slowed	Decreased	Decreased	Transient depression of left ventricular function; new arrhythmias possibly including heart block.
Amiodarone	Prolongs refractory period throughout heart.	Slowed	Decreased	Decreased	Bradycardia; pulmonary toxicity; neurotoxicity; hypothyroidism.
Atropine	Blocks effects of vagus nerve stimulation.	Hastened	Increased	No change	Antimuscarinic effects: dry mouth, dry skin, blurred vision.
Bretylium	Lowers sympathetic input to heart.	No change	No change or slightly increased	No change or slightly increased	Bradycardia, hypotension, and precipitation of anginal attacks.
Digoxin	Slows conduction through AV node.	Slowed	Increased at high doses	Increased	Bradycardia, premature ventricular beats, AV block, anorexia, nausea.
Disopyramide	Suppresses automaticity, especially in ectopic foci.	No change or slightly slowed	Decreased	Decreased	Anticholinergic effects: dry mouth, constipation, urinary retention, blurred vision; hypoglycemia.
Esmolol	Cardioselective beta-1 adrenergic receptor blockade; slows SA node rate.	Slowed	Decreased	Decreased	Bradycardia; confusion; hypotension; impaired peripheral circulation.
Flecainide	Prolongs refractory period in conductive fibers.	Slowed	Decreased	Slightly decreased	New ventricular arrhythmias; AV block; bradycardia; congestive heart failure.
Lidocaine	Increases electrical threshold for ventricular stimulation.	No change	Decreased	No change	Anxiety, drowsiness, convulsions.
Mexiletine	Increases threshold of excitability in conductive fibers.	No change	Decreased	No change	Ventricular arrhythmias; shortness of breath; hepatic necrosis.
Moricizine	Decreases excitability, conduction velocity, automaticity in conductive tissue.	Slowed	Decreased	Decreased	Dizziness, congestive heart failure, new arrhythmias.
Procainamide	Prolongs refractory period.	Slowed	Decreased	No change	Hypotension, ventricular tachycardia, gastrointestinal distress; lupuslike syndrome with chronic use.
Propafenone	Slows conduction in AV node and ventricular tissue.	Slowed	Decreased	Decreased	Congestive heart failure, new ventricular arrhythmias, AV blockade.
Quinidine	Prolongs refractory period.	Slowed	Decreased	Decreased	Hypotension, new arrhythmias, cinchonism, allergy.
Tocainide	Increases threshold of excitability in conductive fibers.	No change	Decreased	No change	Pulmonary toxicity, allergic reactions, blood dyscrasias.
Verapamil	Blocks calcium channels, slowing conduction through AV node.	Slowed	No change or slightly decreased	Decreased	Hypotension, bradycardia, asystole; headache.

AV, Atrioventricular; *SA*, sinoatrial.

TABLE 19-3 Drugs Used to Control Cardiac Arrhythmias

GENERIC NAME	TRADE NAME	ADMINISTRATION/DOSAGE	COMMENTS
Adenosine	Adenocard	INTRAVENOUS: *Adults*—6 mg given rapidly over 1-2 sec. If not effective, 12 mg may be given 1-2 min later. FDA pregnancy category C.	Extremely short half-life, thus side effects are usually self-limiting.
Amiodarone	Cordarone*	ORAL: *Adults*—800 mg-1.6 gm daily in divided doses; reduce dose when control is adequate or side effects occur, 600-800 mg daily for 1 mo; maintain with lowest effective dose. FDA pregnancy category D. *Children*—10 mg/kg body weight or 800 mg/1.72 m^2 daily until control is adequate or side effects occur; reduce to 5 mg/kg or 400 mg/1.72 m^2 for several weeks; maintain with lowest effective dose.	Very long duration of action (weeks or months) and very slow onset (2 days-2 mo). Persists in the body for months after the drug is discontinued.
Atropine		INTRAVENOUS: *Adults*—0.4-1 mg every 1-2 hr as needed, up to a maximum of 2 mg. FDA pregnancy category C. *Children*—0.01-0.03 mg/kg body weight.	Rapidly effective; excreted by the kidney within 12 hr of administration.
Bretylium	Bretylol Bretylate†	INTRAMUSCULAR: *Adults*—5-10 mg/kg repeated in 1-2 hr, then every 6-8 hr. FDA pregnancy category C. INTRAVENOUS: *Adults*—5-10 mg/kg repeated every 15-30 min to a maximum dose of 30 mg/kg.	Excreted unchanged by the kidneys.
Digoxin	Lanoxin*	ORAL: *Adults*—tablets or elixir, 0.375-0.625 mg repeated at 6-8 hr; maintain with 0.125-0.5 mg daily. Capsules, 0.4 to 0.6 mg once; maintain with 0.05 to 0.35 mg divided into 2 doses. FDA pregnancy category C. *Children*—doses are individualized for age and body weight.	Effective serum level 1-2 ng/ml and toxic at 3 ng/ml. Bioavailability with capsules is higher so that 0.1 mg dose is equivalent to 0.125 mg in tablets.
Disopyramide	Norpace* Rythmodan†	ORAL: *Adults*—150 mg every 6 hr. Maintenance with extended-release forms, 300 mg every 12 hr. FDA pregnancy category C. *Children*—6-30 mg/kg body weight daily divided into 4 doses.	Serum half-life 74 hr; kidneys eliminate 80% of active drug and metabolites.
Esmolol	Brevibloc	INTRAVENOUS: *Adults*—0.5 mg/kg body weight in 1 min, then 0.05 mg/kg/min for 4 min. Increase maintenance dose as necessary up to 0.2 mg/kg/min. FDA pregnancy category C. *Children*—0.05 mg/kg body weight/min, titrated up to 0.3 mg/kg/min as needed.	This very short-acting drug must be given by continuous infusion. May be used up to 48 hr.
Flecainide	Tambocor*	ORAL: *Adults*—100 mg every 12 hr, increasing in increments of 50 mg twice daily every 4 days as needed. Maximum daily dose 300 mg. FDA pregnancy category C.	Toxicity increases at plasma concentrations above 0.7-1 μg/ml.
Lidocaine	Xylocaine HCl* (for cardiac arrhythmias) Xylocard†	INTRAMUSCULAR: *Adults*—emergency use, 4.3 mg/kg. FDA pregnancy category B. INTRAVENOUS: *Adults*—up to 300 mg in any 1 hr period. *Children*—continuous infusion, 20-50 μg/kg body weight/min.	Effective serum level 1-5 μg/ml; serum half-life 15-20 min; metabolized in liver.
Mexiletine	Mexitil*	ORAL: *Adults*—200 mg every 8 hr; adjust up or down by 50-100 mg per dose every 2-3 days. Doses not to exceed 1200 mg daily. FDA pregnancy category C.	Effective plasma concentrations are 0.5-2 μg/ml, but toxicity may occur even at these levels.
Moricizine	Ethmozine	ORAL: *Adults*—200-300 mg every 8 hr, not to exceed 900 mg daily. FDA pregnancy category B.	New ventricular arrhythmias may be fatal.
Procainamide	Procan* Promine Pronestyl*	ORAL: *Adults*—6.25 mg/kg body weight every 3 hr. FDA pregnancy category C. *Children*—12.5 mg/kg every 6 hr. INTRAMUSCULAR: *Adults*—6.25 mg/kg every 3-6 hr. INTRAVENOUS: *Adults*—initially 20 mg/min; maintain with 2-6 mg/min.	Effective serum level 4-8 μg/ml; serum half-life about 3 hr.

*Available in Canada and United States.
†Available in Canada only.

Continued.

TABLE 19-3 Drugs Used to Control Cardiac Arrhythmias—cont'd

GENERIC NAME	TRADE NAME	ADMINISTRATION/DOSAGE	COMMENTS
Procainamide extended release	Procan SR* Pronestyl-SR*	ORAL: *Adults*—12.5 mg/kg every 6 hr.	For maintenance only.
Propafenone	Rhythmol*	ORAL: *Adults*—initially 150 mg every 8 hr, increasing gradually to a maximum of 300 mg every 8 hr. FDA pregnancy category C.	Adverse cardiac effects occur in many patients. Careful monitoring is essential.
Quinidine gluconate	Duraquin Quinaglute* Quinalan Quinate†	ORAL: *Adults*—325-650 mg every 6 hr. FDA pregnancy category C. INTRAMUSCULAR: *Adults*—initially 600 mg; 200-400 mg every 2-6 hr. INTRAVENOUS: *Adults*—20 mg/min.	More slowly absorbed than quinidine sulfate; IV doses require ECG and blood pressure monitoring.
Quinidine polygalacturonate	Cardioquin*	ORAL: *Adults*—275 mg every 3-12 hr. *Children*—8.25 mg/kg 5 times daily.	Less GI irritation than other forms of quinidine.
Quinidine sulfate	Cin-Quin Quinora	ORAL: *Adults*—200-300 mg 3 or 4 times daily. *Children*—6 mg/kg 5 times daily.	Effective serum level 3-6 μg/ml.
Tocainide	Tonocard*	ORAL: *Adults*—400 mg every 8 hr, adjusted as necessary; maintenance 400-600 mg every 8 hr. FDA pregnancy category C.	Bioavailability is high and is unaffected by food.
Verapamil	Calan Isoptin*	ORAL: *Adults*—80-120 mg every 8 hr. FDA pregnancy category C. *Children*—4-8 mg/kg daily in divided doses. INTRAVENOUS: *Adults*—initially 5-10 mg over 2-5 min, repeated if necessary at 30 min. *Children*—0.1-0.3 mg/kg over 2 min, repeated if necessary at 30 min.	Therapeutic serum levels are 0.08-0.3 μg/ml. Monitor ECG and blood pressure continuously with intravenous doses.

Disopyramide is avoided in patients with AV block because of the risk of complete heart block. Disopyramide also worsens cardiogenic shock and is avoided in patients with this condition.

Toxicity
Overdose causes pronounced widening of the QRS complex and the QT interval of the ECG tracing. Cardiac arrhythmias may ensue. Apnea, loss of spontaneous respirations, and unconsciousness precede death by cardiovascular collapse.

Interactions
Disopyramide may worsen conduction in patients who have received other arrhythmics. Disopyramide is avoided for 48 hours before and 24 hours after a dose of verapamil; deaths from conduction blockade have occurred. Arrhythmias may be provoked in patients receiving pimozide with disopyramide.

Moricizine

Mechanism of Action
In addition to blocking sodium channels, moricizine also has potent local anesthetic activity and membrane-stabilizing activity. It may also have anticholinergic effects. The AV node and the His-Purkinje system are most sensitive to moricizine. Conduction through these tissues is slowed considerably, but there is little effect on the SA node.

Pharmacokinetics
Moricizine is extensively biotransformed by the liver and has a half-life of about 2 hours. The drug is well absorbed orally but is subject to first-pass effects (see Chapter 1) that lower absolute bioavailability to about 38%. The onset of action is usually within 2 hours. Elimination is by the biliary or fecal route and by the kidneys, but little unchanged drug is eliminated.

Adverse Reactions and Contraindications
Moricizine, like other antiarrhythmics, can induce new arrhythmias in some patients. About 4% of patients receiving the drug in controlled trials suffered new or exacerbated ventricular arrhythmias. Other patients developed signs of congestive heart failure, AV block, or sinus arrest. Dizziness and other central nervous system (CNS) effects may also be observed with long-term administration.

Moricizine is avoided in patients with AV block or right bundle branch block because risk of total heart block is substantial.

Toxicity
Overdoses of moricizine have been fatal, producing cardiotoxicity, coma, and respiratory failure. Most of the side effects are dose related and become more pronounced as doses exceed the normal therapeutic range.

Interaction
Moricizine may hasten the metabolism of theophylline. If the drugs must be used together, theophylline concentrations should be monitored in blood and dosages should be adjusted accordingly to maintain effective control of pulmonary disease.

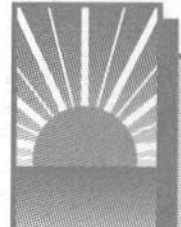

GERIATRIC CONSIDERATION

Antiarrhythmics

THE PROBLEM

Older adults often respond differently to antiarrhythmic agents than do younger adults. Procainamide and tocainide are more likely to cause dizziness or hypotension in older persons. Amiodarone is more likely to cause ataxia or other neurologic problems in older adults. Older adults are more sensitive to the antimuscarinic effects (dry mouth, urinary retention) of disopyramide. Clearance of drugs like verapamil, flecainide, or the beta-adrenergic blockers is lower, and these drugs may accumulate. Especially with flecainide, higher serum levels may lead to development of dangerous drug-induced arrhythmias. Older persons may be more susceptible to hypothermia if they take beta-adrenergic blockers.

SOLUTIONS

- Lidocaine doses and rates of administration should be cut in half for patients older than 65 years.
- Blood pressure should be carefully monitored.
- Be alert to signs of neurologic toxicity and ataxia.
- Help patients develop strategies to avoid injury from falls if ataxia or dizziness is a problem.
- Watch for signs of urinary retention.
- Watch for hypothermia in older adult patients receiving beta-adrenergic drugs.

Interactions

Moricizine may hasten the metabolism of theophylline. If the drugs must be used together, theophylline concentrations should be monitored in blood and dosages should be adjusted accordingly to maintain effective control of pulmonary disease.

Quinidine and ✣ Procainamide

Mechanism of Action

Quinidine and procainamide have virtually identical mechanisms of action. They alter calcium distribution within cardiac cells, thereby decreasing contractility of heart muscle. They also have atropine-like actions that block the effect of the vagus nerve on the heart. Finally, both drugs alter the membranes of cardiac cells, resulting in a prolonged refractory period. The ability of these drugs to prolong the refractory period of cardiac tissues may explain their ability to suppress ectopic foci. Quinidine and procainamide have equipotent membrane effects; however, quinidine has more potent anticholinergic effects.

Pharmacokinetics

Quinidine sulfate is relatively rapidly absorbed orally. The half-life of quinidine in serum is about 6 hours. Quinidine gluconate is more slowly absorbed orally and hence slightly longer acting. Quinidine polygalacturonate is less irritating to the gastrointestinal (GI) tract than other forms of quinidine. Quinidine is partially metabolized in liver; up to 50% of a dose may be excreted unchanged in urine, and the drug may accumulate in patients in renal failure.

Procainamide reaches effective concentrations in serum (4 to 8 μg/ml) within 1 to 3 hours of an oral dose or within 30 minutes of an intramuscular IM dose. The half-life of the drug in serum is 3 hours, and about half the drug dose is eliminated unchanged in urine.

Adverse Reactions and Contraindications

The anticholinergic effects of quinidine and procainamide may oppose the direct action of the drugs. The dual effects of quinidine have caused serious complications in treating atrial fibrillation. Although the direct effects of quinidine might be expected to slow the atrial rate, the first observed effect may be an anticholinergic action producing increased conduction through the AV node, with the result that ventricular rates soar dangerously high before quinidine can slow atrial rates.

The primary difference between quinidine and procainamide is in their side effects. The most serious reactions to quinidine are allergic responses and cardiovascular toxicity. When the drug is given intravenously, hypotension may result because quinidine is an arteriolar and venous dilator. Quinidine also produces cinchonism, with symptoms of blurred vision, dizziness, headache, and ringing in the ears. The most striking adverse effect with long-term use of procainamide is a syndrome resembling lupus erythematosus, with symptoms such as arthritis, arthralgia, myalgia, fever, and pericarditis.

Both quinidine and procainamide commonly cause GI tract disturbances such as loss of appetite, diarrhea, and stomach pain.

Procainamide worsens torsades de pointes and is avoided in patients with this arrhythmia. Quinidine is avoided in digitalis toxicity or intraventricular conduction defects because the drug further slows conduction. Both quinidine and procainamide are avoided in AV block because of the risk of complete heart block.

Toxicity

At higher doses producing blood levels above 8 μg/ml, quinidine may induce ventricular arrhythmias, including ectopic beats, tachycardia, and fibrillation. Quinidine causes a dose-dependent widening of the QRS complex. This effect can be used to monitor its therapeutic activity and to track the risk of toxicity.

Direct toxicity from procainamide usually relates to changes in conduction, especially in AV nodal tissue and conducting fibers of the ventricles. These direct toxic effects usually occur when blood levels exceed 12 %g/ml. Since normal therapeutic concentrations range from about 4 to 8 μg/ml, this drug, like other antiarrhythmic agents, has a narrow safety margin. Like quinidine, procainamide widens the QRS complex on ECG tracings and lengthens the refractory period.

Interactions

Quinidine serum levels rise when the urine becomes alkaline, as renal reabsorption of drug is enhanced; therefore urinary alkalinizers such as antacids, citrates, or carbonic anhydrase inhibitors must be used with care. Other arrhythmic agents, phenothiazines, rauwolfia alkaloids, or pimozide may have additive cardiac effects with quinidine. Actions of anticoagulants and neuromuscular blockers are enhanced by quinidine.

When used with other antiarrhythmics or pimozide, procainamide may cause increased heart-related side effects. Antihypertensives may produce hypotension if used with procainamide. Antimyasthenic agents are antagonized by procainamide, but neuromuscular blocking agents are enhanced.

CLASS I-B ANTIARRHYTHMIC DRUGS

Class I-B antiarrhythmic drugs depress phase 0 of the action potential (see Figure 19-1), decreasing excitability and automaticity. These drugs have much less effect on atria than class I drugs. Class I-B antiarrhythmic agents are indicated for ventricular arrhythmias, including those caused by myocardial infarction, cardiac surgery, cardiac catheterization, or digitalis toxicity.

✣ Lidocaine

Mechanism of Action

Lidocaine is a local anesthetic (see Chapter 67), as well as an antiarrhythmic agent.

Pharmacokinetics

Over 90% of a dose of lidocaine is rapidly destroyed in the liver. For this reason the drug is useful primarily when administered as a continuous infusion designed to produce therapeutic levels of 1.5 to 5 mg/100 ml in plasma.

Adverse Reactions and Contraindications

Lidocaine may cause anxiety, dizziness, drowsiness, nervousness, numbness, or the sensation of heat or cold. Reactions seldom persist after the infusion is discontinued because the half-life of lidocaine is so short.

Lidocaine is avoided in Adams-Stokes syndrome or severe heart block because the drug may worsen the block.

Toxicity

Lidocaine causes CNS reactions, ranging from muscle twitching and drowsiness to paresthesia, respiratory depression, convulsions, and coma. These reactions may be dose dependent. At serum lidocaine concentrations of 6 to 8 μg/ml, blurred vision, double vision, nausea, ringing in ears, tremors, twitching, or vomiting may occur. When serum concentrations exceed 8 μg/ml, patients may experience bradycardia, difficulty breathing, dizziness, fainting, or seizures. Toxic reactions to lidocaine are more common in patients with reduced hepatic function because the drug may accumulate in these patients.

Interactions

In administering lidocaine, recall that the drug has two separate clinical uses and is packaged differently for each. When intended for use as a local anesthetic, lidocaine is frequently packaged in solution with epinephrine (e.g., Xylocaine or other trade names with epinephrine). When used with the local anesthetic, epinephrine acts as a vasoconstrictor to reduce local blood flow and prolong the action of the anesthetic. If lidocaine with epinephrine were inadvertently administered to treat a cardiac arrhythmia, the epinephrine might trigger a severe arrhythmia by stimulating automaticity of the heart. Lidocaine intended for use in cardiac emergencies is labeled "lidocaine preservative-free" or "Xylocaine for ventricular arrhythmias or continuous infusion."

Mexiletine

Mechanism of Action

Mexiletine is an oral antiarrhythmic drug with a mechanism of action similar to parenteral lidocaine. Both drugs have local anesthetic properties. Mexiletine also has anticonvulsant actions.

Pharmacokinetics

Mexiletine is well absorbed from the GI tract, making oral administration practical and effective. The onset of effect is within 2 hours. Elimination is primarily by hepatic metabolism; the half-life of the drug in the blood may be doubled in severe hepatic disease but only slightly increased in renal impairment.

Adverse Reactions and Contraindications

Side effects of mexiletine increase when plasma concentrations exceed 2 μg/ml. New ventricular arrhythmias may arise, including premature ventricular contractions and torsades de pointes. Heartburn, nausea, and vomiting usually occur within 2 hours of administration. Agranulocytosis, leukopenia, and thrombocytopenia may cause fever, chills, unusual bruising or bleeding. CNS effects include dizziness, trembling, nervousness, and unsteady gait.

Mexiletine is avoided in arrhythmias that respond to other drugs or are not life threatening.

Toxicity

Overdose can cause death from respiratory failure and asystole. Acidifying the urine speeds excretion of mexiletine and may therefore help bring plasma concentrations back into a safe range.

Interactions

Mexiletine may decrease the metabolism of theophylline. As a result, theophylline may accumulate, causing CNS and other toxicity.

Tocainide

Mechanism of Action

Tocainide, like lidocaine, is a type of amide local anesthetic. Its action in the heart is similar to that of lidocaine.

Pharmacokinetics

Tocainide is completely absorbed orally, whether taken with or without food. The onset of action is within 2 hours, and the half-life is about 15 hours. Elimination is nearly equally divided between hepatic metabolism and renal excretion.

Adverse Reactions and Contraindications

The most common side effects include dizziness, loss of appetite, or nausea. Blisters, peeling skin, or skin rashes may signal a rare but dangerous allergic reaction that can culminate in Stevens-Johnson syndrome. After several weeks of therapy, pulmonary damage can occur, with coughing and shortness of breath. Allergic reactions or pulmonary damage can be fatal.

Toxicity

Shaking and trembling are early signs of toxicity. Overdoses may cause respiratory depression or seizures.

Interactions

Mexiletine may worsen cardiac function if it is combined with beta-adrenergic agents.

CLASS I-C ANTIARRHYTHMIC DRUGS

Class I-C antiarrhythmic drugs markedly depress phase 0 of the action potential (see Figure 19-1) and profoundly slow conduction, especially in conductive fibers. These drugs are indicated only for control of life-threatening ventricular arrhythmias.

Flecainide

Mechanism of Action

Flecainide may have greater effects in ischemic than in normal cardiac tissue. It also has local anesthetic action and may decrease contractility of the heart.

Pharmacokinetics

Flecainide is nearly completely absorbed orally, with or without food. The major route of elimination is hepatic metabolism, and the drug has a long half-life of approximately 20 hours.

Adverse Reactions and Contraindications

Blurred vision and dizziness are common side effects. Trembling, chest pain, and arrhythmias can also occur. Flecainide is avoided when AV block or right bundle branch block exists because the risk of complete heart block is increased.

Toxicity

Flecainide has been associated with development of new and potentially fatal arrhythmias, especially when plasma concentrations exceed 1 μg/ml. Ventricular arrhythmias, congestive heart failure, and AV block are most common.

Interactions

Flecainide should not be used with other antiarrhythmic agents because such combinations may lead to fatal arrhythmias.

Propafenone

Mechanism of Action

Propafenone primarily affects the AV node, slowing conduction markedly. The drug also has a weak beta-adrenergic blocking effect (one fortieth as effective as propranolol) and a strong local anesthetic action. Propafenone has a negative inotropic effect that increases the risk for congestive heart failure.

Pharmacokinetics

Propafenone is well absorbed orally, but a first-pass effect (see Chapter 1) reduces absolute bioavailability to 10% or less. The liver converts propafenone to several products, some of which are also active antiarrhythmics. Elimination is mostly by renal mechanisms. The half-life of the drug is 2 to 10 hours in most patients, but up to 10% of the population metabolize propafenone much more slowly. For slow metabolizers the half-life is 10 to 32 hours. Steady-state concentrations of the drug are achieved after 4 or 5 days, but the steady-state plasma concentrations vary widely as a result of variations in metabolism.

Adverse Reactions and Contraindications

Propafenone, like other antiarrhythmics, can induce new arrhythmias in some patients. About 5% of patients receiving the drug in controlled trials experienced new or exacerbated ventricular arrhythmias. Other patients developed signs of congestive heart failure, AV block, or sinus bradycardia. Dizziness and other CNS effects may also be observed with long-term administration. Many patients also report a change in their sense of taste.

Propafenone is avoided when AV block or right bundle branch block exists because the risk of complete heart block is increased.

Toxicity

The side effects of propafenone are dose related; at high doses the cardiotoxic effects can become severe, with dangerous new arrhythmias, heart block, and severe congestive heart failure.

Interactions

Propafenone interferes with metabolism or elimination of digoxin and warfarin and can significantly increase serum concentrations of these drugs. Doses may require reduction and serum concentrations require monitoring when propafenone is also being given.

CLASS II ANTIARRHYTHMIC DRUGS

Class II antiarrhythmic drugs are beta-adrenergic receptor blockers that depress phase 4 depolarization of the action potential (see Figure 19-1). Acebutolol is a relatively cardioselective blocker of beta-1 receptors in the heart and can be used to suppress PVCs. Oxprenolol, propranolol, and sotalol (see Chapter 13) are beta-blockers that have been used for supraventricular arrhythmias and ventricular tachycardia. Esmolol is the only beta-blocker that is used primarily as an antiarrhythmic agent.

Esmolol

Mechanism of Action

Esmolol is a relatively cardioselective blocker of beta-1 receptors, with little sympathomimetic or membrane-stabilizing activity.

Pharmacokinetics

Esmolol is used intravenously, is distributed to tissues within 2 minutes, and achieves therapeutic effects within 5 minutes. The effects last only 10 to 20 min after the infusion is stopped. The drug is rapidly destroyed by esterases in red blood cells.

Uses

It is intended for rapid, short-term control of ventricular rates in atrial flutter or fibrillation. Esmolol is primarily an emergency medication for perioperative or postoperative use.

Adverse Reactions and Contraindications

Hypotension is very common in patients receiving esmolol, causing dizziness and sweating in up to 12% of patients. Reduced peripheral circulation and difficulty breathing may also occur. Esmolol is especially dangerous in patients with heart failure that has been compensated by increased sympathetic stimulation of the heart. Blockade of these sympathetic influences may produce bradycardia or heart arrest, especially if partial AV block already exists. For these reasons esmolol should be avoided in cardiac failure, cardiogenic shock, AV block, or sinus bradycardia.

Toxicity

Overdose may cause slow or irregular heartbeat, dizziness, fainting, difficulty breathing, blue fingernail beds, or seizures. Treatment of overdose includes specific antiarrhythmics to control cardiac symptoms and a beta-2 agonist to halt bronchospasm.

Interactions

Esmolol should not be used with sympathomimetics because the effects of both drugs will be lost. Esmolol also blocks the therapeutic effects of aminophylline and theophylline. Risk of hypertension is increased with monoamine oxidase inhibitors. Esmolol masks signs of hypoglycemia, which can increase risks to patients receiving insulin or oral antidiabetic medications.

CLASS III ANTIARRHYTHMIC DRUGS

Class III antiarrhythmics primarily prolong phase 3, the repolarization phase, of the action potential (see Figure 19-1).

Amiodarone

Mechanism of Action

Amiodarone has many actions on cardiac tissues, which result in prolonging the refractory period and reducing automaticity. Amiodarone also may depress contractility and may cause vasodilation. The drug produces noncompetitive beta-adrenergic blockade and blocks calcium channels.

Pharmacokinetics

Oral absorption is variable, and most patients absorb much less than half the administered dose. Amiodarone is highly lipid soluble and concentrates in adipose tissue, as well as other sites. As a result antiarrhythmic activity is not seen for days or even months. The duration of action is also greatly prolonged. Amiodarone may be detectable in plasma up to 9 months after its use has been discontinued.

Uses

Amiodarone is used for prophylaxis or therapy for life-threatening ventricular arrhythmias.

Adverse Reactions and Contraindications

Sinus bradycardia is common, and arrest or heart block may occur. New arrhythmias may occur in up to 5% of patients. Up to 15% of patients develop significant pulmonary toxicity, which may be fatal. Neurotoxicity, signaled by weakness, numbness, or ataxia, may occur in up to 40% of patients. Sensitivity to sun, ocular toxicity, and hypothyroidism are also expected effects. Reversal of side effects may take months after cessation of therapy.

Amiodarone should be avoided in AV block because the drug may worsen blockade. Amiodarone is also avoided in conditions producing bradycardia because the drug may lower SA node automaticity and create additional bradycardia that is resistant to atropine.

Toxicity

Overdose may result in hypotension, cardiovascular distress, and bradycardia. Because the drug has such a long duration of action, the patient may require monitoring or treatment for weeks after the use of amiodarone is discontinued.

Interactions

Amiodarone significantly increases serum concentrations of digoxin, digitoxin, and phenytoin, which increases the risk of toxicity. Amiodarone inhibits metabolism of coumarin anticoagulants, increasing their concentrations in plasma and thus increasing risk of bleeding. Amiodarone is likely to have additive cardiac effects with other antiarrhythmic agents, which may increase risk of cardiac toxicity.

Bretylium

Mechanism of Action

Bretylium has a mechanism of action different from that of other antiarrhythmic drugs. The drug increases the action potential duration and hence prolongs the refractory period. It does not directly suppress automaticity or conduction velocity. Bretylium accumulates in sympathetic neurons and causes an initial release of norepinephrine that may stimulate contractility, heart rate, and automaticity, but ultimately the drug produces an adrenergic blockade by preventing norepinephrine release.

Pharmacokinetics

Bretylium is administered by intravenous (IV) or intramuscular (IM) injection. The duration of action is 6 to 8 hours, and most of the drug is excreted by the kidneys.

Uses

Bretylium is used primarily for life-threatening ventricular tachycardia, especially episodes refractory to lidocaine or cardioversion, and for ventricular fibrillation.

Adverse Reactions and Contraindications

Major reactions to bretylium are precipitation of anginal attacks, bradycardia, and hypotension. Bretylium does not alter the ECG tracings. There are no specific contraindications to the use of bretylium.

Toxicity

High doses of bretylium may depress respiration by neuromuscular blockade.

Interactions

The early release of norepinephrine caused by bretylium may increase risk of toxicity with digoxin or digitoxin.

CLASS IV ANTIARRHYTHMIC DRUGS

Class IV antiarrhythmic drugs primarily depress phase 4 depolarization and lengthen phase 1 and 2 repolarization. The heart rate may slow significantly.

Calcium Channel Blockers: Diltiazem and Verapamil

Mechanism of Action

Verapamil and diltiazem are used as antiarrhythmic agents and as antianginal agents (see Chapter 15). The slow calcium ion current blocked by these drugs is more important for the activity of the AV node than for many other tissues in the heart. By interfering with this current, the calcium channel blockers achieve some selectivity of action. The major antiarrhythmic effect of these drugs is a delay in conduction through the AV node.

Pharmacokinetics

Verapamil and diltiazem are well absorbed orally but are rapidly metabolized by the liver. This first-pass phenomenon significantly reduces bioavailability (see Chapter 1). Some metabolites may be active. Cirrhosis of the liver significantly diminishes drug elimination. Verapamil or diltiazem may be administered intravenously when the oral route is inappropriate.

Uses

Verapamil and diltiazem are used to control supraventricular arrhythmias.

Adverse Reactions and Contraindications

Side effects related to cardiovascular function include hypotension, peripheral edema, congestive heart failure, and pulmonary edema.

Contraindications include AV block, SA node impairment, bradycardia, heart failure, cardiogenic shock, and hypotension. These conditions are worsened by administration of diltiazem and verapamil. The drugs should also be avoided after MI because they increase the risk of cardiac failure.

Toxicity

Acute overdose may produce bradycardia, progressing to asystole and hypotension. Treatment is symptomatic.

Interactions

Verapamil and diltiazem can increase serum concentrations of digoxin, which can lead to toxicity. Neither verapamil nor diltiazem should be given to patients receiving disopyramide or flecainide because the lower contractility produced by calcium channel blockers is additive with that produced by disopyramide or flecainide. The result can be dangerous cardiac failure.

UNCLASSIFIED ANTIARRHYTHMIC DRUGS

Adenosine

Adenosine is a naturally occurring metabolite that acts as an autocoid. Receptors for adenosine exist on the outer surface of many cells in the body, including cells in blood vessels and organs such as the brain, heart, and kidneys. Large doses of adenosine given by rapid IV injection are effective in terminating supraventricular tachycardia and returning the heart to normal sinus rhythm. Adenosine slows conduction in the SA and AV nodes and can interrupt reentry. In addition, adenosine may impair ventricular function, but because the drug has a half-life of about 10 seconds, this undesired action is considered minor and transient for most patients. The antiarrhythmic effect persists after the drug has been metabolized and removed.

Atropine

Atropine, a blocker of muscarinic cholinergic receptors (see Chapter 11), may also be used to treat certain arrhythmias. Its action as an antiarrhythmic drug depends on its ability to reduce the effects of vagal nerve stimulation, primarily on the SA node. Since stimulation of the vagus nerve slows heart rate, atropine increases heart rate by blocking that effect. Because it also speeds conduction through the AV node, atropine may lessen heart block in certain cases.

Cardiac Glycosides: Digoxin and Digitoxin

Cardiac glycosides are primarily cardiotonic agents (see Chapter 18), but in addition to the ability to strengthen contraction of the heart muscle, they also increase vagal tone at the AV node. Through this action and direct effects on nodal tissue, cardiac glycosides slow conduction through the AV node. This action is sought when digoxin is used to treat **atrial flutter** and **fibrillation.** By lowering conduction of impulses through the AV node, digoxin protects the ventricles from overstimulation. The short-term therapeutic goal is not to slow the atrial rate but to produce a partial heart block that allows fewer impulses from the atria to stimulate the ventricles to beat. The patient's condition may therefore be maintained with rapid atrial rates but with ventricular rates from 60 to 80 beats per minute. Many patients spontaneously convert to normal sinus rhythm after a few days of treatment. Digoxin is usually preferred for arrhythmias (see Table 19-3).

As with other antiarrhythmic drugs, higher concentrations of cardiac glycosides may also cause arrhythmias of various types, most characteristically bradycardia and PVCs. Bradycardia may be a sign of impending heart block (no impulse passes through the AV node to the ventricles). PVCs arise because cardiac glycosides increase the spontaneous rate of ventricular depolarization (phase 4 of the action potential). The first step in controlling these reactions is to discontinue the cardiac glycoside. If the arrhythmia is not severe, no further therapy may be required. However, cardiac glycosides are relatively long-acting drugs, and treating the arrhythmia while the cardiac glycoside is being eliminated from the system may be necessary (see Table 18-1). Potassium levels should be assessed in these patients because a low potassium level increases the sensitivity of the heart to digoxin or digitoxin and may predispose it to arrhythmias. Potassium supplements may be given if required.

NURSING PROCESS OVERVIEW

Antiarrhythmic Therapy

Assessment

Antiarrhythmic therapy is used in patients with cardiac arrhythmias. An arrhythmia is diagnosed by use of the ECG tracings, although the patient may complain of missed beats, fluttering in the chest, pounding in the chest, or irregular heart rates or patterns. Perform a thorough cardiovascular assessment, and question the patient about previous cardiac problems.

Nursing Diagnoses

- Risk for arrhythmias
- Risk for activity intolerance related to insufficient knowledge of adaptive techniques needed related to impaired cardiac function

Patient Outcomes

The nurse will manage and minimize complications associated with arrhythmias. The patient will identify factors that increase cardiac workload, will identify modifications needed in activities of daily living, and will modify activities to maintain pulse, blood pressure, and respirations in normal range.

Planning/Implementation

Treatment may take place in the coronary care unit or in the outpatient care setting if the arrhythmia is less serious. Perform periodic or continuous ECG monitoring as needed. Monitor vital signs and blood pressure, weight, fluid intake and output, serum electrolyte levels, and laboratory work appropriate for the drug prescribed. Observe the general physical condition of the patient and watch for the appearance of side effects.

Evaluation

Before discharge, determine that the patient can explain interactions among prescribed drugs, plan meals within prescribed dietary restriction, state how to manage persistent side effects, describe side effects and the signs and symptoms of toxicity, and understand when to notify the physician.

NURSING IMPLICATIONS SUMMARY

General Guidelines: Antiarrhythmic Therapy

Drug Administration

- Monitor the vital signs and blood pressure. Although a change in the heart rate is frequently a desired outcome of therapy, a heart rate <60 beats per minute or >120 beats per minute in an adult should be avoided.
- Establish specific guidelines for each patient in consultation with the physician.
- Monitor the ECG patterns continuously in the short-term care setting and periodically thereafter.
- Monitor other indicators of cardiovascular functioning as appropriate, including blood pressure, pulse, intake and output, weight, and heart and lung sounds. Assess for edema, especially in dependent areas, and jugular venous distention. Assess for activity tolerance with daily activities. Monitor other available data: central venous pressure, pulmonary capillary wedge pressure.
- Monitor the blood urea nitrogen (BUN) level, liver function studies, and serum drug levels if available.
- For IV administration, use microdrip tubing and/or an electronic infusion monitor. Usually, monitor the ECG during IV administration. Monitor the blood pressure and pulse. Keep the patient in the supine position after IV doses until vital signs are stable. Keep siderails up. Have available emergency equipment and drugs to treat toxicity or to resuscitate the patient.

Patient and Family Education

- Instruct the patient about the desired effects and common side effects of prescribed drugs. Emphasize that it is important to report the development of any unexpected sign or symptom. Point out that drugs or doses may require changing or adjustment if unusual side effects develop and so the patient should not hesitate to contact the health care provider.
- Review with the patient the importance of taking medications as ordered. Antiarrhythmic drugs are most effective when taken on a regular basis, with doses spread evenly throughout the 24-hour day, as prescribed. If a dose is missed, the patient should not double up for it. Refer the patient as appropriate to community-based nursing care agencies.
- Instruct the patient not to discontinue antiarrhythmic medications without first consulting the physician.
- Stress the importance of concomitant therapies, if ordered, including modifying diet; losing weight; restricting sodium; using potassium replacements, diuretics, and antihypertensives; limiting caffeine intake; stopping smoking; and exercising regularly. Emphasize the importance of returning for follow-up visits as scheduled to monitor drug effectiveness.
- Assess the need for the patient to monitor weight, pulse, blood pressure, or other parameters in the home. Consider the patient's medical condition, prescribed medication, ability, and resources when making this decision.
- Suggest that the patient carry a medical identification tag or bracelet indicating that antiarrhythmics are being used. Remind the patient to keep all health care providers, including dentists, informed of all drugs being used.
- Instruct the patient to avoid drinking alcoholic beverages unless approved by the physician.
- Remind the patient to keep all medications out of the reach of children.
- Digoxin is discussed in Chapter 18.
- Beta-adrenergic receptor blockers are discussed in Chapter 13.
- Calcium channel blockers are discussed in Chapter 15.
- Phenytoin is discussed in Chapter 55.

Disopyramide

Drug Administration

- See the general guidelines for antiarrhythmic therapy.
- Assess for urinary retention. Monitor intake and output, question the patient about hesitancy or difficulty voiding; palpate the bladder.
- Monitor blood glucose since dysopyramide can cause hypoglycemia.

Patient and Family Education

- See the general guidelines for antiarrhythmic therapy.
- Instruct the patient to take a missed dose as soon as remembered, unless within 4 hours of the next scheduled dose, then omit the missed dose and resume the regular dosing schedule.
- Disopyramide may cause the patient to sweat less. Instruct the patient to avoid becoming overheated or exercising excessively during hot weather.
- Instruct the patient to avoid driving or operating hazardous equipment if dizziness, light-headedness, or blurred vision develop.
- Emphasize to patients with diabetes that it is important to monitor blood glucose carefully at the start of therapy and during periods of dosage adjustment. A change in diet or insulin may be required; check with the physician. Review with the patient the signs of hypoglycemia, including fast heart rate, cold sweats, headache, hunger, nausea, nervousness, shakiness, unsteady walk, and anxious feeling. Instruct the patient to eat or drink a food containing sugar if any of these symptoms develop and to notify the physician.
- Instruct patients taking extended-release capsules or tablets to swallow the dose whole, without chewing, crushing, or breaking the medication.
- See the patient problem boxes on dry mouth (xerostomia) (p. 300), orthostatic hypotension (p. 157), and constipation (p. 304). Instruct the patient to report any difficulty urinating.

Continued.

NURSING IMPLICATIONS SUMMARY—cont'd

Moricizine

- See the general guidelines for antiarrhythmic therapy.
- Caution the patient to avoid driving or operating hazardous equipment if dizziness develops. Instruct the patient to notify the physician if dizziness develops.
- Instruct the patient to take a missed dose as soon as remembered if within 4 hours of when the dose was due; otherwise the patient should omit the missed dose and resume the regular dosing schedule.

Quinidine

Drug Administration

- See the general guidelines for antiarrhythmic therapy.
- Read medication labels carefully; do not confuse quinidine with quinine.
- Monitor liver function tests, blood count, platelet count, serum electrolyte levels, and prothrombin time.
- A test dose may be ordered before the full dose is given to test for possible idiosyncrasy to quinidine.
- Assess for rash or skin changes.
- IM injections may be painful and may increase serum creatine phosphokinase (creatine phosphokinase [CPK] or creatine kinase [CK]) levels.

Intravenous Administration

- Dilute 800 mg (10 ml) in at least 40 ml of 5% dextrose in water (D5W). Do not add to IV solutions or mix with other drugs in a syringe. Administer at a rate of 1 ml (16 mg)/min. Monitor ECG changes and blood pressure.
- IV quinidine may be used in treatment of life-threatening malaria; see Chapter 48.

Patient and Family Education

- See the general guidelines for antiarrhythmic therapy.
- Instruct the patient to take doses with full (8 ounce) glass of water on an empty stomach, 1 hour before or 2 hours after meals. If gastric irritation develops, instruct the patient to take doses with meals. Encourage the patient to take all doses the same way, either with or without food and to notify the physician if diarrhea develops.
- Remind patients taking extended-release tablets to swallow the tablet whole without breaking, chewing, or crushing it.
- Review with the patient the symptoms of cinchonism such as ringing in the ears, headache, nausea, or changes in vision. Instruct the patient to notify the physician if these occur.
- Warn the patient to avoid driving or operating hazardous equipment if visual changes occur and to notify the physician if these symptoms occur.
- Patients may develop a bitter taste in the mouth. There is little that can be done for this, but caution the patient not to discontinue the drug without consulting with the physician.
- Review the patient problem boxes on bleeding tendencies (p. 586) and depressed white blood cell count (leukopenia) (p. 585) with the patient.
- Instruct the patients to report the development of any unexpected sign or symptom.
- Instruct the patient to take a missed dose as soon as remembered if within 2 hours of when scheduled; otherwise the patient should omit the missed dose and resume the regular dosing schedule.

Procainamide

Drug Administration

- See the general guidelines for antiarrhythmic therapy.
- Monitor antinuclear antibody (ANA) test and complete blood count.

Intravenous Administration

- For direct IV injection, dilute each 100 mg with 5 to 10 ml of D5W or sterile water. Administer at a rate of 20 mg/min. For infusion, add 1 gm to 500 ml D5W for a dilution of 2 mg/ml; other dilutions may be used. Use microdrip tubing and/or an infusion control device, and infuse at a rate of 2 to 6 mg/min.

Patient and Family Education

- See the general guidelines for antiarrhythmic therapy.
- Doses are best taken on an empty stomach with a full (8 ounce) glass of water 1 hour before or 2 hours after meals. Instruct the patient to take doses consistently with meals or on an empty stomach. However, if GI symptoms are severe, instruct the patient to take doses with meals.
- Instruct patients taking extended-release formulations to swallow the medication whole without crushing or breaking it.
- Instruct the patient to report the development of arthritis, polyarthralgia, pleuritic pain, myalgia, skin lesions, fever, or any other new sign or symptom.
- Caution the patient to avoid driving or operating hazardous equipment if dizziness develops and to notify the physician if dizziness occurs.
- Instruct the patient to take a missed dose as soon as remembered if within 2 hours of when the dose was scheduled (4 hours for sustained-release preparations); otherwise the patient should omit the missed dose and resume the regular dosage schedule.

NURSING IMPLICATIONS SUMMARY—cont'd

- Caution the patient that the matrix from extended-release tablets may be seen in the stool and that this situation is normal.

Lidocaine

Drug Administration

- See the general guidelines for antiarrhythmic therapy.
- Lidocaine is rarely used outside of the short-term care setting. Keep the patient and family informed of the patient's condition.
- Assess for the side effects noted in the text. Instruct the patient to report any subjective changes.

Intramuscular Administration

- Read drug labels carefully. Lidocaine with epinephrine is not given as an antiarrhythmic. Administer IM doses into the deltoid muscle. IM injection may cause elevations in the CPK or CK levels.

Intravenous Administration

- Read drug labels carefully. Lidocaine with epinephrine is not used as an antiarrhythmic. Label must state "for IV use." Bolus doses may be given undiluted at a rate of 50 mg/min; too rapid administration may cause seizures. For continuous infusion, dilute per agency protocol or consult manufacturer's literature. Premixed forms are available. Use microdrip tubing and/or an infusion control device, and adjust dose to patient response.

Patient and Family Education

- Selected patients may be discharged with lidocaine for self-injection. A patient instruction leaflet is provided with the drug. Review this carefully with the patient. If used correctly, the patient will remove the protective cap, place the device against the thigh, and press the device against the thigh. The medication will be injected. Verify that the patient knows the symptoms of heart attack and when to call the physician. The self-injection should not be used unless the patient is instructed to use it by the physician. After using the device, the patient should go to the physician's office or emergency department. The patient should not drive, but a family member or friend should drive the patient.

Mexiletene

Drug Administration

- See the general guidelines for antiarrhythmic therapy.
- Monitor aspartate transaminase (AST, serum glutamic-oxaloacetic transaminase [SGOT]) white blood cell count, white blood cell differential, and platelet count.
- Assess the patient for ataxia, slurred speech, ringing in the ears, and development of CNS side effects.

Patient and Family Education

- See the patient problem boxes on bleeding tendencies (p. 586) and depressed white blood cell production (p. 585). Instruct the patient to report the development of these rare but serious side effects.
- Caution the patient to avoid driving or operating hazardous equipment if dizziness or blurred vision develop and to notify the physician if these symptoms occur.
- Remind the patient to take doses with meals or a snack to lessen gastric irritation.
- Instruct the patient to take a missed dose as soon as remembered if within 4 hours of when the dose was due; otherwise the patient should omit the missed dose and resume the regular dosing schedule.

Tocainide

Drug Administration

- See the general guidelines for antiarrhythmic therapy.
- Assess regularly for skin changes or rashes. Auscultate breath sounds and assess respiratory rate. Assess for tremor.

Patient and Family Education

- See the general guidelines for antiarrhythmic therapy.
- Instruct the patient to take doses with food or milk to lessen gastric irritation.
- Explain that the patient should notify the physician immediately if rashes, skin changes, peeling or scaling of skin, blisters on skin or mouth, cough, or shortness of breath develops.
- Caution the patient to avoid driving or operating hazardous equipment if dizziness, light-headedness, confusion, or visual changes develop; instruct the patient to notify the physician if these symptoms occur.
- Instruct the patient to take missed dose as soon as remembered if within 4 hours of when scheduled; otherwise the patient should omit the missed dose and resume the regular dosage schedule.
- See the patient problem box on bleeding tendencies (p. 586).

Flecainide

Drug Administration/Patient and Family Education

- See the general guidelines for antiarrhythmic therapy.
- Caution the patient to avoid driving or operating hazardous equipment if dizziness or visual changes develop and to notify the physician if these symptoms occur.
- Instruct the patient to take a missed dose as soon as remembered if within 6 hours of when scheduled; otherwise the patient should omit the missed dose and resume the regular dosing schedule.
- Instruct the patient to notify the physician if jaundice, trembling, or chest pain develops.

Continued.

Nursing Implications Summary—cont'd

Propafenone

Drug Administration/Patient and Family Education

- See the general guidelines for antiarrhythmic therapy.
- Caution the patient to avoid driving or operating hazardous equipment if dizziness, blurred vision, or lightheadedness develop and to notify the physician if these symptoms occur.
- Review the patient problem boxes on dry mouth (p. 300) and constipation (p. 304).
- Some patients develop a metallic taste in the mouth. If the patient is unable to tolerate this side effect, consult the physician. Remind the patient not to discontinue medication without consulting the physician. Monitor weight.
- Instruct the patient to take a missed dose as soon as remembered if within 4 hours of the scheduled time; otherwise the patient should omit the missed dose and resume the regular dosage schedule.

Esmolol

Drug Administration/Patient and Family Education

- See the general guidelines for antiarrhythmic therapy.
- Esmolol is rarely used outside of the short-term care setting. Keep the patient and family informed of the patient's condition.

Intravenous Administration

- Esmolol may be given undiluted for the loading dose; use only the 10 mg/ml concentration. Administer the dose as ordered (there may be one dose for the first minute, followed by a lower dose for 4 minutes.)
- For infusion, dilute 5 gm with 20 ml of compatible IV fluid (see manufacturer's instructions) then further dilute with 480 ml of the same fluid. This makes a concentration of 10 mg/ml. Use microdrip tubing or an infusion control device to prevent overdose and keep administration rate steady. Monitor ECG changes and blood pressure.
- Monitor the patient for signs of toxicity described in text.

Amiodarone

Drug Administration

- See the general guidelines for antiarrhythmic therapy.
- Assess breath sounds and respiratory rate for signs of pulmonary toxicity.
- Assess visual acuity at the start of therapy.

Patient and Family Education

- See the general guidelines for antiarrhythmic therapy. Review the common side effects. Instruct the patient to report the development of respiratory difficulties, weakness, numbness, or ataxia.
- Review the patient problem box on photosensitivity (p. 649). Patients receiving amiodarone who develop photosensitivity may be sensitive to sunlight coming through windows.
- Instruct the patient to report subjective visual or eye changes. Encourage patients who wear glasses to continue periodic ophthalmic examinations.
- Warn the patient that the skin may turn a bluish gray color but the discoloration should fade when therapy is discontinued. Instruct the patient to notify the physician if skin color begins to change.
- Review the patient problem box on constipation (p. 304).
- Some patients develop a metallic taste in the mouth. If the patient is unable to tolerate this side effect, consult the physician. Remind the patient not to discontinue medication without consulting the physician. Monitor weight.
- Instruct the patient not to take a missed dose and not to double the next one but to go back to the regular dosing schedule. If two or more doses are missed, the patient should contact the physician.

Bretylium

Drug Administration

- See the general guidelines for antiarrhythmic therapy.

Intramuscular Administration

- Administer in large muscle masses. Record and rotate injection sites. Do not dilute. Do not administer more than 5 ml into a single injection site; if a larger volume is ordered, divide the dose into two equal volumes for injection into two sites.

Intravenous Administration

- Bretylium may be given undiluted, one dose over 1 minute or less.
- For intermittent infusion, dilute drug in at least 50 ml of diluent or use commercially prepared diluted solutions. Administer dose over 10 to 30 minutes. Too rapid an infusion may contribute to nausea and vomiting.
- For constant infusion, use microdrip tubing and/or an infusion control device.
- Monitor continuous ECG recording and blood pressure. Nausea and vomiting may occur with rapid IV administration.
- Bretylium is rarely used outside of the short-term care setting. Keep the patient and family informed of the patient's condition.

Diltiazem and Verapamil

Drug Administration/Patient and Family Education

- See the general guidelines for antiarrhythmic therapy.
- For additional information about diltiazem and verapamil, see Chapter 15.

Adenosine

Drug Administration/Patient and Family Education

- See the general guidelines for antiarrhythmic therapy.

NURSING IMPLICATIONS SUMMARY—cont'd

Intravenous Administration

- Read drug labels carefully. Do not confuse adenosine with adenosine phosphate.
- Adenosine may be given undiluted and should be given in an injection site as close to the IV insertion site as possible. Administer as a rapid bolus over 1 to 2 seconds. Follow with a rapid normal saline flush (±50 ml) if given via IV line.
- Monitor ECG changes and blood pressure.
- A variety of side effects have been reported but usually last less than 1 minute. These include chest pressure or pain, hyperventilation, hypotension, metallic taste in the mouth, neck or back pain, tight throat, nausea, and premature atrial complex (PACs) or PVCs. Notify the physician of side effects that last longer than 1 minute. Because side effects are short lived, overdose is rarely a problem; however, xanthines are competitive antagonists that may be used if necessary.
- Adenosine is rarely used outside of the short-term care setting. Keep patient and family informed of the patient's condition.

Atropine

Drug Administration/Patient and Family Education

- See the general guidelines for antiarrhythmic therapy, and review the patient care implications for anticholinergic drugs at the end of Chapter 23.
- See the patient problem boxes on dry mouth (p. 300) and constipation (p. 304).

Intravenous Administration

- Atropine may be given undiluted or diluted in at least 10 ml of sterile water. Do not add to infusing fluids or drugs. Administer at a rate of 1 mg or less over 1 minute.

CRITICAL THINKING

APPLICATION

1. What is an action potential?
2. What tissues in the heart are normally automatic?
3. What is the normal pacemaker of the heart?
4. What is the effect of vagus nerve stimulation on the heart?
5. What is the effect of sympathetic stimulation on the heart?
6. What is the refractory period?
7. What is reentry?
8. What is the mechanism of action of quinidine and procainamide?
9. What secondary action do both quinidine and procainamide share?
10. What is the mechanism of action of disopyramide?
11. Flecainide is reserved for what clinical indication? Why?
12. What is the antiarrhythmic effect shared by acebutolol and esmolol?
13. What is the mechanism of action of amiodarone?
14. What are the uses of amiodarone?
15. What is the mechanism of action of bretylium as an antiarrhythmic agent?
16. What is the mechanism of action of verapamil as an antiarrhythmic agent?

CRITICAL THINKING

1. Describe how the waves on an ECG tracing are related to electrical activity of different portions of the heart.
2. What are the classes of antiarrhythmic drugs? On what is the classification based? How would you include this information in teaching plans?
3. How do the toxic effects of quinidine and procainamide differ? How would you assess the patient for them?
4. How does the use of lidocaine differ from that of mexiletine and tocainide?
5. What are the side effects of amiodarone? How would you assess for them?

SECTION V

Drugs Modifying the Blood

CHAPTER 20 *Agents Affecting Blood Coagulation* details blood coagulation and the agents that affect this important process: anticoagulants, antiplatelet drugs, thrombolytic agents, and both local and systemic hemostatic agents. It includes a discussion of hemostatic replacement therapy for hemophilia.

CHAPTER 21 *Drugs to Lower Blood Lipid Levels* focuses on agents used to lower blood cholesterol levels. This subject is important because epidemiologic studies have supported a direct relationship between the level of total serum cholesterol and the rate of coronary heart disease.

CHAPTER 22 *Drugs to Treat Anemia* highlights the medications and other agents used in the prevention and treatment of anemia: iron, vitamin B_{12}, folic acid, and epoetin alpha.

CHAPTER 20

Agents Affecting Blood Coagulation

OBJECTIVES

After studying this chapter, you should be able to do the following:

- *Discuss the groups of drugs used in anticoagulation.*
- *Develop a nursing care plan for patients receiving an anticoagulant.*
- *Identify the antidotes for hemorrhage caused by drug overdose.*
- *Describe the use of antiplatelet therapy, thrombolytic therapy, and hemostatic therapy.*
- *Differentiate between treatments for hemophilia.*
- *Develop nursing care plans, including teaching plans, for patients receiving drugs affecting blood coagulation.*

KEY TERMS

anticoagulant drugs
antiplatelet drugs
antithrombic drugs
blood coagulation
embolus
hemophilia
hemostatic drugs
in vitro
in vivo
thrombocytes
thrombus
transient ischemic attack (TIA)

CHAPTER OVERVIEW

Blood can quickly produce plugs and clots when blood loss is threatened. This chapter describes blood coagulation and drugs and agents used to control it. Anticoagulants interfere with the process of coagulation. Antiplatelet drugs inhibit the aggregation of blood platelets and play a prophylactic role against heart attacks and strokes. Thrombolytic drugs degrade blood clots and can limit the damage of a heart attack. Hemostatic agents aid in promoting blood coagulation.

Therapeutic Rationale: Anticoagulation

Steps in Blood Coagulation

The process of **blood coagulation** is diagrammed in Figure 20-1. The initial step can be in the intrinsic pathway with the activation of the blood component factor XII (the Hageman factor) by contact with exposed collagen or an event in the extrinsic pathway (e.g., the release of tissue factor by damaged tissue). Either pathway results in the activation of factor X. Factor Xa (activated factor X) forms a complex with platelet phospholipids, calcium, and factor V. This complex, which is sometimes called *thromboplastin,* catalyzes the conversion of prothrombin (factor II) to thrombin. Thrombin then catalyzes the conversion of fibrinogen to fibrin. After cross-linking of fibrin by factor XIIIa, fibrin becomes insoluble, forming a mesh that is the blood clot, also called a **thrombus.**

Blood clots in the arterial system are initially composed largely of platelets with a fibrin mesh (white thrombus). Blood clots in the venous system have only a few platelet aggregates and are composed largely of fibrin with trapped red blood cells (red thrombus). A thrombus in the arterial or venous system may dislodge, becoming an **embolus.** Venous emboli often lodge in the small arteries of the pulmonary circulation, thereby markedly blocking the oxygenating capacity of the lungs and increasing the blood pressure in the pulmonary system, a life-threatening situation. Thrombi form in veins in which blood flow is low, favoring the accumulation of activated clotting factors. Patients at risk for experiencing venous thrombosis include those immobilized as a result of trauma or surgery and those with a history of thromboembolism.

Role of Calcium in Blood Coagulation

Calcium is a cofactor for each of the steps through the activation of prothrombin. The removal of calcium prevents the coagulation of blood. Citrate and ethylenediaminetetraacetic acid (EDTA) are compounds that complex calcium, making calcium unavailable for blood coagulation. When blood is drawn for testing or storage, citrate or EDTA may be used to keep the blood from clotting in the container. Since calcium is essential for many biochemical events, anticoagulants that complex calcium can be used only in storage containers (**in vitro**), not in a patient (**in vivo**).

Mechanisms for Anticoagulant and Antiplatelet Drugs

Anticoagulant drugs interfere with any of the steps depicted in Figure 20-1, leading to the formation of fibrin. Blood coagulation is often referred to as a *cascade phenomenon,* since the process becomes magnified at every step. Each activated factor is a catalyst leading to the formation of many molecules of the next activated factor. The earlier in the process that a step can be blocked, the more efficient is the inhibition of blood coagulation.

Therapeutic Agents: Anticoagulant and Antiplatelet Drugs

Anticoagulant drugs prevent clot formation; they do not affect existing clots. They can be classified into two groups: the drug heparin and oral anticoagulants. Antiplatelet drugs inhibit the aggregation of platelets and inhibit coagulation in the arterial system.

HEPARIN

Heparin (Calciparine; Liquaemin) is an anticoagulant that can either be administered to the patient (Table 20-1) or added to a storage container.

Mechanism of Action

Heparin activates a plasma protein, antithrombin III, which neutralizes thrombin. However, antithrombin III also neutralizes factor Xa, the step before the activation of prothrombin to thrombin. This inhibition of factor Xa, rather than the inhibition of thrombin, appears to be primarily responsible for the effective anticoagulant action of heparin in low doses. Heparin is also an antiplatelet drug. In vitro, heparin stimulates platelet aggregation. In vivo, however, heparin appears to coat the endothelial lining of the vessels. Since heparin is a highly negatively charged polymer, it adds a negative charge to the endothelium that keeps platelets from attaching and forming a thrombus.

Pharmacokinetics

Heparin is administered intravenously or by deep subcutaneous injection. Heparin is active within minutes and has a plasma half-life of 1 to 2 hours. Low doses of heparin are taken up by mast cells. High doses are excreted in the urine.

Uses

The clinical uses of heparin differ in dose and route of administration. It achieves anticoagulation (in high doses), prevents postoperative thromboembolism (in low doses), and prevents coagulation of laboratory samples and stored blood in vitro.

High-dose administration. Heparin is used in the hospital to prevent the further growth of venous thrombi. Large doses (35 to 100 U/kg) must be administered intravenously to achieve this anticoagulation. Heparin cannot be taken orally, since it is not absorbed and causes a painful hematoma if administered intramuscularly. Heparin may be given as an intravenous (IV) injection, achieving immediate anticoagulation, with the same or lesser dose repeated every 4 to 6 hours. Blood levels of heparin decrease by half every 1½ hours. Intermittent IV administration results in virtual incoagulability after administration and is associated with a higher risk of bleeding than continuous IV infusion. Thus an initial IV injection followed by continuous infusion at approximately 1000 U/hr is commonly given. An IV drip must be carefully

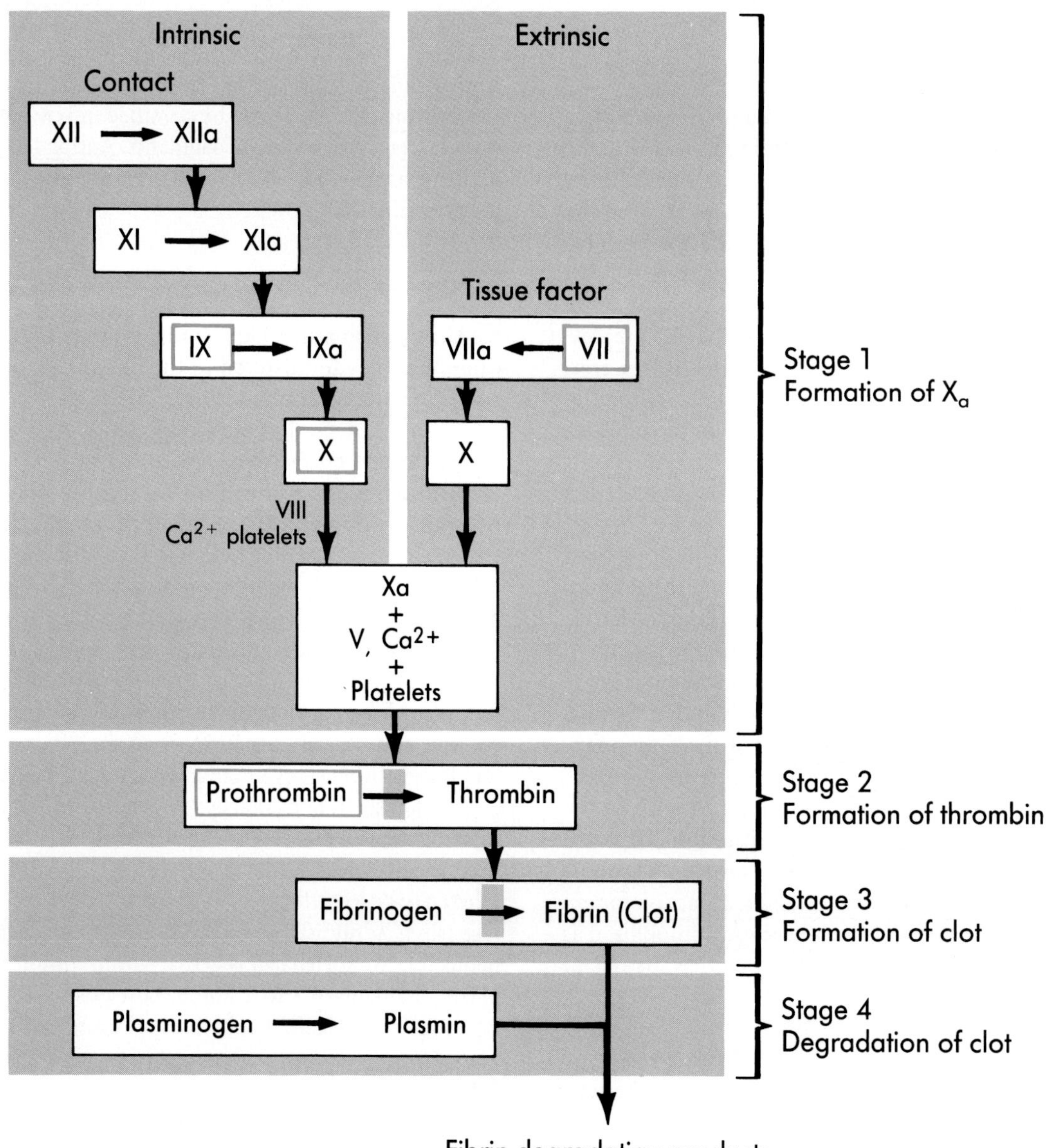

FIGURE 20-1

Stages of blood coagulation. Actions of drug classes include four stages: *Stage 1,* Antiplatelet drugs inhibit platelet aggregation in intrinsic pathway. Citrate and EDTA, which chelate calcium, prevent formation of factor Xa. Heparin, by activating antithrombin III, neutralizes factor Xa and stops coagulation at stage 1. Oral anticoagulants prevent synthesis of factors VII, IX, and X, which are necessary for stage 1. Local hemostatic agents provide contact to activate intrinsic pathway. *Stage 2,* Oral anticoagulants prevent synthesis of prothrombin. *Stage 3,* Heparin activates antithrombin III to prevent thrombin activity. *Stage 4,* Aminocaproic acid inhibits activation of profibrinolysin and thus inhibits clot degradation. TPA, streptokinase, and urokinase activate profibrinolysin to aid clot digestion.

TABLE 20-1 Anticoagulant Drugs

GENERIC NAME	TRADE NAME	ADMINISTRATION/DOSAGE	COMMENTS
Heparin	Calciparine* Calcilean† Liquaemin Hepalean†	SUBCUTANEOUS: *Adults*—10,000-20,000 U, then 8000-10,000 U every 8 hr or 15,000-20,000 U every 12 hr. INTRAVENOUS: *Adults—Intermittent*—10,000 U then 5000-10,000 U every 4-6 hr. *Continuous*—20,000-40,000 U daily in 1000 ml. SUBCUTANEOUS: *Adults*—5000 U 2 hr before surgery, then every 8-12 hr until ambulatory. FDA pregnancy category C.	High dose is for therapeutic anticoagulation. Low dose is for prophylaxis of postoperative thromboembolism.
Enoxaparin	Lovenox*	SUBCUTANEOUS: *Adults*—30 mg twice a day for 7-10 days.	Drug is for prophylaxis for postsurgical thrombosis; administer within 24 hr of surgery.
Oral Anticoagulants			
Anisindione	Miradon*	ORAL: *Adults*—300 mg on day 1; 200 mg on day 2; 100 mg on day 3; 25-250 mg daily for maintenance.	Half-life is 3-5 days. Peak effect occurs in 2-3 days. Anticoagulant effect persists 1-3 days after discontinuance. Dermatitis is a side effect. Drug imparts orange color to alkaline urine.
Dicumarol (bishydroxycoumarin)	Generic	ORAL: *Adults*—200-300 mg on day 1; 25-200 mg daily for maintenance.	Dicumarol is prototype oral anticoagulant. Half-life is 1-2 days. Peak effect occurs in 1-4 days. Anticoagulant effect persists 2-10 days after discontinuance. This coumarin is poorly and erratically absorbed.
Warfarin	Coumadinn* Panwarfin Warfilone* Sofarin	ORAL, INTRAMUSCULAR, INTRAVENOUS: *Adults*—10-15 mg daily until prothrombin time is in therapeutic range; 2-10 mg daily for maintenance. Loading dose of 40-60 mg (20-30 mg in older adult patients) may be given initially.	Half-life is 2 days. Peak effect occurs in 1-3 days. Anticoagulant effect persists 4-5 days after discontinuance.

*Available in Canada and United States.
†Available in Canada only.

monitored if used to deliver heparin, or overdosing may result; an infusion monitor is usually used.

Low-dose administration. Heparin may also be given subcutaneously to achieve a slow, continual administration over 8 to 12 hours. Low-dose heparin is used for patients older than 40 years of age undergoing thoracoabdominal surgery who are at increased risk for thrombosis. (Heparin is not used in brain, spinal cord, or eye surgery, in which even minor hemorrhage could be catastrophic. It is not effective in hip replacement surgery.) Heparin is administered subcutaneously (5000 U) 2 hours before thoracoabdominal surgery, and then 5000 U is administered every 8 to 12 hours until the patient is walking. This regimen can reduce the incidence of deep leg vein thrombosis by 50% in thoracoabdominal surgical patients without significantly affecting their bleeding or clotting times. The effectiveness of this therapy results from heparin activating antithrombin III, which in turn rapidly inactivates newly formed factor Xa. After antithrombin III has inactivated factor Xa, the heparin can dissociate from this inactive complex and act again to cause further inactivation.

In vitro use. Heparin prevents the coagulation of blood after it leaves the body. Tubing used to shunt blood can be pretreated with heparin to prevent clotting. The negative charge of the heparin coating on the wall of the tubing that prevents platelet adherence is probably the effective anticoagulant mechanism. Heparin is also added to containers used for blood collection. For transfusions, 4 to 6 U of heparin per milliliter of blood is used. For laboratory samples, 7 to 15 U of heparin per milliliter of blood is used.

Adverse Reactions and Contraindications

Heparin is a natural compound, extracted from animal lungs or intestines. Some patients become allergic to heparin. The usual symptoms of heparin hypersensitivity are chills, fever, and urticaria, but other allergic reactions such as asthma, rhinitis, lacrimation, or anaphylaxis have been reported. In some patients heparin has caused thrombocytopenia; thus the platelet count should be measured daily after therapy.

Toxicity

The major side effect of heparin is hemorrhage. Since the half-life of intravenously administered heparin is only 1½ hours, discontinuing heparin therapy is usually sufficient to reverse a hemorrhagic episode. If hemorrhaging must be stopped immediately, protamine sulfate may be given by slow IV infusion. Protamine sulfate is a highly positively charged molecule that complexes the negatively charged heparin. It is an anticoagulant and has a longer half-life than heparin. Protamine sulfate may persist and cause bleeding after heparin is eliminated. One milligram of protamine sulfate neutralizes 100 U of heparin. No more than 50 mg of protamine sulfate should be administered in 10 minutes.

Enoxaparin

Enoxaparin (Lovenox) is a new, low molecular weight version of heparin that is used to prevent postoperative deep vein thrombosis after hip replacement surgery. Deep subcutaneous injections are begun just after surgery and repeated every 12 hours for 7 to 10 days. Enoxaparin is longer lasting than heparin.

ORAL ANTICOAGULANT DRUGS: GENERAL CHARACTERISTICS

Only three oral anticoagulant drugs are currently in use: dicumarol, warfarin, and anisindione. The first two drugs, dicumarol and warfarin, belong to the coumarin drug class and are often referred to as coumarins.

Coumarins are well tolerated but have two very distinctive features. One is that they bind very tightly to plasma proteins from which they are only slowly released, thereby greatly prolonging their action. The second is that coumarins have a large number of interactions with other drugs that calls for careful monitoring of any drugs the patient is taking.

The third oral anticoagulant is anisindione, which belongs to the indandione drug class. Indandiones can cause a number of side effects and are not widely used.

Mechanism of Action

Clotting factors II (prothrombin), VII, IX, and X are synthesized in the liver, with vitamin K as a necessary cofactor. If vitamin K is deficient, these clotting factors are synthesized in a functionally inactive state, impairing blood coagulation. The coumarins and the indandiones interfere with the regeneration of active vitamin K in the liver and thereby produce vitamin K deficiency. Since the synthesis of functional clotting factors II, VII, IX, and X is inhibited, the anticoagulant effect does not appear until preexisting factors II, VII, IX, and X are removed by normal degradation. This takes 1 day or longer. Factor II, prothrombin, is the longest lived of these clotting factors, and 24 hours are required to deplete half the existing prothrombin. A one-stage prothrombin test frequently determines if the dose of oral anticoagulants is appropriate. Therapeutic doses of the oral anticoagulants increase the prothrombin time (PT) by 1½ to 2½ times the baseline values. Anticoagulant therapy must be individualized for each patient (see Table 20-1).

Pharmacokinetics

Warfarin is the most widely used coumarin. It is the only coumarin that can be administered intramuscularly or intravenously. Warfarin is well absorbed orally. Its peak effect occurs 36 to 72 hours after administration, and the duration of action is 4 to 5 days.

Dicumarol is longer acting than warfarin. The peak action is 3 to 5 days after administration, and the duration of action is up to 10 days. Dicumarol is not well absorbed and causes flatulence and diarrhea.

Anisindione is well absorbed orally. The onset of action is 2 to 3 days, and duration of action after discontinuing therapy is 1 to 3 days.

Protein binding is important to the pharmacokinetics of coumarins. The coumarins stay in the body a long time because they are bound tightly to plasma albumin. This tight binding has several consequences. Only a small amount of the total drug in the body is free to diffuse to the site of action in the liver. The liver also degrades the coumarin to inactive forms that are then excreted in the urine so that only a small amount of the total coumarin is available for degradation. Other drugs can displace coumarins from albumin. This displacement dramatically increases the effective concentration of coumarin. For example, if only 1% of the total coumarin is not bound and displacement causes another 1% to be free, the concentration of free coumarin drug has doubled. The albumin-bound coumarin acts as a reservoir for the drug. After administration is discontinued, several days are required for the drug to dissociate from the albumin and to be degraded by the liver.

Uses

The major indication for the oral anticoagulants is the prophylaxis or treatment for a deep venous or pulmonary thrombus. However, low-dose heparin administered during surgery has significantly reduced the risk of thrombus formation. The oral coumarins were widely used as prophylaxis against myocardial reinfarction, a use never well substantiated by controlled studies. Recently, the number of available oral anticoagulants has dropped to two coumarins, warfarin and dicumarol, and one indandione, anisindione. Anticoagulants that are vitamin K antagonists do not prevent coagulation of blood after it is drawn, because the clotting factors are already synthesized and present.

Adverse Reactions and Contraindications

The principal side effect of oral anticoagulant therapy is hemorrhage, commonly first seen as bleeding of the gingiva. Other signs of overdose include blood in the urine or stools, causing them to turn red, orange, smoky, or black. The drug can be discontinued temporarily when minor hemorrhaging occurs. When hemorrhaging is severe, fresh or frozen plasma may be transfused to replace clotting factors immediately. Less severe hemorrhage can be treated by administering 10 mg (up to 50 mg) of vitamin K_1 phytonadione. This adds excess vitamin K to overcome the block caused by the coumarins. Clotting factors are then again synthesized by the liver, returning the PT to normal in about 24 hours. Side effects other than hemorrhaging are rare.

Anisindione more frequently causes other side effects, including rashes, depression of the bone marrow, hepatitis, and renal damage.

Interactions

Drug interactions are not prominent with anisindione. However, drug interactions are especially numerous with the coumarins, dicumarol and warfarin. Many drugs alter the effectiveness of dicumarol and warfarin. No drug should be added to or deleted from a therapeutic regimen that includes a coumarin without considering drug interactions and appropriately modifying dosages.

The anticoagulant action of both heparin and coumarins is enhanced by drugs that decrease platelet adhesion (e.g., aspirin, clofibrate, dextran, dipyridamole, hydroxychloroquine, ibuprofen, indomethacin, and phenylbutazone). The anticoagulant action of coumarins is enhanced by drugs that inhibit coumarin degradation, such as clofibrate, disulfiram, metronidazole, oxyphenbutazone, phenylbutazone, and trimethoprim; drugs that displace bound anticoagulant, such as chloral hydrate, oxyphenbutazone, and phenylbutazone; and drugs that interact by unknown mechanisms, such as anabolic steroids, cimetidine, D-thyroxine, glucagon, quinidine, and sulfinpyrazone. The anticoagulant action of coumarins is diminished by drugs that accelerate coumarin degradation, such as barbiturates, ethchlorvynol, glutethimide, griseofulvin, and rifampin; drugs that decrease gastrointestinal (GI) tract absorption of coumarins, such as cholestyramine; and drugs that interact by unknown mechanisms, such as 6-mercaptopurine. Dicumarol enhances the action of phenytoin. This list summarizes the major drug interactions but is not exhaustive.

ANTIPLATELET DRUGS: GENERAL CHARACTERISTICS

Mechanism of Action

Platelets (**thrombocytes**) are the small cell fragments in blood derived from giant bone marrow cells called *megakaryocytes*. Ordinarily, platelets do not stick to each other or to the endothelial lining of the blood vessels. When there is a break in the endothelial lining, however, platelets readily attach to the collagen in the exposed tissue. This attachment causes the platelets to aggregate, rapidly forming a plug that stops the bleeding and aids in the formation of a thrombus. This aggregation of platelets in the presence of abnormal surfaces is the initial step in the normal repair system for the blood vessels. Drugs that interfere with this process are termed **antiplatelet** or **antithrombic drugs** (Table 20-2).

In the late 1970s, it was discovered that when the platelets adhere to a surface, they synthesize thromboxane A_2, a substance related to the prostaglandins. Thromboxane A_2 is a potent stimulus for the further aggregation of platelets and thereby accelerates the formation of the platelet plug. Therefore drugs blocking the synthesis of thromboxane A_2 inhibit the aggregation of platelets to form a plug. Aspirin and sulfinpyrazone (Anturane) are inhibitors of thromboxane A_2 synthesis. Dipyridamole (Persantine) and sulfinpyrazone prolong the survival of platelets in persons with thromboembolic diseases so that platelets do not initiate thrombus formation as readily.

Uses

The role of platelet aggregation as the initial step leading to blood coagulation is well established. In particular, the blood clots forming in the arterial system, as opposed to the venous system, are highly linked to conditions promoting platelet aggregation. Patients at risk for developing arterial clots are those who have already had a myocardial infarction (MI) or a stroke. Another established clinical use of antiplatelet drugs is for heart valve prostheses, disorders, and shunts.

SPECIFIC ANTIPLATELETS

Aspirin

Aspirin is the most widely studied antiplatelet drug. It provides effective prophylactic treatment for the following:

- Patients who have experienced a **transient ischemic attack (TIA,** a ministroke) have a decreased incidence of further TIAs, strokes, or death. This is a dramatic effect in men but probably not in women. Sulfinpyrazone and dipyridamole were not effective.
- Patients who have had an MI or who have stable or unstable angina have a decreased incidence of subsequent heart attacks. These results are from studies in men and may not apply to women.

Primary prevention of heart attacks has been demonstrated. Large scale studies in both men and women have shown that taking 325 mg aspirin (1 adult tablet) or less per day is effective in preventing MI, especially in those individuals over 50 years old who have risk factors for atherosclerotic cardiovascular disease (high blood pressure, high cholesterol levels, smoking).

The dose of aspirin may be important to its effectiveness in preventing thrombus formation. A low dose of aspirin (80 to 180 mg/day) inhibits the synthesis of thromboxane A_2 by the platelets. A higher dose of aspirin (1000 mg/day) also inhibits the synthesis of prostacyclin (prostaglandin I_2) by the epithelial lining of the blood vessel. Prostacyclin inhibits the aggregation of platelets, an action directly opposite that of thromboxane A_2. Prostacyclin therefore prevents the formation of a platelet plug. For this reason a high dose of aspirin may be less effective than the low dose in preventing the for-

TABLE 20-2 Antiplatelet Drugs

GENERIC NAME	TRADE NAME	ADMINISTRATION/DOSAGE	COMMENTS
✣ Aspirin	Various	ORAL: *Adults—After transient ischemic attack:* 325 mg with each meal and at bedtime or 650 mg twice a day. *Prosthetic heart valve:* 325 mg with each meal. *Atrioventricular shunt or fistula:* 160 mg with each meal and at bedtime. *Graft patency:* 325 mg after each meal. *Prevention of myocardial infarction (MI) or sudden death in patient with unstable angina:* 325 mg with each meal and at bedtime. *Prevention of recurrent MI or coronary death post-MI:* 325-1300 mg/day.	Taken with a coumarin for prosthetic heart valve. Taken with dipyridamole for graft patency.
✣ Dipyridamole	Persantine* Apo-Dypridamole†	ORAL: *Adults*—400 mg daily. FDA pregnancy category B.	Taken to prevent thrombi formation with prosthetic heart valve or to maintain graft patency. Taken with warfarin for prosthetic heart valve. May also be taken with aspirin for prosthetic heart valve or graft patency.
Sulfinpyrazone	Anturan† Anturane Apo-sulfinpyrazone† Novopyrazone†	ORAL: *Adults*—200 mg 4 times/day.	Taken to prevent thrombi formation with prosthetic heart valve, AV shunt or fistula, mitral stenosis, or to prevent sudden death after MI. Taken with a coumarin for prosthetic heart valve or mitral stenosis.
Ticlopidine	Ticlid*	ORAL: *Adults*—250 mg 2 times/day with food.	Used as prophylaxis for stroke.

*Available in Canada and United States.
†Available in Canada only.

mation of a thrombus. However, for prophylaxis following a TIA, only high doses have been found effective.

✣ Dipyridamole

Dipyridamole (Persantine) combined with warfarin is used for patients with artificial heart valves. It has not been shown effective as prophylaxis in preventing heart attacks or strokes.

Sulfinpyrazone

The effectiveness of sulfinpyrazone (Anturane) as prophylaxis in preventing heart attacks or strokes is not clear.

Ticlopidine

Ticlopidine (Ticlid) is a new drug approved as prophylactic therapy for strokes. It inhibits platelet aggregation irreversibly. The onset of action is about 2 days, and the inhibition of platelet aggregation persists for 1 to 2 weeks. Ticlopidine is somewhat more effective than aspirin but also causes more adverse effects. The most common adverse effects include nausea, vomiting, cramps, or diarrhea. Occasionally a rash or urticaria develops during the first month of therapy. The most serious side effects include bleeding complications, agranulocytosis, leukopenia, or thrombocytopenia.

NURSING PROCESS OVERVIEW

Anticoagulant and Antiplatelet Drugs

Assessment

Anticoagulation *prevents* clot formation; it does not dissolve existing clots. Obtain a history of problems with clots. Assess the patient's mental status, vital signs, and ability to perform activities of daily living. Assess the general physical condition of the patient, including bruising or easy bleeding. Monitor blood coagulation studies, including PT, partial thromboplastin time (PTT), platelet count, and clotting times. Document the presence of any bleeding.

Nursing Diagnoses

- Risk for hemorrhage
- Risk for altered health maintenance related to insufficient knowledge of the implication of anticoagulant or antiplatelet therapy

Patient Outcomes

The patient will not have a TIA, stroke, thromboembolism, or other vascular problem while taking one or more of these drugs as prescribed. The patient will not have side effects caused by any of these drugs.

Planning/Implementation

Assess for bleeding from any site and check stools for occult blood. Evaluate any symptoms signaling possible thrombus formation such as chest or leg pain or any symptom of internal bleeding such as headache. Monitor blood coagulation studies carefully. Use an infusion monitoring device for infusions of heparin and check dosages carefully. Keep antidotes readily available for the drugs being used.

Evaluation

Before discharge, determine that the patient can explain why the drug is needed, how to take or administer the drug, what signs and symptoms of bleeding should be reported, how to avoid injury and bruising, what side effects may be related to the drug but do not involve bleeding, and which additional side effects require notification of the physician. Finally, verify that the patient can state which other drugs, such as aspirin, to avoid while taking anticoagulants.

Therapeutic Rationale: Thrombolytic Drugs

As shown in Figure 20-1, the plasma contains the enzyme plasmin, which degrades the fibrin network of a clot into small, soluble fragments. Plasmin normally exists in an inactive form, plasminogen. Plasminogen is activated to plasmin by various factors in the plasma, primarily tissue plasminogen activator (TPA), which originates in the blood vessel wall. Plasminogen and TPA bind to fibrin, and TPA converts plasminogen to plasmin and plasmin digests fibrin. Degradation products of fibrin act as anticoagulants, thereby limiting further clot formation.

Although the steps in coagulation occur very rapidly, the dissolution of a blood clot may take several days. Drugs to speed the clot dissolution process are widely used. The treatment of choice for an acute MI has become the injection of a clot-dissolving drug as quickly as possible, which prevents the myocardial ischemia that leads to tissue death. Patients can leave the hospital after 3 days instead of 10 and may not require prolonged recovery at home. The drugs available are streptokinase, TPA, and anistreplase (Table 20-3). Thrombolytic therapy is also used in acute pulmonary embolism, deep vein thrombosis, or peripheral arterial occlusion. This therapy helps locally to clear atrioventricular (AV) shunts in patients receiving long-term renal dialysis; however, clotting often recurs.

Therapeutic Agents: Thrombolytic Drugs

Thrombolytic agents are used to dissolve thrombi. They are administered following a heart attack to prevent prolonged myocardial ischemia and are also used to treat pulmonary emboli and deep vein thrombosis. The thrombolytic agents are proteins and must be infused. Except for anistreplase, they are relatively short-acting, 30 minutes or less. Bleeding or its complications are potential side effects of thrombolytic drugs.

✣ Alteplase Recombinant

Alteplase (Activase) is a naturally occurring product produced by recombinant DNA technology. Alteplase is an en-

TABLE 20-3 Thrombolytic Drugs

GENERIC NAME	TRADE NAME	ADMINISTRATION/DOSAGE	COMMENTS
✣ Alteplase, recombinant	Activase Activase rt-PA*	INTRAVENOUS: *Adults*—Initially, bolus of 6-10 mg over 1-2 min, followed by infusion of 60 mg for 1 hr and 20 mg for next 2 hr. For patients weighing <65 kg, total dose is 1.25 mg/kg.	Monitor for arrhythmias, reocclusion.
Antistreplase (APSAC)	Eminase	INTRAVENOUS: *Adults*—30 U injected for 2-5 min.	Monitor for bleeding.
✣ Streptokinase	Kabikinase Streptase*	INTRAVENOUS: *Adults*—Loading dose of 250,000 IU in 30 min, then infusion of 100,000 IU/hr. Dosage is continued for 24-72 hr for pulmonary embolism and for 72 hr for deep vein embolism. *For coronary thrombosis:* INTRAVENOUS: *Adults*—1.5 million IU, administered within 1 hr. INTRAARTERIAL (via coronary artery catheter)—20,000 IU initially, followed by 2000 IU/min for 1 hr.	Monitor thrombin times every 12 hr. Allergic reactions are common (15% of patients); usually of milder variety (itching, flushing, nausea, headache). Treat with antihistamines.
Urokinase	Abbokinase* Open-Cath	INTRAVENOUS: *Adults*—Loading dose of 4400 IU/kg in 10 min by infusion, then 4400 IU/kg for 12 hr. FDA pregnancy category B.	Isolated from human urine. Not as allergenic as streptokinase.

*Available in Canada and United States.

zyme that binds to fibrin, is activated, and catalyzes conversion of plasminogen to plasmin. Plasmin is the enzyme that degrades fibrin, dissolving a thrombus (clot). Alteplase is most effective if administered within 6 hours of a heart attack. It is effective in promoting thrombus reduction in 2 hours. Unbound alteplase is rapidly cleared by the liver.

Anistreplase

Anistreplase (APSAC [anisoylated plasminogen-streptokinase activator complex], Eminase)is a complex of streptokinase and human plasminogen. The human plasminogen has been modified with a blocking group so that it is not readily activated. The injected complex binds to the fibrin of a clot, and the plasminogen slowly loses its blocking group and is activated by streptokinase. This happens at a controlled rate and at the fibrin network of the clot. Anistreplase is active for about 6 hours.

✣ Streptokinase

Streptokinase (Streptase) is isolated from group C beta-hemolytic streptococci; it acts by forming a complex with plasminogen to activate it. Streptokinase is antigenic and may cause allergic reactions. The cost of streptokinase treatment is about one tenth that of alteplase or anistreplase and appears to be as effective in treating coronary thrombosis.

Urokinase

Urokinase (Abbokinase) is isolated from human urine; it is an enzyme that cleaves plasminogen to plasmin. Urokinase treats thromboembolisms but not coronary thrombosis.

NURSING PROCESS OVERVIEW

Thrombolytic Drugs

Thrombolytic drugs have revolutionized the treatment of MI and other problems caused by clots. They promote the digestion of fibrin, thereby dissolving the clot.

Assessment

Anticoagulant therapy prevents clots, and thrombolytic therapy dissolves clots. Both alter the normal coagulation mechanism to cause anticoagulation. Obtain a history of the presenting problem. Assess vital signs and blood pressure. Assess mental status and neurologic status. Assess the size and location of the clot and the signs and symptoms caused by the clot. Assess for a recent patient history of streptococcal infection since this would influence the choice of agents.

Nursing Diagnoses

- Risk for arrhythmias (reperfusion arrhythmias)
- Risk for hemorrhage/excessive bleeding

Patient Outcomes

The nurse will manage and minimize arrhythmic episodes or hemorrhage. The clot will be successfully lysed, and the patient will experience no lasting side effects from the clot or the medications used to lyse it.

Planning/Implementation

Use systemic thrombolytic drugs only in short-term care settings. Monitor patients for signs of clot dissolution and hemorrhage.

Monitor the usual tests for blood coagulation and check the hematocrit level daily because it may drop even when bleeding is not present. Use an infusion monitoring device for infusions. Have available appropriate drugs to control bleeding, such as aminocaproic acid.

Evaluation

If effective, a thrombolytic drug dissolves the existing clot without causing hemorrhage. Patients are not discharged while still receiving systemic thrombolytic therapy.

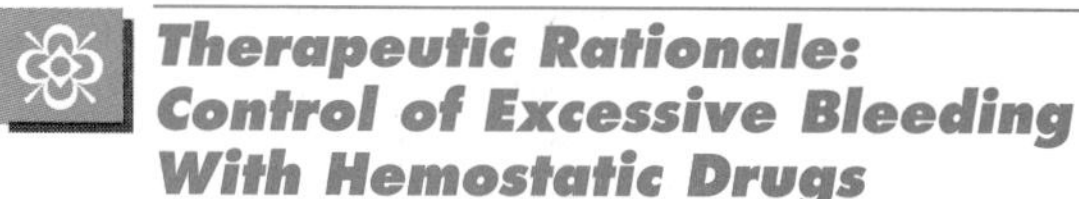

Therapeutic Rationale: Control of Excessive Bleeding With Hemostatic Drugs

Hemostatic drugs are systemic or local agents used to control excessive bleeding. Specialized biologic hemostatics are used to control bleeding episodes in individuals with hemophilia (see Table 20-4).

Therapeutic Agents: Systemic Hemostatic Drugs

Aminocaproic Acid

Aminocaproic acid (Amicar) inhibits the activation of profibrinolysin (plasminogen) to the active enzyme fibrinolysin (plasmin). The lack of fibrinolysin inhibits dissolution of blood clots. Aminocaproic acid is used in instances in which it is desirable to protect blood clots, such as surgery on the prostate, after a ruptured cerebral aneurysm, or for patients with hemophilia after a tooth extraction.

Aminocaproic acid can be given orally or intravenously. It is rapidly excreted in the urine. Side effects are transient and minor and include nausea, cramps, dizziness, headache, ringing in the ear, or stuffy nose. When IV therapy is used, aminocaproic acid can irritate the veins and give rise to thrombophlebitis. This effect may be minimized by diluting the drug before use and by carefully placing the needle.

Tranexamic Acid

Tranexamic acid (Cyklokapron), like aminocaproic acid, inhibits the activation of plasminogen to the active enzyme plasmin. Tranexamic acid also directly inhibits plasmin. As an antifibrinolytic agent, it is 5 to 10 times more potent than aminocaproic acid. The major indication for the drug is in patients with hemophilia undergoing dental surgery.

Patients receiving tranexamic acid should be monitored for signs of thromboembolic complications. If they are to receive the drug for more than a few days, they should also receive an ophthalmologic examination; animal studies have indicated that high doses of the drug can cause focal areas of retinal degeneration. More frequent side effects are GI tract upsets, including diarrhea, nausea, and vomiting. Tranexamic acid is eliminated largely unchanged in the urine.

Vitamin K

Vitamin K is a fat-soluble vitamin required for the synthesis of clotting factors II, VII, IX, and X in the liver. Vitamin K is contained in many foods. Humans cannot synthesize vitamin K, but bacteria in the GI tract can synthesize vitamin K for absorption by the host. Conditions that can produce vitamin K deficiency include the following:

- Long-term IV feeding
- Debilitation resulting from poor diet
- Prolonged oral antibiotic therapy
- Malabsorption syndrome
- Acute diarrhea in infants
- Biliary disease

In addition, the oral anticoagulant drugs produce a relative vitamin K deficiency by inhibiting the reactivation of vitamin K.

Vitamin K is available as vitamin K_1 (phytonadione) and vitamin K_4 (menadiol) for replacement therapy, but only phytonadione is effective as an antidote for severe bleeding episodes caused by an overdose of one of the oral anticoagulants. Vitamin K is safest when taken orally. IV injection must be made slowly with a dilute solution and even then may cause a severe reaction. Reactions to IV injection include flushing, a heavy feeling on the chest, sweating, vascular collapse, and an anaphylactic reaction. Intramuscular (IM) and subcutaneous administration may cause pain and bleeding at the injection site.

In infants and anyone with a deficiency of the enzyme, glucose-6-phosphate dehydrogenase, menadiol can produce hemolysis but phytonadione does not. These vitamins do not promote clotting in a patient with liver disease or a hereditary deficiency of one of the vitamin K–dependent clotting factors.

Therapeutic Agents: Local Absorbable Hemostatic Drugs

Local absorbable hemostatics provide a surface that promotes platelet adhesion and thereby promotes blood clotting where the agent is applied (Table 20-4).

Absorbable Gelatin Sponge: Gelfoam

Gelfoam is a sterile absorbable gelatin sponge that is moistened with sterile saline solution and applied to bleeding capillary beds that cannot be readily sutured. It is absorbed in 4 to 6 weeks.

Absorbable Gelatin Film: Gelfilm

Gelfilm is a thin, sterile absorbable gelatin film used in neurologic, thoracic, and ocular surgery to repair membrane surfaces. Reabsorption may take from 1 week to 6 months, depending on the size and site of the film.

Oxidized Cellulose

Oxidized cellulose (Oxycel) and oxidized regenerated cellulose (Surgicel) are used much like the absorbable gelatin sponge. They interfere with bone regeneration and therefore cannot be packed around fractures. Oxycel retards formation of new skin and cannot be used as a surface dressing. Small implants are reabsorbed in 1 week, but large ones may require 6 weeks for reabsorption.

Microfibrillar Collagen Hemostat

Microfibrillar collagen hemostat (Avitene)is a water-insoluble powder that is applied to a bleeding surface to activate natural clotting. The collagen is absorbed in 7 weeks. Microfibrillar collagen is used during surgery to control bleeding in capillary beds, liver, and skin graft sites. It does not interfere with the healing of skin or bone. Microfibrillar collagen must be kept dry and cannot be resterilized after the container is opened.

Thrombin

Thrombin is an activated clotting factor (see Figure 20-1). Thrombin is applied topically only as a sterile protein powder to bleeding surfaces. It must be kept cold and dry until use or it becomes inactive. Thrombin can be applied topically as a solution; however, it is important to note that it must not be injected.

Therapeutic Agents: Hemostatic Drugs for Replacement Therapy for Hemophilia

Hemophilia is an inherited disorder in which there is a deficiency of one of the factors necessary for coagulation of the blood. Hemophilia A, or classic hemophilia, is a deficiency of factor VIII, which is important in the activation of factor X. Hemophilia A is inherited as an X-linked recessive disorder and is seen almost exclusively in boys and men. Hemophilia B, or Christmas disease, is an inherited X-linked recessive disorder characterized by a deficiency of factor IX. Von Willebrand's disease is a non–sex-linked (autosomal) codominant disorder in which von Willebrand's factor is decreased or abnormal. Von Willebrand's factor is important for the adhesion of platelets to the blood vessels and as a carrier for factor VIII.

Antihemophilic Factor

There are several methods of isolating factor VIII from human plasma. A unit of antihemophilic factor (AHF) may represent a pool from as many as 25,000 donors because of the viral inactivation steps now needed. (It is estimated that 80% of patients with severe hemophilia are human immunodeficiency virus [HIV] positive because of contaminated supplies of antihemophilic factor from the early 1980s.) Cryoprecipi-

TABLE 20-4 Hemostatic Agents

GENERIC NAME	TRADE NAME	ADMINISTRATION/DOSAGE	COMMENTS
Systemic Hemostatic Agents			
Aminocaproic acid	Amicar*	ORAL, INTRAVENOUS: *Adults*—5-6 gm initially orally or by slow IV infusion, then 1 gm hourly or 6 gm every 6 hr. Maximum in 24 hr is 30 gm. Reduced dosage is used with low renal output or renal disease. *Children*—100 mg/kg body weight every 6 hr for 6 days.	Prevents activation of plasminogen (fibrinolysis) so that blood clots are not broken down. Used in special surgical situations.
Phytonadione (vitamin K_1)	AquaMEPHYTON Konakion* Mephyton	ORAL, INTRAMUSCULAR, SUBCUTANEOUS: *Adults and children*—2.5-25 mg. INTRAMUSCULAR, SUBCUTANEOUS, INTRAVENOUS: *Newborns*—0.5-1 mg immediately after birth. Alternatively, mother is given 1-5 mg 12-24 hr before delivery.	IV route can be dangerous. Use only in emergencies for oral anticoagulant overdose, and dilute so that no more than 1 mg is given per min. Subcutaneous and IM injection may be painful.
Menadiol sodium diphosphate (vitamin K_4)	Synkayvite*	ORAL, INTRAMUSCULAR, SUBCUTANEOUS, INTRAVENOUS: *Adults*—5-15 mg once or twice daily. *Children*—5-10 mg once or twice daily.	Used to correct secondary hypoprothrombinemia. Converted to menadione (vitamin K_3) in body.
Tranexamic acid	Cyklokapron*	ORAL: *Adults and children*—25 mg/kg 3 or 4 times day before surgery and 2-8 days after surgery. INTRAVENOUS: *Adults and children*—10 mg/kg before surgery, administered with factor VIII or IX, and 10 mg/kg 3 or 4 times daily for 2-8 days after surgery. FDA pregnancy category B.	Indicated use is for patients with hemophilia who are undergoing dental surgery.
Local Hemostatic Agents			
Absorbable gelatin sponge	Gelfoam	Blocks and cones of various sizes. Also sterile (surgical) and nonsterile (dental) powder.	Used to control bleeding in wound or at operative site.
Absorbable gelatin film	Gelfilm	Thin film strips.	Used to repair membranes in neural, thoracic, and ocular surgery.
Oxidized cellulose	Oxycel*	Type of gauze pads or strips. Also as sponges 2 × 1 × 1 inch.	Used to control hemorrhage and absorb blood. May be left in wound. Not for packing around bone fractures or to be left on skin.
Oxidized regenerated cellulose	Surgicel	Knitted fabric strips.	Used like oxidized cellulose, but may be left on skin.
Microfibrillar collagen hemostat	Avitene	Sterile powder. 1 gm should cover 50 × 50 cm (20 × 20 inches) to control light bleeding.	Used to control bleeding in wound or at operative site. May be used on skin. Discard unused material since it cannot be resterilized.
Thrombin	Fibrindex Thrombin, topical	Sterile powder. Packaged by units. May be dissolved in sterile saline solution and applied in absorbable gelatin sponge.	Used to control bleeding in wound or at a operative site. Discard unused material since it cannot be resterilized and solution is unstable.
Replacement Therapy for Hemophilia			
Antihemophilic factor—human	Hemofil M Koate-HP Profilate OSD Others	INTRAVENOUS: *Adults and children*—Usually single dose of 15-20 U/kg given at rate of 10-15 ml/min maintains activities sufficient for clotting.	There are four different methods of purifying factor VIII from plasma.
Cryoprecipitated antihemophilic factor—human		INTRAVENOUS: *Adults and children*—Usually single dose of 15-20 U/kg given at rate of 10-15 ml/min maintains activities sufficient for clotting.	This product is prepared by hospital blood bank. Thaw in water bath at 37°C; keep at room temperature and use within 3 hr.
Antihemophilic factor (AHF)—porcine	Hyate:C	INTRAVENOUS: *Adults and children*—Initially, 100-150 U/kg. If this is insufficient, second larger dose should then be given, followed by third dose if necessary.	This product is purified freeze-dried concentrate of AHF from pig. It can be used for patients who have developed antibodies to human product.

*Available in Canada and United States.

TABLE 20-4 Hemostatic Agents—cont'd

GENERIC NAME	TRADE NAME	ADMINISTRATION/DOSAGE	COMMENTS
Replacement Therapy for Hemophilia—cont'd			
Antithrombin III	ATnativ Thrombate III	INTRAVENOUS: *Adults and children*—Initially, 50-100 U/min is administered over 5-10 min. Final dosage is determined by level of deficiency, response, and weight of patient.	Anticoagulant to treat thromboembolism associated with hereditary antithrombin III deficiency. It is prepared from human plasma to be free of human immunodeficiency virus and hepatitis B and is heat treated.
✣ Desmopressin	DDAVP Stimate	INTRAVENOUS: *Adults and children*—0.3 μg/kg is infused slowly over 15-30 min. Dosage should not be repeated within 24 hr.	This synthetic analogue of arginine vasopressin is used for short-term hemostatic control in patients with mild or moderate factor VIII deficiency and in those with type I von Willebrand's disease.
Factor IX complex human	Konyne-80 Profilnin, heat treated	INTRAVENOUS: *Adults and children*—For non–life-threatening bleeding in patients with hemophilia who have factor VIII inhibitors, 75 U/kg is initial dose, repeated in 8-12 hr if necessary.	Factor IX complex treats bleeding associated with Christmas disease or deficiency of one or more of the other factors in this preparation (factors II, VII, and X).

tated AHFs are made from the plasma of one unit of whole blood. This product may be kept frozen for about 1 year.

Factor VIII, produced by recombinant DNA technology, is currently being tested clinically. Availability of factor VIII from a source other than the blood supply would eliminate the risk of blood-transmitted diseases such as HIV and hepatitis.

Antithrombin III, Human

A deficiency of antithrombin III is seen in several thousand Americans and results in an increased risk of thromboembolic diseases and venous thrombosis, especially after surgery and obstetric procedures. Antithrombin III (AT-III) is now prepared from plasma tested and treated to exclude viruses.

✣ Desmopressin

Desmopressin (DDAVP, Stimate) temporarily increases the concentrations of factor VIII and von Willebrand's factor. This action controls mild-to-moderate bleeding. Desmopressin is a synthetic analogue of the pituitary hormone, vasopressin.

Adverse reactions to desmopressin may be seen in patients who have certain blood disorders that predispose them to reactions. For this reason, desmopressin should not be used for patients with type IIB of von Willebrand's disease and should be used with caution for patients with coronary artery disease, hypertension, or atherosclerosis or for older adult patients.

Factor IX Complex, Human

Factor IX is derived from human plasma and used to treat bleeding episodes in hemophilia B or factor IX deficiency (Christmas disease). Patients receiving factor IX may experience transient fever, chills, itching, nausea, vomiting, headache, flushing, or tingling. Slow administration can reduce these reactions. Patients, particularly those undergoing surgery, may experience thromboembolic complications.

NURSING PROCESS OVERVIEW

Hemostatic Drugs

Assessment

Assess the type, location, and amount of bleeding; the symptoms related to the bleeding, such as pain, swelling, and level of consciousness; appropriate blood coagulation tests such as PTT, PT, clotting time, platelet count, and hematocrit; and general physical condition of the patient.

Nursing Diagnoses

- Altered health maintenance related to insufficient knowledge of how to manage injectable antihemophilic agent

Patient Outcomes

The patient will become adept at preparing and administering the prescribed injectable agent, will use it appropriately, and will experience less severe bleeding episodes.

Planning/Implementation

Observe the patient for signs that bleeding is stopping and for side effects of the drugs. Overdose with the systemic hemostatic agents is possible; ensure that the patient receives the correct dose. Monitor the appropriate coagulation studies and the hematocrit.

Evaluation

The goal of therapy with hemostatic agents is to stop bleeding without causing side effects resulting from the drug therapy. Many hemostatic agents are discussed in this section. Some are used only in the hospital setting, whereas others would be prescribed for short-term or long-term management by the patient.

NURSING IMPLICATIONS SUMMARY

General Guidelines: Patient Receiving Anticoagulants

Drug Administration

- Inspect the patient twice daily for the appearance of bruising and bleeding.
- Check the patient's stool for guaiac or blood.
- Monitor vital signs at regular intervals. Be alert for signs of hemorrhage such as hypotension, rapid pulse, pale color, or weakness. In pregnant women hemorrhage occurs most often in the third trimester or immediate postpartum period.
- Avoid the use of restraints. If necessary to use them, pad the extremities well and remove the restraints frequently to inspect the area.
- Handle the patient carefully to avoid bruising.
- Have experienced personnel perform venipuncture. Apply pressure to the venipuncture site for 10 minutes after blood is drawn to help prevent bruising.

Patient and Family Education

- Instruct the patient to notify the physician if nosebleeds, bleeding gums, blood in stool or urine, unexplained or severe bruising, severe headache, or stiff neck occurs.
- Suggest that patients wear a medical identification tag or bracelet indicating they are taking anticoagulants.
- Instruct the patient to keep all health care providers, including dentists and oral surgeons, informed of anticoagulant use.
- Tell the patient to avoid using razors with blades and to use electric shavers instead.
- Instruct the patient not to take any medications (except those prescribed) without checking with the physician. This precaution applies especially to aspirin or over-the-counter drugs that might contain aspirin.
- Emphasize to the patient that it is important to brush teeth with a soft-bristle brush if bleeding from gums is prolonged and to avoid flossing. Remind the patient to use water-spray oral care devices on low settings only.
- Instruct the patient not to go barefoot.
- Caution the patient to avoid rough contact activities or sports while taking anticoagulants.

ANTICOAGULANT AND ANTIPLATELET DRUGS

Heparin

Drug Administration

- Review the general guidelines for the patient receiving anticoagulants.
- It is recommended that patients with a history of allergies or asthma receive a test dose of 1000 U before a full dose.
- Monitor blood work before administering doses, especially with high-dose heparin (>15,000 U/24 hr). Some agencies have protocols for monitoring blood work in patients receiving heparin. Monitor activated PTT (aPTT); the goal of anticoagulation therapy is 1.5 to 2.5 times the control in seconds. Other tests that may be monitored include the Lee-White whole blood clotting time (desired level is 2½ to 3 times the control value in minutes) and the activated clotting time (ACT; the desired level is 2 to 3 times the control value). Blood specimens for these tests are usually obtained shortly (½ hour) before an ordered dose is to be administered with intermittent therapy. If laboratory work indicates anticoagulation above the desired range, notify the physician before administering the dose. There will be little or no change in coagulation studies when low-dose heparin is used. With constant infusion, blood will be drawn 1½ to 2 hours after the infusion is begun, and again every 4 hours until stable, then at least daily. Notify the physician immediately if laboratory work indicates anticoagulation above the desired range.
- Monitor platelet count and hematocrit.
- If the patient is receiving heparin and an oral anticoagulant, monitor laboratory work appropriate to both drugs.
- For mild heparin overdose, the physician may simply discontinue heparin until the laboratory findings return to the therapeutic range. Keep protamine sulfate available for treatment of severe overdose (see discussion of toxicity, p. 256). Transfusion of whole blood or plasma may also be ordered for severe overdose; the transfusion dilutes the heparin in the patient's body but does not neutralize it.
- Read medication labels carefully. There are several strengths of heparin available. Check calculations carefully; some institutions require that two nurses check doses of heparin before administration.
- Place a note above the patient's bed (or as is customary in the institution) stating that the patient is receiving heparin therapy so that laboratory personnel will use care to avoid excessive bleeding after venipuncture.
- Avoid IM injections in patients receiving high-dose heparin.

Subcutaneous Administration, Intermittent Doses

- Use any subcutaneous site (see Chapter 5), but the abdomen is preferred because it contains few muscles and bruising is less of a cosmetic problem. Avoid using the arms.
- Keep a record of sites used and rotate sites, even if the abdomen is used for all doses. Avoid the area 2 inches around the umbilicus and any abdominal scars.
- Use careful technique to avoid bruising, but be aware that bruising may occur with even the best technique. Avoid areas that are already bruised. Use a concentrated heparin solution because the smaller volume is less likely to cause bruising.

NURSING IMPLICATIONS SUMMARY—cont'd

- After drawing up the dose, change needles. Pinch the skin and create a subcutaneous "pocket." After careful assessment to avoid injection into a muscle, inject dose into the pocket with a ⅝- to ½-inch 25- to 28-gauge needle at a 45- to 90-degree angle. Do not aspirate the needle before injecting the drug. Do not rub the area after injecting the drug.

Continuous IV Infusion of Heparin

- Use microdrip tubing and/or an electronic infusion monitoring device.
- Prepackaged dilutions of heparin suitable for constant infusion are available, or they may be prepared by the pharmacy. Read medication labels carefully.
- Many drugs are incompatible with heparin. If other IV drugs must be administered, establish a second IV infusion line for these medications, or flush the tubing containing heparin with normal saline before and after administering other medications. Heparin blood levels will be erratic if the heparin infusion is interrupted frequently or for long periods.

Intermittent IV Heparin via Heparin Well or Other Infusion Access Devices

- Insert the heparin well (heparin lock) into the vein with an accepted venipuncture technique and secure the well in place.
- Prime the well with a small amount (1 to 2 ml) of heparin of the same strength that will be used for anticoagulation.
- Inject each dose of heparin into the heparin well. The injected dose displaces the heparin remaining in the well each time a dose is given, so flushing the well after the dose is administered is not necessary. Follow agency procedures if different from those listed.

Other IV Medications via Heparin Well or Heparin-Primed Infusion Access Devices

- Insert the heparin well into the vein with an accepted venipuncture technique, and secure the well in place.
- Prime the heparin well with 1 ml of a solution of normal saline containing 10 or 100 U of heparin per milliliter (as agency policy dictates). Implanted ports may require up to 5 ml; consult the manufacturer's literature. These solutions are available in prepackaged syringes and multiple-dose vials or can be prepared by the nurse or pharmacist. Some institutions use only normal saline for flushing.
- Each time a dose of medication is given, flush the heparin well with 1 to 2 ml of saline (unless there is only saline in the heparin well); administer the prescribed medications via IV push or infusion; flush the well again with 1 to 2 ml of normal saline; finally, flush with 1 ml of the dilute heparin solution. Follow agency procedures if different from those listed.
- Check for patency and correct location of the heparin well before administering heparin or other medications. Assess for pain, tenderness, swelling, or redness. It should be possible to gently aspirate blood from the heparin well. It should be possible to smoothly but slowly inject drugs via the well with no patient discomfort or resistance. If in doubt that the heparin well is patent and in the vein, it should be removed and another one inserted elsewhere.

Patient and Family Education

- See the general guidelines for the patient receiving anticoagulants.
- If heparin is prescribed for home management, instruct the patient in the necessary techniques involved (subcutaneous injection or injection via implanted ports, heparin well, or catheter, and safe disposal of syringes). Provide positive reinforcement and encouragement. Supervise return demonstrations. Refer the patient to a community-based nursing care agency.
- Inform the patient that a variety of side effects may occur and that the physician should be notified immediately if any of the following develop: fast or irregular breathing, shortness of breath, tightness in the chest, skin rash, hives, itching, frequent or persistent erection, or fever. Other side effects include alopecia (hair loss), burning sensation of the feet, myalgia, and bone pain. Encourage the patient to notify the physician of any unusual sign or symptom.
- Instruct the patient to take a missed dose as soon as remembered, unless almost time for the next dose, and then omit the missed dose and resume the regular dosing schedule; do not double up for missed doses since it may cause bleeding. Suggest that the patient keep a record of drug doses and times administered and take the record to the physician at each visit.
- Emphasize the importance of returning for follow-up visits to monitor blood work.

Enoxaparin

Drug Administration

- Review the general guidelines for the patient receiving anticoagulants.
- Monitor baseline blood work before administering the first dose: aPTT, hemoglobin, hematocrit, and platelet count. Enoxaparin should not alter these test results.
- For mild enoxaparin overdose, the physician may simply discontinue the drug until the laboratory findings return to the therapeutic range. Keep protamine sulfate available for treatment of severe overdose (see p. 256).

Continued.

Nursing Implications Summary—cont'd

- Place a note above the patient's bed (or as is customary in the institution) that the patient is receiving enoxaparin therapy so that laboratory personnel will use care to avoid excessive bleeding after venipuncture.

Subcutaneous Administration, Intermittent Doses

- Use any subcutaneous site (see Chapter 5), but the abdomen is preferred because it contains few muscles, and bruising is less of a cosmetic problem. Avoid the arms.
- Keep a record of sites used and rotate sites, even if the abdomen is used for all doses. Avoid the area 2 inches around the umbilicus and any abdominal scars.
- After drawing up the dose, change needles. Pinch the skin and create a subcutaneous "pocket." After careful asessment to avoid injection into a muscle, inject the dose into the pocket with a ⅜- to ½-inch, 25- to 28-gauge needle at a 45- to 90-degree angle. Do not aspirate the needle before injecting the drug. Do not rub the area after injecting the drug.

Patient and Family Education

- See the general guidelines for the patient receiving anticoagulants.
- If enoxaparin is prescribed for home management, instruct the patient in the necessary techniques involved for subcutaneous injection and safe disposal of syringes. Provide positive reinforcement and encouragement. Supervise return demonstrations. Refer patients to a community-based nursing care agency.
- Inform the patient that a variety of side effects may occur and that the physician should be notified immediately if any of the following develop: shortness of breath, tightness in the chest, and fast or irregular heartbeat. Other side effects include increased menstrual bleeding, nausea, and vomiting. Encourage the patient to notify the physician of any unusual sign or symptom.
- Instruct the patient to take a missed dose as soon as remembered, unless within 4 hours of the next dose, and then omit the missed dose and resume the regular dosing schedule; do not double up for missed doses.
- Emphasize the importance of returning for follow-up visits to monitor blood work.

Protamine Sulfate

Drug Administration

- The dose of protamine sulfate is based on the amount of heparin or enoxaparin administered during the preceding 3 to 4 hours. Protamine sulfate injection USP may be given undiluted. Administer intravenously at a rate of 5 mg or less over 1 minute. Do not exceed 50 mg in 10 minutes. The solution may be further diluted for infusion in 5% dextrose in water (D5W) or normal saline.
- Monitor vital signs; protamine sulfate may cause hypotension.
- Warn the patient that flushing and a feeling of warmth may occur.
- Patients receiving protamine zinc insulin may be sensitized to protamine and may experience a severe reaction.
- Keep available appropriate drugs and equipment to treat anaphylactic shock.
- Continue to assess the patient and monitor blood work because the effects of heparin or enoxaparin may persist longer than the protamine, necessitating additional doses of protamine. Monitor the aPTT, ACT, and thrombin time (TT). These tests may not be useful with enoxaparin overdose.
- Protamine sulfate is rarely used outside of a hospital setting. Keep the patient and family informed regarding the patient's condition.

Anticoagulant Drugs: Coumarins and Indandiones

Drug Administration

- See the general guidelines for the patient receiving anticoagulants.
- Monitor the PT. A guideline for the desired therapeutic range is 1.3 to 1.5 times the control value, unless there is an especially high risk of thromboembolism, when the therapeutic range may be 1.5 to 2 times the control value. In recent years the World Health Organization instituted a standardized system based on the international normalized ratio (INR). PT values of 1.3 to 1.5 times the control value are equivalent to INR values of 2 to 3 times the control value; PT values of 1.5 to 2 times the control value are equivalent to INR values of 3 to 4.5 times the control value. The specific desired therapeutic range for PT or INR varies with the patient's medical problem and should be prescribed by the physician. Laboratory work will be done before the first dose is administered and daily until the patient's condition is stable. Check laboratory results before administering each dose. If laboratory results indicate excessive anticoagulation, withhold the dose and contact the physician.
- If the patient is receiving heparin and an oral anticoagulant, monitor the appropriate blood work for both drugs.
- Monitor the white blood cell differential and platelet count.
- For mild overdose, the physician will withhold the anticoagulant until the blood results return to the therapeutic range. Keep phytonadione available to treat severe overdose with the oral anticoagulants.
- Pregnant women requiring anticoagulants are usually treated with heparin because the oral agents cross the pla-

NURSING IMPLICATIONS SUMMARY—cont'd

centa and may cause birth defects. Anticoagulation is usually discontinued at about the 37th week of pregnancy in anticipation of labor and delivery.

Parenteral Administration of Warfarin

- Reconstitute by adding 2 ml of sterile water for injection to the vial containing 50 mg of warfarin. May be given intramuscularly or intravenously. Administer IV doses at a rate of 25 mg/min, direct IV push. Do not mix with IV fluids.

Patient and Family Education

- See the general guidelines for the patient receiving anticoagulants.
- Inform the patient that anisindione may turn alkaline urine orange, which may be mistaken for blood. If in doubt, the patient should consult the physician.
- Rare side effects may develop in patients taking oral anticoagulants. Emphasize the importance of notifying the physician if unexpected signs or symptoms develop.
- Instruct patients to avoid drinking alcoholic beverages while taking anticoagulants.
- Instruct the patient to take a missed dose as soon as remembered if it is during the same day, otherwise omit the missed dose and resume the regular dosing schedule; do not double up for missed doses since doing so may contribute to bleeding.
- Emphasize the importance of returning for follow-up visits to monitor laboratory studies.
- Anticoagulant drugs act by creating a vitamin K deficiency (see text). Instruct patients not to change their diet significantly while taking an oral anticoagulant; they should not begin a weight-reduction diet, begin nutritional or vitamin supplements, or otherwise change their diet without consulting with the physician because the dose of anticoagulant may require alteration. Encourage patients to maintain a well-balanced diet and not to make changes in the amount of vitamin K in the diet. Sources of vitamin K are listed in the dietary consideration box on vitamins (p. 215). Also instruct patients to notify physician if persistent GI tract upset, fever, or diarrhea develops.

Aspirin

- For a detailed discussion of aspirin, see Chapter 30.

Dipyridamole

Drug Administration

- Dipyridamole may also be used for some diagnostic studies such as myocardial perfusion imaging.
- For IV administration, dilute the dose in sufficient 0.45% or 0.9% sodium chloride injection or D5W to make a volume of 20 to 50 ml. The dose is determined by the patient's weight. Administer at a rate of 142 μg/kg/min for 4 minutes. Monitor vital signs, especially blood pressure, and electrocardiographic changes.

Patient and Family Education

- Instruct the patient to take doses with a full glass (8 ounce) of water. It is best to take doses on an empty stomach, 1 hour before or 2 hours after meals. However, if gastric irritation is a problem, instruct the patient to take doses with meals, milk, or a snack.
- Dipyridamole may be prescribed with aspirin or another anticoagulant. Review with the patient the importance of taking both drugs as ordered and not increasing the dose of either drug without consulting the physician.
- Remind the patient to keep all health care providers informed of all drugs being taken. Instruct the patient not to take aspirin or any blood thinner (anticoagulant) unless prescribed by the same physician who prescribed the dipyridamole.
- Instruct the patient to avoid over-the-counter medications, especially aspirin-containing products, unless approved by the physician.
- Tell the patient to space doses evenly throughout the day. Instruct the patient to take a missed dose as soon as remembered, unless within 4 hours of the next dose, then omit the missed dose and resume the regular dosing schedule; do not double up for missed doses.
- Instruct the patient to notify the physician if bruising, bleeding gums, nosebleeds, or bleeding in the stool occurs. Also notify the physician if skin rash or itching, tightness in the chest, or chest pain develops.

Sulfinpyrazone

- For a detailed discussion of sulfinpyrazone, see Chapter 30.

Ticlopidine

Patient and Family Education

- Instruct the patient to take doses with meals or snack.
- Emphasize the importance of returning for scheduled follow-up visits. It is especially important during the first 3 months of therapy to monitor for side effects.
- Remind the patient to keep all health care providers informed of all medications being used. Ticlopidine may increase the risk of bleeding from surgery or dental procedures, so the drug may need to be stopped for a week or two before scheduled procedures.
- Notify the physician if bleeding, unexplained or excessive bruising, blood in urine or stool, black tarry stools, severe headache, bleeding gums, excessively heavy menstrual periods, or nosebleeds develop.
- Review the signs of agranulocytosis with the patient (see box on p. 268).

Continued.

PATIENT PROBLEM

Agranulocytosis

Agranulocytosis, also called malignant neutropenia, is characterized by very low granulocyte levels. It can develop during the course of some diseases, but is most often caused by drug toxicity or hypersensitivity. While rare, it is potentially fatal if not recognized. Symptoms include the following:

- High fever and chills
- Sore throat
- Ulcers or sores in the mouth and pharynx and difficulty swallowing
- Weakness, severe fatigue
- Cough or hoarseness, lower back or side pain, painful or difficult urination

Laboratory work indicates leukopenia (low white blood cell count) with extremely low polymorphonuclear (PMN) cell count of 0% to 2%.

Treatment involves discontinuing the suspected causative drug, placing the patient in protective isolation or protecting the patient from infection, treating any existing infection, and providing supportive care.

NURSING IMPLICATIONS SUMMARY—cont'd

- Advise the patient to check with the physician before discharge regarding any possible restrictions in activities while taking ticlopidine.

Thrombolytic Drugs

Drug Administration

- Monitor vital signs and temperature. Be alert to signs of hemorrhage such as hypotension, rapid pulse, or other signs of shock. Monitor mental status and neurologic status. Assess for nosebleeds, bleeding gums, blood in urine, stool, vomitus, or bleeding at IV sites; notify physician. Heparin may also be prescribed, which puts the patient at even greater risk for hemorrhage.
- Assess the patient systematically. Many other side effects have been reported, including nausea, vomiting, rash, fever, muscle aches, and dyspnea. Sometimes it is difficult to distinguish drug side effects from symptoms of the underlying medical condition.
- Monitor laboratory work, including complete blood count (CBC), TT, aPTT, PT, creatine phosphokinase (CPK), fibrinogen level, and platelet count.
- Monitor continuous electrocardiogram (ECG). Reperfusion arrhythmias occur frequently.
- Check stools daily for presence of blood.
- Use caution in handling and moving the patient to avoid excessive bleeding or bruising. Do not restrain the patient.
- If arterial puncture is necessary, apply pressure to the puncture site for 30 minutes after the procedure. Check the site regularly for signs of bleeding.
- For continuous infusion, use microdrip tubing and an electronic infusion monitoring device. Use a separate infusion line from the one being used for other medications; do not mix medications with anistreplase or alteplase.
- Do not administer IM injections to patients receiving these drugs.
- Avoid venipuncture unless absolutely necessary. Apply pressure to the site for at least 15 minutes after venipuncture. Label the bed (or as agency custom dictates) so that personnel from the laboratory use appropriate technique to minimize bleeding after venipuncture.
- Anaphylaxis has been reported. Keep available appropriate drugs and equipment to treat acute allergic reactions.
- For systemic infusion these drugs are used only in short-term care settings. Keep the patient and family informed of the patient's condition.
- For arteriovenous cannula occlusion clearance, try to clear the cannula by using a heparinized saline solution. If that is not successful, wait until the effects of the heparin have diminished. Inject the thrombolytic agent into the cannula, and then clamp cannula for 2 hours. Assess the patient for side effects during that period. After 2 hours, aspirate the contents of the affected cannula; then flush the cannula with saline.

Intravenous Alteplase

- Dilute as directed by the manufacturer. Use the diluent provided to make a concentration of 1 mg/ml. Intravenous alteplase may be given undiluted or further diluted with an equal volume of 0.9% sodium chloride injection or 5% dextrose injection to make a concentration of 0.5 mg/ml. No other diluents should be used.

Intravenous Anistreplase

- Assess for history of allergic response to streptokinase or anistreplase or previous administration of either of these drugs within the past 12 months.
- Have available appropriate drugs, equipment, and personnel to treat acute allergic reactions.
- Reconstitute anistreplase as directed by the manufacturer. Roll vial to mix powder and diluent; avoid shaking because

NURSING IMPLICATIONS SUMMARY—cont'd

foaming may occur. There is no preservative. Use each vial for 1 dose then discard vial. Administer the dose within 30 minutes of reconstitution. Administer the dose over 2 to 5 minutes; 4 to 5 minutes is the usual time.

Intravenous Streptokinase

- Assess the patient for history of allergic response to streptokinase or anistreplase or previous administration of either of these drugs within the past 12 months.
- Have available appropriate drugs, equipment, and personnel to treat acute allergic reactions.
- Reconstitute as directed by the manufacturer.

Intravenous Urokinase

- Reconstitute as directed by the manufacturer. When mixing, roll vial; avoid shaking.
- For clearing occluded IV catheters, see the manufacturer's insert. Before disconnecting a central venous catheter, instruct the patient to exhale and hold breath until the catheter is disconnected and reconnected to the tubing or syringe. Avoid excessive pressure when injecting the dose. Because catheters may be occluded by material that will not be dissolved by the injected thrombolytic, urokinase may not be successful in clearing obstruction. Be careful not to force precipitate substance into the circulation.

SYSTEMIC HEMOSTATIC DRUGS

Aminocaproic Acid and Tranexamic Acid

Drug Administration

- Aminocaproic acid and tranexamic acid may be used to treat overdose with fibrinolytic drugs.

Intravenous Aminocaproic Acid

- Dilute the 250 mg/ml concentration with sterile water for injection, normal saline, D5W, or lactated Ringer's injection. See the manufacturer's directions. Do not dilute with sterile water for injection if it is to be used for subarachnoid hemorrhage.
- Because aminocaproic acid can cause clot formation, be alert to signs of possible thrombosis such as pain in extremities, one extremity cooler than the other, loss of pulse in an extremity, shortness of breath, chest pain, slurred speech, changes in vision, and Homans' sign. When aminocaproic acid is used after urologic surgery, the bladder should be free of clots before aminocaproic acid is administered or the drug may accumulate in the clots, preventing them from dissolving. This situation could lead to bladder obstruction, manifested by decreased urination and eventually bladder pain.
- Monitor vital signs.

Intravenous Tranexamic Acid

- Dilute a single dose to at least 50 ml with normal saline, 5% dextrose in normal saline, D5W, Ringer's solution, amino acids, or dextran. Heparin may be added to the solution if needed. Do not mix tranexamic acid with penicillin or blood. Administer a dose over at least 1 minute. Monitor blood pressure. Too rapid administration may cause hypotension.
- Because tranexamic acid can cause clot formation, be alert to signs of possible thrombosis such as pain in extremities, one extremity cooler than the other, loss of pulse in an extremity, shortness of breath, chest pain, slurred speech, changes in vision, and Homans' sign.
- Other routes of administration being investigated include using diluted tranexamic acid as a bladder irrigant, applying the drug topically to the nasal mucosa as a spray, or soaking gauze that is then packed into the nasal cavity. See the manufacturer's insert.

Patient and Family Education

- Review the goals of therapy with the patient. Therapy is usually short term, but side effects may develop. Review the symptoms of clot development described under IV forms, above. The development of clots is rare, but instruct the patient to notify the physician if any of the symptoms develop. Encourage the patient to notify the physician if any unexpected sign or symptom develops.
- Instruct the patient to take a missed dose of aminocaproic acid as soon as remembered, unless almost time for next dose, then omit the missed dose and resume the regular dosing schedule; do not double up for missed doses.
- Instruct the patient to take a missed dose of tranexamic acid as soon as remembered then space remaining doses evenly through the rest of the day; do not double up for missed doses; contact the physician with questions.
- For long-term use of tranexamic acid, the physician may recommend regular ophthalmic examinations to check for side effects.

Phytonadione

Drug Administration

- Assess for history of allergy before administering. Monitor vital signs and blood pressure. Remain with the patient for 5 to 10 minutes after administration. Have available appropriate drugs, equipment, and personnel to treat an acute allergic response.
- IM injection is painful, and the injection site may be tender. Use large muscle masses. Record and rotate injection sites.
- Monitor the PT.
- Read labels carefully. Konakion is for IM injection only. AquaMEPHYTON may be given intramuscularly, intravenously, or subcutaneously.

Continued.

NURSING IMPLICATIONS SUMMARY—cont'd

Intravenous Phytonadione

- Dilute with sodium chloride injection, 5% dextrose injection, or 5% dextrose in normal saline. Diluents containing benzyl alcohol should not be used in neonates or infants. Administer diluted solution at a rate of 1 mg or less over 1 minute. The IM route is preferred. Solution is light sensitive; prepare dose just before administration.

Menadiol

Drug Administration

- Assess for glucose-6-phosphate dehydrogenase deficiency before administering; if present, do not administer.
- IM injection is painful, and the injection site may be tender. Use large muscle masses. Record and rotate injection sites.
- Monitor the PT.

Intravenous Menadiol

- May be given undiluted or added to most infusion solutions. Administer undiluted dose over at least 1 minute.

Patient and Family Education for Phytonadione or Menadiol

- Review with the patient the expected benefits of therapy.
- Dietary deficiency of vitamin K is rare in adults. For dietary sources of vitamin K, see the dietary consideration box on vitamins (p. 215).
- Instruct the patient to take a missed dose as soon as remembered, unless almost time for next dose, and then omit the missed dose and resume the regular dosing schedule; do not double up for missed doses. Encourage the patient to keep a record of missed doses and to inform the physician of these omissions on the next visit.
- Emphasize to the patient the importance of follow-up visits to monitor drug effectiveness.
- Remind the patient to keep all health care providers, including dentists, informed of all drugs being used.

HEMOSTATIC DRUGS FOR REPLACEMENT THERAPY FOR HEMOPHILIA

Antihemophilic Factor and Cryoprecipitated Antihemophilic Factor

Drug Administration

- Monitor vital signs and remain with the patient for 5 to 10 minutes after beginning drug administration to watch for allergic reaction. Symptoms include fast or irregular breathing, tightness in the chest, swelling of eyelids, skin rash, hives or itching, and hypotension. If allergic reaction occurs, discontinue use of the remaining AHF, but keep the IV line patent. Notify the physician.
- For the dry form, bring the concentrate and diluent to room temperature. Use plastic disposable syringe and filter needle to prepare dose. Reconstitute with the diluent provided by the manufacturer, adding diluent to the vial by directing the stream against the side of the vial to prevent foaming. Do not shake the vial. Administer within 1 to 3 hours after reconstitution (see the manufacturer's instructions with the preparation being used).
- Cryoprecipitated AHF is handled like all blood products (see Chapter 17). Thaw in a water bath at 30° to 37°C (86° to 98.6°F) for up to 15 minutes.
- Administer through a separate IV line; do not mix with other IV fluids or medications (except for 0.9% sodium chloride with cryoprecipitated form).

Patient and Family Education

- Some patients may be candidates to learn how to administer AHF at home. Review the directions for reconstitution. Have the patient give return demonstration. In addition to teaching how to reconstitute and administer a dose, demonstrate the appropriate disposal technique for used syringes, needles, and equipment. Review the side effects.
- Patients recently diagnosed with hemophilia should be immunized against hepatitis B; consult the physician.
- Instruct patients with hemophilia to wear a medical identification tag or bracelet indicating their condition and treatment.
- Instruct the patient to contact the physician for missed doses. If unable to contact the physician, instruct the patient to take a missed dose as soon as remembered, unless almost time for next dose, then omit the missed dose and resume the regular dosing schedule; do not double up for missed doses.

Antithrombin III

Drug Administration

- Review the manufacturer's instructions provided with the preparation. Reconstitute as directed. Roll the vial to mix. Do not shake the vial because foaming may occur.
- Administer ATnativ at a rate of 50 IU of less over 1 minute; do not exceed 100 IU/minute. Administer a single dose of Thrombate III over 10 to 20 minutes.

Desmopressin

Drug Administration

- Desmopression is also discussed in Chapter 59.
- For treatment of hemophilia A and von Willebrand's disease, dilute a single dose in 10 ml of normal saline for children weighing <10 kg and in 50 ml for children weighing >10 kg and adults. Administer a dose over 15 to 30 minutes.
- Monitor blood pressure and pulse. Other side effects include headache, nausea, flushing, abdominal cramps, and pain at the injection site.
- Desmopressin has an antidiuretic effect. Monitor intake and output. Caution the patient to limit fluid intake.

NURSING IMPLICATIONS SUMMARY—cont'd

- Monitor blood work such as factor VIII coagulant, factor VIII–related antigen, and ristocetin cofactor, depending on diagnosis.

Factor IX complex

Drug Administration

- Review the manufacturer's instructions provided with the preparation. Reconstitute as directed. Roll the vial to mix. Do not shake the vial because foaming may occur. Use plastic syringes and filter needles.
- Administer at a rate of 2 to 3 ml/min or 100 U/min, although it may vary according to patient's condition. Slow the infusion rate if chills, fever, flushing, headache, tingling, or pain at the injection site develops. Monitor blood pressure and pulse.
- Administer through a separate line; do not mix with other drugs or IV fluids.

Patient and Family Education

- Some patients may be candidates to learn how to administer factor IX at home. Review the directions for reconstitution, and have the patient give a return demonstration. In addition to teaching how to reconstitute and administer dose, demonstrate the appropriate disposal technique for used syringes, needles, and equipment. Review the side effects.
- Patients recently diagnosed with hemophilia should be immunized against hepatitis B; consult the physician.
- Instruct patients with hemophilia to wear a medical identification tag or bracelet indicating their condition and treatment.
- For missed doses, instruct the patient to notify the notify physician as soon as possible.

CRITICAL THINKING

APPLICATION

1. Describe the major steps in blood coagulation.
2. What are the groups of anticoagulants you see in clinical practice? What is the mechanism of action of each group?
3. Which anticoagulants would you expect to see in test tubes when blood is drawn for storage or testing?
4. How does protein binding affect the pharmacodynamics of the coumarins?
5. What are the therapeutic limitations of the indandiones?
6. How do platelets initiate clot formation?
7. What drugs might you see prescribed to inhibit platelet aggregation?
8. What roles do thromboxane A_2 and prostacyclin play in platelet aggregation?
9. What is the action of thrombolytic drugs? Name the thrombolytic drugs.
10. What is the mechanism of action of aminocaproic acid? Of vitamin K? When would these drugs be used?
11. List the agents used as local hemostatics. What is their mechanism of action?

CRITICAL THINKING

1. Differentiate between nursing care activities required to administer heparin in high-dose and low-dose therapy.
2. Compare and contrast how protamine sulfate and vitamin K function as antidotes for drug-induced hemorrhage.
3. Compare and contrast heparin with warfarin; consider action, side effects, ease of administration, and contraindications.
4. How do the actions of thromboxane$_2$ and prostacyclin influence the dose of aspirin used to prevent thrombus formation?
5. Compare and contrast the four thrombolytics. Call the pharmacy and include cost in your discussion.
6. Compare and contrast hemophilia A, hemophilia B, and von Willebrand's disease.
7. What drugs are used to treat hemophilia? What are the nursing care implications of these drugs?

CHAPTER 21

Drugs to Lower Blood Lipid Levels

OBJECTIVES

After studying this chapter, you should be able to do the following:

- *Differentiate between the two main types of lipids in the blood and the four major classes of lipoprotein.*
- *State the normal blood level of cholesterol.*
- *Discuss the four types of lipoproteins.*
- *Develop a teaching plan for a patient who needs to decrease cholesterol intake.*
- *Develop a nursing care plan for a patient who is taking one of the drugs discussed in this chapter.*

KEY TERMS

atherosclerosis
cholesterol
enterohepatic circulation
lipids
lipoprotein

CHAPTER OVERVIEW

Atherosclerosis is the gradual blocking of arteries by a buildup of plaque. This clogging of the arteries is the major factor behind heart attacks, strokes, and peripheral vascular disease. Lipids, particularly cholesterol, are a major component of atherosclerotic plaques. The association of high blood levels of cholesterol with atherosclerosis has led to preventive measures to control **cholesterol.** This chapter reviews the current pharmacologic approaches to controlling blood cholesterol.

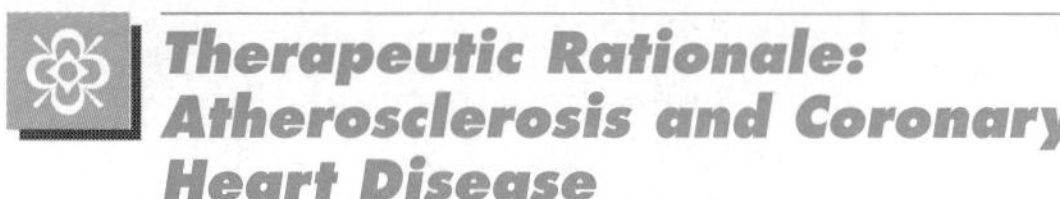

Therapeutic Rationale: Atherosclerosis and Coronary Heart Disease

Origin of Blood Lipids and Their Role in Atherosclerosis

The **lipids** in the blood are triglyceride and cholesterol. Triglyceride is an energy source for muscle and is stored in fat. Cholesterol is a fatlike substance that is present in cell membranes and is a precursor of bile acids and steroid hormones. Triglycerides and cholesterol are bound to special proteins to form soluble **lipoprotein.**

The major classes of lipoprotein are chylomicrons, very-low-density lipoprotein (VLDL), low-density lipoprotein (LDL), and high-density lipoprotein (HDL). Chylomicrons and VLDL are largely composed of triglycerides; they transport triglycerides to tissues for metabolic use or storage. LDL and HDL transport cholesterol. The role and composition of lipoprotein are summarized in Figure 21-1.

Chylomicrons

Chylomicrons are very large lipoprotein that contain about 90% triglyceride by weight. After a meal the ingested fat is processed by the intestine into chylomicrons, which are transported through the lymphatic system to the plasma. Chylomicrons are normally found in the blood only during the 8 to 12 hours after a meal. Because chylomicrons represent dietary fat, patients who are evaluated for triglyceride abnormalities should not eat for 12 to 16 hours before a blood sample is drawn.

Very-Low-Density Lipoprotein

VLDLs are 60% triglyceride by weight. This triglyceride pool is synthesized by the liver from carbohydrate sources for export as fuel to other tissues. Triglycerides cannot be transported directly into cells for use. Tissues that require triglycerides, particularly muscle and fat tissues, secrete an enzyme called *lipoprotein lipase,* which breaks down the triglycerides to fatty acids and glycerol, compounds that can be taken into the cells.

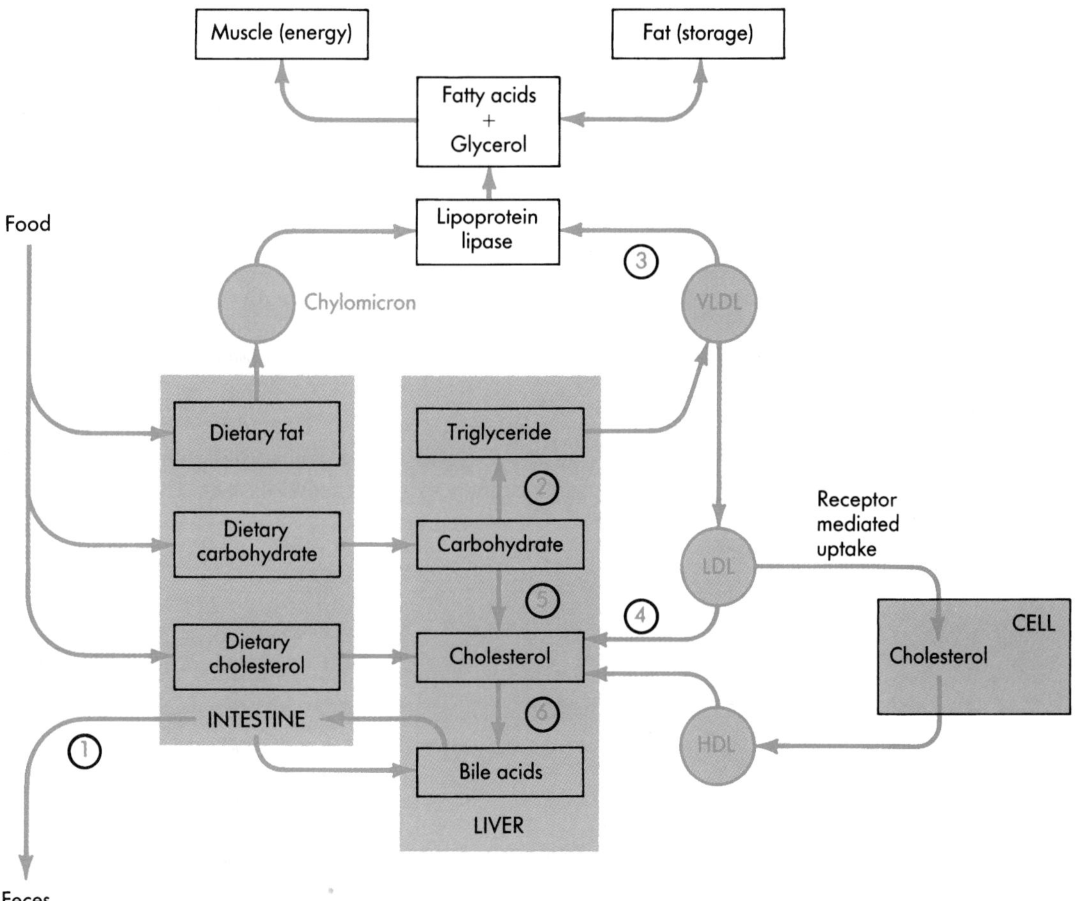

FIGURE 21-1

Diagram of origin and fate of lipids. Sites of action of drugs that can lower excessive plasma concentrations of lipids include (1) drugs that lower cholesterol by increasing excretion of bile acids (cholestyramine and colestipol); (2) drugs that lower triglycerides by inhibiting hepatic triglyceride synthesis (gemfibrozil and niacin); (3) drug that lowers VLDL, inhibiting its release and activating lipoprotein lipase (clofibrate); (4) drug that lowers cholesterol by stimulating LDL degradation (probucol); (5) drug that lowers cholesterol by inhibiting cholesterol synthesis (HMG CoA reductase inhibitors [statins]); and (6) drug that lowers cholesterol by increasing cholesterol excretion into bile (clofibrate, probucol).

Low-Density Lipoprotein

LDLs ("bad cholesterol") are only 5% triglyceride but are 50% cholesterol by weight. About 60% to 70% of the total serum cholesterol in a fasting serum sample is found in LDLs. When triglyceride values are <400 mg/dl, the calculation for LDL-cholesterol is made from the following formula:

$$\text{LDL-cholesterol} = \text{Total cholesterol} - \text{HDL-cholesterol} - (\text{triglyceride}/5)$$

The desirable level of LDL is <130 mg/dl. LDLs are the remains of the VLDLs after removal of triglycerides and some protein. When cells need cholesterol, they synthesize receptors for LDL. LDLs bind to these receptors and are taken into the cell by pinocytosis and degraded. Most cells can synthesize cholesterol, but this synthesis is turned off when the cholesterol from LDL is used. When the cell has sufficient cholesterol, it stops making LDL receptors.

High-Density Lipoprotein

HDLs ("good cholesterol") are 50% protein, 20% cholesterol, and 5% triglyceride by weight. Only about 20% of the total plasma cholesterol is found in HDL. The HDLs help remove excess cholesterol from peripheral tissues. HDL can also remove cholesterol from cells and can inhibit the uptake of LDL by cells. Recent studies indicate that persons with high concentrations of HDL (>65 mg/dl) have a lower incidence of atherosclerosis and the related problems of heart disease and strokes. Higher HDL levels can be promoted by exercise, weight reduction, and smoking cessation. On the other hand, individuals with a very low HDL level (<35 mg/dl) have an increased risk for atherosclerosis even if the LDL level is in the "normal" range.

Degradation of Cholesterol

The liver degrades cholesterol to bile acids, which are excreted into the small intestine. Bile acids emulsify lipids to aid in fat absorption. Some bile acids are absorbed into the portal vein for transport back to the liver. This circulation between the liver and small intestine is called **enterohepatic circulation.**

Atherosclerosis and Blood Cholesterol

Role of LDL in Atherosclerosis

Research has focused on the role of LDL in atherosclerosis because the concentration of LDL reflects the total cholesterol concentration. Increased total plasma cholesterol concentration is linked to increased incidence of atherosclerosis. When there is injury to the epithelial cells of arteries or when the amount of circulating LDL becomes high, the receptor mechanism controlling LDL uptake no longer operates properly, and the cell becomes overwhelmed with cholesterol. This situation is believed to be an origin of atherosclerotic plaques.

Atherosclerotic Plaques

Platelets may also initiate atherosclerosis. Aggregated platelets release factors that stimulate smooth muscle growth. This stimulation of growth heals the minute breaks in the normal blood vessel. When the epithelial cells are overloaded with cholesterol and aggregated platelets stimulate an overgrowth of smooth muscle cells, an atherosclerotic plaque is formed. The outcome of atherosclerosis is the narrowing of an artery so that the blood flow is reduced and may not be sufficient to maintain tissue function (Figure 21-2). Reduced blood flow also favors the formation of a clot that may completely obstruct flow. A stroke may result when the cerebral arteries are involved, or a myocardial infarction may result when the coronary arteries are involved. When the legs are affected, limbs may be lost to gangrene. Renovascular hypertension is associated with atherosclerosis.

Risk Factors for Coronary Heart Disease

High blood cholesterol has been shown to be a major risk factor for coronary heart disease. The classification of total cholesterol levels is:

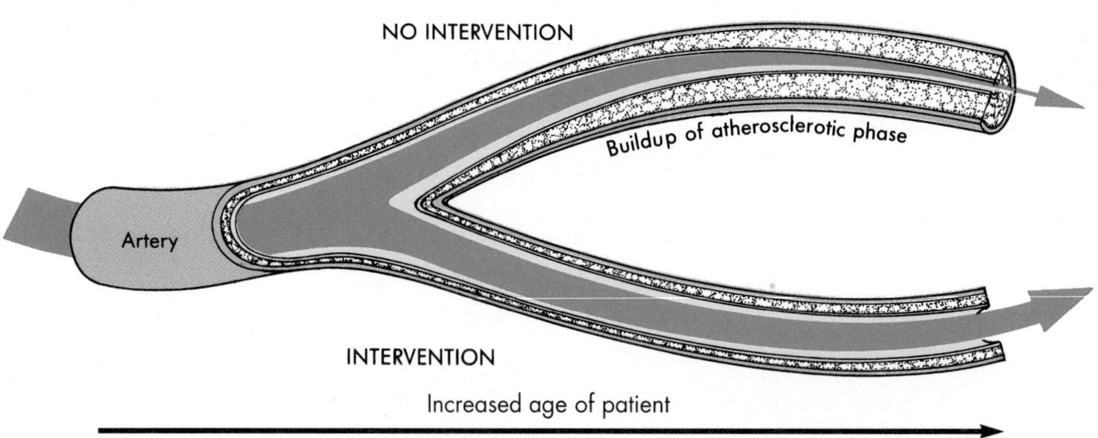

FIGURE 21-2
Diagram of increasing blockage of artery caused by atherosclerotic plaque. Buildup of plaque is shown as time-dependent phenomenon. Intervention, through diet, exercise, or drugs, can slow buildup. Recent studies have shown that some interventions can reverse atherosclerosis.

<200 mg/dl	Desirable total blood cholesterol
200-239 mg/dl	Borderline-high total blood cholesterol
≥240 mg/dl	High total blood cholesterol

Epidemiologic studies support a direct relationship between the level of total serum cholesterol and the rate of coronary heart disease. Migration studies show that within one generation of moving, a population adopts both the blood cholesterol levels and the coronary heart disease rate of the new country. The risk for death from coronary heart disease in men rises fivefold over the range of blood cholesterol levels. In recent years studies have examined the outcome of lowering high blood cholesterol levels in individuals with established coronary heart disease. Lowering cholesterol levels reduces rates of recurrent coronary heart disease events along with a strong trend toward decreased total mortality rates.

The emphasis today for preventing coronary heart disease is twofold: first, to identify individuals at high risk who will benefit from intensive intervention efforts (see box below) and, second, to promote lower blood cholesterol levels in the whole population by encouraging changes in dietary habits (see box, p. 276) and physical activity levels.

Genetic Factors in Atherosclerosis

The fact that atherosclerosis runs in families has prompted searches for the genetic factors underlying unusually high blood lipid levels. Hypercholesterolemia in its severest form is due to mutations in the gene responsible for producing a functional LDL receptor. Without a functional LDL receptor, LDL cannot be taken into cells and cholesterol cannot be used. Instead, cholesterol remains circulating while bound to LDL. Individuals monozygous for this trait are 1 in a million and suffer severe atherosclerosis by their twenties. Far more common (1 in 500) are individuals who are heterozygous for a defective LDL receptor but still have about 50% of the normal number of LDL receptors. These individuals show premature atherosclerosis. Most cases of hypercholesterolemia have no specific genetic abnormality, however. Multiple genetic and environmental factors are being identified.

High levels of total cholesterol combined with elevated levels of triglycerides are designated as combined hyperlipidemia and reflect elevated LDL and VLDL. This condition is commonly found to run in families, although specific genetic factors have not been determined and in fact may be multiple. Combined hyperlipidemia is also caused by obesity, diabetes mellitus, and nephrotic syndrome.

RISK FACTORS IDENTIFIED FOR CORONARY HEART DISEASE

- Age: Men older than 45 years; women older than 55 years or those who have undergone premature menopause without estrogen replacement therapy.
- Family history of premature coronary heart disease (myocardial infarction or sudden death before 55 years of age in a male first-degree relative or 65 years of age in a female first-degree relative)
- Current cigarette smoking
- Hypertension
- Low HDL cholesterol (<35 mg/dl)
- Diabetes mellitus

A negative risk factor is:

- High HDL cholesterol (≥60 mg/dl)

An individual with two or more risk factors should be given dietary consultation and drug therapy if needed to bring and keep cholesterol levels in the desirable range.

Dietary Modification and Physical Activity

Dietary modification, weight reduction in overweight individuals, and increased physical activity are important lifestyle modifications for lowering blood cholesterol levels. Weight reduction may be important in itself or through its beneficial effect in reducing hypertension or moderating diabetes mellitus. Physical activity increases HDL cholesterol.

Diet modification is always the first therapeutic intervention (see box, p. 277). A trial of at least 6 months can determine whether diet modification alone is sufficient to lower blood cholesterol without addition of drug therapy. The goal of a step I diet is to reduce saturated fat intake to <10% of calories, total fat to 30% or less of total calories, and cholesterol to <300 mg/day. The goal of a step II diet is to reduce saturated fat to <7% of total calories, total fat to 30% or less of total calories, and cholesterol to <200 mg/day.

Therapeutic Agents: Drugs to Lower Blood Cholesterol

Drugs that are used to reduce blood lipid concentrations are listed in Table 21-1. The major drugs used include the bile acid sequestrants, the 3-hydroxy-3-methylglutaryl coenzyme A (HMG CoA) reductase inhibitors ("statins"), and nicotinic acid. Other drugs include the fibric acid derivatives, probucol, and estrogens.

BILE ACID SEQUESTRANTS

Cholestyramine (Questran) and colestipol (Colestid) are the bile acid sequestrants used to treat high LDL cholesterol levels. They have been shown in prevention trials to reduce the risk for coronary heart disease while having a long-term safety record.

Mechanism of Action

The bile acids sequestrants are resins that are not absorbed systemically. In the intestine they bind bile acids, which are then excreted, interrupting the enterohepatic circulation of bile acids. This action causes the liver to convert more cholesterol to bile acids. With hepatic cholesterol lowered, more LDL receptors are formed on cells, and LDL removal is enhanced. The overall result is a lowering of LDL cholesterol levels.

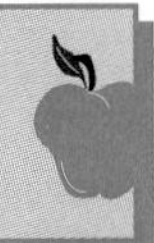

DIETARY CONSIDERATION

Reducing Cholesterol

Dietary changes to lower serum cholesterol levels usually involve decreasing cholesterol intake, lowering the intake of saturated fat, and increasing the intake of polyunsaturated fat. As with all major dietary prescriptions, refer patients to a dietitian for more extensive teaching and explanation if necessary.

FOODS ALLOWED	FOODS TO AVOID OR LIMIT
Meat	
Lean, well-trimmed meat; poultry, fish (not shrimp), and veal preferred, with occasional ham, pork, lamb, beef	Fatty meat, regular ground beef, bacon, sausage, luncheon meat, fried meat, meat in gravy, shrimp, organ meats, fish roe
Eggs and Other Meat Alternatives	
Egg white only, no-cholesterol egg substitutes, legumes, soy protein, peanut butter, nuts (e.g., walnuts, pecans, almonds)	Egg yolk, canned pork and beans, cashews, macadamia nuts
Milk and Cheese	
Skim milk and skim milk products, buttermilk, low-fat cheese, cottage cheese, yogurt containing up to 1% milkfat, sherbet	Whole milk and milk products, malted milk and milkshakes, cream (sweet and sour), ice cream and ice milk, nondairy substitutes for cream, whipped toppings containing coconut or palm oil, cheese made from cream or whole milk
Vegetables and Fruits	
Fresh, canned, frozen, or dried fruits or vegetables; juices; vegetables prepared without animal fat; vegetarian baked beans	Buttered, creamed, or fried vegetables; pork and beans, avocado (use sparingly)
Fat	
Vegetable oils, soft margarine listing allowed liquid oil as first ingredient, mayonnaise, salad dressings not containing sour cream or cheese	Other margarines, including low-calorie; butter, hydrogenated vegetable shortening, bacon, lard, meat drippings, salt pork, suet, cream; coconut, palm, and peanut oils; gravies (unless made with allowed fat and skim milk)
Breads and Cereals	
Cooked and dry cereal; rice; flour; pasta; breads made with minimum of saturated fat; white, whole-wheat, rye, pumpernickel, raisin, Italian, and French breads; English muffins; hard rolls; matzo; pretzels; saltines; homemade breads made without whole milk, egg yolk, or saturated shortening	Egg noodles; egg bread; commercial biscuits, muffins, donuts, pancakes, waffles, and butter rolls; mixes for preceding; corn chips, potato chips, and other deep-fried snacks; cheese crackers
Soup	
Bouillon; clear broths; fat-free vegetable soup and pot liquor; cream soups made with skim milk and allowed fat; packaged dehydrated soup	All other soups
Desserts and Sweets	
Angel food cake; fruit ices; sherbet (1%-2% fat); gelatin desserts; meringues; homemade pastries made with allowed fat, skim milk, and egg white; pure sugar candies; jam; jelly; honey; syrup made without fat; molasses; sugar	Commercial pies, cakes, mixes; desserts and candy containing nonallowed fat, egg yolk, and whole milk; chocolate; coconut
Miscellaneous	
Coffee, tea, caffeine-free coffee, carbonated beverages, relishes, fat-free barbecue sauce, catsup, chili sauce, spices, herbs, extracts, lemon juice, vinegar	

Pharmacokinetics

Bile acid sequestrants are powders mixed with water or fruit juice. They are taken in one or two doses daily with meals. Alternatively, they may be given in one large dose after the evening meal in order not to absorb other drugs that must be taken earlier in the day. A lowering of LDL cholesterol is usually seen within 2 weeks of beginning therapy. Cholestyramine and colestipol are not absorbed and are excreted in the feces.

Uses

Cholestyramine and colestipol are especially effective in lowering LDL-cholesterol levels. A 15% to 30% reduction is

TREATMENT DECISIONS BASED ON LDL-CHOLESTEROL AND CORONARY HEART DISEASE

Dietary Therapy	Initiation level	LDL goal
Without CHD and with fewer than 2 risk factors	≥160 mg/dl	<160 mg/dl
Without CHD and with 2 or more risk factors	≥130 mg/dl	<130 mg/dl
With CHD	>100 mg/dl	≤100 mg/dl
Drug Therapy	**Consideration level**	**LD goal**
Without CHD and with fewer than 2 risk factors	≥190 mg/dl	<160 mg/dl
WIthout CHD and with 2 or more risk factors	≥160 mg/dl	<130 mg/dl
With CHD	>130 mg/dl	≤100 mg/dl
Drug Selection	**Single drug**	**Combination drug**
Elevated LDL-cholesterol and triglycerides <200 mg/dl	Bile-acid sequestrant (BAS)	BAS + Statin
	HMG CoA reductase inhibitor (statin)	BAS + NA
	Nicotinic acid (NA)	Statin + NA*
Elevated LDL-cholesterol and triglycerides 200-400 mg/dl	Nicotinic acid	NA + Statin*
	HMG CoA reductase inhibitor	Statin + GEM†
		NA + BAS
	Gemfibrozil (GEM)	NA + GEM

From Second Report of the Expert Panel on Detection, Evaluation, and Treatment of High Blood Cholesterol in Adults, National Institutes of Health Publication No. 93-3095, September 1993, U.S. Department of Health and Human Services, Public Health Service.
*Possible increased risk of myopathy and hepatitis.
†Increased risk of myopathy; must be used with caution.

commonly seen. Because of their safety and proven effectiveness, these drugs are the first to be prescribed when diet therapy alone is not sufficient and the patient is younger and has moderate hypercholesterolemia (men <45 years and women <55 years, LDL-cholesterol 160 to 220 mg/dl). These drugs are also effective in combination of the HMG CoA reductase inhibitors in treating patients with severe hypercholesterolemia.

Adverse Reactions and Contraindications

Gastrointestinal (GI) symptoms are the major side effects of the bile acid sequestrants. Symptoms include constipation, bloating, epigastric fullness, nausea, and flatulence. Serum triglyceride levels may increase in some patients as a result of increased hepatic VLDL production. For this reason bile acid sequestrants are not recommended for patients with triglyceride levels about 200 mg/dl.

Interactions

Bile acid sequestrants may bind other drugs and prevent their absorption. Other drugs should be taken at least 1 hour before or 4 hours after cholestyramine or colestipol. In particular, decreased absorption of digitoxin, warfarin, thyroxine, thiazide diuretics, and beta-blockers has been shown. It may be advisable to administer some drugs early in the day and to administer cholestyramine or colestipol with the evening meal.

FIBRIC ACID DERIVATIVES

Gemfibrozil (Lopid) and clofibrate (Abitrate, Atromid-S, Claripex, Novofibrate) are the two fibric acid derivatives available in the United States. Other fibric acid derivatives not currently available include bezafibrate, ciprofibrate, and fenofibrate.

Mechanism of Action

Fibric acid derivatives primarily lower triglycerides. They act in a complex manner to increase lipoprotein lipase activity, thereby enhancing catabolism of VLDL and LDL and reducing triglyceride levels. They also decrease the synthesis of VLDL triglycerides and partially inhibit the synthesis of cholesterol and bile acids to increase the secretion of cholesterol in bile.

Pharmacokinetics

Both clofibrate and gemfibrozil are administered orally and are well absorbed from the GI tract. Gemfibrozil is metabolized by the liver. Clofibrate is also metabolized in the GI tract to an active form, clofibric acid. The drugs and metabolites are excreted in the urine.

A measurable onset of action is seen in 2 to 5 days with continuous administration. The peak effect is seen in 3 weeks for clofibrate and in 4 weeks to several months for gemfibrozil. VLDL levels will return to pretreatment values about 3 weeks after therapy is discontinued.

TABLE 21-1 Drugs to Lower Blood Cholesterol

GENERIC NAME	TRADE NAME	ADMINISTRATION/DOSAGE	COMMENTS
Bile Acid Sequestrants			
✣ Cholestyramine	Questran*	ORAL: *Adults and children*—4 gm 1 or 2 times/day before meals. Maintenance: 8-24 gm in 2-6 doses.	Valuable for isolated elevations of LDL-cholesterol. Stays in intestine, removing bile acids and thereby increasing cholesterol degradation by liver.
Colestipol	Colestid*	ORAL: *Adults*—15-30 mg/day before meals in 2-4 divided doses.	Valuable for isolated elevations of LDL-cholesterol. Stays in intestine, removing bile acids and thereby increasing cholesterol degradation by liver.
Fibric Acid Derivatives			
Clofibrate	Abitrate Atromid-S Claripex Novofibrate	ORAL: *Adults*—1.5-2 gm/day in 2-4 divided doses.	Inhibits triglyceride synthesis in liver and inhibits breakdown of triglycerides in fat tissue. Triglycerides are lowered; HDL concentration may be increased.
Gemfibrozil	Lopid*	ORAL: *Adults*—1.2 gm/day in 2 divided doses 30 minutes before morning and evening meals.	Inhibits triglyceride synthesis in liver and inhibits breakdown of triglycerides in fat tissue. Triglycerides are lowered; HDL concentration may be increased.
HMG-CoA Reductase Inhibitors (Statins)			
✣ Lovastatin	Mevacor*	ORAL: *Adults*—20 mg once a day with evening meal. May adjust at 4-week intervals. Maintenance: 20-80 mg/day, as single dose or in divided doses with meals.	Lowers LDL-cholesterol levels by inhibiting cholesterol synthesis.
Pravastatin	Pravachol*	ORAL: *Adults*—10-20 mg once a day at bedtime. May adjust at 4-week intervals. Maintenance: 10-40 mg/day, as single dose at bedtime.	Lowers LDL-cholesterol levels by inhibiting cholesterol synthesis.
Simvastatin	Zocor*	ORAL: *Adults*—5-10 mg once a day in evening. May adjust at 4-week intervals. Maintenance: 5-40 mg/day, as single dose in evening.	Lowers LDL-cholesterol levels by inhibiting cholesterol synthesis.
Other Agents			
Nicotinic acid	Niacor Novo-Niacin†	ORAL: *Adults*—1 gm 3 times/day. May increase by 500 mg a day every 2-4 weeks as needed.	Reduce VLDL production by liver. Useful in most lipid and lipoprotein abnormalities.
Probucol	Lorelco*	ORAL: *Adults*—500 mg 2 times/day with morning and evening meals.	Generally used for patients not tolerating or responding to other drugs. Lowers LDL-cholesterol, but HDL-cholesterol is also decreased.

*Available in Canada and United States.
†Available in Canada only.

Uses

Clofibrate and gemfibrozil reduce triglycerides by 20% to 50% and increase HDL by 10% to 15%. The primary use of clofibrate is to treat severe hyperlipidemia in persons with a significant risk of coronary artery disease or at risk for pancreatitis. Gemfibrozil is used for primary prevention of coronary heart disease in those with elevated LDL, high triglycerides, and low HDL. Gemfibrozil is also used to treat severe hyperlipidemia.

Adverse Reactions, Contraindications, and Toxicity

The fibric acid derivatives are generally well tolerated. The most common side effects are GI complaints. Patients with impaired renal or hepatic function may require a reduced dose. This drug class increases the likelihood of developing cholesterol gallstones.

A large trial by the World Health Organization found an increase in overall mortality associated with clofibrate therapy that may be associated with gallstone disease. The Helsinki Heart Study did not find an increased overall mortality associated with gemfibrozil. Clofibrate is not recommended for use during pregnancy because it crosses the placenta. Clofibrate is also excreted in breast milk and should therefore not be taken by nursing mothers. Gemfibrozil may significantly increase LDL values in patients with type IV hyperlipidemia (relatively normal cholesterol but elevated triglycerides) and therefore is not recommended.

Interactions
Clofibrate and gemfibrozil can significantly increase the anticoagulant effect of coumarin and indanedione anticoagulants. Clofibrate displaces several drugs from albumin, including coumarins, phenytoin, and tolbutamide. The concurrent use of lovastatin with gemfibrozil is associated with an increased risk for myopathy, leading to elevated creatine kinase levels and myoglobinuria.

HMG-CoA REDUCTASE INHIBITORS (STATINS)

Lovastatin (Mevacor), pravastatin (Pravachol), and simvastatin (Zocor) are the HMG CoA reductase inhibitors currently available. They are referred to as the "statins."

Mechanism of Action
The HMG CoA reductase inhibitors block an early step in the synthesis of cholesterol by the liver. This inhibition leads to an overall reduction in LDL production and lowers LDL-cholesterol 20% to 40%, whereas HDL-cholesterol increases 5% to 15%.

Pharmacokinetics
Administered once a day, lovastatin should be taken with a meal to maximize absorption, but pravastatin and simvastatin may be taken with a meal or on an empty stomach. Lovastatin and simvastatin are metabolized to an active metabolite, whereas pravastatin is active as administered. Excretion is primarily fecal. The duration of action persists 4 to 6 weeks after therapy is discontinued.

Uses
Statins are used to treat hypercholesterolemia caused by elevated LDL. At therapeutic doses they reduce, but do not completely block, synthesis of cholesterol. As a result, liver cells produce more LDL receptors to capture LDL from the plasma, thereby clearing excess LDL from the blood. A long-term study of patients taking simvastatin showed that those with both high blood cholesterol and heart disease cut their risk of dying by about 30% over 5 years. This patient population tends to be older. The long-term safety among middle-aged adults is not known.

Adverse Reactions, Contraindications, and Toxicity
Statins are well tolerated. Unlike the fibric acids, they do not increase the risk of gallstones. The most common side effects include dyspepsia, flatulence, constipation, and abdominal pain or cramps. High doses very occasionally increase hepatic transaminase levels. An infrequent severe side effect is myopathy with muscle aches, soreness, weakness, and elevated creatine kinase values.

These drugs are contraindicated in patients with allergies or active liver disease. They pose potential harm to the fetus and should not be used during pregnancy or by nursing mothers.

Interactions
Concurrent administration of cyclosporine, gemfibrozil, or niacin with a statin is associated with an increased risk for muscle damage (rhabdomyolysis) and acute renal failure. Creatine kinase values may also be higher.

NICOTINIC ACID

Mechanism of Action
Nicotinic acid is a B vitamin for which the minimum daily requirement (MDR) is 20 mg. At doses 10 to 20 times higher than the MDR, niacin is a vasodilator. At doses 100 to 200 times higher than the MDR, niacin depresses the synthesis of VLDL by the liver and thereby reduces LDL. Serum total and LDL cholesterol are lowered by 10% to 25%, triglyceride levels are lowered by 20% to 50%, and HDL cholesterol levels are raised by 15% to 35%.

Pharmacokinetics
Nicotinic acid is readily absorbed from the GI tract and has a short half-life; it is readily excreted unchanged in the urine. A reduction in triglyceride concentration is seen in a few hours, but a reduction in cholesterol concentration is seen only after several days.

Uses
Nicotinic acid is effective in treating most hyperlipidemias. Nicotinic acid or a bile acid sequestrant is the initial medication recommended to lower LDL cholesterol when dietary and other lifestyle modifications have failed to be effective. LDL cholesterol is usually lowered by 10% to 25%, triglycerides by 20% to 50%, and HDL cholesterol is usually raised by 15% to 35%.

Adverse Reactions, Contraindications, and Toxicity
The high doses of nicotinic acid needed as an antilipemic agent produce troublesome side effects in most patients, and only a few patients can tolerate continued use of nicotinic acid. Most patients experience marked flushing because of its vasodilator action. Itching and GI upset are also frequent side effects. Tolerance to these symptoms may develop; thus the dosage is usually low at first and increased gradually to avoid severe reactions. Niacin can cause or aggravate peptic ulcer, glucose intolerance (diabetes), and high plasma uric acid (gout). Chronic liver disease is a contraindication for use of nicotinic acid. An extended-release form of nicotinic acid is available but is associated with a greater prevalence of hepatotoxicity.

CONJUGATED ESTROGENS

Conjugated estrogens have been shown to decrease the risk for coronary heart disease in postmenopausal women by about 50%. The levels of LDL are decreased by 15%, and the levels of HDL are increased by 15%. Triglycerides are also increased. Estrogen may be given alone if the woman has had a hysterectomy. However, women with a uterus should also receive a progestin either cyclically or continuously to reduce the risk of endometrial cancer (see Chapter 64). Although there is concern that estrogen administration may increase the risk for breast cancer, this association has not been substantiated in clinical trials to date. The National Institutes of Health is addressing this concern in the Women's Health Initiative. Estrogen also protects postmenopausal women against osteoporosis. Estrogen given to men not only causes feminization but also increases the incidence of heart attacks.

PROBUCOL

Probucol (Lorelco) enhances the uptake of LDL by the liver and increases fecal bile acid excretion. Serum LDL-cholesterol is lowered by 5% to 15%, HDL-cholesterol is lowered by 20% to 30%, and triglycerides are generally unchanged. Because of the lowering of HDL, probucol has limited use. The combination of probucol and a bile acid sequestrant (cholestyramine or colestipol) produces an additive lowering of LDL, whereas the HDL lowering effect is decreased. A clinical response to probucol occurs after 1 to 3 months of therapy.

Probucol is very lipid soluble and accumulates in the adipose tissue, where it remains for about 6 months after therapy is discontinued. Probucol is not recommended for pregnant or nursing mothers because of its accumulation in adipose tissue, although specific problems have not been documented. The most common side effects of probucol are GI upset, including diarrhea, gas, abdominal pain, nausea, and vomiting. Some cardiac effects have been demonstrated in animal tests, so patients with a history of cardiac arrhythmias should be monitored.

NURSING PROCESS OVERVIEW

Blood Lipid Levels

Assessment

Baseline assessment should include a general physical assessment and weight, serum cholesterol and triglyceride levels, blood pressure, and dietary history. Be sure to include exercise and smoking patterns in the assessment.

Nursing Diagnoses

- Altered health maintenance related to insufficient knowledge of effects of tobacco use
- Altered nutrition: more than body requirements related to lack of knowledge of nutritional needs and exercise
- Altered bowel elimination: diarrhea related to antilipemic therapy
- Health-seeking behaviors: low cholesterol diet, available smoking cessation clinics, or age-appropriate exercise programs

Patient Outcomes

The patient will lose weight to ideal body weight by limiting fat and caloric intake and adhering to a low-fat, low-cholesterol diet. The patient will achieve a lower serum cholesterol level through dietary modification, exercise, and the use of medications, with no intolerable side effects due to the medications. The patient will stop smoking.

Planning/Implementation

These drugs have few side effects in usual doses. Evaluate new signs or symptoms. Discharge planning should include instruction by the dietitian, particularly if the type of hyperlipidemia can be better treated by dietary restriction or weight loss.

Evaluation

By discharge, ascertain that the patient can explain why and how to take the prescribed drug, when to take it in relation to meals, what anticipated side effects to expect and what to do about them, which symptoms should be reported immediately to the physician, and how to plan meals within prescribed dietary restrictions.

NURSING IMPLICATIONS SUMMARY

General Guidelines: Drugs to Lower Blood Lipid Levels

Patient and Family Education

- Many of the drugs cause GI side effects. Forewarn the patient about this. Provide emotional support as needed. Instruct the patient about the importance of taking the drug as prescribed for best effect.
- Review the patient problem box on constipation (p. 304).
- Tell the patient to report persistent or severe diarrhea to the physician.
- Teach the patient about necessary changes in diet to lower fat, carbohydrate, and cholesterol intake, as needed; see the dietary consideration box on cholesterol (p. 276). Refer the patient to the dietitian as needed. Teach the patients that these drugs must be taken for weeks to months before their full benefit can be seen. If the drugs prove to be beneficial, they may then be prescribed on a long-term basis.
- Remind the patient not to discontinue taking the drug without consulting the physician. Doses of other medications may be prescribed based on their effect when the patient is taking the prescribed antilipemic agent. Discontinuing the antilipemic therapy may result in incorrect doses of other drugs being taken. Because antilipemic agents may interfere with absorption of other prescribed drugs, remind the patient to keep all health care providers informed of all drugs being taken.
- Emphasize the importance of all prescribed activities, including drug therapy, ceasing smoking, exercise, and modifying diet in lowering cholesterol and reducing the risk of heart and vascular disease.
- For missed doses: take the missed dose as soon as remembered unless almost time for the next dose, then omit missed dose and resume regular dosing schedule. Do not double up for missed doses.
- It may be appropriate to screen children for the presence of familial hyperlipidemias; if necessary, place them on therapeutic diets to lower lipid levels.

Cholestyramine and Colestipol

Drug Administration

- Monitor intake and output, weight, urinalysis, and vital signs. Assess the patient for skin changes and rashes.
- Schedule drug administration times to allow as much time as possible between cholestyramine or colestipol and other drugs taken orally. At minimum, other drugs should be taken 1 hour before or 4 hours after cholestyramine or colestipol.

Patient and Family Education

- Review the general guidelines.
- GI side effects are the most common. Instruct the patient to report the development of any unexpected sign or symptom.
- Review all the drugs the patient is taking. Plan a dosing schedule to allow as much time as possible to elapse between the administration of the antilipemic and other medications.
- For the chewable bar form, instruct the patient to chew each bite well before swallowing.
- Instruct the patient not to take the powder in dry form. Always mix it with fluid or food or fruit with a high fluid content such as applesauce, crushed pineapple, or thin soups, or with milk in hot or regular breakfast cereals. Fill a glass with 2 ounces of chosen fluid. Put the correct dose of medication on top of the fluid and mix thoroughly. Add an additional 2 to 4 ounces of fluid and again mix thoroughly. Instruct the patient to stir and drink the mixture while the drug is still suspended. The drug will not dissolve in the fluid. Add a little more of the selected beverage to rinse the glass, and drink this also. If a carbonated beverage is chosen, use a large glass to prevent spillover, because the mixture will foam up. To prevent swallowing air, especially if a carbonated beverage is chosen, drink the mixture slowly. Take doses before meals and at bedtime as ordered.
- Because these drugs interfere with absorption of fat-soluble vitamins, supplemental vitamins may be necessary; consult the physician.
- If these drugs are used to treat the pruritus of biliary stasis, the pruritus may reappear if the drug is discontinued.

Clofibrate

Patient and Family Education

- See the general guidelines.
- Nausea and diarrhea are the most common side effects, but others occasionally occur. Tell the patient to report the development of any unexpected sign or symptom. Impotence and decreased libido have occurred; the patient may be reluctant to mention these effects. Assess the patient carefully for sexual side effects. Provide emotional support. It may be possible to change the dose or the drug; consult the physician.
- Take doses with meals to lessen gastric irritation. Nausea may diminish with continued use of the drug.

Gemfibrozil

Patient and Family Education

- Review the general guidelines.
- Instruct the patient to take doses 30 minutes before breakfast and the evening meal.

Continued.

NURSING IMPLICATIONS SUMMARY—cont'd

- GI upset is the most common side effect, but others occasionally occur. Tell the patient to report the development of any unexpected sign or symptom.

Lovastatin, Pravastatin, and Simvastatin

Patient and Family Education

- Review the general guidelines.
- GI discomfort may occur, and a variety of other side effects have been reported. Instruct the patient to report the development of any unexpected sign or symptom.
- Warn the patient to avoid driving or operating hazardous equipment if blurred vision or weakness develops and to notify the physician of these effects.
- For pravastatin and simvastatin, take doses in the evening or at bedtime. For lovastatin, take doses with the evening meal if ordered once a day; if ordered more than once a day, take each dose with a meal or snack.

Nicotinic Acid (Niacin)

Patient and Family Education

- Review the general guidelines.
- Most patients experience flushing of the face and neck after taking the high dose needed for the antilipemic effect. This effect usually diminishes with continued use of the drug. Starting with low doses and gradually increasing them may also help reduce flushing and pruritus. Flushing may be ameliorated by taking one 300 mg or a single 300 mg or one regular (300 mg) aspirin tablet 30 minutes before the niacin dose (check with physician). GI discomfort may occur, and a variety of other side effects have been reported. Instruct the patient to report the development of any unexpected sign or symptom. Taking doses with meals or milk may reduce GI irritation.
- For information about dietary sources of niacin, see the dietary consideration box on vitamins (p. 215).
- Instruct the patient to swallow extended-release forms whole, without chewing or crushing. Scored tablets may be broken in half. Contents of capsules may be poured into a small amount of food and swallowed but should not be chewed.
- Caution patients with diabetes to monitor blood glucose levels carefully during periods of dosage adjustment while on niacin.

Probucol

Patient and Family Education

- Review the general guidelines.
- Instruct the patient to report the development of a fast or irregular heartbeat or fainting. GI discomfort may occur, and a variety of other side effects have been reported. Instruct the patient to report the development of any unexpected sign or symptom.
- Instruct the patient to take doses with meals for best effect.

CRITICAL THINKING

APPLICATION

1. List the four categories of lipoprotein and describe the role of each.
2. What is hyperlipidemia? What causes it?
3. Name drugs and their mechanism of action for lowering triglyceride levels.

CRITICAL THINKING

1. Compare and contrast the bile acid sequestrants, fibric acid derivatives, and HMG-CoA reductase inhibitors. Consider actions, side effects, and potential for patient compliance. Call the pharmacy and find the cost for a 30-day supply of each drug.
2. Develop a teaching plan for the patient who needs to decrease dietary intake of cholesterol.
3. Consider the risk factors identified for coronary heart disease (see box, p. 275). Which ones can be influenced by the patient? Who can you help the patient lower the risk for heart disease?

CHAPTER 22

Drugs to Treat Anemia

OBJECTIVES

After studying this chapter, you should be able to do the following:

- *Explain the role of iron in normal body functioning.*
- *Develop a nursing care plan for the patient receiving iron therapy.*
- *Describe the treatment of iron toxicity.*
- *Explain the treatment of pernicious anemia and develop a nursing care plan for patients who receive vitamin B_{12}.*
- *Outline dietary sources of iron, folic acid, and vitamin B_{12}.*
- *Explain the use of epoetin alpha and develop a nursing care plan for patients receiving it.*

KEY TERMS

hemochromatosis
hemosiderosis
intrinsic factor
iron
iron deficiency anemia
megaloblastic macrocytic anemia
pernicious anemia

CHAPTER OVERVIEW

This chapter discusses iron, vitamin B_{12}, folic acid, and related agents used to treat anemia. These agents are most commonly associated with anemia of nutritional origin. They play a major role in the production of new red blood cells—the process of *hematopoiesis.*

Erythropoietin, a growth factor produced by the kidney, promotes hematopoiesis. Erythropoietin is a new product available through recombinant DNA technology.

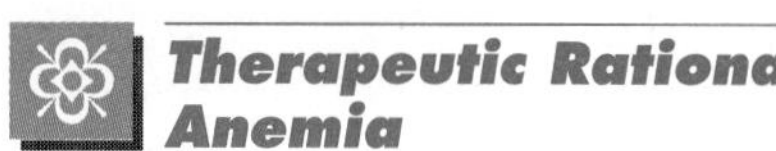

Therapeutic Rationale: Anemia

Iron, vitamin B_{12}, and folic acid are essential for the production of new blood cells. A deficiency results in anemia.

Iron Deficiency Anemia

When the intake of iron is inadequate to meet the demand, iron is first taken from the iron stores in hemosiderin and ferritin. Absorption of iron from the gastrointestinal (GI) tract can increase twofold when the ferritin within the mucosal cells is no longer saturated with iron. When iron stores are exhausted and the intake of iron is still inadequate, the newly made red blood cells are small (microcytic) and do not have much color (hypochromic) because there is not enough iron to make an adequate amount of hemoglobin to fill the cells. **Iron deficiency anemia** is therefore a microcytic hypochromic anemia.

Iron deficiency anemia commonly results from blood loss or rapid growth. This condition is reflected in the varying requirements for dietary iron. The average American diet contains about 6 mg of iron per 1000 calories, and only 10% of dietary iron is actually absorbed, although up to 20% may be absorbed in iron-deficient individuals. Adult men and postmenopausal women have the lowest daily requirement for dietary iron (5 to 10 mg). Menstruating women have a higher daily requirement, depending on the amount of blood loss during menstruation (7 to 20 mg). Pregnant women have the highest daily requirement (20 to 58 mg) because of the added demand of the placenta and developing fetus. Children and adolescents have a higher requirement per unit weight (4 to 20 mg total) than adults because of their rapid growth.

Megaloblastic Macrocytic Anemia

Both vitamin B_{12} and folic acid are required for a key reaction in the synthesis of thymidylate, a component of DNA. Whereas folic acid is the immediate cofactor in this synthesis, vitamin B_{12} regenerates the active form of folic acid. Deficiency of folic acid or vitamin B_{12} results in the release of too few red blood cells. Those red blood cells that are released are large and immature because of the deficiency of DNA synthesis required for cell division and maturation. This condition is a **megaloblastic macrocytic anemia,** or immature large cell anemia. Other tissue cells that turn over rapidly and require active DNA synthesis include some white and mucosal cells of the GI tract. A deficiency in white cell counts and GI upset can appear in vitamin B_{12} or folic acid deficiency.

Vitamin B_{12} and Pernicious Anemia

Vitamin B_{12} is unique because it requires a special binding protein for transport into the intestinal cells. This binding protein is called **intrinsic factor,** which is produced and released by the parietal cells of the stomach. (Parietal cells also release hydrochloric acid.) **Pernicious anemia** is the relative or complete lack of intrinsic factor so that vitamin B_{12} is no longer absorbed. The body has a large store of vitamin B_{12}, 4 to 5 mg, and a deficiency will not occur for 2 to 5 years after intrinsic factor is no longer released. Stomach atrophy is a normal part of the aging process, and pernicious anemia appears more frequently in patients older than 50 years of age than in younger patients. Any condition that damages the stomach can also cause pernicious anemia.

Anemia Related to Kidney Failure

Chronic renal failure is associated with underproduction of red blood cells. This happens because the kidney is the major producer of the growth factor, erythropoietin, which is critical to the production of red blood cells. When the kidneys fail, erythropoietin is not produced in sufficient quantity to maintain adequate red blood cell production in the bone marrow.

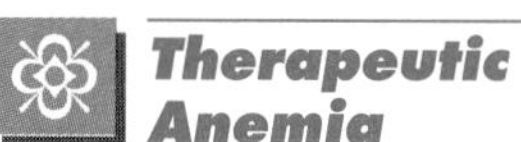

Therapeutic Agents: Anemia

✣ Iron

Mechanism of Action

Iron is an essential component of several key proteins that carry or use oxygen. Over 70% of body iron is part of hemoglobin, the protein of red blood cells that transports oxygen to tissues and carbon dioxide away from tissues. The red color of blood is caused by the iron-oxygen complex in the heme portion of hemoglobin. Iron is also part of several of the electron transport enzymes of the mitochondria responsible for the oxidation-reduction reactions essential to functioning cells.

Pharmacokinetics and Uses

Recycling of the body's iron. Given the importance of iron, it is not surprising that the body uses iron efficiently. The total iron content of a 70 kg man is about 4 gm, yet iron is reused so efficiently that less than 1 mg of iron is lost daily. Not only is the iron of the red blood cell reused after cell degradation, but 10% to 35% of the iron is in a storage form for use when required. Iron is lost only as body cells are lost through shedding of cells from the GI tract, skin, fingernails, and hair and in fluids such as bile, urine, and sweat.

Absorption of iron from food. Iron is available in many foods (see box, p. 285). The absorption of iron from food is regulated. Iron is taken up by active transport into the mucosal cells of the duodenum and upper jejunum in the small intestine. These cells contain the protein ferritin that binds the iron. When ferritin is saturated with iron, further absorption of iron is limited. It remains in the mucosal cells unless transferred to the plasma protein transferrin. Iron not transferred within 5 days is lost in the feces when the mucosal cell is sloughed. Iron bound to transferrin is carried in the plasma and transferred to the proteins ferritin and hemosiderin, which act as storage forms of iron within the liver, spleen, and bone marrow.

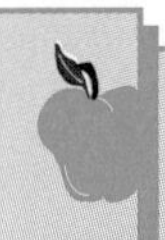

DIETARY CONSIDERATION

Iron

Inadequate iron intake contributes to iron deficiency anemia, the most common nutritional deficiency in the United States. Good dietary sources of iron include the following:

- Red meats
- Legumes and nuts
- Whole grains
- Molasses
- Dried fruits
- Organ meats
- Green leafy vegetables
- Enriched bread and cereal
- Brewer's yeast
- Oysters

Administration of iron. Iron for replacement therapy is most commonly given orally as a ferrous salt. Iron preparations are listed in Table 22-1. Ferrous sulfate is the standard for these preparations. The usual daily dose of iron in iron deficiency anemia is 50 to 100 mg. The amount of iron per tablet depends on the ferrous salt used. A 300 mg tablet of ferrous sulfate contains 60 mg of iron and 240 mg of sulfate; a 300 mg tablet of ferrous gluconate contains 37 mg of iron and 263 mg of gluconate; and a 300 mg tablet of ferrous fumarate contains 99 mg of iron and 201 mg of fumarate.

Iron in the ferrous form is absorbed most readily in the presence of acid. Therefore optimum absorption occurs when a tablet of ferrous sulfate or other soluble ferrous salt is taken before meals. However, iron is also highly irritating to the GI tract; many patients cannot tolerate iron tablets taken on an empty stomach and have to take iron with meals. Enteric forms are not satisfactory because they generally dissolve past the duodenum, where there is little capacity for the absorption of iron. Infants and children given iron-supplemented formula or vitamins may develop acute diarrhea from the GI irritation.

Patients with iron deficiency anemia respond to iron therapy in the first 2 days with increased energy and appetite. Because this is too soon to correct the hemoglobin deficiency, the response may be due to restoration of the cellular enzymes containing iron. After 1 week there is an increase in the number of reticulocytes (immature red blood cells) and the rate of hemoglobin synthesis. Although the microcytic anemia of iron deficiency is eliminated after a few weeks of therapy, at least 6 months of therapy is necessary to restore iron storage sites.

Iron may also be given parenterally as iron dextran when oral administration is not possible. Slow intravenous (IV) injection is preferred. Deep intramuscular (IM) injection is painful and can discolor the injection site. An anaphylactic response is more common after IM than after IV injection.

Adverse Reactions and Contraindications

Iron taken orally can cause GI discomfort. Infants are especially sensitive to the iron in infant formulas and vitamins. Liquid dosage forms can stain the teeth. More seriously, iron can occasionally cause an allergic reaction with skin rash or hives and trouble breathing. This reaction is more common after parenteral administration. Iron is contraindicated for persons with hemochromatosis or hemosiderosis and for those with hemolytic anemia or thalassemia.

Toxicity

Acute toxicity. Acute toxicity from iron is uncommon in adults and is primarily seen in young children. The population most likely to take iron tablets includes pregnant women who may also have small children. Many iron tablets are brightly colored and look like candy, leading young children to swallow many tablets at once. Commonly the child experiences acute nausea and vomiting 30 to 60 minutes after ingesting the tablets. Treatment is gastric lavage with sodium phosphate or sodium bicarbonate to remove undissolved tablets, to create an alkaline environment that retards absorption, and to complex the ferrous iron into insoluble salts.

Within a few hours of ingestion, metabolic acidosis is common and cardiovascular collapse can occur. If supportive treatment carries the child through these stages, the next stage originates from tissue injury. The high concentration of iron overloads the uptake capacity of the mucosal cells so that a high concentration of free ferrous iron enters the portal circulation. Signs of extensive damage to the liver and kidney are evident in children who die of iron toxicity after 24 hours.

Deferoxamine. To avoid damage from high plasma concentrations of iron, a specific antidote, deferoxamine mesylate (Desferal), is given as soon as possible and concurrently with lavage and supportive measures. Deferoxamine is given IM or IV and combines with iron in the plasma to form a water-soluble complex that is excreted in urine (67%) and in bile (33%). This complex gives a pink to red color to urine, which shows elevated concentrations of iron in the plasma. The free deferoxamine imparts no color to urine.

Chronic toxicity. Because the body has no mechanisms to remove excess iron, excess intake can cause iron overload, called **hemosiderosis** (after the storage protein for iron). Chronic iron overload can occur in patients treated with parenteral iron who receive frequent blood transfusions because each milliliter of blood contains 0.5 mg of iron. Some patients have a genetic tendency to store excess iron; this genetic disorder is called **hemochromatosis.** Iron overload traditionally imparts a bronze color to the skin of the face, neck, upper chest, genitalia, hands, and forearms. The pancreas is especially sensitive to damage, and diabetes mellitus can result. Liver damage is seen on biopsy but is generally not serious unless superimposed on liver disease. Patients with iron overload generally die of heart failure. Treatment for iron overload is weekly bleeding (phlebotomy).

Interactions

Absorption of iron salts is increased with ingestion of large doses of ascorbic acid (vitamin C). Cereal and eggs decrease absorption, as do antacids, particularly magnesium trisilicate,

TABLE 22-1 Drugs to Treat Nutritional Anemias

GENERIC NAME	TRADE NAME	ADMINISTRATION/DOSAGE	COMMENTS
Iron Salts for Iron Deficiency Anemia			
Ferrous fumarate (33% elemental iron)	Femiron Fumerin Palafer† Various others	Replacement therapy requires 90-300 mg of elemental iron daily in divided doses before meals if tolerated or with meals.	Timed-release or enteric coated forms considered less effective because of poor iron absorption beyond duodenum.
Ferrous gluconate (11.6% elemental iron)	Fergon Fertinic† Various others	See above.	See above.
✣ Ferrous sulfate (20% elemental iron)	Feosol Fer-In-Sol* Fero-Gradumet Various others	See above.	See above.
Iron-dextran injection	Imferon* Various others	INTRAVENOUS: *Adults and children*—no more than 100 mg daily, no faster than 50 mg (1 ml)/min of undiluted solution, or dilute in 500-1000 ml normal saline solution and administer by drip over 10 hr. FDA pregnancy category C.	Reserved for use in severe iron deficiency anemia when oral iron is contraindicated (GI disease) or unsuccessful. Serious toxic effects, including anaphylaxis, may accompany parenteral administration and are more common with IM than with IV administration.
Iron-polysaccharide complex	Hytinic Niferex	See above.	Not well absorbed. May be milder to stomach than other formulations.
Antidote for Iron Toxicity			
Deferoxamine mesylate	Desferal*	INTRAMUSCULAR: Preferred route; 1 gm followed by 0.5 gm at 4 hr and 8 hr. INTRAVENOUS: In face of cardiovascular collapse; as IM but infused at 15 mg kg/hr. Not to exceed 6 gm in 24 hr.	A specific chelator for iron. To manage acute iron intoxication. Will turn urine pink to red. Can be administered long term to manage secondary hemochromatosis.
Vitamin B_{12} (Cyanocobalamin) for Pernicious Anemia			
Hydroxocobalamin	Alphamine Acti-B_{12}† Various others	As for cyanocobalamin.	Like cyanocobalamin. Somewhat longer acting.
Vitamin B_{12} (cyanocobalamin)	Betalin 12 Redisol Rubramin PC* Various others	INTRAMUSCULAR: 30-50 μg daily for 5-10 days, then 100-200 μg monthly.	For pernicious anemia, only IM injection effective. Oral forms taken for dietary deficiency.
Folic Acid for Anemia			
Folic acid	Apo-Folic† Folvite*	ANY ROUTE: *Adults and children*—1 mg daily.	Solutions of sodium salt used for parenteral administration.
Leucovorin calcium	Wellcovorin Generic	For megaloblastic anemia, 1 mg daily. To counter folic acid antagonists, give in amounts equal to weight of antagonist.	Metabolically active form of folic acid. Expense does not justify use for anemia, but protects normal tissue when given with methotrexate (antineoplastic drug) or pyrimethamine (antimalarial drug).
Hormone for Anemia			
✣ Epoetin Alpha	Epogen EPO	INTRAVENOUS, SUBCUTANEOUS: *Adults and children*—initially, 50-100 units/kg 3 times weekly. Dosage is adjusted to reach hematocrit of 30% to 33%.	Epoetin is protein hormone, erythropoietin, produced by recombinant DNA technology. Used to treat anemia of chronic renal failure.

*Available in Canada and United States.
†Available in Canada only.

and tetracyclines, because all these bind to iron and prevent its uptake by the mucosal cells in the small intestine.

Vitamin B_{12}

Mechanism of Action

Vitamin B_{12} is required for the synthesis of thymidylate, a component of DNA. Deficiency of vitamin B_{12}, like folic acid, affects the maturation of red blood cells and results in a megaloblastic macrocytic anemia. In addition, vitamin B_{12} is required for maintenance of the myelin sheath of nerves.

Pharmacokinetics

A diet that includes animal protein, eggs, and dairy products contains adequate vitamin B_{12}. The usual American diet contains 5 to 15 μg of vitamin B_{12}, although the minimum daily requirement is only 1 to 2 μg. Only strict vegetarians may develop dietary vitamin B_{12} deficiency over a period of several years. Vitamin B_{12} bound to intrinsic factor is absorbed in the distal ileum, the part of the small intestine just ahead of the large intestine, and this absorption requires a slightly alkaline pH. Conditions in which the distal ileum is damaged or removed or in which the pancreas fails to secrete sufficient bicarbonate to keep the intestine at a slightly alkaline pH slow absorption of vitamin B_{12}. After absorption, vitamin B_{12} is carried to storage sites. Some vitamin B_{12} is excreted in the bile but is later reabsorbed.

The IM injection of vitamin B_{12} to bypass the intestine for systemic absorption is the treatment for pernicious anemia. Initial therapy is administered daily for about 1 week, then monthly throughout life. Oral vitamin B_{12} is indicated only for the rare dietary deficiency of vitamin B_{12} when there is an adequate amount of intrinsic factor released.

Uses

Vitamin B_{12} is indicated for the treatment of pernicious anemia. Neurologic damage may result from deficiency of vitamin B_{12}. This damage arises because vitamin B_{12} is a cofactor for an enzymatic step necessary for producing the myelin sheath of nerves. A frequent initial neurologic symptom of vitamin B_{12} deficiency is a tingling sensation of the extremities (paresthesia) from neurologic damage. Neurologic damage becomes irreversible if vitamin B_{12} deficiency persists.

Vitamin B_{12} injections have been given indiscriminately to older adult patients as a general tonic, which it is not. Vitamin B_{12} injections are also not of therapeutic value for general neurologic disorders, psychiatric disorders, general malnutrition, or loss of appetite.

Adverse Reactions, Contraindications, and Toxicity

Vitamin B_{12} injections are virtually free of side effects. Patients who receive vitamin B_{12} injections for pernicious anemia must understand that injections must be continued for the rest of their lives to avoid irreversible neurologic damage.

Interactions

Folic acid taken in large doses will overcome the block in DNA synthesis caused by the deficiency of vitamin B_{12}. Folic acid will thereby cure the anemia, but folic acid cannot affect the vitamin B_{12}–dependent reaction necessary for myelin synthesis. If folic acid is taken indiscriminately, the anemia of vitamin B_{12} deficiency will never appear, but neurologic damage may proceed until it is irreversible.

Folic Acid

Mechanism of Action

Like vitamin B_{12}, folic acid is required for the synthesis of thymidylate, a component of DNA. Deficiency of folic acid, like vitamin B_{12}, affects the maturation of red blood cells and results in a megaloblastic macrocytic anemia.

Pharmacokinetics

Folic acid is found in most meats, fresh vegetables, and fresh fruits, but it is destroyed when these foods are cooked for longer than 15 minutes. Folic acid preparations are listed in Table 22-1. The minimum daily requirement is 50 gm, and the average American diet contains 200 to 300 gm. Unlike vitamin B_{12}, stores of folic acid are not large and can be depleted in a few weeks when the diet is deficient in folic acid. It is readily absorbed in the intestine and administered orally. Individuals with poor diets and chronic alcoholics may be deficient in folic acid.

Uses

Pregnant women and nursing mothers have increased requirements for folic acid, and this agent is commonly given as a routine supplement to these women. Studies have shown that folic acid taken during pregnancy reduces the incidence of neurologic defects in newborn infants.

Adverse Reactions, Contraindications, and Toxicity

Some drugs interfere with the use of folic acid; examples include phenytoin, oral contraceptives, glucocorticoids, and aspirin. Methotrexate, antineoplastic drugs, and pyrimethamine (an antimalarial drug) are folic acid antagonists. When these drugs are used, folinic acid (leucovorin), the metabolically active form of folic acid, can be given to protect normal tissues from folic acid deficiency.

Folic acid is nontoxic. The greatest danger associated with the indiscriminate ingestion of folic acid is that it may correct the anemia of pernicious anemia but leave the neurologic damage untreated.

✣ Epoetin Alpha

Mechanism of Action

Epoetin alpha (Epogen and EPO) is the human hormone erythropoietin, manufactured by recombinant DNA technology, that stimulates the production of red blood cells.

Pharmacokinetics

Epoetin alpha is a protein and must be administered intravenously or subcutaneously. It is commonly administered three times a week. The effect is seen in 1 to 2 weeks. The dosage should not be adjusted for 8 weeks, and it should not be changed more frequently than every 4 weeks. The dosage should be discontinued gradually by lowering the dose by 25 units/kg body weight every 4 weeks.

Uses

Epoetin counteracts the anemia associated with chronic renal failure. This effect eliminates the need for transfusion of red blood cells and greatly improves the patient's quality of life. Patients should be evaluated to ensure that they have adequate iron stores to support red blood cell production. Epoetin is being evaluated for treatment of anemia resulting in a number of other conditions, including azathioprine (AZT) treatment and cancer.

Adverse Reactions, Contraindications, and Toxicity

Side effects of epoetin are minimal. Occasional headaches or joint pain are reported. About one third of patients have elevated blood pressure that may require drug therapy. However, renal function does not worsen. Epoetin should not be administered to individuals with uncontrolled hypertension.

Abuse of epoetin has been reported among athletes in high-endurance sports, especially cyclists. The increased production of red blood cells enhances athletic performance by increasing the blood's ability to carry oxygen. The increased number of red blood cells makes the blood more viscous, and this viscosity is enhanced by the dehydration of performance. Death from heart blockage was reported in one young athlete who was taking epoetin.

NURSING PROCESS OVERVIEW

Iron Therapy

Assessment

Patients who require iron therapy may have fatigue, pallor, and lethargy. Folic acid and vitamin B_{12} deficiency are usually diagnosed from blood studies but may be seen in patients with iron deficiency anemia. Assess vital signs, weight, and diet history; blood studies, including hemoglobin level, peripheral blood smear, and reticulocyte count; and any neurologic symptoms such as tingling in the fingers or toes.

Nursing Diagnoses

- Altered bowel elimination: constipation related to iron therapy
- Fatigue related to anemia

Patient Outcomes

The patient will display increased energy and less pallor as anemia is treated. The patient will state that his or her energy level is better.

Planning/Implementation

At usual dosages there are few side effects with these drugs. If the source of anemia is diet related, provide dietary instruction about iron-rich foods. If pernicious anemia is diagnosed, instruct the patient about the need for continued treatment.

Evaluation

Determine that the patient can explain what kind of anemia is present, what the goals of drug therapy are, how to take the prescribed medications correctly, what anticipated side effects are and what to do about them, and which symptoms can be expected to improve and which will not. (The neurologic damage in pernicious anemia may be permanent.) Verify that the patient can identify dietary sources of needed iron or folic acid.

NURSING IMPLICATIONS SUMMARY

General Guidelines: Patient Receiving Iron Therapy

Drug Administration

- Parenteral and oral iron preparations should not be given at the same time because this combination increases the incidence of toxic reactions.
- Parenteral doses of iron may cause anaphylactic reactions. Before giving the first dose of IM or IV iron dextran, administer a test dose of 25 mg. Monitor the vital signs. Wait at least 1 hour before administering the remaining dose. Have available appropriate equipment, drugs, and personnel to treat anaphylactic reactions. Other reactions may include febrile reactions, arthralgias, myalgia, headache, transitory paresthesia, nausea, shivering, and rash.

Intramuscular Iron Dextran

- Use large muscle masses, preferably the buttocks. The drug may stain the skin, which is cosmetically unacceptable on the thigh. Consult the physician when administering this drug to small children and infants. Draw up the prescribed dose. Put a fresh needle on the syringe. Use the Z-track method of administration (see Chapter 5).

Intravenous Iron Dextran

- Read the vial carefully; use preparations labeled "for IV use." The drug may be given undiluted or diluted in 50 to 250 ml normal saline solution. Administer a test dose over at least 5 minutes. Administer other doses at a rate of 50 mg/minute. Flush the IV line with normal saline solution before and after administering dose. Keep the patient in a supine position for 30 minutes after IV doses; monitor vital signs and blood pressure.

Patient and Family Education

- Review the dietary sources of iron with the patient (see the dietary consideration box on iron (p. 285). Remind the patient to keep all medications out of the reach of children. Instruct the family to have ipecac available when iron preparations are in use but always to call the poison control center or emergency department before using ipecac to induce vomiting. Tell the patient to notify the physician immediately if overdose with iron is suspected.
- Instruct the patient to take liquid iron preparations through a straw to avoid staining the teeth. Teach the patient to dilute the preparation well with water or fruit juice and to rinse the mouth thoroughly after taking the dose. Advise the patient to brush teeth with baking soda or hydrogen peroxide 3% to remove stains.
- Ideally, instruct the patient to take the iron preparation on an empty stomach, 1 hour before or 2 hours after meals, although this may cause significant GI upset. Teach the patient to take doses with a full glass (240 ml) of fluid for an adult or one half glass (120 ml) of fluid for children. Teach the patient to take drug with meals or snack to reduce gastric irritation. Take iron 2 hours after or 1 hour before eating cheese and yogurt, eggs, milk, spinach, tea, coffee, or whole-grain breads and cereals, and bran. Do not take iron at the same time as antacids or calcium supplements; space doses of these 1 to 2 hours apart. Ascorbic acid (vitamin C) increases the absorption of iron; some patients may wish to take the iron with orange or other citrus juice.
- Inform the patient that regular use of iron will cause the feces to turn dark green or black and to become more tarry in consistency. Patients who have *no* change in stool should notify the physician. If there is doubt about whether the cause of a change in color or consistency in stools is due to blood or ingestion of iron, test the stool for the presence of blood.
- Most patients experience constipation while taking iron preparations; some experience diarrhea. See the patient problem box on constipation (p. 304). If diarrhea is severe or persistent, notify the physician. To decrease gastric irritation, suggest that the patient take smaller but more frequent doses of iron (check with the physician).

Deferoxamine Mesylate

Drug Administration

- See Chapter 9.
- Deferoxamine may be administered via IM, IV, or subcutaneous injection, usually by subcutaneous pump. IM or subcutaneous injection may cause swelling, irritation, pain, and itching at the injection site.
- Deferoxamine has been associated with allergic reactions, including anaphylactic reactions. Monitor vital signs. Have equipment and drugs available to treat acute allergic reactions.

Intravenous Deferoxamine

- Dilute as directed in the manufacturer's literature. Administer at a rate not exceeding 15 mg/kg/hour. Monitor the blood pressure and vital signs. Treatment of acute iron overdose should be done in the acute care setting.

Continued.

NURSING IMPLICATIONS SUMMARY—cont'd

Vitamin B_{12}

Drug Administration

- Administer parenteral doses via the IM route only.
- Allergic reactions have been reported. Monitor vital signs and blood pressure. Have available drugs and equipment to treat acute allergic responses.

Patient and Family Education

- Teach patients with pernicious anemia about their disease. It may be difficult for them to understand why the vitamin B_{12} cannot be taken orally and why it must be continued for life.
- Review dietary sources of vitamin B_{12} (see the dietary consideration box on vitamins (p. 215) with patients in whom vitamin B_{12} deficiency is due to dietary causes. Strict vegetarians may require vitamin supplements that contain vitamin B_{12}.
- Limit the use of alcohol while taking vitamin B_{12}.

Folic Acid

Drug Administration

- In addition to the more common oral administration, folic acid may be given by the IM, IV, or subcutaneous route.
- IV folic acid may be given undiluted or added to most IV solutions and given as an infusion. For direct IV administration, administer at a rate not to exceed 5 mg/minute.
- Allergic reactions, though rare, have been reported. Monitor vital signs after parenteral administration. Have drugs and equipment available to treat acute allergic reactions.

Patient and Family Education

- Review the dietary sources of folic acid (see the dietary consideration box on vitamins, p. 215).
- Warn the patient that self-treatment with large doses of vitamins is unwise and may mask some health problems. Large doses of vitamins should be taken only under the direction of a physician.

Leucovorin

Drug Administration/Patient and Family Education

- Leucovorin is the calcium salt of folinic acid, a metabolite of folic acid. Read the physician's orders carefully. The drug may be given orally, IM, or IV. Parenteral administration is usually used when the drug is given to counteract some of the toxic effects of the folic acid antagonists, especially some cancer chemotherapy drugs (called leucovorin rescue). (See Chapter 49.)

Parenteral Administration

- Reconstitute as directed on the vial. For total doses <10 mg/m^2, dilute with bacteriostatic water that contains benzyl alcohol as a preservative for injection. For doses >10 mg/m^2, use sterile water without a preservative. Further dilute in 100 to 500 ml of common IV fluid. Administer dilute volume at a rate not exceeding 160 mg/minute because of the calcium content. Monitor vital signs.
- For leucovorin rescue/folinic acid rescue several protocols may be used. The dose is based on the dose of methotrexate and the body surface area of the patient. Monitor the serum creatinine level.
- Review with the patient and family the reason leucovorin is being used. Instruct them to report the development of any unexpected sign or symptom.

Epoetin Alpha

Drug Administration

- This drug may be given undiluted as an IV bolus. Read the accompanying literature. Do not shake the vial. Prepare only 1 dose per vial. Administer the dose over at least 1 minute. For dialysis patients, it may be administered via the venous line at the end of dialysis. This agent may also be administered IV or subcutaneously in patients not receiving dialysis. Monitor blood pressure, and report increases to the physician.
- Dose and length of therapy are based on patient response. Monitor the complete blood cell count with differential, platelet counts, blood urea nitrogen, uric acid, serum creatinine, phosphorus, and serum electrolytes.

Patient and Family Education

- Although usually given by a nurse, this drug may be prescribed for self-administration at home by some patients. Instruct the patient in how to administer and have the patient give a return demonstration of the injection technique.
- This drug may cause seizures, especially during the first 90 days. This side effect is rare, but caution the patient to avoid driving or operating hazardous equipment during this period until the effects of the medication are known.
- Review the reasons for epoetin therapy. Instruct the patient to report the development of any new sign or symptom. Emphasize the importance of returning for scheduled follow-up visits and taking doses as ordered, even if the patient is feeling better. Emphasize the importance of prescribed therapies, including other medications and special dietary restrictions.

CRITICAL THINKING

APPLICATION

1. What is the role of iron?
2. Describe factors governing the absorption of iron.
3. What are the symptoms of iron toxicity?
4. How does deferoxamine function as an antidote for iron toxicity?
5. What is pernicious anemia?
6. Why does vitamin B_{12} have to be injected intramuscularly to treat pernicious anemia?
7. What role do vitamin B_{12} and folic acid play in red blood cell maturation?
8. Why is folic acid contraindicated for treatment of pernicious anemia?
9. Why is chronic renal failure associated with underproduction of red blood cells?

CRITICAL THINKING

1. Why is iron poisoning so dangerous in young children?
2. What are important teaching points about epoetin alpha?
3. How would you respond to a student athlete colleague who wants to know about epoetin to increase athletic endurance?

SECTION VI

Drugs Affecting the Gastrointestinal System

The gastrointestinal system processes food and water and eliminates undigestible material. The parasympathetic (cholinergic) nervous system stimulates the digestive processes by increasing digestive secretions and the tone and motility of the smooth muscle of the stomach and intestines. The sympathetic (adrenergic) nervous system plays a minor role in the digestive processes. Although the parasympathetic nervous system acts on all parts of the digestive tract, current research is uncovering a complex system in which activities in each segment of the digestive tract are further regulated by a variety of peptide hormones, prostaglandins, and the biogenic amines histamine and serotonin. The roles of only a few of these factors are well characterized.

This section focuses on specific conditions affecting the gastrointestinal tract for which there are pharmacologic interventions. The four chapters of Section VI cover drugs that alter gastrointestinal tone and motility (Chapter 23), control diarrhea and relieve constipation (Chapter 24), control vomiting (Chapter 25), and are used to treat ulcers (Chapter 26).

CHAPTER 23

Drugs Affecting Motility: Cholinergic Stimulants and Anticholinergics/ Antispasmodics

OBJECTIVES

After studying this chapter, you should be able to do the following:

- *Discuss the use of drugs that alter gastrointestinal tone and motility.*
- *Develop a nursing care plan for patients receiving the following drugs or drug groups: bethanechol, cisapride, metoclopramide, neostigmine, belladonna alkaloids, atropine and related drugs, and antispasmodics.*
- *Develop a teaching plan for patients who have xerostomia.*

KEY TERMS

anticholinergic drugs
antispasmodic
belladonna alkaloids
xerostomia

CHAPTER OVERVIEW

Motility of the gastrointestinal system is controlled locally as well as by the autonomic nervous system (Figure 23-1). Two major nerve plexuses provide the intrinsic control and use acetylcholine as the neurotransmitter. These two intrinsic nerve plexuses are the myenteric plexus, located between the longitudinal and circular layers of the intestinal smooth muscle, and the submucous nerve plexus, located in the submucosal region. These local nerve complexes not only respond to local events but are subject to regulation by the autonomic nervous system. The cholinergic nervous system stimulates gastrointestinal activity. The release of acetylcholine from the cholinergic neurons to the ganglia of the intrinsic nerve plexuses is controlled by dopaminergic presynaptic receptors.

Drugs that mimic acetylcholine or stimulate its release promote gastrointestinal motility. Drugs that antagonize acetylcholine or its release inhibit gastrointestinal motility.

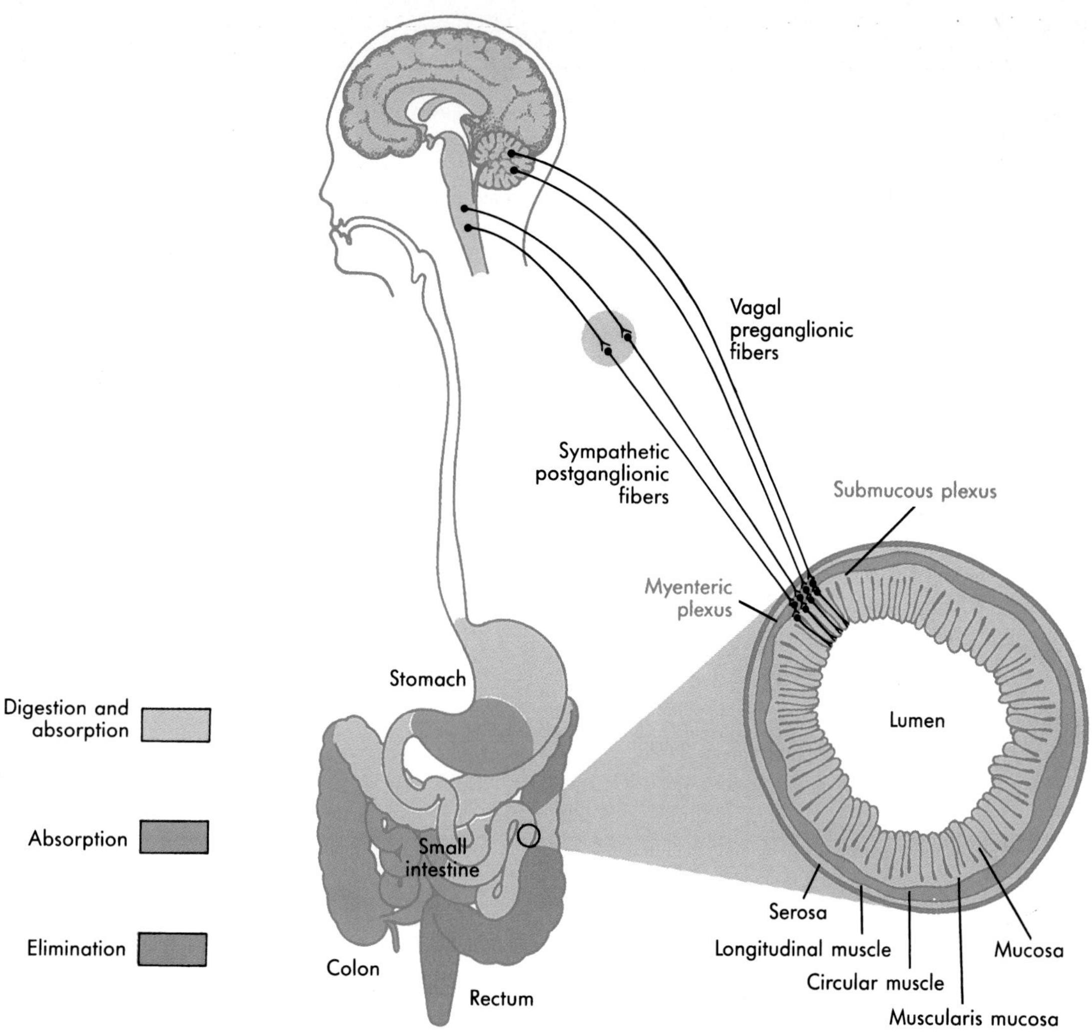

FIGURE 23-1

Overall functions of GI tract. Autonomic nervous system modulates longitudinal musculature of small intestine. Small intestine also has complex intrinsic autonomic system controlling circular musculature and secretion.

Therapeutic Rationale: Atonic Intestine

Hypomotility of the intestine can arise after surgery or result from conditions such as gastroesophageal reflux disease, diabetic gastroparesis, or gastric stasis. Atonic conditions of the intestine include intestinal atony, pseudoobstruction, and adynamic colon.

Therapeutic Agents: Gastrointestinal Stimulants

Drugs used to treat an atonic gastrointestinal (GI) tract act directly or indirectly to stimulate the muscarinic receptors of the intrinsic nervous system that control motility in the intestine. The cholinomimetic drugs bethanechol and neostigmine act at the level of the smooth muscle. Metoclopramide, a dopaminergic antagonist, acts at presynaptic dopamine receptors of the parasympathetic nervous system to promote release of acetylcholine. Cisapride stimulates the release of acetylcholine by an action on the myenteric plexus. These drugs are listed in Table 23-1.

GASTROINTESTINAL STIMULANTS

Bethanechol

Mechanism of Action

Bethanechol (Urecholine) is the only direct-acting cholinomimetic drug with sufficient tissue specificity to be administered systemically. It directly stimulates muscarinic receptors in the intestinal smooth muscle.

Pharmacokinetics

Bethanechol may be administered orally or subcutaneously. Absorption is rapid and complete. The onset of action is 30 to 60 minutes with a half-life of 7 to 10 hours. Bethanechol is metabolized by the liver and excreted in the urine.

TABLE 23-1 Drugs to Increase Gastrointestinal Tone and Motility

GENERIC NAME	TRADE NAME	ADMINISTRATION/DOSAGE	COMMENTS
Bethanechol chloride	Duvoid* Urabeth Urecholine*	ORAL: *Adults*—10-30 mg every 6-8 hr. SUBCUTANEOUS: *Adults*—2.5-5 mg every 6-8 hr; maximum, 10 mg/day. Never give intravenously or intramuscularly. Onset: 30 min.	Direct-acting cholinomimetic that stimulates atonic bladder and GI tract.
Cisapride	Propulsid*	ORAL: *Adults—Prophylaxis for gastroesophageal reflux:* 10 mg 2 times/day, before breakfast and at bedtime or 20 mg at bedtime. *Treatment:* 5-10 mg every 6-8 hr, 15 min before meals and at bedtime. *Children*—0.15-0.3 mg/kg body weight every 6-8 hr, before meals.	Serotonin antagonist; stimulates GI tract.
Domperidone†	Motilium†	ORAL: *Adults*—10 mg 3 or 4 times daily before meals, bedtime. *Children*—0.3 mg/kg 3 or 4 times daily before meals, bedtime.	Dopamine antagonist that hastens gastric emptying in diabetic gastroparesis and after barium administration. Related to metoclopramide but does not cross blood-brain barrier.
✣ Metoclopramide	Apo-Metoclop† Clopra Emex† Maxeran† Octamide Reclomide Reglan*	INTRAVENOUS: *Adults—Peristaltic stimulant:* 10 mg injected over 1-2 min. *Children*—1 mg/kg body weight; may repeat one time after 60 min. ORAL: *Adults*—10 mg 30 min before each meal and at bedtime. *Children 6-14 yr*—2.5-5.0 mg 3 times/day 30 min before meals. Onset: 1-3 min IV; 30-60 min orally.	Dopamine antagonist that hastens gastric emptying in diabetic gastroparesis and after barium administration.
Neostigmine methylsulfate	Prostigmin methylsulfate*	SUBCUTANEOUS, INTRAMUSCULAR: *Adults*—0.25-0.5 mg every 3-4 hr to stimulate bladder or GI tract. Onset: 10-20 min.	Acetylcholinesterase inhibitor that stimulates atonic bladder and GI tract.

*Available in Canada and United States.
†Available in Canada only.

Uses

At therapeutic doses bethanechol is relatively specific for the urinary and GI tracts. The stimulation it produces is useful for situations in which the bladder or intestine has lost its tone, such as after childbirth, surgery, or other abdominal trauma.

Adverse Reactions and Contraindications

Side effects of bethanechol are expected from muscarinic stimulation such as salivation, flushing of the skin, sweating, diarrhea, nausea and belching, and abdominal cramps. Because of these widespread side effects, the use of bethanechol has decreased with the introduction of newer agents.

Bethanechol should never be administered if there is any mechanical obstruction of the GI or urinary tract, such as stones or adhesions, because the hypermotility caused by the drug could lead to rupture of the tissue in the presence of an obstruction. Also, bethanechol is never administered intravenously or intramuscularly because the rate of absorption is so fast that toxic plasma concentrations of the drug are reached, resulting in possible heart block or a severe drop in blood pressure. Bethanechol may be administered subcutaneously if the oral route is not effective.

Interactions

Bethanechol interferes with anticholinergic or ganglionic blocking drugs. Bethanechol synergizes the action of cholinergic agents, especially cholinesterase inhibitors.

Cisapride

Mechanism of Action

Cisapride (Propulsid) is a serotonin receptor antagonist that increases the release of acetylcholine from the myenteric plexus. This action increases several activities, including esophageal clearance, tone of the lower esophageal sphincter, gastric emptying, and propulsion in the small intestine and colon.

Pharmacokinetics

Cisapride is absorbed rapidly and completely after oral administration. The onset of action is 30 to 60 minutes with a half-life of 7 to 10 hours. Cisapride is metabolized by the liver and excreted in the urine and feces.

Uses

Cisapride is used to manage gastroesophageal reflux disease, diabetic gastroparesis, intestinal atony, and adynamic colon. Treatment may continue for 2 to 3 months, but tolerance will often develop, limiting effectiveness.

Adverse Reactions and Contraindications

The most common side effect is diarrhea, which is dose dependent. Abdominal cramping, nausea, headache, or fatigue are other side effects sometimes reported. Rarely, seizures have been reported in patients with a history of seizures.

Cisapride is contraindicated for patients with GI hemorrhage, mechanical obstruction, or perforation. Dosage should be reduced for patients with hepatic or renal insufficiency because of the reduced clearance of cisapride. Nursing mothers should not take the drug because small amounts appear in breast milk.

Interactions

The absorption of cimetidine and ranitidine is accelerated because of the increased gastric emptying. The sedative effects of benzodiazepines and alcohol are enhanced. Anticholinergic drugs antagonize the effect of cisapride.

Metoclopramide

Mechanism of Action

Metoclopramide (Reglan, others) is a dopamine antagonist that promotes the release of acetylcholine from the myenteric plexus. It stimulates motility of the upper GI tract without stimulating gastric, biliary, or pancreatic secretions. The tone and amplitude of gastric contractions are increased, as is peristalsis of the small intestine, so that gastric emptying and intestinal transit times are increased.

Pharmacokinetics

Metoclopramide may be administered intramuscularly, intravenously, and orally. The onset of action is 10 to 15 minutes after intramuscular injection and 30 to 60 minutes after oral administration. The half-life is 4 to 6 hours. Metoclopramide crosses the blood-brain barrier and can produce effects in the central nervous system (CNS). The drug is excreted in the urine as unchanged drug and sulfate and glucuronide conjugates.

Uses

The gastrostimulatory action of metoclopramide is useful in treating diabetic gastroparesis, a condition in which stomach tone is lost and contents are not emptied readily into the intestine. Metoclopramide also facilitates intubation of the small intestine for biopsy and stimulates gastric emptying and intestinal transit of barium in radiologic examinations.

Metoclopramide is also effective as an antiemetic, probably through a CNS action in the chemoreceptor trigger zone and vomiting center. The antiemetic effect is especially helpful in controlling emesis that occurs during cancer chemotherapy, especially with cisplatin or cyclophosphamide (see Chapter 25).

Adverse Reactions and Contraindications

About 10% of patients experience the side effects of metoclopramide, including restlessness, drowsiness, fatigue, and lassitude. Metoclopramide is contraindicated in patients with mechanical obstruction, perforation, or possible hemorrhage of the GI tract. An increase in GI motility poses danger for such patients.

Interactions

Anticholinergic drugs and narcotic analgesics inhibit GI tone and thereby antagonize the action of metoclopramide. Sedation is intensified with the concurrent use of alcohol, tranquilizers, sleeping medications, or narcotic analgesics.

ADDITIONAL GASTROINTESTINAL STIMULANTS

Domperidone

Domperidone (Motilium) is related to metoclopramide. It is similar to that drug except that domperidone does not cross the blood-brain barrier and is not effective as metoclopramide an antiemetic. Domperidone is available in Canada but not in the United States.

Erythromycin

Erythromycin is an antibiotic with GI side effects (see Chapter 41). Recently the ability of erythromycin to stimulate GI motility has been shown directly. Erythromycin appears to stimulate the receptor for motilin, a GI hormone. Erythromycin is being used to improve gastric emptying and increase propulsion throughout the GI tract for such conditions as gastroparesis and intestinal hypomotility.

Neostigmine

Neostigmine (Prostigmin) is a reversible acetylcholinesterase inhibitor prescribed for its muscarinic and neuromuscular effects (see Chapter 38). Neostigmine may be given subcutaneously or intramuscularly in place of bethanechol to restore bladder or intestinal tone. If urination does not occur within 1 hour, a catheter should be inserted.

NURSING PROCESS OVERVIEW

Drugs to Increase Gastrointestinal Tone and Motility

Assessment

Drugs to increase GI tone and motility are used following trauma, after surgery to treat atonic intestines or bladder, and when barium is used for radiologic examination. They are also used to treat diabetic gastroparesis. Assess the patient to rule out any obstruction of the bladder or intestine. Also assess vital signs, check for the presence of bowel sounds, check intake and output, palpate the bladder for distention, and check the patency of urinary catheters.

Nursing Diagnoses

- Altered comfort related to abdominal cramps or diarrhea
- Diarrhea related to drug action or side effect

Patient Outcomes

The patient will have a bowel movement and return to usual defecation pattern. The patient having difficulty voiding will be able to void and will return to usual elimination pattern. The patient who has undergone a diagnostic test will expel the barium without difficulty.

Planning/Implementation

After administering bethanechol or neostigmine, remain at the patient's bedside for 15 minutes to observe for side effects. Side effects often occur with subcutaneous bethanechol. Have the antidote atropine readily available before bethanechol is administered. After the drug is administered, monitor vital signs and measure output. If side effects become serious, notify the physician or consider administering atropine (0.6 mg). If metoclopramide is administered intravenously, remain at the bedside; oral administration produces much slower effects.

Evaluation

These drugs are effective if they enhance the patient's ability to defecate or urinate. Some patients require only one or two doses, whereas other patients require continued use of these drugs. Before discharging a patient, assess the patient's knowledge of how to take the drug correctly, the anticipated effects, the possible side effects and what to do about them, and the symptoms requiring medical attention.

Therapeutic Rationale: Decreasing Gastrointestinal Secretions, Tone, and Motility

At one time treatment of peptic ulcers included anticholinergic drugs to decrease acid secretions. The H_2 blockers are much more effective and have fewer side effects. These new agents have replaced anticholinergics for the treatment of peptic ulcers (see Chapter 26).

Selected anticholinergic agents are used as preanesthetic medications to block salivation and respiratory tract secretions during surgery.

The irritable bowel syndrome, also called spastic colitis, is a common GI disorder characterized by hyperactivity of the colon. Abdominal pain coincides with hypermotility of the colon. Constipation or diarrhea are characteristic. There are also psychologic or emotional factors commonly associated with the irritable bowel syndrome. Some patients have had a previous bout of infectious diarrhea; others may have laxative abuse as a predisposing factor.

Behavioral and dietary therapy are the first treatments for irritable bowel syndrome. Anticholinergic drugs administered alone or with an antianxiety agent may be helpful.

Therapeutic Agents: Atropine and Antispasmodic Agents

A number of anticholinergic and antispasmodic drugs have been developed to decrease GI tone and motility. **Anticholinergic drugs** (drugs that block muscarinic receptors) inhibit gastric acid secretion and depress GI motility. These drugs are listed in Table 23-2.

ATROPINE AND RELATED DRUGS

Atropine was originally derived from the plant *Atropa belladonna*, or deadly nightshade. Other **belladonna alkaloids** include hyoscyamine and scopolamine. Charged derivatives of atropine include homatropine and methscopolamine. These are listed in Table 23-2.

Mechanism of Action

Atropine is the prototypic anticholinergic agent, blocking acetylcholine at the muscarinic receptors. This action blocks the parasympathetic nervous system at various end organs (see Chapter 11).

Pharmacokinetics

Atropine may be administered orally, intramuscularly, subcutaneously, or intravenously. The duration of action is 4 to 6 hours. About 30% to 50% of the drug is excreted unchanged in the urine. See Table 23-2 for information on other atropine-like drugs.

Uses

Atropine and related drugs are used as anticholinergic agents for the treatment of irritable bowel syndrome and as a treatment adjunct for peptic ulcer. Atropine is also used as an antidote for the toxicity of cholinesterase inhibitors including organophosphate pesticides and for muscarinic mushroom poisoning.

Scopolamine is occasionally used as a preanesthetic medication to reduce salivation and respiratory secretions.

Atropine and related drugs are used in ophthalmology (see Chapter 71). Atropine is used to treat selected arrhythmias (see Chapter 19).

Adverse Reactions and Contraindications

Common side effects of anticholinergic drugs include dry mouth (**xerostomia**) (see box, p. 300), photophobia from dilated pupils (mydriasis), blurred vision (cycloplegia), fast heart rate (tachycardia), constipation, and acute urinary retention. If patients do not have dry mouth, they are not getting a dose large enough to suppress acid secretion.

Toxicity

Toxic doses of the uncharged anticholinergic drugs atropine (and its L-isomer, hyoscyamine) and oxyphencyclimine reach the CNS and produce CNS stimulation such as restlessness, tremor, irritability, delirium, or hallucinations. Infants and children are especially susceptible. Toxic doses of the charged anticholinergic drugs that do not reach the CNS cause ganglionic blockade (usually seen as orthostatic hypotension) or neuromuscular blockade. Death can result from respiratory arrest related to neuromuscular blockade.

Interactions

Atropine and related drugs give additive anticholinergic effects with phenothiazines, amantadine, antiparkinson drugs,

TABLE 23-2 Drugs to Decrease Gastrointestinal Tone and Motility

GENERIC NAME	TRADE NAME	ADMINISTRATION/DOSAGE	COMMENTS
Beladonna Alkaloids (uncharged)			
Atropine sulfate		ORAL, SUBCUTANEOUS: *Adults*—0.3-1.2 mg every 4-6 hr. SUBCUTANEOUS: *Children*—0.01 mg/kg every 4-6 hr.	Atropine sulfate reduces GI motility and gastric acid secretion and reduces tone of bladder and ureter.
Belladona tincture		ORAL: *Adults*—0.6-1 ml every 6-8 hr. *Children*—0.03 ml/kg in 3 or 4 divided doses.	As above. Atropine is active ingredient.
Hyoscyamine sulfate	Anaspaz Levsin Cytospaz	ORAL: *Adults*—0.125-0.25 mg every 4-6 hr. *Children 2-10 yr:* ½ adult dosage; *children <2 yr:* ¼ adult dosage. INTRAMUSCULAR, INTRAVENOUS, SUBCUTANEOUS: *Adults*—0.25-0.5 mg every 4-6 hr.	As above. Atropine is active ingredient.
Scopolamine butylbromide	Buscopan†	ORAL: *Adults*—10-20 mg 3 or 4 times/day. INTRAMUSCULAR, INTRAVENOUS, SUBCUTANEOUS: *Adults*—10-20 mg 3 or 4 times/day.	Older adult patients are more sensitive to scopolamine.
Scopolamine hydrobromide		INTRAMUSCULAR, INTRAVENOUS, SUBCUTANEOUS: *Adults*—0.3-0.6 mg as single dose.	
Charged Derivatives of Atropine			
Homatropine methylbromide	Homapin	ORAL: *Adults*—2.5-10 mg every 6 hr. *Children*—3-6 mg every 6 hr. *Infants*—0.3 mg dissolved in water every 4 hr.	Homatropine methylbromide reduces GI hypermotility and gastric acidity.
Methscopolamine bromide	Pamine	ORAL: *Adults*—2.5-5 mg every 6 hr. *Children*—0.2 mg/kg every 6 hr. INTRAMUSCULAR, SUBCUTANEOUS: *Adults*—0.25-1 mg every 6-8 hr. Onset: 1 hr.	Methscopolamine bromide reduces GI hypermotility and gastric acidity.
Synthetic Substitutes for Atropine			
Anisotropine methylbromide	Valpin	ORAL: *Adults*—50 mg 3 times/day. Onset: 1 hr.	Anisotropine methylbromide is used to treat GI spasms and control gastric acid secretion.
Clidinium bromide	Quarzan	ORAL: *Adults*—2.5-5 mg 3 or 4 times/day before meals and at bedtime. Reduce dosage to 2.5 mg 3 times/day before meals for older adult patients.	Clidinium bromide controls gastric acidity and hypermotility.
Glycopyrrolate	Robinul*	ORAL: *Adults*—1-2 mg 3 times/day initially; then 1-2 mg 2 times/day for maintenance. Onset: 1 hr. INTRAMUSCULAR, SUBCUTANEOUS, INTRAVENOUS: *Adults*—0.1-0.2 mg every 4 hr. Onset: 10 min.	Glycopyrrolate treats GI hypermotility and controls gastric acidity.
Isopropamide iodide	Darbid*	ORAL: *Adults and children >12 yr*—5 mg every 12 hr; may increase to 10 mg every 12 hr for severe symptoms.	Mepenzolate bromide controls gastric acidity and hypermotility.
Mepenzolate bromide	Cantil	ORAL: *Adults*—25 mg 4 times/day. Increase to 50 mg if necessary.	
Methantheline bromide	Banthine	ORAL: *Adults*—50-100 mg every 6 hr initially; reduce by ½ for maintenance. *Children*—6 mg/kg/day in 4 doses. Onset: 30 min. INTRAMUSCULAR: *Adults*—50 mg every 6 hr. *Children*—6 mg/kg/day in 4 doses. Onset: 30 min.	Methantheline bromide is used like atropine.
Oxyphencyclimine hydrochloride	Daricon	ORAL: *Adults*—10 mg 2 times/day; can be increased to 50 mg if tolerated.	Oryphencyclimine hydrochloride treats gastric acidity or hypermotility of GI, genitourinary, or biliary tract.
Propantheline bromide	Norpanth Pro-Banthine* Propanthel†	ORAL: *Adults*—15 mg 3 times/day plus 30 mg at bedtime or 30 mg timed-release every 8-12 hr. *Children*—1.5 mg/kg daily every 6 hr. INTRAMUSCULAR, INTRAVENOUS: *Adults*—30 mg every 6 hr.	Propantheline bromide controls gastric acidity and hypermotility of GI, genitourinary, and biliary tracts.

*Available in Canada and United States.
†Available in Canada only.

Continued.

TABLE 23-2 Drugs to Decrease Gastrointestinal Tone and Motility—cont'd

GENERIC NAME	TRADE NAME	ADMINISTRATION/DOSAGE	COMMENTS
Synthetic Substitutes for Atropine—cont'd			
Tridihexethyl chloride	Pathilon	ORAL: *Adults*—25 mg 3 times/day before meals and 50 mg at bedtime; timed-release, 75 mg every 6-12 hr. INTRAMUSCULAR, SUBCUTANEOUS, INTRAVENOUS: *Adults*—10-20 mg every 6 hr.	Tridihexethyl chloride controls gastric acidity and hypermotility of GI tract.
Antispasmodic Drugs			
Dicyclomine hydrochloride	Antispas Bentyl Bentylol† Others	ORAL, INTRAMUSCULAR: *Adults*—10-20 mg 3 or times daily. *Children*—10 mg 3 or 4 times/day. *Infants*—5 mg 3 or 4 times/day.	Dicyclomine hydrochloride controls hypermotility of colon.
Pirenzepine†	Gastrozepin†	ORAL: *Adults*—50 mg 2 times/day. May be increased to 3 times/day if needed.	This antimuscarinic is relatively specific for GI tract.

PATIENT PROBLEM
Dry Mouth (Xerostomia)

THE PROBLEM

Some drugs produce an excessively dry mouth. This effect may cause discomfort, trauma to the mouth, bad breath, irritation from dentures, potential for the development of dental caries, and potential for injury to the oral mucosa.

SIGNS AND SYMPTOMS

Dry oral mucous membranes; bad breath; mouth feels dry and sticky.

MEASURES TO DECREASE PATIENT DISCOMFORT

- Perform thorough, regular oral hygiene, with teeth brushing.
- Rinse mouth with a pleasant tasting rinse or normal saline solution (dissolve 1 tsp of salt in 1 pt water).
- Sip water frequently.
- Suck on sugarless hard candy or chew sugarless gum.
- Avoid drying mouthwashes (those containing alcohol).
- Avoid lemon-glycerin swabs for oral hygiene.
- Keep lips moist with lip moisturizer.
- Keep environmental air moist with a humidifier.
- Consider using a commercially available saliva substitute.
- Have regular dental check-ups.

glutethimide, meperidine, tricyclic antidepressants, quinidine, disopyramide, and some antihistamines. Levodopa absorption is decreased, but digoxin absorption is increased. Antacids will decrease the absorption of anticholinergics when taken concurrently.

SYNTHETIC SUBSTITUTES FOR ATROPINE

A number of synthetic substitutes for atropine were developed as antiulcer medications: anisotropine, clidinium, glycopyrrolate, isopropamide, mepenzolate, methantheline, oxyphencyclimine, propantheline and tridihexethyl chloride (see Table 23-2). They are no longer commonly used in the treatment of ulcers. Glycopyrrolate is used as preanesthetic medication to prevent or reduce salivation and respiratory tract secretions.

ANTISPASMODIC AGENTS

In addition to atropine and related drugs, dicyclomine and pirenzepine have **antispasmodic** but not anticholinergic effects (see Table 23-2). These drugs relax the smooth muscle of the GI tract and are used to treat hyperactivity or spasm of the intestine. Their side effects are not as prominent as those reported for the anticholinergic drugs. Side effects reported include constipation or diarrhea, rash, euphoria, dizziness, drowsiness, headache, nausea, and weakness.

NURSING PROCESS OVERVIEW

Drugs to Decrease Gastrointestinal Secretion, Tone, and Motility

Assessment

Assess the patient with attention to vital signs, any subjective complaints, frequency and character of stools, and presence of occult blood in the stool.

Nursing Diagnoses

- Colonic constipation related to drug side effects
- Altered oral mucous membranes related to dry mouth produced as a drug side effect

Patient Outcomes

The patient will have symptomatic relief of ulcer pain without constipation. The patient with irritable bowel disease will have less pain and decreased frequency of bowel movements. The patient who is nauseous will have relief of nausea without vomiting. The patient treated for poisoning will have reversal of the effects of the poisons.

Planning/Implementation

These drugs are used with dietary management and other therapies. Continue to monitor the patient's subjective complaints and vital signs and to assess the patient for side effects. Anticholinergic drugs and related compounds produce side effects if administered in effective dosages. Assist the patient in dealing with unpleasant side effects (e.g., sucking on hard candy for treatment of dry mouth). Monitor intake and output and assess for constipation. Watch for CNS effects such as restlessness, tremor, or irritability, which may indicate a need to reduce the drug dose.

Evaluation

These drugs are effective if the patient complains of fewer symptoms or the signs of ulcer disease disappear. Before discharge, the patient should be able to explain why and how to take the medications, which side effects will probably occur, how to treat these side effects, which symptoms warrant medical attention, and how to carry out related therapies such as dietary modification for treatment of ulcer disease.

NURSING IMPLICATIONS SUMMARY

Cholinomimetics: Bethanechol and Neostigmine

Drug Administration

- Have atropine sulfate (0.5 to 1.0 mg for adults; 10 μg/kg for infants and children) on hand to counteract excessive cholinergic side effects when administering cholinomimetics subcutaneously.
- Check doses carefully. The oral dose of bethanechol may be as high as 50 mg, whereas the subcutaneous dose should not exceed 5 mg.
- Remain at the bedside of patients for the first 10 minutes after administering subcutaneous bethanechol to assess for side effects.
- The physician may order a test dose of half or less of the usual dose to check for patient response. Monitor vital signs.
- Check the pulse before administering neostigmine. Notify the physician if the rate is <80 beats/minute, and withhold the dose pending physician approval. For additional information about neostigmine, see Chapter 37.

Patient and Family Education

- Teach the patient to take oral doses of bethanechol on an empty stomach 1 hour before or 2 hours after eating.
- If a dose is missed, instruct the patient to take the missed dose if within 2 hours of the scheduled time. If close to the next dosing time, omit the missed dose and resume the usual dosing schedule. Do not double up for missed doses.
- Remind the patient to keep these and all medications out of the reach of children.

Cisapride

Patient and Family Education

- Instruct the patient to take doses 15 minutes before meals and at bedtime with a beverage. Shake suspensions well before preparing dose.
- For missed doses, teach the patient to take the missed dose as soon as remembered, unless almost time for the next dose, then omit missed dose and resume regular schedule.
- Alcohol intake should be avoided unless first approved by the physician.
- Driving or operating hazardous equipment should be discontinued if drowsiness occurs.

Metoclopramide

Drug Administration

- Administer undiluted intravenous doses over 1 to 2 minutes. The drug may be diluted in 50 ml of solution and administered slowly, over at least 15 minutes. Give doses administered in conjunction with cancer chemotherapy 30 minutes before chemotherapy is begun. A second dose may be given in 2 hours and a third dose in 3 hours. Doses for this purpose may be as high as 2 mg/kg body weight. Other regimens are also in use.

Patient and Family Education

- Instruct the patient to take oral doses 30 minutes before meals; doses may also be taken at bedtime.
- Metoclopramide may produce extrapyramidal reactions (see Table 52-3). Instruct the patient to report any unusual side effects, especially protrusion of the tongue, puffing of the cheeks, chewing movements, and involuntary movements of any body parts. Although rare, these side effects occur more often in children and older adults.
- Caution the patient to avoid drinking alcohol or operating hazardous equipment until the effects of the medication can be evaluated.
- Caution the patient to avoid alcohol intake while taking this drug, as well as any drug that may depress the CNS such as sleeping medications, tranquilizers, narcotic analgesics, or other drugs that cause drowsiness.

Continued.

NURSING IMPLICATIONS SUMMARY—cont'd

- Agranulocytosis occurs rarely. Assess the patient for chills, fever, sore throat, and fatigue (see box, p. 268).

Anticholinergics and Antispasmodics

Drug Administration

- Use anticholinergics and antispasmodics cautiously in patients with prostatic hypertrophy, pyloric obstruction, obstruction of the bladder neck, or serious cardiac disease. Assess for preexisting glaucoma because anticholinergics may precipitate an attack of acute angle closure glaucoma.
- Assess for urinary retention, especially in older men with preexisting prostatic hypertrophy. Monitor intake and output. Instruct the patient to report inability to void, increasing difficulty in initiating urination, or a sensation of incomplete bladder emptying. Instruct the patient to void before taking each dose.
- Monitor the patient's pulse before administering doses. Withhold the dose if the pulse exceeds 90 to 100 beats/minute in an adult. Administer anticholinergics with caution in patients with a history of heart disease characterized by tachycardia. Auscultate bowel sounds. Keep a record of bowel movements. Treat overdose with neostigmine.
- Administer intramuscular doses into a large muscle mass, such as the dorsogluteal site or rectus femoris muscle in adults or the vastus lateralis muscle in infants and small children. Use careful technique; aspirate before administering the dose to avoid inadvertent intravenous administration.
- Tincture of belladonna may be prescribed by number of drops. Dilute the dose in 15 to 30 ml of water before administering. If drowsiness or disorientation develops, supervise ambulation, keep siderails up, and use night lights.

Patient and Family Education

- Instruct the patient to take doses 30 minutes to 1 hour before meals and at bedtime unless a timed-release form is used. If antacids are also prescribed, take doses 30 minutes before or 2 hours after antacid doses.
- Inform the patient that constipation is a common side effect. Instruct the patient to increase the daily fluid intake to at least 3000 ml, to increase dietary intake of fruits and fiber, and to get regular exercise. Tell the patient to record bowel movements; if a bowel movement has not occurred in 3 days, consult the physician. Teach the patient to avoid cathartics or laxatives unless instructed to use specific ones by the physician, because they may be contraindicated in certain medical conditions that require anticholinergics. Remind the patient to avoid drugs for diarrhea while taking these drugs, unless approved by the physician.
- Caution the patient to avoid driving or operating hazardous equipment until the effects of the medication can be evaluated; drowsiness and blurred vision may occur. Encourage the patient to wear sunglasses and avoid bright sunlight if photophobia develops; keep room lights dim.
- Teach the patient to suck on sugarless hard candy or chew sugarless gum to relieve dry mouth. Refer the patient to the pharmacist for commercially available saliva substitutes (see the patient problem box on dry mouth, p. 300).
- Instruct the patient to be careful about undertaking strenuous activities on warm days because these drugs inhibit the body's ability to perspire. Tell the patient to take frequent rest periods to cool off. Inform the patient that atropine may produce a fever, especially in children.
- Because these drugs often produce side effects when taken in therapeutic doses, patient compliance may be poor. Provide emotional support as needed. Teach the patient the importance of taking drugs as prescribed. Reinforce the importance of keeping all drugs out of the reach of children. If combination products are prescribed, review the side effects of each drug with the patient.
- Patients using scopolamine should avoid the use of alcohol.
- Review the correct use of suppositories or transdermal patches if these drug forms are prescribed. Scopolamine transdermal patches are applied behind the ear; review the patient instruction sheet supplied by the manufacturer.

CRITICAL THINKING

APPLICATION

1. How do cholinomimetic drugs act on the GI tract? Name two cholinomimetic drugs that are used for their activity on the GI tract.
2. How do the mechanisms of metoclopramide and cisapride differ from direct acting cholinomimetic drugs?
3. What actions do anticholinergic drugs have on the GI tract?

CRITICAL THINKING

1. What is the antidote for bethanechol? Under what circumstances should you consider administering the antidote? What symptoms would you see with excessive bethanechol dosage?
2. The drug atropine is classically given as a preoperative medication. What are the desired effects? For the patient using atropine on a regular (chronic) basis, what are the side effects, and how would you suggest the patient manage them?

CHAPTER 24

Laxatives and Antidiarrheals

OBJECTIVES

After studying this chapter, you should be able to do the following:

- *Discuss the use of laxatives and antidiarrheals.*
- *Develop a nursing care plan for patients receiving laxatives or antidiarrheals.*
- *Develop a teaching plan for patients who have constipation or diarrhea.*

KEY TERMS

constipation
diarrhea
laxative
wetting agents

CHAPTER OVERVIEW

The major muscular activity of the large intestine is a contraction of circular smooth muscle, which decreases the diameter to segment and knead the fecal mass without moving it along. About 8 L of fluid travel through the intestines of the average adult in 24 hours. Water ingested in food or drink accounts for about 2 L, and secretions (salivary, gastric, biliary, and pancreatic) account for about 6 L. Since only 100 to 200 ml of water is normally excreted daily in feces, the intestines are highly efficient in reabsorbing water and electrolytes.

About 2 L of water are removed from the fecal mass in the large intestine. Bulk in the large intestine stimulates stretch receptors to cause a reflex peristalsis, which moves the fecal mass forward. Usually 3 to 4 times daily strong propulsive contractions occur spontaneously to move the fecal mass through the large intestine. The strongest movements usually occur after the first meal of the day, and the perception of the need to defecate follows the filling of the rectum. The relaxation of the external anal sphincter is a voluntary act, as are the straining movements to expel the feces. The pattern of defecation described implies that defecation is a regular morning event, but the timing of defecation is highly individual and may occur more or less frequently.

Therapeutic Rationale: Constipation

A *normal bowel movement* refers to whatever pattern of defecation results in readily passed feces for a given individual. **Constipation** arises when the frequency of bowel movements decreases and defecation yields hard stools that are difficult to pass (see box).

Therapeutic Agents: Laxatives

Laxative, cathartic, and *purgative* describe agents that act on the large intestine (colon, bowel) to promote defecation, but these terms have evolved to represent different degrees of action. A **laxative** produces soft stools with a minimal incidence of abdominal cramping. A cathartic produces a soft to fluid stool and may also cause abdominal cramping. A purgative produces a watery stool and violent cramping to such an extent that shock and hemorrhaging may result. Purgatives are no longer used in medical practice, and only some cathartics, also called *stimulant cathartics,* are commonly used.

Table 24-1 lists the drugs used as laxatives. Traditionally, laxatives are classified as bulk-forming, stimulant (irritant) cathartic, saline (osmotic) cathartic, wetting agent (stool softener), and lubricant. Laxatives are indicated for patients with true constipation. Causes of constipation include poor bowel habits, narcotic analgesics, drugs with anticholinergic side effects, and intestinal muscle tone loss because of surgery, bed rest, or age. Laxatives are also indicated when straining is painful or risky, such as in women with episiotomies and patients with hemorrhoids, hernias, or aneurysms. Laxatives are also used to clean out the large intestine before surgery or examination. With the exception of mineral oil, laxatives act by providing a greater bulk to the fecal mass, primarily by keeping water in the large intestine. The large, hydrated fecal mass can fill the rectum to stimulate defecation, which is then accomplished with minimal irritation or strain.

Bulk-Forming Laxatives

This class of laxatives includes bran, methylcellulose, polycarbophil, and psyllium hydrophilic mucilloid. They act by retaining water so that the stool remains large and soft. Bulk-forming laxatives provide what should be a part of good nutrition. It is generally believed that people in developed countries eat a diet containing too little fiber that favors the formation of small, hard stools. Including bran, whole grain products, and fibrous fruits and vegetables in the diet promotes the formation of large, soft stools that readily stimulate the large intestine and the rectum (see box, p. 306).

In a patient who does not regularly use laxatives, bulk-forming laxatives are effective in 12 to 24 hours. Bulk-forming laxatives can also relieve a mild watery diarrhea by absorbing water to produce a soft stool.

Stimulant Cathartics

Stimulant (irritant) cathartics include bisacodyl, cascara, castor oil, glycerin, phenolphthalein, and senna. These drugs usually form a soft to fluid stool in 6 to 12 hours (see box, p. 306). Stimulant cathartics were believed to act only by directly stimulating the motility of the large intestine; however, newer research indicates that these drugs also inhibit the reabsorption of water in the large intestine.

Stimulant cathartics are the most abused laxatives. When a stimulant cathartic is used for more than 1 week, the large intestine loses its tone and becomes less responsive to any stimulation. Continued use of a stimulant cathartic can produce diarrhea severe enough to cause dehydration and to lower blood concentrations of sodium and potassium.

PATIENT PROBLEM

Constipation

THE PROBLEM

The patient is not having bowel movements as often as necessary.

SIGNS AND SYMPTOMS

Abdominal discomfort; feeling a need to defecate but inability to do so; dry, firm, hard stools when bowel movements do occur; infrequent defecation (The meaning of *infrequent* may vary with each patient.)

ASSOCIATED OR CONTRIBUTING FACTORS

Dehydration or inadequate fluid intake; constipating medications; misuse or overuse of antidiarrhea medications or improper use of cathartics, causing the patient to move from constipation to diarrhea; and immobility.

MEASURES TO HELP ELIMINATE CONSTIPATION

Keep a record of bowel movements to help verify the problem, and note any associated factors.

- Increase daily fluid intake to 2500 to 3000 ml.
- Increase dietary intake of fruit and fruit juices.
- Increase dietary intake of fiber (see box on p. 306).
- Increase level of exercise.
- Examine use of drugs causing diarrhea or constipation.

ADDITIONAL NURSING CARE MEASURES

Keep a record of bowel movements for all hospitalized, immobilized, or institutionalized patients since constipation is easier to prevent than treat.

Auscultate bowel sounds in patients complaining of constipation.

TABLE 24-1 Drugs to Relieve Constipation

GENERIC NAME	TRADE NAME	ADMINISTRATION/DOSAGE	COMMENTS
Bulk-Forming Agents			
Methylcellulose; carboxymethyl cellulose	Cologel Citrucel	ORAL: *Adults*—4-6 gm daily. *Children <6 yr*—1-1.5 gm daily.	Drug is nonprescription.
Polycarbophil	Mitrolan† Fibercon	ORAL: *Adults*—4-6 gm daily. *Children 6-12 yr*—1.5-3 gm daily; *children 2-5 yr*—1-1.5 gm daily.	Drug is nonprescription.
Psyllium hydrocolloid Psyllium hydrophilic mucilloid	Fiberall Konsyl Metamucil* Modane Bulk Serutan	ORAL: *Adults*—1 round tsp (7 gm) or 1 packet. Add to glass of water and drink rapidly and then follow with second glass of water. Repeat 1 to 2 times daily if necessary.	Drug is nonprescription.
Stimulant (Irritant) Cathartics			
Bisacodyl	Bisco-Lax† Dulcolax* Others	ORAL: *Adults*—10 mg. Up to 30 mg may be given to clear gastrointestinal tract. *Children >6 yr*—5 mg. RECTAL: *Adults and children >2 yr*—10 mg. *Children <2 yr*—5 mg.	Drug is nonprescription. Initial response occurs in 6-12 hr. Patient should not take it within 60 min of milk or antacids. Rectal administration is effective in 15 min.
Cascara sagrada		ORAL: *Adults*—200-400 mg of extract, 0.5-1.5 ml of fluid extract, or 5 ml of aromatic extract.	Drug is nonprescription. It is one of mildest of stimulant cathartics.
Castor oil		ORAL: *Adults*—15-60 ml. *Children >2 yr*—5-15 ml; *children <2 yr*—1-5 ml.	Drug is nonprescription. Castor oil is degraded to ricinoleic acid, which is active drug.
Castor oil, emulsified	Neoloid	ORAL: *Adults*—30-60 ml. *Children >2 yr*—7.5-30 ml; *children <2 yr*—2.5-7.5 ml.	Drug is nonprescription. This emulsion is mint flavored. It turns alkaline urine pink.
Glycerin suppositories		RECTAL: *Adults*—3 gm. *Children <6 yr*—1-1.5 gm.	Drug is nonprescription. It is effective in 15-30 min.
Phenolphthalein	Ex-lax* Feen-A-Mint Phenolax Others	ORAL: *Adults*—30-270 mg daily. *Children >6 yr*—30-60 mg daily; *children 2-6 yr*—15-20 mg daily.	Drug is nonprescription. It turns alkaline urine pink.
Senna concentrate	Senokot suppositories	RECTAL: *Adults*—1 suppository. *Children >60 lb*—½ suppository.	
Senna pod	Senokot Others	ORAL: *Adults*—twice daily give 1-2 tsp (granules), 2-3 tsp (syrup), or 2-4 tablets. *Children, pregnant or postpartum women, or geriatric patients*—½ adult dose. *Children 1 mo-1 yr*—1.25-2.5 ml (syrup).	Drug is nonprescription. Not all preparations are recommended for children.
Senna, whole leaf		ORAL: *Adults*—0.5-2 gm or 2 ml of senna fluid extract. *Children 6-12 yr*—½ adult dose; *children 2-5 yr*—¼ adult dose; *children <2 yr*—⅓ adult dose.	Drug is nonprescription.
Sennosides A and B	Glysennid† Gentle Nature	ORAL: *Adults*—12-24 mg at bedtime. *Children >10 yr*—same as adult; *children 6-10 yr*—12 mg at bedtime.	Drug is nonprescription.
Saline (Osmotic) Cathartics			
Magnesium citrate	Citroma Citro-Mag†	ORAL: *Adults*—1 glassful (about 240 ml). *Children*—0.5 ml/kg body weight.	Drug is nonprescription.
Magnesium hydroxide	Phillips' Milk of Magnesia	ORAL: *Adults*—10-15 ml (concentrated) or 15-30 ml (regular). *Children*—0.5 ml (regular)/kg body weight.	Drug is nonprescription.
Magnesium sulfate	Epsom salt	ORAL: *Adults*—15 gm in glass of water. *Children*—0.25 gm/kg.	Drug is nonprescription.
Monosodium phosphate	Sal Hepatica	ORAL: *Adults*—5-20 ml with water.	Drug is nonprescription.

*Available in Canada and United States.
†Available in Canada only.

Continued.

TABLE 24-1 Drugs to Relieve Constipation—cont'd

GENERIC NAME	TRADE NAME	ADMINISTRATION/DOSAGE	COMMENTS
Saline (Osmotic) Cathartics—cont'd			
Sodium phosphate		ORAL: *Adults*—5 gm in glass of warm water. *Children*—0.25 gm/kg.	Drug is nonprescription.
Sodium phosphate with biphosphate	Phospho-Soda	ORAL: *Adults*—20-40 ml in glass of cold water. *Children*—5-15 ml.	Drug is nonprescription.
✣ Wetting Agents (Stool Softeners)			
Docusate calcium	Surfak	ORAL: *Adults*—50-360 mg daily. *Children*—50-150 mg daily.	Drug is nonprescription.
Docusate sodium	Colace D-S-S Others	ORAL: *Adults*—50-360 mg. *Children 6-12 yr*—40-120 mg; *children 3-6 yr*—20-60 mg; *children <3 yr*—10-40 mg.	Drug is nonprescription.
Lubricants			
Mineral oil	Agoral, Plain Kondremul, Plain* Neo-Cultol Petrogalar, Plain	ORAL: *Adults*—15-30 ml at bedtime.	Drug is nonprescription. It eases strain of passing hard stools. It should not be used regularly because fat-soluble vitamins (A, D, E, and K) are not absorbed. Response occurs in 1-3 days.
Miscellaneous			
Lactulose	Chronulac* Constilac Others	ORAL: *Adults*—15-30 ml, increased to 60 ml/day if necessary (15 ml = 10 gm).	Drug is nonprescription. It works by osmotic effect in 1-3 days.

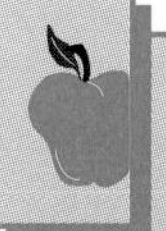

DIETARY CONSIDERATION

Fiber

Adequate amounts of dietary fiber may help prevent constipation and colon diseases, may help maintain blood glucose levels, and may lower blood cholesterol levels. Good sources of dietary fiber include fruits and vegetables, especially raw, unpeeled, or with edible seeds; whole grains and whole-grain products; such as bread, cereals, pastas, bran, oats, peas, beans, and lentils.

Bisacodyl

Bisacodyl is a synthetic compound available in suppositories and tablets. As a suppository, bisacodyl is effective in 15 minutes and as a tablet, in 6 hours. Since bisacodyl irritates the stomach, the tablet is coated to dissolve only in the intestine. This enteric-coated tablet should not be taken within 1 hour of ingestion of milk products or antacids, which neutralize stomach acid. Bisacodyl is often used to clear the large intestine for proctoscopic or colonoscopic examination.

Cascara and Senna

Cascara and senna are extracted from plants. Cascara is the milder and senna the more potent. They should not be used by breast-feeding mothers, since these laxatives are excreted in the milk. Senna and cascara turn acid urine yellow-brown and alkaline urine red.

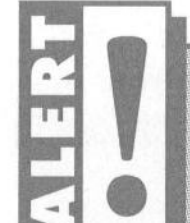

DRUG ABUSE ALERT

Cathartics

BACKGROUND

Cathartics are subject to two types of abuse. Individuals may fixate on being regular. Individuals with eating disorders may use cathartic laxatives in excess to get rid of ingested food.

PHARMACOLOGY

Cathartics are laxatives that produce a soft to fluid stool in 6 to 12 hours. They directly stimulate the colon.

HEALTH HAZARDS

The colon becomes unresponsive when cathartics are used for more than 1 week. Persistent diarrhea may result that in its most severe form causes dehydration and produces electrolyte imbalances. Therapy is supportive as the cathartic is discontinued.

Castor Oil

Castor oil is an old remedy for constipation and is still used medically. Castor oil is the most potent of the stimulant cathartics, producing a watery stool in 2 to 6 hours, which thoroughly removes gas and feces from the intestine. Castor oil has an unpleasant taste and is best disguised by chilling and administering with fruit juice.

Glycerin

Glycerin is used only as a suppository. It acts by stimulating the rectum and attracting water to increase bulk. It is effective in 15 to 30 minutes.

Phenolphthalein

Phenolphthalein is found in many over-the-counter laxative preparations. Phenolphthalein enters the enterohepatic circulation and may be effective for several days. In alkaline urine, phenolphthalein is pink.

Saline Cathartics

Saline (osmotic) cathartics are poorly absorbed salts of magnesium or sodium such as magnesium carbonate, oxide, citrate, hydroxide, or sulfate; sodium phosphate or sulfate; and potassium and sodium tartrate. Concentrated solutions of these salts attract water osmotically into the lumen of the large intestine, and the resulting bulk stimulates peristalsis. Saline cathartics empty the bowel in 2 to 6 hours.

Patients with poor kidney function should not use saline cathartics since they cannot excrete the small fraction of the salt that is absorbed systemically.

Wetting Agents

Wetting agents, or stool softeners, are detergents that inhibit the absorption of water so that the fecal mass remains large and soft. This class of laxatives is indicated when the objective is to avoid straining to pass the stools. Such laxatives include dioctyl sodium sulfosuccinate (docusate sodium) and dioctyl calcium sulfosuccinate (docusate calcium).

Lubricants

The only lubricant laxative still used is mineral oil, which is indigestible and acts to soften the feces, thus easing the strain of passing stools and lessening irritation to hemorrhoids. Long-term use of mineral oil interferes with the absorption of fat-soluble vitamins A, D, E, and K. Mineral oil can cause a lipid pneumonia if accidentally aspirated. Wetting agents are regarded as superior to mineral oil in softening the stools for easy passage.

Miscellaneous Agents

Lactulose is a synthetic disaccharide that is not hydrolyzed by intestinal enzymes and is not absorbed. Instead, lactulose is degraded by bacteria in the colon to short-chain organic acids that are not absorbed and act as osmotic agents. The net effect is a moderate fluid accumulation in the colon and the formation of a soft stool. Lactulose may initially produce gas and cramps. Lactulose has reduced the incidence of fecal impaction in older adults. However, older adult patients should have serum electrolyte levels monitored after treatment for more than 6 months.

NURSING PROCESS OVERVIEW

Drugs to Relieve Constipation

Assessment

Assess vital signs, fluid intake and output, and presence of bowel sounds. Perform a digital rectal examination to determine the presence of impacted stools. Obtain a history of previous constipation and its treatment, the patient's perception of constipation, and any recent change in lifestyle, diet, or medications.

Nursing Diagnoses

- Diarrhea related to drug side effects
- Perceived constipation

Patient Outcomes

The patient will have relief of constipation and will learn how to avoid constipation in the future.

Planning/Implementation

The treatment of uncomplicated constipation is usually simple. If constipation is persistent, the physician must rule out serious causes such as cancer. Administer ordered medications and teach the patient about other factors that influence the frequency of stools such as diet, fluid intake, and exercise.

Evaluation

Drugs to relieve constipation are effective if they produce a bowel movement. Before a patient is discharged, verify that the patient can explain how to take the ordered medications and what the desired effects of the medications are.

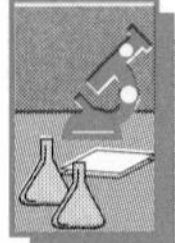

RESEARCH HIGHLIGHT

Managing Constipation Using a Research-Based Protocol

— GR Hall, M Karstens, B Rakel, E Swanson, A Davidson: Medsurg Nursing 4(1):11, 1995.

PURPOSE

This study was designed to develop a nursing care protocol for the management of constipation in postoperative vascular surgery patients.

METHODOLOGY

Many older adult patients on a vascular surgery unit were immobilized or had decreased mobility, which contributed to constipation. A team of nurses, dietitians, and clinical specialists did a retrospective chart review to document the severity of the problem and then reviewed the research literature about constipation to develop a treatment protocol for the unit.

The protocol that was developed included four interventions: increasing dietary fiber, encouraging a fluid intake of 1500 to 2000 ml/day, ensuring privacy and assisting patients to be upright for defecation, and using abdominal strengthening exercises that could be performed in bed. The nurses tried several different fiber sources, including high-fiber cereals, bran added to milkshakes and puddings, bran muffins, and high-fiber cookies. The article includes two recipes that the nurses, and later the patients, found palatable as sources of fiber.

SAMPLE

All patients admitted to the unit were assessed to see if they were at high risk for constipation. Assessment data included age >55 years, insulin-dependent diabetes, immobility, diet, and medications. High-risk patients were counseled about dietary fiber and encouraged to choose from a selection of high-fiber foods. The nurses were taught the protocol and how to implement the exercises with the patient. This was a quality assurance study, so results were measured quarterly for 9 months, then for one quarter each year thereafter. The staff felt that a reasonable goal was 85% of patients should have usual or normal bowel function, 85% should have no requests for laxatives or enemas, and 85% of patients should not have fecal impactions.

FINDINGS

Prior to the study, the records of 16 patients were evaluated. Of these, 41% indicated subjective report of normal bowel function, 66% indicated no impaction, and 41% had no patient request for laxatives or enemas. By the end of the third quarter, 95% of 19 patients at high risk for constipation reported normal bowel function, 95% had no impaction, and 100% of the patients had no requests for laxatives or enemas. By the third year, 88% of 17 patients reported normal bowel function, 100% had no impaction, and 94% had no requests for laxatives or enemas. These results were based on regular use of three interventions; the nurses failed to teach or encourage the abdominal exercises with any regularity.

IMPLICATIONS

Quality assurance studies have a slightly different focus than empirical studies. In this study the nurses identified a problem, researched the literature, designed a protocol that involved a team approach, and after all staff members were educated in the use of the protocol, implemented nursing care measures to address the problem. Improvement was sustained more than three years.

Therapeutic Rationale: Diarrhea

Diarrhea has no precise definition but refers to bowel movements that are frequent (more than three per day), fluid (unformed stools), or large (>200 gm/day). Acute diarrhea lasts for hours or days, whereas chronic diarrhea lasts for more than 3 to 4 weeks. A patient with chronic diarrhea must be thoroughly examined to establish a cause, which can then be specifically treated. Acute diarrhea rarely requires treatment beyond avoidance of food and maintenance of adequate liquid intake.

The primary treatment of diarrhea is replacement of lost fluids and electrolytes. Glucose is required for the intestinal absorption of water and electrolytes. Mild dehydration can be treated with carbonated drinks, which add glucose and bicarbonate, and broths or clear soups, which add sodium and chloride. Infants and older adults can become seriously dehydrated if adequate intake of glucose and salts is not maintained to replace the fluid and electrolytes lost. Commercially available drinks for replacement of glucose and electrolytes include Gatorade and Lytren. A similar drink can be made at home with ½ teaspoon of corn syrup or honey and a pinch of table salt added to 1 cup (8 ounces) of fruit juice (to provide potassium), alternating with a drink made by adding ¼ teaspoon of baking soda (sodium bicarbonate) to 1 cup (8 ounces) of water. A simpler drink is made with the following recipe: 1 teaspoon table salt, 1 teaspoon baking soda, and 4 teaspoons of sugar in a quart of boiled water. Since the latter recipe does not provide needed potassium, ½ teaspoon of potassium chloride should be added to a quart of the solution.

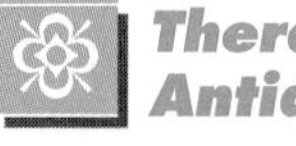

Therapeutic Agents: Antidiarrheals

Table 24-2 lists the drugs used to treat diarrhea. The most effective nonspecific antidiarrheal agents are the opioids, which decrease the tone of the small and large intestines in a manner that slows the transit of material. The longitudinal contractions propelling the contents (peristalsis) are inhibited by the opioids, but the circular contractions, which cause the

TABLE 24-2 Drugs to Control Diarrhea

GENERIC NAME	TRADE NAME	ADMINISTRATION/DOSAGE	COMMENTS
Opioids and Related Drugs			
Codeine phosphate; codeine sulfate		ORAL: *Adults and children >12 yr*—15-60 mg every 4-8 hr as needed. INTRAMUSCULAR: *Adults and children >12 yr*—15-30 mg every 2-4 hr.	Codeine phosphate and sulfate and schedule II drugs.
Diphenoxylate hydrochloride with atropine	Lomotil* Lofene Others	ORAL: *Adults*—5 mg 3-4 times daily. *Children 8-12 yr*—10 mg daily in 5 divided doses; *children 5-8 yr*—8 mg daily in 4 divided doses; *children 2-5 yr*—6 mg daily in 3 divided doses.	Diphenoxylate hydrochloride with atropine is schedule V drug.
Difenoxin with atropine	Motofen	ORAL: *Adults*—2 mg initially, then 1 mg after each loose stool or every 3-4 hr as needed.	Difenoxin with atropine is schedule IV drug.
✣ Loperamide	Imodium	ORAL: *Adults*—4 mg initially, then 2 mg with each diarrheal episode, up to 16 mg daily.	Drug is also available as nonprescription drug. It is in FDA pregnancy category B.
Opium tincture		ORAL: 0.6 ml 4 times daily. Maximum single dose is 1 ml. Maximum daily dose is 6 ml.	Opium tincture is schedule II drug.
Paregoric		ORAL: *Adults*—5-10 ml 1-4 times daily. *Children*—0.25-0.5 ml/kg 1-4 times daily.	Paregoric is schedule III drug.
Bismuth Salts			
Bismuth subsalicylate	Pepto-Bismol	ORAL: *Adults*—30 ml. *Children 10-14 yr*—20 ml; *children 6-10 yr*—10 ml; *children 3-6 yr*—5 ml.	This nonprescription drug is effective for "traveler's" diarrhea. It may turn stools gray-black.

*Available in Canada and United States.

segmental activity that mixes the intestinal contents, are stimulated by the opioids. The treatment of diarrhea with opioids is nonspecific, and when diarrhea is caused by poisons, infections, or bacterial toxins, opioids can make the condition worse by delaying the elimination of these agents. Opioids that are used to control diarrhea include opium tincture, paregoric, codeine, difenoxin, and diphenoxylate (Lomotil). The effective antidiarrheal dose is lower than that which can cause euphoria or analgesia. Toxic doses produce respiratory depression, which can be reversed with a narcotic antagonist.

Opioid-Related Drugs

Codeine

Codeine can be given orally, or the drug can be administered intramuscularly.

Diphenoxylate and Difenoxin

Diphenoxylate (Lomotil) is an opioid that has a lower potential than codeine or opium tincture for causing drug dependence. Difenoxin (Motofen), an active metabolite of diphenoxylate, has about 5 times greater activity than diphenoxylate. These drugs are combined with atropine to diminish abdominal cramping while reducing the loss of water and electrolytes.

✣ Loperamide

Loperamide (Imodium) is a relatively new antidiarrheal drug that depresses longitudinal and circular contractions of the intestinal smooth muscles and decreases the release of acetylcholine. Loperamide has a broader spectrum of actions on the intestine than the opioids. Loperamide is structurally related to diphenoxylate but has no effects on the central nervous system (CNS) and does not appear to produce physical dependence. Originally available as a schedule V drug, loperamide is now available over the counter. Loperamide is concentrated by the liver and excreted into the bile. Its use is contraindicated in liver disease.

Opium Tincture

Opium tincture is a 10% solution of opium containing 10 mg/ml morphine. The antidiarrheal dose of opium tincture is measured in drops (usually 6 to 20 drops), and such a dose does not usually produce euphoria or analgesia.

Paregoric

Paregoric (Camphorated Opium Tincture) contains only 0.4 mg/ml morphine and is administered by the teaspoonful. Paregoric has an unpleasant taste.

Other Antidiarrheal Agents

Bismuth Salts

In addition to opioids that depress intestinal motility, many agents have been used as antidiarrheal drugs in the belief that they absorb toxins and thus remove the cause of diarrhea. Of these, only bismuth salts have been proved effective.

Bismuth subsalicylate (Pepto-Bismol) is effective in controlling traveler's diarrhea, apparently by binding the bacterial toxins. Bismuth causes the feces to become black, which does not indicate the presence of blood. Use in infants or older adults may produce feces that cannot be expelled (impacted feces).

Nursing Process Overview

Drugs to Control Diarrhea

Assessment

Assess patients, focusing on vital signs, intake and output of solids and liquids, presence and character of bowel sounds, and the character of diarrhea. Question patients about recent exposure to new water or dietary sources, infectious agents, international travel, and any medications taken recently. Appropriate laboratory studies include culturing a stool specimen and testing stools for ova, parasites, and occult blood.

Nursing Diagnoses

- Altered thought processes related to drowsiness produced as a drug side effect
- Colonic constipation related to drug side effects

Patient Outcomes

The patient will have no diarrhea and will return to normal bowel patterns.

Planning/Implementation

Diarrhea treatment aims to provide symptomatic relief and identify and treat the cause. Monitor vital signs and intake and output and observe the frequency and character of bowel movements. Limit the diet to clear liquids. If the diarrhea results from milk intolerance or other dietary cause, refer the patient to a dietitian for instruction. Observe the patient for drug side effects, especially constipation and sedation. If diarrhea is severe, monitor serum electrolyte levels and provide replacement fluids as ordered (see box on p. 210 and Table 17-1).

Evaluation

Drugs to control diarrhea are effective if the frequency of bowel movements is decreased to the patient's normal range. Before discharge patients should be able to explain when and how to take the medication prescribed, symptoms that may indicate too high a dose, and what to do if drugs do not relieve the symptoms.

Nursing Implications Summary

Drugs to Relieve Constipation

Drug Administration

- Keep a record of bowel movements on all institutionalized, immobilized, or incapacitated patients. Prevention, early detection, and treatment of constipation are much easier and less time consuming than treatment of severe constipation or impaction. Assess bowel sounds before administering any drug to relieve constipation. If bowel sounds are absent, withhold drug dose and notify the physician.
- Read medication orders and labels carefully. Many drugs have similar names. Be alert to the action of each component drug in combination products. For example, Colace contains the stool softener docusate sodium, whereas Peri-Colace contains docusate and casanthranol, a mild stimulant laxative.
- Physicians also sometimes prescribe bulk-forming agents to treat diarrhea, especially diarrhea associated with tube feedings. If the agent is to be given through a feeding tube, dilute the solution with sufficient fluid to prevent clogging of the tube and flush the tube with water after administration. Large-bore tubes are better suited to administer these agents.
- Castor oil does not mix with a water-based diluent. Add a small amount of baking soda (less than ¼ teaspoon) immediately before administering to cause the mixture to fizz, and the castor oil will be partially suspended in the juice for 1 or 2 minutes. Patients may find it easier to drink castor oil this way. In an institution, the routine use of baking soda for this purpose must be cleared by the pharmacy or physician.
- Monitor the serum electrolyte levels of patients receiving lactulose, especially older adult patients.
- Lactulose is also used to treat elevated serum ammonia levels.

Patient and Family Education

- Instruct the patient that a daily bowel movement is not necessary for normal bowel function. Review with parents the inadvisability of encouraging laxative dependence in small children. To help keep a regular bowel schedule, teach the patient to increase daily fluid intake to 2500 to 3000 ml. If necessary, suggest that the patient drink a full (8 ounce) glass of water before each meal and a full glass with each meal.
- Instruct the patient to increase daily dietary intake of bran in cereals and other foods; fruits and vegetables, fruit juices, or foods known by the patient to be stimulating to defecation (e.g., hot chocolate or coffee). Encourage the patient to exercise regularly to promote bowel regularity.
- Remind the patient to use laxatives only as directed. Many laxatives are available without prescription. They may be

NURSING IMPLICATIONS SUMMARY—cont'd

misused or abused by patients who do not understand that increasing dependence on these drugs can develop with regular use.

- Review with the patient using laxatives in preparation for gastrointestinal (GI) tract diagnostic procedures the importance of following the prescribed regimen. The major reason that many studies of the GI tract are poor in quality or must be repeated is that the preparation of the gut or colon was inadequate.
- Inform women who are pregnant or lactating that drugs to relieve constipation should be used only under the direction of a physician.
- Inform the patient that sudden or persistent changes in bowel habits should be thoroughly evaluated by a physician.
- Special points about bulk-forming laxatives include teaching the patient to stir the prescribed dose into an 8-ounce glass of fluid and drink the mixture while the drug is still suspended in the liquid. For best results the patient should follow the first glass with a second full glass of water. The patient should never take these drugs dry since they can cause obstruction. Pills should be swallowed whole and not chewed. Under most circumstances, use these agents regularly, 1 to 3 times daily, to promote regular defecation.
- Remind the patient to take daily doses of stimulant (irritant) cathartics, but not castor oil, at bedtime to promote regular defecation in the morning. Swallow enteric-coated preparations, such as bisacodyl, whole and do not chew them. The patient should not take bisacodyl preparations within 1 hour of drinking milk or taking antacids.
- Castor oil has an unpleasant taste; inquire whether the patient would like it mixed with fruit juice. Some patients prefer to take castor oil straight and then drink juice as a follow-up so that the taste of the juice is not ruined by the medication. Encourage the patient to chill the castor oil to help lessen the unpleasant taste and to take doses early in the day since results usually occur within 2 to 6 hours.
- Inform the patient that storing suppositories in the refrigerator will make them firmer and easier to insert.
- Note in Table 24-1 that many of these drugs change the color of urine. Warn the patient about these changes.
- Encourage the patient to chill magnesium citrate before drinking to make it more palatable. The patient should drink the entire prescribed amount at once for best results.
- Instruct patients adhering to a sodium-restricted diet to avoid saline cathartics.
- Saline cathartics are often used to eliminate parasites after antihelminthic therapy if the trophozoites are not destroyed and can be found in the laboratory.
- The patient should be warned that when mineral oil is used on a regular basis there may be leakage of the oil or fecal material from the anus. Mineral oil stains clothing. Suggest that the patient wear a perianal pad or incontinence shield to protect clothing and sheets. Regular mineral oil use is associated with increased incidence of lipid pneumonia, especially in older adult patients. Encourage the patient to always sit upright or stand when taking this medication. For long-term treatment of constipation, drugs other than mineral oil are preferred. Warn the family not to use mineral oil or any oil-based substance to lubricate the nose or mouth of an immobilized patient since the patient may inadvertently aspirate small amounts. Instruct the patient not to take doses of mineral oil within 2 hours of meals because the mineral oil may interfere with absorption of fat-soluble vitamins and other nutrients.
- Explain the action of fecal softeners to the patient. Many patients misunderstand their function and expect defecation to occur a few hours after taking a single dose. Inform the patient that best results are achieved by using fecal softeners on a daily basis as prescribed. The patient may take liquid forms in milk or fruit juice, if desired.
- Encourage the patient taking saline cathartics or lactulose to follow doses with an additional glass of water, if possible, to facilitate laxative action. If the laxative leaves an unpleasant taste in the mouth, the patient should drink a glass of fruit juice or carbonated beverage after the dose, rather than water.
- Caution patients with diabetes to monitor blood glucose levels carefully when taking lactulose since the drug contains high concentrations of lactose and galactose. Warn patients taking lactulose that flatulence and abdominal cramps are common initially but will subside with continued therapy.
- Review with the patient how to administer suppositories or enemas if these routes of administration are prescribed.

Drugs to Control Diarrhea

Drug Administration

- Assess the patient with diarrhea for a history of recent travel, especially international travel; recent antibiotic use; recent cancer chemotherapy; and recent work with children in day care centers or other settings where harmful microorganisms are easily spread.
- Monitor intake and output, daily weight, skin turgor, level of consciousness, blood pressure, and pulse. Monitor serum electrolyte level.
- Dilute opium tincture in 15 to 30 ml of water to ensure that the patient receives the entire dose.
- Codeine is discussed in greater detail in Chapter 31.
- Paregoric tastes unpleasant. Many patients find combination drugs such as Parepectolin more palatable. (Parepectolin 30 ml contains paregoric 2.7 ml, pectin 162 mg, and kaolin 5.5 gm. Note that combination drugs subject the patient to additional ingredients that may or may not be helpful.)

Continued.

NURSING IMPLICATIONS SUMMARY—cont'd

- Theoretically, addiction to diphenoxylate or difenoxin is possible. Overdose with this drug resembles an overdose with a narcotic analgesic and is treated in a similar manner (see Chapter 31).
- Diphenoxylate and difenoxin preparations contain a small amount of atropine. A single dose of these preparations causes few side effects from the atropine, but the accumulated dose after 1 or 2 days of treatment might cause problems. Review the side effects of and contraindications to atropine use (Chapter 23).

Patient and Family Education

- Review side effects with the patient. Note that loperamide is now available over the counter but caution the patient that side effects may be associated with excessive or long-term use.
- Encourage the patient to keep a record of bowel movements. After several days of treatment for diarrhea, the patient may become constipated.
- Instruct patients with diarrhea to switch to a clear liquid diet and increase daily intake to 3000 ml of fluid but to avoid full-strength fruit juices. Homemade (see recipe on p. 308) or commercially available electrolyte solutions or products such as Gatorade may be helpful.
- Many cases of diarrhea are self-limiting. Instruct the patient to consult the physician if diarrhea persists longer than 3 to 5 days; prescribed antidiarrheal medications are not affording relief; stools are especially foul smelling or contain flecks of blood or large amounts of mucus; or the patient is unable to take in sufficient replacement fluids. Review with the patient the symptoms of hypokalemia such as muscle weakness, fatigue, anorexia, vomiting, drowsiness, irritability, and eventually coma and death. Review with the patient the symptoms of hypochloremia, including hypertonic muscles, tetany, and depressed respiration.
- Caution the patient to avoid drinking alcohol and to avoid driving or operating hazardous equipment if drowsiness develops. This effect may be dose related.
- Remind the patient to keep the perianal area clean to avoid anal irritation and to wash hands carefully after defecating to avoid spreading infectious organisms.
- Caution the patient to avoid the use of bismuth salts in infants or children who are recovering from the flu or chickenpox. If nausea and vomiting are present, the patient should check with the physician since these symptoms may indicate Reye's syndrome.

CRITICAL THINKING

APPLICATION

1. List some teaching points about ways to prevent constipation without using medications.
2. What drugs might you use for the treatment of diarrhea? What is their mechanism of action?

CRITICAL THINKING

1. List the five classes of laxatives. How do they differ in the time for a laxative effect to be produced and in the type of stool produced?
2. Why does the continued use of the stimulant (irritant) cathartics not help establish regular bowel habits?
3. What is diarrhea? Why do you need to monitor fluid and electrolyte replacement for the patient with diarrhea?

CHAPTER 25

Antiemetics

OBJECTIVES

After studying this chapter, you should be able to do the following:

- *Discuss the use of antiemetic drugs.*
- *Develop a care plan for patients receiving one of the various antiemetic drugs.*

KEY TERMS

antiemetics
cannabinoids
chemoreceptor trigger zone
emesis
nausea
vomiting

CHAPTER OVERVIEW

Nausea and vomiting are most commonly associated with motion sickness, anesthesia, radiation therapy, and cancer chemotherapy. A variety of agents with different mechanisms of action are effective against selected causes of nausea and vomiting.

Therapeutic Rationale: Vomiting

Antiemetics are drugs to control vomiting. **Vomiting (emesis)** is an involuntary act of regurgitating the contents of the stomach and is coordinated by an area in the medulla called the *vomiting center* (Figure 25-1). **Nausea** is the unpleasant sensation that usually precedes vomiting. Input from three major neural sites can stimulate the vomiting center. The first input is controlled by the higher central nervous system (CNS) functions, with vomiting being secondary to emotion, pain, or disequilibrium (motion sickness). The second pathway arises from peripheral stimuli, with vomiting related to injury or disease of a body tissue or organ. In particular, irritation of the mucosa of the gastrointestinal (GI) tract or bowel or biliary distention stimulates the vomiting center by way of the autonomic neurons carrying information to the CNS (afferent neurons). A third pathway is from the **chemoreceptor trigger zone,** a medullary center sensitive to stimulation by circulating drugs and toxins.

Nausea and vomiting are not necessarily treated with drugs. For instance, since antiemetic drugs have caused fetal abnormalities in experimental animals, the recommended treatment for the nausea and vomiting of pregnancy is by having patients sip water or tea and eat small meals. Many drugs cause nausea and vomiting because they act directly on the chemoreceptor trigger zone. Examples of such drugs include levodopa, digitalis, opiates (narcotic analgesics), and aminophylline. The effective treatment is to lower the dose of the offending drug or to increase the dose slowly. Drugs may also irritate the gastric mucosa, thus causing a reflex stimulation of nausea and vomiting. Aspirin is an example of an irritant drug. To dilute the drug, patients should take it with a large volume of liquid or with a meal.

Therapeutic Agents: Antiemetics

Drugs used to prevent nausea and vomiting are listed by drug class in Table 25-1. These drugs include antagonists of acetylcholine, histamine and dopamine, as well as drugs whose actions are not yet determined. Drugs for treating nausea and vomiting are most effective when administered before nausea and vomiting have begun rather than after.

The choice of an antiemetic is determined by the cause of the nausea and vomiting. Motion sickness and vertigo are most effectively treated prophylactically with scopolamine or antihistamines, including buclizine, cyclizine, meclizine, promethazine, and trimethobenzamide. Diphenidol also acts on the aural vestibular apparatus to control nausea and vomiting. The drugs effective in reducing the vomiting of chemotherapy and radiation therapy are dopamine antagonists, including thiethylperazine, chlorpromazine, perphenazine, promazine, triflupromazine, trimeprazine, and the serotonin antagonists granisetron and ondansetron. The cannabinoids (active ingredients in marijuana) dronabinol and nabilone are used for cancer chemotherapy. For the severely emetic chemotherapeutic agents, cisplatin, dacarbazine, and mechlorethamine, the serotonin receptor antagonists, granisetron and ondansetron, are effective antiemetic agents.

ANTICHOLINERGIC ANTIEMETIC: ✣ SCOPOLAMINE

Mechanism of Action

Scopolamine is an anticholinergic agent. Its effectiveness in preventing motion sickness is attributed to blockade of muscarinic receptors in the vestibular system.

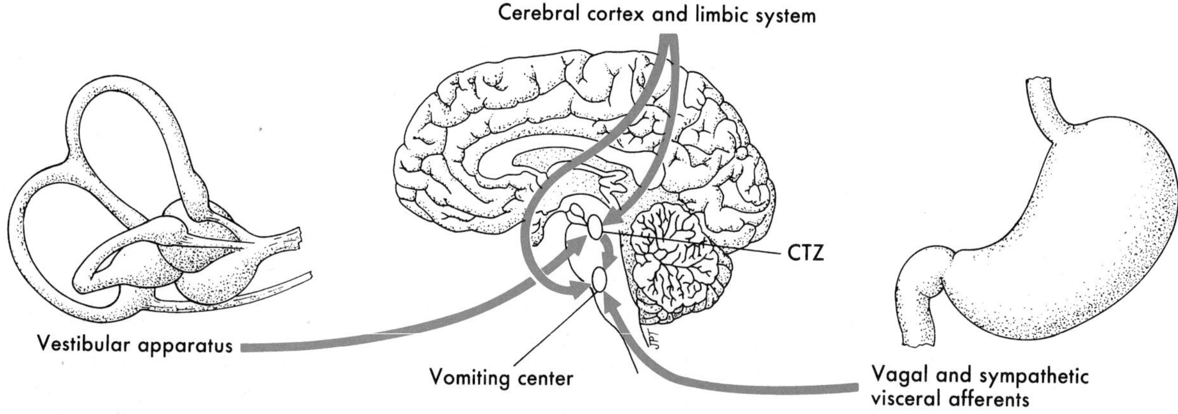

FIGURE 25-1
Vomiting action. Once stimulated, vomiting center acts on cranial nerves, spinal nerves to diaphragm, and abdominal muscles, which results in autonomic response of vomiting. *CTZ,* Chemoreceptor trigger zone. *(From Beare PG, Myers JL: Principles and practice of adult health nursing, St Louis, 1990, Mosby.)*

TABLE 25-1 Drugs to Control Vomiting

GENERIC NAME	TRADE NAME	ADMINISTRATION/DOSAGE	COMMENTS
Anticholinergic Drugs			
✣ Scopolamine	Transdermscop Transderm-V†	TOPICAL: *Adults*—1 adhesive unit is placed behind ear several hours before travel. Duration is 72 hr.	Sustained release protects most patients from motion sickness while greatly reducing anticholinergic side effects (blurred vision, sensitivity to light, dry mouth, and drowsiness).
Scopolamine hydrobromide		ORAL, SUBCUTANEOUS: *Adults*—0.6-1.0 mg. *Children*—0.006 mg/kg body weight.	Drug is one of most effective drugs in preventing motion sickness, but side effects (dry mouth, drowsiness) limit its use.
Antihistaminic Drugs			
Buclizine hydrochloride	Bucladin-S	ORAL: *Adults*—50 gm 30 min before traveling and 4-6 hr later. For vertigo, 50 mg 2 times daily.	Drug is effective for preventing motion sickness.
Cyclizine hydrochloride; cyclizine lactate	Marezine Marzin†	ORAL: *Adults*—50 mg 30 min before traveling and 4-6 hr later; maximum, 300 mg daily. *Children 6-10 yr*—3 mg/kg body weight divided into 3 doses daily.	Drug is effective for preventing motion sickness and vertigo.
Dimenhydrinate	Dramamine* Gravol† Others	INTRAMUSCULAR: *Adults*—50 mg as needed. *Children*—5 mg/kg body weight divided into 4 doses daily; maximum, 300 mg daily. INTRAVENOUS: *Adults*—50 mg diluted in 10 mg saline solution, injected over 2 min. ORAL: *Adults*—50-100 mg every 4 hr. *Children*—5 mg/kg body weight divided into 4 doses; maximum, 150 mg daily. RECTAL: *Adults*—100 mg 1-2 times daily.	Drug is effective for preventing vertigo, motion sickness, and nausea and vomiting of pregnancy. It also causes drowsiness.
✣ Diphenhydramine hydrochloride	Benadryl Hydrochloride*	DEEP INTRAMUSCULAR: *Adults*—10 mg increased to 20-50 mg every 2-3 hr if needed; maximum, 400 mg daily. *Children*—5 mg/kg body weight divided into 4 doses; maximum, 300 mg daily. INTRAVENOUS: *Adults*—same as deep intramuscular. ORAL: *Adults*—50 mg 30 min before traveling, then 50 mg before each meal. *Children*—5 mg/kg body weight divided into 4 doses; maximum, 300 mg daily.	Drug causes sedation. It is effective for preventing vertigo, motion sickness, and nausea and vomiting of pregnancy.
Hydroxyzine hydrochloride	Vistaject*	INTRAMUSCULAR: *Adults*—25-100 mg. *Children*—1 mg/kg body weight.	Antianxiety drug is effective for preventing motion sickness and postoperative nausea and vomiting.
Hydroxyzine pamoate	Vistaril	ORAL: *Adults*—25-100 mg 3-4 times daily. *Children >6 yr*—50-100 mg daily divided into 4 doses; *children <6 yr*—50 mg daily divided into 4 doses.	
Meclizine hydrochloride	Antivert* Bonine* Others	ORAL: *Adults*—25-50 mg once daily, taken 60 min or longer before traveling; 25-100 mg daily in divided doses for vertigo or radiation sickness.	Drug is effective for preventing motion sickness, vertigo, and nausea and vomiting of radiation therapy. It is longer acting than most antihistamines.

*Available in Canada and United States.
†Available in Canada only.

Continued.

TABLE 25-1 Drugs to Control Vomiting—cont'd

GENERIC NAME	TRADE NAME	ADMINISTRATION/DOSAGE	COMMENTS
Antihistaminic Drugs—cont'd			
Promethazine hydrochloride	Phenergan* Remsed	INTRAMUSCULAR, RECTAL: *Adults*—25 mg, then 12.5-25 mg as needed every 4-6 hr. *Children <12 yr*—no more than half the adult dose. ORAL: *Adults*—25 mg 2 times daily. *Children*—12.5-25 mg twice daily.	Drug is effective for preventing motion sickness and vertigo and postoperative nausea and vomiting.
Antidopaminergic Drugs			
Chlorpromazine hydrochloride	Thorazine	RECTAL: *Adults*—50-100 mg every 6-8 hr. *Children*—1 mg/kg body weight every 6-8 hr. INTRAMUSCULAR: *Adults*—25 mg, then 25-50 mg every 3-4 hr to stop vomiting. *Children*—0.5 mg/kg body weight every 6-8 hr; maximum, 40 mg (up to 5 yr or 50 lb), 75 mg (5-12 yr or 50-100 lb) daily. ORAL: *Adults*—10-25 mg every 4-6 hr. *Children*—0.5 mg/kg body weight every 4-6 hr.	Nurse watches for hypotension with initial injection. Drug is effective for postoperative nausea and vomiting and that caused by toxins, radiation therapy, or chemotherapy. It may cause considerable drowsiness.
Droperidol	Inapsine	To prevent postoperative nausea: INTRAVENOUS: *Adults*—1.25-2.5 mg. *Children*—0.05 mg/kg. Administer 5 min before termination of anesthesia. To control nausea of cancer chemotherapy: administer 30-60 min before treatment. Same or half dose may be given intramuscularly after therapy on request but not more than once every hour. INTRAVENOUS: *Adults*—2.5-5 mg. *Children*—1.25 mg/20 kg. For nausea of cisplatin or other potent emetic agents: INTRAVENOUS: *Adults*—15 mg loading dose followed by 7.5 mg every 2 hr for 7 doses.	Drug is effective for postoperative nausea and vomiting and that caused by toxins, radiation therapy, or chemotherapy. With large doses, incidence of dystonic reactions may be high.
Fluphenazine hydrochloride	Permitil* Prolixin Others	INTRAMUSCULAR: *Adults*—1.25 mg every 6-8 hr as needed.	Drug is effective for postoperative nausea and vomiting and that caused by toxins, radiation therapy, or chemotherapy.
Haloperidol	Haldol*	INTRAMUSCULAR, ORAL: *Adults*—1, 2, or 5 mg every 12 hr as needed.	Drug is effective for postoperative nausea and vomiting and that caused by toxins, radiation therapy, or chemotherapy.
Metoclopramide	Emex† Maxolon Maxeran† Reclomide Reglan*	INTRAVENOUS: *Adults*—10-20 mg, administered over 2 min. *Children up to 6 yr*—0.1 mg/kg body weight; *children 6-14 yr*—2.5-5 mg. ORAL: *Adults*—5-10 mg 3 times daily 15-30 min before meals.	Drug acts centrally to block stimulation of chemoreceptor trigger zone and peripherally to enhance GI tone. High-dose therapy is effective in reducing nausea and vomiting caused by cisplatin therapy.
Perphenazine	Trilafon*	ORAL: *Adults*—8-24 mg daily in 2 or more divided doses. INTRAMUSCULAR: *Adults*—5 mg daily.	Drug is effective for postoperative nausea and vomiting and that caused by toxins, radiation therapy, or chemotherapy.
Prochlorperazine	Compazine	RECTAL: *Adults*—25 mg 2 times daily. *Children ≤10 kg*—0.4 mg/kg body weight daily divided into 3-4 doses.	Drug is effective for postoperative nausea and vomiting and that caused by toxins, radiation therapy, or chemotherapy.
Prochlorperazine edisylate	Compazine	DEEP INTRAMUSCULAR: *Adults*—5-10 mg every 3-4 hr; maximum, 40 mg daily. *Children ≤10 kg*—0.2 mg/body weight daily.	

TABLE 25-1 Drugs to Control Vomiting—cont'd

GENERIC NAME	TRADE NAME	ADMINISTRATION/DOSAGE	COMMENTS
Antidopaminergic Drugs—cont'd			
✚ Prochlorperazine maleate	Compazine	ORAL: *Adults*—5-10 mg every 3-4 hr; maximum, 40 mg daily. *Children >10 kg*—0.2 mg/body weight daily.	
Promazine hydrochloride	Sparine*	ORAL: *Adults*—25-50 mg every 4-6 hr as needed. INTRAMUSCULAR: *Adults*—50 mg.	Drug is effective for postoperative nausea and vomiting and that caused by toxins, radiation therapy, or chemotherapy. Nurse watches for hypotension after intramuscular injection. Sedation and anticholinergic effects are common.
Thiethylperazine malate (injection) or maleate (oral)	Torecan	INTRAMUSCULAR: *Adults*—10 mg 1-3 times daily. ORAL: *Adults*—10 mg 1-3 times daily.	Drug is effective for postoperative nausea and vomiting and that caused by toxins, radiation therapy, or chemotherapy.
Triflupromazine hydrochloride	Vesprin	ORAL: *Adults*—25-30 mg daily. *Children*—0.2 mg/kg body weight divided into 3 doses; maximum daily dose, 10 mg. INTRAMUSCULAR: *Adults*—5-15 mg every 4 hr as needed; maximum daily dose, 60 mg. *Older adults*—2.5-15 mg daily. *Children*—0.2-0.25 mg/kg body weight; maximum daily dose, 10 mg.	Drug is effective for postoperative nausea and vomiting and that caused by toxins, radiation therapy, or chemotherapy.
Cannabinoids			
Dronabinol	Marinol	ORAL: *Adults*—5-7.5 mg/m^2 every 3-4 hr. Begin 4-12 hr before chemotherapy and continue 8-24 hr after. Dose may be increased by 2.5 mg/m^2 if necessary.	Dronabinol is delta-9-tetrahydrocannabinol, major active ingredient in marijuana. It is particularly effective antiemetic when combined with phenothiazine. It is schedule II drug.
Nabilone	Cesamet†	ORAL: *Adults*—1 mg twice daily, increasing to 2 mg twice daily if necessary.	Drug is especially effective antiemetic for cisplatin chemotherapy. Controlled substance in Canada.
Miscellaneous Drugs			
Benzquinamide hydrochloride	Emete-Con	INTRAMUSCULAR: *Adults*—0.5-1 mg/kg body weight at least 15 min before chemotherapy or emergence from anesthesia. Repeat in 1 hr, then every 3-4 hr as required. INTRAVENOUS: *Adults*—0.2-0.4 mg/kg body weight diluted in 5% dextrose, sodium chloride injection, or lactated Ringer's injection and administered over 1-3 min. Additional doses are given IM.	This rapidly acting antiemetic with a short duration of action is effective in controlling postoperative nausea and vomiting. It acts by inhibiting the chemoreceptor trigger zone.
Diphenidol hydrochloride	Vontrol*	ORAL: *Adults*—25-50 mg 4 times daily. *Children >6 mo and ≥12 kg*—5 mg/kg body weight daily divided into 4 doses.	Drug acts on vestibular apparatus to prevent vertigo after surgery on middle ear. It is effective for postoperative nausea and vomiting and that caused by toxins, radiation therapy, or chemotherapy.
Granisetron	Kytril	INTRAVENOUS: *Adults and children ≥ 2 yr*—10 μg/kg 30 min before chemotherapy, administered over 5 min.	This serotonin receptor blocker controls nausea and vomiting with chemotherapy.

Continued.

TABLE 25-1 Drugs to Control Vomiting—cont'd

GENERIC NAME	TRADE NAME	ADMINISTRATION/DOSAGE	COMMENTS
Miscellaneous Drugs—cont'd			
✣ Ondansetron	Zofran*	INTRAVENOUS: *Adults*—150 μg/kg 30 min before chemotherapy, administered over 15 min.	This serotonin receptor blocker controls nausea and vomiting with chemotherapy.
Trimethobenzamide hydrochloride	Tigan*	INTRAMUSCULAR: *Adults*—200 mg 3-4 times daily. For preventing postoperative nausea and vomiting, give 1 dose before or during surgery and another 3 hr after surgery. ORAL: *Adults*—250 mg 3-4 times daily. *Children*—15 mg/kg body weight divided into 3-4 doses or 100-200 mg divided into 3-4 doses.	Drug relieves nausea and vomiting of radiation therapy, in immediate postoperative period, and in gastroenteritis.

Pharmacokinetics

Scopolamine is well absorbed and readily crosses the blood-brain barrier. When administered orally, scopolamine causes significant anticholinergic side effects. For preventing motion sickness, a transdermal patch is preferred to decrease side effects. The patch is applied at least 4 hours in advance of travel and delivers scopolamine over a 3-day period. The patch should not be used by children because of their sensitivity to the anticholinergic effects. Administered orally, scopolamine is effective in 30 minutes and has a duration of action of 4 to 6 hours. It is metabolized by the liver and excreted in the urine.

Uses

Scopolamine is considered the most effective agent available for prophylactic treatment of motion sickness. Scopolamine is also administered as a preanesthetic agent to depress respiratory secretions and salivation.

Adverse Reactions and Contraindications

Anticholinergic effects of scopolamine include dry mouth, blurred vision, decreased sweating, urinary hesitancy, and constipation. Drowsiness, amnesia, and fatigue may also be experienced. Because vagal tone is depressed, patients with cardiac disease may experience an undesirable increase in heart rate. Children are sensitive to the anticholinergic effects and with the reduced sweating may run significant fevers. Children and older adults are more sensitive to the effects of urinary retention, constipation, and disorientation. Men with prostatic hypertrophy are also likely to have difficulty with urination. Lactation may be inhibited by scopolamine. Moreover, scopolamine is secreted in breast milk and should be avoided by nursing mothers since infants may be quite sensitive to the anticholinergic effects. Patients with glaucoma should be given scopolamine cautiously because of the increase in intraocular pressure resulting from the anticholinergic effect.

Interactions

Scopolamine causes additive anticholinergic effects with other agents having this activity. In particular, antiparkinsonian drugs, disopyramide, glutethimide, opioids, phenothiazines, tricyclic antidepressants, quinidine, and some antihistamines have significant anticholinergic activity.

ANTIHISTAMINIC ANTIEMETICS

Mechanism of Action

Selected antihistamines have been developed that help prevent motion sickness and vertigo. Stimulation of receptors in the labyrinth of the ear from which signals governing the sense of equilibrium arise is suppressed. A central anticholinergic action depresses the chemoreceptor trigger zone.

Pharmacokinetics

Most antihistamines are taken orally 30 minutes before travel and every 4 to 6 hours as needed. Metabolites are excreted in the urine within 24 hours.

Uses

Antihistamines are primarily effective for treating motion sickness and vertigo. Therapy is most effective when given prophylactically, a half hour before travel.

Adverse Reactions and Contraindications

The most common side effects are drowsiness and dry mouth. Headache and jitters may also occur. Older adults tend to be more sensitive to the anticholinergic effects of dryness of mouth and urinary retention. Older adults are also more likely to become sedated, confused, or dizzy.

Antihistamines can worsen the symptoms of urinary retention, prostatic hypertrophy, bladder neck obstruction, and pyloroduodenal obstruction. Therapy for glaucoma may require alteration.

Interactions

Antihistamines cause additive depression with concurrent use of CNS depressants and alcohol. Anticholinergic effects are enhanced with concurrent administration of other drugs that have anticholinergic activity.

SPECIFIC ANTIHISTAMINIC ANTIEMETICS

Buclizine

Buclizine (Bucladin) is primarily used to prevent motion sickness. It is available as a chewable tablet.

Cyclizine

Cyclizine (Marezine) is effective for motion sickness, vertigo, and symptoms of vestibular disorders.

Dimenhydrinate

Dimenhydrinate (Dramamine) is effective in treating vertigo and motion sickness. It is also effective in treating nausea and vomiting during pregnancy. Dimenhydrinate can be administered intramuscularly, intravenously, or orally.

✣ Diphenhydramine

Diphenhydramine (Benadryl) has actions and uses similar to those of dimenhydrinate. When given intravenously, diphenhydramine is especially effective in treating dystonic reactions caused by dopaminergic blockers such as metoclopramide.

Hydroxyzine

Hydroxyzine (Atarax, Vistaril) is used for preventing motion sickness. Given intramuscularly, it also reduces postsurgical nausea and vomiting.

Meclizine

Meclizine (Antivert, Bonine) has a slower onset (60 minutes) and longer duration (24 hours) than other antihistamines. It is especially useful in treating the nausea of vestibular disorders such as labyrinthitis and Meniere's disease. It is also used to prevent motion sickness.

Promethazine

Promethazine (Phenergan) is a phenothiazine with pronounced antihistaminic activity in addition to strong central cholinergic blocking activity. It is effective in preventing both motion sickness and postoperative nausea.

ANTIDOPAMINERGIC ANTIEMETICS: GENERAL CHARACTERISTICS

Mechanism of Action

Antidopaminergic antiemetics act at the chemoreceptor trigger zone. They are antagonists of dopamine, the major neurotransmitter of the chemoreceptor trigger zone. Most of these dopamine antagonists are drugs that are used as antipsychotic drugs (see Chapter 52).

Pharmacokinetics

In addition to oral administration, most of these drugs are available for intramuscular or intravenous injection. In general, the drug is metabolized by the liver and excreted in the urine.

Uses

Antidopaminergic drugs are effective in reducing vomiting from chemotherapy and radiation therapy of cancer. They also control postoperative vomiting, although they do not prevent motion sickness.

Adverse Reactions and Contraindications

Occasionally, extrapyramidal symptoms are seen with the antidopaminergics. Extrapyramidal symptoms are disorders of motor control associated with too little dopamine in a certain area of the brain.

The side effects of the antidopaminergics are more fully discussed in Chapter 52.

Interactions

The major drug interaction of antiemetics is a synergistic depression with drugs depressing the CNS, particularly when respiratory depression is involved. For instance, vomiting that is related to alcohol intoxication or ingestion of narcotic analgesics can be relieved with an antidopaminergic, but the resultant respiratory depression makes this treatment undesirable.

SPECIFIC ANTIDOPAMINERGIC ANTIEMETICS

Chlorpromazine

Chlorpromazine (Thorazine) is used to prevent nausea and vomiting associated with use of chemotherapeutic agents that are not highly emetic. Chlorpromazine causes considerable sedation and orthostatic hypotension, actions that limit its use.

Droperidol

Droperidol (Inapsine) is used for prophylactic treatment of postsurgical nausea and vomiting. It is effective in low doses and has a long duration of action.

Fluphenazine

Fluphenazine (Permitil, Prolixin) is used principally for treatment of nausea and vomiting associated with surgery and use of toxins and radiation.

Haloperidol

Haloperidol (Haldol) is used to treat nausea and vomiting associated with use of opioids and surgery, radiation therapy, cancer chemotherapy, and GI tract disorders. Chemically related to droperidol, haloperidol has a longer duration of action.

Metoclopramide

Metoclopramide (Octamide PFS, Maxolon, Reglan) stimulates the GI system, which counteracts the loss of tone in vomiting. In addition, metoclopramide acts at the chemoreceptor trigger zone to prevent vomiting.

Perphenazine

Perphenazine (Trilafon) is effective in treating nausea and vomiting associated with surgery and use of opioids and radiation.

✣ Prochlorperazine

Prochlorperazine (Compazine) is widely used to prevent nausea and vomiting associated with use of mildly emetic chemotherapeutic agents, toxins, and radiation. Prochlorperazine does not produce the profound sedation associated with chlorpromazine. Hypotension is minimized by administering prochlorperazine in a slow intravenous infusion over 15 to 20 minutes.

Promazine

Promazine (Sparine) is used primarily to prevent postoperative nausea and vomiting.

Thiethylperazine

Thiethylperazine (Torecan) is considered very effective to prevent postoperative nausea and vomiting. It is also effective in treating nausea and vomiting caused by the use of mildly emetogenic chemotherapeutic drugs, radiation, and toxins.

Triflupromazine

Triflupromazine (Vesprin) is used primarily to prevent postoperative nausea and vomiting.

OTHER ANTIEMETIC DRUGS

Benzquinamide

Benzquinamide (Emete-Con) inhibits stimulation of the chemoreceptor trigger zone and prevents vomiting. It is used primarily to treat postoperative nausea and vomiting.

Diphenidol

Diphenidol (Vontrol) acts on the aural vestibular apparatus to prevent nausea associated with surgery on the middle and inner ear. It is also effective in treating postoperative nausea and vomiting as well as that associated with toxins, radiation therapy, and some chemotherapeutic agents.

Dronabinol

Dronabinol (Marinol) is the major active substance in marijuana and appears to be an especially effective antiemetic when combined with a phenothiazine. **Cannabinoids** are new additions to antiemetic therapy for cancer chemotherapy. Patients who smoked marijuana before receiving cancer chemotherapy reported a decreased incidence of nausea and vomiting. Research revealed that the active ingredients, cannabinoids, appeared to depress the chemoreceptor trigger zone.

Granisetron

Granisetron (Kytril) is a new drug that like ondansetron blocks the serotonin receptor. Both drugs are effective in preventing nausea and vomiting from use of severely emetic chemotherapeutic agents such as cisplatin.

Nabilone

Nabilone (Cesamet) is an active cannabinoid-like dronabinol that appears to be especially effective for relieving the nausea from low-dose cisplatin therapy (see box below). It is available in Canada but not in the United States.

✣ Ondansetron

Ondansetron (Zofran), like granisetron, is a serotonin receptor blocker effective against nausea-inducing anticancer drugs. Some anticancer drugs, such as cisplatin, trigger the release from the gut of the transmitter serotonin that stimulates the vagal nerve, resulting in nausea. Ondansetron is a selective blocker of the serotonin receptor.

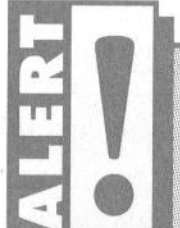

DRUG ABUSE ALERT

Marijuana

BACKGROUND

Tetrahydrocannabinols are the active ingredients found in the marijuana plant. The leaves and tops of the marijuana plant are smoked or eaten. Users seek relaxation and feeling of heightened perception. The only medical use of cannabinols, however, is for their antiemetic effect during cancer chemotherapy.

PHARMACOLOGY

Cannabinols impair memory and judgment and raise blood pressure. Characteristically, the user's eyes are bloodshot. When cannabinols are smoked, effects are felt after a few inhalations and reach a maximum about 20 minutes after the last inhalation. Intoxication includes euphoria, depersonalization, and uncontrollable laughter. Acute effects last about 3 hours.

HEALTH HAZARDS

Acute intoxication may impair judgment; thus the intoxicated individual should not drive or perform potentially dangerous tasks. Anxiety, paranoia, loss of concentration, slower movements, and time distortion are effects of overdose. Long-term health effects have not been clearly shown. Addiction is psychologic. There is no major withdrawal syndrome, although insomnia, hyperactivity, and decreased appetite have been reported.

Trimethobenzamide

Trimethobenzamide (Tigan) inhibits stimulation of the chemoreceptor trigger zone and prevents vomiting.

NURSING PROCESS OVERVIEW

Drugs to Treat Nausea and Vomiting

Assessment

Patients develop nausea with associated vomiting from a variety of causes. Assess the patient, focusing on the vital signs, character and quantity of any emesis, presence of bowel sounds, and intake and output. Perform a brief neurologic examination. Obtain a history of precipitating factors, exposure to recent infectious processes, and recent changes in diet or medications.

Nursing Diagnoses

- Altered thought processes related to drowsiness produced as a drug side effect
- Risk for injury related to impaired vision related to drug side effect (e.g., scopolamine)

Patient Outcomes

The patient will have relief of nausea, without vomiting.

Planning/Implementation

Antiemetics are used to relieve symptoms. Continue to monitor the vital signs and intake and output and assess the subjective complaints of nausea and vomiting. Observe the patient for side effects, although these are usually not severe. CNS depression, hypotension, and dry mouth are seen frequently. Limit odors in the patient's environment, limit intake to clear liquids, and provide backrubs or cool washcloths to the forehead to aid comfort.

Evaluation

Success is measured by a reduction in the subjective complaint of nausea and by less vomiting. Before discharge, patients should be able to explain why and how to take the drug, the frequency of drug administration, the anticipated side effects of the medication, and what to do if nausea and vomiting are unrelieved by the medication.

NURSING IMPLICATIONS SUMMARY

Antiemetics

Drug Administration

- Measure emesis as part of fluid intake and output.
- Use antiemetics with caution in children who may be suffering from Reye's syndrome. This syndrome is characterized by an abrupt onset of persistent severe vomiting, lethargy, irrational behavior, progressive encephalopathy, convulsions, coma, and death.
- Be alert to patient response to the cannabinoids; some patients may hesitate to use drugs derived from marijuana. Inform the patient that psychologic or physical dependence is unlikely at therapeutic doses and with short-term use of these drugs. Since the gelatin capsule form of dronabinol contains sesame seed oil, check for allergy to this oil before administering the first dose.
- Intravenous benzquinamide has been associated with an increase in blood pressure and cardiac arrhythmias. The intramuscular route is preferred. For intravenous use, dilute 50 mg with 2.2 ml of sterile water for injection. Monitor the blood pressure and pulse, and administer intravenous doses slowly, a single dose over 1 minute.
- Avoid intramuscular use of trimethobenzamide in children.
- Dilute dose of ondansetron in 50 ml of 5% dextrose in water (D5W) or 0.9% sodium chloride. Administer dose over 15 minutes.
- Dilute dose of granisetron in 20 to 50 ml of D5W or 0.9% sodium chloride. Administer dose over 5 minutes, 30 minutes before chemotherapy or radiotherapy.

Intravenous Dimenhydrinate

- Dilute 50 mg of drug in 10 ml of 0.9% sodium chloride injection. Administer at 25 mg/min.

Intravenous Promethazine

- Dilute with normal saline to at least 25 mg/ml, preferably to 2.5 to 5 mg/ml. Administer at 25 mg/min. Slightly yellow solutions may be safely used; discard highly discolored solutions. Avoid spilling on hands because it may cause contact dermatitis.
- Other antihistamines are discussed in detail in Chapter 28. The antidopaminergic drugs are discussed in detail in Chapter 52. Scopolamine is also discussed in Chapter 23.

Patient and Family Education

- Review the side effects of antiemetics with the patient. Warn the patient to use antiemetics only as prescribed and not to self-medicate with leftover doses. The use of these drugs in pregnant women is contraindicated unless the benefit outweighs the risk. Warn the patient to avoid drinking alcohol or operating hazardous equipment when

Continued.

NURSING IMPLICATIONS SUMMARY—cont'd

taking antiemetics since sedation and drowsiness are common side effects. Caution the patient to avoid other drugs that may depress the CNS while using antiemetics. These drugs include alcohol, tranquilizers, sleeping medications, and narcotic analgesics.

- For treatment of motion sickness, suggest that the patient ride in the front seat of the car if possible, facing forward. Suggest that the patient take prophylactic drugs 1 to 2 hours before a trip rather than when nausea develops.
- For sustained-release transdermal drugs, emphasize the importance of reading the manufacturer's instructions. Instruct the patient to wash hands before and after applying the device. The disk is usually applied behind the ear, in front of the hairline. The patient should avoid cut or denuded skin and should replace the disk every 3 days or as directed by the physician. If the disk falls off, the patient should apply a new one. Instruct the patient to apply the disk 4 hours before a trip.
- For dry mouth, suggest that the patient chew sugarless gum or suck sugarless hard candy. Provide frequent mouth care, but avoid drying, alcohol-containing mouthwashes, or lemon and glycerin swabs. See the patient problem box on dry mouth (p. 300). For the person who can have nothing by mouth (NPO) or who has vomited, provide frequent mouth care. Suggest that the patient suck ice chips; consult the physician for the NPO patient.
- Encourage the family to keep the environment free of odors and to keep food out of sight of the nauseated person. The patient should try clear liquids in small amounts before progressing to a more complete diet.
- If dry eyes are a problem, suggest that the patient use artificial tears on a regular basis; consult the physician. Warn the patient that intramuscular antiemetics often produce burning at the injection site. Remind the patient to keep these and all drugs out of the reach of children.
- Review the drug administration technique that the patient is to use at home. If the patient is to inject the medication intravenously or intramuscularly, have the patient give a return demonstration before discharge.

CRITICAL THINKING

APPLICATION

1. What are the three major pathways that stimulate vomiting?

CRITICAL THINKING

1. What are some nonpharmacologic treatments of nausea and vomiting you might recommend?
2. Differentiate between antihistamines vs. the antidopaminergic drugs for types of nausea and vomiting, actions, and effectiveness.

CHAPTER 26

Drugs to Treat Ulcers

OBJECTIVES

After studying this chapter, you should be able to do the following:

- *Discuss the use of drugs to treat ulcers.*
- *Develop a nursing care plan for patients receiving the following drugs or drug groups: antacids, histamine H_2-receptor antagonists, omeprazole, sucralfate, and misoprostol.*

KEY TERMS

esophageal ulcer
H_2 antagonists
hydrochloric acid
peptic ulcer
secretin
ulcer

CHAPTER OVERVIEW

Peptic ulcers occur when the mucosal defense system of the gastroduodenal tract fails to protect the tissue from erosive effects of acid and pepsin. The treatment of ulcers has changed dramatically in recent years with the introduction of H_2 antagonists that effectively suppress acid secretion. The demonstration that a bacterium, *Helicobacter pylori,* may be a significant risk factor for ulcer formation will further change the treatment of ulcers.

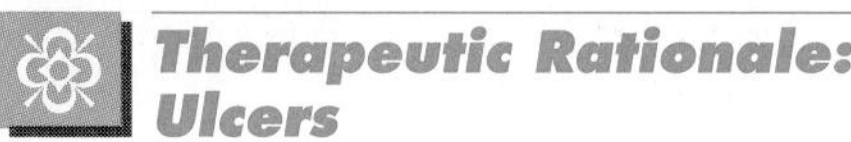

Therapeutic Rationale: Ulcers

Definitions

An **ulcer** is the loss of the skin or mucosal tissue that provides the protective layer of cells normally surrounding an organ. A **peptic ulcer** occurs in the esophagus, stomach, or duodenum after the mucosal barrier is destroyed, exposing the underlying tissue to stomach acid; as a result, the anatomic structure of the stomach and the regulation of stomach secretions are affected. The goal in treating an ulcer is to depress or neutralize stomach acid, thereby allowing the ulcer to heal and preventing the recurrence of the ulcer.

An **esophageal ulcer** results when there is reflux of stomach acid into the esophagus because of a defective esophageal sphincter. An ulcer in the duodenum results from overactive secretion of acid in the stomach so that stomach contents cannot be neutralized in the duodenum. The acidic contents then damage the duodenal mucosa. Stomach ulcers are most frequently caused by a tumor, but a nonmalignant cause of stomach ulcers is the reflux of duodenal contents back into the stomach because of a faulty pyloric sphincter. The duodenal contents contain bile acids that disrupt the mucosal barrier normally protecting the stomach from acid and pepsin.

Control of Acid Secretion

Factors controlling the secretion of hydrochloric acid by the parietal cells of the stomach are diagrammed in Figure 26-1. The neurotransmitter acetylcholine (released from a branch of the vagus nerve), the hormone gastrin, and histamine stimulate the secretion of acid. **Hydrochloric acid** aids in the breakdown of connective tissue in food, activates pepsinogen to pepsin (which degrades protein), and kills any bacteria ingested in food. The acidic digest leaves the stomach to enter the duodenum. This movement of digested food lessens stomach distention and thereby removes a stimulus for the release of gastrin and for vagal activity. In response to acidity the duodenum releases **secretin,** a hormone that stimulates the release of bicarbonate and digestive enzymes from the pancreas. Secretin also depresses the release of hydrochloric acid by the parietal cells and depresses the motility of the stomach. The bicarbonate released by the pancreas neutralizes the acidity of the partially digested food entering the duodenum. This neutralization is also necessary for the digestive enzymes in the intestine to be active.

Bacterial Cause of Ulcers

Recent attention has focused on a bacterial cause of ulcers. The bacterium, *Helicobacter pylori,* may account for 80% of all stomach ulcers and all duodenal ulcers. This bacterium may

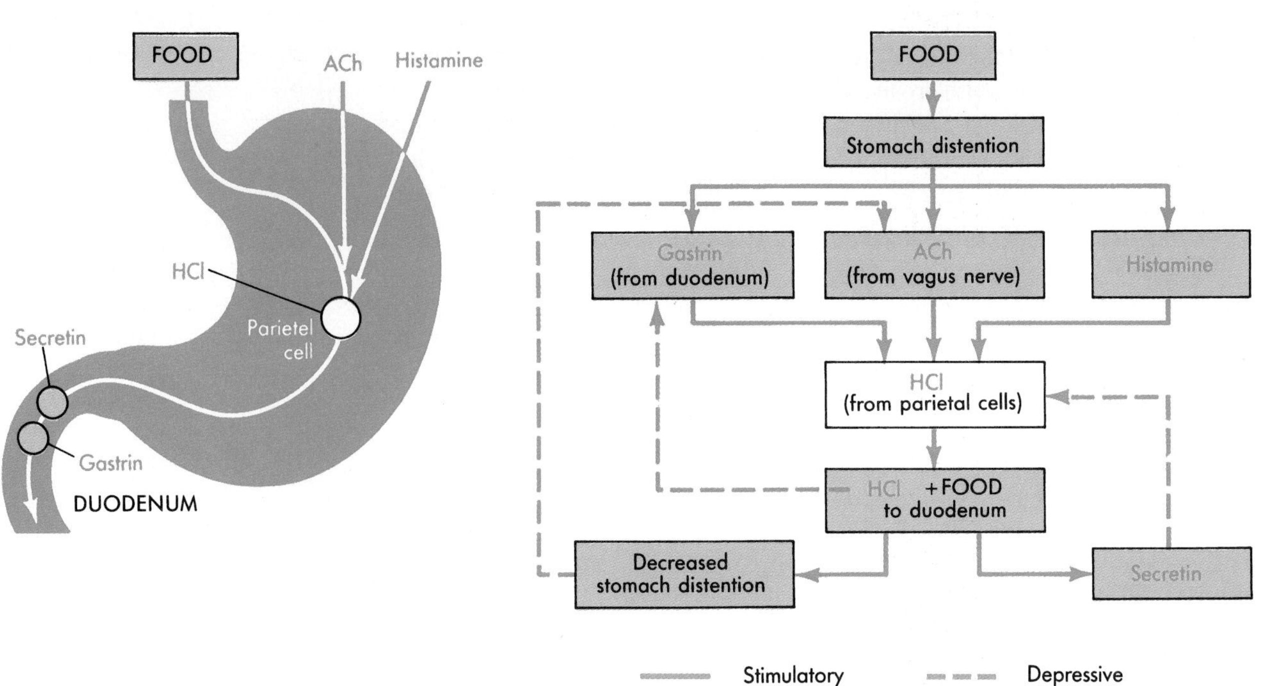

FIGURE 26-1
Secretion of acid parietal cells of stomach is controlled by duodenally released hormone, gastrin; parasympathetic nervous system, via neurotransmitter acetylcholine *(ACh)*; and histamine. Histamine is most effective stimulant of gastric acid secretion. Acid secretion is discontinued when food reaches duodenum, where hydrochloric acid (HCl) inhibits gastrin release and stimulates secretin release, and distention of stomach is lessened, decreasing vagal stimulation.

burrow into the duodenum and digest the layer of mucus that protects the lining of the stomach and duodenum from acid. However, most persons infected with this organism do not develop an ulcer, so other risk factors also play a role.

Eradication of *H. pylori* can be achieved with a combination therapy. A major study showed success with 5 to 8 tablets (262 mg each) of bismuth subsalicylate daily, 250 mg metronidazole 3 times daily, and 500 mg tetracycline 4 times daily, with ranitidine given daily during the first 2 weeks of therapy. However, resistance can develop to metronidazole, and this complicated therapy causes gastrointestinal tract disturbances. Increased attention will be paid in the future to developing better regimens to eradicate *H. pylori.*

Risk Factors for Ulcers

Nonsteroidal antiinflammatory drugs (NSAIDs) inhibit prostaglandin synthesis. Since prostaglandins are important in maintaining the gastric mucosal system, use of NSAIDs is associated with upper gastrointestinal tract bleeding, and prolonged use can cause peptic ulcers. Older adults are especially sensitive to this effect. Corticosteroids enhance the incidence of ulcer formation in patients, especially those also taking NSAIDs.

In the past, much attention was given to dietary and emotional factors. However, these are exacerbating factors and not causal factors. Smoking is also an aggravating factor.

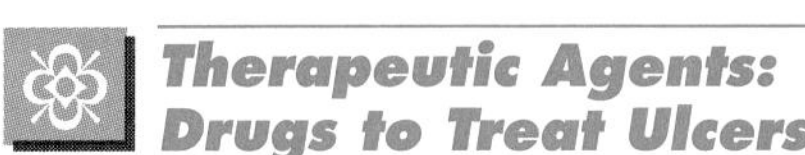

Therapeutic Agents: Drugs to Treat Ulcers

Drugs to treat an ulcer are listed in Table 26-1. Ulcers were once treated with antacids and anticholinergic drugs; today, these drugs play a secondary role. The introduction of H_2 receptor antagonists and mucosal protective agents has dramatically improved the treatment of ulcers. The identification of *H. pylori* as a major risk factor for ulcers will stimulate development of new treatment regimens designed to eradicate this bacterium in patients with ulcers.

Histamine H_2-Receptor Antagonists

Mechanism of Action

The **H_2 antagonists** specifically block the H_2 receptors that control the basal and stimulated secretion of hydrochloric acid by the parietal cells (see Figure 26-1). (H_1 receptors are blocked by the antihistamines discussed in Chapter 28.) Gastrin and acetylcholine are believed to act through histamine to cause the release of hydrochloric acid because H_2 antagonists are so effective in decreasing acid secretion stimulated by pentagastrin (an active analogue of gastrin) or bethanechol (an agonist of acetylcholine), as well as by food, insulin, and caffeine.

Pharmacokinetics

The H_2 antagonists are taken orally and absorbed rapidly. They are effective within an hour. Cimetidine has a duration of action of up to 6 hours, whereas other H_2 antagonists have a duration of up to 12 hours. They are metabolized by the liver and excreted in the urine. Patients with severe renal disease should receive reduced doses.

Uses

Because H_2 antagonists dramatically decrease stomach acid, they alleviate many conditions in which stomach acid impedes therapy, including the following:

1. Duodenal ulcer: A duodenal ulcer usually heals within 8 weeks of therapy with H_2 antagonists, but maintenance therapy is necessary to prevent recurrence.
2. Gastric ulcer: H_2 antagonists increase the healing rate of gastric ulcers. Long-term therapy is moderately effective in preventing recurrences.
3. Reflux esophagitis: H_2 antagonists tend to reduce the frequency of symptoms. Long-term therapy may yield sustained improvement.
4. Zollinger-Ellison syndrome: A tumor secretes excessive gastrin that stimulates excessive acid production. H_2 antagonists depress this acid production.
5. Gastrointestinal hemorrhage: Stomach acid intensifies inflammation of the stomach, worsening the hemorrhaging.
6. Pancreatic insufficiency: Digestive enzymes must be administered orally. Without H_2 antagonists, stomach acid inactivates most of the administered enzymes.

Adverse Reactions and Contraindications

H_2 antagonists are remarkably free of general side effects. Central nervous system (CNS) effects include mental confusion, agitation, and hallucinations; these symptoms are reversible when the drug is discontinued. CNS effects are more frequent in patients with liver or renal disease.

Interactions

All H_2 antagonists decrease the gastric acidity that can alter the absorption of other drugs. The absorption of ketoconazole in particular is reduced unless it is taken at least 2 hours before the H_2 antagonist. The absorption of the H_2 antagonists is slowed by concurrent administration of antacids.

Cimetidine inhibits the liver cytochrome P-450 system that metabolizes many drugs. Some of the drugs whose metabolism is inhibited include warfarin, theophylline, and phenytoin. The doses of these drugs should be reduced. Cimetidine also inhibits the gastric metabolism of alcohol. The other H_2 antagonists do not affect drug metabolism.

Cimetidine given in high doses over a long time has a feminizing effect on men, producing gynecomastia, impotence, and loss of libido. These effects are not characteristic of the other H_2 antagonists.

Specific Histamine H_2-Receptor Antagonists

✣ Cimetidine

Cimetidine (Tagamet) was the first histamine H_2-receptor antagonist released for commercial use. It has a shorter dura-

TABLE 26-1 Drugs to Treat an Ulcer

GENERIC NAME	TRADE NAME	ADMINISTRATION/DOSAGE	COMMENTS
H_2-Receptor Antagonists			
✣ Cimetidine	Tagamet* Apo-Cimetidine† Novocimetidine†	ORAL: *Adults*—300 mg with meals and at bedtime until ulcer is healed (3-6 wk), then 300 mg at bedtime to inhibit nocturnal secretion.	Nurse should administer with meals because food slows absorption and prolongs action of cimetidine. Nurse should administer at least 1 hr after antacids or metoclopramide, which reduces absorption of cimetidine if taken concurrently.
Cimetidine hydrochloride	Tagamet Hydrochloride*	INTRAVENOUS: *Adults*—1-4 mg/kg/hr or 300 mg diluted and infused over 15-20 min. INTRAMUSCULAR: *Adults*—300 mg every 6 hr. ORAL, INTRAVENOUS: *Children*—20-40 mg/kg in divided doses.	Nurse should switch to oral doses when ulcer bleeding has stopped.
Famotidine	Pepcid*	ORAL: *Adults*—40 mg daily at bedtime, or in 2 divided doses. INTRAVENOUS: *Adults*—20 mg every 12 hr.	Famotidine acts longer than cimetidine.
Nizatidine	Axid*	ORAL: *Adults*—300 mg daily at bedtime to heal ulcer, then 150 mg daily to prevent recurrence.	Nizatidine acts longer than cimetidine.
Ranitidine hydrochloride	Zantac* Apo-Ranitidine†	ORAL: *Adults*—150 mg every 12 hr. INTRAMUSCULAR/SLOW INTRAVENOUS: *Adults*—50 mg every 6-8 hr. Maximum daily dose is 400 mg.	Ranitidine hydrochloride acts longer than cimetidine.
Mucosal Protective Agents			
Lansoprazole	Prevacid	*For erosive esophagitis:* ORAL: *Adults*—30 mg/day before eating, for up to 12 wk. *For ulcer:* ORAL: *Adults*—15 mg/day before eating, for 4 wk. *For hypersecretion:* ORAL: *Adults*—60 µg/day before eating.	Like omeprazole, lansoprazole blocks acid secretion.
✣ Misoprostol	Cytotec	ORAL: *Adults*—100-200 mg 4 times daily at meals and bedtime.	Misoprostol protects against ulcers from nonsteroidal antiinflammatory drugs used for arthritis. It is also effective for healing peptic ulcer.
Omeprazole	Losec† Prilosec	ORAL: *Adults*—20 mg once a day for 4-8 wk.	Omeprazole is used for gastroesophageal reflux.
Sucralfate	Carafate Sulcrate†	ORAL: *Adults*—1 gm 4 times daily taken 1 hr before meals and 1 hr before bedtime.	If antacids are prescribed for pain relief, they should not be taken 30 min before or after sucralfate.
Antacids			
Aluminum hydroxide gel	AlternaGEL Amphojel*	ORAL: *Adults*—5-30 ml up to 40 ml every 30 min if pain is severe.	Aluminum hydroxide gel is constipating. Long-term use may cause hypophosphatemia. The drug complexes with tetracycline and can interfere with absorption of warfarin, digoxin, quinine, and quinidine.
Aluminum carbonate gel	Basaljel	ORAL: *Adults*—5-20 ml or 2 capsules every 2 hr up to 12 times daily.	See above.

*Available in Canada and United States.
†Available in Canada only.

TABLE 26-1 Drugs to Treat an Ulcer—cont'd

GENERIC NAME	TRADE NAME	ADMINISTRATION/DOSAGE	COMMENTS
Antacids—cont'd			
Calcium carbonate	Dicarbosil Titralac Tums Others	ORAL: *Adults*—1-4 gm 1 and 3 hr after meals and at bedtime. (Tablets should be chewed before swallowing.)	Calcium carbonate is constipating. It can be used hourly to keep acid neutralized, but some patients become hypercalcemic.
Magnesium carbonate Magnesium hydroxide Magnesium oxide Magnesium phosphate Magnesium trisilicate	Milk of Magnesia Others	ORAL: *Adults*—Check individual product label for information.	These magnesium salts are laxatives and must be taken with aluminum or calcium antacid to maintain normal stool consistency.

tion of action than the other H_2 antagonists. Cimetidine is also available without a prescription.

Famotidine

Famotidine (Pepcid) can be taken once a day. Famotidine is also available without a prescription.

Nizatidine

Nizatidine (Axid) can be taken once a day and is also available without a prescription.

Ranitidine

Ranitidine (Zantac) can be taken once a day and is also available without a prescription.

Mucosal Protective Agents

Lansoprazole Omeprazole

Lansoprazole (Prevacid) and omeprazole (Losec) are new drugs for inhibiting acid secretion with a mechanism different than the histamine H_2-receptor antagonists. These drugs directly inhibit the hydrogen ion pump in the parietal cells of the stomach. Gastric acid secretion can be completely blocked. Lansoprazole and omeprazole have not caused toxicity with long-term use. These drugs are powerful antiulcer agents and are effective in healing peptic ulcer or reflux esophagitis unresponsive to histamine H_2-receptor antagonists.

Misoprostol

Misoprostol (Cytotec) is an ester of prostaglandin E_1 and represents a new drug class for treating ulcers. Prostaglandin E_1 is normally synthesized in the stomach, where it blocks gastric acid secretion. NSAIDs, including aspirin, inhibit the synthesis of naturally occurring prostaglandin E_1 when they dissolve in the stomach. For this reason, bleeding from gastric ulcers is a significant problem with long-term use of NSAIDs. Patients with arthritis who must take NSAIDs to relieve inflammation and pain are a major market for misoprostol. Misoprostol replaces the prostaglandin E_1 that is not produced in the stomach when NSAIDs are present. With the protection of misoprostol, excess acid secretion is blocked, and therefore stomach mucosa is protected. Misoprostol is also used to treat duodenal and peptic ulcers.

Minor effects such as diarrhea, mild nausea, abdominal discomfort, and dizziness are occasionally reported. Serious side effects are bleeding and abortion in pregnant women, an action expected of a prostaglandin E_1 analogue. In one study there was bleeding in 50% of pregnant women and a 7% incidence of abortion. Therefore misoprostol is contraindicated for pregnant women and should be used cautiously by women of childbearing age.

Sucralfate

Sucralfate (Carafate) is a complex of sulfated sucrose and aluminum hydroxide that is changed by stomach acid into viscous material that binds to proteins in ulcerated tissue. This action protects the ulcer from the destructive action of the digestive enzyme pepsin. Sucralfate is used in the initial treatment (first 1 to 2 months) of a duodenal ulcer. Sucralfate does not neutralize stomach acid or inhibit acid secretion. Give sucralfate alone 30 to 60 minutes before mealtime so that it can be activated by stomach acid and coat the ulcer. Sucralfate binds digoxin and tetracycline; thus these drugs should be taken at different times.

Antacids

Antacids are weak bases that can be ingested to neutralize the hydrochloric acid secreted by the stomach.

Sodium bicarbonate (baking soda) reacts with hydrochloric acid to yield water and carbon dioxide. Carbon dioxide is a gas that causes the frequent belching associated with the ingestion of sodium bicarbonate. Sodium bicarbonate is the only common antacid that is readily absorbed from the gastrointestinal tract. Taken in excess, sodium bicarbonate also makes the blood slightly alkaline, thus making urine alkaline. Excess bicarbonate stimulates the stomach to secrete more acid (rebound hypersecretion). This hypersecretion can persist after the bicarbonate has been absorbed. For these reasons, sodium bicarbonate is not an antacid of choice when prolonged therapy is required.

Nonsystemic antacids include alkaline salts of aluminum, magnesium, and calcium, which neutralize acid but are not readily absorbed into the bloodstream. Aluminum and calcium salts tend to cause constipation, whereas magnesium salts tend to loosen the bowels. Therefore most antacids combine a magnesium salt or hydroxide and an aluminum or calcium salt or hydroxide. Nonsystemic antacids are most effective when taken hourly. This regimen neutralizes acid without causing the rebound secretion of acid.

Nonsystemic antacids are available as liquids or chewable tablets. The most common side effect is diarrhea or constipation, even with a combination antacid. The patient must then add more aluminum or calcium antacid to correct diarrhea or more magnesium antacid to correct constipation. Antacids can impede the absorption of drugs, notably tetracyclines (antibiotics), digoxin (a cardiac glycoside), and quinidine (a cardiac antiarrhythmic drug).

Anticholinergic Drugs

Anticholinergic drugs used to treat an ulcer were discussed with antispasmodic drugs in Chapter 23. Anticholinergic drugs are taken before meals so that they can depress the secretion of acid that occurs while eating. Anticholinergic drugs should not be taken with antacids, since antacids slow their absorption. Moreover, the acid would already have been released in response to the meal and neutralized by the antacid, making the anticholinergic drugs useless.

Nursing Process Overview

Drugs to Treat Ulcers

Assessment

Patients with suspected ulcer disease may have a variety of symptoms. Obtain a baseline patient assessment, focusing on the vital signs, level of consciousness, and character or quality of any emesis or stool, including the presence of occult blood. Monitor the patient's intake and output. Question the patient about relevant history, such as recent alcohol intake or previous ulcer disease. Monitor the hematocrit and hemoglobin levels.

Nursing Diagnoses

- Altered thought processes related to drug side effect (H_2 antagonists)
- Altered health maintenance related to complicated dosing regimens when patient is taking several drugs

Patient Outcomes

The patient will state there is relief of gastrointestinal discomfort.

Planning/Implementation

The goal of treating an ulcer is to stop blood loss and to promote the healing of the ulcerated area. Monitor the patient's vital signs, intake and output, level of consciousness, and character of any emesis or stool. Monitor hematocrit, hemoglobin, and serum electrolyte levels. Prepare the patient for ordered diagnostic studies. Teach the patient about any ordered dietary restrictions.

Evaluation

Before discharge, the patient should be able to explain why the drugs have been ordered, how to take them correctly, how to treat side effects, which side effects require medical attention, and how to implement dietary or other restrictions prescribed by the physician.

NURSING IMPLICATIONS SUMMARY

HISTAMINE H_2-RECEPTOR ANTAGONISTS

Cimetidine

Drug Administration

- For direct intravenous injection, dilute 300 mg in at least 20 ml of normal saline. Administer at a rate of 300 mg or less over 5 minutes. For intermittent intravenous infusion, dilute 300 mg of drug in at least 50 ml of compatible intravenous solution. Do not add to continuously infusing fluids. Administer over 15 to 20 minutes. The solution may also be diluted and administered over 24 hours; use an infusion control device. Warn the patient that there may be discomfort associated with intramuscular administration.
- Read medication labels carefully. Prefilled syringes are intended for intramuscular use or for diluting for intermittent infusion. Prefilled syringes are not for direct intravenous injection. This drug is incompatible with many other drugs for infusion. Do not add other drugs to infusions of cimetidine.
- Administer once-daily doses before bedtime, twice-daily doses in the morning and at bedtime, and more frequent doses with meals and at bedtime. If antacids or metoclopramide are also ordered, they should be administered 1 hour before or after the cimetidine dose.
- The action of many drugs, including aminophylline, caffeine, anticoagulants, and some heart medications, may be potentiated when the patient is also receiving cimetidine since cimetidine is metabolized by the liver and excreted through the kidney. Assess the patient carefully for side effects and monitor appropriate laboratory tests carefully since dosages of other drugs may require adjustment.
- Monitor level of consciousness, blood pressure and pulse, intake and output, and complete blood count. Assess the patient for skin changes and gynecomastia.

Famotidine, Nizatidine, and Ranitidine

Drug Administration

- Administer once-daily doses before bedtime, twice-daily doses in the morning and at bedtime, and more frequent doses with meals and at bedtime. If antacids or metoclopramide are also ordered, they should be administered 1 hour before or after the histamine H_2-receptor antagonists.
- For direct intravenous use of famotidine, dilute 20 mg with 5 to 10 ml of compatible solution, and administer over at least 2 minutes. For intermittent infusion of famotidine, dilute 20 mg in 100 ml of compatible solution, and administer dose over 15 to 30 minutes.
- For direct intravenous use of ranitidine, dilute 50 mg with 20 ml of compatible intravenous solution, and administer over at least 5 minutes. For intermittent infusion of ranitidine, dilute 50 mg in 50 to 100 ml of compatible intravenous solution, and administer over 15 to 20 minutes. The solution may also be diluted and administered over 24 hours; use an infusion control device.
- Be alert when administering ranitidine intravenously; too rapid administration has been associated with bradycardia, tachycardia, and premature ventricular contractions (PVCs).
- Monitor pulse and blood pressure. Monitor level of consciousness, blood pressure, and pulse; assess for constipation or diarrhea and monitor complete blood count. With famotidine, monitor blood urea nitrogen (BUN), serum creatinine level, and urinalysis.

Patient and Family Education

- Review with the patient the side effects associated with the prescribed drug and instruct the patient to report the development of these side effects to the physician. Review all prescribed medications with the patient, and help the patient develop a dosing schedule that is consistent with the therapy goals and possible drug interactions.
- Warn the patient to avoid alcohol and smoking while taking these drugs, especially after the final dose of the day. Emphasize the importance of all aspects of therapy, which may include modifying the diet, taking other drugs, and limiting caffeine intake. Warn the patient to avoid using over-the-counter preparations while taking histamine H_2-receptor antagonists.
- *Note:* This Patient and Family Education information also applies to cimetidine.

MUCOSAL PROTECTIVE AGENTS

Lansoprazole and Omeprazole

Patient and Family Education

- Instruct the patient to take doses immediately before meals. Instruct the patient to swallow capsules whole, not to break or chew them. Omeprazole may be taken with antacids if ordered.

Misoprostol

Drug Administration/Patient and Family Education

- Question female patients about possible pregnancy before administering first dose. Ensure that women of childbearing age are informed of the possible side effects of bleeding and abortion before administering first dose.
- Instruct the patient to report severe or persistent diarrhea. Instruct the patient to avoid concurrent use of magnesium-containing antacids; they may aggravate diarrhea. Encourage the patient to take misoprostol with or after meals and at bedtime for best effect. Instruct the patient to report any new sign or symptom.

Continued.

NURSING IMPLICATIONS SUMMARY—cont'd

Sucralfate

Drug Administration/Patient and Family Education

- Instruct the patient to take antacids 30 minutes before or 1 hour after sucralfate. For best effects, instruct the patient to take sucralfate with water on an empty stomach 1 hour before meals and at bedtime.
- Review with the patient the complete list of medications prescribed, and develop a dosing schedule that is suitable considering known drug interactions. The patient should take cimetidine, digoxin, phenytoin, tetracyclines, and fat-soluble vitamins at different times than sucralfate.
- Instruct the patient to keep a record of bowel movements. If constipation develops, instruct the patient to increase daily intake of fluids to 2500 to 3000 ml, increase level of activity, and increase dietary intake of fruit and fiber. If the patient is taking antacids, changing the brand of antacid may also help; consult the physician.

ANTACIDS

Patient and Family Education

- Instruct the patient to avoid administering antacids with tetracyclines, digoxin, or quinidine. Review with the patient the complete list of medications, and schedule home drug administration that prevents the antacids from interfering with absorption of any other drugs. Try to schedule antacids for 30 minutes before or 1 hour after sucralfate; try to schedule histamine H_2-receptor antagonists 1 hour before or after antacids.
- Remind the patient to chew antacid tablets, not to swallow them whole.
- Instruct the patient to take a small amount of water after doses of antacid liquid to ensure that the antacid dose is carried to the stomach.
- Instruct the patient to alternate aluminum or calcium salts with magnesium salts to prevent diarrhea or constipation unless a specific antacid is ordered. Also instruct the patient to increase fluid intake to 2500 to 3000 ml/day and increase dietary intake of fruits and fiber to prevent constipation.
- Patients with renal failure should not increase fluid intake and may require concomitant stool softeners.
- Instruct the patient to read labels carefully. Antacids vary in their strength, acid-neutralizing ability, and sodium content, especially if other drugs are included in the formulation. Frequently included drugs are magaldrate, another antacid, and simethicone, an antigas drug.
- Instruct the patient taking aluminum carbonate or aluminum hydroxide products for hyperphosphatemia not to substitute other antacids. Doses of antacids used to bind phosphates are often administered with meals. Refer the patient to a dietitian for instruction in following a low-phosphate diet if indicated.
- Antacids used to treat ulcers are often administered 1 and 3 hours after meals and at bedtime; review prescription orders with patients. Instruct the patient taking antacids to prevent kidney stones to increase daily fluid intake to 3000 ml.
- Instruct the patient requiring sodium restriction for heart disease or other health problems to avoid antacids high in sodium; consult the physician or pharmacist. Low-sodium or sodium-free products include Advanced Formula Di-Gel, Maalox Plus Extra Strength Oral Suspension, magaldrate, and Mi-acid. Products relatively high in sodium include Gaviscon-2 chewable tablets (36.8 mg) and Genaton Extra Strength tablets (35 mg). Instruct the patient to use antacids as prescribed and avoid frequent self-medication with over-the-counter products unless advised to do so by a physician.

ANTICHOLINERGIC DRUGS (PIRENZEPINE)

- Anticholinergics are discussed in Chapter 23.

CRITICAL THINKING

APPLICATION

1. What three factors stimulate the secretion of stomach acid?
2. How do ulcers arise? What does the location of the ulcer indicate?
3. What do antacids do?
4. Name the major side effects you might expect with the use of sodium bicarbonate, aluminum and calcium alkaline salts, and magnesium alkaline salts.

CRITICAL THINKING

1. Why does cimetidine inhibit gastric acid secretion, whereas antihistamines used to treat hay fever do not?
2. Differentiate among lansoprazole and omeprazole, misoprostol, and sucralfate. Would two of these be ordered concurrently?
3. Patients with renal failure may take antacids to bind phosphate. Give an example of a phosphate-binding antacid. When should you administer it? Why do you administer these phosphate-binding antacids at those times?

SECTION VII

Drugs Affecting the Respiratory System

This section presents the pharmacologic basis of treating respiratory conditions, especially those arising from asthma, allergies, and colds.

CHAPTER 27 *Bronchodilators and Other Drugs to Treat Asthma and Other Pulmonary Diseases* deals with the therapeutics of asthma, for which pharmacologic intervention is primarily the use of inhaled glucocorticoids and inhaled adrenergic bronchodilators.

CHAPTER 28 *Antihistamines* discusses those antihistamines effective in treating allergies and other conditions.

CHAPTER 29 *Drugs to Control Bronchial Secretions* covers the medications commonly used in treating cold symptoms.

CHAPTER 27

Bronchodilators and Other Drugs to Treat Asthma and Other Pulmonary Diseases

OBJECTIVES

After studying this chapter, you should be able to do the following:

- *Discuss the role of the nonselective and selective beta-adrenergic bronchodilators, xanthines, cromolyn, ketotifen, glucocorticoids, and ipratropium in treating asthma.*
- *Describe the alpha-, beta-1, beta-2, and central nervous system (CNS) effects of sympathomimetic bronchodilators.*
- *Discuss the role of alpha-1 proteinase inhibitor in the treatment of chronic obstructive pulmonary disease.*
- *Discuss the role of surfactant in infants with respiratory distress syndrome.*
- *Develop a nursing care plan for patients receiving one or more of the groups of drugs discussed in this chapter.*

KEY TERMS

asthma
bronchodilators
chronic obstructive pulmonary disease (COPD)
extrinsic asthma
intrinsic asthma
respiratory distress syndrome

CHAPTER OVERVIEW

Drugs that dilate the bronchioles (**bronchodilators**) and other drugs that are used to treat asthma are discussed in this chapter. Asthma affects about 12 million Americans. Treatment has focused on dilating the constricted bronchioles and relieving the wheezing, difficult breathing, and coughing that occur during an asthma attack. Theophylline or a beta-adrenergic bronchodilator has been used. Recently attention has focused on inflammation in asthma. Inhaled steroids or cromolyn sodium decreases inflammation. This chapter also introduces the new surfactant drugs used to prevent lung collapse in premature infants.

Therapeutic Rationale: Asthma and Obstructive Lung Diseases

Asthma

Asthma is a disease of reversible obstruction of the bronchioles. About 12 million Americans have asthma, and about 5000 die of severe asthma attacks each year. An asthma attack involves not only constriction of the bronchioles but also edema of the bronchial mucosa and excess secretion of mucus, combining to restrict the caliber of the airway, as diagrammed in Figure 27-1. Asthma is classified as **extrinsic asthma** if an allergic response is the primary stimulus for bronchial constriction. When no such response can be identified, asthma is classified as **intrinsic asthma.**

Mechanisms in Extrinsic Asthma

Extrinsic asthma involves an immunologic mechanism. The mast cells play a major role in precipitating the attack. In the lung, mast cells are primarily located in the epithelial layer and exposed to the surface. Immunoglobulin E (IgE) antibodies bind to mast cells; when an antigen appears, it binds to the IgE. The formation of the antigen-antibody complex causes the mast cells to degranulate, releasing several substances, including histamine and leukotrienes C and D.

The leukotrienes are potent bronchoconstrictors, chemically related to the prostaglandins. Histamine, also a bronchoconstrictor, additionally induces vasodilation and increased capillary permeability, which results in the mucosal edema characteristic of asthma.

Factors Triggering an Asthma Episode

Why some individuals become asthmatic is not known. Those who are asthmatic have airways that become overly responsive to environmental factors. Some of the agents that trigger an asthma episode include the following:

- Allergens such as pollens, foods, dust, mold, feathers, or animal dander
- Irritants in the air such as dirt, cigarette smoke, gases, and odors
- Respiratory infections such as colds, flu, sore throats, and bronchitis
- Too much exertion such as running upstairs too fast or carrying heavy loads
- Emotional stress such as excessive fear or excitement
- Very cold or windy weather or sudden changes in weather
- Some medications such as aspirin and related drugs and some drugs to treat glaucoma and high blood pressure

Since each person with asthma reacts differently, each should learn to identify individual triggers and either avoid the trigger or be prepared to take prophylactic medication.

Adrenergic Mechanisms in Asthma

There is little, if any, direct innervation of the bronchioles by the sympathetic nervous system. However, there is indirect involvement since sympathetic nerve terminals in pulmonary blood vessels release norepinephrine, which can act on the beta-2 receptors in the bronchioles. Norepinephrine is not a potent stimulant of beta-2 receptors. The beta-2 receptors are activated by epinephrine released from the adrenal medulla in response to stress.

As diagrammed in Figure 27-2, the beta-adrenergic system affects relaxation of bronchial smooth muscle and inhibits degranulation of the mast cells. Activation of the beta-2 receptor stimulates an enzyme, adenylate cyclase, to synthesize more cyclic adenosine monophosphate (cyclic AMP), which is a second messenger for the beta-2 receptor (see Chapter 12). Cyclic AMP activates intracellular pathways, resulting in relaxation of smooth muscle, inhibition of mast cell degranulation, and stimulation of the ciliary apparatus to remove secretions more effectively.

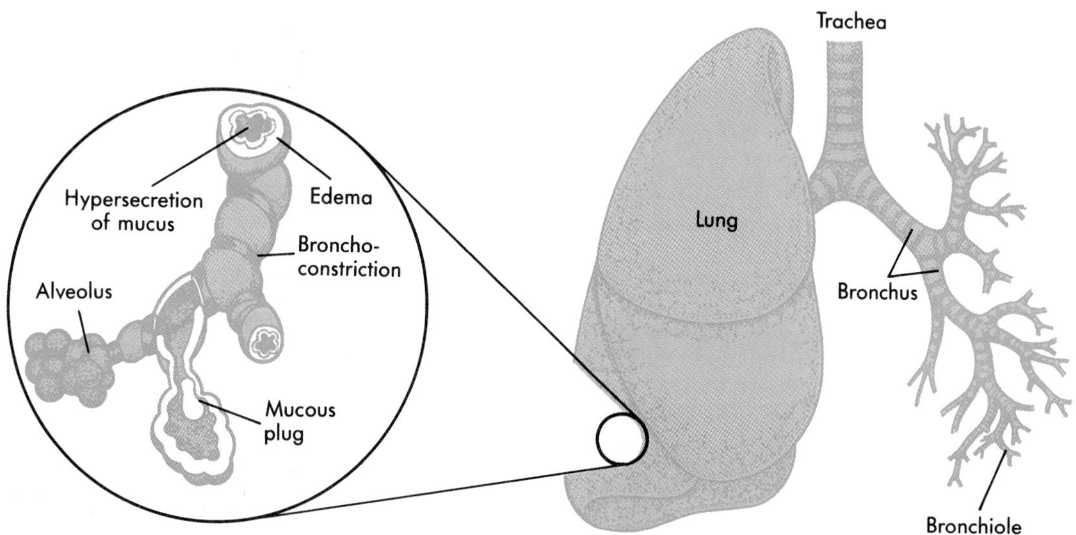

FIGURE 27-1
Factors restricting airway include hypersecretion of mucus, mucosal edema, and bronchoconstriction. Mucous plugs may form in alveoli.

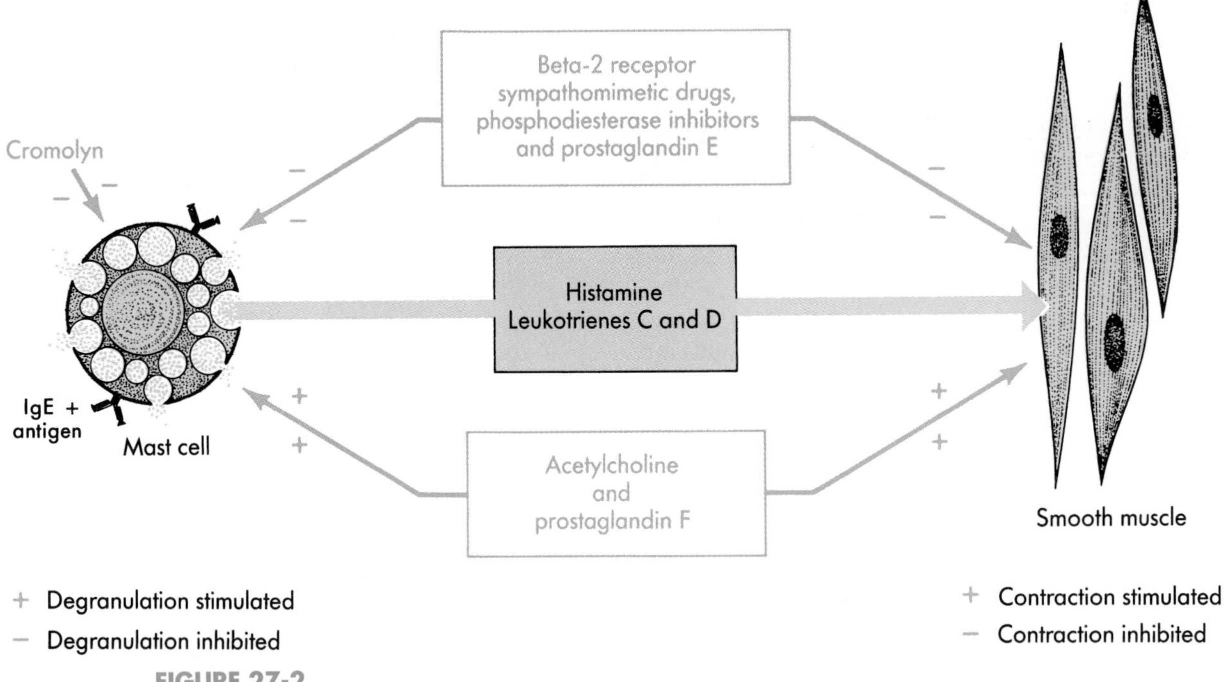

FIGURE 27-2

Histamine and leukotrienes C and D released from mast cells stimulate smooth muscle contraction to produce bronchoconstriction. Mast cell degranulation and smooth muscle contraction are stimulated by acetylcholine and prostaglandin F. Smooth muscle relaxation and inhibition of mast cell degranulation are promoted by beta-2 receptor agonists, phosphodiesterase inhibitors, and prostaglandin E.

Drugs that increase cyclic AMP are bronchodilators, inhibitors of mast cell degranulation, and promoters of secretion flow in the bronchioles. These drugs include beta-adrenergic agonists, which stimulate the beta-2 receptor, and phosphodiesterase inhibitors, which inhibit the breakdown of cyclic AMP. Xanthine compounds are used clinically as bronchodilators because they inhibit phosphodiesterase.

Cholinergic Mechanisms Controlling Bronchioles

Acetylcholine, the neurotransmitter of the parasympathetic nervous system, acts on muscarinic receptors to cause bronchoconstriction through the intracellular second messenger, cyclic guanosine monophosphate (cyclic GMP). Mast cell degranulation is also promoted by agents that stimulate the formation of cyclic GMP. Intrinsic asthma is believed to arise from direct stimulation of the enzyme guanylate cyclase, which synthesizes cyclic GMP. Irritants such as noxious gases can stimulate guanylate cyclase. Asthmatic individuals respond to low doses of inhaled methacholine, a cholinomimetic drug, with bronchospasm, whereas high doses are required to induce bronchospasm in nonasthmatic individuals. Intrinsic asthma may therefore primarily involve a parasympathetic response, mediated by cyclic GMP, to inhaled bronchial irritants. Blocking the muscarinic receptor with atropine or scopolamine causes bronchodilation. The atropine-like drug, ipratropium, is used for bronchodilation.

Other Airflow Obstructive Lung Diseases

Obstruction of airflow is a component of other pulmonary diseases. Chronic bronchitis and emphysema are referred to as **chronic obstructive pulmonary disease (COPD).** Patients with COPD commonly have some degree of reversible airflow obstruction. As with asthma, bronchodilators and corticosteroids play a major role in supportive therapy. In long-standing pulmonary disease, irreversible changes take place so that the elastic smooth muscle tissue is replaced with inelastic scar tissue. This can occur in the bronchioles in chronic bronchitis or in the alveoli in emphysema. These irreversible changes cannot be modified with drugs. The drug, alpha-1 antitrypsin, can slow these changes. However, since the early stages of chronic bronchitis and emphysema often involve reversible bronchospasm, bronchodilators can provide some relief.

About 60,000 to 70,000 American premature infants develop respiratory distress syndrome each year, with 6000 to 10,000 of those affected dying. In addition, about half of the 150,000 adult Americans who develop respiratory distress syndrome as a result of injuries or blood infections die. **Respiratory distress syndrome,** also called *hyaline membrane disease,* is caused by a collapse of the tiny air sacs of the lung related to a deficiency of surfactant. Surfactant is a lipoprotein material coating the air sacs in mature lungs, lowering the surface tension, and thereby allowing ready inflation of the lungs. Synthetic surfactant preparations are available to treat respiratory distress syndrome.

Therapeutic Agents: Asthma

Drug therapy for asthma aims to prevent bronchospasm and to control the hyperactivity of the bronchioles. Mild asthma involves brief episodes of wheezing. These episodes are commonly managed with a beta-adrenergic inhalant bronchodilator for prompt relief. Cromolyn sodium is of value as a prophylactic treatment since it prevents the mast cells from degranulating to start an asthma attack. Moderate asthma is characterized by wheezing and difficulty in breathing to a degree that interferes with daily activities. Inhaled steroids have become the preferred therapy for moderate-to-severe asthma and have replaced theophylline, a long-acting oral bronchodilator. Inhaled steroids have fewer side effects. An inhalant beta-adrenergic bronchodilator is used for acute attacks.

Beta-Adrenergic Agonists

Mechanism of Action

The most widely used beta-adrenergic bronchodilators are relatively specific beta-2 receptor agonists. The beta-receptors of the bronchial smooth muscle are beta-2 receptors, whereas cardiac beta-receptors are beta-1 receptors. The goal has been to develop drugs that are selective in stimulating only beta-2 receptors since stimulation of the heart is not desirable and can limit the use of the drug.

The nonselective beta-adrenergic bronchodilators are sometimes combined with either cyclopentamine or phenylephrine, alpha-adrenergic agonists. Stimulation of alpha-receptors causes vasoconstriction of the blood vessels around the bronchioles, limiting systemic absorption of the bronchodilator and also limiting the edema of asthma. However, systemic constriction of alpha-receptors can cause an undesirable increase in blood pressure. Alpha-receptors may also constrict bronchiolar smooth muscle, at least in disease states.

Table 27-1 summarizes the alpha, beta-1, and beta-2 activities of the adrenergic drugs used as bronchodilators.

TABLE 27-1 Bronchodilators' Specificity for Adrenergic Receptors

DRUG	ALPHA EFFECTS	BETA-1 EFFECTS	BETA-2 EFFECTS
✣ Albuterol	0	0	+
Bitolterol	0	0	+
Cyclopentamine	+	0	0
Ephedrine	+	+	+
✣ Epinephrine	+	+	+
Ethylnorepinephrine	0	0	+
Fenoterol	0	0	+
Isoetharine	0	0	+
Isoproterenol	0	+	+
Metaproterenol	0	(±)	+
Phenylephrine	+	0	0
Pirbuterol	0	0	+
Procaterol	0	0	+
Terbutaline	0	0	+

Alpha Effects

Vasoconstriction

1. Systemic: increased blood pressure.
2. Inhaled: decreased bronchial congestion, increased duration of action for coadministered beta-2 drug.

Beta-1 Effects

1. Stimulation of heart, increasing rate, force of contraction, and rate of repolarization. Overstimulation causes palpitations and arrhythmias.
2. Increased breakdown of fat (lipolysis).
3. Relaxation of gastrointestinal tract.

Beta-2 Effects

1. Bronchiole dilation.
2. Stimulation of skeletal muscle to cause a tremulous or shaky feeling.
3. Vasodilation (mainly in blood vessels supplying muscle).
4. Breakdown of stored glucose (glycogenolysis).

CNS Effects

Stimulation, causing nervousness, anxiety, insomnia, irritability, dizziness, and sweating.

0, No stimulation; +, stimulation; ±, modest stimulation.

Pharmacokinetics

The route of administration and the onset and duration of action are important in selecting a beta-adrenergic bronchodilator. Table 27-2 summarizes these points. Inhalation is a particularly effective route of administration for the bronchodilators since most are degraded if swallowed. Inhalation also places the drug near the site of action.

Many bronchodilators are available in metered aerosol form so that one inhalation delivers a given amount of a drug. These include bitolterol, fenoterol, isoetharine, metaproterenol, pirbuterol, procaterol, and terbutaline (Table 27-3). If more than one inhalation is administered, patients should wait a minute or so between inhalations. The metered-dose inhaler has emerged as the standard for aerosol therapy. The correct use of the inhaler is illustrated in Figure 27-3. Since only about 10% of the delivered drug is deposited in the lung, the likelihood of overdosing is small. However, recent studies indicate that overuse of inhalers (more than one incident per month) may be associated with an increased death rate.

Another inhalation technique is to put a solution of the drug into a nebulizer, which disperses the drug solution in tiny drops to be taken into the lungs by deep inhalation.

Albuterol, fenoterol, metaproterenol, and terbutaline are available in oral forms. Although oral administration is convenient, especially for children, the patient is exposed to more side effects with oral administration than with aerosol administration.

In a severe attack, patients may not be able to inhale the drug. Subcutaneous injection of epinephrine or terbutaline is then appropriate. An orally or subcutaneously administered bronchodilator is preferred if there is a great deal of mucosal

TABLE 27-2 Bronchodilators: Onset and Duration of Action

GENERIC NAME	TRADE NAME	ADMINISTRATION	ONSET (MIN)	DURATION (HR)
✚ Albuterol	Proventil	Inhalation	30	4-6
	Ventolin	Oral		
Bitolterol	Tornalate	Inhalation	3	5-8
Ephedrine	[Generic]	Oral	15	2-4
Epinephrine	Primatene	Inhalation	2	2-3
✚ Epinephrine suspension	Sus-Phrine	Subcutaneous	15	Up to 8
Ethylnorepinephrine	Bronkephrine	Subcutaneous	10	1-2
Fenoterol	Berotec	Inhalation	5	2-3
		Oral	30-60	6-8
Isoetharine	Bronkosol	Inhalation	2	1
Isoproterenol	Isuprel	Inhalation	2	½-2
Isoproterenol and phenylephrine	Duo-Medihaler	Inhalation	2	3½
Metaproterenol	Alupent	Inhalation	2	2-4
	Metaprel	Oral	15	3-4
Pirbuterol	Maxair	Inhalation	5	5
Procaterol	Pro-Air	Inhalation	5	6-8
Terbutaline	Bricanyl	Oral	10	4-7
	Brethine	Subcutaneous	15	2-4

TABLE 27-3 Bronchodilators and Other Drugs to Treat Asthma

GENERIC NAME	TRADE NAME	ADMINISTRATION/DOSAGE	COMMENTS
Beta-Receptor Agonists			
✚ Albuterol (salbutamol) sulfate	Airet Novo-Salmol Proventil Ventolin*	INHALATION: *Adults and children >12 yr*—1 or 2 inhalations every 4-6 hr. ORAL: *Adults and children >12 yr*—2-4 mg 3 or 4 times daily. FDA pregnancy category C.	Relatively selective for beta-2 (bronchial) receptors. May cause fine finger tremor. Injectable form available in Canada.
Bitolterol	Tornalate	INHALATION: *Adults*—2 inhalations every 8 hr for prophylaxis. To treat an attack, 1 inhalation followed by a second after 1-3 min; then 2 inhalations every 4 hr or 3 inhalations every 6 hr. FDA pregnancy category C.	Selective for beta-2 (bronchial) receptors.
Ephedrine sulfate	[Generic]	ORAL: *Adults*—25-50 mg every 3-4 hr as needed. FDA pregnancy category C. *Children 6-12 yr*—6.25-12.5 mg every 4-6 hr; *children 2-6 yr*—0.3-0.5 mg/kg every 4-6 hr.	Oral or parenteral administration only. CNS stimulation is a common side effect. Not selective for beta-2 receptors.
✚ Epinephrine (base)	Sus-Phrine* (1:200)	INTRAMUSCULAR, SUBCUTANEOUS: *Adults*—For 1:200 solutions, 0.1-0.3 ml not more often than every 4 hr, maximum test dose, 0.1 ml. FDA pregnancy category C. *Children*—For 1:200 solutions, 0.005 ml/kg body weight not more than every 4 hr, maximum test dose, 0.15 ml.	Long-acting suspension. Effect may persist for 8-10 hr.
	Asmolin (1:400)	For 1:400 solutions, double above volumes.	
Epinephrine bitartrate	Asthma Haler Medihaler-Epi* Primatene Mist Various others	INHALATION: Aerosol nebulizers metered to deliver 0.2 mg epinephrine (0.1 mg for Medihaler-Epi) with each inhalation. Allow 1-2 min between inhalations.	Overuse can cause serious adverse effects, leading to death. Reduce dose if bronchial irritation or CNS stimulation arises. For symptomatic relief only.
Epinephrine (racemic)	Vaponefrin*	As for epinephrine bitartrate.	
✚ Epinephrine hydrochloride	Adrenalin Chloride* (1:1000)	SUBCUTANEOUS: *Adults*—0.2-0.5 mg every 2 hr as needed for an acute asthma attack. *Children*—0.01 mg/kg body weight, maximum, 0.5 mg, every 4 hr as needed for an acute asthma attack. For severe acute attacks, may repeat initial dose every 20 min for 3 doses.	Short-acting injection. Do not expose drug to light. Do not use if brown or contains a precipitate. Reacts with many compounds.

*Available in Canada and United States.
†Available in Canada only.

TABLE 27-3 Bronchodilators and Other Drugs to Treat Asthma—cont'd

GENERIC NAME	TRADE NAME	ADMINISTRATION/DOSAGE	COMMENTS
Beta-Receptor Agonists—cont'd			
	Adrenalin Chloride (1:100)* Vaponephrin (2.25%)*	INHALATION: Solutions for nebulization. Allow 1-2 min between inhalations.	Excessive use causes bronchial inflammation and stimulation of heart and CNS.
Ethylnorepinephrine	Bronkephrine	INTRAMUSCULAR, SUBCUTANEOUS: *Adults*—1-2 mg. FDA pregnancy category C. *Children*—0.2-1 mg.	A beta-2 selective bronchodilator.
Fenoterol	Berotec†	INHALATION: *Adults*—1 or 2 inhalations every 6 hr as needed.	A beta-2 selective bronchodilator. Not available in United States.
Isoetharine hydrochloride	Bronkosol Various others	INHALATION: Nebulized solution; 3-7 inhalations. FDA pregnancy category C.	A beta-2 selective drug. Phenylephrine is included to relieve congestion and prolong duration of action.
Isoetharine mesylate	Bronkometer	INHALATION: Aerosol; 1-4 inhalations every 3-6 hr, maximum 12 inhalations daily.	
Isoproterenol hydrochloride	Isuprel Glossets Various others	SUBLINGUAL: *Adults*—10 mg initially. No more than 15 mg 4 times daily or 20 mg 3 times daily. FDA pregnancy category C. *Children*—5-10 mg, not exceeding 30 mg daily.	Sublingual absorption is unreliable. Patients should not swallow saliva until tablet has completely disintegrated.
		INTRAVENOUS: *Children only*—initial infusion rate is 0.1 μg/kg/min. Increase by 0.1 μg/kg/min every 15 min until heart rate exceeds 180 bpm or clinical improvement is seen or infusion rate is 0.8 μg/kg/min.	This route of administration is used only in pediatric intensive care units for children in respiratory failure.
	Isuprel Mistometer*	INHALATION (solution for nebulization, 0.5% to 1%): *Adults*—1 or 2 deep inhalations, repeated no more than every 4 hr.	Excessive use has caused refractory bronchial obstruction and tolerance to drug. In some individuals inhalation precipitates a severe, prolonged asthma attack.
Isoproterenol sulfate	Medihaler-Iso*	INHALATION (aerosol metered dose): *Adults*—1 or 2 deep inhalations repeated once or twice at 5 to 10 min intervals if necessary. Repeat after 4 hr. *Children*—5 to 15 deep inhalations of 1:200 aerosol repeated in 10-30 min if necessary.	
Metaproterenol sulfate	Alupent* Metaprel	ORAL: *Adults*—20 mg 3 or 4 times daily. FDA pregnancy category C. *Children 6-9 yr*—10 mg 3 or 4 times daily; *children >9 yr or ≥ 60 lb*—20 mg 3 or 4 times daily.	Longer acting than isoproterenol. Patients are less likely to develop tolerance to metaproterenol than to isoproterenol.
		INHALATION (metered aerosol): *Adults and children ≥12 yr only*—2-3 inhalations every 3-4 hr, not to exceed 12 inhalations daily.	
Pirbuterol	Maxair	INHALATION: *Adults*—1 or 2 inhalations every 6 hr as needed. FDA pregnancy category C.	Beta-2 selective bronchodilator.
Procaterol	Pro-Air†	INHALATION: *Adults*—2 inhalations 3 times daily.	Beta-2 selective bronchodilator.
Terbutaline sulfate	Brethine Bricanyl*	SUBCUTANEOUS: *Adults*—0.25 mg repeated in 15-30 min if necessary, with no more than 0.5 mg administered in any 4 hr period. FDA pregnancy category B. *Children*—0.01 mg/kg body weight to maximum of 0.25 mg.	Shakiness is the most frequent side effect.

Continued.

TABLE 27-3 Bronchodilators and Other Drugs to Treat Asthma—cont'd

GENERIC NAME	TRADE NAME	ADMINISTRATION/DOSAGE	COMMENTS
Beta-Receptor Agonists—cont'd			
		ORAL: *Adults*—initially 2.5 mg every 8 hr, increased to 5 mg every 8 hr 3 times daily over 2-4 wk. Dose may be lowered to 2.5 mg if side effects are too disturbing. *Children* ≤12 *yr*—1.25-2.5 mg 3 times daily during waking hours.	
	Brethaire	INHALATION (metered aerosol): *Adults and children* <12 *yr*—2 inhalations 1 min apart, every 4-6 hr.	Side effects are mild. Headache, nausea, and GI upset are the most common.
Xanthines			
Aminophylline (theophylline ethylenediamine)	Sold mainly under generic name	*For acute asthma attack:* INTRAVENOUS: Solutions should be diluted to 25 mg/ml and injected no more rapidly than 25 mg/min to avoid circulatory collapse. Loading dose, 5.6 mg/kg over 30 min. Maintenance dose, no more than 0.9 mg/kg/hr by continuous infusion. Dose is determined by age, cardiac and liver status, and smoking history. RECTAL: *Adults*—250-500 mg 1 to 3 times daily. FDA pregnancy category C. *Children*—5 mg/kg not more often than every 6 hr. ORAL: *Adults*—500 mg for acute attack. Maintenance dose, 200-250 mg every 6-8 hr. *Children*—7.5 mg/kg for acute attack. Maintenance dose, 5 mg/kg every 6 hr. INTRAMUSCULAR: *Adults*—250-500 mg.	85% theophylline, so 116 mg of aminophylline is equivalent to 100 mg theophylline. Watch for nausea, wakefulness, restlessness, and irritability as early symptoms of toxicity. Serious toxic effects of IV include delirium, convulsions, hyperthermia, and circulatory collapse.
Oxtriphylline	Choledyl* Novotriphyl†	ORAL: *Adults*—200 mg every 6 hr. FDA pregnancy category C. *Children 2-12 yr*—100 mg/60 lb every 6 hr.	64% theophylline, so 156 mg is equivalent to 100 mg theophylline.
✚ Theophylline	Many names, elixirs, syrups, tablets, capsules, timed-release preparation, and suppositories	ORAL: *Adults*—initial dose, 3-5 mg/kg every 6 hr. For maintenance: *Adults*—100-200 mg every 6 hr. FDA pregnancy category C. *Children*—50-100 mg every 6 hr. RECTAL: *Adults*—250-500 mg every 8-12 hr. *Children*—10-12 mg/kg/24 hr. Administered no more frequently than every 6 hr.	Headache, dizziness, nervousness, nausea, vomiting, and epigastric pain are most common side effects of oral administration. Therapeutic levels are 10-20 mg/ml serum.

edema and bronchoconstriction limiting the access of the inhaled drug.

Uses

Beta-adrenergic bronchodilators are used prophylactically for asthma and other conditions with reversible bronchospasm. They are also used for the acute treatments of asthma.

Adverse Reactions and Contraindications

The older beta-adrenergic bronchodilators, ephedrine, epinephrine, and isoproterenol, are not selective for the beta-2 adrenergic receptor. They have a range of side effects resulting from their nonselective action. Side effects are related to stimulation of the heart and include palpitation, tachycardia, and arrhythmias. CNS activity can cause tremors, headache, nervousness, and hypotension. Beta-1 adrenergic activity promotes the breakdown of glycogen to glucose, which impairs control in patients with diabetes mellitus.

The newer beta-adrenergic bronchodilators are relatively selective for the beta-2 receptor, the adrenergic receptor mediating bronchodilation. Because of this selective action, these drugs are less likely to cause unwanted cardiac effects or breakdown of liver glycogen to glucose. Patients with hypertension, cardiac disease, or diabetes can better tolerate the selective beta-adrenergic bronchodilators. Occasionally, nervousness or restlessness are side effects.

Toxicity

Overdose with beta-adrenergic drugs can cause chest discomfort and pain with an irregular heartbeat and irregular

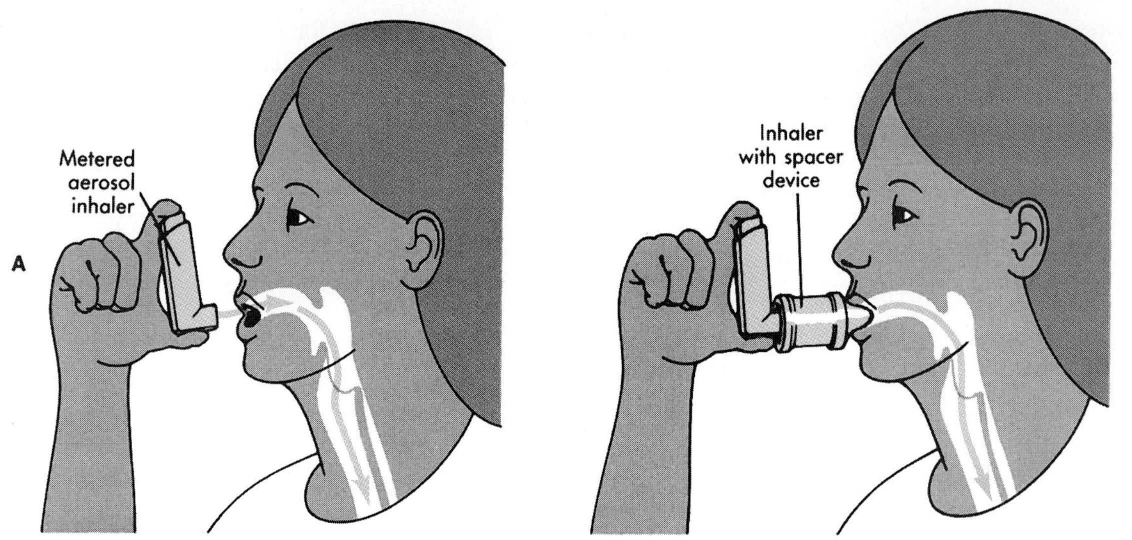

FIGURE 27-3
Inhaled drugs commonly used in asthma treatment include beta-adrenergic bronchodilators, cromolyn sodium, and aerosol glucocorticoids. Metered aerosol inhaler **(A)** should not be put in mouth but held about two finger widths (1½ inch) in front of mouth. Alternatively, inhaler with spacer device **(B)** can be used. Patients should breathe deeply once before activating the inhaler and then continue breathing in for about 5 seconds. Patients should then hold the breath for 10 to 15 seconds before breathing out slowly. If second dose is needed, patients should wait 1 to 2 minutes before taking another dose.

blood pressure. Chills, fever, light-headedness, and dizziness may be experienced. Other symptoms of overdose include nervousness, restlessness, unusual anxiety, and trembling. Inhalation medication should be discontinued and supportive therapy given.

Interactions

Beta-adrenergic drugs are potentiated by drugs that have direct or indirect sympathomimetic activity, including monamine oxidase inhibitors, tricyclic antidepressants, and other sympathomimetic agents. This interaction may aggravate cardiovascular conditions such as arrhythmias and hypertension. Thyroid hormones may also aggravate cardiovascular conditions when taken with beta-adrenergic drugs.

Selective Beta-Adrenergic Bronchodilators

The second generation of beta-adrenergic bronchodilators are relatively selective for the beta-2 receptor, the adrenergic receptor mediating bronchodilation. These drugs are available in metered aerosol inhalers for easy administration. Albuterol, fenoterol, metaproterenol, and terbutaline are also available in oral forms.

Albuterol

Albuterol (Proventil, Ventolin) is available in forms for oral and inhalation administration for treatment of acute asthma or for prophylaxis in chronic asthma. The inhalation forms include a metered aerosol and a solution. The solution is administered by nebulizer or intermittent positive pressure breathing (IPPB). The onset of action is 5 to 15 minutes, and the duration of action 3 to 6 hours. For oral administration, albuterol is available as a syrup, tablets, or extended-release tablets. The onset of action is 15 to 30 minutes, and the duration of action is 8 hours. In Canada an injectable form is also available with a duration of action of 12 hours. Albuterol is metabolized by the liver to an inactive form and excreted in the urine.

Bitolterol

Bitolterol (Tornalate) is available in metered aerosol form for treatment of acute asthma or for prophylaxis in chronic asthma. The onset of action is 3 to 4 minutes, and the duration of action is 5 to 8 hours. Bitolterol is conjugated and excreted in the urine.

Fenoterol

Fenoterol (Berotec) is available in metered aerosol form, solution, and as tablets for the treatment of acute asthma or for prophylaxis in chronic asthma. Although available in Canada, fenoterol is not available in the United States.

Isoetharine

Isoetharine (Arm-a-Med, Isoetharine, Bronkosol, others) is available in metered aerosol form and as a solution for the treatment of acute asthma or for prophylaxis in chronic asthma. The onset of action is 1 to 6 minutes, and the duration of action is 1 to 4 hours. Isoetharine is metabolized by the liver and excreted in the urine.

Metaproterenol

Metaproterenol (Alupent, Metaprel) is available as a metered aerosol and as a solution for inhalation administration and as a syrup and tablet for oral administration. Metaproterenol is used for treatment of acute asthma or for prophylaxis in chronic asthma. The aerosol form has an onset of action of 1 minute and a duration of action of 1 to 5 hours. The solution, administered by hand-bulb nebulizer or IPPB, has a slower onset of action, 5 to 30 minutes, and a duration of action of 2 to 6 hours. Oral forms are effective in 15 to 30 minutes for up to 4 hours. Metaproterenol is metabolized by the liver and excreted in the urine.

Pirbuterol

Pirbuterol (Maxair) is available as a metered aerosol for the treatment of acute asthma or for prophylaxis in chronic asthma. The onset of action is 5 minutes, and the duration of action is 5 hours. Pirbuterol is conjugated and excreted in the urine.

Procaterol

Procaterol (Pro-Air) is available as a metered aerosol for asthma but is available only in Canada. The onset of action is 5 minutes, and the duration of action is 6 to 8 hours.

Terbutaline

Terbutaline (Brethine, Bricanyl) is available as metered aerosol, tablets, and an injection for the treatment of acute asthma or for prophylaxis in chronic asthma. Inhaled terbutaline is effective in 5 to 30 minutes and has a duration of action of 3 to 6 hours. With oral administration, the onset of action is 1 to 2 hours and the duration of action 4 to 8 hours. When injected, onset of action is within 15 minutes, and the duration of action is ½ to 4 hours. Terbutaline is metabolized by the liver and excreted in the urine.

Nonselective Beta-Adrenergic Bronchodilators

The older beta-adrenergic bronchodilators, ephedrine, epinephrine, and isoproterenol, are not selective for the beta-2 adrenergic receptor. They have a range of side effects resulting from their nonselective action. These drugs are listed in Table 25-3.

✣ Epinephrine

Epinephrine (Adrenalin, Asmolin, Medihaler-Epi, others) can be administered subcutaneously to relieve an acute asthmatic attack. The drug causes bronchodilation and vasoconstriction to relieve bronchial edema. Given subcutaneously, an aqueous suspension of epinephrine (Sus-Phrine) lasts 8 hours; the hydrochloride salt lasts only 3 hours. Epinephrine is also available in metered-dose inhalers as an aerosol or in solution for use in a nebulizer.

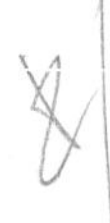

Ephedrine

Ephedrine (generic) acts like epinephrine but is effective orally. Ephedrine is a weaker bronchodilator than epinephrine and is of no use for an acute asthma attack. It is used as a prophylactic for patients with mild-to-moderate asthma. Several formulations combine ephedrine with theophylline and a sedative in a single pill.

Ephedrine releases stored norepinephrine from sympathetic neurons, an indirect sympathomimetic effect that explains the weak bronchodilator action. The major metabolite is phenylpropanolamine, an active alpha-adrenergic drug frequently used as a decongestant.

Ethylnorepinephrine

Ethylnorepinephrine (Bronkephrine) acts on beta-1 and beta-2 adrenergic receptors. It also exerts some vasoconstrictive activity that reduces bronchial congestion. Ethylnorepinephrine is available only for subcutaneous or intramuscular (IM) administration.

Isoproterenol

Isoproterenol (Isuprel Hydrochloride, Medihaler-Iso) was the first widely used adrenergic drug with selectivity for beta- rather than alpha-receptors. It is not selective for beta-2 receptors and therefore stimulates the heart. Isoproterenol is primarily given by inhalation and relieves bronchoconstriction for up to 2 hours. If swallowed, it is degraded in the gut wall. It is available as a sublingual tablet, but absorption is so erratic that this route is not often used.

✣ Theophylline and Related Xanthines

Theophylline and related drugs are listed in Table 27-3. They were once widely used as a prophylactic drug for asthma. Inhaled steroids are now preferred as prophylaxis for moderate-to-severe asthma because of the side effects associated with theophylline.

Mechanism of Action

Theophylline is the prototype of the xanthines used to treat asthma. Like beta-adrenergic agonists, theophylline acts by increasing cellular cyclic AMP concentrations, which relaxes bronchial smooth muscle and inhibits mast cell degranulation. Theophylline and the other xanthines accomplish this by inhibiting the degradation of cyclic AMP by the enzyme phosphodiesterase. This action complements that of the beta-agonists, and the two kinds of agents may be included in therapy when the effect of either drug alone is insufficient to control bronchospasm.

Pharmacokinetics

Theophylline can be given intravenously (as aminophylline) to control acute bronchospasm in status asthmaticus or orally to control the bronchospasm of mild, moderate, or severe asthma. Theophylline is not highly water soluble, and there are many formulations to improve the solubility. Studies have shown that theophylline tablets are well absorbed, with more than 96% of the drug appearing in the plasma within 2 hours. Aminophylline, the most common soluble form of theophylline, is the only form that can be administered intravenously.

Several soluble salts of theophylline are available, and dosage is determined by the theophylline content. The drug is also available in slow- and fast-release preparations, alcoholic or aqueous solutions, and suppositories. Only the suppository is erratically absorbed and therefore unreliable. Rectal solutions are well absorbed. Theophylline is combined with ephedrine and a sedative in several combination products for treating asthma. Most clinicians prefer to individualize doses of each ingredient to minimize side effects while maximizing therapeutic effects and therefore do not favor combination drugs. Theophylline is not effective when administered by inhalation. IM injections of theophylline are not used because they are painful.

Theophylline is metabolized by the liver into inactive compounds excreted in the urine. There is a wide variability among individuals as to the plasma half-life of theophylline. In normal, nonsmoking adults the plasma half-life is about 6 hours but can vary from 3 to 12 hours. In smokers and children the plasma half-life is shorter, whereas in older adult patients, premature infants, and patients with liver disease or congestive heart failure with pulmonary edema, the plasma half-life is prolonged.

Uses

Theophylline and related drugs are used for the prophylaxis and treatment of asthma. They relieve the shortness of breath, wheezing, and dyspnea of asthma. Stimulation of the medullary centers of respiration may occur, which is beneficial if the asthmatic patient is hypoxic. Theophylline treats Cheyne-Stokes respiration, in which the medullary sensitivity to hypoxia is decreased. Theophylline stimulates respiration in newborns who do not breathe well.

Adverse Reactions, Contraindications, and Toxicity

The most common side effects of theophylline after oral administration are nausea and epigastric pain. Headache, dizziness, and nervousness are also common. The effectiveness of theophylline is determined by its plasma concentrations, and the therapeutic range is 10 to 20 μg/ml. Agitation, exaggerated reflexes, and mild muscle tremors (fasciculations) are often seen when plasma levels are 20 to 30 μg/ml. Seizures and cardiac arrhythmias may occur when plasma levels exceed 30 μg/ml but occasionally occur with plasma concentrations between 20 and 30 μg/ml.

Other actions of theophylline seen in the therapeutic dose range are dilation of blood vessels and mild diuresis resulting from the increased renal blood flow and glomerular filtration. Stomach acid secretion is increased, which may be a problem for a patient with an ulcer.

Interactions

Phenobarbital increases the metabolism of theophylline so that larger doses are required. The serum concentration of theophylline is increased by cimetidine, erythromycin, influenza virus vaccine, and troleandomycin. Sympathomimetic drugs enhance CNS stimulation. Theophylline decreases the effects of phenytoin, lithium nondepolarizing muscle relaxants, and beta-blockers.

Cigarette or marijuana smoking induces hepatic metabolism of theophylline. Smokers may require a 50% to 100% increase in the dose of theophylline.

Other Agents

For information related to drugs in this category, refer to Table 27-4.

Cromolyn Sodium

Cromolyn sodium (Intal) is a prophylactic drug that acts by inhibiting mast cell degranulation and the release of bronchospastic agents caused by immunologic (antigen IgE) or nonimmunologic (exercise or hyperventilation) stimulation. Cromolyn does not treat an ongoing asthma attack or prevent asthma attacks brought on by vagal reflexes rather than by mast cell degranulation. By itself, cromolyn does not have bronchodilator or antiinflammatory activity.

Cromolyn is available as a metered inhalation aerosol. Cromolyn was originally administered with a "spinhaler," a hand-held, hand-operated device that when activated punctures a capsule, releasing a dry powder. This powder is dispersed by the air current from a small rotor blade and enters the lungs during deep inhalation. In addition, cromolyn is formulated for nasal administration (Nasalcrom and Rynacrom), as prophylaxis for allergic rhinitis, and for ophthalmic administration (Opticrom and Vistacrom) for allergic conjunctivitis.

Given orally or parenterally, cromolyn is so rapidly excreted in the urine that effective drug levels cannot be maintained. Because of this rapid clearance, cromolyn is practically nontoxic. The major side effect that can limit use is bronchospasm caused by the dry powder in sensitive individuals. Some individuals become allergic to cromolyn.

Cromolyn is usually added to bronchodilator therapy to avoid the use of glucocorticoids, especially in children, or to allow the gradual reduction in the dose of glucocorticoids. No tolerance develops to the drug. Cromolyn is more effective in treating children than adults for asthma.

Glucocorticoids

Aerosol glucocorticoids have been developed that can be inhaled daily without producing adrenal suppression or Cushing's syndrome. Asthma specialists now advocate the use of aerosol glucocorticoids over theophylline in the daily management of moderate-to-severe asthma. As with other aerosol medications, the patient must be carefully instructed in the administration of the aerosol glucocorticoids (see Figure 27-3). The aerosol cannot be used during an episode of acute bronchospasm because the powder causes further irritation and the bronchospasm prevents adequate inhalation. An oral glucocorticoid is indicated instead. Patients using these aerosols should gargle after use to prevent the drug trapped in the throat from being swallowed and absorbed systemi-

TABLE 27-4 Other Asthma Drugs

GENERIC NAME	TRADE NAME	ADMINISTRATION/DOSAGE	COMMENTS
✚ Beclomethasone dipropionate	Beclovent* Becotide† Vanceril*	INHALATION (metered dose inhaler): Each dose is 50 μg. *Adults*—2 inhalations 3 to 4 times daily. *Children 6-12 yr*—1-2 inhalations 3-4 times daily.	Inhaled glucocorticoid. Patients transferring from oral glucocorticoids to beclomethasone must be carefully monitored because adrenal function is impaired and may require months to begin functioning adequately.
Budesonide	Rhinocort Turbohaler† Rhinocort Aqua†	INHALATION: *Adults and adolescents* (metered dose inhaler, 100 μg/inhalation)—2 inhalations in each nostril once daily in morning; (metered dose spray, 100 μg/spray)—2 sprays in each nostril once daily.	
✚ Cromolyn sodium	Intal*	INHALATION: *Adults and children >5 yr*—20 mg capsule inhaled 4 times daily (Spinhaler); 2 inhalations 4 times daily (inhalation aerosol). FDA pregnancy category B.	Prophylactic drug used to inhibit mast cell degranulation. Cough or bronchospasm is occasionally experienced after inhaling dry powder.
Dexamethasone sodium	Decadron Respihaler*	INHALATION (metered dose inhaler): Each dose is 84 μg. *Adults*—3 inhalations 3 or 4 times daily. *Children*—2 inhalations 3 or 4 times daily.	Inhaled glucocorticoid. See comments for beclomethasone.
Flunisolide	AeroBid*	INHALATION (metered dose inhaler): Each dose is 250 μg. *Adults and children >6 yr*—2 inhalations 2 times daily initially. Patients >15 yr may increase dose to 4 inhalations twice daily if necessary.	Inhaled glucocorticoid. See comments for beclomethasone.
Ipratropium	Atrovent*	INHALATION (metered dose inhaler): Each dose is 18 μg. *Adults*—1 or 2 inhalations 3 or 4 times daily. FDA pregnancy category B.	Anticholinergic bronchodilator.
Ketotifen	Zaditen†	ORAL: *Children ≥3 yr*—1 mg 2 times daily with morning and evening meals.	Prophylactic for asthma in children
Triamcinolone	Azmacort*	INHALATION (metered dose inhaler): Each dose is 100 μg. *Adults*—2 sprays 3 or 4 times daily, up to 12-16 sprays daily. *Children 6-12 yr*—1 or 2 sprays 3 or 4 times daily, up to 12 sprays daily for severe cases.	Inhaled glucocorticoid. See comments for beclomethasone.

*Available in Canada and United States.
†Available in Canada only.

cally and to avoid a *Candida* infection (a fungal infection) in the mouth or throat. Glucocorticoids available as aerosols include beclomethasone, dexamethasone, flunisolide, and triamcinolone.

Oral glucocorticoids (corticosteroids) treat asthmatic patients with severe symptoms that are not controlled by bronchodilator therapy. Initially, very high doses (up to 1 gm of methylprednisolone) of a glucocorticoid may be administered for as long as 5 days to bring a severe asthma attack under control when intravenous (IV) aminophylline and sympathomimetics have proved inadequate. High doses of glucocorticoids can be tolerated for short periods but cause many severe side effects when used on a long-term basis. Few patients with asthma require glucocorticoids even after an acute attack. The mechanisms by which these drugs act to alleviate asthma are not known, but they do potentiate the action of the bronchodilators. To minimize the long-term toxic effects of glucocorticoids, they are administered in small doses (20 mg) every other day. This schedule minimizes suppression of adrenal function and also avoids excessive use, which could cause Cushing's syndrome (characteristic of excessive glucocorticoid administration; see Chapter 60).

Ipratropium

Ipratropium bromide (Atrovent) was the first anticholinergic drug available to treat asthma and conditions such as chronic bronchitis and emphysema in which bronchoconstriction is present. It opens narrowed breathing passages by blocking vagal nerve impulses that tighten the muscles in the walls of the bronchial tubes. Mucus secretion is also reduced. Ipratropium is not appropriate for treating acute asthma. The onset of action is 5 to 15 minutes, and the duration of action is 3 to 6 hours. The drug is primarily excreted unchanged in the feces. It has negligible cardiovascular effects. Atropine-like side effects are rare with inhalation administration.

Ketotifen

Ketotifen (Zaditen) is an antihistamine with cromolyn-like activity. It can be taken orally and has a duration of action of 12 to 24 hours. This drug may be prophylactic for asthma and relief of the sneezing and eye irritation from allergies. Side effects include sedation, dizziness, nausea, headache, and dry mouth. Asthma and bronchospasm may be aggravated.

Therapeutic Agent: Chronic Obstructive Pulmonary Disease

Alpha-1 Proteinase Inhibitor

Lung damage in COPD results from the destruction of elastin, a major structural protein of the lung. Elastin is destroyed when there is an imbalance between the lung proteinase, elastase, which breaks down elastin, and alpha-1 proteinase inhibitor (Prolastin) (also called alpha-1 antitrypsin), a protein that inhibits elastase. Smoking depresses alpha-1 proteinase inhibitor, which can account for the high association between smoking and COPD. Some people have a genetic defect that results in low levels of alpha-1 proteinase inhibitor (Table 27-5). Alpha-1 proteinase inhibitor (Prolastin) is available for replacement therapy in patients with a congenital deficiency of alpha-1 proteinase inhibitor. This drug is currently purified from human plasma and administered intravenously. The recommended dosage is 60 mg/kg body weight administered once weekly.

Therapeutic Agents: Respiratory Distress Syndrome

Surfactant Preparations

Surfactant preparations that diminish the mortality from respiratory distress syndrome in infants (see Table 27-5) have become available recently. It is not clear whether it is preferable to give surfactant for prophylaxis or as treatment only. Dosing schedules are still being refined.

Beractant or surfactant TA (Survanta) is derived from cow's lungs. For high-risk infants weighing 600 to 1250 gm, beractant is administered prophylactically in a single 100 mg dose immediately after birth. For infants with respiratory distress syndrome, 100 mg doses are given no more than every 6 hours, up to 4 doses. All doses are administered intratracheally.

The combination of colfosceril palmitate, cetyl alcohol, and tyloxapol (Exosurf) is a synthetic mixture. The colfosceril palmitate is the lipid and active ingredient. Cetyl alcohol is a spreading agent, and tyloxapol is a nonionic detergent that serves as a dispersing agent. For high-risk infants weighing less than 1350 gm, 80 mg/kg is given shortly after birth and again at 12 and 24 hours. For infants with respiratory distress syndrome, two doses of 80 mg/kg are given at 12-hour intervals. All doses are administered intratracheally.

NURSING PROCESS OVERVIEW

Bronchodilators

Assessment

Perform a general assessment of the patient. The focus is often on the respiratory system. Check the vital signs, the amount and characteristics of secretions, and the level of fatigue; auscultate breathing sounds; determine arterial blood gas levels and vital capacity; assess subjective complaints and patient's ability to perform and tolerate activities of daily living; and obtain relevant history regarding issues such as smoking, exposure to irritants, infection, and stress. Assess history of medications used and their effect (see box, p. 344).

Nursing Diagnoses

- Anxiety related to difficult breathing, air hunger, tachycardia, and drug side effects
- Possible complication: hypertension secondary to bronchodilator use

Patient Outcomes

The patient will state a subjective feeling of less anxiety. Pulse rate will be lower, and breathing will be subjectively easier. Hypertension will be diagnosed if it occurs, and appropriate measures to lower blood pressure will be developed by nurse and physician.

Planning/Implementation

Monitor vital signs; a short-term care unit may be appropriate for the patient in acute respiratory distress. Monitor fluid intake and output, level of consciousness, blood gas levels, vital capacity, and treatment of any infectious process. Use an infusion control device for IV drugs. Monitor serum xanthine levels and blood glucose level in patients receiving xanthine therapy.

Evaluation

Bronchodilators are successful if the patient's condition is subjectively and objectively improved. The vital capacity should increase, arterial blood gas levels should be closer to normal values, the respiratory rate should decrease, and the patient should appear to be in less respiratory distress. Subjectively, the patient should report easier breathing, less shortness of breath, less fatigue, and better tolerance for activities of daily living.

Before discharge, verify that the patient can explain which drugs are to be taken and how to take them correctly, what situations require notification of the physician because of exacerbation of the disease process or because of effects resulting from drug therapy, how to perform measures such as exercises for respiratory management, and how to use oxygen correctly. Determine that the patient can demonstrate correct use of any equipment such as IPPB machines or drug administration devices such as inhalers or nebulizers. Finally, check that the patient can explain which respiratory irritants should be avoided.

TABLE 27-5 Miscellaneous Drugs for Pulmonary Conditions

GENERIC NAME	TRADE NAME	ADMINISTRATION/DOSAGE	COMMENTS
Alpha-1 proteinase inhibitor, human	Prolastin*	INTRAVENOUS: *Adults*—60 mg/kg body weight, administered at rate of 0.08 m/kg body weight per min, once a week.	For emphysema caused by a deficiency of alpha-1 antitrypsin.
Beractant	Survanta	INTRATRACHEAL: *Neonates*—100 mg immediately after birth. Doses may be repeated every 6 hr, up to 4 doses.	Pulmonary surfactant for respiratory distress syndrome of neonates.
Colfosceril palmitate, cetyl alcohol, and tyloxapol	Exosurf	INTRATRACHEAL: *Neonates*—80 mg/kg just after birth and again at 12 and 24 hr for high-risk infants. For infants with respiratory distress syndrome, 2 doses of 80 mg/kg at 12 hr intervals.	Pulmonary surfactant for respiratory distress syndrome of neonates.

*Available in Canada and United States.

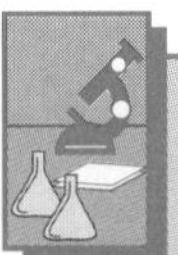

RESEARCH HIGHLIGHT

Medication Compliance of Patients With COPD

—*SG Powell: Home Healthcare Nurse, 12(3):44, 1994.*

PURPOSE

It is estimated that 30 million people have chronic obstructive pulmonary disease (COPD), which includes asthma, emphysema, and chronic bronchitis. These patients are taking multiple medications and are usually trying to manage at home. This study was designed to provide information about how COPD patients manage so that home health care nurses could better understand the needs of these patients.

SAMPLE

Thirty home health care patients aged 35 to 98 years (average age 72) with COPD were included in the study. There were 13 men and 17 women. The mean number of years of education was 10.4, with a range of 8 to 18 years. Medicare was the payor source for 22 patients. The sample consumed 297 prescribed medications (mean of 9.9 per person).

METHODOLOGY

The Taking Prescribed Medication Scale tool developed by Lalonde was used to help collect data. Patients were interviewed in their homes regarding medication use during the 24 hours preceding the interview. There was a score sheet for calculating the percentage of medications taken as prescribed (AP), not as prescribed with extenuating circumstances (NAPE), and not as prescribed (NAP). An example of an NAPE situation would be if the medication was held pending laboratory work.

Each medication taken was scored. If all criteria were met for AP, the drug was scored AP. If the medication was part AP and part NAPE, the score for the drug was NAPE. If any criterion for a drug was NAP, the score for that drug was NAP.

FINDINGS

Five patients, all women, were taking medications AP 100% of the time. There were 25 patients taking medications NAP (13 men and 12 women). Five patients were found to have noncompliance with prednisone, and three of these were intentional. Eleven of the 30 patients were receiving prednisone. Two patients were not taking theophylline as prescribed. Medications and the number of patients having problems with them included inhalers (16), prednisone (5), antibiotics (2), cardiac medications (8), theophylline (2), controlled substances (4), and miscellaneous (7).

Factors contributing to medications not being taken as prescribed and the number of patients affected included knowledge deficit (14), poor memory (4), patient believed he or she needed more (7), patient could not find the medication or had an inadequate supply (5), and living in chaotic environment (3).

IMPLICATIONS

This study had a small sample size, but each patient had many medications to manage. Side effects associated with many of these medications (steroids, theophylline, cardiac drugs, diuretics, and others) may be severe. Nurses working with patients in the home must frequently reevaluate the patient's understanding and ability to carry out the prescribed drug regimen.

CRITICAL THINKING: What are some ways the hospital nurse or nurse in the outpatient clinic or physician's office can teach patients about complex medication regimens and assess compliance?

NURSING IMPLICATIONS SUMMARY

General Guidelines: Bronchodilator Therapy

Drug Administration

- Review the side effects discussed in the text and the information in Tables 27-1 to 27-3.
- Monitor pulse, blood pressure, and respiratory rate. Auscultate lung sounds. The frequency of monitoring varies with the drug, dose, route of administration, and patient condition. During IV administration, monitor vital signs every 5 to 15 minutes until stable. With subcutaneous and inhalation administration, monitor every 15 minutes.
- Carefully monitor all patients requiring bronchodilators but especially older adult patients and those with cardiovascular or hypertensive disease or diabetes mellitus.
- Monitor acutely ill patients in the intensive care setting. Monitor electrocardiographic (ECG) changes.
- Anxiety, insomnia, fear, and other emotional responses may aggravate bronchospasm and air hunger. Maintain a calm but efficient attitude in caring for patients. Do not leave patients unattended for long periods. Keep the call bell within easy reach.
- With subcutaneous or IM injection, perform aspiration before administering dose to avoid inadvertent IV administration.
- For continuous IV infusion, use an infusion control device and (usually) microdrip tubing. Monitor intake and output and vital signs.
- Carefully monitor blood glucose levels of patients with diabetes since bronchodilators may produce hyperglycemia.

Patient and Family Education

- After the acute respiratory distress episode is over, review with the patient the common side effects of the prescribed drugs.
- Many bronchodilators are dispensed with patient instruction leaflets; review the leaflets with the patient.
- Encourage patients with respiratory problems to stop smoking. Provide them with information about local resources available to help smokers quit.
- Before discharge, the patient should be able to describe or demonstrate the correct way to take ordered medication including frequency, route of administration, and use of inhalation devices, and know under what circumstances to return to the physician or emergency room if the drugs are not effective. Caution the patient to use these drugs only as prescribed and not to increase the dose or frequency unless directed to do so by the physician. Patients who find relief with metered-dose inhalers may begin using them more often than prescribed. These drugs soon become ineffective, or patients will suffer significant side effects.
- Warn patients with diabetes to monitor blood glucose levels carefully, especially when changing doses of a bronchodilator.
- The patient should let sublingual tablets dissolve under the tongue. Instruct the patient not to swallow saliva until the tablet is completely dissolved.
- Instruct the patient to take oral doses with meals or snacks to lessen gastric irritation.
- Ensure that the patient can use the metered-dose inhaler correctly when using it for the first time. Review manufacturer's instruction sheet with the patient. Have the patient assemble the inhaler and shake the canister. The patient should exhale deeply, then put the mouthpiece into the mouth with the opening directed to the back of the throat. The patient should grasp the mouthpiece with the teeth and lips. The patient should inhale deeply while depressing the aerosol container or activating the spray mechanism. Then the patient should hold the breath as long as possible before exhaling. Instruct the patient to wait several minutes before taking a second dose (if prescribed). For children, it may be necessary to hold the nose shut. When finished, tell the patient to wash and dry the mouthpiece (see Figure 27-3). For additional information about drugs via inhalation, see Chapter 5.
- Special devices can help children use inhalation medications if they are having difficulty using the metered-dose inhaler; examples include the Inhal-Aid and InspirEase devices. The patient should consult the pharmacist.
- When two drugs are ordered via inhalation, the patient should use the bronchodilator first, then take the second drug such as beclomethasone.
- Some of these drugs contain sulfites. If the patient is allergic to sulfites, instruct him or her to read carefully all literature provided with the prescriptions to see if any contain sulfites and to work with the pharmacist to obtain sulfite-free brands.
- If tachycardia is a problem, suggest that the patient limit caffeine intake.
- Instruct the patient to check the supply of drug on hand to avoid running out at inopportune times. To check the amount in a canister, drop the canister into water (without mouthpiece). Full containers sink to the bottom, and half-full containers float with part of the container out of the water. The empty container floats on its side, half submerged (see Figure 5-24) . Consult the manufacturer's literature for additional information.
- Remind the patient to inform all health care providers of all drugs being taken. Remind the patient to avoid over-the-counter (OTC) drugs unless first approved by the physician. Many decongestants and cold remedies contain products that duplicate the effects of the bronchodilators, causing increased side effects.
- Instruct the patient to keep these and all drugs out of the reach of children.
- No drugs should be used during pregnancy or lactation unless first approved by the physician.

Continued.

NURSING IMPLICATIONS SUMMARY—cont'd

Beta-Adrenergic Bronchodilators

Patient and Family Education

- Review the general guidelines for bronchodilator therapy.
- Review the patient problem boxes on dry mouth (p. 300) and orthostatic hypotension (p. 157).
- Isoproterenol may cause saliva to turn pinkish to red; this effect is harmless.
- Ephedrine may cause trouble sleeping. Instruct the patient to take the last dose of this drug several hours before bedtime.
- Sustained-release formulations should be swallowed whole, without chewing or crushing. If there is a question about a specific product, instruct the patient to consult the pharmacist.

Epinephrine

Drug Administration

- Epinephrine hydrochloride (adrenalin chloride) is used via subcutaneous injection or IM injection to treat anaphylactic allergic reactions. The dose is 0.1 to 0.5 mg (0.1 to 0.5 ml) of 1:1000 injection.
- Epinephrine can be administered via endotracheal tube if the patient is intubated, at the same dose used for IV injection.
- To use epinephrine inhalation solution, place about 10 drops of a 1% solution in the reservoir of the nebulizer.
- See the general guidelines for bronchodilator therapy. Monitor the pulse and blood pressure carefully.
- Sus-Phrine is a suspension. Rotate the vial between the hands to mix the suspension before preparing the dose and administer immediately so the drug does not settle out of suspension.
- See Chapter 16 for a discussion of use of epinephrine in shock.

Xanthines to Treat Asthma

Drug Administration

- Review the general guidelines for bronchodilator therapy.
- Monitor the vital signs and blood pressure, and auscultate lung sounds. Hypotension may be pronounced. Supervise ambulation. Keep siderails up.
- Monitor serum theophylline levels.
- When using oral liquid forms of aminophylline or theophylline to treat neonatal apnea, use the less concentrated form (5 mg/ml) to reduce the possibility of error in measuring the small volumes needed of the more concentrated solution. It may be preferable to use the parenteral form administered orally; check with the pharmacist.

Intravenous Aminophylline

- Read labels carefully; the label must state for IV use. Only the concentration of 25 mg/ml may be given undiluted, by direct IV push, at a rate of 20 mg/minutes. Usually, aminophylline is diluted in at least 100 to 200 ml of 5% dextrose in water and given as an infusion, based on serum levels or patient's response, 1 dose over 20 to 30 minutes. Even when diluted, do not administer at a rate faster than 20 mg/min. It is available prediluted. It is incompatible with many drugs, so do not administer it "piggyback;" start and maintain a separate IV for replacement fluids and other drugs.

Patient and Family Education

- Review the general guidelines for bronchodilator therapy.
- Take oral doses on an empty stomach with a full (8-ounce) glass of water, 1 hour before meals or 2 hours after meals. Doses can also be taken with meals or snack to lessen gastric irritation. Whichever way the patient takes the medication, it should be taken the same way each day to decrease fluctuations in serum levels.
- Inform the patient taking once-a-day doses to take the dose after fasting through the night and 1 hour before eating or in the evening with or without food, depending on the product.
- Instruct the patient to notify the physician if fever, diarrhea, or symptoms of the flu develop. Encourage the patient to return for follow-up visits to have blood work done to monitor serum drug levels.
- Instruct the patient to avoid having charcoal-broiled foods on a daily basis since this will interfere with the effectiveness of xanthines.
- Review the patient problem box on orthostatic hypotension (p. 157).
- Warn the patient to avoid driving or operating hazardous equipment if dizziness, light-headedness, or vertigo develop; if these symptoms occur, the patient should notify the physician.
- Instruct the patient to read drug prescriptions and labels carefully. Many xanthines are available in regular and sustained-release formulations; they cannot be interchanged on the same dosing schedule. See Chapter 5 for a discussion of sustained-release products. In addition, various brands are not interchangeable. Inform the patient not to switch brands without checking with physician.
- Inform patients who have difficulty swallowing extended-release capsules that the contents may be sprinkled on a small amount of food such as jam, jelly, or applesauce and swallowed without chewing.

NURSING IMPLICATIONS SUMMARY—cont'd

- Instruct the patient to limit or avoid the use of coffee, tea, chocolate, and other methylxanthines since they may affect xanthine metabolism.
- Instruct the patient to avoid smoking cigarettes or marijuana, which may alter serum levels.

OTHER AGENTS TO TREAT ASTHMA

Cromolyn

Patient and Family Education

- See the general guidelines for bronchodilator therapy for a discussion of metered-dose inhalers. Unlike other drugs administered via inhalation, the cromolyn canister cannot be floated to estimate the number of doses remaining. Teach patients using this form to keep a record of doses used. There are about 200 doses in a canister. The drug may also be administered with a Spinhaler or a Halermatic device; the drug is packaged with detailed instructions, which should be reviewed with the patient.
- Inform the patient of the importance of taking cromolyn as ordered, on a regular basis. Spreading doses out evenly throughout the day is more beneficial than erratic use. Cromolyn is useful for prophylactic treatment of asthma but will not control an acute attack of asthma. Several weeks of therapy may be required to see full benefit of cromolyn therapy. Instruct the patient to continue all concomitant therapy, even if he or she begins to feel better.
- See the patient problem box on dry mouth (p. 300).
- Side effects are rare, but encourage the patient to report unexpected signs or symptoms.
- There are also cromolyn capsules, eyedrops, nasal powder for inhalation, and nasal solution. All should be dispensed with patient instruction leaflets. Review these instructions with the patient.

Inhaled Glucocorticoids

Drug Administration/Patient and Family Education

- See Chapters 36 and 60 for a detailed discussion of glucocorticoid therapy.
- Systemic side effects with inhaled forms are uncommon but may occur. See the general guidelines for bronchodilator therapy for a discussion of the use of metered-dose inhalers.
- For best effect, glucocorticoids should be used at evenly spaced intervals, daily as prescribed. Several weeks of therapy may be required to see full benefit of therapy.
- Glucocorticoids for inhalation are dispensed with an inhaler and a patient instruction leaflet. Review this leaflet with the patient.
- Instruct the patient to gargle and rinse the mouth after each use of the inhaler to help prevent fungal infections.
- Instruct the patient to notify the physician if they experience unusual stress such as surgery or illness, have an asthma attack that does not respond to usual treatment, develop an infection of the mouth or throat, or their general physical condition worsens. Also, instruct patients taking glucocorticoids on a regular basis to wear a medical identification tag or bracelet. Finally, instruct patients not to discontinue any medications prescribed for asthma without consulting with physician.

Ipratropium

Patient and Family Education

- See the general guidelines for bronchodilator therapy for a discussion of metered-dose inhalers. Ipratropium is usually dispensed with a patient instruction leaflet; review the leaflet with the patient.
- Review the patient problem boxes on dry mouth (p. 300) and constipation (p. 304). See Chapter 23 for a detailed discussion of anticholinergics.
- Instruct patients to notify the physician if they do not have the usual response to ipratropium or their condition worsens.
- Ipratropium is also prescribed in an inhalation solution form. If used concurrently with cromolyn inhalation solution, inform patients that only solution from the ipratropium 2 ml single-dose vials should be used.
- Ipratropium is also available as a nasal aerosol.

Ketotifen

Patient and Family Education

- Inform the patient of the importance of taking this drug as ordered, on a regular basis. This drug is useful for prophylactic treatment of asthma.
- Instruct the patient to avoid driving or operating hazardous equipment if sedation or dizziness occur and to notify the physician.
- See the patient problem box on dry mouth (p. 300).

DRUG TO TREAT CHRONIC OBSTRUCTIVE PULMONARY DISEASE

Alpha-1 Proteinase Inhibitor

Drug Administration

- Consult the manufacturer's literature for current guidelines.
- Store the drug in the refrigerator before reconstitution and at room temperature after reconstitution and administer within 3 hours. Use diluent supplied by the manufacturer to prepare the dilution.
- Patients should be immunized against hepatitis B because the drug is prepared from pooled human plasma.
- Monitor vital signs. Administer intravenously at 0.08 ml/kg/min.

Continued.

NURSING IMPLICATIONS SUMMARY—cont'd

Patient and Family Education

- This drug is administered intravenously. If used by the patient for self-administration, teach the patient how to store drug and prepare doses, manage infusion, and dispose of contaminated needles, tubing, and equipment.

DRUGS TO TREAT RESPIRATORY DISTRESS SYNDROME

Surfactant Preparations

Drug Administration

- Protocols for administration of these agents are being developed and refined. Check the hospital protocol for guidelines.
- Rotate vial to suspend or resuspend drug in diluent.
- Dosage is based on weight. Inject drug intratracheally via an endotracheal tube. The manufacturer of Exosurf provides an endotracheal tube adapter to permit injection.
- Aspirate an infant's lungs before administration of surfactant; avoid suctioning if possible for at least 2 hours after administration of the drug and for as long as 6 hours, if tolerated by infant.
- To distribute the drug throughout the lungs, it may be necessary to gently rotate the infant's body from side to side or to ventilate the infant's lungs manually with a resuscitation bag after administration of the drug.
- Monitor clinical appearance, pulse oximetry, partial pressure of oxygen (PO_2), carbon dioxide partial pressure (PCO_2), arterial blood gases, lung sounds, and cardiac monitoring.
- Keep the mother and family informed of the infant's condition.

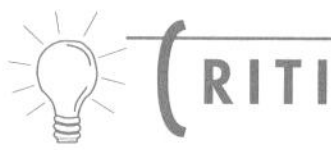

CRITICAL THINKING

APPLICATION

1. What three components restrict the airway in extrinsic asthma?
2. Which beta-adrenergic agonists used as bronchodilators are relatively specific for the beta-2 receptor?
3. What side effects are associated with bronchodilators?
4. How does cromolyn treat extrinsic asthma? What is its mechanism of action?
5. For what purpose are surfactant preparations used? How would you administer them?

CRITICAL THINKING

1. Compare and contrast the mechanisms responsible for extrinsic and intrinsic asthma.
2. What is the mechanism of action of the bronchodilators (beta-adrenergic receptor agonists and theophylline)? List three beneficial responses attributed to this mechanism.
3. How do beclomethasone and other glucocorticoids treat extrinsic asthma? What is their mechanism of action?
4. How does alpha-1 proteinase inhibitor treat COPD? What are the nursing considerations in its administration?

CHAPTER 28

Antihistamines

OBJECTIVES

After studying this chapter, you should be able to do the following:

- *Describe localized and generalized allergic responses.*
- *Discuss the role of histamine in allergic responses.*
- *Describe the common side effects of antihistamines, including the anticholinergic effects.*
- *Develop a nursing care plan for a patient taking an antihistamine.*

KEY TERMS

anaphylaxis
angioedema
antihistamine
asthma
eczema
histamine
purpura
rhinitis
urticaria

CHAPTER OVERVIEW

Histamine is a naturally occurring amine that is formed from the amino acid histidine. Histamine is found in mast cells, which are numerous in the lung and skin, and basophils, the counterparts of mast cells in the blood. The histamine released from the mast cells causes many of the symptoms associated with allergic reactions. It is also found in the gastrointestinal (GI) tract, where histamine is a potent stimulant for the secretion of acid in the stomach. Histamine is also found in parts of the brain, where it is believed to be a neurotransmitter. At present, the role of histamine in the brain is speculative but may involve regulating the level of arousal. This chapter focuses on the role of histamine in allergic reactions and the drugs available to treat these reactions. The role of histamine in the stomach is discussed in Chapter 26.

Therapeutic Rationale: Allergies

Histamine Release and Metabolism

Histamine in mast cells and basophils is complexed with heparin and stored in granules. The typical allergic reaction such as hay fever or contact dermatitis involves the release of these granules in response to an antigen. Antibodies of the immunoglobulin E (IgE) class fix to the mast cells and basophils. When an antigen binds to the fixed IgE, the cells degranulate, releasing histamine, heparin, and other compounds, which alter capillary permeability and attract phagocytes to degrade the bound antigen. This process is illustrated in Figure 28-1.

In addition to antigen-induced degranulation, many drugs and venoms cause degranulation. These include drugs and dyes that carry a positive charge, large molecules that occur in animal sera and dextran solutions, and venoms and enzymes that damage tissue.

Once histamine is released, it is metabolized to inactive compounds in 5 to 15 minutes. One of the degradative pathways is inhibited by aspirin so that histamine may persist. This is the mechanism for one type of aspirin sensitivity.

Allergic Responses Explained by the Action of Histamine

Local allergic responses involving histamine are as follows:

- **Anaphylaxis:** Systemic; onset is usually indicated by a generalized itching and tingling sensation and a feeling of apprehension; profound hypotension leading to shock may follow, and the bronchioles are constricted, causing a choking sensation.
- **Angioedema:** Swelling caused by plasma leakage and blood vessel dilation in the skin or mucous membranes ("giant hives").
- **Asthma:** Spasm of the bronchial smooth muscle.
- **Eczema:** Inflamed areas of skin.
- **Purpura:** Red spots on the skin caused by the leakage of blood from small vessels.
- **Rhinitis:** Inflammation of the nasal mucous membranes that allows fluid to escape.
- **Urticaria:** Hives, which are large wheals caused by leakage of plasma and are accompanied by severe itching.

Two actions of histamine are prominent in explaining allergic responses. Histamine is a potent dilator of arterioles and renders the capillaries more permeable so that fluid and protein are lost into the extravascular space. This explains the bump that appears after an insect sting. Initially, a red spot reflects the dilation of the small blood vessels; as fluid leaks into the extravascular space, the bump, representing local edema, appears. Histamine also stimulates the contraction of smooth muscle, particularly the bronchial smooth muscle. When mast cells are degranulated in the lung, as in asthma, the airway is narrowed and patients have difficulty breathing.

Histamine released systemically causes anaphylaxis, characterized by a profound fall in blood pressure resulting from vasodilation and severe constriction of the bronchioles making breathing difficult. The loss of fluid from circulation resulting from the increased capillary permeability causes the

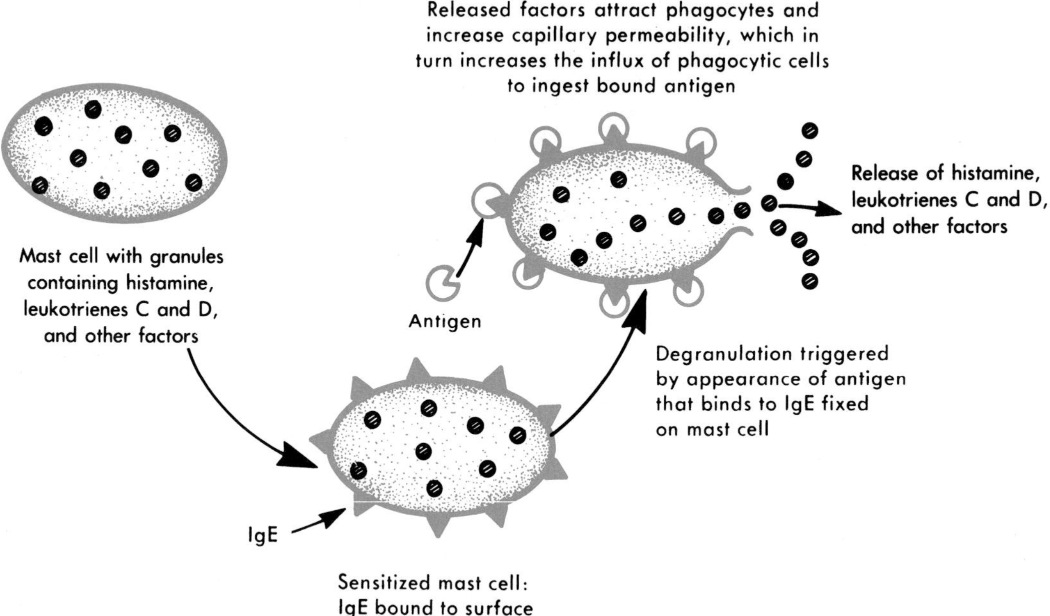

FIGURE 28-1
Immunologic mechanism underlying release of histamine from mast cells. Antibodies of immunoglobulin E (IgE) class are bound to surface of mast cells. Binding of antigen to IgE triggers degranulation of mast cell, releasing histamine and leukotrienes C and D. Histamine is responsible for many allergy and asthma symptoms.

shock that develops in an untreated anaphylactic response. Edema in the mucous tissue of the upper windpipe (laryngeal edema) can block the airway altogether. Epinephrine is the drug of choice for anaphylactic shock. Epinephrine constricts blood vessels to raise the blood pressure and relieve laryngeal edema and dilates the bronchioles, actions that reverse those of histamine (see Chapter 16).

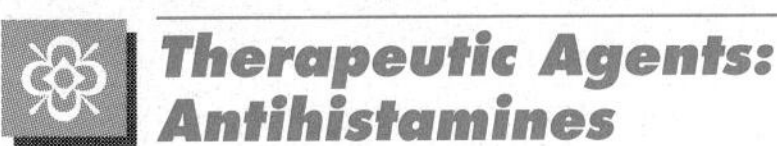

Therapeutic Agents: Antihistamines

Mechanism of Action

Antihistamines (Table 28-1) have been available for over 50 years. Although these drugs block some actions of histamine, they do not block the histamine-mediated secretion of acid in the stomach. There are two types of histamine receptors, the H_1 receptors, acting principally on blood vessels and the bronchioles, and the H_2 receptors, acting mainly on the GI tract. The older antihistamines described in this chapter are specific antagonists for the H_1 receptors. Antagonists specific for the H_2 receptor are cimetidine (Tagamet), famotidine (Pepcid), nizatidine (Axid), and ranitidine (Zantac). These drugs, used primarily to decrease stomach acid, are discussed in Chapter 26. In this chapter, the term **antihistamine** refers to drugs that specifically block the H_1 receptors.

Pharmacokinetics

Antihistamines are given orally and are well absorbed. Their action is seen in 10 to 30 minutes and lasts for 4 to 6 hours. Timed-release forms are active for 8 to 12 hours. Antihistamines are metabolized to inactive compounds by the liver and kidneys.

Uses

Antihistamines and allergic reactions. Antihistamines used to control allergic reactions are described in the previous discussion. Antihistamines are primarily effective in decreasing the discomfort of acute allergic reactions that involve the upper respiratory system, such as hay fever, or the skin, such as hives. Hay fever is most successfully treated when the anti-

TABLE 28-1 Antihistamines for Allergies

GENERIC NAME	TRADE NAME	ADMINISTRATION/DOSAGE	COMMENTS
Astemizole	Hismanal*	ORAL: *Adults*—10 mg once a day, taken on empty stomach. *Children*—2 mg/10 kg body weight once a day, taken on empty stomach.	New nonsedating antihistamine.
Azatadine maleate	Optimine*	ORAL: *Adults*—1-2 mg twice daily. *Children*—not established. FDA pregnancy category B.	Drowsiness is most common side effect.
Brompheniramine maleate	Dimetane*‡ Various others	ORAL: *Adults*—4-8 mg 3-4 times daily or 8-12 mg of sustained-release form 2-3 times daily. *Children >6 yr*—½ adult dose; *children <6 yr*—0.5 mg/kg daily divided into 3-4 doses. FDA pregnancy category B.	Drowsiness is most common side effect.
Carbinoxamine maleate		ORAL: *Adults*—4-8 mg 3-4 times daily or 8-12 mg of sustained-release form 2-3 times daily. *Children >6 yr*—4 mg 3-4 times daily; *children 3-6 yr*—2-4 mg 3-4 times daily; *children 1-3 yr*—2 mg 3-4 times daily. FDA pregnancy category B.	Low incidence of drowsiness. Anticholinergic effect is weak. Commonly combined with pseudoephedrine or dextromethorphan.
Cetirizine hydrochloride	Reactine† Zyrtec	ORAL: *Adults and children 6-11 yr*—5-10 mg once a day. *Children 2-6 yr*—5 mg once a day.	New, nonsedating antihistamine.
Chlorpheniramine maleate	Aller-Chlor‡ Chlortab Chlor-Trimeton‡ Teldrin‡ Various others	ORAL: *Adults*—4 mg 3-4 times daily or 8-12 mg of sustained-release form 2-3 times daily. *Children 6-12 yr*—2 mg 3-4 times daily or 8 mg of sustained-release form once daily; *children 2-6 yr*—1 mg 3-4 times daily.	Low incidence of drowsiness. A common ingredient in cold remedies.
Clemastine fumarate	Tavist*	ORAL: *Adults*—2.68 mg 3 times daily. Not intended for children.	Low incidence of drowsiness. Very weak anticholinergic effects.
Cyproheptadine hydrochloride	Periactin	ORAL: *Adults*—4-20 mg daily, not more than 0.5 mg/kg. Dose is started at 4 mg 3 times daily. *Children 7-14 yr*—4 mg 2-3 times daily to maximum of 16 mg daily; *children 2-6 yr*—2 mg 2-3 times daily to maximum of 12 mg daily. FDA pregnancy category B.	Used to relieve itching. Drowsiness is most common side effect.

*Available in Canada and United States.
†Available in Canada only.
‡Not available without a prescription.

Continued.

TABLE 28-1 Antihistamines for Allergies—cont'd

GENERIC NAME	TRADE NAME	ADMINISTRATION/DOSAGE	COMMENTS
Dexchlorpheniramine maleate	Polaramine*	ORAL: *Adults*—1-2 mg 3 or 4 times daily or 4-6 mg 2 times daily or 6 mg of time-released form 3 times daily. *Children <12 yr*—0.15 mg/kg daily divided into 4 doses. FDA pregnancy category B.	Drowsiness is most common side effect.
✚ Diphenhydramine hydrochloride	Benadryl Hydrochloride‡ Various others	ORAL: *Adults*—25-50 mg 3-4 times daily. *Children >20 lb*—2.5-25 mg 3-4 times daily; *children <12 yr*—5 mg/kg in 4 divided doses each day.	High incidence of drowsiness with little paradoxical stimulation in children. Also used to treat motion sickness and mild parkinsonism. Also used as antitussive. May be used with epinephrine in treating anaphylactic reaction.
Diphenylpyraline hydrochloride	Hispril	ORAL: *Adults*—2 mg every 4 hr or 5 mg of sustained-release form every 12 hr. *Children >6 yr*—2 mg every 6 hr or 5 mg of sustained-release form once daily; *children 2-6 yr*—1-2 mg every 8 hr.	Commonly combined with phenylephrine and other agents.
Doxylamine succinate	Unisom	ORAL: *Adults*—12.5-25 mg every 4-6 hr. *Children 6-12 yr*—75 mg divided into 4-6 doses daily; *children <6 yr*—2 mg/kg body weight divided into 4-6 doses daily. Decapryn available without prescription.	High incidence of drowsiness. Often included in nonprescription sleeping aids.
Loratadine	Claritin*	ORAL: *Adults*—10 mg once a day.	New nonsedating antihistamine for seasonal rhinitis.
Methdilazine hydrochloride	Tacaryl	ORAL: *Adults*—8 mg 2-4 times daily. *Children >3 yr*—4 mg 2-4 times daily.	A phenothiazine derivative used primarily to relieve itching. Incidence of drowsiness is less than with other phenothiazines.
Phenindamine tartrate	Nolahist	ORAL: *Adults*—25 mg every 4-6 hr as needed. *Children 6-12 yr*—12.5 mg every 4-6 hr.	Used for seasonal rhinitis.
Pyrilamine maleate	Nisaval	ORAL: *Adults*—25-50 mg 4 times daily. *Children 6-12 yr*—½ adult dose. Available without prescription.	Low incidence of drowsiness.
✚ Terfenadine	Seldane*	ORAL: *Adults*—60 mg every 8-10 hr as needed. FDA pregnancy category C.	New nonsedating antihistamine.
Trimeprazine tartrate	Panectyl† Temaril	ORAL: *Adults*—2.5 mg 4 times daily or 5 mg of sustained-release form every 12 hr. *Children >3 yr*—2.5 mg at bedtime or up to 3 times daily (children >6 yr can take 5 mg of sustained-release form once a day); *children 6 mo-3 yr*—1.25 mg at bedtime or up to 3 times daily.	A phenothiazine derivative. Drowsiness is most common reaction. Used primarily to relieve itching of neurodermatitis, contact dermatitis, and chickenpox.
Tripelennamine citrate or hydrochloride	PBZ-SR Pyribenzamine† Various others	ORAL: *Adults*—25-50 mg every 4-6 hr or 100 mg of sustained-release form every 12 hr. *Children >5 yr*—50 mg of sustained-release form every 12 hr; *children and infants*—5 mg/kg daily divided into 4-6 doses.	Dizziness is common side effect.
Triprolidine hydrochloride	Myidil	ORAL: *Adults*—2.5 mg 3-4 times daily. *Children >6 yr*—½ adult dose; *children <6 yr*—0.3-0.6 mg 3-4 times daily. FDA pregnancy category B.	Low incidence of side effects, with drowsiness being most common.

histamine therapy is begun while the pollen count is still low. Sneezing, runny nose, and swollen eyes are reduced in more than 70% of patients. Antihistamines reduce the swelling and itching (pruritus) of urticaria and related conditions.

The most recently developed antihistamines are those that blunt allergic reactions effectively but without the sedation commonly associated with the older antihistamines. The newer antihistamines include astemizole (Hismanal), cetirizine (Zyrtec), loratadine (Claritin), and terfenadine (Seldane). These drugs are available by prescription only at present.

Antihistamines do not prevent or treat colds effectively, although they are present in many over-the-counter (OTC) cold remedies. Because most antihistamines have anticholinergic actions, they can dry up a runny nose and relieve the symptoms of a cold. Antihistamines do not treat asthma, probably because substances other than histamine are responsible for the prolonged bronchiole constriction characteristic of asthma. Since the drugs have a drying effect because they inhibit bronchial secretions, they can aggravate asthma.

Antihistamines only block histamine receptors. Because of this, some allergic responses are not effectively treated with antihistamines. Anaphylaxis represents a true emergency for which an antihistamine is inadequate because it neither acts fast enough nor reverses the histamine reactions. Epinephrine acts rapidly, and its pharmacologic actions reverse those of histamine.

Antihistamines as sedatives. Sedation is a common side effect of antihistamines, some of which are used principally for this purpose. Many OTC sleeping aids use an antihistamine as the active agent. The antihistamines approved as sleep-aid ingredients are pyrilamine, doxylamine succinate, and diphenhydramine. Hydroxyzine (Atarax, Vistaril) is an antihistamine often used as an antianxiety agent (see Chapter 51).

Antihistamines as antiemetics and antiparkinsonism agents. Selected antihistamines have other uses. Some antihistamines prevent nausea and vomiting, particularly from motion sickness and vertigo. These antihistamines are discussed in Chapter 28. Antihistamines that suppress the tremors of parkinsonism are discussed in Chapter 56.

Adverse Reactions and Contraindications

Although the antihistamines are so named because they specifically compete with histamine for the H_1 receptors, they have other pharmacologic properties. The main secondary action is an anticholinergic or atropine-like action. This is the origin of side effects such as inhibition of secretions, blurred vision, urinary retention, fast heart rate (tachycardia), and constipation. In the central nervous system (CNS) the anticholinergic effect can cause insomnia, tremors, nervousness, and irritability. These effects are particularly predominant in children. Sedation and drowsiness, the central antihistaminic effects, are more common in adults. The spectrum of antihistaminic and anticholinergic properties depends on the drug, the dose, and the individual. Most antihistamines have a local anesthetic effect, which might relieve the itching of skin rashes. Antihistamines are rarely used for this purpose because they tend to be good antigens, thereby causing skin rashes themselves.

Antihistamines are contraindicated for nursing mothers because the drugs are secreted in milk. Antihistamines taken by young children can cause paradoxical excitement, whereas older adult patients are sensitive to the sedative actions.

Toxicity

Antihistamine overdose can cause CNS depression or stimulation, the latter being more common in children. The atropine-like symptoms (i.e., a flushed skin and fixed, dilated pupils) are also prominent. Management maintains an airway and treats hypotension. In children a high temperature is common, which can be reversed with ice packs and sponge baths. If the antihistamine is not a phenothiazine, vomiting is induced, gastric lavage is carried out, and cathartics are used to empty the GI tract of remaining drug. Vomiting should not be induced with phenothiazines since they can cause uncoordinated movements of the head and neck, which would cause aspiration of vomitus. Antihistamines that are phenothiazine derivatives are identified in the drug tables.

Interactions

The main drug interaction associated with antihistamines is the additive depression of the CNS when taken with alcohol, hypnotics, sedatives, antipsychotics, antianxiety drugs, or narcotic analgesics. Because of their atropine-like effects, antihistamines should be used with caution in patients with glaucoma, hyperthyroidism, cardiovascular disease, or hypertension.

NURSING PROCESS OVERVIEW

Antihistamines for Allergic Reactions

Assessment

Assess vital signs, respiratory and cardiovascular status, relevant history of previous allergy, exposure to possible allergens, subjective symptoms, and objective data such as the extent and type of rash, or nasal exudate, difficulty breathing through nose, headache, and sore throat for respiratory allergy. Anaphylaxis is an emergency; the more delayed and chronic responses may represent a source of annoyance to the patient but may never progress to an acute phase.

Nursing Diagnoses

- Risk for injury related to drowsiness related to antihistamine therapy
- Possible altered bowel elimination: constipation related to antihistamine use

Patient Outcomes

The patient will state subjective improvement in symptoms of allergy and will not experience serious side effects.

Planning/Implementation

Anaphylaxis requires immediate diagnosis and treatment, usually with 1:1000 epinephrine injected subcutaneously or intramuscularly, followed by parenteral antihistamines. Supportive care is symptomatic and based on rapid assessment of the cardiovascular and respiratory response. Management of the less acute allergic response is not an emergency. Monitor the vital signs, respiratory status, cardiovascular status, platelet count, and white blood cell count. Observe for side effects of drug therapy, especially drowsiness; monitor fluid intake and output to check for urinary retention; and monitor the frequency of bowel movements to assess for constipation.

Evaluation

Before discharge, determine that patients can explain why and how to take the prescribed medication, what side effects may appear and which of these to report immediately, and what to do for specific side effects such as dry mouth, constipation, hypotension, and drowsiness. If specific allergens are identified, patients should be able to name them. Verify that patients understand the importance of wearing a medical identification tag or bracelet listing specific allergens.

Nursing Implications Summary

Antihistamines

Drug Administration

- Monitor blood pressure, pulse, and intake and output. Auscultate breath sounds. Inspect for development of rash. Monitor complete blood count, white blood cell count and differential, and platelet count. Supervise ambulation, especially of older adult patients. Keep siderails up and a night light on. Monitor smoking. Assess for urinary retention (difficulty initiating voiding and feeling of incomplete bladder emptying). Palpate the bladder.

Intramuscular Administration

- Use large muscle masses (see Chapter 5). Record and rotate injection sites. Aspirate before injecting medication to prevent accidental intravenous (IV) administration. Warn the patient that intramuscular (IM) injection of antihistamines may burn as the medication is injected.
- Read drug labels carefully. Some forms are for IM use only and should not be used for IV administration. Antihistamines may be prescribed with narcotic analgesics for pain relief. They may decrease nausea and may potentiate CNS depression, but they do not enhance the analgesic effect of the narcotic. It may be necessary to lower the dose of one of the drugs because of the hypotension, sedation, and other side effects that may occur when both drugs are used.

Intravenous Brompheniramine

- IV brompheniramine may be given undiluted, but further dilution is preferred. Do not use the concentrated solution (100 mg/ml) for IV administration. Check with the pharmacist regarding compatibility with other drugs. Administer a single bolus injection over at least 1 min.

Intravenous Chlorpheniramine

- IV chlorpheniramine may be given undiluted. Do not use the concentrated solution (100 mg/ml) for IV administration. Administer at a rate of 10 mg over 1 minute or longer if possible.

Intravenous Diphenhydramine

- IV diphenhydramine may be given undiluted. Administer at 25 mg/min or longer if possible.

Patient and Family Education

- Warn the patient to avoid driving or operating hazardous equipment if drowsiness, blurred vision, or dizziness occurs. Instruct the patient to notify the physician if blurred vision develops.
- Review the patient problem boxes on constipation (p. 304), dry mouth (p. 300), orthostatic hypotension (p. 157), and photosensitivity (p. 649).
- Instruct the patient to report fever, sore throat, rash, unexplained bleeding, or bruising since these may be signs of rare but serious hematologic side effects. Instruct the patient to take oral doses with meals or a light snack to decrease gastric irritation.
- Instruct the patient to swallow sustained-release forms whole, without crushing or chewing. Scored tablets may be broken before swallowing. Capsules may be opened and contents poured into soft food for ease in taking. The patient should chew gum forms for 15 minutes or longer (see manufacturer's literature). Review administration technique for patients using suppository forms.
- Instruct the patient on correct IM administration technique if this route is prescribed for self-administration.
- For motion sickness, doses should be taken 30 to 60 minutes before beginning travel. Patients traveling by car should face forward in the center of the front seat if possible.
- Instruct the patient to avoid the use of alcohol and other CNS depressants.
- Remind the patients to keep all health care providers informed of all medications being used, even OTC preparations. Regular use of antihistamines may mask side effects developing from other drugs, such as ringing in the ears from salicylates.
- Instruct the patient to read labels of OTC preparations carefully. Patients using remedies for colds, hay fever,

NURSING IMPLICATIONS SUMMARY—cont'd

insomnia, and other problems may be taking unnecessary drugs or taking the same drug in two or more combination products and should consult the pharmacist for assistance.

- Remind the patient that antihistamines may also cause allergies. Encourage the patient to report any unexpected sign or symptom to the physician.
- Encourage patients with allergies to wear a medical identification tag or bracelet indicating the nature of the allergies. Pregnant women should not take any medication without the approval of the physician. Remind patients to keep these and all drugs out of the reach of children.
- A potentially fatal drug interaction exists between astemizole, loratadine, or terfenadine, and itraconazole or ketoconazole. Remind the patient to inform all health care providers of all medications being used.

CRITICAL THINKING

APPLICATION

1. Describe the origin, location, and role of histamine.
2. What factors mediate histamine release?
3. What are five pharmacologic actions of antihistamines?
4. What are the drug interactions and contraindications for the antihistamines?
5. Describe three clinical uses of the H_1 receptor antihistamines.
6. How does cimetidine differ from the H_1 receptor antihistamines?
7. Give examples of five situations in which patients may manifest allergic reactions or require antihistamines. One example is when a transfusion reaction occurs; name four others.

CRITICAL THINKING

1. Ideally, all antihistamines would be effective, without side effects. Yet, many antihistamines are in common use with known side effects such as drowsiness and dry mouth. Why are antihistamines that cause these side effects still in common use?
2. Antihistamines can be found in OTC sleep remedies. Older adults are more sensitive to the side effects of antihistamines than younger individuals. As a home health nurse, you learn that your older adult patient is taking a sleeping aid containing an antihistamine. What suggestions can you give the patient to try that might help the patient get to sleep without relying on medication?

CHAPTER 29

Drugs to Control Bronchial Secretions

OBJECTIVES

After studying this chapter, you should be able to do the following:

- *Discuss the action of the alpha-adrenergic agonists, the imidazolines, and the antihistamines in relieving nasal congestion.*
- *Differentiate between expectorants, antitussives, and mucolytic agents in treating a cough.*
- *Develop a nursing care plan for a patient receiving a nasal decongestant or a drug to treat a cough.*

KEY TERMS

antitussive
cough
expectorant
mucociliary escalator
mucolytic
rebound congestion
respiratory tract fluid

CHAPTER OVERVIEW

Many of the drugs covered in this chapter are available over-the-counter (OTC) for treatment of colds and coughs. Nasal decongestants are covered in the first section, and drugs to treat a cough are covered in the second section.

Therapeutic Rationale: Nasal Congestion

Nasal congestion results when the blood vessels in the nasal passage become dilated as a result of infection, inflammation, allergy, or emotional upset. Dilation increases capillary permeability and allows fluid to escape into the nasal passage.

Therapeutic Agents: Nasal Decongestants

Alpha-Adrenergic Agonists

Mechanism of Action

Nasal decongestants are alpha-adrenergic agonists and mimic the action of the neurotransmitter norepinephrine (see Chapter 12). These agents stimulate alpha receptors and cause blood vessels to constrict, thereby relieving the congestion.

Pharmacokinetics and Uses

Several alpha-adrenergic agonists are applied topically as drops or sprays. Because these nasal decongestants have immediate and direct contact with the nasal mucosa, they act rapidly and provide temporary symptomatic relief by opening the nasal passages.

When a nasal decongestant is applied as drops into the nostril, the patient should be lying on a bed with the head hanging over the edge and turned to one side. The drops are instilled into the upper nostril. After a few seconds the head is turned to allow administration to the other nostril. Use of this lateral, head-low position allows the drops to coat the nasal mucosa without being immediately swallowed.

Orally active alpha-adrenergic agonists commonly found in cold remedies include phenylpropanolamine, phenylephrine, and pseudoephedrine. Cold remedies are syrups, tablets, or capsules that may also include an antihistamine, an analgesic, or other miscellaneous ingredients. Cold remedies are discussed in Chapter 7.

Adverse Reactions, Contraindications, and Toxicity

Nasal decongestants may cause a stinging or burning sensation or induce sneezing when sprayed into the nose. **Rebound congestion** is a common side effect. This occurs when the effect of the drug wears off. If nasal decongestants are used with increasing frequency, they have less and less effect. The drug ultimately irritates the nasal passages and causes the congestion to become worse rather than better. For this reason, decongestants are most effective when used only occasionally and for no longer than 3 to 5 days. Nasal decongestants are available without a prescription.

With repeated use of a nasal decongestant, more of the drug is absorbed, and systemic effects become possible. The symptoms of an overdose are those expected from a sympathomimetic drug (see Chapter 12), including nervousness, dizziness, palpitation, and transient high blood pressure readings. Children are especially vulnerable to overdoses of nasal decongestants and may have reactions that include sweating, drowsiness, shock, or coma.

Interactions

Patients with hyperthyroidism, diabetes mellitus, hypertension, or heart disease are vulnerable to the sympathomimetic side effects of nasal decongestants and should avoid these drugs. A hypertensive reaction to a nasal decongestant may occur in patients taking a monoamine oxidase inhibitor. Patients receiving tricyclic antidepressants are vulnerable to the cardiac effects of sympathomimetic agents.

Specific Sympathomimetic Drugs

Summary information on sympathomimetic drugs is presented in Table 29-1.

Phenylephrine

Phenylephrine (Coricidin, Neo-Synephrine, others) is a potent alpha-adrenergic agonist that is administered orally or topically. It is available both alone and in many combination cold preparations.

Phenylpropanolamine

Phenylpropanolamine (Prolamine) is used mainly in oral combination cold remedies. An alpha-adrenergic agonist, it acts indirectly, releasing norepinephrine from nerve terminals.

Propylhexedrine

Propylhexedrine (Benzedrex) is a volatile drug that stimulates alpha-receptors. It causes little stimulation of the central nervous system (CNS) and is therefore generally safer than some of the other nasal decongestants.

Pseudoephedrine

Pseudoephedrine (Novafed, Sudafed, others) is included in many oral combination cold remedies. It is a beta- and an alpha-agonist.

Imidazolines

The imidazolines include four chemically related nasal decongestants (see Table 29-1). These drugs stimulate the alpha-adrenergic receptors to produce vasoconstriction. They are potent, and only xylometazoline is considered safe for young children. All are used topically. Naphazoline and xylometazoline react with aluminum and should not be used in atomizers with aluminum parts.

Naphazoline

Naphazoline (Privine) is an effective nasal decongestant but can produce a severe rebound congestion resulting from irritation and swelling of the nasal mucosa. Overdosage of naphazoline has reportedly produced coma in children and systemic effects such as hypertension, sweating, cardiac arrhythmias, and drowsiness in adults.

TABLE 29-1 Nasal Decongestants

GENERIC NAME	TRADE NAME	ADMINISTRATION/DOSAGE	COMMENTS
Naphazoline hydrochloride	Privine Hydrochloride*	TOPICAL: 0.05% and 0.1% solutions. Two drops in each nostril no more than every 3 hr or 2 sprays every 4-6 hr.	An imidazoline. Can cause rebound congestion. Systemic effects from overuse include arrhythmias, transient hypertension, slowing of the heart rate, and drowsiness. Do not use in an atomizer with aluminum parts.
Oxymetazoline hydrochloride	Afrin* Nafrine†	TOPICAL: *Adults*—2-4 drops or 2-3 sprays of 0.05% solution in each nostril at morning and at bedtime. *Children >6 yr*—as for adults; *2-5 yr*—0.025% solution is used as above.	An imidazoline. Long acting. Side effects are mild and generally safe.
✚ Phenylephrine hydrochloride	Coricidin Decongestant Nasal Mist Neo-Synephrine hydrochloride* Super-Anahist Nasal Spray	TOPICAL: *Adults*—drops of 0.25%-1% solution in each nostril (head in lateral, head-low position) every 3-4 hr. Nasal spray or jelly may be used. *Children >6 yr*—as for adults. *Infants and young children*—0.125% solution is used as above.	Less potent and longer action than epinephrine. No CNS stimulation but can cause transient hypertension, headaches, and palpitations.
Phenylpropanolamine hydrochloride	Various combination drugs	ORAL: *Adults*—25 mg every 3-4 hr or 50 mg every 6-8 hr. *Children 8-12 yr*—20-25 mg 3 times daily. Not recommended for children <8 yr.	Similar to ephedrine but with less CNS stimulation.
Propylhexedrine	Benzedrex	TOPICAL (inhalation): 2 inhalations in each nostril as needed.	A volatile drug safe for adult use; children should be supervised. Inhaler should be warmed with hands if cold.
Pseudoephedrine hydrochloride	Novafed Sudafed* Robidrine†	ORAL: *Adults*—60 mg every 6-8 hr. *Children*—4 mg/kg body weight in 4 divided doses.	Steroisomer of ephedrine with lesser incidence of CNS stimulation and hypertension than ephedrine. Useful for relief of runny nose or congestion leading to earache.
Pseudoephedrine sulfate	Afrinol Repetabs	As for pseudoephedrine hydrochloride.	
Tetrahydrozoline hydrochloride	Tyzine	TOPICAL: *Adults*—2-4 drops of 0.1% solution in each nostril. Do not repeat more frequently than every 3 hr. *Children ≥6 yr*—as for adults; *children 2-6 yr*—2-3 drops of 0.05% solution in each nostril every 4-6 hr.	An imidazoline. Adverse reactions can be severe and include hypertension, drowsiness, sweating, rebound hypotension, bradycardia, and cardiac arrhythmias. May cause high fever and coma in young children. Rebound congestion may persist a week after discontinuing.
Xylometazoline hydrochloride	Neo-Synephrine II Long-acting Otrivin-Spray* Sinutab Long-Lasting Sinus Spray	TOPICAL: *Adults*—2-3 drops of 0.1% solution or 1-2 inhalations of 0.1% spray in each nostril every 8-10 hr. *Children 6 mo-12 yr*—2-3 drops of 0.05% solution in each nostril every 4-6 hr. *Infants*—1 drop of 0.05% solution in each nostril every 6 hr.	An imidazoline. A relatively safe, long-acting decongestant but should not be used excessively or for more than a few days. Do not use in atomizers with aluminum parts.

*Available in Canada and United States.
†Available in Canada only.

Oxymetazoline

Oxymetazoline (Afrin) is a relatively long-lasting nasal decongestant that has not been implicated in as many severe systemic effects as naphazoline. However, rebound congestion occurs with repeated use.

Tetrahydrozoline

Tetrahydrozoline (Tyzine) is an effective nasal decongestant similar to naphazoline in its adverse effects.

Xylometazoline

Xylometazoline (Neo-Synephrine II, Sinutab Long-Lasting Sinus Spray, others) is similar to oxymetazoline in its effects.

Other Drugs to Relieve Nasal Congestion

Nasal congestion is common in allergies such as hay fever. As discussed in Chapter 28, antihistamines treat hay fever because they block the receptors for histamine on the blood vessels and thereby prevent the dilation that causes nasal congestion. Antihistamines are also frequently included in cold remedy preparations. The anticholinergic action characteristic of antihistamines aids in reversing the vasodilation of the nasal blood vessels.

Therapeutic Rationale: Expectorants, Antitussives, and Mucolytic

Origin of Secretions

Respiratory secretions in the trachea, bronchi, and bronchioles originate from the goblet cells and bronchial glands (Figure 29-1). The goblet cells lie on the surface, making up part of the epithelial layer. The tracheal epithelium consists of about 20% goblet cells, and the bronchiolar epithelium consists of 2% goblet cells. These cells produce a gelatinous mucus that they periodically secrete. It is not known what factors normally control the goblet cells, but chronic exposure to irritants increases their size, number, and activity. An example is the phlegm coughed up by smokers. The bronchial glands lie several layers beneath the epithelium. The grapelike (acinar) cells are controlled by the cholinergic nervous system; when stimulated, acinar cells secrete a plentiful watery fluid into a duct that empties onto the surface.

The secretions of the goblet cells and bronchial glands combine to form a mucus called the **respiratory tract fluid.** Much of the water in the respiratory secretions evaporates to humidify the air taken into the lungs. If too much water is lost to humidification, the mucus forms thick plugs that cannot be readily eliminated. Normally, the respiratory tract fluid forms a lining that is swept upward by the action of the ciliary hairs into the throat (pharynx), where it is swallowed. This activity, the **mucociliary escalator,** provides a cleansing mechanism for the lungs since any foreign particles or bacteria are trapped in this viscous layer and eliminated. If the ciliary hairs are paralyzed by tobacco smoke or alcohol, secretions cannot be cleared naturally and give rise to the "smoker's cough."

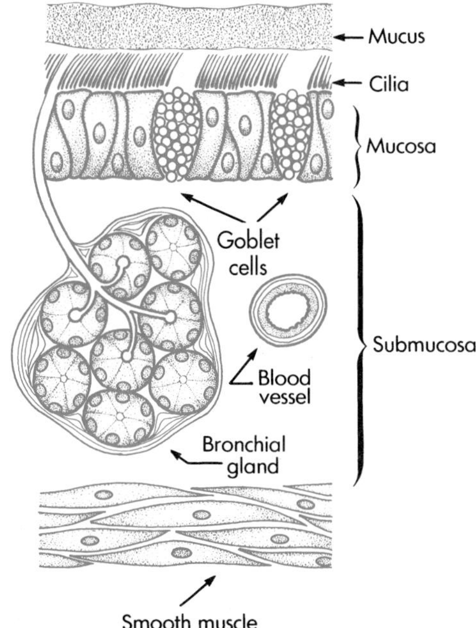

FIGURE 29 -1
Mucous layer at top is lumen of airway. Relative position of goblet cells and bronchial glands, secretions of which make up mucus, are shown. Mucous layer is normally swept up toward throat by cilia to cleanse airway.

Cough

A **cough** is a protective reflex initiated by irritation in the airway. As long as material is being brought up by the cough, it is beneficial. Several situations cause an unproductive cough. The air of heated rooms can dry the airway enough to cause irritation. A sore throat can produce an unproductive cough and can be self-perpetuating when the cough further irritates the throat. A cough can result from irritants responsible for asthma or pulmonary edema, which also stimulate the cough receptors. Congestion of the nasal mucosa results in postnasal drip, which irritates the throat and produces the cough associated with a cold or the flu.

When a cough is not productive and disrupts sleep and rest, relief is sought. Therapy for a cough depends on the cause. If the air is dry, a vaporizer or steamer may sufficiently liquefy the secretions so that they do not become irritating. A dehydrated state limits respiratory secretions, so having the patient drink plenty of fluids prevents or overcomes the dehydration that accompanies common illnesses. Patients with sore throats can suck hard candies to increase saliva flow to coat the throat. If these simple measures do not eliminate the cough, expectorants may be used. An **expectorant** increases the output of respiratory tract fluid to coat the trachea and bronchi. In addition, a cough suppressant or **antitussive** drug may be taken. Expectorants and antitussive drugs are widely available as OTC drugs.

Therapeutic Agents: Expectorants, Antitussives, and Mucolytic

Expectorants

Although many drugs are used as expectorants (Table 29-2), no expectorant has been proven effective. The following agents are commonly used as expectorants.

Iodide

Iodide, usually given as potassium iodide, was once widely used as an expectorant. After entering the bloodstream, potassium iodide is believed to stimulate the bronchial glands to secrete more fluid. Use of iodides is associated with a high incidence of adverse effects. Potential side effects include skin rash, hypothyroidism, and a mumpslike swelling of the parotid glands, presumably a result of stimulation of the glands. Iodides are seldom used today as expectorants.

TABLE 29-2 Expectorants

GENERIC NAME	TRADE NAME	ADMINISTRATION/DOSAGE	COMMENTS
✣ Guaifenesin (glyceryl guaiacolate)	Anti-tuss Glycotuss Nortussin Robitussin* Various others	ORAL: *Adults*—200-400 mg every 3-4 hr. *Children 6-12 yr*—100 mg every 3-4 hr; *children 2-6 yr*—50 mg every 3-4 hr.	Use for symptomatic relief of dry, unproductive cough. Occasionally causes nausea or drowsiness. Available without prescription.
Potassium iodide	Potassium Iodide SSKI Pima Iodo-Niacin	ORAL: *Adults*—300 mg every 4-6 hr. *Children*—60-500 mg daily, divided in 2-4 doses.	Contraindicated for patients with hyperkalemia, hyperthyroidism, or hypersensitivity to iodide. Symptoms of hypersensitivity include skin rash. Iodism (overdose of iodide) causes metallic taste in mouth, fever, skin eruptions, nausea, vomiting, mucous membrane ulcerations, and salivary gland swelling.

NOTE: Only those expectorants available alone are listed. Other drugs included in cough or cold mixtures as an expectorant include potassium guaiacolsulfonate, ammonium chloride, terpin hydrate, ipecac, calcium iodide, and citric acid.
*Available in Canada and United States.

✣ *Guaifenesin*

One mechanism that stimulates the secretion of respiratory tract fluid is the reflex activity carried by the vagal nerve and characteristic of nausea. Some drugs used as expectorants are believed to initiate this reflex by irritating the stomach when swallowed. One such drug is guaifenesin (glyceryl guaiacolate), a widely used expectorant for which there is some evidence of efficacy.

Syrup of Ipecac

Like guaifenesin, syrup of ipecac stimulates the vagal nerve and increases secretion. Syrup of ipecac is more commonly used to induce vomiting (emesis) than as an expectorant.

Miscellaneous Expectorants

Other agents added as expectorants to cough suppressant mixtures include terpin hydrate, citric acid, sodium citrate, and calcium iodide.

Antitussives

Tussis is the Latin word meaning cough, and cough suppressants are called antitussives. These drugs are listed in Table 29-3. Opioids are effective antitussives, but only codeine and hydrocodone are used for this effect. Nonopiate antitussives include chlophedianol, dextromethorphan, and diphenhydramine.

Codeine and Hydrocodone

Codeine and hydrocodone are good antitussives, but they are opiates and therefore are capable of producing drug dependence. Hydrocodone has a greater potential for producing drug dependence than codeine. Most preparations containing codeine or hydrocodone are prescription drugs. Some preparations are available as Schedule V drugs and may be obtained by signing for them with a registered pharmacist. The opiates suppress a cough by directly inhibiting the medullary center for the cough reflex. The doses required to suppress a cough are less than those to produce analgesia or respiratory depression. Side effects at antitussive doses are uncommon but include nausea, dizziness, and constipation.

Chlophedianol

Chlophedianol (Ulone) is a centrally acting antitussive with some local anesthetic and anticholinergic action. Use of this drug may cause some patients to become excited and hyperirritable. Large doses cause sedation. Chlophedianol is available in Canada but not the United States.

✣ *Dextromethorphan Hydrobromide*

Dextromethorphan hydrobromide is the most widely used antitussive in OTC cough mixtures. It is related to the opiates but has no analgesic effect and causes no drug dependence.

Dextromethorphan is an effective cough suppressant that inhibits the medullary center for the cough reflex. It is well tolerated and only occasionally causes drowsiness or dizziness.

Diphenhydramine

Diphenhydramine (Benylin) is an antihistamine with antitussive action. Adverse effects include drowsiness common to the antihistamines and the anticholinergic drying effect that hinders a productive cough.

Mucolytic

Water, taken as liquid or inhaled as vapor, keeps the mucus from becoming too viscous. An expectorant stimulates the watery secretion of the bronchial glands. A **mucolytic**

TABLE 29-3 Antitussives

GENERIC NAME	TRADE NAME	ADMINISTRATION/DOSAGE	COMMENTS
Chlophedianol	Ulo† Ulone†	ORAL: *Adults*—25 mg 3-4 times daily. *Children 6-12 yr*—12.5-25 mg 3-4 times daily; *children 2-6 yr*—12.5 mg 3 or 4 times daily.	Prescription drug. Side effects include drowsiness and nausea.
Codeine, codeine phosphate, codeine sulfate		ORAL: *Adults*—10-20 mg every 4-6 hr; no more than 120 mg in 24 hr. *Children 6-12 yr*—½ adult dose; *children 2-6 yr*—¼ adult dose.	Schedule II drug. Codeine is included in some schedule III and schedule V combination formulations, usually including a decongestant, an antihistamine, and an expectorant. For adverse effects, see Chapter 31.
Dextromethorphan hydrobromide	Benylin† Robitussin DM Various others	ORAL: *Adults*—10-20 mg every 4 hr or 30 mg every 6-8 hr. *Children 6-12 yr*—½ adult dose; *children 2-6 yr*—¼ adult dose.	Nonnarcotic, available without prescription. No tolerance develops. Has no analgesic or hypnotic effect and does not depress respiration. Does not cause constipation as readily as codeine.
Diphenhydramine hydrochloride	Benylin Cough Syrup† Benadryl*	ORAL: *Adults*—25 mg every 4 hr, no more than 100 mg in 24 hr. *Children 6-12 yr*—½ adult dose; *children 2-5 yr*—¼ adult dose.	An antihistamine. Side effects include drowsiness and a drying effect.
Hydrocodone bitartrate	Adatus D.C. Codan Others	ORAL: *Adults*—5-10 mg every 6-8 hr. *Children*—0.6 mg/kg body weight daily in divided doses.	Schedule II drug. Hydrocodone is included in some schedule III and schedule V combination formulations, usually including a decongestant, an antihistamine, and an expectorant. For adverse effects, see Chapter 31.

*Available in Canada and United States.
†Available in Canada only.

TABLE 29-4 Mucolytic

GENERIC NAME	TRADE NAME	ADMINISTRATION/DOSAGE	COMMENTS
Acetylcysteine	Mucomyst* Airbron†	NEBULIZATION (using face mask, mouthpiece, or tracheostomy): 1-10 mg of 20% solution or 2-20 ml of 10% solution every 2-6 hr. DIRECT INSTILLATION: 1-2 ml of 10% or 20% solution as often as every hour.	Has odor of rotten eggs, which may cause GI upset. Solutions can be diluted with sterile water for nebulization. Reacts with iron, copper, and rubber, so nebulization equipment should not contain these materials.

*Available in Canada and United States.
†Available in Canada only.

breaks up viscous mucus so that it can be coughed up or otherwise drained. Viscous mucus is most likely to occur in the patient with a pulmonary infection or with chronic obstructive lung disease in which the normal mechanisms for clearing the lungs are compromised. Table 29-4 lists dosages and administration of the mucolytic drug currently available.

Acetylcysteine (Mucomyst)

Acetylcysteine is a sulfhydryl compound that can break disulfide bonds. Viscous mucus has long molecules linked by disulfide bonds; when these disulfide bonds are broken, the molecules separate, reducing the viscosity.

Acetylcysteine is administered by nebulizer through a face mask, mouthpiece, or tracheostomy. Acetylcysteine has a rotten egg odor and may irritate the nasal passages.

Nursing Process Overview

Drugs Modifying Respiratory Secretions

Assessment

Perform a general assessment of the patient in addition to focusing on subjective complaints. An appropriate history asks about the onset of symptoms, possible irritants for symptoms, times of the day when symptoms are worse (e.g., a cough that is more troublesome at night), therapies used by the patient that have successfully relieved the symptoms, and the history of irritants or environmental conditions that may aggravate the symptoms. Objective data include the respiratory rate, vital signs, character and quantity of secretions, assessment of the lungs, and examination of the nose, throat, and ears.

Nursing Diagnoses

- Ineffective airway clearance related to suppressed ability to cough
- Altered health maintenance related to misuse or overuse of nasal decongestants

Patient Outcomes

The patient will successfully clear airway by learning to cough effectively; any infection present will be resolved. The patient will use nasal decongestants only 3 to 5 days and only as frequently as ordered.

Planning/Implementation

Monitor symptoms, vital signs, and in some patients fluid intake and output. Identify nonmedical solutions for troublesome symptoms. For patients receiving the mucolytic agent, have a suction machine at the bedside if there is doubt that the patient can adequately handle secretions.

Evaluation

These drugs are successful if symptoms are relieved. Before discharge, patients should be able to explain how to take the drugs correctly, what side effects might occur that would require notification of the physician, why the drugs should be discontinued after symptoms have improved, and what actions to take if the symptoms return or do not improve.

Nursing Implications Summary

Nasal Decongestants

Drug Administration

- Monitor blood pressure and pulse. Monitor blood glucose levels in diabetic patients.
- Assess for gastrointestinal (GI) symptoms. Persistent or severe GI tract symptoms indicate a need to change drug or dose.

Patient and Family Education

- Review side effects with the patient. Instruct the patient to choose OTC remedies appropriate for their symptoms and to read product labels. There are hundreds of OTC products, containing two or more of the following: antihistamines, antitussives, analgesics, expectorants, and decongestants. The patient should use products only as directed and should consult the pharmacist in choosing an appropriate remedy for a specific problem.
- Remind the patient to keep all health care providers informed of all drugs being used, even OTC preparations. In particular, patients with thyroid disease, diabetes mellitus, hypertension, or heart disease should use nasal decongestants only with physician approval.
- Remind the patient to keep all drugs out of the reach of children, even nasal sprays and drops. Only pediatric preparations and pediatric doses should be used for children.
- Review Chapter 5 for information about using nosedrops and nose sprays correctly. To prevent contamination of equipment, family members should not share droppers or spray applicators. Instruct the patient to rinse and dry applicators after each use.
- To prevent insomnia, instruct the patient to take the last dose of the day around the time of the evening meal. If photophobia occurs, instruct the patient to avoid brightly lit areas and to wear sunglasses.
- Instruct the patient how to use nasal jelly (phenylephrine and others): First, blow the nose. Wash hands. Place a pea-sized amount of jelly in each nostril. Sniff well to move jelly back into nose. Wipe off the tip of the tube with a tissue and replace the cap.

Expectorants and Antitussives

Patient and Family Education

- Instruct the patient about the difference between an antitussive and an expectorant.
- Remind the patient to read labels carefully on OTC preparations to avoid taking unnecessary medications and to consult the pharmacist for assistance as needed.
- Remind the patient to keep these and all drugs out of the reach of children. Only products for pediatric use and in pediatric doses should be administered to children.

NURSING IMPLICATIONS SUMMARY—cont'd

- Remind the patient to avoid driving or operating hazardous equipment if drowsiness is a problem.
- Instruct patients with a cough to stay well hydrated (daily fluid intake of at least 2500 ml for an adult), avoid smoking, and keep the room air moist by using a vaporizer or humidifier.
- For preparations containing iodide, question the patient about history of allergy to iodine or shellfish before administering. Instruct the patient to swallow enteric-coated tablets whole, without chewing or crushing, and take them with a full glass (8-ounce) of liquid. Liquid preparations should be diluted with water, milk, or juice. Teach patients to take doses with meals or a snack to reduce gastric irritation. Discuss signs of chronic iodine poisoning such as headache, swelling of eyelids, metallic taste in the mouth, nausea, vomiting, diarrhea, skin changes, and mouth ulcers. Remind the patient to report any unexpected sign or symptom to the physician.
- Codeine and hydrocodone have the same potential for side effects as all narcotics; see Chapter 31.

Mucolytic

Drug Administration/Patient and Family Education

- Supervise the patient receiving acetylcysteine during and after treatment to see that the airway is still patent in the presence of increased pulmonary secretions. Have a suction machine at the bedside of patients who are older adults, immobilized, or intubated or anyone who may not be able to handle secretions.
- Before using a mucolytic agent with a patient for the first time, review the purpose and desired effects of the drug. Instruct the patient to cough up and expectorate loosened secretions.
- Supervise patients with asthma who are receiving acetylcysteine since the drug may cause bronchospasm. If bronchospasm develops, discontinue nebulization; if severe, notify the physician. Assess for other common side effects including stomatitis, rhinorrhea, and nausea.
- Acetylcysteine is administered orally to treat acetaminophen overdose. The dose is based on the time since acetaminophen ingestion and the serum level of acetaminophen. The regimen involves a loading dose, followed by 17 doses at 4-hour intervals. Dilute doses in juice or cola beverages before administering. The drug has an unpleasant odor. Chill diluted dose by pouring over ice and administer it from a covered container through a straw. If the patient vomits within 1 hour after receiving a dose, the dose should be repeated; consult the physician. For additional information, see the manufacturer's insert.

CRITICAL THINKING

APPLICATION

1. Explain how alpha-adrenergic agonists relieve nasal congestion.
2. Describe the technique for administering topical nasal decongestants.
3. What are the side effects, drug interactions, and contraindications for nasal decongestants?
4. What is rebound congestion?
5. Describe the origin and function of mucus.
6. List expectorants and their mechanisms of action.
7. Describe the mucolytic drug and its mechanism of action.
8. List antitussives and their mechanisms of action.
9. What are the nonmedicinal approaches for treating a cough?

CRITICAL THINKING

1. Categorize the drugs used as nasal decongestants as topical sympathomimetics, oral sympathomimetics, and imidazolines.
2. As a home health nurse, you determine that your patient is using an OTC nasal spray 6 to 8 times per day. What more should you assess? If your patient states inability to stop using the nasal spray, what should you do next?
3. Many OTC cough and cold remedies contain both an expectorant and an antitussive. What are advantages or disadvantages to such a combination?

Section VIII

Drugs Used to Manage Pain

Section VIII is devoted to the control of pain. Chapter 30 discusses aspirin, acetaminophen, and NSAIDs and their uses in treating acute and chronic pain. Drugs to treat gout are also covered in Chapter 30. Chapter 31 discusses the opioids and their uses for moderate to severe pain. Chapter 32, a new chapter, describes the management of the patient who is in pain.

CHAPTER 30

Aspirin, Acetaminophen, NSAIDs, and Drugs for Treating Gout

OBJECTIVES

After studying this chapter, you should be able to do the following:

- *Differentiate between the actions, side effects, and uses of aspirin and acetaminophen.*
- *Discuss drug therapy with nonsteroidal antiinflammatory drugs (NSAIDs) and differentiate between individual drugs.*
- *Discuss drug therapy for gout.*
- *Develop a nursing care plan for a patient receiving one of the drugs discussed in this chapter.*

KEY TERMS

analgesia, analgesic
antipyresis, antipyretic
gout
Reye's syndrome
salicylism

CHAPTER OVERVIEW

This chapter covers analgesic-antipyretic drugs, including the nonsteroidal antiinflammatory drugs (NSAIDs), and drugs to treat gout. Aspirin is the prototype for analgesic-antipyretic drugs as well as for NSAIDs. Aspirin is used to reduce a fever (antipyresis), to provide analgesia for mild-to-moderate pain, and to reduce inflammation.

Therapeutic Rationale: Analgesia and Antipyresis

Analgesia refers to the relief of pain. The analgesics discussed in this chapter, also called the nonnarcotic analgesics, inhibit the enzyme cyclooxygenase. This enzyme is key to the synthesis of local mediators, prostaglandin endoperoxides, PGG and PGH, released in damaged tissue to stimulate nerve endings. In the presence of the nonnarcotic analgesics, the nerves are not stimulated. Objective pain, pain arising from stimulation of peripheral nerve endings, is therefore not felt. This mechanism contrasts that of the narcotic analgesics, which interfere with subjective pain at the level of the central nervous system (CNS) (see Chapter 31).

Antipyresis refers to the reduction of fever. The balance between heat production and heat dissipation is regulated by the brain. An area of the preoptic anterior hypothalamus is the thermostat of the body. Fever results from an increase in the set point of this hypothalamic center. An endogenous fever-producing agent (pyrogen) is released by white cells engulfing foreign matter (phagocytic leukocytes). This pyrogen enters the CNS and stimulates the synthesis of prostaglandin E_2. This prostaglandin is the mediator elevating the temperature set point in the hypothalamus. The cyclooxygenase inhibitors prevent the synthesis of prostaglandin E_2.

Therapeutic Agents: Analgesic-Antipyretic Drugs

Acetaminophen (Datril, Tylenol, Panadol, and others) and several salicylates, including aspirin, are so widely available and generally used by the public that a patient may not mention them when asked, "What drugs have you taken recently?" Acetaminophen and the salicylates produce analgesia and antipyresis and are safe enough to be available without a prescription. However, they do have side effects and can interact with other drugs. Aspirin and acetaminophen are frequently found in over-the-counter (OTC) and prescription combination drugs that are marketed for relief of colds and allergies.

Like acetaminophen and the salicylates, the NSAIDs are also antipyretics and analgesics. Except for ibuprofen and naproxen, NSAIDs are prescription drugs used primarily to treat inflammation and resulting pain.

✣ ACETAMINOPHEN

Mechanism of Action

Acetaminophen (Datril, Tylenol, Panadol, and others) is believed to act principally by inhibiting prostaglandin synthesis in the CNS and to a lesser extent in the periphery. The peripheral action of acetaminophen involves both a blocking of pain-impulse generation and an inhibition of the synthesis of factors that sensitize pain receptors to mechanical or chemical stimulation.

Pharmacokinetics

Unlike aspirin, acetaminophen can be formulated as a liquid for infants and young children. Elixirs, solutions, suspensions, chewable tablets, wafers, tablets, caplets, and capsules are available. Acetaminophen is rapid and completely absorbed from the gastrointestinal (GI) tract. Analgesia is usually apparent within 20 minutes and peak plasma concentrations are reached in 30 to 60 minutes. The duration of action is 3 to 4 hours. Acetaminophen is metabolized in the liver to glucuronide and sulfate conjugates, which are eliminated in the urine.

Uses

Acetaminophen is a drug of choice for mild pain and fever. It is also an effective analgesic for tension-type headache, muscle and joint pain, postpartum pain, postoperative pain, and the chronic pain of cancer. Acetaminophen is frequently combined with codeine to provide analgesia for moderate to severe pain. (Table 30-1).

The advantages of acetaminophen are that it does not interfere with blood coagulation and platelet function or irritate the stomach. In addition, acetaminophen is not associated with Reye's syndrome when administered to children or adolescents with flu or chickenpox.

Acetaminophen has minimal antiinflammatory activity and therefore is not useful for dysmenorrhea, sunburn, rheumatic diseases, or juvenile arthritis.

Adverse Reactions and Contraindications

Persons with a known glucose-6-phosphate dehydrogenase deficiency can develop hemolytic anemia if they take acetaminophen. Chronic daily ingestion of acetaminophen is reportedly associated with an increased risk of renal disease.

Toxicity

In adults overdose of acetaminophen causes liver damage. Alcoholics are especially prone to this problem. Children rarely suffer permanent liver damage from the drug, but adults who take more than 2.6 gm in 24 hours may show mild symptoms of liver damage such as loss of appetite, nausea, vomiting, and slight jaundice. In deliberate overdoses of 10 gm or more, adults are highly susceptible to severe liver damage; death has been reported after ingestion of 15 gm. This toxicity arises because the liver normally conjugates toxic metabolites of acetaminophen with a sulfhydryl compound, glutathione, to produce an inactive readily excreted compound. The amount of glutathione available for conjugation is exceeded when large amounts of acetaminophen are ingested. The unconjugated metabolites then bind to and destroy liver cells. Acetylcysteine is most effective if administered within 8 hours of an acetaminophen overdose. Cimetidine, which inhibits hepatic metabolism of acetaminophen, is being tested as an additional antidote for overdose.

Acetylcysteine (Mucomyst) prevents liver damage caused by excessive acetaminophen. Acetylcysteine degrades bronchial mucus in respiratory therapy (see Chapter 29). When

TABLE 30-1 Analgesic-Antipyretic Drugs

GENERIC NAME	TRADE NAME	ADMINISTRATION/DOSAGE	COMMENTS
✣ Acetaminophen	Tylenol* Datril Panadol* Liquiprin Various others	ORAL: *Adults*—325-650 mg every 6-8 hr. No more than 2.6 gm in 24 hr. *Children 7-12 yr*—½ adult dose; *3-6 yr*—⅙ adult dose. Available without prescription.	Acts as analgesic and antipyretic only. Has little antiinflammatory action and no inhibition of platelets. Contraindicated in patients with glucose 6-phosphate dehydrogenase deficiency. Nonprescription.
✣ Aspirin (acetylsalicylic acid)	A.S.A. Aspergum Bayer Aspirin Children's Aspirin Ecotrin* Measurin	*For analgesia or antipyresis:* ORAL, RECTAL: *Adults*—650 mg every 4 hr, or 1.3 gm of timed-release form every 8 hr. *Children*—65 mg/kg over 24 hr in divided doses, every 4-6 hr.	Oral doses should be taken with large glass of water or milk to decrease stomach irritation. Some patients may need to take aspirin after a meal to avoid GI distress. Nonprescription.
Aspirin, buffered	Aluprin Ascriptin Bufferin Alka-Seltzer Various others	Same as for aspirin. There are no smaller dose tablets for children.	Alka-Seltzer contains 1.9 gm sodium bicarbonate and 1 gm citric acid per tablet. To avoid acid-base disturbances, limit ingestion to occasional use only. Remaining products contain magnesium and aluminum antacid salts. These salts are not absorbed systemically to any great extent. Nonprescription.
Sodium salicylate	Dodd's Pills† Uracel	Same as for aspirin. Injectable form is available by prescription.	Less effective than equal dose of aspirin. May be tolerated by patients who are allergic to aspirin. Does not affect platelet function but does retain vitamin K antagonist effect, which can increase prothrombin time. Nonprescription.

*Available in Canada and United States.
†Available in Canada only.

given to counteract acetaminophen, it provides the sulfhydryl groups needed to conjugate and inactivate the toxic metabolites of acetaminophen. Treatment should begin within 12 hours after overdose. The stomach is first emptied by lavage or induced vomiting. An initial dose of 140 mg/kg is given as a 5% solution; doses of 70 mg/kg are then administered every 4 hours for approximately 17 doses. Because acetylcysteine has the pervasive flavor of rotten eggs, it must be disguised in a flavored iced drink and preferably drunk through a straw to minimize contact with the mouth.

✣ ACETYLSALICYLIC ACID

Mechanism of Action

Acetylsalicylic acid (aspirin) is the prototype of the NSAIDs. Aspirin inhibits the enzyme cyclooxygenase, the key enzyme regulating the formation of prostaglandins. Prostaglandins are involved in inflammatory pathways and can cause pain, fever, edema, and erythema.

Pharmacokinetics

Aspirin is rapidly absorbed from the stomach and upper small intestine. Once aspirin is absorbed, 50% to 90% binds loosely to plasma albumin. Aspirin is rapidly hydrolyzed in the blood. The acetyl group of aspirin is readily transferred to the enzyme cyclooxygenase of the blood platelets.

Salicylic acid is the other product of the hydrolysis of aspirin. Salicylate (the basic salt to which salicylic acid dissociates at the pH of blood) is an analgesic-antipyretic and a reversible inhibitor of prostaglandin synthesis. Salicylate does not affect platelet aggregation, and therefore a salicylate salt is sometimes used in place of aspirin.

In acidic urine, salicylic acid is uncharged and therefore diffuses back into the blood. Vitamin C (ascorbic acid) maintains an acidic urine when taken in large doses and can therefore delay the excretion of salicylic acid. This interaction can be dangerous if large doses of aspirin are being taken, such as for arthritis. In alkaline urine, salicylic acid dissociates to salicylate, which is charged, cannot diffuse back into the blood, and is therefore eliminated in the urine. Salicylate is metabolized to inactive salicyluric acid by the liver. However, a 325 mg aspirin tablet saturates this liver inactivation system, thus the liver cannot readily metabolize large doses of aspirin.

Buffering agents are present in several aspirin brands to hasten dissolution of the tablet and to reduce gastric irritation from the tablet. The advantages of buffering agents are minimal, and if several doses are taken, the buffering agents may cause loose stools. Alka-Seltzer contains so much sodium and bicarbonate that it should be used only on a short-term basis.

Uses

Aspirin in low doses (325 to 650 mg or 1 to 2 adult tablets) reduces fever and relieves mild pain. Two aspirin tablets are the analgesic equivalent of 60 mg of codeine. Aspirin is an effective analgesic for most common mild-to-moderate headaches and generalized mild muscular aches. Aspirin or aspirin-codeine combinations also treat mild-to-moderate pain of tooth extractions, episiotomies, cancer, and bone fractures. A dose of 1.2 gm/day of aspirin produces the maximum analgesic effect. At much higher doses (3 to 6 gm/day) aspirin treats the inflammation of rheumatoid arthritis. At this concentration, aspirin is the prototype for the NSAIDs (see Table 30-1).

Aspirin is also widely taken as a prophylactic agent to prevent myocardial infarction (MI) and stroke and other thromboembolic conditions because aspirin inhibits platelet aggregation. A unique property of aspirin is that it irreversibly acetylates cyclooxygenase of blood platelets, an effect that persists for the 3- to 7-day lifetime of the platelet. Acetylated cyclooxygenase is inactive, and synthesis of the prostaglandin thromboxane A_2 is therefore blocked. Thromboxane A_2, a potent agent promoting platelet aggregation, is normally synthesized by platelets as they begin to aggregate. Even one aspirin tablet inhibits blood clotting by inhibiting platelet aggregation.

Aspirin in high doses is frequently the initial treatment to control the symptoms of inflammatory arthritis. Doses of 2.6 to 7.8 gm/day are required to produce the plasma concentrations of 20 to 30 mg/dl needed for an effective antiinflammatory response. These doses are associated with considerable gastric irritation with or without bleeding, salicylism, decreased platelet aggregation, and interactions with other drugs. Aspirin must be taken continuously for at least 2 weeks before an improvement may be noted. Timed-release or enteric-coated formulations may improve patient compliance by decreasing the number of times aspirin must be taken each day and by bypassing the stomach, thereby reducing gastric irritation (Table 30-2).

Adverse Reactions and Contraindications

Approximately 2% to 10% of those taking an occasional aspirin tablet experience GI upset. This effect may be felt as heartburn or nausea. Aluminum and calcium-urea salts of aspirin have been formulated to be less irritating to the stomach than aspirin. When aspirin is taken regularly in large doses for arthritis, this incidence becomes 30% to 50% and may be the factor limiting the use of aspirin. Sometimes antacids are prescribed to minimize stomach irritation, but antacids also raise the pH of the urine and increase the rate of excretion of salicylic acid. Alternatively, enteric-coated or timed-release preparations may be tried to decrease gastric irritation.

Aspirin is directly irritating and damaging to gastric mucosal cells. Because alcohol also has these gastric effects, aspirin should not be taken when alcohol is in the stomach. The combination of alcohol and aspirin is greater than additive in producing gastric bleeding. Advise patients with active peptic ulcers not to use aspirin.

Long-term aspirin ingestion can cause the loss of 10 to 30 ml of blood daily from GI irritation. This loss may lead to iron deficiency anemia in women with heavy menses. Rarely, massive GI bleeding occurs in patients who take aspirin on a long-term basis.

Some people develop an allergy to aspirin. The most common form of aspirin intolerance is manifested as a rash. Patients with a skin rash caused by aspirin may tolerate other salicylates. A few people develop nasal polyps and sometimes later develop an asthma that is triggered by aspirin.

Patients sensitive to aspirin may be sensitive to a variety of other compounds. Most commonly, individuals sensitive to aspirin may show cross-sensitivity to the following: salicylin-containing foods (e.g., apples, oranges, and bananas); processed foods or drugs containing tartrazine dye or sodium benzoate; iodide-containing substances; various other NSAIDs; or tartrazine (see box, p. 372).

As can be seen from these items, the origin of these cross-sensitivities is not always the classic cross-reactivity caused by structural similarities of the agents.

Aspirin is contraindicated to treat children and teenagers who have an acute febrile illness such as flu or chickenpox because aspirin puts them at increased risk for contracting **Reye's syndrome.** Reye's syndrome is rare but serious. It is characterized by vomiting and rapidly progressive encephalopathy. Acetaminophen and other NSAIDs have not been so implicated. Nonprescription aspirin products now contain a warning against administration to children and teenagers who manifest chickenpox or flu symptoms.

Toxicity

Mild intoxication with aspirin is called **salicylism** and is commonly experienced when the daily dosage is more than 4 gm. Tinnitus (ringing in the ears) is the most frequent effect and may be accompanied by a degree of reversible hearing loss. Because salicylate stimulates the respiratory center, hyperventilation (rapid breathing) may occur. Fever may result because salicylate interferes with the metabolic pathways coupling oxygen consumption and heat production.

Acute overdose of aspirin causes serious disturbances in the body's acid-base balance. A child is more likely to die from a large overdose of aspirin than an adult. Fatalities among children have been dramatically reduced since 1970, when the Poison Prevention Packaging Act required that orange-flavored baby aspirin (81 mg tablets) be limited to 36 tablets per bottle and that safety caps be used. If a child has ingested more than 150 mg/kg (36 baby tablets [one bottle] or 9 adult tablets for a 45 lb child), vomiting may be induced, or gastric lavage may be used to eliminate undissolved tablets. Because charcoal absorbs about half its weight in aspirin, it is given orally to reduce absorption of aspirin.

Children, particularly those younger than 4 years of age, can rapidly develop metabolic acidosis. This condition may result because of the acidic nature of aspirin and its metabolites and because salicylate inhibits metabolism in a manner that favors the accumulation of organic acids, which would normally have been metabolized to carbon dioxide and water. The hyperthermia that is also produced with this metabolic block must be treated with sponge baths. Profuse sweating

TABLE 30-2 Nonsteroidal Antiinflammatory Drugs

GENERIC NAME	TRADE NAME	ADMINISTRATION/DOSAGE	COMMENTS
Aspirin and Salicylates			
Aspirin	Bayer Timed-Release Bufferin, Arthritis Strength Measurin Various others	ORAL: *Adults*—arthritis: 2.6-5.2 gm daily in divided doses (every 8 hr for timed-release forms). For acute rheumatic fever, up to 7.8 gm daily in divided doses. *Children*—65 mg/kg over 24 hr in divided doses every 6 hr. Available without prescription.	Dose needed to achieve blood levels for antiinflammatory activity of 20%-30 mg% may vary from person to person. Doses given are average ones. Children who have viral illness and are given aspirin have increased risk of developing Reye's syndrome.
Choline salicylate	Arthropan	ORAL: *Adults and children >12 yr*—870 mg (1 teaspoon) every 3-4 hr, up to 6 times daily. Available without prescription.	Mint-flavored liquid formulated for patients with arthritis.
Diflunisal	Dolobid*	ORAL: *Adults*—500-1000 mg daily, taken as 2 doses. Maximum dose is 1.5 gm daily. Prescription drug.	Long-acting salicylic acid derivative. Has lower incidence of same side effects as aspirin.
Magnesium salicylate	Doan's* Magan Mobidin	Same as aspirin. No pediatric forms. Prescription drug. FDA pregnancy category C.	Contains no sodium; low incidence of GI upset. Contraindicated in renal failure.
Olsalazine	Dipentum	ORAL: *Adults and adolescents*—1 gm daily divided in 2 doses.	Prophylaxis for inflammatory bowel disease for patients intolerant to sulfasalazine.
Salsalate	Amigesic* Disalcid*	ORAL: *Adults only*—1 gm 3 times daily. Prescription drug. FDA pregnancy category C.	Dimer of salicylate. Absorption is from intestine only after hydrolysis to salicylic acid. Delayed onset compared to free salicylic acid.
Sodium salicylate	Dodd's Pills† Uracel	Same as aspirin. Available without prescription. Injectable form is available by prescription.	Less effective than equal dose of aspirin. May be tolerated by patients with allergic reaction to aspirin. Does not affect platelet function but does retain vitamin K antagonist effect, which can increase prothrombin time.
Other Nonsteroidal Antiinflammatory Drugs			
Diclofenac	Voltaren*	ORAL: *Adults*—150-200 mg daily divided into 2-4 doses. Also available in extended release form for once-daily administration. Available in Canada in suppository form. FDA pregnancy category B.	For rheumatoid arthritis, osteoarthritis, and ankylosing spondylitis.
Etodolac	Lodine	ORAL: *Adults*—800-1200 mg daily for osteoarthritis. For pain, 400 mg, then 200-400 mg every 6-8 hr as needed. Daily dose should not exceed 20 mg/kg of body weight or 1200 mg, whichever is less.	New drug for management of pain in patients with osteoarthritis.
Fenoprofen	Nalfon*	ORAL: *Adults*—300-600 mg 3 or 4 times daily for rheumatoid arthritis. For pain or dysmenorrhea, 200 mg every 4-6 hr.	For mild-to-moderate pain, dysmenorrhea, and rheumatoid arthritis.
Floctafenine	Idaract†	ORAL: *Adults*—200-400 mg every 6-8 hr.	For mild-to-moderate pain and inflammation.
Flurbiprofen	Ansaid* Froben†	ORAL: *Adults*—for arthritis, 100-200 mg daily in 3 or 4 divided doses. For dysmenorrhea, 50 mg 4 times daily. FDA pregnancy category B.	For arthritis or dysmenorrhea.
✚ Ibuprofen	Advil Motrin* Nuprin Various others	ORAL: *Adults*—for mild pain, fever, or dysmenorrhea, 200-400 mg every 4-6 hr. For antiinflammatory response, 1.2-3.2 gm daily in 3 or 4 divided doses.	Nonprescription for mild pain, fever, or dysmenorrhea. Higher doses available in prescription form for arthritis.

*Available in Canada and United States.
†Available in Canada only.

TABLE 30-2 Nonsteroidal Antiinflammatory Drugs—cont'd

GENERIC NAME	TRADE NAME	ADMINISTRATION/DOSAGE	COMMENTS
Other Nonsteroidal Antiinflammatory Drugs—cont'd			
Indomethacin	Apo-Indomethacin† Indocid† Indocin Novomethacin†	ORAL: *Adults*—25 mg 2-3 times daily. If necessary, total daily dose can be increased by 25-50 mg daily at weekly intervals, but total daily dose should not exceed 200 mg. *Children*—1.5-2.5 mg/kg body weight per day, divided into 3 or 4 doses. Maximum dose is 4 mg/kg of body weight daily or 200 mg daily, whichever is less. *Premature infants*—0.3-0.6 mg/kg/24 hr to close ductus arteriosus. Available in capsules, extended-release capsules, oral suspension, and suppositories.	Administer with meals or with antacids to minimize gastric irritation. For acute inflammatory episodes. Also given to premature infants to close ductus arteriosus.
Ketoprofen	Orudis*	ORAL: *Adults*—150-300 mg daily divided into 3 or 4 doses. Available in capsules, delayed-release capsules, and suppositories. FDA pregnancy category B.	For rheumatoid arthritis and dysmenorrhea.
✣ Ketorolac tromethamine	Toradol	ORAL: *Adults*—10 mg every 4-6 hr, up to maximum of 40 mg/day. INTRAMUSCULAR: *Adults*—60 mg initially, followed by 30 mg every 6 hr. Maximum 150 mg first day, then 120 mg daily thereafter.	NSAID with analgesia equivalent to morphine. Useful for outpatient surgery.
Meclofenamate	Meclomen	ORAL: *Adults*—200 mg daily divided into 3 or 4 doses. May be increased up to 400 mg daily if necessary.	For rheumatoid arthritis. Not available in Canada.
Mefenamic acid	Ponstel Ponstan†	ORAL: *Adults*—500 mg initially, then 250 mg every 6 hr as needed. FDA pregnancy category C.	For mild-to-moderate pain. Administer after meals to avoid gastric irritation.
Nabumetone	Relafen	ORAL: *Adults*—initially 1000 mg a day, taken as single dose. May increase dose to 1500 or 2000 mg, taken as single dose or in 2 divided doses.	New drug for rheumatoid arthritis and osteoarthritis.
Naproxen	Anaprox* Naprosyn* Various others	ORAL: *Adults*—250-750 mg 2 times daily for rheumatoid arthritis; 500 mg initially, then 250 mg every 6-8 hr for mild-to-moderate pain, including dysmenorrhea; 750 mg initially, then 250 mg every 8 hr for acute gout. FDA pregnancy category B.	For dysmenorrhea, mild to moderate pain, acute gout, and rheumatoid arthritis.
Oxaprozin	Daypro	ORAL: *Adults*—1200 mg/day initially, then adjust according to patient tolerance and response.	For rheumatoid arthritis and osteoarthritis. Patients with renal impairment should be started at half dose.
Phenylbutazone	Butazolidin* Butazone Novobutazone Various others	ORAL: *Adults*—initially, 300-600 mg daily divided into 3 or 4 doses. Maintenance dose is 100 mg 1-4 times daily. For acute gout, 400 mg initially, then 100 mg every 4 hr for 4 days or a maximum of 1 week. Available in capsules, tablets, and delayed-release and buffered tablets. FDA pregnancy category C.	For rheumatoid arthritis and acute attacks of other arthritic conditions, including gout. Administer after meals to avoid gastric irritation.
Piroxicam	Apo-Piroxicam† Feldene* Novopirocam†	ORAL: *Adults*—20 mg once a day or 10 mg twice a day.	For rheumatoid arthritis and osteoarthritis. Administer after meals to avoid gastric irritation.
Sulindac	Apo-Sulin† Clinoril* Novo-Sundae†	ORAL: *Adults*—150-200 mg twice a day.	For rheumatoid arthritis, acute gout, and bursitis.
Tiaprofenic acid	Surgam†	ORAL: *Adults*—600 mg daily divided into 2 or 3 doses.	For rheumatoid arthritis and osteoarthritis.
Tolmetin	Tolectin*	ORAL: *Adults*—initially, 400 mg every 8 hr, then 600-1800 mg daily, divided into 3 or 4 doses. FDA pregnancy category C.	For rheumatoid arthritis and osteoarthritis.

Patient Problem

Tartrazine Allergy

THE PROBLEM

Tartrazine (FD & C yellow dye #5) is used by many drug companies in manufacturing their drugs. Ingestion of this dye may cause an allergic reaction in susceptible individuals. This rare reaction is seen more often in persons with aspirin hypersensitivity. Example drugs containing tartrazine include Pronestyl procainamide film-coated tablets, Choloxin 2 mg dextrothyroxine tablets, and Nicolar 500 mg niacin tablets.

SOLUTIONS

- Instruct patients with a known allergy to tartrazine to wear a medical identification tag or bracelet.
- Assess patients with an allergy to aspirin for associated allergy to tartrazine before giving medications that contain tartrazine.
- Instruct patients to warn the pharmacist of tartrazine allergy before prescriptions are filled so that tartrazine-containing products can be avoided. Instruct patients with this allergy not to switch brands of a drug without consulting the pharmacist to avoid accidental exposure to tartrazine.

Tartrazine is known to be associated with allergic reactions, but there are many other dyes, fillers, and preservatives used in the manufacture of drugs. Patients who experience an unusual reaction to a drug may be manifesting an allergic response to an ingredient used in its manufacture. Read ingredient labels carefully. Take a thorough drug history. Consult the pharmacist.

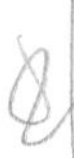

can produce dehydration. The supportive treatment of aspirin toxicity therefore consists of careful monitoring of the acid-base and electrolyte levels and appropriate fluid administration. Intravenous (IV) sodium bicarbonate can counter the tendency toward metabolic acidosis and produce an alkaline urine that hastens the excretion of salicylate. Osmotic diuretics or dialysis may be necessary in extreme cases to remove salicylate. Salicylate is a weak vitamin K antagonist and in large doses acts like an oral anticoagulant. A day or two after massive aspirin ingestion, increased bleeding tendency and signs of minor hemorrhaging may be noted (see box).

Interactions

The drug interactions characteristic of aspirin are especially important because of its widespread and uncritical use. Drug interactions arise because aspirin enhances the potential for GI bleeding and ulcers with glucocorticoids, alcohol, and phenylbutazone. Aspirin can displace oral anticoagulants, oral hypoglycemic drugs, phenytoin, and methotrexate. Because the unbound drug is the effective concentration, free drug may reach toxic levels when displaced by aspirin. Aspirin also antagonizes the uricosuric effect of probenecid and sulfinpyrazone.

Patient Problem

Aspirin Toxicity

TOXIC SALICYLATE PLASMA CONCENTRATIONS

Mild	45-65 mg/dl
Moderate	65-90 mg/dl
Severe	90+ mg/dl
Usually fatal	>120 mg/dl

TREATMENT STEPS

1. Undissolved tablets are removed through induced vomiting or absorption with charcoal.
2. Plasma salicylate, acid-base, glucose, sodium, and potassium concentrations are determined every 4 to 5 hours.
3. Hyperthermia is treated with sponge baths, and dehydration is treated with fluid replacement.
4. Fluids are administered as required to treat electrolyte imbalances and acidosis.
5. If salicylate concentration is dangerously high or does not fall with supportive treatment, dialysis or exchange transfusions may be used.

OTHER OTC SALICYLATES

Salicylamide

Salicylamide is a chemically modified form of salicylate and is not hydrolyzed to salicylic acid. It is used only in combination with other drugs.

Sodium Salicylate

Sodium salicylate (Uracel, Dodd's Pills) does not alter platelet function as does aspirin. Salicylates bind to plasma albumin and displace other drugs, particularly the oral anticoagulants (see Table 30-1).

Methyl Salicylate

Methyl salicylate (oil of wintergreen) is only used topically. It causes vasodilation in the applied areas and thereby creates a warmth that relieves muscle or joint stiffness.

NURSING PROCESS OVERVIEW

Analgesic-Antipyretic Drugs

An analgesic-antipyretic drug relieves pain and reduces fever. Aspirin and acetaminophen are the major analgesic-antipyretic drugs. They are available without a prescription as OTC drugs.

Assessment

The patient who requires a drug to reduce fever is one who has a temperature above 38.5°C (101°F) or above the locally accepted limit of normal. Fever is not a disease; it is a symptom. Monitor temperature and other vital signs; note the presence of diaphoresis, chills, or seizures; assess the level of consciousness and the fluid intake and output. Assess the patient for possible causes of fever such as pulmonary infections, wound infection, and urinary tract infection.

Nursing Diagnoses

- Risk for impaired home maintenance management related to knowledge deficit of safe use of antipyretic agents

Patient Outcomes

The patient will self-medicate appropriately with antipyretics and will not experience drug side effects.

Planning/Implementation

The treatment of fever is twofold: to reduce the fever and to determine its cause. Administer antipyretics when the temperature exceeds the ordered upper limit or every 4 hours around the clock, as ordered. Monitor the patient's temperature every 4 hours, ensure adequate fluid intake, monitor fluid intake and output, and monitor blood counts and other vital signs. Maintain patient comfort. Use additional measures if needed such as cool water baths and hypothermia mattresses. If aspirin is used, monitor the patient for bruising or bleeding.

Evaluation

Verify that the patient knows the correct dose and frequency of administration and the possible side effects of antipyretics. The patient should also know when to seek medical assistance for fever, and what other drugs and substances to avoid during antipyretic therapy.

Therapeutic Rationale: Pain and Inflammation

Prostaglandin production is associated with a variety of conditions characterized by pain and inflammation. These conditions include inflammatory arthritic conditions and musculoskeletal injury. How prostaglandins affect pain receptors is not known. The actions of prostaglandin E_2 include vasodilation and increased bone resorption. Large amounts of prostaglandin E_2 have been present in the synovial fluid of affected joints in patients with rheumatoid arthritis, synthesized by cells in the mesenchymal synovial lining. Presumably this production of prostaglandin E_2 contributes to the swelling and eventual bone erosion of rheumatoid arthritis. In addition, inflammation at other sites may involve prostaglandin E_2 synthesis.

Dysmenorrhea (menstrual cramps) appears to be caused by the overproduction of prostaglandins by the uterus at the time of menstruation. The prostaglandins can cause the uterus to contract to the point of cramping, producing dysmenorrhea.

Therapeutic Agents: Nonsteroidal Antiinflammatory Drugs

Nonsteroidal Antiinflammatory Drugs

Mechanism of Action

The primary mechanism of action of the NSAIDs is the inhibition of the enzyme cyclooxygenase so that prostaglandins are not formed.

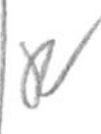

Recent studies have clarified other mechanisms of the NSAIDs that contribute to their action. These include inhibition of various enzymes, inhibition of transmembrane ion fluxes, and inhibition of the chemoattractant binding that affects the inflammatory process.

Pharmacokinetics

NSAIDs are generally well absorbed after oral administration and effective for the relief of pain in 30 to 60 minutes. When used to treat arthritis, significant relief of other inflammatory symptoms may take several days. The duration of action depends on the NSAID, generally from 4 to 12 hours. Metabolism by the liver is the common route of degradation, with elimination of metabolites in the urine.

Uses

NSAIDs are widely used as first-line therapy for inflammatory types of arthritis, including rheumatoid arthritis, ankylosing spondylitis, and juvenile arthritis. Osteoarthritis is not characterized by inflammation, and lower analgesic doses of NSAIDs can be used to treat pain associated with osteoarthritis. NSAIDs are also useful in treating pain and inflammation in athletic injuries, bursitis, synovitis, and other soft tissue injuries involving strains and sprains.

NSAIDs are effective analgesics for mild-to-moderate pain from a variety of conditions, including dental, obstetric, or orthopedic surgery.

NSAIDs are effective in averting menstrual cramps, particularly if therapy is begun a few days before the start of menses.

Ibuprofen and naproxen are used to reduce a fever.

Adverse Reactions and Contraindications

The major side effect of the NSAIDs is gastric irritation leading to an increase in peptic ulcers. Prostaglandins protect the gastric mucosa by inhibiting gastric acid secretion. GI irritation commonly caused by aspirin and other NSAIDs may arise because this protection is absent when these drugs, which inhibit prostaglandin synthesis, are present in the stomach. These effects can be minimized by taking the drugs with meals. All prescription NSAIDs now carry a warning to reflect concern about the GI side effects seen with their chronic use.

Misoprostol (Cytotec) controls gastric irritation associated with aspirin and other NSAIDs. Misoprostol, an analog of prostaglandin E_1, is protective by inhibiting excessive gastric acid secretion. Thus it replaces the prostaglandin that is suppressed by the NSAIDs (see Chapter 26 and Table 26-2).

Inhibition of platelet aggregation is another common side effect of the NSAIDs. Although this effect is irreversible with aspirin, it is reversible with the other NSAIDs. The inhibition of prostaglandin synthesis is responsible also for the platelet phenomenon.

Patients who develop a rash or other allergic reactions to one of the NSAIDs may be intolerant of the others. This is especially true of patients who have experienced bronchospasm that results from aspirin ingestion or who are sensitive to aspirin because they have asthma.

Older adult patients are more likely to develop GI distress, liver toxicity, or renal damage while taking NSAIDs and should be carefully monitored. In addition, patients with clinical conditions such as congestive heart failure, cirrhosis, and renal insufficiency are at risk for impaired renal function when taking NSAIDs. These patients require the local synthesis of vasodilating prostaglandins to maintain renal perfusion. NSAIDs, by inhibiting these prostaglandins, can allow unopposed vasoconstriction. This renal ischemia can lead to a deterioration of renal function.

Interactions

In general, the NSAIDs are protein bound and displace other drugs, particularly hydantoins, sulfonamides, sulfonylureas, and calcium channel blockers, leading to exacerbation of side effects because of these drugs. NSAIDs may increase the risk of renal damage if acetaminophen is used concurrently over long periods. The risk of GI complications, especially ulceration or hemorrhage, is increased if NSAIDs are taken concurrently with alcohol, anticoagulants, thrombolytics, or glucocorticoids. NSAIDs may diminish the effectiveness of diuretics and intensify the risk of renal failure. They potentiate drugs that inhibit platelet aggregation. NSAIDs should be discontinued when a gold compound or methotrexate is administered to treat rheumatoid arthritis because of their potential for renal damage.

Specific Nonsteroidal Antiinflammatory Drugs: Salicylates

In addition to aspirin, a number of salicylates are used as antiinflammatory agents.

Diflunisal

Diflunisal (Dolobid) is a fluoridated derivative of salicylic acid with a long duration of action. It relieves the symptoms of rheumatoid arthritis and osteoarthritis. Diflunisal has fewer side effects than aspirin; they include GI reactions, dizziness, edema, and tinnitus.

Olsalazine

Olsalazine (Dipentum) is an alternative to sulfasalazine in patients with ulcerative colitis. Olsalazine does not have the sulfa component that causes intolerance in some patients. Currently, olsalazine is only indicated for patients in remission from ulcerative colitis.

Salicylate Salts

Sodium salicylate, magnesium salicylate, and choline salicylate are all salicylate salts that produce less GI upset than aspirin.

Salsalate

Salsalate (Disalcid) is a dimer of salicylic acid. It is slowly hydrolyzed to two molecules of salicylic acid in the small intestine and absorbed into the bloodstream.

Nonsalicylate Nonsteroidal Antiinflammatory Drugs

Although indomethacin and phenylbutazone have been available for several years, many NSAIDs have been introduced into clinical practice in the past 20 years (see Table 30-2).

Diclofenac

Diclofenac (Voltaren) is relatively new to the U.S. market. It treats rheumatoid arthritis, osteoarthritis, and ankylosing spondylitis.

Etodolac

Etodolac (Lodine) is a new drug introduced to control the pain of osteoarthritis.

Ibuprofen and Related NSAIDs

About half the NSAIDs are propionic acid derivatives. These include fenoprofen (Nalfon), floctafenine (Idarac), flurbiprofen (Ansaid), ibuprofen (Advil, Mediprin, Motrin, Nuprin, and others), ketoprofen (Orudis), naproxen (Anaprox, Naprosyn), oxaprozin (Daypro), and tiaprofenic acid (Surgam). They provide good analgesic and antiinflammatory action. They often treat dysmenorrhea, rheumatoid arthritis, osteoarthritis, and gout (see Table 30-2).

Ibuprofen (Motrin) is available OTC. It is rapidly absorbed and has a plasma half-life of 2 hours. It appears to be well tolerated. GI irritation and bleeding occur less frequently than with aspirin and may be decreased by taking the drug with meals.

Naproxen (Aleve) is available OTC. It is longer acting than aspirin or ibuprofen and can be taken twice a day.

Indomethacin

Indomethacin (Indocin, Indocid, and others) is prescribed for its analgesic and antiinflammatory actions. GI disturbances such as nausea, vomiting, loss of appetite, indigestion, or diarrhea are common but can be reduced by taking the drug after meals. Occasionally, indomethacin can cause ulceration along the GI tract that may become serious if bleeding or perforation results.

Headaches and dizziness are the most common side effects. These can often be minimized if the dose is lowered and then increased gradually. Other CNS disturbances that can limit the use of indomethacin include confusion, light-headedness, fainting, or drowsiness.

Ketorolac Tromethamine

Ketorolac tromethamine (Toradol) is a new NSAID. However, it is being used principally as an analgesic, equivalent in potency to morphine. It is given by intramuscular (IM) injection for the short-term management of moderate-to-severe pain, particularly in postoperative patients. The lack of mental effects is especially beneficial in outpatient surgery.

Meclofenamate and Mefenamic Acid

Meclofenamate (Meclomen) and mefenamic acid (Ponstel, Ponstan) are fenamate derivatives. Mefenamic acid is prescribed for mild-to-moderate pain. However, therapy with this drug is limited to 1 week because of the frequent occurrence of toxicity associated with the GI, kidney, and blood-forming systems. Side effects may include GI upset, diarrhea, and rash.

Meclofenamate is prescribed for rheumatoid arthritis and osteoarthritis. Side effects are similar to those of mefenamic acid.

Nabumetone

Nabumetone (Relafen) is a relatively new drug for the treatment of rheumatoid arthritis and osteoarthritis. This is a prodrug that undergoes hepatic biotransformation to the active substance.

Phenylbutazone

Phenylbutazone (Azolid, Butazolidin, and Butazone) is a potent antiinflammatory drug with a long plasma half-life of 2 to 3 days. It binds strongly to plasma albumin and can displace other bound drugs, particularly oral anticoagulant and oral hypoglycemic drugs. Phenylbutazone causes fluid retention and gastric irritation and prolongs platelet function, thereby inhibiting blood clotting. Occasionally, phenylbutazone causes liver damage or bone marrow suppression. Because of these problems, it is commonly prescribed for only 1 to 2 weeks to treat an acute inflammatory response.

Piroxicam

Piroxicam (Feldene) is well absorbed and has a long half-life of 45 hours, making once-a-day dosing adequate. Piroxicam is rapidly excreted in the urine as a glucuronide. Piroxicam is prescribed principally for rheumatoid arthritis and osteoarthritis.

Sulindac and Tolmetin

Sulindac (Clinoril) and tolmetin (Tolectin) are chemically related to indomethacin. In general, their side effects are similar to those of aspirin, although the incidence is less than with aspirin. Sulindac has a plasma half-life of 8 hours and can be taken less frequently than indomethacin or tolmetin. It is a pro-drug, activated after conversion by the liver. The active drug is excreted in the bile and reabsorbed from the intestine. Tolmetin induces fewer side effects in the CNS than does indomethacin. Tolmetin is absorbed rapidly and has a plasma half-life of only 1 hour.

NURSING PROCESS OVERVIEW

Nonsteroidal Antiinflammatory Drugs

Assessment

Assess temperature, pulse, respiration, blood pressure, blood counts, and other laboratory data relevant to the possible or probable diagnosis. Perform a brief neurologic examination. Assess the patient's ability to perform activities of daily living to assist in planning for discharge.

Nursing Diagnoses

- Risk for GI distress or bleeding
- Potential complication: hematologic disorders

Patient Outcomes

The patient will not experience GI distress or bleeding. The nurse will minimize and manage complications of hematologic disorders.

Planning/Implementation

For individualized care, develop a plan with the patient to reach the goals of drug therapy. Reinforce the importance of other therapies including other medications, heat or cold application, immobilization, special exercises, and restricted activity. Monitor vital signs and subjective and objective data related to the specific problem and the laboratory data appropriate to the problem and the drug therapy.

Evaluation

Check that the patient can explain why and how to take the prescribed drugs and what other therapies are being used to treat the problem, which other drugs should be avoided while receiving therapy, whether alcohol should be avoided, what are reasonable expectations of the regimen (e.g., will joint pain disappear or only diminish), what are possible side effects and what to do if they occur, how to implement a plan for prophylactic treatment, and when to return for follow-up or assistance.

Therapeutic Rationale: Gout

Gout is a metabolic disease in which total body pools of uric acid (a product of DNA and RNA degradation) are elevated. The uric acid crystallizes in joints or, less commonly, in tendons or bursae. The joint at the base of the big toe is most commonly affected. During an attack of acute gouty arthritis there is a marked inflammation of the joint accompanied by significant pain. This acute attack is treated with the drug colchicine, which acts (in an unknown manner) to relieve the pain, with one of the NSAIDs already discussed, or in special circumstances with adrenocorticotropic hormone (ACTH) (see Chapter 61).

Some patients develop a tophus in a joint (crystals of uric acid with fibrous tissue surrounding them). Patients with tophi or recurrent attacks of gouty arthritis must receive long-term treatment, often for the rest of their lives, with drugs that will reduce uric acid levels in the body. With drug therapy, tophi, if present, often regress with long-term therapy, restoring the joint to a normal range of function. About 25% of such patients overproduce uric acid. These patients are treated with the drug allopurinol, which prevents the formation of uric acid from xanthine and hypoxanthine, the purine metabolites of DNA and RNA metabolism. Other patients are treated with a uricosuric drug, probenecid or sulfinpyrazone. These drugs increase the renal excretion of uric acid by inhibiting its reabsorption from the proximal kidney tubule.

Therapeutic Agents: Gout

Gout is a type of arthritis caused by a specific metabolic disorder. If gout is diagnosed early and therapy begun promptly, the disease can be arrested and complications of the disease prevented. Drugs used to treat gout are listed in Table 30-3.

Colchicine

Colchicine provides relief from the pain of an acute attack of gouty arthritis, usually within 24 hours. The earlier in an episode colchicine is taken, the more effective it is. (Similarly, antiinflammatory drugs are similarly more effective if taken early in an acute episode). Colchicine taken orally at the doses required to treat an acute gouty attack may cause nausea and vomiting followed by diarrhea. These effects limit the amount of colchicine that can be taken. Alternatively, the drug may be given intravenously to minimize these side effects. Because it causes severe tissue inflammation, it is diluted before IV administration to minimize the effect of any drug leakage.

Colchicine may be continued at reduced dosages once the acute episode is over. Continuance of colchicine is most common if a drug to reduce uric acid is begun. A sudden change in body uric acid concentration often precipitates a new acute attack of gouty arthritis. This effect can often be avoided with prophylactic colchicine.

✣ Allopurinol

Allopurinol (Zyloprim) inhibits the formation of uric acid from xanthine or hypoxanthine so that xanthine or hypoxanthine is excreted instead. A patient whose morning urine has a ratio of uric acid to creatinine greater than 0.75 or whose 24-hour urine contains more than 600 mg of uric acid is classified as an overproducer of uric acid. These overproducers and patients with renal uric acid crystals or impaired renal function are those for whom allopurinol will be most effective. It is also effective for patients with gout resulting from drug therapy that increases uric acid production, particularly cancer therapy. Side effects are rare; they appear to be allergic reactions (see box, p. 377).

TABLE 30-3 Drugs to Treat Gout

GENERIC NAME	TRADE NAME	ADMINISTRATION/DOSAGE	COMMENTS
✣ Allopurinol	Lopurin Zyloprim*	ORAL: *Adults*—200-300 mg daily as single dose; maximum, 800 mg daily. Dose is reduced if there is renal insufficiency. FDA pregnancy category C.	Inhibits formation of uric acid from hypoxanthine or xanthine; these are excreted instead.
Colchicine	Generic	ORAL: *Adults*—0.5-0.6 mg hourly or 1-1.2 mg initially and 0.5-0.6 mg every 2 hr. This is regimen for acute gouty attack and is continued until pain subsides or GI symptoms appear. Maximum dose, 7-8 mg. For prophylaxis, 0.5-1 mg daily.	Terminates acute gouty attack. Appearance of GI distress usually limits amount given.
		INTRAVENOUS: for acute attack, 1-2 mg initially, then 0.5 mg every 3-6 hr or 1 dose of 3 mg; maximum dose, 4 mg. FDA pregnancy category D.	Dilute drug 10-fold with sterile saline solution before injecting to minimize tissue damage.
Probenecid	Benemid* Benuryl† Various others	ORAL: *Adults*—250 mg 2 or 3 times daily in first week, 500 mg twice daily thereafter. May increase to 2.0 gm daily if necessary.	Inhibits reabsorption of uric acid by kidney. Prophylactic drug to reduce existing tophi and to prevent recurrence of gouty attack.
Sulfinpyrazone	Anturan† Anturane	ORAL: *Adults*—100-200 mg 2 times daily with meals or with milk at bedtime. Dosage is raised as needed to control blood urate levels (400-800 mg daily). Dose is then reduced to minimum effective level, usually 300-400 mg daily.	Acts like probenecid. May also prevent recurrence of MI.

*Available in Canada and United States.
†Available in Canada only.

Probenecid and Sulfinpyrazone

Probenecid (Benemid) and sulfinpyrazone (Anturane) inhibit the reabsorption of uric acid by the kidney tubules and thereby promote the excretion of uric acid in the urine. The patient should drink at least eight glasses of water daily to keep the uric acid dilute so that it does not crystallize in kidney tubules or the bladder. Because these drugs flood the kidney tubules with uric acid, they are contraindicated in patients with renal failure or with a history of renal stones.

Probenecid is generally well tolerated but occasionally causes GI upset or an allergic reaction. It interferes with the renal excretion of many compounds.

Sulfinpyrazone is also well tolerated. The incidence of GI upset is higher with sulfinpyrazone than with probenecid. Recent studies show that sulfinpyrazone decreases the incidence of sudden death in the first 8 months after an MI. This effect is believed to be due to decreased platelet aggregation. Because many patients with gout also have conditions such as diabetes, hypertension, or coronary artery disease (high-risk factors for MI), sulfinpyrazone may be more desirable than probenecid despite the higher incidence of GI upset.

Drug Interactions in the Therapy of Gout

Factors that diminish the effectiveness of the uricosuric drugs probenecid and sulfinpyrazone include the following:

1. A diet high in purines produces too much uric acid (see box).
2. Inhibition of uric acid secretion counteracts the block in reabsorption by the uricosuric drugs.
   a. Heavy alcohol consumption produces enough lactic acid to inhibit uric acid secretion.
   b. Aspirin and other salicylates at low doses (300 to 650 mg) inhibit uric acid secretion. Acetaminophen should be substituted for simple pain relief.
   c. Diuretics, particularly the thiazides, furosemide, ethacrynic acid, triamterene, and spironolactone inhibit uric acid secretion. Drugs used to treat gout can potentiate other drugs.

The uricosuric drugs inhibit the secretion or degradation of several medications:

1. Probenecid inhibits the renal secretion of penicillin, indomethacin, methotrexate, sulfonylureas (oral hypoglycemics), sulfinpyrazone, salicylates, and rifampin keeping their plasma levels high.
2. Sulfinpyrazone inhibits the degradation of sulfonamides, particularly sulfadiazine and sulfisoxazole, sulfonylureas, and coumarins.
3. Allopurinol inhibits the degradation of azathioprine, 6-mercaptopurine, antipyrine, coumarins, and cyclophosphamide.

DIETARY CONSIDERATION

Purine

Uric acid is produced when purine is catabolized. Gout is a problem of elevated uric acid. Formerly, a mainstay of gout therapy was purine restriction in the diet. With better drug therapy, purine restriction is a less significant component of therapy. Patients should probably modify their diets to limit excessive purine intake, unless more severe restriction is indicated on an individual basis. High purine foods to avoid or limit include the following:

- Organ meats
- Roe
- Sardines
- Scallops
- Anchovies
- Broth and consomme
- Mincemeat
- Herring
- Shrimp
- Mackerel
- Gravy
- Yeast

NURSING PROCESS OVERVIEW

Gout

Assessment

Assess vital signs, weight, history of previous attacks, family history of gout, subjective complaints, and objective data. Monitor blood work, including the serum uric acid level. X-ray films and joint aspiration may be required.

Nursing Diagnoses

- Risk for impaired home maintenance management related to the need to increase daily fluid intake to 2500 ml
- Risk for GI distress

Patient Outcomes

The patient will successfully incorporate an increased fluid intake into daily life. The patient will not experience GI distress.

Planning/Implementation

Encourage a high urinary output (2000 to 3000 ml/day) to prevent the formation of kidney stones; this requires a high fluid intake. Monitor fluid intake and output until certain that the high fluid output is being maintained. Monitor vital signs, blood pressure, condition of affected joints, subjective complaints, objective signs, and appropriate laboratory work.

Evaluation

Before discharge, check that the patient can describe the disease, the medications that have been prescribed and their actions, the administration of the drugs to achieve maximum benefit, and the possible side effects and the ones that should be reported immediately. In addition, verify that the patient can demonstrate how to plan meals within any prescribed dietary restrictions and explain how to maintain a fluid intake that will ensure adequate urinary output.

Nursing Implications Summary

Acetaminophen

Patient and Family Education

- When used in usual doses, there are few side effects associated with this drug. Notify the physician if jaundice, diarrhea, nausea or vomiting, blood in the stools, unusual bleeding or bruising, or pinpoint red spots develop on the skin. Instruct the patient to report the development of any new sign or symptom to the physician.
- Remind the patient to keep these and all drugs out of the reach of children. Never encourage children to take medications by telling them that drugs are candy. Do not give children younger than 12 years of age more than 5 doses a day. Tell parents to seek medical help immediately if overdose is suspected, even if there are no apparent symptoms. Tell the patient to be alert to signs of acute toxicity such as nausea, vomiting, and abdominal pain. Severe poisoning may result in CNS stimulation, excitement, and delirium followed by CNS depression, stupor, hypothermia, rapid shallow breathing, tachycardia, hypotension, and circulatory failure.
- Teach the patient to read labels of all medications carefully. Many OTC products for pain and sinus problems or colds contain acetaminophen alone or in combination with other drugs, including caffeine or aspirin. Tell the patient to avoid taking several drugs simultaneously unless necessary.
- Fever that persists beyond 3 days, pain that persists longer than 10 days in an adult or 5 days in a child, or sore throat that persists longer than 2 days or worsens may signal a more serious health problem. Instruct the patient to seek medical help rather than to self-medicate indefinitely. Remind the patient to take only the recommended dose; too much may cause liver damage.
- Review with parents the dosages appropriate for children of various sizes and ages. Assist the parents in finding a drug form that is easy to administer. Note that absorption from a rectal suppository is variable and there may be rectal irritation; this route may be the least desirable.
- To take effervescent preparations, pour the granules into a glass. Fill the glass with 4 ounces of cool water. Drink all of the contents of the glass, whether still fizzing or not.
- To take oral powders, open the number of capsules needed for the prescribed dose, and pour the contents into 1 teaspoon water or other liquid. Drink all of the liquid and follow with more. The contents of the capsules may also be mixed with a small amount of applesauce, pudding, ice cream, or other soft food.
- Teach the patient to avoid taking aspirin-containing products or NSAIDs while taking acetaminophen unless specifically directed to do so by the physician.
- Teach diabetic patients that acetaminophen may cause false results with blood glucose tests. Check with the physician before changing diet or insulin dose if test results change, especially if diabetes is not well controlled.
- Emphasize the importance of avoiding alcoholic beverages while taking acetaminophen.
- Remind patients to inform all health care providers of all drugs they take.
- Acetylcysteine is discussed in Chapter 29.

Aspirin and Related Drugs

Drug Administration

- Monitor platelet count and hematocrit level. Regularly check stools for presence of blood or guaiac.

Patient and Family Education

- Instruct the patient about the signs of aspirin toxicity.
- Instruct the patient to report the development of tinnitus, unexplained bleeding or bruising, severe or persistent gastric irritation, or blood in the stool. Salicylates other than aspirin do not affect platelet aggregation.
- Warn parents to avoid the use of aspirin and other salicylates to treat fever and discomfort of the flu or chickenpox in children and teenagers because aspirin is associated with the development of Reye's syndrome. Acetaminophen is preferred over aspirin to treat childhood flu and chickenpox symptoms.
- Remind the patient to keep these and all drugs out of the reach of children. Never encourage children to take medications by telling them that drugs are candy. Instruct parents to seek medical help immediately if overdose is suspected, even if symptoms are not apparent.
- Teach the patient to read labels of all medications carefully. Many OTC products for pain and for sinus problems or colds contain salicylates alone or in combination with other drugs, including caffeine or acetaminophen. Instruct the patient to avoid taking several drugs simultaneously unless necessary.
- To reduce gastric irritation, teach the patient to take oral doses with a full glass of fluid or with meals or a snack.
- Pain or fever that persists beyond 3 to 5 days may signal a more serious health problem. Instruct the patient to seek medical help rather than self-medicate indefinitely. Teach the patient to take only the recommended dose; too much medication may result in salicylism or other complications.
- Remind the patient to keep all health care providers informed of all medications being taken, including aspirin; this includes dentists and oral surgeons. In addition, avoid the use of aspirin for 7 days after tonsillectomy or oral surgery.

NURSING IMPLICATIONS SUMMARY—cont'd

- Instruct the patient not to take aspirin products that smell strongly of vinegar because they may have broken down and may not be effective.
- To take effervescent preparations, pour the granules into a glass. Fill the glass with 4 ounces of cool water. Drink all the contents of the glass, whether still fizzing or not.
- Instruct the patient to swallow enteric-coated preparations whole, without chewing or crushing. Chewable aspirin tablets may be crushed, chewed, or swallowed whole. Chew aspirin-chewing gum for several minutes (or as directed on the package label) for the best effect. Break extended-release preparations along scored lines; some should not be chewed or crushed; consult the pharmacist about specific brands. Mix choline and magnesium salicylates oral solution with fruit juice just before taking, and follow dose with a full glass (8 ounces) of water.
- Instruct the patient to avoid alcoholic beverages while taking aspirin or salicylates. Do not take buffered aspirin and choline and magnesium salicylates at the same time as tetracyclines. Patients who take one of these drugs and tetracycline should allow 1 to 2 hours between doses. Do not take doses of ketoconazole within 3 hours of doses of buffered aspirin. Do not take laxatives containing cellulose within 2 hours of doses of salicylates.
- Patients on long-term therapy may find extended-release preparations helpful, particularly at night, because morning blood levels of aspirin may not be so low.
- Teach patients who take aspirin for arthritis and other musculoskeletal conditions that the best effect is achieved through regular use of the drug as prescribed.
- Warn patients with diabetes that chronic or excessive use of aspirin-containing products may cause false urine sugar results. Monitor blood glucose levels. Consult the physician or pharmacist.
- Low-dose aspirin may be used for its antiplatelet effect. It may be prescribed to decrease the incidence of thromboembolism in immobilized patients and postoperative orthopedic patients. It is also used to prevent other vascular problems; see Chapter 20.
- Teach women to avoid the use of aspirin during the last trimester of pregnancy unless first approved by the physician.
- Encourage patients who are allergic to aspirin to wear a medical identification tag or bracelet indicating this.

Nonsteroidal Antiinflammatory Drugs

Drug Administration

- Monitor vital signs, blood pressure, and weight. Monitor the complete blood cell count, differential, platelet count, blood urea nitrogen level (BUN), serum creatinine level, and liver function tests. Check stools for presence of blood or guaiac. If diarrhea or vomiting is severe or persistent, monitor intake and output.
- Question the patient about a possible history of allergy to other drugs before administering the drug. If unsure that an allergy to an NSAID exists, consult the physician before administering the first dose.
- In patients with cardiovascular, renal, or hypertensive disease, assess for possible fluid retention. Auscultate lung sounds. Assess for jugular venous distention. Monitor daily weight.

Patient and Family Education

- Review anticipated benefits and possible side effects of drug therapy. Instruct the patient to report the development of bruising, bleeding gums, nosebleeds, blood in stool, fever, rash, sore throat, mouth ulcers or irritation, jaundice, right upper quadrant abdominal pain, and malaise. Instruct the patient to notify the physician if unexpected symptoms develop.
- Tell patients with long-term musculoskeletal problems that several weeks of therapy may be necessary before full benefit is seen. Best effects are seen if the drugs are taken regularly, as ordered. Instruct patients not to discontinue or increase therapy without consulting the physician.
- Teach the patient to take doses with meals, a snack, or milk to reduce gastric irritation. Doses are taken with a full glass (8 ounces) of fluid. Tell the patient not to lie down for at least 15 to 30 minutes after an oral dose.
- The physician may want the patient to take doses with an antacid. This practice is especially important with indomethacin, mefenamic acid, phenylbutazone, or piroxicam. The best kind of antacid is one containing magnesium and aluminum hydroxides. Do not mix liquid forms of NSAIDs with the liquid antacid.
- Teach patients taking mefenamic acid to notify the physician if diarrhea develops.
- Review the other medications and drug interactions noted in the text; counsel patients as appropriate. Remind the patient to keep all health care providers, including dentists and oral surgeons, informed of all drugs they take. Tell the patient not to take OTC products without consulting the physician. This applies especially to products that contain aspirin or acetaminophen.
- Warn the patient to avoid driving or operating hazardous equipment if visual changes, dizziness, fatigue, confusion, drowsiness, or weakness occur and to notify the physician.
- Instruct the patient to avoid drinking alcoholic beverages while taking NSAIDs.

Continued.

NURSING IMPLICATIONS SUMMARY—cont'd

- NSAIDs may cause photosensitivity. Warn the patient to limit time in the sun or under sun lamps until the effects of the drug can be evaluated. (See the patient problem box on photosensitivity, p. 649.)
- NSAIDs may be used to treat fever, even in children.
- Long-term use of these drugs is associated with visual changes. Encourage the patient to have recommended ophthalmic examinations.
- Instruct the patient to swallow enteric-coated forms whole, do not chew or crush them. Capsules may be opened and the contents mixed with food. Some tablets may be crushed and mixed with food. Work with the patient to find a form that he or she can take. Consult the pharmacist for information about crushing, breaking, or mixing an individual product.
- Instruct patients taking nonprescription NSAIDs to review the manufacturer's literature supplied with the package. Emphasize the importance of continuing with other prescribed therapies, which might include other medications, a prescribed exercise program, weight reduction, application of heat and cold, and physical therapy.
- Some of these drugs cause fluid retention. Assess the patient's ability, resources, and other health problems (e.g., hypertensive, cardiovascular, or renal disease). If appropriate, teach the patient to monitor and record weight on a daily basis. Report weight gain in excess of 2 lb/day or 5 lb/week to the physician.
- Remind pregnant or lactating women to avoid all drugs unless prescribed by the health care provider.

Allopurinol

Drug Administration

- Inspect the patient to detect rash and skin changes. Assess vision. Monitor serum creatinine level, BUN level, uric acid levels, complete blood cell count, differential, platelet count, and liver function tests.

Patient and Family Education

- Review anticipated benefits and possible side effects of drug therapy. Instruct the patient to report bruising, bleeding, nosebleeds, blood in stool, fever, sore throat, malaise, jaundice, or abdominal pain. GI discomfort is common. Encourage the patient to notify the physician of GI discomfort.
- Tell the patient to maintain daily fluid intake sufficient to ensure a daily urinary output of at least 2 L; this may require an intake of 2500 ml/day (about 10 8-ounce glasses of water)
- Caution the patient to avoid analgesics containing salicylates unless approved by the physician.
- Remind patients to inform all health care providers of all drugs they take. Allopurinol may interfere with the effects of other drugs.
- Instruct the patient to take oral doses with meals or a snack to reduce gastric irritation.
- Review the dietary consideration box on purine, p. 377.
- Teach the patient to limit the intake of alcoholic beverages. Tell the patient not to take vitamin C concurrently with allopurinol because it may increase urine acidity and promote the formation of kidney stones.
- Avoid driving or operating hazardous equipment if drowsiness or dizziness develops.
- For missed doses, take missed dose as soon as remembered, unless it is almost time for the next dose, then omit missed dose and resume regular dosing schedule.

Colchicine

Drug Administration

- Inspect the patient to detect hair loss and skin changes. Assess for GI discomfort. Monitor serum creatinine level, BUN level, complete blood cell count, differential, platelet count, liver function tests, and uric acid levels.

Intravenous Colchicine

- Dilute with 10 to 20 ml of 0.9% sodium chloride without a bacteriostatic agent. Administer over 2 to 5 minutes. Avoid extravasation or IM administration. Check that IV line is patent before administering.

Patient and Family Education

- Review anticipated benefits and possible side effects of drug therapy. Review dosage instructions, which are different for prophylactic treatment of gout and for treatment of an acute attack. Toxicity depends on the total dose given over a period of time, so it is important to teach patients who take the higher doses needed for an acute attack to take the drug only as prescribed and not to increase the dose or change the dosage regimen without checking with physician.
- Instruct the patient to report change in the color of urine (hematuria), bruising, bleeding, nosebleeds, blood in stool, fever, sore throat, malaise, jaundice, or abdominal pain. GI discomfort is common. Encourage the patient to notify the physician of any GI discomfort.
- Instruct the patient to maintain daily fluid intake sufficient to ensure daily urinary output of at least 2 L; this may require an intake of 2500 ml/day (about 10 8-ounce glasses of water).
- Instruct the patient to take oral doses with meals or a snack to reduce gastric irritation.

NURSING IMPLICATIONS SUMMARY—cont'd

- Caution the patient to avoid the use of analgesics that containing salicylates without approval of the physician.
- Remind patients to inform all health care providers of all drugs they take. Colchicine may interfere with the desired effect of other drugs.
- Review the dietary consideration box on purine, p. 377.
- Remind the patients to limit intake of alcoholic beverages.

Probenecid

Drug Administration

- Inspect for development of skin changes. Monitor blood pressure. Monitor liver function tests and serum creatinine, BUN, and uric acid levels.
- Probenecid is sometimes used concurrently with some antibiotics such as penicillins and cephalosporins; the probenecid helps increase the plasma and tissue antibiotic concentration.

Patient and Family Education

- Review the anticipated benefits and possible side effects of drug therapy. Instruct the patient to report malaise, jaundice, or abdominal pain. GI discomfort is common. Encourage the patient to notify physicians of GI discomfort.
- Tell the patient to maintain daily fluid intake sufficient to ensure a daily urinary output of at least 2 L; this may require an intake of 2500 ml per day (about 10 8-ounce glasses of fluid).
- Warn the patient to avoid driving or operating hazardous equipment and to notify the physician if dizziness occurs. Warn the patient that flushing may occur after drug ingestion. Caution the patient to avoid analgesics that contain salicylates without the physician's approval. In addition, avoid alcoholic beverages while taking probenecid.
- Remind patients to inform all health care providers of all drugs they take. Probenecid may interfere with the desired effect of other prescribed drugs.
- Alkalinization of urine helps prevent crystallization of uric acid. Sodium bicarbonate, potassium citrate, or other alkalinizing agent may be prescribed concurrently.
- Review the dietary consideration box on purine, p. 377.
- Remind the patient to limit intake of alcoholic beverages.
- Some products contain colchicine and probenecid. Review side effects of both drugs with patients.

Sulfinpyrazone

Drug Administration

- Assess for development of tinnitus and changes in hearing or GI distress. Inspect for skin changes or rash.

Patient and Family Education

- Review the anticipated benefits and possible side effects of drug therapy. Instruct the patient to report bruising, bleeding, nosebleeds, blood in stool, fever, sore throat, malaise, or tinnitus. GI discomfort is common. Encourage the patient to notify the physician of any GI discomfort. Administer oral doses with milk, meals, or snacks to reduce gastric irritation.
- Tell the patient to maintain daily fluid intake sufficient to ensure daily urinary output of at least 2 L; this may require an intake of 2500 ml/day (about 10 8-ounce glasses of fluid).
- Caution the patient to avoid the use of analgesics that contain salicylates without obtaining the physician's approval.
- Remind patients to inform all health care providers of all drugs they take. Sulfinpyrazone may interfere with the desired effect of other drugs taken.
- Review the dietary consideration box on purine, p. 377.
- Remind the patient to limit intake of alcoholic beverages.

CRITICAL THINKING

APPLICATION

1. List the three pharmacologic actions characteristic of aspirin.
2. How do the nonnarcotic analgesics produce analgesia?
3. What is the mechanism of antipyresis?
4. What are the side effects of acetaminophen?
5. What is the mechanism of acetaminophen toxicity?
6. What is the dosage difference between aspirin taken for analgesia-antipyresis and for an antiinflammatory response?
7. What factors determine the metabolism and excretion of salicylate?
8. Describe salicylism. Describe aspirin toxicity.
9. What pharmacologic actions are characteristic of the NSAIDs?
10. Why is phenylbutazone used for 2 weeks or less?
11. What are the major side effects of indomethacin?
12. Describe the uses of NSAIDs.
13. Describe the role of colchicine in treating gout.
14. Describe the mechanisms of allopurinol, probenecid, and sulfinpyrazone for lowering the uric acid concentration of the body.

CRITICAL THINKING

1. Why is acetaminophen considered safer than aspirin? Why should children not take aspirin?
2. How does aspirin affect the stomach? How does aspirin affect platelets? Describe nursing care considerations related to these effects.
3. Develop a nursing care plan for a patient receiving one or more of the drugs in this chapter.

CHAPTER 31

Opioids (Narcotic Analgesics)

OBJECTIVES

After studying this chapter, you should be able to do the following:

- *Explain the action of morphine in the central nervous system and the periphery.*
- *Describe the role of endogenous opioid peptides and the four types of opioid receptors in providing pain relief.*
- *Discuss tolerance and dependence with opioids.*
- *Describe the symptoms and treatment of acute opioid toxicity.*
- *Develop a nursing care plan for the patient receiving a narcotic analgesic.*

CHAPTER OVERVIEW

Analgesics are drugs that relieve pain. Nonnarcotic analgesics are covered in Chapter 30. This chapter presents the opioids (narcotic analgesics). The nature of pain and its treatment with opioids are described. The pharmacology of morphine, the prototype for the opioids, is reviewed, followed by a discussion of the specific characteristics of clinically used opioids and the narcotic antagonists. The chapter concludes with an examination of the nature and treatment of opioid tolerance and dependence.

KEY TERMS

chemoreceptor trigger zone
cough center
drug dependence
drug tolerance
dynorphins
endorphins
enkephalins
opioids
respiratory center

Therapeutic Rationale: Pain and the Use of Opioids

History of Opioids

Analgesics are drugs that relieve pain. Opium has been used to produce analgesia and euphoria throughout history. The word *opium* comes from the Greek *opion,* meaning poppy juice, and the source of morphine today is still the sticky brown gum (opium) collected from the seed pod of *Papaver somniferum,* a variety of poppy. About 10% of the content of opium is morphine. Codeine can also be extracted from opium, although in such small amounts that most medicinal codeine is derived by chemically modifying morphine. Morphine was isolated in 1803 by a German pharmacist and named after Morpheus, the Greek god of sleep. Morphine was the first pure chemical substance that mimicked the pharmacologic effects of the natural product after extraction from the natural product.

Drug dependence as a property of morphine was not realized in the United States until the Civil War, when morphine was widely used to treat wounded soldiers, whose addiction subsequently became a significant social problem. Opium and morphine were readily available and were often ingredients of patent medicines. By the late 1800s attempts were made to modify the structure of morphine to keep the analgesic property but eliminate the addictive potential. The first semisynthetic drug was heroin, but heroin produces drug dependence more readily than morphine. Today heroin is not a legal drug in the United States or Canada, although it is in other countries. Most narcotic analgesics come under the Controlled Substances Act (United States) or are listed as controlled substances (schedule G) under the Canadian Food and Drugs Act (see Chapter 2). Morphine is the prototype for the narcotic analgesics, a class of drugs more properly called the **opioids.** Some narcotic analgesics are chemical modifications of morphine. The first purely synthetic morphinelike compound was meperidine (Demerol), which came into clinical use in the 1940s. Because meperidine was not a chemical modification of morphine, widespread belief held that meperidine did not cause drug dependence. Today, meperidine is considered a drug with high abuse potential (schedule II) similar to morphine. The most recent examples of opioids with abuse potential that was not originally recognized are pentazocine (Talwin) and propoxyphene (Darvon), which are now classified as drugs of low abuse potential (schedule IV). The characteristics of opioid dependence and its treatment are discussed later in this chapter.

Overview of Pain

Pain is classified into two major components. Objective pain represents the stimulation of peripheral nerve endings when tissue is damaged. Nonnarcotic analgesics such as aspirin and acetaminophen (Nuprin and Tylenol) act by inhibiting the synthesis of local mediators, the prostaglandins, that are released in damaged tissue to stimulate the nerve endings. In the presence of nonnarcotic analgesics, pain is not felt because the nerves are not stimulated, and the pain message therefore is never delivered to the central nervous system (CNS). Nonnarcotic analgesics are discussed in Chapter 30. Subjective pain represents how a person reacts to pain, usually with fear, anxiety, and withdrawal. The subjective level of pain involves the spinal cord and brain, which collect and process the painful stimuli. The narcotic analgesics blunt this subjective pain, allowing the individual to tolerate pain. With high doses of these drugs, individuals become unaware of pain and become indifferent to all unpleasant stimuli.

Acute Pain

The major use of opioids is for the short-term treatment of severe acute pain such as that associated with trauma, surgery, or burns. Opioids are commonly classified by the level of pain they can relieve: severe, severe-to-moderate, and mild pain (Table 31-1). These are not specifically defined categories, however.

The pain of some specific conditions is effectively treated with opioids. These conditions include myocardial infarction, pulmonary edema, labor, preanesthesia and postanesthesia, and sickle-cell crisis. Under some circumstances pain associated with gastrointestinal (GI) and urinary tract disorders may be treated with an opioid.

In treating acute pain, opioids are administered in sufficient doses to relieve pain and at intervals frequent enough to prevent the recurrence of pain. Each patient must be evaluated frequently to determine the need for dosage adjustment. There is little danger of producing drug addiction in treating acute pain because psychologic dependence on opioids is unlikely under most medical circumstances. Most patients are able to discontinue medication with little difficulty. A more common problem is the undermedication of patients in acute pain by health care providers unduly concerned about causing addiction. The usual 10 mg dose of morphine produces effective analgesia in only two thirds of patients.

Chronic Pain

Opioids treat the chronic pain associated with cancer. Special care must be used to keep the dose as low as possible to prolong the effectiveness of the drug and to keep the patient alert. Nonmedical aspects of patient comfort should be considered, including physical, social, mental, and spiritual measures. Often, aspirin, acetaminophen, or nonsteroidal antiinflammatory drugs (NSAIDs) are effective analgesics. The treatment of chronic pain associated with cancer requires an individualized regimen that should be evaluated frequently. If opioids are used, increasing the dosage is usually preferable to increasing the frequency of administration. Because cross-tolerance of opioids is limited, a different opioid may be tried if the one being used must be discontinued because of adverse effects associated with increased dosage.

Anesthesia

Additional uses of opioids include preanesthetic medication and surgical anesthesia. As preanesthetic medication, opioids

TABLE 31-1 Comparison of Opioids (Narcotic Analgesics)

LEVEL OF PAIN	DRUG	EQUIVALENT ANALGESIC DOSE (MG) GIVEN IM OR SC	TIME FOR PEAK EFFECT (MIN)	DURATION (HR)	SCHEDULE	
					U.S.	CANADA
Severe	Morphine	10	30-90	3-7	II	N
	Buprenorphine (Buprenex)	0.5	15	4-6	V	†
	Dezocine (Dalgan)	10	60-120	3-6	*	†
	Hydromorphone hydrochloride (Dilaudid)	1.5	30-90	4-5	II	N
	Levorphanol tartrate (Levo-Dromoran)	2-3	60-90	5-8	II	N
	Methadone (Dolophine)	7.5-10	60-120	3-6	II	N
	Oxymorphone (Numorphan)	1-1.5	30-90	3-6	II	N
Moderate-to-severe	Butorphanol (Stadol)	1.5-3.5	30	3-4	*	C
	Meperidine (Demerol)	75-100	30-60	2-4	II	N
	Nalbuphine (Nubain)	10	30	3-6	*	C
	Oxycodone (Roxicodone)	15	60	3-4	II	N
	Pentazocine (Talwin)	40-60	30-60	2-3	IV	N
Mild-to-moderate	Codeine phosphate	120	60-90	4-6	II	N
	Propoxyphene (Darvon)	180-240	60	4-6	IV	N

*Not scheduled as a controlled substance.
†Not available.

relieve anxiety and provide sedation so that the patient is not in a fearful state before surgery. More potent analgesics—morphine, meperidine, fentanyl, and hydromorphone—are widely used as components of surgical anesthesia with nitrous oxide. Nitrous oxide by itself is not potent enough for surgical anesthesia but is potentiated by a narcotic analgesic. A muscle relaxant such as tubocurarine is also used. This combination of opioid, nitrous oxide, and muscle relaxant is called *balanced anesthesia* (see Chapter 68). Duration of anesthesia is controlled by the duration of action of the opioid used.

Therapeutic Agents: Opioids

Pharmacology of Opioids

The pharmacology of morphine provides the standard for describing and comparing the actions of all opioids. The general activities of morphine are described in depth, including the biochemical basis of action and the central and peripheral physiologic effects. The clinical use of morphine and other opioids are detailed separately, and the chapter concludes with a discussion of opioid dependence and its treatment.

Mechanism of Action

Opioid receptors. In the early 1970s scientists demonstrated that specific receptors for opioids exist in the brain, spinal cord, and gut. These receptors did not recognize any of the known neurotransmitters. This finding suggested that a previously unknown, naturally occurring substance exists in the brain, spinal cord, and gut that is mimicked by morphine. Such compounds have now been found. So far, three classes of naturally occurring neuropeptides have been characterized. These are **endorphins, enkephalins,** and **dynorphins.**

Beta endorphin is a large peptide derived from the prohormone for adrenocorticotropic hormone (ACTH) and is found in the pituitary gland. The dynorphins are also peptides derived from a larger peptide and found in the pituitary. The enkephalins are pentapeptides (five amino acids) and seem to be neurotransmitters associated with (1) mediation of pain and analgesia; (2) release of growth hormone, prolactin, and vasopressin from the pituitary; (3) modulation of locomotor activity; (4) regulation of mood; and (5) regulation of gut motility.

Four types of opioid receptors have been characterized. The μ (mu) receptor mediates central analgesia, euphoria, respiratory depression, and physical dependence. The μ receptor is associated with classic morphine effects and with endorphins. The κ (kappa) receptor mediates spinal analgesia, miosis, sedation, and appetite regulation. The receptor appears sensitive to opioids with mixed agonist-antagonist activity and to the naturally occurring dynorphins. The δ (delta) receptor is thought to be the primary receptor for the enkephalins and endorphins. The σ (sigma) receptor mediates the dysphoric, hallucinogenic, and cardiac-stimulant effects. The σ receptor appears sensitive to opioid-antagonist activity. The σ receptor may also respond to nonopioid agents such as the hallucinogen phencyclidine. Other opioid receptor types have also been postulated.

These recent discoveries should clarify the nature of analgesia and the development of the opioid type of drug dependence and provide the basis for understanding the role of these opioid peptides in mental disorders, seizure activity, and behavior patterns involving the reward system, eating, and drinking.

With the characterization of opioid receptors, it is clear that opioids such as pentazocine and nalbuphine, which have the least dependence potential, not only have agonistic properties (mimicking effects) but also antagonistic properties (blocking effects). The search for a nonaddicting opioid may depend on finding the drug that has the right combination of agonist-antagonist properties without causing unpleasant side effects.

Central nervous system actions

Analgesia. The analgesia produced by morphine has three characteristics. Morphine raises the threshold for pain perception, making patients less aware of pain. It also reduces anxiety and fear, the emotional reactions to pain. Finally, morphine induces sleep, even in the presence of severe pain.

The biochemical mechanism of pain relief by the opioids is their ability to mimic endogenous compounds, the endorphins, which act at many sites in the brain to modify the perception of and reaction to pain. Support for this concept has come from studies of naloxone (Narcan), which is a specific opioid antagonist. Naloxone blocks the placebo response and reduces the effectiveness of acupuncture anesthesia, processes believed to reflect the activity of endorphins. The interpretation of these effects of naloxone is that naloxone blocks the effect of endorphins, which are released in response to pain to minimize its perception. These studies also provide a biochemical explanation for the effectiveness of the acupuncture technique to reduce pain.

Medullary actions. Morphine affects several medullary centers. The most important is the **respiratory center**, which becomes less sensitive to carbon dioxide in the presence of morphine. Tolerance develops to this effect so that individuals who abuse one of the opioids can tolerate doses of opioids that would cause fatal respiratory depression in nondependent individuals. Death from an opioid overdose is frequently caused by respiratory arrest; the victim stops breathing. Similarly, the most important drug interactions with morphine are those arising from a synergistic depression of the respiratory center such as with any of the sedative-hypnotic drugs, antianxiety agents, alcohol, general anesthetics, or phenothiazines. Tolerance does not develop to the respiratory depression produced by these latter drug classes. An individual abusing an opioid and a drug of another class such as alcohol or one of the other sedative-hypnotic drugs can readily succumb to drug-induced respiratory depression.

The **cough center** is the second medullary center depressed by morphine. Morphine seldom is prescribed as a cough suppressant, as is a related drug such as codeine. Cough suppressants (antitussive drugs) are described in Chapter 29. The **chemoreceptor trigger zone** is the third major medullary center affected by morphine. Morphine stimulates this center to produce nausea and vomiting. This effect is transient, so repeated doses do not usually cause nausea and vomiting. Individuals vary in their sensitivity to this emetic action.

Mental state. The effect of morphine on behavior depends on the mental state of the individual. Euphoria may be experienced if the individual has been in pain or has been fearful and anxious. Therapeutic doses produce minimum sedation, but larger doses cause drowsiness, sleep, or in large doses, coma. A few individuals become excited rather than depressed.

Peripheral actions

Gastrointestinal system. Morphine has a profound depressant effect on the GI tract; constipation is a common side effect of morphine administration. Although morphine is not used to treat nonspecific diarrhea, related drugs such as codeine or diphenoxylate are. The common medicinal use of opium historically was to stop diarrhea.

Gastric, biliary, and pancreatic secretions are inhibited by morphine. Morphine treats the pain associated with biliary colic but may exacerbate rather than relieve the pain in some patients because the biliary tract may go into painful spasms in the presence of morphine.

Urinary retention. Urinary retention is another side effect of morphine. Morphine stimulates the release of vasopressin (an antidiuretic hormone); therefore more water is absorbed in the kidney tubules, decreasing urine volume. The drug also reduces perception of the need to void.

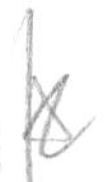

Cardiovascular effects. Morphine commonly causes hypotension. This effect may be a result of depression of the vasomotor center in the medulla. In addition, morphine causes histamine release, and histamine is a potent vasodilator. The concurrent administration of a phenothiazine or atropine can intensify the hypotension. In large doses morphine slows the heart rate.

Ocular effect. A classic effect of morphine is to reduce pupillary size. A pinpoint pupil is one characteristic of a narcotic overdose. However, if the victim is near death, hypoxia causes the release of epinephrine, which dilates the pupil.

Adverse Reactions and Contraindications

The common adverse reactions of morphine and the other opioids are those predicted by the pharmacologic actions of morphine, including nausea and vomiting, constipation, urinary retention, itching, and hypotension resulting from histamine release.

Some actions characteristic of morphine are undesirable in certain patients, including the respiratory depression caused by opioids. Patients with impaired respiratory function may be severely compromised by an opioid because their respiratory drive is already impaired. Although in general the opioids relax bronchial smooth muscle, a few patients with asthma experience severe bronchoconstriction and die. These drugs also pass into the milk of a nursing mother and affect the infant.

Patients with a head injury should not be given an opioid because the decreased respiration increases carbon dioxide retention and carbon dioxide dilates the intracranial blood vessels, worsening the situation. In addition, sedative and behavioral effects obscure evaluation of the CNS. Because opioids can cause hypotension, they must be used cautiously in patients with shock or blood loss, conditions worsened by a hypotensive action.

Acute Toxicity

Respiratory depression is the usual cause of death from an acute overdose of an opioid. An overdose is likely to occur in an individual who buys drugs on the street. Since street drugs have an unknown purity and concentration, occasionally the drug content is higher than anticipated.

The overdosed individual is stuporous or in a deep sleep and initially is warm and has flushed wet skin. The next stage is coma, in which respiration is depressed. As the individual becomes hypoxic (starved for oxygen), the skin becomes cold, clammy, and mottled, and the pupils dilate. Death is then imminent.

Clinical Use of Opioids: Severe Pain

The narcotic analgesics currently in use are compared with respect to efficacy, dose, onset, and duration of action in Table 31-1. In addition to these drugs, alfentanil (Alfenta), fentanyl (Sublimaze), and sufentanil (Sufenta) are short-acting narcotic analgesics used primarily in anesthesia.

The major use of the opioids is for the relief of moderate-to-severe pain. These drugs are most effective in relieving the constant dull pain associated with trauma, surgery, heart attack, biliary or ureteral colic, inflammation, or cancer. Isolated sharp pain is not as effectively relieved by opioids.

A summary of the most commonly used opioids is presented in Table 31-2.

✣ Morphine

Morphine has already been described as the prototype for the opioids. Chemically, morphine is a base that is positively charged at the pH in the GI tract and therefore is not readily abosrbed when taken orally. Because it is readily metabolized within the gut and by the liver, morphine is given by intramuscular (IM) or subcutaneous routes. Older adult patients usually require a smaller dose because they do not metabolize morphine as readily as do younger patients.

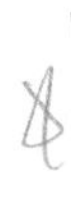

Morphine or meperidine treats the pain of an acute myocardial infarction. At analgesic doses, morphine not only relieves the pain but also reduces the anxiety without altering the cardiovascular system. If undue reduction in respiration, heart rate, or blood pressure occurs as a result of morphine administration, it can be reversed by administering naloxone, the narcotic antagonist.

Morphine is the drug of choice in pulmonary edema. The beneficial actions of morphine include relief of anxiety and vasodilation, which reduces the workload of the heart so that it pumps more efficiently. This increased cardiac efficiency relieves the pulmonary edema that arises when the left side of the heart cannot adequately pump the blood being supplied by the pulmonary veins. This inefficiency gives rise to hypertension and edema in the pulmonary system.

Dezocine

Dezocine (Dalgan) is a new chemically different opioid that relieves pain as effectively as morphine. It is administered by IM or intravenous (IV) routes. Dezocine does not seem to have the dysphoria side effects characteristic of pentazocine. Dezocine does not adversely affect cardiac performance. When dezocine is given at higher doses, respiratory depression is not as severe as with morphine.

Hydromorphone

Hydromorphone (Dilaudid) is a semisynthetic derivative of morphine. It is more potent but shorter acting than morphine. Oral doses require more time to become effective but are longer acting than parenteral doses. The actions of hydromorphone are identical to those of morphine.

Levorphanol

Levorphanol (Levo-Dromoran) is an opioid that has actions identical to those of morphine. The effective dose is about one fourth that of morphine.

Methadone

Methadone (Dolophine) is an opioid with actions similar to those of morphine. Methadone can be taken orally. Although the onset of action for a single analgesic dose is similar to that for morphine, methadone is highly protein bound and is not readily metabolized. Methadone has a half-life of 25 hours.

Methadone, 40 to 120 mg daily, substitutes for other opioids in drug-dependent individuals and prevents withdrawal symptoms. Methadone currently is used in the treatment of opioid dependence because it is effective orally and only one dose/day is necessary. In addition, the long plasma half-life more easily allows the gradual reduction in dose without side effects.

Oxymorphone

Oxymorphone (Numorphan) is a semisynthetic derivative of morphine that has all the actions of morphine except the antitussive action. Oxymorphone is more potent than morphine but must also be given by injection.

Clinical Use of Opioids: Moderate-to-Severe Pain

Summary information about opioids is presented in Table 31-2.

Buprenorphine

Buprenorphine (Buprenex) is an opioid with agonist and antagonist properties. Its abuse potential appears low; it is a schedule V drug in the United States. Buprenorphine is administered intramuscularly. The onset of action is 15 minutes, and the duration of action is about 6 hours. Buprenorphine is effective for moderate-to-severe pain associated with surgery, cancer, neuralgias, labor, renal colic, or myocardial infarction.

TABLE 31-2 Opioids (Narcotic Analgesics)

GENERIC NAME	TRADE NAME	ADMINISTRATION/DOSAGE	COMMENTS
Buprenorphine hydrochloride	Buprenex	INTRAMUSCULAR: *Adults*—0.3-0.6 mg, repeat every 6-8 hr as required.	Possesses agonist and antagonist properties. Schedule V substance.
Butorphanol tartrate	Stadol*	INTRAMUSCULAR: *Adults*—1-4 mg every 3-4 hr. INTRAVENOUS: *Adults*—0.5-2 mg every 3-4 hr.	Possesses agonist and antagonist properties. Not a scheduled drug.
Codeine sulfate, codeine phosphate		ORAL, INTRAMUSCULAR, SUBCUTANEOUS: *Adults*—30-60 mg every 4-6 hr. FDA pregnancy category C. *Children*—0.5 mg/kg body weight every 4-6 hr.	Schedule II substance.
Dezocine	Dalgan	INTRAMUSCULAR: *Adults*—5-20 mg every 3-6 hr as needed. Maximum daily dose: 120 mg. INTRAVENOUS: *Adults*—2.5-10 mg every 2-4 hr.	New opioid with agonist and antagonist properties. Not a scheduled drug.
Hydromorphone hydrochloride	Dilaudid*	ORAL: *Adults*—2 mg every 4-6 hr. FDA pregnancy category C. INTRAMUSCULAR, SUBCUTANEOUS: *Adults*—1-1.5 mg every 4-6 hr. May be given by slow IV injection or as a suppository.	Schedule II substance.
Levorphanol tartrate	Levo-Dromoran*	ORAL, SUBCUTANEOUS: *Adults*—2 mg.	Schedule II substance.
✣ Meperidine hydrochloride	Demerol*	ORAL, INTRAMUSCULAR, SUBCUTANEOUS, SLOW INTRAVENOUS: *Adults*—50-150 mg every 3-4 hr. *Children*—1-1.5 mg/kg body weight, maximum 100 mg, every 3-4 hr.	Schedule II substance.
Methadone hydrochloride	Dolophine	ORAL, INTRAMUSCULAR, SUBCUTANEOUS: *Adults*—2.5-10 mg. For pain relief, repeat every 6 hr.	Used as replacement drug for opiate dependence or to facilitate withdrawal. Schedule II substance.
✣ Morphine sulfate	MSIR Statex† Astramorph* Generic	ORAL: *Adults*—5-15 mg every 4 hr. FDA pregnancy category C. INTRAMUSCULAR, SUBCUTANEOUS: *Adults*—5-20 mg every 4 hr. *Children* (subcutaneous only)—0.1-0.2 mg/kg body weight, maximum 15 mg. INTRAVENOUS: *Adults*—2.5-15 mg in 5 ml water, injected over 4-5 min. *Children*—0.1-0.2 mg/kg.	Not well absorbed orally. Schedule II substance.
Nalbuphine hydrochloride	Nubain*	INTRAMUSCULAR, SUBCUTANEOUS, INTRAVENOUS: *Adults*—10 mg every 3-6 hr, maximum single dose 20 mg, and maximum daily dose 160 mg.	Possesses agonist and antagonist properties. Not a scheduled drug.
Oxycodone	Roxicodone Supeudol†	ORAL: *Adults*—5 mg every 3-6 hr or 10 mg 3 or 4 times a day as needed. May be increased for severe pain.	Schedule II substance.
Oxymorphone hydrochloride	Numorphan*	INTRAMUSCULAR, SUBCUTANEOUS: *Adults*—1-1.5 mg every 6 hr. INTRAVENOUS: *Adults*—0.5 mg. RECTAL: *Adults*—5 mg every 4-6 hr.	Schedule II substance.
Pentazocine hydrochloride	Talwin 50*	ORAL: *Adults*—50 mg every 3-4 hr, maximum daily dose 600 mg.	Possesses agonist and antagonist properties. Schedule IV substance.
Pentazocine lactate	Talwin Lactate*	INTRAMUSCULAR, SUBCUTANEOUS, INTRAVENOUS: *Adults*—30 mg every 3-4 hr. Subcutaneous route is not recommended (tissue damage may occur).	
Propoxyphene hydrochloride	Darvon Dolene Novopropoxen†	ORAL: *Adults*—65 mg every 6-8 hr.	Schedule IV substance.
Propoxyphene napsylate	Darvon-N*	ORAL: *Adults*—100 mg every 6-8 hr.	Schedule IV substance.

*Available in Canada and United States.
†Available in Canada only.

Butorphanol

Butorphanol (Stadol) has agonist and antagonist properties. Its abuse potential appears low, and it is not a scheduled drug in the United States. Administered intramuscularly, butorphanol has an onset of action of 10 to 30 minutes with a duration of action of about 4 hours. In general, its actions resemble those of morphine, except that butorphanol increases pulmonary arterial pressure and the cardiac workload, which makes it undesirable for treating the pain of a myocardial infarction.

Hydrocodone

Hydrocodone (Hycodan, Robidone) is a semisynthetic derivative of morphine. In Canada it is available as a syrup for cough suppression and in tablet form for analgesia or cough suppression. In the United States hydrocodone is commercially available only in combination with aspirin or acetaminophen.

Meperidine

Meperidine (Demerol) was the first of the synthetic narcotic analgesics. It is shorter acting than morphine and does not have an antitussive effect. Meperidine is widely used for obstetric analgesia. Meperidine is also available in the United States as a combination product with acetaminophen.

Nalbuphine

Nalbuphine (Nubain) is a semisynthetic derivative of morphine that has agonist and antagonist properties. The uses and limitations of nalbuphine are primarily those of meperidine or morphine. Nalbuphine may be preferable for treating the pain of a myocardial infarction, because it appears to reduce the oxygen needs of the heart without reducing blood pressure. Nalbuphine is a stronger antagonist than pentazocine, which suggests that the degree of tolerance and drug dependence should be low. However, withdrawal symptoms are seen when nalbuphine is abruptly discontinued, and it causes withdrawal symptoms when administered to an individual already dependent on one of the more common narcotic analgesics.

Oxycodone

Oxycodone (Roxicodone) is a semisynthetic derivative of morphine. It is taken orally. Oxycodone has an onset of action in 10 to 15 minutes and a duration of action of 3 to 6 hours. In the United States and Canada oxycodone is also available as a combination product with aspirin or acetaminophen.

Pentazocine

Pentazocine (Talwin) is an opioid with weak antagonist properties. For several years after pentazocine was introduced, it was believed not to produce drug dependence. Pentazocine is now a schedule IV drug, reflecting a low potential for producing drug dependence. Pentazocine causes respiratory depression in the fetus. Unlike morphine, pentazocine increases blood pressure and cardiac workload, making it less desirable than morphine for treating the pain of myocardial infarction or pulmonary hypertension. Pentazocine causes dysphoria rather than euphoria. Dysphoria can include nightmares, feelings of depersonalization, and visual hallucinations. Large doses induce seizures. Although there are reports of individuals with drug dependence for pentazocine, its administration to a person dependent on the other narcotic analgesics results in withdrawal symptoms because of its antagonistic properties. In the United States pentazocine is also available as a combination product with aspirin or acetaminophen.

Clinical Use of Opioids: Mild Pain

A summary of information about opioids is presented in Table 31-2.

Codeine

Codeine is not administered in doses large enough to be as effective as morphine because the high dose required to produce an equal degree of analgesia results in a high incidence of side effects. An oral dose of 32 or 65 mg of codeine is equivalent to 2 aspirin tablets (650 mg). At these low doses codeine seldom produces side effects. At high doses the side effects of codeine are similar to those of morphine. In the United States and Canada codeine is available as a combination product with acetaminophen or aspirin.

Because codeine causes significant histamine release if given intravenously, it is given only intramuscularly or orally. A portion of codeine dose is metabolized to morphine in the liver. Codeine is a schedule II drug when given in analgesic doses. It is also formulated with the nonnarcotic analgesics for pain relief, and these are usually schedule III drugs. Codeine is an effective cough suppressant at low doses, and it is available for this purpose in dilute solutions as a schedule V drug.

Propoxyphene

Propoxyphene (Darvon), an opioid related to methadone, is not a very potent analgesic. Propoxyphene at a dose of 65 mg is the analgesic equivalent of 2 tablets (650 mg) of aspirin or acetaminophen. Propoxyphene is commonly prescribed in combination with one of the nonnarcotic analgesics. Alone or in combination, propoxyphene is a schedule IV drug. Side effects are not common at analgesic doses. Propoxyphene has low abuse potential but has been implicated as a cause of death when abused in combination with alcohol and other CNS depressant drugs. In the United States propoxyphene is available as a combination product with acetaminophen or aspirin. In Canada a combination product with aspirin is available.

Therapeutic Agents for Opioid Overdose

Narcotic antagonists produce few effects when used by themselves under usual circumstances. Their clinical use is to treat an opioid overdose. A summary of information about opioid antagonists is presented in Table 31-3.

TABLE 31-3 Opioid Antagonists

GENERIC NAME	TRADE NAME	ADMINISTRATION/DOSAGE	COMMENTS
Naloxone hydrochloride	Narcan*	INTRAVENOUS, INTRAMUSCULAR, SUBCUTANEOUS: *Adults—for respiratory depression caused by narcotic overdose:* 0.4 mg. Repeat in a few minutes if necessary, up to 3 doses. *For narcotic depression of respiration after surgery:* 0.1-0.2 mg every few minutes as necessary. FDA pregnancy category B. INTRAVENOUS: *Neonates*—0.01 mg/kg body weight.	Pure narcotic antagonist used to reverse respiratory depression from narcotic overdose. Unlike levallorphan, naloxone produces no respiratory depression of its own.
Naltrexone	ReVia	ORAL: *Adults*—initial dose 25 mg. If there are no symptoms of withdrawal, rest of daily dose may be given. Usual daily dose is 50 mg, but it may also be administered as 100 mg every other day or 150 mg every third day. FDA pregnancy category C.	Adjunctive therapy for drug rehabilitation from opioids. Patients should have completed a withdrawal program and should be free of opioids for 7-10 days.

*Available in Canada and United States.
†Available in Canada only.

Naloxone

Naloxone (Narcan) is a pure antagonist for the opioid receptor, which makes it especially useful in the emergency room. When a comatose patient is brought to the emergency department because of a drug overdose, the first goal is to support respiration and the second is to determine which drug was used. If an opioid is suspected, a specific test is used. Naloxone is administered intravenously, and if the overdose is a result of an opioid, the patient will respond in 2 to 3 minutes with improved respiration and will return to consciousness. Naloxone displaces the opioid from the receptor but produces no effect of its own. The result is a dramatic reversal of the drug overdose. The patient must still be monitored carefully, however, because naloxone has a short duration of action and its effect may wear off before the overdosed drug has been sufficiently eliminated. If the patient again becomes comatose, naloxone must be given again.

Multiple drug abuse is common, and naloxone only reverses the depression resulting from the narcotic analgesic. Naloxone has no effect when the overdose is not caused by a narcotic analgesic.

Naltrexone

Naltrexone (ReVia) is an opioid antagonist. It has little pharmacologic activity but reverses opioid activity. Naltrexone is orally effective and long acting. It is prescribed for individuals detoxified of opioids. Because naltrexone blocks the effects of opioids, it is used in behavioral therapy to discourage resumption of opioid use. Naltrexone precipitates withdrawal symptoms when administered to an individual addicted to opioids.

Therapeutic Agents for Opioid Tolerance and Dependence

Drug Tolerance

Drug tolerance occurs when repeated use of a drug results in a lesser response unless the dose is increased. Tolerance to the euphoric effect of the opioids develops rapidly. Individuals who abuse narcotic analgesics keep increasing the dose to maintain the good feeling associated with the drug. Patients who receive an opioid for severe pain over a limited period may also develop tolerance. Patients are unlikely to become drug dependent because as the pain subsides, so will the need and use of the drug. Tapering the dose of the drug is usually sufficient for a patient to discontinue opioid therapy. However, individuals who abuse an opioid to achieve its euphoric effect increase the dose and become drug dependent rapidly. Daily use of an opioid can produce drug dependence in 3 weeks. Little or no tolerance develops to the pupillary constriction or to the constipating effect of the opioids.

Drug Dependence

Drug dependence has complex psychologic and social components. In addition to the physical dependence produced by drug tolerance, there is a psychic dependence characterized by a continued desire or craving for the drug. Detoxification of addicted individuals is rarely sufficient to prevent relapse. Medications such as methadone may help in a drug rehabilitation program, but educational and psychosocial interventions are also needed (see box, p. 390).

Symptoms of Withdrawal Syndrome

Drug-dependent persons experience distinct physical reactions if the drug is suddenly discontinued. Opioid withdrawal syndrome after the sudden cessation of morphine or heroin use is predictable. The individual has a runny nose (rhinorrhea), gooseflesh (piloerection), tearing (lacrimation), sweating, and yawning 16 hours after the last dose. The pupils do not react readily to light. Over the next 20 hours the individual becomes restless, cannot sleep, and experiences muscle twitching. Hot and cold flashes and abdominal cramping occur. By 36 hours the individual feels nauseous, vomits, and has diarrhea. Withdrawal symptoms are generally the reverse

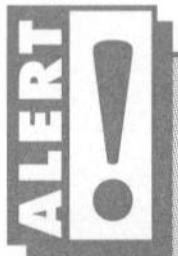

Drug Abuse Alert

Heroin and Other Opioids (Narcotic Analgesics)

BACKGROUND

Heroin and other opioids are abused to achieve euphoria. Heroin is injected intravenously.

PHARMACOLOGY

Heroin is an illegal opioid in the United States and Canada. Side effects include restlessness, vomiting, and drowsiness.

HEALTH HAZARDS

Heroin causes a high degree of physical and psychologic dependence. An overdose produces slow, shallow breathing, clammy skin, convulsions, and coma. Death can result. Withdrawal symptoms include nausea, cramps, chills and sweating, panic, tremors, irritability, and loss of appetite. Repeated injections may lead to infection of heart tissues, skin abscesses, and congested lungs.

Because of needle and syringe sharing, IV drug abuse is associated with a high incidence of transmission of human immunodeficiency virus (HIV) and has become a major risk factor for contracting acquired immunodeficiency syndrome (AIDS).

of the drug effects described for the opioids. The body overcompensates when the drug is removed.

Clonidine for Withdrawal Treatment

Clonidine is an antihypertensive drug that activates central alpha-2 adrenergic receptors (see Chapter 13). This activity reduces sympathetic overactivity. Because of this reduction in centrally mediated sympathetic activity, clonidine is useful in treating opioid withdrawal symptoms, reducing symptoms without producing a withdrawal syndrome.

Methadone for Maintenance and Detoxification

In the United States the most widely used treatment for addiction to opioids is to substitute methadone, which can be given orally in a daily dose. Because tolerance already has developed to the "kick" from heroin in these individuals, the methadone maintains this tolerance while protecting against withdrawal symptoms. The goal of maintenance is to discourage the individual from continuing to seek drugs and to participate instead in rehabilitation programs. If detoxification (elimination of drug) is the goal, methadone is administered first when withdrawal symptoms appear, and then the dose of methadone gradually is reduced to zero over 1 to 3 weeks. Because methadone has a long half-life in the body, the withdrawal symptoms are not as severe as with morphine or heroin.

Nursing Process Overview

Opioids

Assessment

Assess the history, nature, and location of pain. Use an objective tool such as a visual analog scale or a numerical rating such as 1 to 10, with 1 = mild pain and 10 = the worst possible pain. Include objective data on the patient's position, facial expression, medical history, vital signs, and age. Perform a brief neurologic examination. Pay close attention to the subjective complaints of pain.

Nursing Diagnoses

- Altered bowel elimination: constipation as drug side effect
- Altered comfort: nausea and vomiting as drug side effect
- Altered thought processes related to drug side effect

Patient Outcomes

The patient will have regular bowel elimination. The patient's nausea and vomiting will resolve. The patient's drug regimen will be manipulated until the patient's mentation is not clouded by the medications.

Planning/Implementation

Regular use of opioids at identified intervals usually provides better relief of pain than use on a prn (as needed) basis. No patient who needs medication for pain should be denied it, but augment medication use with nursing care measures to promote comfort, including positioning, distracting, and touching the patient, and introducing relaxation techniques. Monitor vital signs, level of consciousness, and frequency of bowel movements; check for nausea, vomiting, and urinary retention. Some side effects necessitate discontinuing therapy, decreasing the dose, or using additional kinds of treatments. Have narcotic antagonists available. If antiemetics or other drugs are ordered, monitor side effects; also check compatibilities before administering two or more drugs in the same syringe. Use a microdrip administration set and an infusion monitoring device for constant IV infusion.

Evaluation

Before discharge, verify that the patient can explain the name and dose of drugs to be taken, the possible side effects and how to treat them, the signs indicating too large a dose, what to do if the pain worsens, and what drugs to avoid. Determine that the patient knows to avoid alcohol while these drugs are being taken.

NURSING IMPLICATIONS SUMMARY

Opioids

Drug Administration

- Analgesics, especially narcotic analgesics, constitute one of the most useful classes of medications because they permit individuals to tolerate short- and long-term pain and thus tolerate surgery and trauma and perhaps to face death more peacefully. Failure of the health care team members to be knowledgeable about adequate drug doses, frequency of drug administration, and choice of appropriate medication results in patients receiving inadequate treatment for pain.
- Assess the patient thoughtfully before administering pain medication. If the decision is made to use a narcotic analgesic, use adequate doses and administer frequently enough to maintain a therapeutic blood level of medication. Administer medications 30 to 60 minutes before painful activities such as dressing changes, physical therapy, or whirlpool.
- Although narcotic analgesics are useful, they should be used as adjuncts to other nursing measures such as massage, distraction, deep breathing and relaxation exercises, application of heat or cold, or just being there to provide care and comfort. Include effective nursing measures in the nursing care plan, and keep the care plan updated.
- Monitor respiratory rate as an indicator of CNS depression. If the rate is <12 breaths/minute in an adult, withhold additional doses unless ventilatory support is being provided.
- Monitor pulse. If bradycardia develops (pulse <60 beats/minute in an adult or 110 beats/minute in an infant), withhold the dose and notify the physician.
- Monitor blood pressure. Hypotension is more common in older adults, the immobilized, and patients receiving other medications that have hypotension as a side effect. It may also be a sign of sepsis or shock.
- Auscultate breath sounds every 2 to 4 hours. Because narcotic analgesics suppress the cough reflex, continue activities to prevent atelectasis and pneumonia such as turning, deep breathing, and incentive spirometry.
- Have narcotic antagonists, oxygen, and resuscitation equipment available in settings in which narcotic analgesics are administered.
- Monitor level of consciousness and mental status. Evaluate findings carefully. For example, restlessness may be due to pain, hypoxia, shock, or an unusual reaction to the analgesic.
- Keep siderails up, keep a night light on, supervise ambulation, and discourage smoking.
- Monitor intake and output and weight. If nausea and vomiting occur, a switch to another analgesic may be appropriate; consult the physician. If nausea occurs, it may be appropriate to administer an antiemetic concomitantly with the narcotic. The peak effect of many antiemetics occurs at a different time from that of the narcotic; if so, the drugs should be on a different dosing schedule. In addition, antiemetics may potentiate CNS depression, but they do not potentiate analgesic effects. Sedation and hypotension may be pronounced.
- Assess for urinary retention. It may be more pronounced in older adult patients, the immobilized, and men with preexisting prostatic hypertrophy. Question the patient about difficulty in voiding, pain in the bladder area, or sensations of inadequate bladder emptying. Palpate the bladder for distention. Suggest that the patient void before each dose of narcotic.
- Although the theoretic possibility of narcotic addiction exists for all patients who receive narcotic analgesics, only a very small percentage of them do become dependent. Patients who persist in requesting frequent or large doses of pain medication beyond the average time postoperatively should not be automatically characterized as becoming addicted. Pain is a warning signal, and its unexpected persistence should be investigated.
- Some postoperative patients fear requesting any medication for pain because they fear addiction. Reassure the patient that the use of narcotics in decreasing amounts over a typical postoperative course will not cause addiction and that recovery will be easier if the pain is reduced.
- Use of aspirin, acetaminophen, or a nonsteroidal antiinflammatory drug (NSAID) along with narcotic analgesics may increase pain relief. Consult the physician.
- Record carefully the patient's response to pain and the response to narcotic administration.
- Check the physician's orders carefully. Observe agency policy regarding expiration date of controlled substances.
- In addition to the standard oral, intramuscular (IM), intravenous (IV), and subcutaneous (SC) routes, narcotics may be administered via the intrathecal or intraspinal route, with patient-controlled analgesia (PCA) devices, and with implanted pumps. Become familiar with the equipment in use. Consult the current literature for additional information. Review the manufacturer's directions and patient instruction information. Ascertain that the patient understands the advantages and uses of the various routes and equipment being used.
- For PCA use, the initial loading dose, continuous rate of infusion, patient self-administered dose, lock-out interval, and total doses per hour must be ordered by the physician.
- Transdermal dosage forms are now available for some drugs (see Fentanyl, Chapter 68). This route is not appropriate for relief of acute pain. See the manufacturer's insert.

Continued.

NURSING IMPLICATIONS SUMMARY—cont'd

- Use preservative-free morphine for intrathecal and intraspinal or epidural use.
- Dilute doses of meperidine syrup in at least a half-glass of water. When taken undiluted, it may cause temporary mucous membrane anesthesia.
- Dilute doses of methadone oral concentrate with water to a volume of at least 90 ml. Dilute dispersible tablets in at least 120 ml of water, orange juice, citrus flavor (Tang brand) drink, or other acidic fruit beverage. Complete dispersion occurs in about 1 minute.
- For continuous infusion, use microdrip tubing and an infusion-controlling device to keep the rate of administration steady.

Intravenous Butorphanol

- May be given undiluted. Administer at a rate of 2 mg or less over 3 to 5 minutes.

Intravenous Dezocine

- May be given undiluted. Administer at a rate of 5 mg over 2 to 3 minutes.

Intravenous Hydromorphone

- Dilute dose with 5 ml of sterile water or normal saline solution for injection. Administer at a rate of 2 mg or less over 3 to 5 minutes.

Intravenous Levorphanol

- Dilute dose with 5 ml of sterile water or normal saline for injection. Administer at a rate of 3 mg or less over 4 to 5 minutes.

Intravenous Meperidine

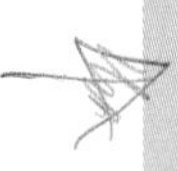

- Must be diluted. Dilute in at least 5 ml of sterile water or normal saline for injection. Administer dose over 4 to 5 minutes. For infusion in a narcotic syringe infuser system, dilute each 10 mg in at least 1 ml compatible IV fluid. May also be diluted to 1 mg/ml and given as a constant infusion under the observation of an anesthesiologist.

Intravenous Morphine Sulfate

- Dose should be diluted in at least 5 ml of sterile water or normal saline for injection, or other IV solutions. Administer at a rate of 15 mg or less over 4 to 5 minutes (direct injection). May also be diluted for infusion.

Intravenous Nalbuphine

- May be given undiluted. Administer 10 mg or less over 3 to 5 minutes.

Intravenous Oxymorphone

- Dilute dose with 5 ml of sterile water or normal saline for injection. Administer dose over 2 to 5 minutes.

Intravenous Pentazocine

- May be given undiluted, but dilution is preferable. Dilute each 5 mg with at least 1 ml of sterile water for injection. Administer 5 mg or less over 1 minute.

Patient and Family Education

- Review the anticipated benefits and possible side effects of drug therapy. Encourage the patient to phone with any questions that arise.
- Review the patient problem boxes on constipation (p. 304) and orthostatic hypotension (p. 157).
- Patients should take oral doses with milk or a snack to reduce gastric irritation.
- If the patient is to self-administer via injection, infusion, transdermal patch, or other route, teach the administration technique and have the patient give a return demonstration.
- Instruct the patient to avoid drinking alcoholic beverages while taking narcotic analgesics.
- Teach the patient to avoid the use of other medications that may also cause CNS depression such as barbiturates, antiemetics, antihistamines, or tranquilizers, unless first approved by the physician.
- Warn the patient to avoid driving or operating hazardous equipment if dizzy or drowsy.
- If a combination drug product has been prescribed, review the side effects associated with each of the drugs in the combined product.
- Remind the patient to keep these and all medications out of the reach of children. Accidental overdose with narcotic analgesics in children may quickly lead to death.

Opioid Antagonists: Naloxone

Drug Administration

- Monitor blood pressure, pulse, and respiratory rate every 5 minutes initially, tapering to every 15 minutes, then every 30 minutes until stable. Attach acutely ill or comatose patients to electrocardiogram (ECG) monitor. Have a suction machine available.
- Auscultate breath sounds. If respiratory symptoms are severe or persistent, notify the physician.
- Monitor intake and output; auscultate bowel sounds.
- Have drugs, equipment, and personnel available for resuscitation if needed. Do not leave the patient unattended until stable.
- Continue to monitor the patient closely for several hours after initial treatment, because the effects of the narcotic antagonist may wear off before the effects of the narcotic wears off, causing the patient to again display signs of narcotic overdose.

NURSING IMPLICATIONS SUMMARY—cont'd

Intravenous Naloxone

- May be given undiluted, diluted with sterile water for injection, or diluted for infusion with NS or D5NS or D5W. Administer at a rate of 0.4 mg over 15 seconds. Infusion is usually titrated to patient response. These drugs are rarely used outside of the acute care setting.

Opioid Antagonist: Naltrexone

Drug Administration

- Assess for CNS effects. It may be difficult to differentiate between effects caused by naltrexone and those caused by the emotional effect of narcotic withdrawal. If insomnia is present, administer doses in the morning.
- Obtain baseline measurement of blood pressure, pulse, and ECG tracing, then monitor pulse and blood pressure daily, tapering to monthly if no abnormalities are noted.
- Monitor bowel sounds, and keep a record of bowel movements. If abdominal discomfort is severe or persistent, notify the physician.
- Monitor respiratory rate, and auscultate breath sounds. If respiratory symptoms are severe or persistent, notify the physician.
- Inspect for rash.
- Monitor liver function tests.
- Naltrexone therapy should not be initiated until the patient has completed detoxification and has been free of opioids for 7 to 10 days.
- Before administering oral naltrexone, the patient may be given a naloxone challenge test. In this test a subcutaneous or IV dose of naloxone is administered, and the patient then is observed for signs of opiate withdrawal including nasal stuffiness, rhinorrhea, tearing, sweating, tremor, abdominal cramps, vomiting, goose flesh, and myalgia. If symptoms of withdrawal appear, the patient is not sufficiently drug free to begin naltrexone therapy. The challenge test may be repeated daily until the patient is opiate free.
- Monitor the patient carefully for at least 1 hour after the first dose of naltrexone for withdrawal symptoms.
- Naltrexone should be used only as a component of a medically supervised behavior modification program designed to help the patient maintain an opioid-free state.

Patient and Family Education

- Review with the patient the anticipated benefits and possible side effects of therapy. Instruct the patient to report unexpected side effects.
- Emphasize the importance of returning to the physician for follow-up visits and the importance of other aspects of treatment, including individual therapy and support groups.
- Tell the patient to take oral doses with meals or a snack to lessen gastric irritation.
- Review with the patient the need to avoid ingestion of opioids via any route of administration while taking naltrexone; this may include antidiarrheal medications and cough syrups.
- Remind patients to inform health care providers of all medications they are taking, including naltrexone.
- Instruct the patient to wear a medical identification tag or bracelet indicating that he or she is receiving naltrexone.

CRITICAL THINKING

APPLICATION

1. What are the two components of pain? Which is affected by opioids?
2. Which diseases are associated with chronic pain that the nurse might administer opioids to treat?
3. What are endorphins, enkephalins, and dynorphins? Which actions do enkephalins mediate?
4. What are the three characteristics of the analgesia produced by morphine?
5. What are the three major actions of morphine in the medulla?
6. What actions does morphine have on tissues outside the CNS?
7. What five common adverse reactions to morphine should you monitor?
8. What opioids might you administer to relieve severe pain?
9. What opioids might you administer to relieve moderate-to-severe pain?
10. What opioids are used to relieve mild pain?
11. Which opioids have antagonist and agonist activity?
12. Which opioids are significant in treating pulmonary edema? Pain of a heart attack?

CRITICAL THINKING

1. Why is naloxone a good drug for treating acute opioid toxicity?
2. What properties of methadone make it useful for maintaining or withdrawing from opioid dependence?
3. What role do opioids have in anesthesia?

CHAPTER 32

Management of the Patient in Pain

OBJECTIVES

After studying this chapter, you should be able to do the following:

- *Describe methods for assessing a patient's pain.*
- *Discuss selected nonpharmacologic therapies for pain relief.*
- *Discuss the use of medications in pain relief.*
- *Describe challenges to assessment and management of pain in children and older adults.*
- *Develop a plan of care for the patient in pain.*

KEY TERMS

epidural analgesia
patient-controlled analgesia (PCA)

CHAPTER OVERVIEW

Nursing management of the patient in pain can be challenging and complicated. Drugs are an important part of the treatment plan for many kinds of pain. Nonnarcotic drugs for pain were discussed in Chapter 30, and opioids (narcotic analgesics) were discussed in Chapter 31. This chapter covers assessment of the patient with pain and a selection of nursing measures for pain relief, but the major emphasis is the use of medications with the patient in pain.

IS PAIN A PROBLEM?

Most people experience pain at times during their lifetime. Many kinds of pain disappear without treatment. Other kinds of pain resolve after treatment of the associated infection, obstruction, or other cause. Nevertheless, there are many patients who seek assistance from the health care team for help in pain relief. The health care team has many strategies available to help patients in pain, including medications, surgery, exercises, traction, nerve blocks, surgery to alleviate pain, massage, and application of heat or cold. Despite this list of treatments, there are many times when patients do not receive adequate pain relief.

Unrelieved pain may contribute to a variety of problems. The patient in pain is less likely to remain active and so may develop decreased mobility. The patient may be reluctant to cough and may retain secretions, which can lead to pneumonia. Immobility may contribute to slowed gastric function and constipation. Since the patient in pain may not wish to be around others, the pain may contribute to the patient developing social isolation.

The Meaning of Pain to the Patient

Pain may mean many things to patients. For an athlete, muscle or joint pain may signal that the athlete will be removed from the game or competition. A soldier wounded in action may not even notice pain until the battle is over, then may recognize the pain as a legitimate reason for leaving the high-stress battlefield. For a weekend sportsman, pain may be the signal that it is time to stop playing basketball, soccer, or football. For some patients the occurrence of pain may remind them they are aging or signal a recurrence of cancer or other chronic problem.

Patients may also have different expectations of pain and its expression. Some patients may feel it is "unmanly" to complain of pain, whereas others may come from a background where free expression of pain is the norm. Some may fear pain and therefore ignore it, whereas others fear that if they do *not* express pain they will be ignored. Patients are also influenced by personal experiences with pain in themselves or in those around them.

Factors That May Interfere With Pain Relief

Even when the health care team is working with the patient to help produce pain relief, certain factors may interfere. Patients may not have the same goal as the health care team has. For example, the patient may assume that complete pain relief is possible in a given situation, whereas the health care team may assume that the patient is willing to tolerate a degree of short-term discomfort in an effort to achieve a long-term goal.

Sometimes patients do not understand how a specific therapy is expected to work, so the patients do not use it correctly. A few patients sometimes feel that they "deserve" pain or that there is a religious meaning to pain. These patients may feel that they are not "permitted" to experience pain relief, so they refuse to carry out prescribed therapies. Other patients may not understand how a prescribed activity could help, so they do not use it.

Pain and the Nurse

Research continues to document that some nurses, physicians, and other members of the health care team are inadequately prepared to help patients with pain relief (see box on p. 396). Studies have shown that some nurses hold misconceptions about patients and their pain. These misconceptions include the belief that many patients exaggerate their pain, that all patients with the same medical diagnosis have the "same amount" of pain and should all require the same treatment, that men should be stoic and women may freely show pain, or that individuals from a specific ethnic or racial group respond to pain the same way.

The nurse's personal life experiences influence the view of pain. A nurse who had a difficult, painful labor and childbirth may feel everyone has an equally painful one, or conversely, that no one's could be as bad as her own. A nurse who had a pain-free arthroscopic examination of a knee may be intolerant of patients who complain of pain after a similar examination. Health care workers may also have misconceptions about a patient's behavior. For example, it is incorrect to assume that if a patient is sleeping, the patient is not experiencing pain, or that if a child can enjoy playing, the child is not in pain.

ASSESSMENT OF PAIN

Objective Assessment

Objective data are important in defining changes in the patient's situation and in providing additional information about problems that the patient may have. Obtain baseline vital signs and blood pressure, and monitor these periodically. Pain may cause an increase in respiratory rate, blood pressure, and pulse. The patient may perspire or have dilated pupils. In time, as the patient adapts to pain, these observable signs will return to normal. Assess the patient's mood: crying, grimacing, calm, agitated, pacing, or restless. Does the patient have full range of movement, or is the patient guarding or protecting a joint, limb, or other area of the body? Assess the patient's gait.

Observe the area of pain, if localized, for redness or discoloration, swelling, temperature differences. Is there any exudate or drainage? If there is a recent incision, is it healing as anticipated? Assess for other objective indicators of pain that the patient might have. For example, some patients with migraine headaches will develop reddened, swollen eyes as the headache continues. Do the results of diagnostic tests provide information?

Assessment of Subjective Data

McCaffery, one of the leading nurse researchers in the field of pain, taught that "Pain is whatever the experiencing person

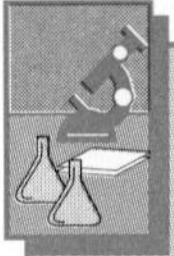

RESEARCH HIGHLIGHT

Cancer Pain: Knowledge, Attitudes of Pharmacologic Management

—P Ryan, R Vortherms, S Ward: J Gerontol Nurs 20(1):7-16, 1994.

PURPOSE

To compare oncology nurses with nurses who practice in long-term care facilities (LTCFs) in three areas: level of knowledge about cancer pain, opioids, and scheduling regimens; attitudes toward cancer pain management; and adequacy of and perceived barriers to pain management in their work setting.

METHODS

Subjects were a convenience sample of nurses who belonged to oncology nursing specialty organizations (128 participants) and all nurses who practiced in LTCFs who responded from a questionnaire sent to a random sample of all registered nurses in Wisconsin (72 participants). Oncology nurses had an average age of 40.1 years, had been in nursing an average of 15.8 years, and 44.5% held national certification in oncology nursing. LTCF nurses had an average age of 44.8 years and had been in practice an average of 18.2 years.

The instrument was constructed in part from previous questionnaires. There were three subscales: knowledge, attitudes supportive of effective pain management, and perceived barriers. The questionnaire was mailed to participants.

RESULTS

Oncology nurses performed significantly better in the area of overall knowledge and on the subtests of opioids, pain, and scheduling. In the area of attitudes, oncology nurses were no more liberal in their attitude toward cancer pain management than LTCF nurses. Liberalness refers to "a tendency to advocate maximum tolerated analgesia early in the disease course and to advocate for patient control of analgesia" (p. 10). Oncology nurses reported the quality of pain management in their work settings as significantly better than LTCF nurses. A large percentage of both groups of nurses identified one or more of nine factors as important barriers to pain management in their settings. These barriers included inadequate staff knowledge of pain management, patients' reluctance to take opioids, patients' reluctance to report pain, inadequate assessment of pain and pain relief, and medical staff reluctance to prescribe opioids.

IMPLICATIONS

The nurses in this study had positive attitudes toward assessing and relieving patients' pain but lacked knowledge about the drugs, pain, and medication scheduling. Nurses also identified their own assessment skills for pain and pain relief as inadequate. This study is one of many done over the years that indicate that nurses' knowledge about how to manage pain is still inadequate.

CRITICAL THINKING: How can student nurses prepare themselves to manage pain needs in their patients?

EXAMPLE PAIN RATING SCALES

There are several tools that are variations of the visual analog scale (VAS). The VAS is a straight line marked or calibrated to represent increasing pain. For example, a 10 cm line on a paper could be drawn, as shown below.

No pain ________________________________ Worst possible pain

The patient is asked to mark on the line at the point that represents the current level of pain. That point is measured, and a "level" can be attached to it. For example, a mark at 4.2 cm from the left is a pain level of 4.2 out of a possible 10.

Sometimes, the VAS is marked at 1 or 2 cm intervals, with or without accompanying descriptors:

|——|——|——|——|——|

No pain | Mild pain | Moderate pain | Severe pain | Very severe pain | Worst possible pain

Another variation is to ask patients to rate their pain from 1 to 10, with 0 representing "No pain" and 10 representing the "Worst possible pain," but no visual scale is shown to the patient. Variations of VAS are available to measure distress and pain intensity.

says it is and exists whenever he says it does."* This guideline continues to be appropriate. Ask the patient about the pain: Where is it? How long has it been there? Are there any aggravating factors? Ask the patient to describe the pain. Typical descriptors of pain include sharp, dull, throbbing, stabbing, and crushing. Ask the patient if there is a pattern to the pain: time of day or month, duration, frequency. Are there other accompanying symptoms, such as nausea and vomiting, itching, numbness?

What does the patient think the cause of the pain may be? Has the patient experienced this pain before, and what has the patient done about it? Question the patient about interventions used to relieve the pain and determine if they were successful.

Several tools for assessing a patient's pain have been developed. One is described in the box on p. 396, and another is shown in Figure 32-1. There are several advantages to using a pain assessment tool. The patient's ratings over time can be compared. The nurse can record the level of the patient's pain. Finally, using a tool or scale gives both the nurse and the patient a way to communicate about current pain and goals for pain alleviation.

The Pediatric Patient

Assessing the pediatric patient can be difficult. Objective data include crying, changes in vital signs, fretfulness, or general changes in behavior. On physical examination, the infant may indicate apparent pain or discomfort on movement of extremities or systematic palpation. As the infant grows older, the ability of the child to provide more specific indicators improves. Observe the child for clues about pain, for example, that the child avoids certain movements, pulls at one or both ears, or refuses to do certain activities that were previously done. Question parents and caregivers about changes in the child's behavior.

As a child grows older, assessment becomes gradually easier. The child can begin to answer simple questions or respond to directions. The nurse may ask "Does it hurt?" followed by asking the child to point to where it hurts. Certain assessment tools can be used with children (see box on p. 399). Some of these tools may be used with children as young as 4 years of age.

In working with children, remain calm and unhurried. Children may need more time to develop some trust with the nurse and to feel comfortable in talking with the nurse, who is frequently a stranger to the child. Some children respond better with a parent present, whereas other children should be assessed without parents present. Offering a young child a toy to hold or play with during assessment may cause the child to relax so that examination of the child is easier. Some children may respond if dolls or puppets are used.

The Older Adult

Avoid making assumptions about older adults. Reported assumptions about this age group include assuming that older adults do not experience pain to the degree that younger adults do or assuming that older adults do not mind pain. Other misconceptions include assuming that pain is a natural part of the aging process or assuming that approaches used with younger patients (exercises, relaxation, narcotics) cannot be used with older individuals.

Assessing older adults may pose special challenges. Some older adults have communication problems because of hearing or vision loss. Older adults who have had strokes or have some aphasia may not be able to communicate clearly. Patients with Alzheimer's disease or other dementias may not be able to provide accurate subjective data. Careful objective assessment may provide important data. Ask family members or caregivers about changes in the patient's behavior, activity level, and ability to perform activities of daily living. Do not assume that patients immediately think to complain of pain, depending on their own expectations about discomfort.

Many of the strategies suggested for children are helpful in working with some older adults. Remain calm and unhurried. If possible, sit down with the patient. Some older adults respond better if questions are kept simple and sufficient time is allowed to formulate an answer. Try to eliminate background noise by turning off the television or radio or shutting the door. Remain within the patient's vision. Of course, these strategies are appropriate with all patients but may be especially helpful with older adult patients.

NURSING DIAGNOSES AND PATIENT OUTCOMES

Once the initial assessment is completed, develop the nursing diagnoses appropriate for the patient. Analysis of the data may indicate several appropriate diagnoses for the patient. "Pain related to . . ." may be the primary diagnosis, but other diagnoses are frequently seen when a patient has pain: (1) anxiety (potential or actual), (2) altered health maintenance, (3) impaired physical mobility, (4) sleep pattern disturbance, (5) fatigue, and (6) fear.

Work with the patient and/or family to develop appropriate outcomes. It would seem obvious that the goal is for the patient to be pain free, but that may not be immediately possible. One advantage of a pain rating scale is that the nurse and patient can share a common language about pain. If the patient currently describes a pain level of 5 out of a possible 10, the nurse can determine the level that is satisfactory to the patient. Together the patient and nurse can develop specific strategies to achieve this.

In the course of developing outcomes, the nurse may also be able to provide some guidance, based on the nurse's expertise and experience. For example, the nurse may conclude that a patient's nausea may be caused by an analgesic currently being used by the patient, so the nurse could explain to the patient that changing the current medication may be helpful in relieving pain *and* relieving nausea. For another patient, the nurse may conclude that nausea is actually a manifestation of the patient's pain, and relieving the pain will help in relieving the nausea.

*McCaffery M: *Nursing management of the patient with pain,* Philadelphia, 1972, JB Lippincott, p. 219.

INITIAL PAIN ASSESSMENT TOOL

Date ____________

Patient's Name ____________ Age ____________ Room ____________

Diagnosis ____________ Physician ____________

Nurse ____________

I. LOCATION: Patient or nurse mark drawing.

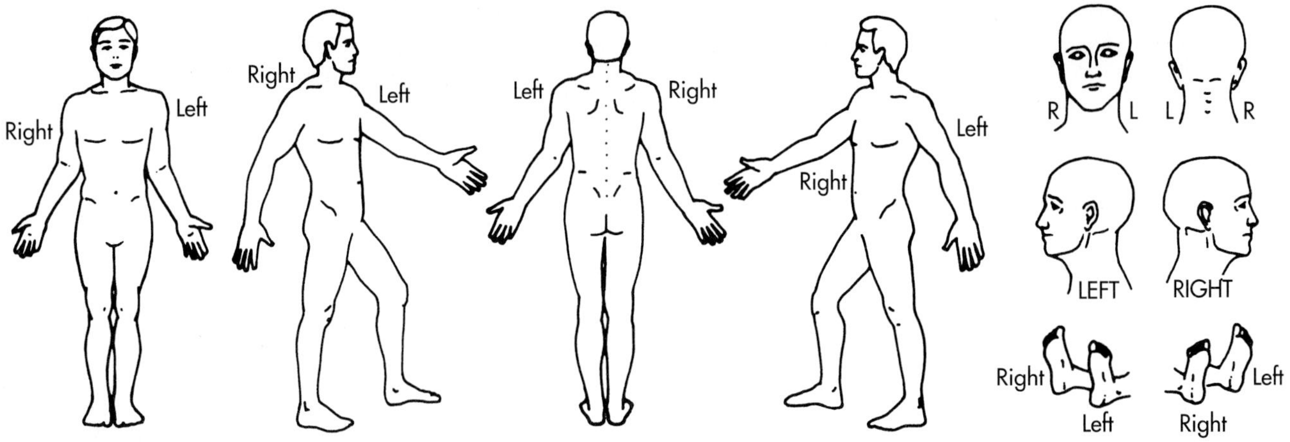

II. INTENSITY: Patient rates the pain. Scale used ____________

Present: ____________

Worst pain gets: ____________

Best pain gets: ____________

Acceptable level of pain: ____________

III. QUALITY: (Use patient's own words, e.g., prick, ache, burn, throb, pull, sharp) ____________

IV. ONSET, DURATION VARIATIONS, RHYTHMS: ____________

V. MANNER OF EXPRESSING PAIN: ____________

VI. WHAT RELIEVES THE PAIN? ____________

VII. WHAT CAUSES OR INCREASES THE PAIN? ____________

VIII. EFFECTS OF PAIN: (Note decreased function, decreased quality of life.) ____________

Accompanying symptoms (e.g., nausea) ____________

Sleep ____________

Appetite ____________

Physical activity ____________

Relationship with others (e.g., irritability) ____________

Emotions (e.g., anger, suicidal, crying) ____________

Concentration ____________

Other ____________

IX. OTHER COMMENTS: ____________

X. PLAN: ____________

FIGURE 32-1

Initial pain assessment tool. *(From McCaffery M, Beebe A: Pain: clinical manual for nursing practice, St Louis, 1989, Mosby, p 21. Used with permission.)*

EXAMPLE TOOLS TO ASSESS PAIN IN CHILDREN

In working with children and some adults, it may be necessary to use a rating scale that does not depend on the ability to read. Below is the Wong/Baker Faces Rating Scale,* with accompanying instructions.

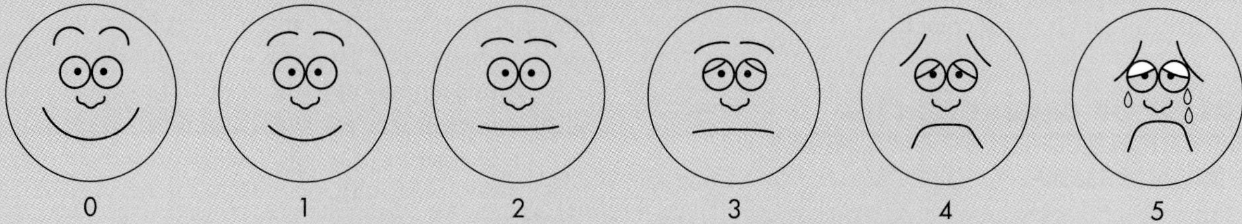

1. Explain to the child that each face is for a person who feels happy because he has no pain (hurt, or whatever word the child uses) or feels sad because he has some or a lot of pain.
2. Point to the appropriate face and state, "This face is . . .":
   0—"very happy because he doesn't hurt at all."
   1—"hurts just a little bit."
   2—"hurts a little more."
   3—"hurts even more."
   4—"hurts a whole lot."
   5—"hurts as much as you can imagine, although you don't have to be crying to feel this bad."
3. Ask the child to choose the face that best describes how he feels. Be specific about which pain (e.g., "shot" or incision) and what time (e.g. now? earlier before lunch?).

*From Wong D: *Whaley and Wong's Nursing Care of Infants and Children*, ed. 5, 1995, p. 1085. Copyrighted by Mosby–Year Book, Inc. Reprinted by permission.

Another way to assess pain in children as young as 4 years old is to use the Hester Poker Chip Scale.†

1. Use four red poker chips.
2. Align the chips horizontally in front of the child on the bedside table, a clipboard, or other firm surface.
3. Tell the child, "These are pieces of hurt." Beginning at the chip nearest the child's left side and ending at the one nearest the right side, point to the chips and say, "This (the first chip) is a little bit of hurt and this (the fourth chip) is the most hurt you could ever have."

For a young child or for any child who does not comprehend the instructions, clarify by saying, "That means this (the first chip) is just a little hurt; this (the second chip) is a little more hurt; this (the third chip) is more hurt; and this (the fourth chip) is the most hurt you could ever have."

4. Ask the child, "How many pieces of hurt do you have right now?" Children without pain will say they don't have any.
5. Clarify the child's answer by words such as "Oh, you have a little hurt? Tell me about the hurt."
6. Record the number of chips selected on the bedside flow sheet.

Regardless of the tool used in an agency, better results will be obtained if everyone uses the same tool and the results of the assessment are recorded and used for planning purposes.

†Developed in 1975 by Nancy O. Hester, University of Colorado Health Sciences Center, Denver, Colo. Reproduced from AHCPR Publ No 92-0032. Used with permission of Dr. Hester.

PATIENT EDUCATION

The nurse must include patient education throughout the development and implementation of the plan of care. First, acknowledge the patient's pain. Then let the patient know that the health care team will work with the patient to relieve the patient's pain. As more data are obtained about the patient's specific situation, the nurse may be able to explain the cause(s) of some or all of the pain. Knowing the cause of the pain does not relieve the pain, but it may help decrease a patient's anxiety. Keep the patient informed as the physical examination continues, diagnostic tests are performed, and medications are administered.

Present each therapy used for pain relief in a positive way. A nurse who suggests "I don't really think this will help much, but . . ." will not elicit the same outcome as a statement like "Some of my patients have found this helpful, and I would like to try it with you. . . ." Most patients are not interested in the physiologic explanation of pain relief strategies but would like to know the following: what will happen; how long will the therapy, treatment, or intervention take; if it works, how soon will relief begin; and if it does not work, what next? Reassure patients that the health care team will continue to work together with the patient as long as needed to help problem-solve.

Anxiety often accompanies pain, but the patient may not identify anxiety as a problem. Strategies to relieve pain may help lessen anxiety, and efforts to lessen anxiety may also result in more effective pain relief. Keeping the patient informed of what is going on and what will happen to the patient will help lessen his or her anxiety.

THE PLAN OF CARE: SELECTED NONPHARMACOLOGIC MEASURES FOR PAIN RELIEF

As the data are analyzed, the diagnoses determined, and the hoped-for patient outcomes decided, the plan begins to emerge. As with all care plans, this one should be specific and be developed by the health care team working together. The more the team shares common goals and common understanding about pain and its management, the more likely the plan will succeed. If one member of the team believes primarily in cognitive-behavioral approaches and another prefers medicinal approaches, then implementation of the plan may be uneven.

Once the plan is developed, it is important to monitor its effectiveness. One way to do this is to use a flow sheet to record the patient's response, as shown in Figure 32-2. The column headings can be modified to meet the patient's individual situation.

Many patients profit from an approach that combines several approaches such as combining a cognitive-behavioral approach with medication or combining two kinds of physical agents. Cognitive-behavioral measures for pain relief are especially helpful in giving patients a sense of involvement and control over their pain. Patients can become active in personal pain assessment and can become knowledgeable about how to control their own pain. These strategies may help patients alter their pain behavior. Some of these strategies are well suited for patients who have long-term pain or who do not want or should not have strong or sedating drugs. Some patients, however, will be resistant to these measures, even after efforts to present them in a positive, therapeutic manner. Cognitive behavioral measures include relaxation (see box), distraction, music therapy, imagery, and prayer.

In addition to cognitive-behavioral approaches to pain control and management, there are many physical agents or approaches that can be used. One physical agent is heat, including hot compresses, soaking in warm water, application of a hot water bottle, heating pad, or heat lamp. Another physical agent is cold, which can be applied in moist forms (e.g., soaking foot or hand in ice water; towels dipped in ice water, wrung out, and applied) or dry forms (waterproof bag filled with ice, frozen gel packs, bag of frozen green peas or corn). Other forms of physical agents include massage, exercise, and transcutaneous electrical nerve stimulation (TENS).

USE OF MEDICATIONS FOR PAIN RELIEF

Medications remain a mainstay of pain relief. Usually, begin with less potent drugs before moving to more potent. Thus the beginning drug should be aspirin, acetaminophen, or a nonsteroidal antiinflammatory drug (NSAID) (see Chapters 30 and 31). There are other situations in which it is not appropriate to begin with any of these drugs. In many postoperative situations, oral nonnarcotics are not a satisfactory choice for the immediate postoperative period because the patient is not yet ready to resume oral intake.

Next, use an adequate dose and decide on the frequency of doses. Recommended doses are based on studies done on large numbers of patients and reflect the dose that is effective for the *average* patient. Any individual patient may require more or less. Use an appropriate pain assessment tool and monitor the effectiveness of the dose. Work with the physician to determine if prn (as necessary) or around-the-clock doses are better for the specific patient and situation.

Anticipate pain rather than waiting until the patient is obviously uncomfortable. Assess the patient frequently. If it appears that the patient's pain level is increasing, medicate the patient. Anticipate that the patient will experience pain during certain activities, and medicate the patient before activities such as physical therapy or postoperative ambulation.

The usual approach is to begin with a nonnarcotic and then to change to oral narcotics when nonnarcotics are no longer effective. Even if a patient requires a narcotic, a com-

EXAMPLE INSTRUCTIONS FOR A RELAXATION EXERCISE

Help the patient assume a comfortable position. Tell the patient:

1. Clench your fists; breathe in deeply and hold it a moment.
2. Breathe out slowly and go limp as a rag doll.
3. Start yawning.

Yawning becomes spontaneous and is contagious, so others may begin yawning and relaxing too.

From McCaffery M, Beebe A: *Pain: clinical manual for nursing practice,* St Louis, 1989, Mosby, p 199. Used with permission.

FLOW SHEET—PAIN

Patient ______________________________ Date ______________

*Pain rating scale used ______________________________

Purpose: To evaluate the safety and effectiveness of the analgesic(s).

Analgesic(s) prescribed: ______________________________

Time	Pain rating	Analgesic	R	P	BP	Level of arousal	Other†	Plan & comments

**Pain rating:* A number of different scales may be used. Indicate which scale is used and use the same one each time. For example, 0-10 (0 = no pain, 10 = worst pain).

†*Possibilities for other columns:* bowel function, activities, nausea and vomiting, other pain relief measures. Identify the side effects of greatest concern to patient, family, physician, nurses.

FIGURE 32-2

A flow sheet to track the effectiveness of pain management. *(From McCaffery M, Beebe A: Pain: clinical manual for nursing practice, St Louis, 1989, Mosby, p 27. Used with permission.)*

bination of a narcotic and nonnarcotic such as aspirin or acetaminophen is more effective than a low dose of a narcotic alone. This is the logic behind combination products such as Percocet (oxycodone plus acetaminophen), Tylenol #3 (acetaminophen and codeine), or Percodan (oxycodone and aspirin).

Narcotics for Pain Relief

Narcotic analgesics are the most potent drugs for pain, short of general or local anesthesia (see Chapter 31). Even when used in appropriate situations, however, patients are sometimes forced to endure excessive waiting periods between doses, inadequate doses, or insensitivity on the part of members of the health care team (see box, p. 396). Drug addiction or psychologic dependence that develops into drug abuse is very rare in patients receiving medication for pain. Remember that opioid tolerance and physical dependence are predictable consequences of long-term opioid use and are not signs of drug abuse or drug addiction (see Chapter 8). Opioid tolerance may develop in a relatively short period of time and is simply a problem to deal with, not a reason to withhold medication or label a patient inappropriately. When narcotics are used beyond a few days, anticipate the development of some side effects, including constipation, and develop a plan to deal with the side effect.

Many patients who require narcotics for pain relief are initially titrated on intravenous (IV) forms. Once the patient is more comfortable, the health care team can work with the patient to develop a plan for pain relief that relies on routes of administration that are easier to self-administer. An important concept in switching a patient from one drug to another is understanding equianalgesic dosages (Tables 32-1 and 32-2). As the chart illustrates, a patient who requires 10 mg of morphine will require 75-100 mg of meperidine to achieve the same degree of pain relief.

Generally, patients prefer oral drug forms to injectable forms because of the ease of administration. Once a patient achieves pain relief from IV narcotics, the physician usually tries to switch the patient to oral forms. Another approach is to prescribe transdermal fentanyl (see Chapter 68) augmented with oral doses of another drug. This form is effective in providing a constant blood level of drug but is slow to achieve this blood level because it is transdermal.

Patient-Controlled Analgesia

Patient-controlled analgesia (PCA) is a special use of IV narcotics. With PCA, a mechanical pump containing a reservoir of an IV narcotic, usually morphine, is attached to a continuous IV infusion. The patient is given a small control device activated by pressing a button. When the patient is uncomfortable or needs something for pain, the patient pushes the button and a preset dose of the narcotic is infused into the IV line. The pump has controls to set for the minimum time between doses, the maximum number of doses per time period (e.g., 1-hour period), and amount of each dose. The pump may also keep a running record of number of doses used by the patient.

Using PCA has many advantages. The patient controls the frequency of medication administration and does not have to wait for the nurse to prepare and administer a requested dose of medication. Each dose of medication may be low, but the patient can repeat doses within the time limits programmed into the pump. Patients are also given a sense of control over their own pain relief. Currently PCA is widely used for postoperative patients, but it can be used any time IV narcotics are appropriate. The patient in severe pain may be receiving a constant infusion of narcotics, with PCA for breakthrough pain.

Epidural Analgesia

Morphine or other opioids may be administered via epidural catheters. With this approach smaller doses of medication can be used to provide widespread analgesia without motor blockade or excessive central nervous system (CNS) depression. For **epidural analgesia** a catheter is inserted into the thoracic or lumbar epidural space and secured. Intermittent or continuous medication may be administered. Drugs used include morphine, meperidine, fentanyl, or sufentanil (Chapters 31 and 68). A PCA pump may also be attached to allow the patient to control drug delivery. Because of the location of the catheter, it must be inserted by an anesthesiologist or nurse anesthetist.

Assess the patient regularly for side effects and degree of pain relief. Monitor the rate and depth of respirations, pulse oximeter, and degree of sedation. Monitor bladder distension and lower extremity muscle strength.

EMLA for Topical Analgesia

A medication formed from mixing the solid pure bases of lidocaine and prilocaine (eutectic mixture of local anesthetics, or EMLA) is available to provide local anesthesia to the skin before diagnostic tests, venipunctures, or other painful activities. This local anesthetic cream is applied thickly over the prescribed area. The area is then covered with an occlusive dressing and left for an hour or longer. Before the procedure the dressing and cream are removed, and the area is cleaned with an antiseptic solution. Although the agent is applied topically, the same precautions used with injected local anesthetics apply to EMLA.

Special Considerations for the Pediatric Patient

The child may not understand explanations about pain and therapies that are going to be tried. Sometimes the frequent discomfort of repeated tests causes children great distress, and their crying and uncooperative behavior upset the family and the health care team. Other times diagnostic tests or other activities require that the child remain as still as possible for accuracy purposes; however, if the procedure is painful, the child is unlikely to remain still.

TABLE 32-1 Equianalgesic Chart for Opioid Analgesics Commonly Used for Severe Pain

DRUG NAME	EQUIANALGESIC IM DOSE (MG)	EQUIANALGESIC ORAL DOSE (MG)	COMMENTS
Morphine-Like Agonists			
Morphine	10	30 (every 3-4 hr, around the clock) 60 (single dose or intermittent)	Available in sustained-release preparations (MS Contin, Roxanol-SR) and as rectal suppositories.
Codeine	120 (rarely used at this dose)	200 (not recommended)	Doses needed to relieve severe pain may cause nausea, vomiting, severe constipation.
Hydromorphone (Dilaudid)	1.5	7.5	Slightly shorter duration than morphine; available as rectal suppositories.
Levorphanol (Levo-Dromoran)	2	4	Accumulates on days 2-3.
Meperidine (Demerol)	75 (irritating with repeated IM injections)	300 (not recommended)	Normeperidine (toxic metabolite) accumulates with repetitive dosing, causing CNS excitation; avoid in patients with impaired renal function or who are receiving monoamine oxidase inhibitors.
Methadone (Dolophine)	10	20	Accumulates with repetitive dosing and may cause excessive sedation (on days 2-5).
Oxycodone (Roxicodone; also in many combination drugs, e.g., Tylox, Percocet)	Not available	30	
Oxymorphone (Numorphan)	1-1.5	Not available	Available as a rectal suppository; 5 mg rectal suppository = 5 mg morphine IM.
Mixed Agonist: Antagonists			
Butorphanol (Stadol)	2	Not available	Like IM pentazocine.
Dezocine (Dalglan)	10	Not available	Relatively new; not yet classified under Controlled Substances Act.
Nalbuphine (Nubain)	10	Not available	Like IM pentazocine but incidence of psychotomimetic effects lower than with pentazocine.
Pentazocine (Talwin)	60 (irritating to tissues with repeated IM injection)	150-180	Used orally for less severe pain; mixed agonist-antagonists may cause psychotomimetic effects; may precipitate withdrawal in narcotic-dependent patients; contraindicated in myocardial infarction.
Partial Agonist			
Buprenorphine (Buprenex)	0.3-0.4	Not available	Sublingual form not yet in United States; does not produce psychotomimetic effects; may precipitate withdrawal in narcotic-dependent patients.

TABLE 32-2 Comparison Doses of Selected Oral Drugs for Pain

ANALGESIC	ORAL DOSAGE (MG)
Nonopioid Analgesics	
Acetaminophen (Datril, Tylenol)	650-975 (2-3 325 mg tablets)
Aspirin (ASA)	650-975 (2-3 325 mg tablets)
Opioid Analgesics	
Codeine	30-60
Meperidine (Demerol)	50
Hydrocodone (Vicodin, which also contains acetaminophen)	5
Pentazocine (Talwin) (opioid agonist-antagonist)	60
Propoxyphene hydrochloride (Darvon)	65
Propoxyphene napsylate (Darvon-N)	100
Selected Nonsteroidal Antiinflammatory Drugs	
Ibuprofen (Advil, Motrin, others)	200 (superior to ASA in analgesic efficacy at this dose)
Naproxen sodium (Anaprox)	275 (comparable to ASA; 550 is superior)
Indomethacin (Indocin)	25-50 (comparable to ASA)
Ketoprofen (Orudis)	25 (comparable to ASA; 50 superior)
Piroxicam (Feldene)	20 (comparable in efficacy, slower onset, longer duration than ASA)

With children, topical or local anesthetics may be used before painful tests. Oral or IV anxiety-reducing drugs such as benzodiazepines may be given to calm down a child in preparation for procedures. Nitrous oxide or ketamine may be administered (by trained personnel) before procedures. IV drugs for pain may be chosen over intramuscular (IM) or subcutaneous forms to avoid repeated injections. Different routes of administration for drugs may be needed for a child, depending on a child's age.

Special Considerations for the Older Adult Patient

Older adults in pain present special challenges. Since these patients often take many medications for their health problems, the nurse should monitor for drug interactions. Older adults have increased sensitivity to the sedating effects and hypotensive effects of many drugs. In addition, older patients may have diminished liver and/or kidney function, putting them at greater risk for drug toxicity. Finally, although the aging process does not reduce the serum proteins, poor nutrition and chronic disease may contribute to reduced serum albumin, and therefore circulating free-drug levels of protein-bound drugs may be higher, contributing to potential drug toxicity. These factors suggest that frequent assessment, use of lower drug dosages, and less frequent drug administration are appropriate approaches to older adult patients.

Use of Placebos

Occasionally, a physician orders a normal saline injection for a patient in pain. If the patient responds positively to this placebo, the patient may be incorrectly labeled as malingering, or not having real pain, or as addicted to medications. A positive response to a placebo is generally meaningless in the patient with pain because it provides no information about the pain. In addition, it is deceitful to administer a placebo when the patient believes that a different drug is being administered. Placebos are used appropriately in double-blind drug research studies, but in those studies the patient has given informed consent that placebos may be used. For more information about placebos, consult texts about pain and review the American Nurses Association *Code for Nurses.*

Other Drugs Used in Management of the Patient with Pain

Carbamazepine (Chapter 55) is recognized as the drug of choice to treat the pain of trigeminal neuralgia (tic douloureux). Sumatriptan is used in the treatment of migraine headaches. Local anesthetics (Chapter 67) are used to treat many kinds of surface pain. Ergot-derivative containing combination products are used to treat or prevent vascular headaches, including cluster headaches.

Many patients in pain also experience nausea, and antiemetics are often used to control this annoying symptom in patients (see Chapter 25). Some patients in pain have their anxiety treated with an antianxiety agent (Chapter 51). Muscle relaxants may be prescribed to treat muscle spasms (Chapter 58). The antidepressants amitriptyline, doxepin, imipramine, and desipramine may have analgesic properties distinct from their effects on depression. In addition, these drugs may help patients sleep better at night and may reduce anxiety.

PAIN MANAGEMENT PROGRAMS

Sometimes patients do not achieve an acceptable degree of pain relief. These patients may be referred to a pain management program. Pain management programs may be inpatient or outpatient, or comprehensive. There is often a team approach, with physicians, nurses, psychologists, social workers, physical and occupational therapists, rehabilitation counselors, clergy, and others available. The treatment plan may be complex and may include strategies already mentioned and behavioral modification, hypnosis, biofeedback, and acupuncture. Anesthesiologists are available to pain centers to perform nerve blocks, insert spinal catheters, administer intrathecal medications, and so on.

NURSING PROCESS OVERVIEW

The Patient in Pain

Assessment

Perform a complete physical assessment. Monitor vital signs. Observe the behavior and gait of the patient. Use an assessment tool appropriate for the patient and have the patient rate the degree of pain. Obtain the patient's subjective description of pain.

Nursing Diagnoses

- Pain related to (specify)
- Anxiety related to (specify)
- Sleep pattern disturbance related to unrelieved pain

Patient Outcomes

The patient will state that pain is relieved or that the persisting pain is at an acceptable level. The patient will discuss feelings of anxiety and will relate that anxiety is decreased. The patient will state that uninterrupted periods of sleep have increased in length.

Planning/Implementation

Acknowledge that the patient is in pain. Work with the patient to define the goal of pain relief. Combine nursing care measures with drugs or other therapies for pain relief. Present pain relief measures in a positive manner. Administer medications, if prescribed, in doses and frequencies appropriate for the age and condition of the patient and for achieving pain relief. Provide medication to patients in anticipation of painful activities. Anticipate side effects when medications are used and develop interventions to prevent or control them, such as preventing constipation when narcotics are used. Remember that the patient is the greatest authority in the degree of pain the patient has and when pain relief has occurred.

Evaluation

Nursing care of the patient in pain is effective if the patient's pain is relieved to a degree that is satisfactory to the patient. Before discharge, the patients should know how to administer prescribed medications and/or perform other therapies. The patient should know how to treat side effects and when to call the health care team for additional help in pain relief.

CRITICAL THINKING

APPLICATION

1. What are some possible outcomes of unrelieved pain in patients?
2. What are some examples of what pain might mean to a patient?
3. What are some misconceptions the nurse might have about pain? What are misconceptions about pain in children? the older adult?
4. How might a nurse's personal experiences interfere with providing effective pain relief to a patient?
5. What are some objective signs that may indicate that a patient is in pain?
6. What are some subjective signs of pain in a patient?
7. Give examples of tools used for assessing a patient's pain.
8. Give examples of possible nursing diagnoses that might be seen in patients with pain.
9. How does patient education play a role in helping a patient in pain?
10. What groups of drugs are used for pain relief (see also Chapters 30 and 31)?
11. What is EMLA, and when is it used?
12. What is PCA, and when is it used? What are the advantages and disadvantages of PCA?
13. Describe special considerations for pediatric patients or older adult patients.
14. Discuss reasons against the use of placebos except in formal drug testing protocols.
15. Why would antidepressants be used for patients in pain?

CRITICAL THINKING

1. Compare and contrast oral, transdermal, intramuscular or subcutaneous, intravenous, and epidural administration of drugs. Consider the following: ease of administration; ease of preparing the correct dose; speed of achieving therapeutic serum drug levels; degree of sedation; kinds of side effects; ease of self management at home.
2. What is epidural analgesia? What are the advantages and disadvantages of this approach? Is it used in your local agencies? Are there agency protocols in place?
3. Compare and contrast the cost of PCA and epidural analgesia. (Call your local pharmacist and/or hospital for cost information.)
4. Compare and contrast the cost of the following: aspirin, acetaminophen, an NSAID (pick any one), oral and IV morphine, transdermal and epidural fentanyl.

SECTION IX

Drugs Affecting the Immune System

This section presents the pharmacology of the immune system. Chapter 33, *Basic Function of the Immune System,* reviews the immune system so that the rationale for pharmacologic intervention can be understood. Chapter 34, *Immunization,* covers vaccines, immune serum, and antibodies available to prevent or to treat selected infections. Chapter 35 discusses immunomodulators and the care of the patient with altered immune function. Chapter 36 reviews the use of glucocorticoids for the treatment of inflammatory states. Chapter 37 discusses drug therapy to control selected autoimmune diseases.

CHAPTER 33

Basic Function of the Immune System

OBJECTIVES

After studying this chapter, you should be able to do the following:

- *Discuss the organs and cells of the immune system.*
- *Discuss the general function of cytokines.*
- *Describe the classes of immunoglobulins.*
- *Describe the uses of colony-stimulating factors.*

CHAPTER OVERVIEW

The immune system allows us to live safely in a world full of dangerous organisms that could invade the body and cause disease. This chapter describes the components of the immune system. Understanding the function and regulation of the various cells and organs in the immune system creates a foundation for understanding how medical manipulations can influence this vital body system.

KEY TERMS

acquired immunity
antibodies
antigen
antigen-presenting cells
colony-stimulating factors
cytokines
gammopathies
immunoglobulins
innate immunity
interferon γ (IFN-γ)
interleukins
lymphocytes
phagocytosis
primary immune deficiencies
secondary immune deficiencies
tumor necrosis factor (TNF)

IMMUNE SYSTEM

The immune system is a complex and diffuse system that is present throughout the body. It protects the body from damage caused by foreign environmental agents. Foreign agents include invading microorganisms such as bacteria, fungi, parasites, and viruses, as well as foreign tissue such as transplanted kidneys, hearts, and livers. Any foreign agent capable of inducing an immune response is termed an **antigen.** The immune system also protects the body, ridding it of malignant cells as they arise and preventing it from acting against its own tissues. Like all other body systems, the immune system can exhibit pathology and abnormal responses.

Innate and Acquired Immunity

Immunity is innate or acquired. **Innate immunity** is derived from all elements with which a person is born and that are always available on short notice to protect the body from challenges by foreign materials. Innate immunity is conferred by physical, cellular, and chemical barriers. Physical barriers include skin, mucous membranes, and the cough reflex. Phagocytic cells make up the cellular barrier. **Phagocytosis** is ingestion and destruction of foreign particles such as bacteria by individual cells of the immune system. Biologically active substances that include degradative enzymes, toxic free radicals, lipids, and low pH are chemical barriers to invasion by foreign agents.

Acquired immunity is not present at birth but develops as the individual grows and matures. Although a person has the capacity at birth for developing acquired immunity, this immunity is not exhibited until the person has had two sequential exposures to the same foreign agent. Acquired immunity has two main arms, the humoral and the cellular immune response. Humoral immunity involves production of **antibodies,** which are soluble proteins present in normal serum. Cellular immunity consists of responses such as the delayed type of hypersensitivity, which are mediated by cells rather than by soluble substances. **Lymphocytes** are the main providers of acquired immunity.

Organs and Cells of the Immune System

The immune system is comprised of six white blood cell types: lymphocytes, monocytes and macrophages, polymorphonuclear neutrophil leukocytes (PMNs), basophils, mast cells, and eosinophils. All these, as well as red blood cells and platelets, are derived from a common precursor cell type found in the bone marrow. This precursor cell type is the stem cell.

Monocytes and macrophages represent different states of cell maturation. Monocytes circulate freely within the body; with differentiation, they become macrophages. Macrophages may be fixed within the tissues, where they may persist for years; some, however, recirculate through secondary lymphoid organs. Fixed or recirculating macrophages can assist lymphocytes in generating immune responses and can phagocytize foreign particles. Macrophages can become activated to kill tumor cells.

Lymphocytes are subdivided into the thymus-derived cells or T cells and the bone marrow–derived cells or B cells. The B lymphocytes produce antibodies. T lymphocytes are further subdivided into helper T cells and cytotoxic T cells. Helper T cells assist B cells in responding to an antigen and mediate the delayed type of hypersensitivity. Cytotoxic T cells reject grafts and destroy virus-infected cells. The ratio of helper cells to cytotoxic cells normally ranges from 1.2:1 to 2:1. In the acquired immunodeficiency syndrome (AIDS), this ratio is usually reversed and can be as low as 0.2 (1:5).

PMNs are the predominant phagocytes within the circulation. They are usually the first cells to arrive at the site of an infection. Beside phagocytosis, the PMNs have two other means of killing foreign invaders. The oxidative burst of the PMNs leads to release of superoxide dismutase and hydrogen peroxide. Antimicrobial substances including lysozyme, lactoferrin, cathepsin G, and defensins are contained within azurophil granules and are released on activation of the PMNs.

Basophils participate in allergic and inflammatory responses. These cells contain densely staining granules in their cytoplasm. Within these granules are mediators of allergic and inflammatory responses such as histamine, complement components, and leukotrienes C and D. Degranulation occurs when antigen interacts with immunoglobulin E (IgE) molecules bound to the cell surface of the basophil.

Eosinophils participate in allergic reactions but also kill parasites. Contained within the cytoplasmic granules of the eosinophil are some of the same mediators found in basophil granules, such as leukotrienes C and D, and a number of proteins toxic to parasites. Eosinophils can also cause histamine to be released from mast cells and basophils. Eosinophils are also phagocytic, but their role as phagocytes is not as important as is that of the PMNs.

In addition to these circulating white blood cells, mast cells are also important in immunity and especially in certain pathologic disorders. Like basophils, mast cells can participate in allergic reactions and inflammation and are thought to affect asthma. Mast cell granules contain histamine and a number of protease enzymes. Like basophils, mast cells can also synthesize leukotrienes C and D, as well as prostaglandin D_2. Also like basophils, mast cells degranulate when antigen interacts with IgE molecules bound to the cell surface. High numbers of mast cells can be found in the skin, lung, and intestinal mucosa. Subtypes of mast cells have been classified based on the types of proteases found within their granules. The tryptase-containing, or mucosal, mast cells are mainly located in mucosal areas as the name implies. Tryptase-chymase–containing, or connective tissue, mast cells are found in the skin. The connective tissue subtype contains more histamine than the mucosal variety. Depending on the microenvironment, mast cells can interconvert.

Organs of the immune system are classified as primary or secondary. The primary lymphoid organs are the thymus and the bone marrow. Maturation of lymphocytes occurs in these structures. The spleen, lymph nodes, and Peyer's patches are the secondary lymphoid organs. Peyer's patches are clusters of lymphocytes spread throughout the lining of the intestinal wall, tonsils, and appendix. Secondary lymphoid tissues trap and concentrate foreign substances and are the main sites of antibody production and generation of antigen-specific T lymphocytes.

IMMUNE RESPONSES

Antigen-Presenting Cells

Generation of humoral or cellular immunity requires (1) activation, (2) proliferation, and (3) differentiation. Activation of T lymphocytes requires that antigen be processed and presented by specialized cells called **antigen-presenting cells.** The antigen-presenting cells also secrete soluble factors necessary for the proliferation of T cells. The major antigen-presenting cells are monocytes and macrophages. Other cells that can also present antigen include dermal Langerhans' cells, dendritic cells in various locations, and hepatic Kupffer's cells. The antigen-presenting cells take up antigen, process it, and then express it on the cell surface with histocompatibility antigens. T lymphocytes are activated by interaction with this complex of processed and histocompatibility antigen on the surface of the antigen-presenting cells. B lymphocytes are activated by interacting directly with unprocessed antigen via antibody molecules on their surface.

Major Histocompatibility Complex

The major histocompatibility complex (MHC) refers to the genes encoding the molecules that allow the immune system to differentiate self from non-self. Knowledge of the MHC arose from studies of why transplanted tissues are rejected. In humans, MHC is also referred to as HLA for human leukocyte antigen genes. Two classes of MHC gene products play a major role in activation of T cells. Although antigens interact directly with antibody bound to B cells to activate B cells, a T cell receptor must have antigen bound to a MHC class I or class II molecule on another cell, an antigen-presenting cell. The antigen-presenting cell must internalize the antigen, digest it, and process it to peptides that become associated with an MHC molecule and transported in this complex to the cell surface. All nucleated cells have class I MHC. Class II MHC molecules are found primarily on B cells, Langerhans' cells, and dendritic cells. However, endothelial, synovial, and glial cells can present antigen.

T-Cell Subsets

T cells differentiate into two major subsets. The subset of T cells referred to as cytoxic T (T_C) cells are primarily characterized by a surface molecule, CD8. A T_C cell recognizes a cell presenting a foreign antigen by class I MHC molecule on the cell's surface. The T_C cell kills that cell. This is particularly effective in destroying cells infected by viruses or foreign tissue grafts. The subset called helper T (T_H) cells, are distinguished by a surface molecule, CD4. One type of T_H cells, T_{H1} cells, stimulates a macrophage that has ingested a microbe to kill the microbe. Another type of T_H cells, T_{H2} cells, are able to select out B cells with MHC class II molecules presenting an antigen. The T_{H2} cells direct those B cells to make antibodies to the presented antigen.

Activated T and B Cells

Once activated, T and B lymphocytes express receptors for growth factors synthesized and released primarily by activated helper T cells. In response to these growth factors the T and B cells proliferate. Having undergone proliferation, B and T cells can then respond to other soluble mediators secreted by activated helper T cells and will differentiate into functional effector cells. B lymphocytes differentiate into antibody-secreting plasma cells. T lymphocytes differentiate into cells capable of mediating a delayed type of hypersensitivity or killing virus-infected cells. Generation of humoral and cellular immune responses is summarized in Figure 33-1.

Cytokines

Communication within the immune system occurs mainly through release of soluble factors called **cytokines.** Cytokines are primarily released as a means of one immune cell influencing another immune cell. Cytokines are very important in controlling the development of the immune response. Many cytokines have more than one action, and more than one cytokine may be produced depending on the cell type. The result is a complex repertoire for the modulation of the immune response.

The names and major actions of the better characterized cytokines are summarized in Table 33-1. The genes for most of these cytokines have been cloned so that they can be produced outside the body in large amounts. These recombinant DNA techniques have made using those factors in clinical trials in humans possible. **Interleukins** are a diverse series of cytokines allowing one type of leukocyte to influence the function of other leukocytes. Some of these mediators can act on or be produced by cells outside of the immune system. **Tumor necrosis factor** (**TNF**) is the principal mediator produced in response to gram-negative bacteria. TNF is a mediator of both natural and acquired immunity and is also an important link between specific immune responses and acute inflammation. Overproduction of TNF leads to shock. **Interferon γ (IFN-γ)** is produced mainly by activated T cells. IFN-γ activates other immune cells and promotes inflammation. **Colony-stimulating factors** control the differentiation of hematopoietic stem cells to produce new leukocytes. Table 33-2 summarizes the major colony-stimulating factors and the cells that develop from their action. The development of some immune cells can be directed by more than one of these factors.

Antibodies, the soluble mediators of humoral immunity, are specialized proteins called **immunoglobulins.** There are five classes of immunoglobulins: IgM, IgG, IgA, IgE, and IgD (Table 33-3). The immunoglobulin molecule is comprised of two light chains and two heavy chains. Figure 33-2 is a schematic diagram of an antibody molecule.

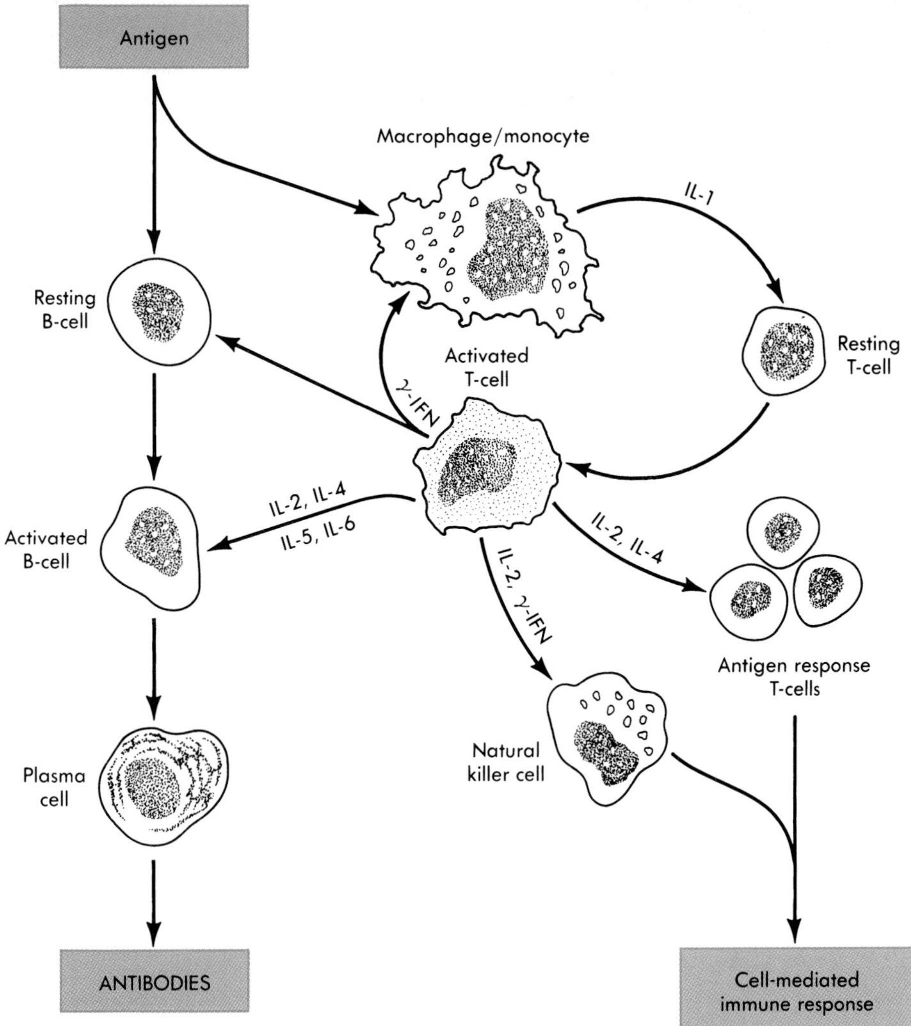

FIGURE 33-1
Generation of immune response. Key features of immune reaction include factors responsible for humoral immunity (shown on left) and factors responsible for delayed, cell-mediated immunity (shown on right).

The light chain is made up of a variable region (V) and a constant region (C). Heavy chains contain three or four constant regions and the variable region. Each variable portion of the immunoglobulin molecule includes three hypervariable regions, which vary widely in amino acid composition. The combination of these hypervariable regions makes up the antibody-combining site of the immunoglobulin molecule. This portion of the molecule binds the antigen against which the antibody was generated. Each antibody molecule has two combining sites. Five different constant regions define the major immunoglobulin classes. IgG is the major immunoglobulin in serum and has four subclasses. Two subclasses of IgA molecules exist. IgG, IgE, and IgD are monomeric, each composed of one antibody molecule. IgM is composed of five antibody molecules, and IgA is composed of two. A protein, the J chain, joins the five basic molecules that make up the IgM molecule. Secretory component, synthesized by epithelial cells, connects the two IgA molecules that compose the dimer. Table 33-3 summarizes the immunoglobulin classes and their functions.

Complement System

The complement system is a group of enzymes found in serum that work together to "complement" the action of antibodies in destroying microorganisms. The major functions of the complement system include mediating inflammatory responses and opsonization, or coating, of antigenic particles (including microorganisms), which causes damage to the membrane of the microorganism and often results in lysis of the microorganism. Nineteen distinct proteins make up the complement system. Proteins of the complement system interact such that the products of one reaction form the enzyme needed for the next step in the enzyme cascade. A

TABLE 33-1 Properties of Human Cytokines

CYTOKINE	BIOLOGIC PROPERTIES
Interleukin-1 (IL-1)	Activates resting T cells; is cofactor for hemopoietic growth factors; stimulates synthesis of cytokines; increases natural killer cell activity; chemotaxin for neutrophils, lymphocytes, and macrophages.
Interleukin-2 (IL-2)	Growth factor for activated T cells; induces cytokine production by T cells; activates cytotoxic T cells; increases natural killer cell activity; induces lymphokine-activated killer cells.
Interleukin-3 (IL-3)	Supports growth of pluripotent bone marrow stem cells; growth factor for mast cells.
Interleukin-4 (IL-4)	Growth factor for activated B cells; induces class II histocompatibility antigens on B cells; growth factor for T cells; growth factor for mast cells; induces IgE synthesis.
Interleukin-5 (IL-5)	Induces differentiation of eosinophils; increases IgM and IgG secretion by activated B cells.
Interleukin-6 (IL-6)	Induces differentiation of activated B cells into plasma cells; with IL-1 activates T cells.
Interleukin-7 (IL-7)	Induces proliferation of immature lymphoid cells; cofactor for T-cell growth with IL-2; induces lymphokine-activated killer cells.
Interleukin-8 (IL-8)	Chemoattraction and activation of PMNs; weak chemoattraction and activation of basophils.
Interleukin-9 (IL-9)	Enhances proliferation of IL-3–dependent mast cells; promotes survival of mast cells; growth factor for T cells.
Interleukin-10 (IL-10)	Inhibits production of IFN-γ and other cytokines by T cells; inhibits production of cytokines by monocytes; cofactor for T-cell growth; cofactor for mast cell growth.
Interferon γ (IFN-γ)	Exerts antiviral activity; induces expression of class II histocompatibility antigens on macrophages; decreases IgE synthesis by B cells; increases natural killer cell activity.
Tumor necrosis factor (TNF)	Directly cytotoxic to some tumor cells; stimulates synthesis of cytokines; activates macrophages; mediates inflammation and septic shock.
Granulocyte-macrophage colony-stimulating factor (GM-CSF)	Stimulates growth of trilineage bone marrow progenitors; inhibits migration of PMNs; induces TNF and IL-1 production by monocytes and macrophages; enhances PMNs, eosinophil, and monocyte- and macrophage-mediated antibody-dependent cellular cytotoxicity.

TABLE 33-2 Colony-Stimulating Factors

FACTOR	PRODUCED BY	COLONY-STIMULATING ACTIVITY
Granulocyte-macrophage colony-stimulating factor (GM-CSF)	T cells; macrophages; fibroblasts; endothelial cells; keratinocytes; thymic epithelium; mesothelium; and uroepithelium	Stimulates colonies of PMNs, monocytes and macrophages, and eosinophils from trilineage bone marrow progenitors.
Granulocyte colony-stimulating factor (G-CSF)	Monocytes; macrophages; fibroblasts; endothelial cells; keratinocytes; thymic epithelium; mesothelium; and uroepithelium	Stimulates colonies of PMNs from trilineage bone marrow progenitors; stimulates early pluripotent stem cells to accelerate entry into the cell cycle; synergizes with IL-3 to support proliferation of early pluripotent stem cells.
Macrophage colony-stimulating factor (M-CSF)	Monocytes; fibroblasts; and endothelial cells	Stimulates colonies of monocyte and macrophage precursors.
Interleukin-3 (IL-3)	T cells and mast cells	Stimulates colonies of pluripotent stem cells; promotes proliferation and maturation of committed granulocyte and macrophage, eosinophil, and basophil progenitors.
Interleukin-5 (IL-5)	T cells and mast cells	Promotes growth and differentiation of eosinophil progenitors.

TABLE 33-3 Major Classes of Immunoglobulins

CLASS	DISTRIBUTION	BIOLOGIC PROPERTIES
IgG	Intravascular and extravascular	Majority of secondary response to most antigens; activation of complement, opsonin; sensitizes target cells for destruction by killer cells; neutralization of toxins and viruses; can pass placenta; immobilization of bacteria.
IgM	Mostly intravascular	First class produced during primary immune response; activates complement well; efficient agglutinating antibodies; natural isohemagglutinins.
IgA	Intravascular and secretions	Most common antibody in secretions, where it protects mucous membranes; bactericidal in presence of lysozyme; efficient antiviral antibody.
IgE	On basophils and mast cells; in saliva and nasal secretions	Mediates hypersensitivity and allergic reactions; protects against parasite infections.
IgD	On surface of B lymphocytes; trace in serum	Serves as antigen-specific receptor on B cells; may be involved in differentiation of B lymphocytes.

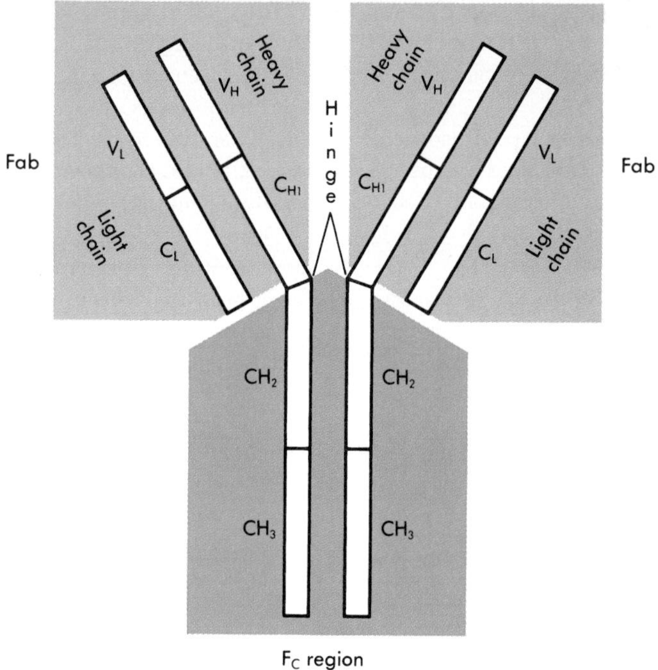

FIGURE 33-2
Schematic diagram of antibody molecule. Heavy and light chains composed of variable (V_H, V_L) regions and constant (C_H, C_L) regions. The Fab portions of molecule are responsible for antigen binding, and F_C portion mediates biologic activity.

small stimulus can be amplified to activate large amounts of complement.

Complement can be activated by the classic and the alternate pathway. The pathways share many components but differ in the ways they become activated. The classic pathway is activated by antigen-antibody complexes. The alternate pathway is activated by suitable surfaces or molecules, including cell walls of some bacteria, cell walls of yeast, endotoxin derived from cell walls of gram-negative bacteria, and aggregated IgA. Several steps in the complement cascade result in the release of a fragment of some of the proteins of the complement system. These small molecules are very potent mediators of a number of reactions. C3a and C5a are chemotaxins and anaphylatoxins. Chemotaxins cause phagocytic cells to migrate from an area where there is less chemotaxin to an area of higher concentration. Anaphylatoxins cause mast cell degranulation, smooth muscle contraction, and increased capillary permeability. C3b opsonizes anything to which it binds. C3b and C5b activate the lytic pathway, leading to the formation of the membrane attack complex, a series of proteins with detergent properties that produce "holes" in the target cell membrane, resulting in lysis of the target cell.

IMMUNE SYSTEM DISORDERS AND PATHOLOGY

The immune system is tightly regulated to ensure optimal function. Disorders in the development of immune cells during the generation of immune responses or in the synthesis of the products of the immune system may cause immunologic disorders ranging in severity from mild to fatal. The disorders can be classified into deficiencies of immune cells or their soluble products and overproduction of immune cells or their products. Immune deficiencies are primary or secondary. **Primary immune deficiencies** are diseases in which the immune deficiency is the cause of the disease; they may be hereditary or acquired. Secondary immune deficiencies result from diseases. Patients with secondary immune deficiencies invariably suffer from recurrent infections; this development often leads to the diagnosis of an immune deficiency.

Primary Immune Deficiencies

B-cell deficiencies can result in the absence of one or all immunoglobulin classes. Persons with B-cell deficiencies suffer mainly from recurrent bacterial infections. Although immunoglobulin replacement therapy may maintain them for as long as 20 to 30 years, the prognosis is poor, and many succumb to chronic lung disease.

T-cell deficiencies affect not only cell-mediated immune responses but also synthesis of antibody since T cells are necessary for most antibody responses. Patients with T-cell disorders are extremely susceptible to fungal, viral, and protozoal infections.

Severe combined immunodeficiencies result from defects in both T and B cells. These disorders are very serious. Untreated infants rarely survive beyond 1 year of age. Patients with combined immunodeficiencies are susceptible to every type of infection. Treatment with drugs alone is ineffective. Infants can be cured by bone marrow transplantation, provided the transplantation is done before irreversible complications of the disease arise.

Phagocytic cell dysfunctions also cause severe disorders because these cells affect both innate and acquired immunity. Defects may result from deficiencies of antibody, lymphokines, or complement deficiencies and can also result from cell defects.

Abnormalities in the complement system can lead to immunodeficiencies. Genetic defects affecting nearly all the individual components of the complement system have been documented.

Secondary Immune Deficiencies

Secondary immune deficiencies occur as complications of other diseases. The most common cause of these disorders is the deliberate immune suppression associated with the use of chemotherapeutic agents in cancer treatment or the immunosuppressive drugs used to prevent rejection of transplanted organs. The best known secondary immune deficiency is AIDS. This disease is caused by infection with human lymphotropic virus III, now called *human immunodeficiency virus* (HIV). The immune deficiency associated with AIDS is largely caused by the loss of helper T cells. These cells are not the only immune cells affected by the virus since the profound immune suppression associated with AIDS cannot be explained only on the basis of loss of helper T cells. Patients with secondary immune deficiencies suffer severe recurrent infections by opportunistic organisms normally not pathogenic.

Autoimmune Diseases

Sometimes the immune system manufactures T cells and antibodies directed against the body's own cells. These T cells and autoantibodies contribute to such diseases as diabetes, rheumatoid arthritis, systemic lupus erythematosus, myasthenia gravis, multiple sclerosis, and Graves' disease (hyperthyroidism). The therapy of selected autoimmune diseases is presented in Chapter 37.

Gammopathies

Several neoplastic diseases arise from abnormal proliferation of B cells and plasma cells. These diseases are termed **gammopathies.** The principal gammopathies are multiple myeloma, macroglobulinemia, and heavy chain disease.

Multiple myeloma is the most common of the gammopathies, resulting from the malignant proliferation of plasma cells. It is characterized by synthesis of large amounts of a given isotype of immunoglobulin and may be accompanied by the production of free light chains (called *Bence Jones proteins*). Multiple myeloma involves multiple organ systems, resulting from infiltration of them by malignant plasma cells. Patients are susceptible to recurrent bacterial and viral infections because of suppression of the synthesis of normal antibodies.

Macroglobulinemia occurs because of synthesis of large amounts of IgM. The excess immunoglobulin leads to increased viscosity of serum, which leads to decreased blood flow, thrombosis, disorders of the central nervous system (CNS), and bleeding. Decreased synthesis of the other immunoglobulin classes is observed, leading ultimately to hypogammaglobulinemia.

Heavy chain disease is characterized by the appearance of large amounts of protein in the serum and urine resembling the Fc portion of the immunoglobulin molecule. This disorder is uncommon. Patients have recurrent bacterial infections, anemias, and enlarged lymphoid organs.

CRITICAL THINKING

APPLICATION

1. What is innate immunity?
2. Define acquired immunity.
3. What are the forms of acquired immunity?
4. What white blood cell types are responsible for phagocytosis?
5. What are T cells? Where are they formed?
6. What are B cells? Where are they formed?
7. What cell type forms antibodies?
8. What cell type produces the delayed type of hypersensitivity?
9. What are interleukins?
10. What are the five classes of antibodies?
11. What are the primary functions of each class of antibody?
12. What is the complement system?
13. What are the two major functions of the complement system?
14. Define primary and secondary immune deficiency.
15. Define gammopathy.

CRITICAL THINKING

1. How does measurement of T cells and B cells provide information about the immune system?
2. How does analysis of a patient's white blood cell differential provide information about the bone marrow, possible infections, and immune status? What does a "shift to the left" mean?
3. Why is AIDS described as a "secondary immune deficiency?"
4. How does information about immunoglobulins relate to allergic reactions to drugs (see Chapter 1 also)?

CHAPTER 34

Immunization

OBJECTIVES

After studying this chapter, you should be able to do the following:

- *Discuss the difference between passive and active immunity.*
- *Develop a nursing care plan for the patient receiving an immunostimulant.*

CHAPTER OVERVIEW

Immunization, a way of modulating the action of the immune system to medical advantage, has been known for a long time. Other ways to alter function of the immune system have been more difficult to develop; only recently have new approaches become available. This chapter describes the classic immunostimulants used for immunization.

KEY TERMS

immunization
immunostimulation
vaccines

Therapeutic Rationale: Immunostimulants

Immunostimulation refers to the activation of T cells and B cells by an antigen. Once an antigen activates the immune system, some of the T cells and B cells become memory cells. The next time that antigen is encountered, the immune system can mount an active and vigorous response.

Immunity varies in its duration and effectiveness depending on how it was acquired. The fetus is protected from bacterial and viral infections and from microbial toxins by maternal immunoglobulin G (IgG) antibodies, which pass to the fetus through the placenta to confer passive immunity. IgG is the only antibody that can cross the placenta. Newborn infants do not have a fully functional immune system; human milk, however, contains factors that aid the newborn response against infectious agents. Some of these factors enhance the growth of beneficial intestinal flora, and others nonspecifically inhibit the growth of harmful microorganisms. The inhibitory factors include lysozyme, lactoferrin, interferon, and leukocytes. Antibodies are also found in breast milk and are especially abundant in colostrum (first milk).

A number of infectious diseases are almost completely preventable through routine childhood immunizations. The recommended childhood immunization schedule in the United States begins when the infant is 2 months of age and can mount an effective immune response on its own. Table 34-1 indicates the recommended schedule for active immunization throughout life. Recommended childhood immunizations include hepatitis B (HB-1); diphtheria, tetanus, and pertussis (DTP); *Haemophilus influenzae* type b (Hib); poliovirus (OPV); and measles, mumps, and rubella (MMR). Immunizations are recommended for adults as well. MMR, if there is no history of disease or active immunization, and tetanus boosters every 10 years are recommended. Adults over 65 years are advised to have an annual influenza vaccination and a pneumococcal vaccination.

Special immunizations are recommended for those at specific risk, as for cholera, meningococcal meningitis, plague, rabies, typhoid, or yellow fever.

Therapeutic Agents: Vaccines, Immune Serum, and Antibodies

Agents for Active Immunity

Mechanism of Action

Active acquired immunity involves **immunization,** administration of substances such as **vaccines** that stimulate the immune system to respond against a foreign material. Vaccines usually contain killed or attenuated bacteria or viruses, but protection can also be conferred with immunogenic proteins (toxoids) from the pathogen in question (Tables 34-2 and 34-3). Once the immune response has occurred, specific cells in the immune system "remember" the response, and a secondary immune response occurs rapidly on a subsequent encounter with the antigen. This principle is illustrated in Figure 34-1. Active immunity usually persists for years.

Pharmacokinetics

Vaccines are administered by either intramuscular (IM) or subcutaneous injection. Oral polio vaccine and an oral typhoid vaccine are exceptions. Duration of protection is usually from 1 to 10 years. Since vaccines stimulate the immune system to respond actively rather than passively, protection persists after the injected agent has disappeared. The fate of vaccines is similar to that of immune globulins. Since vaccines are antigens and not antibodies, they are taken up and processed by antigen-presenting cells (see Chapter 33) for the generation of immune responses. Some of the injected agent is metabolized in this manner. Once antibodies have been produced, any remaining injected material can be complexed with the antibodies and cleared by phagocytes.

TABLE 34-1 Active Immunization Schedule Recommended in United States

AGE	VACCINE
2 mo	DTP-1, HB-1,* OPV-1, Hib-1
4 mo	DTP-2, HB-2, OPV-2, Hib-2
6 mo	DTP-3, OPV-3, Hib-3
6-18 mo	(OPV-3), HB-3
12-15 mo	MMR-1, Hib-4
15 mo	DTP-4 or DTaP
4-6 yr	DTP-5 or DTaP, MMR-2
14-16 yr	Td, (MMR-2)
18-24 yr	MMR if not previously administered
25-64 yr	MMR if not previously administered and no childhood history of the disease; Td every 10 years
65 yr and older	Annual influenza vaccination; single pneumococcal polysaccharide vaccination; Td every 10 years

DTP, Diphtheria, tetanus, and pertussis vaccine; *DTaP,* diphtheria and tetanus toxoids and acellular pertussis vaccine; *HB,* hepatitis B; *, begin within 12 hours of birth if mother is positive for hepatitis B; *OPV,* oral polio vaccine (poliovirus vaccine live oral trivalent); *Hib, Haemophilus influenzae* b conjugate vaccine; *MMR,* measles, mumps, rubella virus live vaccine; *Td,* tetanus and diphtheria toxoids adsorbed for human use.

TABLE 34-2 Vaccines to Prevent Bacterial and Rickettsial Diseases

DISEASE	VACCINE CHARACTERISTICS	VACCINE ADMINISTRATION
Bubonic plague	Inactivated *Yersinia pestis* confers immunity.	Administered during outbreaks or to persons heavily exposed.
Cholera	Killed strains of *Vibrio cholerae* confer resistance.	Used in persons entering a country where cholera exists.
Diphtheria, tetanus, and pertussis (whooping cough)	This combination, known as *DTP,* contains absorbed toxoids and vaccine to protect against all three diseases.	Given routinely to children between ages of 2 mo and 7 yr. In event of injury, additional protection against tetanus may be needed.
Haemophilus influenzae type B	Based on polysaccharide from the organism.	Recommended for all children 2 yr or older.
Meningitis	Meningococcal polysaccharide mixtures give protection against group A, group C, or both.	Used only in outbreaks or in exposed persons who also receive antibiotics to protect against infections by serogroup B.
Plague	Killed *Yersinia pestis* after cultivation on special media; requires 3 doses and boosters at 6 mo to 2 yr intervals.	Recommended for personnel in aerosol experimentation; those in contact with fleas and rodents; or those in plague areas.
Pneumococcal pneumonia	Mixed capsular material from cultured pneumococci confers resistance to lobar pneumonia and bacteremia caused by one of strains used as source of capsular material.	Given only to high-risk patients, weak convalescents, or patients >50 yr.
Tetanus and diphtheria	Mixed absorbed toxoids are used in patients >6 yr.	Used for routine prophylaxis in patients who have not received DTP.
Tetanus toxoid	Absorbed tetanus toxoid confers immunity.	May be used for routine immunization, but DTP is preferred. Most commonly given after injury that poses risk of tetanus infection.
Tuberculosis	Attenuated strain of *Mycobacterium bovis* confers variable temporary immunity.	Given to exposed but uninfected patients who cannot receive drug therapy.
Typhoid	Killed *Salmonella typhosa* gives prolonged protection.	Used in exposed persons or persons traveling where typhoid is endemic.
Typhus	Killed *Rickettsia prowazekii* confers resistance.	Given to persons traveling to areas where exposure to louse-borne disease is likely.

TABLE 34-3 Vaccines to Prevent Viral Diseases

DISEASE	CHARACTERISTICS OF VACCINE
Hepatitis A	Inactivated hepatitis A virus.
Hepatitis B	Developed from surface antigens of hepatitis B virus.
Influenza	Inactivated viruses of types causing recent outbreaks are used; vaccine differs yearly.
Measles (rubeola)	Attenuated live virus vaccine stimulates protective antibodies in 95% of children receiving vaccine.
Mumps	Attenuated live virus vaccine stimulates protective antibodies in 95% of children receiving vaccine.
Poliomyelitis	Oral vaccine containing attenuated live poliovirus mimics natural form of disease without risk of central nervous system involvement.
Rabies	Killed, fixed virus confers resistance to most patients exposed to infection; a newer inactivated, adsorbed virus vaccine is also available.
Rubella (German measles)	Attenuated live rubella vaccine confers long-term resistance.
Varicella (chickenpox)	Live attenuated virus; duration of resistance not yet known.
Yellow fever	Live attenuated virus confers resistance to most persons receiving vaccine.

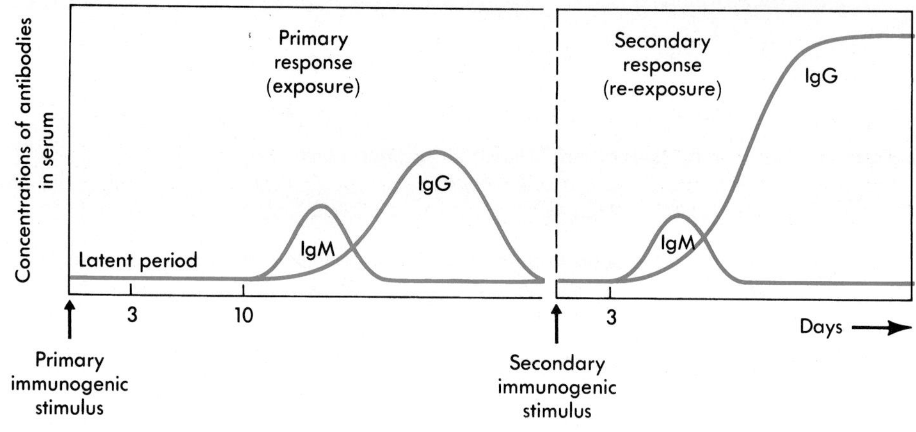

FIGURE 34-1
Time course of antibody release on first exposure vs. subsequent exposure.

Uses

A number of infectious diseases are almost completely preventable through routine childhood immunizations. These include diphtheria, pertussis (whooping cough), tetanus, poliomyelitis, *H. influenzae* type b infection, measles, mumps, and rubella. In adults, pneumococcal vaccine should be administered at least once and influenza vaccine annually to all persons aged 65 years and older. Hepatitis B vaccine should be offered to homosexually active men, intravenous drug users, and others at high risk for infection. All adults should receive tetanus-diphtheria toxoid boosters at least once every 10 years. Vaccination against measles and mumps should be provided to all adults who lack evidence of immunity. Women of childbearing age who do not have rubella immunity should be immunized when they are not pregnant, preferably during the immediate postpartum period.

Currently available agents are included in Table 34-4. Postexposure prophylaxis should be provided with exposures to *H. influenzae* type b, meningococcal infection, hepatitis A, hepatitis B, tuberculosis, and rabies.

Adverse Reactions and Contraindications

Live virus vaccines should not be used in patients receiving immunosuppressive therapy since these vaccines can cause progressive disease in immunocompromised patients. Live virus vaccines are also contraindicated in pregnant women because live virus vaccines can damage the fetus.

Interactions

All immunosuppressive agents can interfere with the generation of active immunity induced by vaccines and toxoids. Corticosteroids, azathioprine, cyclosporine, and some agents used in cancer chemotherapy fall in this category.

Agents for Passive Immunity

Mechanism of Action

Passive acquired immunity involves administration of preformed substances such as immune serum or antibodies that can immediately combine with the foreign agent to which they are directed. Antivenins and antitoxins are prepared from the serum of horses inoculated with the toxin. The passive immunity conferred by immune sera, antibodies, or globulins lasts only weeks.

Pharmacokinetics

IM injection is the usual route of administration of the immune serums and globulins. Oral administration is not usually possible with these agents since the degradative processes in the digestive tract would render them inactive before they could be absorbed. Distribution is fairly rapid after IM injection, but if very rapid therapy is required, these agents can be given intravenously, resulting in immediate distribution. The immunity provided by immune globulins and serums lasts from 1 to 6 weeks. Once injected, the antibodies interact with the entire organism against which they were generated, thus facilitating phagocytosis of the organism by monocytes or macrophages and polymorphonuclear neutrophil leukocytes (PMNs). Antibodies made against toxins of pathogenic microorganisms form complexes with the toxin, and these immune complexes are also cleared by phagocytes. Immunity is lost when the injected antibodies have been cleared from the system.

Uses

Antiserums and immune globulins are used prophylactically and therapeutically to provide temporary immunity against infectious agents, microbial exotoxins, and snake and insect venoms. Examples are antivenins for poisonous bites of snakes and spiders; antitoxins for botulism, diphtheria, and tetanus; and special immune globulin preparations for treatment of tetanus and rabies.

Adverse Reactions and Contraindications

Many side effects of immune serum or globulin injections are dose related. Patients may have pain at the injection site, mild

TABLE 34-4 Agents for Active and Passive Immunity

GENERIC/TRADE NAME	ROUTE	DURATION OF EFFECT	CONTRAINDICATIONS
Antivenin (North American Coral Snake)	INTRAVENOUS: *Adults and children*—IV drip of 250-500 ml with 3-5 vials of antivenin (30-50 ml) added to tubing or reservoir.	Days	After first 1 or 2 ml, administered over 3-5 min; observe for anaphylactic reaction before proceeding.
Antivenin (Crotalidae) polyvalent	INTRAVENOUS: *Adults and children*—dose is based on extent of envenomation; see manufacturer's literature; most effective when given within 4 hr of bite.	Days	Severe hypersensitivity to equine serum.
Bacille Calmette-Guérin (BCG) vaccine	PERCUTANEOUS: *Children with negative tuberculin skin tests, for active immunization against tuberculosis*—see manufacturer's instructions.		Not for individuals with impaired immune response caused by congenital immunodeficiency, Hib infection, leukemia, lymphoma, or generalized malignancy; not for patients taking immunosuppressive agents; not for pregnant women or patients with extensive skin infections.
Black widow spider antivenin	INTRAMUSCULAR: *Adults and children*—one container injected into anterolateral thigh. INTRAVENOUS: *Children <12 yr or in shock*—dilute 1 container into 10-50 ml and administer over 15 min.	Days	Hypersensitivity to horse serum.
Botulism antitoxin trivalent	INTRAVENOUS: *Adults with symptomatic botulism and after sensitivity testing*—2 vials. INTRAMUSCULAR: *Adults after ingestion of contaminated food*—⅕-1 vial.	5-7 days	Sensitivity to equine serum.
Cholera vaccine	INTRAMUSCULAR, SUBCUTANEOUS: *Adults and children >10 yr*—0.5 ml; *children 5-10 yr*—0.3 ml; *children 6 mo-4 yr*—0.2 ml; give second dose 1 wk-1 mo apart. INTRADERMAL: *Adults and children ≥5 yr*—0.2 ml.	6 mo	Previous allergic reaction to vaccine.
Diphtheria and tetanus toxoids adsorbed, pediatric (DT)	INTRAMUSCULAR: *Children <12 mo*—three 0.5 ml injections administered at different sites at 4-8 wk intervals, followed by a fourth dose at 6-12 mo later. *Children >12 mo*—two doses 4-8 wk apart, third dose 6-12 mo later. Booster when child is 4-6 yr.	10 yr	Do not administer to child with fever or if child has history of neurologic or severe hypersensitivity reaction to previous dose; not for primary immunization of child unless pertussis vaccine is contraindicated.
Diphtheria and tetanus toxoids and pertussis vaccine adsorbed (DTP)	INTRAMUSCULAR: *Children 2 mo-6 yr*—0.5 ml, followed by two more doses at 4-8 wk intervals; fourth dose at 15-18 mo and booster at 4-6 yr.	10 yr; boosters required for tetanus toxoid	Do not use after seventh birthday; do not administer to child with fever; do not administer if reaction to earlier DTP administration was severe (fever of 105°F or higher, anaphylaxis, encephalopathy).
Diphtheria antitoxin	INTRAMUSCULAR: *Adults and children*—for prophylaxis of those not immunized who are in contact with patients: 2000-10,000 U. INTRAMUSCULAR OR INTRAVENOUS, SLOW INFUSION: *Adults and children with diphtheria*—20,000-120,000 U.	3 wk	Allergy to serum; pregnancy.

Continued.

TABLE 34-4 Agents for Active and Passive Immunity—cont'd

GENERIC/TRADE NAME	ROUTE	DURATION OF EFFECT	CONTRAINDICATIONS
Diphtheria and tetanus toxoids and pertussis vaccine adsorbed and *Haemophilus influenzae b* conjugate vaccine (Tetramune)	INTRAMUSCULAR: *Children 2-18 mo*—four doses during this period.	See individual vaccines	7 yr or older.
Haemophilus influenzae b polysaccharide vaccines (Hib TITER; PedvaxHIB; ProHIBIT)	INTRAMUSCULAR: *Children 2 mo-5 yr*—initial vaccination for infants at 1-2 mo, two additional doses at 2 mo intervals.	Not known	Febrile illness or active infection.
Hepatitis B vaccine inactivated (HBV vaccine: Engerix-B; Heptavax-B; Recombivax-HB)	INTRAMUSCULAR: dose depends on manufacturer and exposure to hepatitis. See package insert.	At least 5 yr	Severe cardiovascular disease with pulmonary dysfunction; pregnancy.
Hepatitis A vaccine, inactivated (Havrix)	INTRAMUSCULAR: *Adults*—one dose in deltoid region; *children 2-18 yr*—two doses 1 mo apart.	Booster dose after 6-12 mo	Bleeding disorder; febrile illness.
Hepatitis B immune globulin (HBIG: H-BIG, Hep-B-Gammagee, HyperHep)	INTRAMUSCULAR: *Adults and children*—0.06 ml/kg or 5 ml to adults, administered as soon as possible (within 7 days) after exposure; *newborn infants*—0.5 ml as soon as possible after birth.	Weeks; immunization should begin as soon as possible after exposure	Not for treatment of fulminant acute or chronic active hepatitis B.
Immune globulin intravenous (IGIV: Gamimune N; Gammagard; Gammar IV; Sandoglobulin IV)	INTRAVENOUS: *Adults and children—to treat congenital and acquired immunodeficiency disease*—see individual preparation for dosage.	3 wk	History of anaphylactic reaction or severe systemic response to immune globulin.
Immune globulin (IG: Gammar IM)	INTRAMUSCULAR: *Adults and children—for hepatitis A postexposure prophylaxis*—0.02 ml/kg; for travel in areas where hepatitis A is common, 0.02 ml/kg for less than 2 mo length; 0.06 ml/kg repeated every 5 mo for longer visits; also 0.25 ml/kg for prophylaxis against measles.	Months	Not for postexposure prophylaxis of hepatitis B.
Influenza virus vaccine (Fluogen; Fluzone; Influenza Virus Vaccine Trivalent, Subvirion type; Flu-Imune)	INTRAMUSCULAR: *Children 6-35 mo*—0.25 ml; *>3 yr to adult*—0.5 ml. Type of vaccine depends on age, see package insert; *children <8 yr*—require second dose 4 or more weeks later.	1 yr	Allergy to eggs or chicken; history of Guillain-Barré syndrome; pregnancy.
Measles, mumps and rubella virus vaccine live (MMR: M-M-R II)	SUBCUTANEOUS: *Children ≥15 mo*—single dose (0.5 ml) into outer aspect of upper arm.	Years; second dose recommended at entry to grade school or to middle school or high school	Immune deficiencies; pregnancy; women should not become pregnant within 3 mo after vaccination; should not be given to person with anaphylactic reaction to egg products.
Measles and rubella virus vaccine live (M-R-VAX II)	SUBCUTANEOUS: *Adults and children ≥15 mo*—single dose (0.5 ml) into outer aspect of upper arm.	8 yr or longer	Immune deficiencies; pregnancy; women should not become pregnant within 3 mo after vaccination.
Measles virus vaccine live (Attenuvax)	SUBCUTANEOUS: *Children ≥15 mo*—single dose (0.5 ml) into outer aspect of upper arm.	8 yr or longer	Immune deficiencies; febrile seizures or cerebral trauma; pregnancy; women should not become pregnant within 3 mo after vaccination.
Meningococcal polysaccharide vaccines (Menomune A/C/Y/W-135)	SUBCUTANEOUS: *Adults and children >2 yr*—0.5 ml as single injection; *children <4 yr*—may require booster.	Years; young children in endemic areas may require additional injections	Not for routine immunization; patients receiving cancer chemotherapy respond poorly.

TABLE 34-4 Agents for Active and Passive Immunity—cont'd

GENERIC/TRADE NAME	ROUTE	DURATION OF EFFECT	CONTRAINDICATIONS
Mumps virus vaccine live (Mumpsvax)	SUBCUTANEOUS: *Adults and children ≥12 mo*—0.5 ml	Permanent immunity (in 75-90% of patients receiving vaccine)	Immune deficiencies; pregnancy; women should not become pregnant within 3 mo after vaccination.
Pertussis vaccine adsorbed	INTRAMUSCULAR: *Children 2 mo-6 yr*—three doses (0.5 ml) 4-8 wk apart with fourth dose at 15-18 mo of age. Booster given at 4-6 yr of age. *Adults*—0.25 ml booster during pertussis epidemics.	4-6 yr	Adverse reactions are infrequent.
Plague vaccine	INTRAMUSCULAR: *Adults and children >10 yr*—1 ml dose, followed in 4 wk by second dose of 0.2 ml; another 0.2 ml dose at 3-6 mo after first dose. *Children <10 yr*—receive reduced doses, see manufacturer's instructions.	Three booster doses of 0.2 ml at 6 mo intervals; then at 1-2 yr	Sensitivity to constituents of medium (beef, protein, soy, casein)
Pneumococcal polysaccharide vaccine (Pneumovax 23; Pnu-Imune 23)	SUBCUTANEOUS, INTRAMUSCULAR: single 0.5 ml dose.	Months to years	Recent pneumococcal pneumonia; children <2 yr; pregnancy.
Poliovirus vaccine live oral trivalent (OPV: Orimune)	ORAL: *Infants*—administer at 2, 4, and 15-18 mo; *Children and adolescents*—two doses 6-8 wk apart, third dose 1 yr later.	Years	Used in older adult patients and pregnant patients, except single doses may be given when rapid immunization is necessary.
Poliovirus vaccine inactivated (IPV)	SUBCUTANEOUS: *Infants*—initial dose at 6-12 wk, second dose at 4-8 wk; third dose 6-12 mo after second dose.	Years; booster before entering grade school	Acute febrile illness; pregnancy.
Rabies vaccine, adsorbed (RVA)	INTRAMUSCULAR: *Adults and children*—1 ml in deltoid area on days 0, 7, and 28 for preexposure prophylaxis; see package insert for postexposure.	Check antibody levels after 2 yr, give booster if necessary	None.
Rabies vaccine, human diploid cell (HDCV: Immovax Rabies, Immovax Rabies ID)	INTRAMUSCULAR: *Adults and children*—1 ml in deltoid area on days 0, 7, and 28 for preexposure prophylaxis; see package insert for postexposure. INTRADERMAL: *Adults and children*—0.1 ml on days 0, 7, and 28.	Check antibody levels after 2 yr, give booster if necessary	Pregnancy is not a contraindication.
Rabies immune globulin (RIG: Hyperab, Imogam)	INTRADERMAL: 20 IU/kg; with half being infiltrated around wound.	3 wk	Thrombocytopenia.
Rubella virus vaccine live (Meruvax II)	SUBCUTANEOUS: *Adults and children 12 mo or older*—0.5 ml into outer aspect of upper arm.	Years; booster not recommended	Immune deficiencies; recent treatment with blood products or immune globulins; pregnancy; women should not become pregnant within 3 mo after vaccination.
Rubella and mumps virus vaccine live (Biavax-II)	SUBCUTANEOUS: *Children 12 mo-puberty*—single dose (0.5 ml) into outer aspect of upper arm.	Permanent	Immune deficiencies; pregnancy; women should not become pregnant within 3 mo after vaccination.
Tetanus and diphtheria toxoids adsorbed for adult use (Td)	INTRAMUSCULAR: *Adults and children >7 yr*—2 injections of 0.5 ml 4-8 wk apart; reinforcing dose 6-12 mo later.	10 yr; booster required	Reactions are usually mild.
Tetanus toxoid; tetanus toxoid adsorbed	INTRAMUSCULAR: *Adults and children*—three injections (0.5 ml), with 4-6 wk between first two doses and 6-12 mo between last two doses.	10 yr; booster required	Adverse reactions are infrequent; rarely, hypersensitivity.

Continued.

TABLE 34-4 Agents for Active and Passive Immunity—cont'd

GENERIC/TRADE NAME	ROUTE	DURATION OF EFFECT	CONTRAINDICATIONS
Tetanus immune globulin (TIG)	INTRAMUSCULAR: *Adults and children*—for prophylaxis, 250-500 U by deep IM injection; for treatment, *adults*—3000-6000 U; *children*—500-3000 U.	14 wk; for prophylaxis and treatment of persons with wounds	Adverse reactions are infrequent.
Typhoid vaccine	SUBCUTANEOUS: *Adults and children >10 yr*—two 0.5 ml doses 4 or more wk apart or three 0.5 ml doses at weekly intervals; *children 6 mo-10 yr*—two 0.25 ml doses 4 or more wk apart or three doses at weekly intervals.	3 yr; boosters can be given when needed	Severe febrile illness; pregnancy.
Typhoid vaccine live oral TY21a (Virotif Berna)	ORAL: *Adults and children >6 yr*—1 capsule ingested with cold or lukewarm drink 1 hr before meal on days 1, 3, 5, and 7.	5 yr; repeat immunization schedule	Severe febrile illness; pregnancy; known hypersensitivity to vaccine components; not for persons who are immunodeficient or undergoing immunosuppressive therapy.
Vaccinia immune globulin	INTRAMUSCULAR: *Adults and children*—0.3 ml/kg as soon as possible after exposure for prevention or modification of vaccinia infection; doses >10 mg should be injected at two or more sites.	Weeks	No benefit in patients with postvaccinal encephalitis.
Varicella virus vaccine live (Varivax)	SUBCUTANEOUS (DELTOID REGION OF ARM): *Adults and adolescents*—0.5 ml, followed by booster dose of 0.5 ml 4-8 wk later; *children 1-12 yr*—single dose of 0.5 ml.	Unknown, new vaccine	Not recommended for children <12 mo.
Varicella-zoster immune globulin (human) (VZIG)	INTRAMUSCULAR: *Adults*—125 units/10 kg; maximum 626 units, with each vial injected into a different site; for prophylaxis of chickenpox.	10-28 days	Only for individuals with four significant risk factors.
Yellow fever vaccine (YF-Vax)	SUBCUTANEOUS: *Adults and children >6 mo*—0.5 ml.	10 yr	Febrile illness; allergy to eggs; pregnancy; immunodeficient individuals.

chest pain, and chills. Less common side effects include malaise, headache, nausea and vomiting, dyspnea, syncope, and back pain. Hepatitis B immune globulin can also cause urticaria and angioedema. Varicella-zoster immune globulin injections can cause a mild rash, usually observed 10 to 14 days after immunization.

Toxicity

Immune sera, especially those using nonhuman proteins, can cause anaphylaxis in patients with a history of hypersensitivity reactions to immune globulin injections. This serum sickness results from an immune response directed against proteins in the injected serum. Massive immune complex formation occurs, followed by deposition of these complexes in the kidney and circulatory system, leading to nephritis and arteritis. The deposited immune complexes also initiate mediator release from platelets, basophils, and PMNs. This massive mediator release can be life threatening. A local deposition of insoluble immune complexes at the site of injection produces the Arthus reaction, in which redness and edema occur near blood vessels. Use caution when repeating injections of foreign serum. Other signs of serum sickness include arthralgia, lymphadenopathy, and pruritus. In serious cases, abdominal pain, fever, headache, and malaise may occur. Use of immune sera may be contraindicated in patients with thrombocytopenia since excessive bleeding may occur at the injection site.

Interactions

There are no known drug interactions that are associated with the use of passive immunostimulants, immune serum, and globulins.

NURSING PROCESS OVERVIEW

Immunization

Assessment

Perform a baseline assessment based on the age of the patient, severity of presenting problems, acuity level, and planned drug intervention. Assess for history of any problems with previous immunizations.

Nursing Diagnoses

- Potential complication: serum sickness

Patient Outcomes

The patient will experience no side effects related to immunizations.

Planning/Implementation

Most patients receive immunizations as outpatients and have no subjective or objective problems related to the immunization other than a mildly sore arm. Some patients experience low-grade fever and malaise for a few days, depending on the specific immunization. If problems develop, monitor vital signs and assess the patient. For some childhood immunizations, routine use of acetaminophen every 4 hours for 24 hours after the immunization may lessen subjective symptoms; consult the physician.

Evaluation

Before discharge, teach patients about anticipated benefits and possible side effects of immunizations. Encourage patients to call if questions arise or new signs or symptoms develop.

NURSING IMPLICATIONS SUMMARY

Immunizations

Drug Administration

- Any serum product containing proteins can cause acute allergic reactions and serum sickness. Review the signs and symptoms of serum sickness with the patient, and instruct the patient to notify the physician if it develops. Note that serum sickness may not develop for up to 6 to 12 days after immunization.
- Have available epinephrine 1:1000 solution in settings where protein-containing products are administered. Have drugs, equipment, and personnel available to treat acute allergic reactions.
- Question the female patient about the possibility of pregnancy before administering vaccines. Live virus vaccines are contraindicated in pregnant women.
- Assess the patient for human immunodeficiency virus (HIV) or other compromised immune state. Patients with a compromised immune state may require postponement of immunizations or may require an adjusted dose; consult the physician.
- Review the manufacturer's insert for current information about contraindications, cross-sensitivities with other drugs or allergens, and sensitivity testing.
- For IM administration, use anatomic landmarks in selecting injection sites. Use the vastus lateralis muscle in infants and small children. Use the deltoid muscle for administration of most vaccines and similar medications in older children and adults. Usually, avoid injection sites in the gluteal area unless large-volume doses must be divided into two or more injections or the patient is receiving two or more drugs that cannot be administered in the same site. Aspirate before injecting the drug to avoid inadvertent IV administration; if blood is aspirated, withdraw the needle, discard the syringe and needle, and prepare a fresh dose. Record the injection site and rotate sites with subsequent doses.

Patient and Family Education

- Review the anticipated benefits and possible side effects of drug therapy with the patient. With small children, if regular immunizations usually cause a fever, suggest that the mother use acetaminophen to treat this side effect. Instruct the mother to consult the physician.
- Warn the patient to avoid scratching injection sites. Brief application of an ice pack may lessen irritation.
- When appropriate, review with the patient the schedule for additional immunizations.
- Refer the patient to the local health department if appropriate.
- Instruct patients who manifest an allergic response to wear a medication identification tag or bracelet listing the allergic response and to be cautious in taking vaccines or immunomodulators without consulting the physician.

Measles Virus (Live Vaccine), Mumps Virus (Live Vaccine), or Rubella Virus (Live Vaccine)

Drug Administration/Patient and Family Education

- See the general guidelines for immunizations.
- Caution the female patient to avoid pregnancy for 3 months after immunization to prevent possible birth defects.
- Instruct the patient to keep all health care providers informed about immunizations for the next 3 months. The patient should not receive blood transfusions or blood products within 2 weeks of this immunization, gammaglobulin or other globulins within 2 weeks, other live virus vaccines within 1 month, or tuberculin skin test within 6 to 8 weeks of this vaccine.

Critical Thinking

APPLICATION

1. Explain active acquired immunity and how it is achieved. How long does it last?
2. Explain passive acquired immunity and how it is achieved. How long does it last?
3. What immune protection does the fetus have?
4. What is a common side effect of immune serums? How should you assess this and teach patients about it?

CRITICAL THINKING

1. Find out what immunizations are required by your local school system for children to enter public school.
2. What immunizations are required by your hospital for personnel who work with patients?

CHAPTER 35

Immunomodulators and Care of the Patient With Altered Immune Function

OBJECTIVES

After studying this chapter, you should be able to do the following:

- *Describe the clinical uses of immunosuppressants.*
- *Discuss the pharmacology of cyclosporine.*
- *Describe the types of patients who might receive immunostimulants.*
- *Develop a nursing care plan for a patient receiving an immunosuppressant or an immunostimulant.*

KEY TERMS

colony-stimulating factors
granulocyte colony-stimulating factor
granulocyte-macrophage colony-stimulating factor
interleukin-2 (IL-2)
progenitor cells

CHAPTER OVERVIEW

In the preceding chapter we considered the use of vaccines and antibodies for immunostimulation. These substances are mostly used in healthy individuals to prevent disease subsequent to exposure to a pathogen. In this chapter another class of immunostimulants is considered, drugs that are most often used to attempt to stimulate a faltering or failing immmune system. In addition, this chapter discusses specific immunosuppressants that are used primarily in organ transplantation.

Therapeutic Rationale: Immunostimulants

Modern medicine must deal with large numbers of patients whose immune systems are compromised directly by disease or indirectly as a side effect of drugs used to treat neoplastic disease, host-vs.-graft disease, or other conditions. In the past these patients were managed by attempting to protect them from exposure to disease, but little else could be done. Today, recombinant engineering technology coupled with a growing understanding of the immune system has made available a number of agents that can partially restore immune function.

Therapeutic Agents: Immunostimulants

Colony-Stimulating Factors

Colony-stimulating factors are proteins that regulate development of cells that are precursors to specific blood cells. The natural proteins are present in the body in such small amounts that they are difficult to obtain. Recombinant technology allows unlimited quantities of these human proteins to be made in the bacteria, *Escherichia coli.* Two colony-stimulating factors are currently accepted for medical use. One stimulates the production of the granulocyte cell line and the other stimulates the production of both granulocyte and monocyte-macrophage lines. For dosage information see Table 35-1.

Filgrastim

Mechanism of Action

Filgrastim (recombinant **granulocyte colony-stimulating factor**) binds to receptors on specific **progenitor cells** in bone marrow, causing them to increase production of neutrophil granulocytes. Neutrophils are polymorphonuclear leukocytes that play a key role in phagocytosis (Chapter 33). Therefore the end result of treatment with filgrastim is to promote return of cell-mediated immunity.

Pharmacokinetics

Filgrastim is rapidly absorbed from subcutaneous sites and achieves peak concentrations within hours. The effect on neutrophil production can be seen usually within a day.

Uses

The primary use for filgrastim is to treat neutropenia that is induced by cancer chemotherapy. Filgrastim has also been suggested for other conditions such as acquired immunodeficiency syndrome (AIDS)–associated neutropenia or neutropenia arising from genetic defects, but these are not yet approved indications.

Adverse Reactions and Contraindications

The most common adverse reaction to filgrastim is pain in bone, joints, and muscles. Bone pain seems correlated with recovery of the bone marrow and increased production of neutrophils. Headache, skin rash, and redness at the site of

TABLE 35-1 Immunostimulants: Dosages

GENERIC NAME	TRADE NAME	ADMINISTRATION/DOSAGE	COMMENTS
Aldesleukin	Proleukin	INTRAVENOUS: *Adults*—600,000 U/kg infused over 15 min every 8 hr for 14 doses. FDA pregnancy category C.	Recombinant interleukin-2 stimulates immune system at several points.
Filgrastim	Neupogen*	INTRAVENOUS, SUBCUTANEOUS: *Adults*—5 μg/kg starting 24 hr or more after last dose of cytotoxic chemotherapy. FDA pregnancy category C.	Recombinant colony-stimulating factor increases numbers of neutrophils.
Interferon-γ	Actimmune	SUBCUTANEOUS: *Children*—50 μg/m^2 3 times weekly for children >0.5 m^2 surface area; smaller children receive 1.5 μg/kg 3 times weekly. FDA pregnancy category C.	Recombinant protein stimulates phagocyte functions.
Levamisole	Ergamisol*	ORAL: *Adults*—50 mg every 8 hr for 3 days; repeat every 2 wk for a year. FDA pregnancy category C.	Immunostimulant used with fluorouracil for colorectal carcinoma.
Pegademase	Adagen	INTRAMUSCULAR: *Children*—10 U/kg on day 1, 15 U/kg on day 8, 20 U/kg on day 15; then 20 U/kg weekly. FDA pregnancy category C.	Bovine adenosine deaminase corrects enzymatic defect and restores immune function.
Sargramostim	Leukine	INTRAVENOUS, SUBCUTANEOUS: *Adults*—250 μg/m^2 surface area daily for 14-21 days. FDA pregnancy category C.	Recombinant colony-stimulating factor increases numbers of granulocytes and monocyte-macrophages.

*Available in Canada and United States.
†Available in Canada only.

injection are less common. Serious allergic reactions are rare, but patients who are sensitive to proteins derived from *E. coli* are more likely to show signs of allergy.

Patients who have a significant number of leukemic myeloid blasts are at risk for further leukemic progression when treated with filgrastim because filgrastim may promote proliferation of the precursor cells.

Toxicity and Interactions

No specific toxicity or interactions have been documented perhaps because filgrastim tends to be used in complex regimens involving many drugs, each with significant direct and secondary actions.

Sargramostim

Mechanism of Action

Sargramostim (recombinant **granulocyte-macrophage colony-stimulating factor**) binds to receptors on a less differentiated progenitor cell than filgrastim; therefore production of more than one type of cell is promoted. The most important cell types that increase in response to sargramostim are neutrophils and monocyte-macrophages.

Pharmacokinetics

Sargramostim is rapidly absorbed from subcutaneous sites and achieves peak concentrations within hours. The effect on leukocyte production occurs over several days.

Uses

Sargramostim is used primarily for promoting myeloid engraftment after bone marrow transplantation. Sargramostim has also been suggested for other conditions such as AIDS-associated neutropenia or neutropenia arising from genetic defects, but these are not yet approved indications.

Adverse Reactions and Contraindications

The most common adverse reaction to sargramostim is pain in bone, joints, and muscles. Bone pain seems correlated with recovery of the bone marrow and increased production of leukocytes. Headache, skin rash, fever, and redness at the site of injection are less common.

Sargramostim may cause capillary leak syndrome. Symptoms include peripheral edema, pleural effusion, and shortness of breath. Patients may also react to the first dose of sargramostim with an episode of flushing, hypotension, and syncope. This reaction usually does not recur with subsequent doses.

Serious allergic reactions with sargramostim are rare, but patients who are sensitive to proteins derived from *E. coli* are more likely to show signs of allergy.

Patients who have a significant number of leukemic myeloid blasts are at risk for further leukemic progression when treated with sargramostim because sargramostim may promote proliferation of these precursor cells.

Patients with AIDS should not receive sargramostim unless they are also receiving a drug to control human immunodeficiency virus (HIV) proliferation. Some reports have indicated that sargramostim can promote proliferation of the virus.

Toxicity

Capillary leak syndrome and fever are dose-related responses to sargramostim. Overdosages can therefore lead to serious or life-threatening reactions.

Interactions

Specific interactions have not been documented.

CELL-STIMULATING AGENTS

Colony-stimulating factors stimulate progenitor cells in bone marrow to increase the numbers of leukocytes being formed, thus improving immune function. Another class of agents improves immune function by stimulating the activity of cells already formed.

Aldesleukin

Mechanism of Action

Aldesleukin is a recombinant form of **interleukin-2 (IL-2)**, one of the major cytokines regulating function of the immune system (Chapter 33). Multiple effects of aldesleukin contribute to stimulation of cell-mediated immunity.

Pharmacokinetics

Aldesleukin is used only by intravenous routes. The drug distributes well to many sites. Elimination involves hydrolysis of this protein into amino acids in the kidneys. The biological effect of aldesleukin on immune function may persist for months.

Uses

Aldesleukin is indicated only for renal cell carcinoma. The very high risk of side effects limits use for other indications.

Adverse Reactions and Contraindications

Aldesleukin causes a wide array of potentially serious side effects. Central nervous system (CNS) effects include agitation, confusion, depression, dizziness, and fatigue. Pulmonary symptoms may include lung congestion, edema, and shortness of breath. Anemia may require blood transfusions. Arrhythmias are usually transient but may occasionally be life threatening.

A skin rash with redness, itchiness, and peeling commonly appears within 2 or 3 days of the start of treatment and begins to resolve only after the drug is discontinued. Blisters on the skin may signal a more dangerous condition, exfoliative dermatitis, which can be fatal. Dizziness, nausea, and vomiting almost always occur.

Aldesleukin is contraindicated for patients with preexisting impairment of cardiac or pulmonary function. The drug is also avoided in patients with metastatic cancer in the CNS. Aldesleukin is not used in patients with transplanted organs because the immune stimulation produced by the drug may prompt organ rejection.

Toxicity

The reactions to aldesleukin are dose related, which means that they will be worse at higher doses. Capillary leak syndrome is more likely at higher doses. Symptoms of capillary leak syndrome include peripheral edema, pleural effusion, and shortness of breath. This condition may be fatal.

Interactions

Drugs like daunorubicin or doxorubicin may cause dangerous additive cardiotoxicity with aldesleukin. Likewise the toxicity of bone marrow depressants, hepatotoxic drugs, and nephrotoxic medications may be worsened by aldesleukin. Corticosteroids may antagonize the actions of aldesleukin.

Interferon-γ

Mechanism of Action

Interferon-γ promotes the formation of active oxygen species in phagocytes. This and other actions improve phagocytosis.

Pharmacokinetics

The absorption of interferon-γ from injection sites is slow but relatively efficient. Peak concentrations in blood occur in 4 to 7 hours. Mechanisms for biotransformation or elimination are unknown.

Uses

Interferon-γ is used in chronic granulomatous disease, a condition in which oxidative functions of phagocytic cells are impaired. Thus the direct actions of the drug tend to reverse the genetically induced defect, with the result that immune function is improved.

Adverse Reactions and Contraindications

Interferon-γ typically causes a flulike syndrome. Symptoms include achiness, chills, fever, headache, and joint pain. Diarrhea, nausea, or vomiting are also common and may contribute to weight loss.

Rashes and dizziness may occur. Interferon-γ commonly causes leukopenia, but symptoms are rare.

The fever and chills caused by interferon-γ cause stress on the cardiovascular system. Patients with preexisting cardiovascular disease may be unable to tolerate this added load. Patients with CNS disease may be at greater risk for serious reactions with use of interferon-γ.

Toxicity

Leukopenia, CNS effects, and gastrointestinal (GI) tract side effects are dose-related reactions to interferon-γ. These reactions are therefore worse with very high doses.

Interactions

Any drugs that interfere with bone marrow function can influence the activity of interferon-γ.

Levamisole

Mechanism of Action

Levamisole returns leukocyte function to normal levels after chemotherapy or surgery. T cells, monocytes, macrophages, and neutrophils are influenced.

Pharmacokinetics

Levamisole is easily absorbed orally and undergoes extensive biotransformation in the liver. The drug persists in blood for several hours. Elimination of metabolites is primarily in urine.

Uses

Levamisole is used as an adjunct for surgery and chemotherapy of primary colorectal carcinoma. Metastatic disease does not respond.

Adverse Reactions and Contraindications

GI tract effects such as nausea and diarrhea are common with levamisole. Blood dyscrasias can also occur, but usually cause no symptoms. A flulike syndrome may be related to onset of serious blood dyscrasias.

CNS impairment is rare, but when it occurs it includes ataxia, blurred vision, confusion, mental changes, paresthesias, seizures, tardive dyskinesia, or tremors.

Bone marrow depression or infections may be worsened by levamisole; patients with these conditions should be carefully watched for serious reactions.

Toxicity

Many of the potentially serious effects of levamisole are allergic or idiosyncratic reactions and are therefore not dose related.

Interactions

Levamisole is often used in combination with fluorouracil; the drugs may have additive effects on blood cell counts.

Pegademase

Mechanism of Action

Pegademase is bovine adenosine deaminase, an enzyme that is required for removal of toxic metabolites of adenosine. Without this enzyme, lymphocytes die. The absence of this enzyme is the cause of severe combined immunodeficiency disease (SCID).

Pharmacokinetics

Pegademase is designed so that the adenosine deaminase is covalently linked to a larger molecule that allows the material to remain in the blood longer. The material may remain in circulation for several days. The onset of action on immune function is gradual and significant clinical improvement may not occur for as long as a year.

Uses

Pegademase is used only for adenosine deaminase deficiency, or SCID.

Adverse Reactions and Contraindications

Side effects are rare with pegademase but may include headache or pain at the site of injection. Pegademase is avoided in patients with thrombocytopenia because of the risk of bleeding.

Toxicity

Toxicity has not been documented with doses below 30 mg/kg.

Therapeutic Rationale: Immunosuppressants

Organ transplantation has been made possible by the existence of drugs that can successfully control rejection of the transplanted tissue without compromising all immune function in the host. The arm of the immune system that must be controlled is cell-mediated immunity (Chapter 33).

Therapeutic Agents: Immunosuppressants

Several types of agents may be useful to control host-vs.-graft disease. The following section covers cyclosporine, muromonab-CD3, mycophenolate, and tacrolimus, drugs not covered extensively elsewhere in this text. Azathioprine is covered in Chapter 37, and the corticosteroids are covered in Chapter 36. Dosage information is summarized in Table 35-2.

✣ CYCLOSPORINE

Mechanism of Action

Cyclosporine blocks the release of IL-2 from activated helper T cells. This action inhibits induction of cytotoxic T lymphocytes (see Figure 33-1). As a result, cell-mediated immunity is suppressed.

Pharmacokinetics

Oral absorption of cyclosporine is variable and bioavailability is only about 30%. The drug is extensively metabolized by the liver. The half-life of the drug is long in adults, ranging from 10 to 27 hours but tends to be shorter in children. Elimination of the drug is through bile into the feces.

Uses

Cyclosporine is the most widely used drug for prevention of organ rejection following transplantation. It is often combined with corticosteroids.

Adverse Reactions and Contraindications

Cyclosporine commonly causes hypertension and nephrotoxicity, but symptoms are usually absent. These reactions may be monitored by checking blood pressure regularly and by following the blood urea nitrogen (BUN) and creatinine.

Gingival hyperplasia is also common with cyclosporine. This reaction and increased hair growth (hirsutism) are often troublesome to patients because self-image may be impacted.

A variety of potentially serious reactions are possible with cyclosporine, including hepatotoxicity, pancreatitis, and electrolyte imbalances. Alterations in elimination of potassium may lead to confusion, paresthesias, shortness of breath, and muscle weakness. Convulsions may also occur. Anaphylaxis is possible, especially with parenteral dosing. Because cyclosporine suppresses part of the immune system, the risk of serious infection is also increased.

TABLE 35-2 Immunosuppressants: Dosages

GENERIC NAME	TRADE NAME	ADMINISTRATION/DOSAGE	COMMENTS
✣ Cyclosporine	Sandimmune*	ORAL: *Adults and children*—12-15 mg/kg initially, then reduced by 5% weekly to maintenance of 5-10 mg/kg daily. FDA pregnancy category C. INTRAVENOUS: *Adults and children*—2-6 mg/kg daily until oral doses are possible.	IV preparation may be used within 4 hr of transplant, but oral doses should be substituted as soon as possible.
Muromonab-CD3	Orthoclone OKT3*	INTRAVENOUS: *Adults*—5 mg by rapid injection daily for 10-14 days. FDA pregnancy category C. *Children*—0.1 mg/kg by rapid injection daily for 10-14 days.	Monoclonal antibody blocks immune cell activation.
Mycophenolate	CellCept†	ORAL: *Adults*—1 gm 2 times daily, starting within 72 hr of renal transplant. FDA pregnancy category C.	Enzyme inhibitor blocks lymphocyte proliferation.
Tacrolimus	Prograf	ORAL: *Adults*—75 μg/kg every 12 hr. *Children*—150 μg/kg every 12 hr. INTRAVENOUS: *Adults*—50 μg/kg daily by continuous infusion. *Children*—100 μg/kg daily by continuous infusion.	Macrolide with similar actions to cyclosporine but greater potency.

*Available in Canada and United States.
†Available in Canada only.

Cyclosporine is used cautiously in patients with hepatic or renal damage, adjusting doses carefully to avoid drug accumulation. Active infections may be worsened by the drug.

Toxicity

Several of the reactions to cyclosporine are dose related. Irreversible nephrotoxicity may occur with persistently high doses. Tremors are another dose-related symptom that may signal overdose.

Interactions

Many drugs that are metabolized in the liver may interfere with the metabolism of cyclosporine and therefore cause accumulation of cyclosporine, leading to serious side effects. Drugs that may act in this way include androgens, cimetidine, danazol, diltiazem, erythromycin, estrogens, and imidazole antifungal agents.

The risk of hyperkalemia may be increased when potassium-containing medications are used. Other drugs such as potassium-sparing diuretics or succinylcholine may also increase the risk.

Live virus vaccines should not be used with cyclosporine because the immune suppression caused by cyclosporine may allow an uncontrolled proliferation of the virus. Serious generalized disease may result.

Lovastatin may cause cell damage and renal failure in patients with cardiac transplants who receive cyclosporine.

MUROMONAB-CD3

Mechanism of Action

Muromonab-CD3 is a monoclonal antibody that binds to the CD3 receptor on human T helper cells. The binding of the drug prevents the cell from responding to signals from activated macrophages or monocytes. As a result, T-cell function is inhibited and immune responses are blunted.

Pharmacokinetics

Muromonab-CD3 binds directly to helper T cells; therefore its action is almost immediate. Return to normal numbers of fully functional CD3 cells usually occurs within a week after muromonab-CD3 is discontinued.

Uses

Muromonab-CD3 is used to treat episodes of transplant rejection. The drug is usually combined with other immunosuppressants.

Adverse Reactions and Contraindications

Muromonab-CD3 provokes release of cytokines in most patients. Symptoms include chills, diarrhea, dizziness, fainting, spiking fever, headache, malaise, muscle or joint pain, nausea, or vomiting. These symptoms may progress to more serious signs such as arrhythmias, chest pain, shortness of breath caused by pulmonary edema, trembling, and weakness. The cytokine release reaction usually appears 0.5 to 48 hours after injection. Anaphylaxis may also produce similar symptoms but usually appears within 10 minutes of injection.

A variety of CNS signs may occur with muromonab-CD3. These include confusion, headache, hallucinations, sensitivity to light, and tiredness. More serious reactions may include coma or seizures.

Muromonab-CD3 is avoided in patients with fluid overloads or heart failure because of the excessive risk of potentially fatal pulmonary edema. The drug is also avoided in patients with fever or infections.

Muromonab-CD3 is a mouse protein. Patients with strong allergies to mice should not receive the drug because the risk of a serious allergic reaction is increased.

Toxicity

Most of the reactions to muromonab-CD3 are caused by release of cytokines in the body. These effects may worsen with increases in dosage.

Interactions

When muromonab-CD3 is combined with other immunosuppressants, the risk of severe immune suppression is increased; doses of both drugs may require reduction. Serious infections may occur.

Immunosuppressants should not be used with live virus vaccines because the immune suppression caused by the drug may allow an uncontrolled proliferation of the virus. Serious generalized disease may result.

MYCOPHENOLATE

Mechanism of Action

Mycophenolate inhibits inosine monophosphate dehydrogenase, an enzyme required for synthesis of guanine nucleotides needed for DNA synthesis. Both T and B lymphocytes must maintain synthesis of DNA to proliferate normally. Therefore the result of treatment with mycophenolate is to block proliferation of T and B lymphocytes, thereby impairing immune responses that might promote rejection of transplanted organs.

Pharmacokinetics

Mycophenolate is well absorbed orally, but food or cholestyramine may interfere with absorption. The drug is highly bound to plasma proteins and has a half-life of 17 to 18 hours. The drug appears to undergo extensive enterohepatic circulation (Chapter 1). It is converted to mycophenolic acid, the active metabolite, in the body. The liver forms inactive metabolites, including a glucuronide that is eliminated renally.

Uses

The only current indication for mycophenolate is to prevent rejection of allogeneic renal transplants. The drug is combined with cyclosporine and corticosteroids.

Adverse Reactions and Contraindications

GI tract symptoms are common and include abdominal pain, constipation or diarrhea, heartburn, nausea, and vomiting. Headache and general weakness are also common. Common reactions that are more serious include anemia, blood in urine, chest pain, edema, hypertension, and neutropenia. Neutropenia, which exposes the patient to increased risk of infection, peaks 1 to 6 months after transplantation and the start of immunosuppression.

Mycophenolate should be used with caution in patients with serious GI tract disease because the drug may increase the risk of hemorrhage or perforation. Patients with renal impairment may require lower doses.

Toxicity

Overdoses have not been reported. Cholestyramine might be expected to assist in such cases by sequestering mycophenolate and promoting fecal excretion.

Interactions

Mycophenolate is used cautiously in combination with other immunosuppressants; the risk of excessive immunosuppression or development of lymphomas may be increased.

TACROLIMUS

Mechanism of Action

Tacrolimus is a macrolide that suppresses activation of the immune system, blocking production of IL-2. This action is similar to that of cyclosporine, but tacrolimus is many times more potent than cyclosporine.

Pharmacokinetics

Tacrolimus may be absorbed orally or may be used by intravenous infusion.

Uses

Tacrolimus is currently indicated only for treating transplant rejection in patients with transplanted livers. The drug is under investigation for other applications, including use in inflammatory skin lesions.

Adverse Reactions and Contraindications

Nephrotoxicity may arise with tacrolimus. Patients may also experience some allergic reactions.

Toxicity

Toxic reactions are not yet well delineated for this new drug.

Interactions

Cyclosporine may increase the risk of nephrotoxicity. Live virus vaccines may cause dangerous generalized disease in immunosuppressed patients.

NURSING PROCESS OVERVIEW

Immunomodulators

Assessment

Assess vital signs. Perform a complete physical assessment. Obtain a history of previous infections. Monitor weight and assess for recent changes in weight. Auscultate lung sounds. If the patient has received a transplanted organ, take a history appropriate to the transplant.

Nursing Diagnoses

- Potential complication: infection

Patient Outcomes

The patient will not experience an infection, or if one occurs, the nurse will minimize and manage complications associated with the infection.

Planning/Implementation

Monitor vital signs. Assess for signs of infection. If an immunostimulant is prescribed, monitor for improvement in cell counts and subjective improvement. If an immunosuppressant is ordered, review with the patient the potential danger of infection. Teach the patient how to administer prescribed drugs at home.

Evaluation

Immunostimulants are effective if the patient develops more resistance to infections. Immunosuppressants are administered to prevent organ rejection following transplant. Evaluate signs of organ rejection and indicators of continuing function of the transplanted organ(s). The patient should be able to state how to administer ordered medications, the importance of returning for follow-up, and side effects that should be reported to the physician.

NURSING IMPLICATIONS SUMMARY

COLONY-STIMULATING FACTORS

Filgrastim

Drug Administration/Patient and Family Education

- Review side effects. Monitor vital signs. Assess for pain in joints, muscles, and bones.
- If the patient is to self-administer at home, teach injection technique and proper handling of syringes and needles.
- For IV administration, see manufacturer's insert. Administer dose over at least 30 minutes.
- Monitor the complete blood count (CBC) and white blood cell (WBC) differential, platelet count, BUN and serum creatinine, and liver function tests.

Sargramostim

Drug Administration/Patient and Family Education

- Review side effects. Monitor vital signs. Assess for fluid retention and monitor weight. Auscultate lung sounds. Assess for pain in joints, muscles, and bones. Monitor weight and assess hydration.
- Rarely, a first-dose reaction characterized by flushing, hypotension, and fainting may occur.
- If the patient is to self-administer at home, teach injection technique and proper handling of syringes and needles.
- Instruct the patient receiving granulocyte-macrophage colony-stimulating factor (GM-CSF) that fever, chills, headache, nausea and vomiting, weakness, and fatigue may occur. If persistent or severe, instruct the patient to notify the physician.
- For IV administration review the insert supplied by the manufacturer. Administer as a 2-hour infusion via a central venous line. Do not use an in-line filter.
- Monitor the CBC and WBC differential, platelet count, BUN and serum creatinine, and liver function tests.

IMMUNOSTIMULANTS: CELL-STIMULATING AGENTS

Aldesleukin

Drug Administration/Patient and Family Education

- Monitor vital signs. See the patient problem boxes on bleeding tendencies (p. 586) and leukopenia (p. 585). Instruct the patient that side effects are common. The patient should stay in close contact with the physician and report the development of any new sign or symptom.
- Monitor weight and assess for edema. Auscultate lung sounds and assess for shortness of breath. Assess for skin changes.
- Consult the manufacturer's literature for current guidelines about drug administration.
- Monitor CBC, WBC differential, platelet count, thyroid function tests, liver function tests, BUN and serum creatinine, and pulmonary function tests including arterial blood gases.

Gamma Interferon

Drug Administration/Patient and Family Education

- See the patient problem boxes on bleeding tendencies (p. 586) and leukopenia (p. 585).
- Assess vital signs. Monitor weight.
- Fever and flulike symptoms may occur. Some physicians prescribe acetaminophen before doses.
- For self-administration, teach the patient injection technique and proper handling of syringes and needles. Use the deltoid muscle or anterior thigh for injections; see patient instruction leaflet.
- Monitor the WBC differential and platelet count, liver function tests, and lactate dehydrogenase (LDH).

Levamisole

Drug Administration/Patient and Family Education

- See the patient problem boxes on leukopenia (p.585), bleeding tendencies (p. 586), and stomatitis (p. 587).
- Assess vital signs. Assess for CNS effects, including ataxia, tremors, blurred vision, confusion, and numbness or tingling in face, hands, or feet. Assess for tardive dyskinesia: lip smacking, worm-like movements of the tongue, or uncontrolled movements of the arms and legs.
- Caution the patient to avoid driving or operating hazardous equipment if blurred vision occurs.
- Monitor CBC, WBC differential, platelet count, serum electrolytes, carcinoembryonic antigen (CEA), and liver function tests.

Pegademase

Drug Administration/Patient and Family Education

- Monitor trough plasma adenosine deaminase activity and red blood cell (RBC) deoxyadenosine triphosphate concentrations.
- Review with the patient the importance of continuing this medication for life.

IMMUNOSUPPRESSANTS

Cyclosporine

Drug Administration

- See information on side effects.
- Monitor blood pressure and pulse. Monitor intake, output, and weight. Inspect teeth and gums regularly. Assess for skin changes and hair growth.
- Monitor CBC and WBC differential, liver function tests, BUN, serum creatinine levels, serum cyclosporine concentrations, serum uric acid levels, and serum electrolytes.
- Review the manufacturer's instructions when preparing oral doses since doses must be measured with a dropper, then diluted in a glass container. Review instructions with the patient.

NURSING IMPLICATIONS SUMMARY—cont'd

Intravenous Administration

- Review the manufacturer's instructions regarding preparation. Infuse properly diluted doses over 2 to 6 hours. Monitor vital signs.

Patient and Family Education

- Review the anticipated benefits and possible side effects of drug therapy. Encourage the patient to have teeth cleaned and dental caries repaired before starting therapy. Emphasize the importance of thorough teeth brushing and flossing and regular professional teeth cleaning treatment and prevention of gingival hyperplasia.
- Warn the patient that tremor may develop.
- Warn the patient to avoid driving or operating hazardous equipment if confusion develops; the patient should notify the physician.
- See the patient problem box on leukopenia (p. 585). Instruct the patient to avoid having any immunizations while taking cyclosporine. In addition, instruct others living in the patient's household to avoid oral polio vaccine while the patient is taking cyclosporine. If the patient must be near someone who has recently had the oral polio vaccine, have the patient wear a mask that covers the nose and mouth.
- Instruct the patient not to stop therapy without consulting the physician.

Muromonab-CD3

Drug Administration/Patient and Family Education

- Monitor blood pressure and pulse. Remain with the patient for 15 to 30 minutes after the first dose. Chest pain may follow the first dose but is rare thereafter.
- Assess for side effects that commonly occur such as fever, chills, dyspnea, wheezing, nausea, vomiting, tremor, headache, and tachycardia.
- Forewarn the patient that trembling and shaking of the hands after the first dose is common.
- Monitor intake, output, and weight. Auscultate breath sounds.
- See the manufacturer's literature for current guidelines. Administer the prepared dose as a bolus over 1 minute.
- See the patient problem box on leukopenia (p. 585). Instruct the patient to avoid having any immunizations while taking muromonab-CD3. In addition, instruct others living in the patient's household to avoid oral polio vaccine while the patient is taking muromonab-CD3. If the patient must be near someone who has recently had the oral polio vaccine, have the patient wear a mask that covers the nose and mouth.
- Monitor the CBC, WBC differential, platelet count, liver function tests, BUN and serum creatinine, and muromonab-CD3 concentrations.

Mycophenolate

Drug Administration/Patient and Family Education

- See the patient problem boxes on leukopenia (p. 585) and bleeding tendencies (thrombocytopenia) (p. 586).
- Assess for peripheral edema, oral moniliasis (white patches in mouth, throat), and tremor. Monitor weight.
- Advise the patient to take doses on an empty stomach and to swallow capsules whole, without chewing, crushing, or opening. Instruct the patient to take doses with a full glass of water. Do not take doses at the same time as taking antacids.
- Monitor the CBC and WBC differential.
- Emphasize the importance of returning to the physician for regular follow-up. Notify the physician of severe or persistent constipation or diarrhea, headache, nausea and vomiting, skin rash, or weakness.
- Caution the patient to avoid driving or operating hazardous equipment if dizziness develops.

Tacrolimus

Drug Administration/Patient and Family Education

- Review anticipated benefits of drug. Emphasize importance of taking the drug as ordered and not discontinuing the drug without consulting the physician.
- See the patient problem box on leukopenia (p. 585). Instruct the patient to avoid having any immunizations while taking tacrolimus. In addition, instruct others living in the patient's household to avoid oral polio vaccine while the patient is taking tacrolimus. If the patient must be near someone who has recently had the oral polio vaccine, have the patient wear a mask that covers the nose and mouth.
- Monitor the CBC, WBC differential, platelet count, serum electrolytes, liver function tests, BUN, and serum creatinine.

Intravenous Administration

- See the manufacturer's insert for latest information. Remain with the patient for 30 minutes following the first dose to monitor for allergic reaction. Have epinephrine, oxygen, and personnel available to treat acute allergic reactions in settings where this drug is administered.

Critical Thinking

APPLICATION

1. What is the function of colony-stimulating factors? How may they be used clinically?
2. What is the most common adverse reaction to filgrastim?
3. Why is filgrastim avoided in patients with leukemic myeloid blasts?
4. Why does sargramostim increase more types of cells than filgrastim?
5. If a patient with AIDS is to receive sargramostim, what should you confirm before administering the drug?
6. How do the actions of aldesleukin and interferon-γ differ from those of the colony-stimulating factors?
7. What is the most common reaction with interferon-γ?
8. What is the clinical use of levamisole?
9. What is the mechanism of action of pegademase?
10. Why is cyclosporine effective at preventing organ rejection?
11. What organ systems may be affected by cyclosporine?
12. What might tremors signify in a patient receiving cyclosporine? What should you do?
13. Why should a patient taking cyclosporine not receive a live virus vaccine? What vaccines might be included?
14. Why are estrogens and other drugs that are metabolized by the liver usually avoided in patients receiving cyclosporine?
15. What is the mechanism of action of muromonab-CD3?
16. Why are allergies to mice associated with greater risk of allergy to muromonab-CD3?
17. What symptoms associated with cytokine release are caused by muromonab-CD3?
18. Why does mycophenolate interfere with lymphocyte proliferation?
19. What is the mechanism of action of tacrolimus?

CRITICAL THINKING

1. How would you evaluate for capillary leak syndrome in a patient receiving sargramostim?
2. Aldesleukin can be expected to cause skin rashes. What sign would lead you to consider that a patient was experiencing a more serious skin reaction? What should you do?
3. A patient receiving levamisole develops a flulike syndrome. What other potentially more serious reaction would this prompt you to look for in this patient? How would you carry out this evaluation?

CHAPTER 36

Glucocorticoids Used for Inflammatory and Immune Disorders

OBJECTIVES

After studying this chapter, you should be able to do the following:

- *Describe the use of glucocorticoids for inflammatory and immune disorders.*
- *Compare and contrast the antiinflammatory and sodium-retaining activity of the systemic glucocorticoids.*
- *Describe the side effects associated with long-term glucocorticoid use.*
- *Develop a nursing care plan for patients receiving glucocorticoids.*

CHAPTER OVERVIEW

Glucocorticoids are used clinically for a wide variety of clinical inflammatory and immune conditions. The systemic and local uses of glucocorticoids are summarized. The serious toxic effects that limit usage are reviewed.

KEY TERMS

cushingoid symptoms
glucocorticoid activity

Therapeutic Rationale: Inflammatory and Immune Disorders

Inflammation is a nonspecific response of tissues to a stimulus or insult. In this chapter inflammatory conditions for which glucocorticoids are used clinically will be considered.

The inflammatory response includes the migration of various leukocytes to the area and their release of various humoral agents. These humoral agents include complement 5a, leukotrienes, interleukin-8, and transforming growth factor beta. These agents not only have effects of their own but also serve to attract additional leukocytes to the inflammatory site, augmenting the inflammatory response.

Inflammation and an immune response are closely linked. The inflammatory response focuses on the release of humoral agents to affect a given site. The immune response refers to the mobilization and interactions of the various immune cells, such as lymphocytes, macrophages, neutrophils, eosinophils, basophils, and mast cells.

Glucocorticoids inhibit the access of leukocytes to inflammatory sites, interfere with their function, and suppress the production and effects of humoral agents. At high physiologic concentrations, **glucocorticoid activity** suppresses the inflammatory response, whether the initiating event is an infection, physical or chemical injury, or an immune reaction. A number of conditions have an inflammatory or immune response that can be suppressed by glucocorticoids. However, glucocorticoids themselves are rarely curative and their prolonged systemic use leads to serious adverse effects.

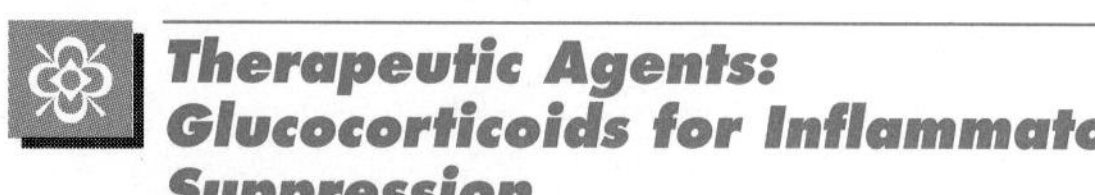

Therapeutic Agents: Glucocorticoids for Inflammatory Suppression

Glucocorticoids: General Characteristics

Mechanism of Action

Glucocorticoids enter a target cell and bind to a steroid receptor in the cell cytoplasm. The binding of the glucocorticoid activates the receptor, which allows the complex to enter the nucleus. In the nucleus the complex binds to selected DNA sites known as glucocorticoid response elements (GREs). This promotes or inhibits the transcription of specific mRNAs. In turn the synthesis of the respective proteins is promoted or inhibited.

There is also a mineralocorticoid receptor with a high affinity for aldosterone. However, cortisol and cortisone, the naturally occurring glucocorticoids, also have low affinity for the mineralocorticoid receptor. A weak or absent affinity for the mineralocorticoid receptor is a characteristic of the intermediate-acting and long-acting glucocorticoids as indicated in Table 36-1.

Glucocorticoids suppress lymphocyte functions, suppressing inflammation and immune reactions. Glucocorticoids are also an important regulator of metabolism in other tissues. In muscle, glucocorticoids decrease the use of glucose and mobilize amino acids from the breakdown of protein. In the liver, glucocorticoids promote the synthesis of glucose and its storage as glycogen. At low or baseline physiologic concentrations, glucocorticoids are important in regulating metabolism of skeletal and connective tissue. At high pharmacologic concentrations, glucocorticoids impair extracellular collagen and matrix formation. This leads to delayed wound healing and tissue maintenance. High pharmacologic concentrations of glucocorticoids also decrease bone formation and increase the urinary excretion of calcium and phosphorus, actions leading to bone loss.

Pharmacokinetics

Oral preparations are commonly used for systemic glucocorticoid therapy because they are well absorbed from the gastrointestinal (GI) tract. Peak plasma concentrations are reached in 1 to 2 hours. Glucocorticoids are lipophilic and readily cross plasma membranes. Cortisone and prednisone are converted to the active forms, hydrocortisone and prednisolone, by the liver. Hydrocortisone and prednisolone bind to a plasma protein, corticosteroid-binding globulin (CBG), and to albumin, which keeps them from being readily cleared from the plasma.

A major factor in the overall potency of the various glucocorticoids is their relative rate of metabolism by the liver. The intermediate- and long-acting glucocorticoids have structural changes that not only decrease their mineralocorticoid activity but also slow their rate of metabolism. Severe liver disease has multiple effects on bioavailability of glucocorticoids. Hydrocortisone and prednisolone are preferred because they do not require hepatic metabolism to an active form. The hypoalbuminemia of severe liver disease increases the free concentration of hydrocortisone and prednisolone. The metabolism of all glucocorticoids may be impaired. In general, severe liver disease increases the biologic and toxic effects of glucocorticoids.

Glucocorticoids are also metabolized by the placenta in pregnant women, limiting exposure of the fetus. However, very high doses of glucocorticoids can suppress fetal adrenal function.

Because the action of glucocorticoids depends on the promotion or inhibition of new protein synthesis, the onset of action is in hours to days and the duration of action is in days to weeks. The eight glucocorticoids used systemically vary in their duration of action depending both on the chemical characteristics of the glucocorticoid and also on the formulation and route of administration. These points are summarized in Table 36-2.

Oral glucocorticoid therapy usually begins with one or more daily doses to control symptoms. When symptoms are under control, treatment can often be continued with alternate-day administration of prednisone, prednisolone, or methylprednisolone. The advantage of alternate-day therapy is the suppression of the hypophysial-pituitary-adrenal axis is less. Growth rate in children is maintained and bone loss in all individuals is less.

TABLE 36-1 Comparison of Systemic Glucocorticoids

DRUG	ACTIVITY RELATIVE TO HYDROCORTISONE		EQUIVALENT DOSE (MG)
	ANTIINFLAMMATORY	SODIUM-RETAINING	
Short-Acting			
✤ Hydrocortisone	1	1	20
Cortisone	0.8	0.9	25
Intermediate-Acting			
Methylprednisolone	5	0	4
Prednisolone	4	0.8	5
Prednisone	3.5	0.8	5
Triamcinolone	5	0	4
Long-Acting			
Betamethasone	25	0	0.6
Dexamethasone	30	0	0.75
Paramethasone	10	0	2

TABLE 36-2 Glucocorticoids Used Systemically

GENERIC NAME	TRADE NAMES*	ROUTE†	ONSET	DURATION
Betamethasone	Celestone	PO	1 hr	3 days
Betamethasone sodium phosphate	Selestoject	IV, IM	Rapid	Short
Betamethasone acetate/sodium phosphate	Celestone soluspan	IM, IA, IL, IS, ST	1-3 hr	1-2 wk
Cortisone acetate	Cortone acetate	PO	Rapid	1-1½ days
		IM	Slow	>2 days
Dexamethasone	Decadron	PO	1 hr	3 days
Dexamethasone acetate	Dalalone LA	IM	<8 hr	6 days
		IA, ST, IL	Slow	1-3 wk
Dexamethasone sodium phosphate	Decadrol	IV, IM	Rapid	Short
		IA, IS, IL, ST	Slow	3-21 days
✤ Hydrocortisone	Cortef	PO	<1 hr	1½ days
		IM	<4 hr	Days
	Cortenema	Rectal	3-5 days	
✤ Hydrocortisone acetate	Hydrocortone acetate	IA, IS, IB, IL, ST	<24 hr	3-28 days
	Cortef	PO	1 hr	
Hydrocortisone sodium phosphate	Hydrocortone phosphate	IV, IM	Rapid	Short
Hydrocortisone sodium succinate	Solu-Cortef	IV, IM	Rapid	Variable
Methylprednisolone	Medrol	PO	<1 hr	1½ days
Methylprednisolone acetate	Depo-Medrol	IM	6-48 hr	1-4 wk
		IA, IL, ST	Slow	1-5 wk
Methylprednisolone sodium succinate	Solu-Medrol	IV, IM	Rapid	Intermed.
Prednisolone	Prelone	PO	<1 hr	1½ days
Prednisolone acetate	Predicort	IM	Slow	
Prednisolone acetate/sodium phosphate	Generic	IM, IB, IS, IA, ST	Slow	3-28 days
Prednisolone sodium phosphate	Predicort-RP	IV, IM	<1 hr	Short
		IA, IL, ST	Slow	3-21 days
Prednisolone tebutate	Predalone TBA	IA, IL, ST	1-2 days	1-3 wk
Prednisone	Meticorten	PO	<2 hr	1½ days
Triamcinolone	Aristocort	PO	<2 hr	2 days
Triamcinolone acetonide	Kenalog	IM	1-2 days	1-6 wk
		IB, IA, IS, IL, ST	Slow	Weeks
Triamcinolone diacetate	Kenacort	PO	<2 hr	Intermediate
	Aristocort forte	IM	Slow	4-28 days
		IL	Slow	1-2 wk
		IA IS, ST	Slow	1-8 wk
Triamcinolone hexacetonide	Aristospan	IA, IL	Slow	3-4 wk

*Representative trade names are given.
†*IA*, Intraarticular; *IB*, intrabursal; *IL*, intralesional; *IM*, intramuscular; *IS*, intrasynovial; *IV*, intravenous; *PO*, oral; *ST*, soft tissue.

A number of glucocorticoids have been developed specifically for local administration. Glucocorticoids formulated for local administration are listed in Table 36-3. Local uses of glucocorticoids include bronchial inhalation for asthma; dental pastes; various creams, ointments, and other preparations for use on the skin; nasal sprays; drops for the eyes and ears; and ointments and suppositories for rectal administration.

Uses

Glucocorticoids are used to treat a number of diseases and conditions, many of which are detailed below. For systemic use in treating inflammatory conditions, the intermediate-acting glucocorticoids (methylprednisolone, prednisone, prednisolone, and triamcinolone) are generally used because they have low mineralocorticoid activity and can be administered in a way to lessen adverse reactions. Prednisone is the most commonly used glucocorticoid of this group because of its long history of reliable use and low cost.

Allergic states. Glucocorticoids may be used as adjunct therapy in treating acute, severe episodes of asthma, angioedema, transfusion reactions, and serum sickness. Inhaled glucocorticoids have become a preferred prophylactic treatment of chronic asthma to suppress inflammation of the bronchioles. Dermatologic reactions such as severe reactions to poison ivy can be blunted with oral glucocorticoids.

Dermatologic disorders. Various types of dermatitis and pemphigus are treated with glucocorticoids. Topical glucocorticoids are used for keloids, lichen planus, lichen simplex chronicus, discoid lupus, and severe psoriasis.

Gastrointestinal disorders. Inflammatory bowel diseases, including ulcerative colitis, regional enteritis (Crohn's disease), and ulcerative proctitis are treated with glucocorticoids.

Hematologic disorders. Large doses of glucocorticoids suppress the immune processes, destroying blood cells in acute phases of autoimmune hemolytic anemia and thrombocytopenia. Lower doses maintain remission.

Joint inflammation. Injection of glucocorticoids into inflamed joints gives symptomatic relief in bursitis.

Neoplastic diseases. Glucocorticoids are administered with antineoplastic agents to produce remissions for leukemias and lymphomas. The antilymphocytic action of glucocorticoids aids in destroying lymphoid cancers.

Ophthalmic diseases. Steroids may be applied directly to the eye to treat allergic conjunctivitis, chorioretinitis, iritis, iridocyclitis, and keratitis. The antiinflammatory action reduces permanent eye damage and controls acute symptoms.

Rheumatic diseases. Acute inflammatory episodes of various types of arthritis (ankylosing spondylitis, psoriatic arthritis, rheumatoid arthritis) respond to glucocorticoids. Modest doses are sometimes used to maintain inhibition of the inflammatory and autoimmune processes. Glucocorticoids are used to control flares of systemic lupus erythematosus.

Adverse Reactions and Contraindications

The adverse actions of glucocorticoids limit their long-term use. High doses of glucocorticoids administered for a few days have relatively few undesirable side effects. However, prolonged therapy with even low doses of glucocorticoids suppresses the hypothalamic-pituitary-adrenal axis regulating the natural production of cortisol (Chapter 59). This means that glucocorticoids cannot be abruptly discontinued. Rather, the dosage must be gradually tapered to allow the adrenal gland to resume functioning, thereby avoiding an adrenal crisis.

Higher than physiologic doses of glucocorticoids leads to altered metabolism of a number of tissues and organs. These changes include muscle wasting from the negative nitrogen balance induced by glucocorticoids and increased fat tissue, especially in the central portion of the body and around the face. The result is a cushingoid appearance: moon face, thin limbs, and fat on the trunk of the body. Other effects of glucocorticoids include changes in behavior and personality, usually marked by euphoria, but occasionally psychotic episodes are seen. Growth is suppressed in children. Long-term use of glucocorticoids leads to osteoporosis. Osteonecrosis is also more common. The metabolic effects of glucocorticoids can lead to impaired glucose tolerance and frank diabetes mellitus.

Glucocorticoids are classified in FDA pregnancy category C. Glucocorticoids are found in breast milk; however, as long as the mother is taking small doses of glucocorticoids, the small amount in the breast milk poses no risk for her infant.

Toxicity

Toxic reactions to long-term glucocorticoid therapy are listed in the box on p. 440. The frequency of side effects is related to the duration of therapy. Common effects, appearing after a relatively short duration of days to weeks, include weight gain, mood changes, glucose intolerance, and transient adrenal suppression. Occasionally hypertriglyceridemia, peptic ulcers, or acute pancreatitis occur. After months of glucocorticoid therapy, weight is redistributed, producing central obesity; the skin becomes fragile; muscle atrophies; the adrenal gland is suppressed; and bone loss occurs. Occasionally, long-term therapy produces cataracts, glaucoma, hypertension, or avascular necrosis. Opportunistic infections are more common.

Interactions

A number of clinically important adverse drug interactions occur with glucocorticoids. Drugs that slow the metabolism or clearance of glucocorticoids include antibiotics, cy-

TABLE 36-3 Glucocorticoid Preparations for Nonsystemic Use

PREPARATIONS	TRADE NAMES
Inhalation: Inflammation, Asthma	
Beclomethasone dipropionate, metered spray	Beclodisk,† Beclofort,† Beclovent*
Budesonide†	Pulmicort† Nubuamp, Turbohaler
Flunisolide, metered spray	AeroBid, Bronalide†
Triamcinolone acetonide, metered spray	Azmacort*
Nasal: Polyps, Rhinitis	
Beclomethasone dipropionate, metered spray	Beconase*
Budesonide,† metered spray	Rhinocort† Turbohaler, Aqua
Flunisolide, metered spray	Nasalide, Rhinalar†
Fluticasone propionate, nasal spray	Flonase
Triamcinolone acetonide, metered spray	Nasacort*
Ophthalmic: Allergic, Inflammation	
Betamethasone sodium phosphate† solution	Betnesol†
Dexamethasone solution, ointment	Maxidex
Dexamethasone sodium phosphate solution, ointment	AK-Dex, Baldex, Decadron, others
Fluorometholone suspension, ointment	FML, Fluor-Op
Fluorometholone acetate suspension	Flarex*
✤ Hydrocortisone acetate ointment†	Cortamed†
Medrysone suspension	HMS Liquifilm*
Prednisolone acetate suspension	Pred Mild,* Pred-Forte,* others
Prednisolone sodium phosphate solution	AK-Pred, Inflamase†
Otic: Inflammation of External Auditory Meatus	
Betamethasone sodium phosphate†	Betnesol†
Dexamethasone	AK-Dex,* Decadron*
Hydrocortisone acetate ointment†	Cortamed†
Topical: Skin Disorders, Rectal Disorders, Oral Lesions	
Alclometasone dipropionate cream, ointment	Aclovate
Amcinonide cream, lotion, ointment	Cyclocort*
Beclomethasone dipropionate† cream, lotion, ointment	Propraderm†
Betamethasone benzoate cream, gel, lotion	Uticort
Betamethasone diproprionate cream, gel, lotion, ointment	Alphatrex, Diprolene,* Diprosone,* Maxivate, Teladar, Topilene,† Topisone†
Betamethasone valerate cream, lotion, ointment	Betaderm,† Betatrex, Valisone, others
Clobetasol propionate cream, solution, ointment	Dermovate,† Temovate
Clobetasone butyrate† cream, ointment	Eumovate†
Clocortolone pivalate cream	Cloderm
Desonide cream, lotion, ointment	DesOwen, Tridesilon*
Desoximetasone cream, gel, ointment	Topicort*
Dexamethasone gel, aerosol	Decaderm, Decaspray
Dexamethasone sodium phosphate cream	Decadron
Diflorasone diacetate cream, ointment	Florone,* Maxiflor, Psorcon
Diflucortolone valerate† cream, ointment	Nerisone†
Flumethasone pivalate cream, ointment†	Locacorten†
Fluocinolone acetonide cream, ointment, topical solution	Bio-Syn, Fluocet, Fluoderm,† Synalar,* others
Fluocinonide cream, gel, ointment, topical solution	Fluocin, Lidex,* Lyderm†
Flurandrenolide cream, lotion, ointment, tape	Cordran, Drenison†
Fluticasone propionate cream, ointment	Cutivate
Halcinonide cream, ointment, topical solution	Halog*
Halobetasol propionate cream, ointment	Ultravate
✤ Hydrocortisone acetate dental paste	Orabase HCA
✤ Hydrocortisone rectal cream, rectal ointment, suppositories	Proctocort, Rectocort†
✤ Hydrocortisone acetate rectal cream, suppositories	Anusol-HC, Corticaine, Cortiment,† Hemril
✤ Hydrocortisone cream, lotion, ointment, topical solution for skin	Allercort, Bactine, Cort-Dome, Cortrate,† many others
✤ Hydrocortisone acetate cream, topical aerosol, lotion, ointment for skin	Cortacet,† Corticaine, Lanacort, many others
✤ Hydrocortisone butyrate cream, ointment for skin	Locoid
✤ Hydrocortisone valerate cream, ointment for skin	Westcort
Mometasone furoate cream, lotion	Elocon*
Triamcinolone acetonide dental paste	Kenalog in Orabase, Oracort, Oralone
Triamcinolone acetonide cream, lotion, ointment topical aerosol for skin	Aristocort,* Kenalog, others

*Available in Canada and United States.
†Available in Canada only.

UNDESIRABLE GLUCOCORTICOID EFFECTS

Common	Sporadic
Early Effects (Days to Weeks)	
Weight gain: from changes in lipid metabolism	*Anaphylactoid reactions:* hypersensitivity reaction
Mood changes: euphoria most common, also increased appetite, insomnia; infrequently, psychoses	*Hypertriglyceridemia:* from changes in lipid metabolism appetite, insomnia; infrequently, psychoses
Glucose intolerance: from gluconeogenic effects; resulting diabetes is usually mild and reversible	*Peptic ulcers:* may be induced or masked by glucocorticoids
Transient adrenal suppression: physiologic feedback on hypothalamic-pituitary-adrenal axis	*Acute pancreatitis:* may result from changes in lipid metabolism
Later Effects (Months to Years)	
Central obesity: classic cushingoid appearance from altered lipid metabolism	*Aseptic necrosis of bone:* most commonly affects femoral head
Skin fragility: from inhibitory effects on synthesis of collagen and extracellular matrix; also, changes in hair	*Cataracts:* cause not known; seen with systemic or local therapy
Myopathy: from protein breakdown; more pronounced with fluoride derivatives such as triamcinolone	*Glaucoma:* from interference with normal aqueous outflow; greater risk in diabetic patients
Osteoporosis: from increased bone resorption; patients with arthritis and postmenopausal women at greatest risk	*Hypertension:* more of a problem with cortisone and hydrocortisone, which have significant mineralocorticoid activity
Growth failure: from inhibition of growth hormone action; limits use in children	*Opportunistic infections:* from suppression of immune functions

closporine, estrogen, isoniazid, and ketoconazole. The dosage of glucocorticoids should be decreased.

Drugs that increase the metabolism or clearance of glucocorticoids include aminoglutethimide, carbamazepine, cholestyramine, phenobarbital, phenytoin, and rifampin. The dosage of glucocorticoids should be increased.

Glucocorticoids affect the metabolism or clearance of some other drugs, requiring adjustment of their dosages. These drugs include antianxiety agents, antipsychotics, anticholinesterases, anticoagulants, antihypertensive agents, cyclosporine, hypoglycemic drugs, liver or killed virus vaccine, pancuronium, salicylates, and sympathomimetic agents.

GLUCOCORTICOIDS: SPECIFIC DRUGS

Betamethasone

Betamethasone (Betnelan, Celestone) is a long-acting glucocorticoid with no mineralocorticoid effect. It is available in preparations for oral and rectal administration. In addition, injectable preparations are available. Long-term use in children inhibits growth.

Cortisone

Cortisone (Cortone) is a short-acting glucocorticoid that is converted by the liver to its more active form, hydrocortisone (cortisol). Cortisone has significant mineralocorticoid activity. It is available in preparations for oral administration and for intramuscular injection.

Dexamethasone

Dexamethasone (Decadron, Deronil, Dexasone, Dexone, others) is a long-acting glucocorticoid with no mineralocorticoid effect. It is used as a diagnostic aid for Cushing's syndrome and for endogenous depression. Dexamethasone can also be effective as an antiemetic for cancer chemotherapy. Long-term use in children inhibits growth.

✣ Hydrocortisone

Hydrocortisone (cortisol) (Cortef, Hydrocortone, Solu-Cortef) is the naturally occurring glucocorticoid. It is short acting and has significant mineralocorticoid activity. Hydrocortisone is available in preparations for oral and rectal administration, as well as in various injectable formulations.

Methylprednisolone

Methylprednisolone (Depo-Medrol, Medrol) has more potent antiinflammatory activity than prednisolone with almost no mineralocorticoid activity. It is available in oral and injectable formulations.

Prednisolone

Prednisolone (Delta-Cortef, Predcor, Prelone, others) has equivalent potency to prednisone with both antiinflammatory and some mineralocorticoid activity. It is available in a variety of salt forms that provide different onset of action and allow various routes of administration. Prednisolone is used in treating multiple sclerosis.

Prednisone

Prednisone (Apo-Prednisone, Deltasone, Meticorten, Orasone, others) is metabolized to prednisolone and has the same antiinflammatory and mineralocorticoid activity. Prednisone is inexpensive and is widely used for replacement therapy and to treat flares of various rheumatic disorders. Prednisone is available only for oral administration.

Triamcinolone

Triamcinolone (Artistocort) is similar to methylprednisolone in being an intermediate-acting glucocorticoid with essentially no mineralocorticoid activity. Salt forms are available for long-acting injections.

NURSING PROCESS OVERVIEW

Glucocorticoids

Assessment

Perform a complete patient assessment. Monitor temperature, pulse, respirations, blood pressure, and weight, and check blood and urine glucose. Assess skin carefully, notice color and characteristics of skin, distribution of body mass, the presence of bruises or petechiae, and the condition of hair and nails. Assess signs and symptoms of other health problems.

Nursing Diagnoses

- Body image disturbance related to weight gain and change in weight distribution related to chronic glucocorticoid administration
- Potential complication: electrolyte abnormalities
- Potential complication: fragile bones resulting in increased susceptibility to fractures

Patient Outcomes

The patient will share feelings related to body image. The nurse will minimize and manage complications associated with electrolyte abnormalities. The patient will not experience fractures related to the effects of glucocorticoids on the bones.

Planning/Implementation

Glucocorticoids are one of the most frequently used groups of drugs. Monitor the blood pressure, weight, serum electrolytes, and blood glucose. Remember that wound healing will be slowed and infection may be masked. Improvement in appetite and sense of well-being may be a result of drug therapy. Drug-induced diabetes mellitus may require treatment with insulin. In planning for discharge, determine with the physician the discharge dose and schedule of drugs, and begin teaching the patient.

Evaluation

Before discharge, ascertain that the patient can explain why the drug has been prescribed, the desired goals of therapy, how to take the drug correctly, and side effects that may occur. Check that the patient can explain additional therapies needed such as antacid therapy, dietary restrictions, and exercise or physical therapy. Ensure that the patient can explain when to notify the physician, for example, if the patient is too sick to take ordered doses. Patients must know not to discontinue or decrease the dose of chronic glucocorticoids without physician approval. Verify that the patient can explain if any parameters should be monitored at home, such as weight, blood pressure, or blood glucose.

NURSING IMPLICATIONS SUMMARY

Glucocorticoids

Drug Administration

- See the box on p. 440 for a list of side effects associated with long-term glucocorticoid therapy.
- Assess vital signs and blood pressure, lung sounds, weight, history of any weight gain or loss, and dependent areas for edema. Assess for nausea and vomiting and perform a mental status examination. Assess skin for striae (reddish-purple lines), thin skin, unusual or excessive bruising, change in skin color, change in amount of hair growth, and acne.
- Monitor height and growth pattern in children receiving long-term therapy.
- With long-term therapy, suggest ophthalmologic examinations at periodic intervals to monitor for cataracts, increased intraocular pressure, and glaucoma.
- Assess for signs of depression including lack of interest in personal appearance, withdrawal, insomnia, and anorexia.
- Check stools for presence of occult blood.
- Monitor complete blood count (CBC) and differential and serum electrolytes and blood glucose. After long-term therapy monitor hypothalamic-pituitary-adrenal (HPA) axis function to determine whether there will be normal adrenal function.
- Use care in moving and positioning immobilized patients receiving long-term therapy to prevent fractures and

Continued.

NURSING IMPLICATIONS SUMMARY—cont'd

bruising. Pad side rails as appropriate. Avoid using adhesive tape on fragile skin.

- Glucocorticoids are given via many routes (see Tables 36-2 and 36-3). Read labels carefully. Ascertain that the preparation can be given via the ordered route.

Intravenous Betamethasone Sodium Phosphate

- May be given undiluted or diluted. Administer undiluted dose over at least 1 minute.

Intravenous Dexamethasone Sodium Phosphate

- May be given undiluted. Administer dose over 1 minute.

Intravenous Hydrocortisone Sodium Phosphate

- May be given undiluted. Always use a separate syringe. Administer 25 mg or less over 1 minute.

Intravenous Hydrocortisone Sodium Succinate

- Reconstitute as directed on label of vial. Administer direct IV at a rate of 500 mg or less over 1 minute.

Intravenous Methylprednisolone Sodium Succinate

- Reconstitute as directed on label of vial. Administer direct IV at a rate of 500 mg or less over 1 minute or longer.

Intravenous Prednisolone Sodium Phosphate

- May be given undiluted at a rate of 10 mg or less over 1 minute.

Patient and Family Education

- Review anticipated benefits and possible side effects of drug therapy. With short-term use (over 7 to 10 days), side effects may be minimal if noticeable. With long-term use, some side effects will usually develop. Instruct the patient to report any new side effects.
- Instruct the patient to take oral doses with meals or a snack to lessen gastric irritation. Some physicians prescribe antacids or other drugs prophylactically to lessen the risk of ulceration. Instruct the patient to avoid alcoholic beverages while taking this medication, as the combination may contribute to increased stomach irritation.
- For missed doses, when the dosage regimen is 1 dose every other day, the patient should take the missed dose as soon as remembered if remembered on the day it was to be taken. If not remembered until the next day, the patient should take the dose, then readjust the dosage schedule to be every other day from the day the most recent dose was taken. Instruct the patient to not double up for missed doses.
- For missed doses, when dose is taken once a day, the patient should take the missed dose as soon as remembered unless not remembered until the next day. In that case the patient should omit the missed dose and resume the regular dosing schedule. Instruct the patient not to double up for missed doses.
- For missed doses, when doses are taken more than once a day, the patient should take the missed dose as soon as remembered. If not remembered until the next dose is due, the patient should take both doses at that time and resume regular dosing schedule.
- See the patient problem box on constipation (p. 304).
- If weight gain is excessive, counsel about weight reduction diets; consult the physician about a change in glucocorticoid or dose. Other dietary modifications may include decreasing sodium intake and increasing potassium intake. See the dietary consideration boxes on potassium sources (p. 170) and sodium and hypertension (p. 150). Encourage the patient to increase protein intake.
- Warn patient with diabetes to monitor blood glucose levels carefully since glucocorticoids increase blood glucose levels. A change in diet or insulin may be necessary.
- Instruct the patient to notify the physician if any of the following develop: blood in stool; black, tarry stools; mood changes, depression, insomnia; changes in vision, headache, weight gain in excess of 2 pounds per day or 5 pounds per week; menstrual irregularities; irregular heartbeat; excessive fatigue; severe or persistent stomach or abdominal pain; or if any serious injury or infection occurs.
- Instruct the patient to avoid rough activities if skin becomes fragile and easily bruised.
- Warn patients receiving long-term therapy to take doses every day as ordered, even if they are sick. Failure to take ordered doses, even for a few days, may result in adrenocortical insufficiency in susceptible patients. Remind the patient not to discontinue long-term steroid therapy without consulting the physician; tapering of the dose may be necessary.
- Remind the patient to inform all health care providers of all medications being used and to not take any medications unless approved by the physician.
- Warn the patient not to increase or decrease dose without consulting the physician.
- Update immunizations before the start of therapy if possible. Instruct the patient to avoid immunizations during therapy and for at least 3 months after therapy and to check with the physician for questions. Instruct the patient to avoid contact with anyone who has received oral polio vaccine recently or to wear a mask covering the nose and mouth if contact is unavoidable.
- Instruct the patient to avoid skin testing unless approved by the physician.
- Instruct the patient to avoid contact with anyone who has measles or chickenpox while taking glucocorticoids.

NURSING IMPLICATIONS SUMMARY—cont'd

- Encourage the patient receiving long-term therapy to wear a medical identification tag or bracelet indicating that glucocorticoids are being used.
- Menstrual difficulties may develop with long-term therapy. Instruct women to keep a record of menstrual periods. Counsel about contraceptive methods as appropriate. Warn the patient to notify the physician if pregnancy is suspected.
- Large doses of glucocorticoids increase susceptibility to infection and mask the symptoms of infection. Warn the patient about this side effect. Instruct the patient to notify the physician of fever, cough, sore throat, malaise, and injuries that do not heal. Instruct the patient to avoid contact with individuals with active infections.
- Review the drug and route of administration prescribed for the patient. Review the manufacturer's instruction for administration. Ascertain that the patient can administer the ordered drug correctly (see Chapter 5).
- Remind the patient not to share medications with others. Remind the patient to keep all medications out of the reach of children.
- If this drug is injected into a joint, remind the patient to use the joint only as directed by physician. Too much use, too soon, may stress the joint.

Nasal Solution

- Review the instruction sheet provided by the manufacturer. The patient should blow the nose. With nosepiece in the nostril, the patient should aim the spray toward the inner corner of the eye, then spray and sniff. Encourage the patient to save the inhaler, which may be reusable.

Aerosol Metered Dose

- Review the instruction sheet provided by the manufacturer. If an adrenergic bronchodilator such as albuterol, metaproterenol, or terbutaline is also prescribed via the inhalation route, instruct the patient to use the bronchodilator first, wait 5 minutes, then use the adrenocorticoid. The patient should not increase the number of sprays unless directed to do so by the physician. Remind the patient to avoid spraying medication in the eyes.
- The aerosol metered dose form of glucocorticoids may cause hoarseness, throat irritation, and infection in the mouth. Gargling or rinsing the mouth after each drug use may help prevent these problems. Warn the patient not to swallow the water after gargling or rinsing. The physician may also want the patient to use a spacer, which is a tube that fits on the inhaler.
- Instruct the patient to rinse the mouth with water after each dose to help prevent dry mouth and clean the mouthpiece of the inhaler every day. See the manufacturer's instructions.
- If the canister is cold, instruct the patient to warm it between the hands before administering the dose.
- Encourage the patient not to discard the inhaler since it may be possible to use it with refill canisters; check with the pharmacist. Remind the patient to use the inhaler for this drug only with this drug, not with any others, even if other canisters fit the inhaler.
- Instruct the patient to use this drug only as prescribed and to not increase the frequency or dose of medication without consulting with the physician.
- Encourage the patient to limit or stop smoking if possible.
- Several weeks of therapy may be needed to see full benefit.

Eyedrops, Eye Ointment

- Emphasize the importance of using the eyedrops or ointment as directed, even if there are no symptoms present.
- Using this drug while wearing contact lenses may increase the chance of infection. The physician may want the patient to avoid contact lenses while using this drug, and for several days after completing the course of eyedrop therapy. Check with the physician.
- See Chapter 5 for information about administering eyedrops or ointment. Instruct the patient to wash hands after administration to keep medication from being absorbed through skin.
- Instruct the patient to apply the missed dose as soon as remembered unless it is almost time for the next dose, then omit missed dose and resume regular dosing schedule. The patient should not double up for missed doses.
- Administration of eyedrops or ointment may make vision blurry or cloudy for a few minutes; warn the patient not to drive or operate hazardous equipment until vision is clear.
- Instruct the patient to notify the physician if any of the following develop: eye pain, irritation.
- Instruct the patient to use eyedrops or ointment as prescribed but not longer than the time ordered since side effects may begin to develop. Also, instruct the patient not to use steroid eyedrops for eye problems that may develop in the future unless directed to do so by the physician.

Otic (Ear) Solutions

- See Chapter 5 to review administration technique. Instruct the patient to put a cotton ball in as a plug if desired. The physician may want eardrops put onto the cotton plug before it is put into the ear. Try to avoid touching the ear with the dropper. The dropper may be wiped off, but should not be rinsed with water.
- Instruct the patient to use the drops as prescribed but not to use leftover medication to treat ear problems that may develop in the future unless directed to do so by the physician.

Continued.

NURSING IMPLICATIONS SUMMARY—cont'd

- Instruct the patient to notify the physician if stinging, itching, or burning of the ear develop.

Otic (Ear) Ointment

- Review administration technique. Instruct the patient to use a finger or piece of gauze to apply a small amount of ointment just inside the ear canal. Instruct the patient not to use a cotton-tipped swab unless directed to do so by the physician. Instruct the patient to use the ointment as prescribed but not to use leftover medication to treat ear problems that may develop in the future unless directed to do so by the physician. Instruct the patient to notify the physician if stinging, itching, or burning of the ear develop.

Enema

- Review the patient instruction leaflet supplied by the manufacturer. Each bottle contains 1 dose; the entire contents of the bottle should be used unless otherwise directed by physician. Inform the patient to use the enema after having a bowel movement. Instruct the patient to lie down on the left side when administering the enema and to insert tip of applicator slowly to prevent injury. After administering the medication, the patient should remain on the left side for 30 minutes to allow the medication to work. If possible, the patient should retain the enema all night.

Rectal Aerosol Form

- Review the patient instruction leaflet supplied by the manufacturer. Instruct the patient to insert the applicator tip only into the rectum and not to insert the aerosol container.

Topical Corticosteroids

- Assess the area being treated for irritation, lesions, redness, and swelling. After beginning use of topical medication, assess for improvement or signs of possible skin irritation caused by the medication.
- Instruct the patient and family to wear gloves to apply the dose or to wash fingers off with soap and water after applying to avoid absorbing medication through the skin or accidentally getting medication in the eyes.
- Instruct the patient to use topical corticosteroids only as prescribed. Several kinds of skin problems should not be treated with topical corticosteroids. Instruct the patient to read the package labels carefully and check with the physician before treating skin problems.
- Instruct the patient not to wrap the skin being treated unless directed to do so by the physician. Also, if used in the diaper area, tight-fitting diapers or plastic pants should not be used unless directed to do so by the physician.
- There may be temporary stinging after gel, solution, lotion, or aerosol forms are applied.
- For aerosol topical forms, see the manufacturer's insert supplied with the medication. Instruct the patient to apply the medication carefully and avoid getting medication in the eyes or breathing in fumes. Instruct the patient to rinse the eyes with copious amounts of water if medication gets in the eyes.
- Instruct the patient to apply a missed dose as soon as remembered unless almost time for next dose; then omit the missed dose and resume the regular dosing schedule. The patient should not double up for missed doses.
- Children or teenagers should not use topical corticosteroids over large areas of skin or for longer than 2 weeks without checking with the physician.
- Instruct the patient to notify the physician if any of the following develop: worsening of skin condition, redness, itching, or blisters.

Flurandrenolide Tape

- Review the manufacturer's instructions supplied with the medication.
- Occasionally, systemic side effects may develop if gel, ointment, creme, lotion, solution, or tape is applied to large areas or at high doses. These side effects range from depression, weight gain, acne, oily skin, blurred vision, stretch marks on skin, increased hair growth, excessive fatigue, to increased blood pressure. Instruct the patient to keep all health care providers informed of all medications being used and to notify the physician if any unusual signs or symptoms develop.

Dental Paste

- Instruct the patient to use a cotton-tipped swab to apply a small amount of the paste to the prescribed area. Instruct the patient not to rub the paste but to press the paste in place until a smooth, slippery film forms. Recommend that the patient apply paste at bedtime, so it can work during the night. Instruct the patient to use the paste as prescribed but not to use leftover medication to treat oral problems that may develop in the future unless directed to do so by the physician. Instruct the patient to notify the physician if stinging, irritation, itching, or burning of the mouth develop.

CRITICAL THINKING

APPLICATION

1. What is the difference between an inflammatory response and an immune response?
2. How do glucocorticoids suppress the inflammatory response?
3. How does liver disease influence the effects of the glucocorticoids?
4. What is the advantage of alternate-day therapy with systemic glucocorticoids?
5. What are some diseases or conditions that may be treated with glucocorticoids?
6. What are the early and late effects of long-term glucocorticoid administration?
7. What are the signs and symptoms of adrenal crisis?

CRITICAL THINKING

1. Why should a patient receiving long-term glucocorticoid therapy consult the physician before discontinuing glucocorticoid therapy?
2. Study Table 36-1. Why is dexamethasone a better choice for treating increased intracranial pressure than cortisone?
3. The patient receiving long-term glucocorticoid therapy should not have allergy skin testing. Why?

CHAPTER 37

Drugs for Selected Autoimmune Diseases

Myasthenia Gravis, Rheumatoid Arthritis, Systemic Lupus Erythematosus, and Multiple Sclerosis

OBJECTIVES

After studying this chapter, you should be able to do the following:

For myasthenia gravis

- *Describe the action of acetylcholinesterase inhibitors.*
- *Develop a nursing care plan for patients receiving drug treatment for myasthenia gravis.*

For rheumatoid arthritis

- *Describe the use and limitations of the various disease-modifying antirheumatic drugs (DMARDs).*
- *Develop a nursing care plan for patients receiving drug treatment for rheumatoid arthritis.*

For systemic lupus erythematosus

- *Describe the drugs used to control symptoms of systemic lupus erythematosus.*
- *Develop a nursing care plan for patients receiving drug treatment for systemic lupus erythematosus.*

For multiple sclerosis

- *Describe the drugs used to control symptoms of multiple sclerosis.*
- *Develop a nursing care plan for patients receiving drug treatment for multiple sclerosis.*

KEY TERMS

anticholinesterase inhibitors
autoimmune disease
disease-modifying antirheumatic drugs (DMARDs)
immunosuppressive agents
multiple sclerosis
myasthenia gravis
rheumatoid arthritis
systemic lupus erythematosus

CHAPTER OVERVIEW

The immune system is normally able to distinguish the body's own components from invading bacteria, viruses, and other foreign organisms. However, autoimmune diseases represent the immune system turned against some component of the host's body. Some of the factors explaining why this happens are beginning to emerge. One component involves the way antigens are handled, with HLA (MHC) molecules presenting antigens to T cells. The antigens picked for presentation may be the same as the body's own naturally occurring antigens (molecular mimicry). Such self-reactive T cells are normally eliminated by the thymus during development, but this elimination may be bypassed by viral or bacterial infection. Certain HLA genes appear to increase the likelihood of certain autoimmune diseases. For instance, HLA-DR4 is associated with an increased prevalence of rheumatoid arthritis, HLA-DR2 with multiple sclerosis, and HLA-DR3, and HLA-DR4 with type one diabetes mellitus.

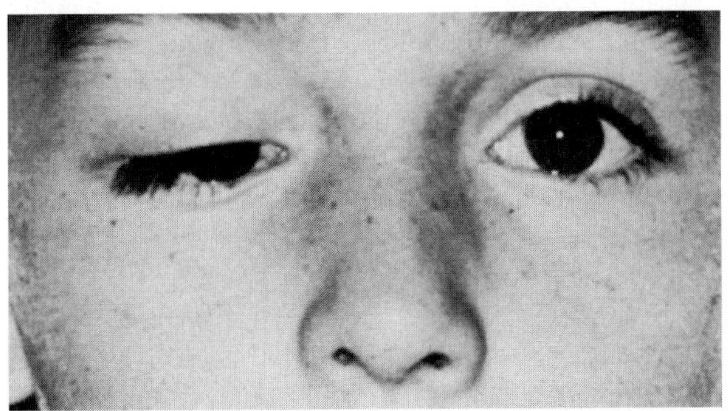

FIGURE 37-1

Myasthenia gravis is often first indicated by a drooping eyelid (paresis of levator palpebrae superioris muscle). Only one upper eyelid may be affected. Disease may stay limited to this muscle group. (From Newell FW: *Ophthalmology: principles and concepts,* ed 7, St Louis, 1992, Mosby.)

Therapeutic Rationale: Myasthenia Gravis

Myasthenia gravis is a disease in which the skeletal muscles quickly show weakness and become fatigued. Muscles controlling facial movements are most commonly involved. One early sign of myasthenia gravis is a drooping eyelid (ptosis) (Figure 37-1). As the disease progresses, chewing and swallowing become increasingly difficult, and the voice becomes less distinct. Death can result if the intercostal muscles and the diaphragm, muscles essential for breathing, become affected.

The basic defect in myasthenia gravis is a reduction by 70% to 90% in the available receptors for acetylcholine at the neuromuscular junction (Figure 37-2). Myasthenia gravis is caused by autoantibodies against the neuromuscular receptors for acetylcholine. These autoantibodies block the active site for acetylcholine of the neuromuscular (nicotinic) receptor and also increase the rate at which the receptors are degraded by the cell.

A number of drugs have weak anticholinergic effects of their own and are contraindicated for the patient with myasthenia gravis. These drugs, listed in the box on p. 448, can dangerously weaken the patient with myasthenia gravis but do not noticeably block the neuromuscular receptor of a healthy person.

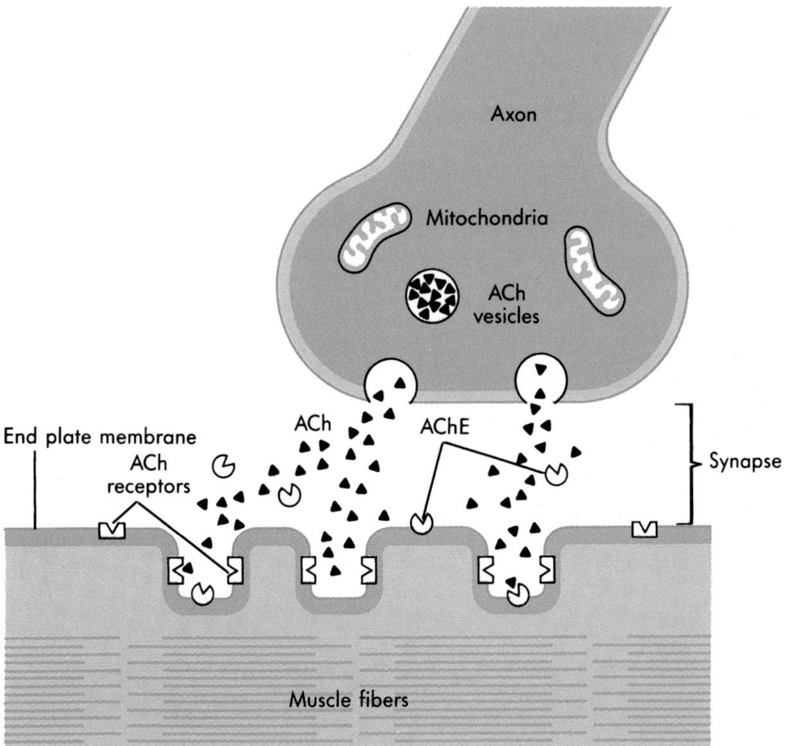

FIGURE 37-2

Acetylcholine is neurotransmitter released by nerve to occupy nicotinic receptors on muscle; it thereby initiates biochemical events causing muscle to contract. Acetylcholine is rapidly degraded by acetylcholinesterase, present throughout synapse. In myasthenia gravis, number of receptors is greatly decreased. Acetylcholinesterase inhibitors prevent rapid breakdown of acetylcholine. With more acetylcholine present, fewer receptors are needed and loss of receptors is partially compensated.

DRUGS THAT MAY WEAKEN A PATIENT WITH MYASTHENIA GRAVIS

Adrenocorticotropic hormone (ACTH) and glucocorticoids
Anesthetics
- Diethyl ether
- Halothane (Fluothane)
- Lidocaine IV (Xylocaine)

Antiarrhythmics
- Procainamide (Pronestyl)
- Propranolol (Inderal)
- Quinidine

Antibiotics
- Bacitracin (Bacitracin)
- Colistimethate (Coly-Mycin M)
- Colistin (Coly-Mycin S)
- Gentamicin (Garamycin)
- Kanamycin (Kantrex)
- Lincomycin (Lincocin)
- Neomycin (Mycifradin, Neobiotic)
- Netilmicin (Netromycin)
- Paromomycin (Humatin)
- Polymyxin B (Aerosporin, Polymyxin B)
- Streptomycin (Streptomycin)
- Viomycin (Viocin)

Anticonvulsants
- Magnesium sulfate

Antimalarials
- Quinine

Diuretics and other drugs or circumstances promoting hypokalemia (low blood potassium concentration)
Muscle relaxants
- Gallamine (Flaxedil)
- Metocurine (Metubine)
- Pancuronium (Pavulon)
- Succinylcholine (Anectine)
- Tubocurarine

Sedatives, especially those with respiratory depressant effects, such as barbiturates, narcotics, and tranquilizers
Thyroid compounds

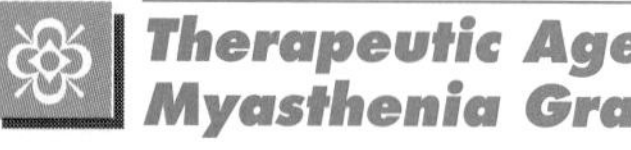

Therapeutic Agents: Myasthenia Gravis

Acetylcholinesterase Inhibitors: General Characteristics

Mechanism of Action

Drugs that inhibit the degradation of acetylcholine, **acetylcholinesterase inhibitors** (anticholinesterases), are the first line of treatment for myasthenia gravis. These drugs are listed in Table 37-1. As seen in Figure 37-2, the enzyme acetylcholinesterase is present throughout the neuromuscular junction, where it rapidly degrades acetylcholine after release. Acetylcholinesterase inhibitors allow acetylcholine to accumulate at the neuromuscular junction, ensuring that available receptors are activated.

Pharmacokinetics

Anticholinesterase drugs are positively charged compounds that are not lipid soluble. These drugs are therefore not readily absorbed orally; the oral dose is 30 times the parenteral dose. The most widely used anticholinesterases are pyridostigmine and neostigmine. The anticholinesterases are metabolized by plasma esterases and by hepatic enzymes to inactive compounds. The drugs and their metabolites are excreted in the urine.

The effective dose must be individualized for each patient. Stress and infection can increase the requirement. Women in the premenstrual part of their cycle may require higher doses. Very ill patients may become unresponsive to their medication, but temporary reduction or withdrawal of the dose over a 3-day period may restore their responsiveness. Parenteral administration may be required.

Uses

Acetylcholinesterase inhibitors used to treat myasthenia gravis are also used to reverse the effects of competitive neuromuscular blocking drugs used in surgery.

Adverse Reactions and Contraindications

Side effects arising from overstimulation of neuromuscular (nicotinic) receptors include muscle cramps, rapid small contractions (fasciculation), and weakness. Acetylcholinesterase inhibitors can also act at sites other than neuromuscular sites. At muscarinic sites, they produce side effects classic for parasympathetic stimulation such as excessive salivation, perspiration, abdominal distress, and nausea and vomiting. Patients frequently develop a tolerance to the muscarinic effects of the anticholinesterases.

Anticholinesterase drugs are contraindicated for patients with intestinal or urinary tract obstruction. These drugs should be used cautiously in patients with bronchial asthma. Persons sensitive to bromide should be given neostigmine methylsulfate or ambenonium chloride instead of more commonly used bromide-containing anticholinesterases.

Acetylcholinesterase Inhibitors: Specific Drugs

Ambenonium

Ambenonium (Mytelase) is slightly longer acting than pyridostigmine or neostigmine. Patients may experience side effects not seen with pyridostigmine or neostigmine, such as jitteriness, headaches, confusion, and dizziness. Ambenonium is not a bromide salt, unlike pyridostigmine and neostigmine. It is therefore the drug of choice for patients allergic to bromides.

Edrophonium

Edrophonium (Tensilon) is a short-acting acetylcholinesterase inhibitor used as a diagnostic agent. When a new patient with suspected myasthenia gravis is given 2 mg of edrophonium intravenously, an increase in muscle strength should be seen in 1 to 3 minutes. If no response occurs, an-

TABLE 37-1 Cholinomimetic Drugs for Myasthenia Gravis

GENERIC NAME	TRADE NAME*	ADMINISTRATION/DOSAGE	COMMENTS
Ambenonium chloride	Mytelase	ORAL: *Adults*—5 mg 3 or 4 times daily increased every 1-2 days as required. *Children*—0.3 mg/kg body weight daily in divided doses, increased gradually if necessary to maximum of 1.5 mg/kg daily.	Mytelase is acetylcholinesterase inhibitor that is rapidly absorbed.
Edrophonium chloride	Tensilon Enlon	*For diagnosis of myasthenia gravis:* INTRAVENOUS: *Adults*—2 mg injected over 15-30 sec. If no response, 8 mg is given. May repeat test after 1 hr. *Children*—2 mg initially as above followed by 5 mg (if under 75 lb) or up to 10 mg (if over 75 lb).	Tensilon is very short-acting acetylcholinesterase inhibitor. Diagnosis is positive if muscle strength increases within 3 min (duration 5-10 min).
		To differentiate myasthenic from cholinergic crisis: 1-2 mg.	Cholinergic crisis if muscle strength decreases (lower medication dose). Patient in cholinergic crisis may require ventilatory assistance after injection.
Neostigmine bromide	Prostigmin bromide	ORAL: *Adults*—15 mg every 3-4 hr initially, then adjust upward as required. *Children*—begin with 2 mg/kg body weight daily in divided doses.	Prostigmin bromide is acetylcholinesterase inhibitor with high incidence of side effects.
Neostigmine methylsulfate	Prostigmin methylsulfate	INTRAMUSCULAR: *Adults*—0.022 mg/kg body weight (atropine, intramuscularly, 0.011 mg/kg may be given to control muscarinic side effects). *Children*—0.01-0.04 mg/kg body weight (with 0.01 mg/kg atropine, IM).	Prostigmin methylsulfate is injectable form for diagnosis of myasthenia gravis.
Pyridostigmine bromide	Mestinon	ORAL: *Adults*—60-120 mg every 3 or 4 hr initially, increased as necessary. *Children*—7 mg/kg in divided doses as required.	Mestinon is acetylcholinesterase inhibitor; it is drug of choice for controlling muscular weakness of myasthenia gravis.
	Regonol	INTRAMUSCULAR, INTRAVENOUS: *Adults*—1/30 of oral dose. *Newborn infants of myasthenic mothers*—0.05-0.15 mg/kg body weight.	

*These drugs are available in Canada and the United States.

other 4 to 10 mg of edrophonium is given over the next 2 minutes, and muscle strength is again tested. If no increase in muscle strength occurs with this higher dose, the muscle weakness is not caused by myasthenia gravis. Patients receiving injections of edrophonium commonly show a drop in blood pressure and feel faint, dizzy, and flushed.

A second diagnostic use for edrophonium is to help physicians determine treatment when a patient being treated for myasthenia gravis becomes weaker. The problem is to identify whether the patient is reacting to an overdose of medication (cholinergic crisis) or an increasing severity of the disease (myasthenic crisis). An edrophonium injection makes the patient in cholinergic crisis temporarily worse (negative Tensilon test) but temporarily improves the condition when the patient is in myasthenic crisis (positive Tensilon test).

Neostigmine

Neostigmine (Prostigmin) can be used to diagnose and treat myasthenia gravis. As a diagnostic tool, an intramuscular injection of neostigmine should improve the patient's muscular strength in 10 minutes, and this improvement should last 3 to 4 hours. Neostigmine is also prescribed to relieve the symptoms of myasthenia gravis. Because neostigmine is irregularly absorbed from the gastrointestinal tract, it can be difficult to establish effective drug levels with oral administration. Muscarinic side effects, particularly salivation, cramps, and diarrhea, are common enough to limit the long-term use of neostigmine. If neostigmine is used, atropine may also be prescribed to block the muscarinic effects.

Pyridostigmine

Pyridostigmine (Mestinon) is the drug of choice for the treatment of myasthenia gravis. Compared with neostigmine, pyridostigmine is better absorbed from the gastrointestinal tract and is longer acting. Adverse effects such as miosis, sweating, salivation, gastrointestinal distress, and slow heart rate are less common with pyridostigmine than with neostigmine.

NURSING PROCESS OVERVIEW

Myasthenia Gravis

Assessment

Patients who have or who are suspected of having myasthenia gravis require acetylcholinesterase inhibitors (anticholinesterases). Symptoms range from mild ptosis and easy fatigue to acute muscular weakness. Assess the temperature, pulse, respiration, blood pressure, vital capacity, ability to swallow, muscle strength, and degree of ptosis. Assess the results of peripheral nerve stimulation. Assess the patient's ability to perform activities of daily living. Finally, assess the patient for additional medical problems that may influence treatment.

Nursing Diagnoses

- Risk for ineffective airway clearance related to medication dosage adjustments
- Risk for impaired swallowing related to inadequate doses of acetylcholinesterase inhibitors
- Anxiety related to frequent swings between myasthenic and cholinergic crises and apparent inability to obtain adequate drug control of myasthenia gravis

Patient Outcomes

The patient will state a decrease in anxiety as the medication treatment plan is developed. The nurse will manage and minimize ineffective airway clearance and impaired swallowing until control by medications is achieved. The patient will learn to self-manage at home.

Planning/Implementation

Monitor signs of myasthenia gravis such as ptosis, ability to swallow, vital capacity, muscle strength, and vital signs. Administer medications on time. Keep a suction machine at the bedside if the patient displays any inability to swallow secretions adequately. Keep edrophonium, pyridostigmine, atropine, neostigmine, and syringes at the bedside. Have equipment for intubation readily available. Teach the patient and family about myasthenia gravis management in the home. Refer the patient to other members of the health care team for physical therapy, home nursing care, or social services. Refer the patient and family to local and national myasthenia support and research groups.

Evaluation

Successful drug therapy helps the patient maintain as normal a lifestyle as possible but does not cure the disease. Patient compliance and understanding are essential to good control of the symptoms. Before discharge the patient should be able to explain how and why the medication should be taken, signs and symptoms of medication overdose and underdose, symptoms that require physician notification, other measures to assist in managing the disease (such as using an alarm clock with battery back-up to awaken the patient for nighttime doses of medication), and medications to avoid.

Therapeutic Rationale: Rheumatoid Arthritis

Rheumatoid arthritis is an **autoimmune disease** that primarily involves the synovial membrane. The synovial membrane is the inner layer of the articular capsule surrounding a freely movable joint, such as the knee and joints of the finger. This tissue, which normally is smooth and shiny and secretes a thick fluid that lubricates the joint, becomes inflamed, painful, and the joint is swollen with fluid. The inflammatory process leads to the production of cytokines such as interleukin-1 and tumor necrosis factor-alpha that trigger the production of proteinases that eventually destroy cartilage and bone.

Rheumatoid arthritis occurs in about 1% of the population (more than 2 million people in the United States), it affects women about three times more often than men. Although the disease can occur at any age, the peak incidence in women is between the ages of 40 to 60 years.

Therapeutic Agents: Rheumatoid Arthritis

Rheumatoid arthritis is a highly variable disease process. It frequently goes into remission for months or years. In early rheumatoid arthritis only the synovial membranes are inflamed, causing painful swelling. Aspirin and the other nonsteroid antiinflammatory drugs (NSAIDs) (Chapter 30) may be sufficient to control symptoms. The antiinflammatory effect added to the analgesic effect eases the pain and increases the mobility of the affected joint.

Disease-modifying antirheumatic drugs (DMARDs) (Table 37-2) were originally reserved for patients with severe, difficult-to-manage rheumatoid arthritis. These drugs include azathioprine, gold therapy, hydroxychloroquine, methotrexate, penicillamine, and sulfasalzine. However, some rheumatologists believe that more aggressive therapy should be initiated earlier in the course of treatment, especially for progressive cases. Hydroxychloroquine has relatively low toxicity and suppresses symptoms in about 50% of patients treated. Methotrexate in low doses has also emerged in recent years as a relatively safe and effective drug for treating progressive rheumatoid arthritis. Glucocorticoids have a restricted role in treating severe exacerbations of rheumatoid arthritis. All antirheumatic drugs have potentially serious side effects that must be monitored carefully.

Although a NSAID may be continued, DMARDs are not generally combined with each other. Many have potentially severe side effects that must be monitored. Some clinicians believe that the disease-modifying drugs should be used

TABLE 37-2 Disease-Modifying Antirheumatic Drugs

GENERIC NAME	TRADE NAME	ADMINISTRATION/DOSAGE	COMMENTS
Auranofin	Ridaura*	ORAL: *Adults*—6 mg once daily or 3 mg twice daily. FDA pregnancy category C.	Dose may be increased to 9 mg daily after 6 mo if inadequate response for another 3 mo. If response is still inadequate, discontinue. CBC and urinalysis should be performed every 2-4 wk. Less toxic than injectable gold.
Aurothioglucose	Solganal	INTRAMUSCULAR: *Adults*—10 mg first week; 25 mg weeks 2 and 3; then 25-50 mg once weekly until total dose of 800-1000 mg has been given. Maintenance: 25 or 50 mg every 2 weeks for 2-20 weeks, then 25 or 50 mg every 3 or 4 weeks. *Children 6-12 yr*—2.5 mg first week, 6.25 mg weeks 2 and 3; then 12.5 mg weekly until total dose of 200-250 mg has been given; then 6.25 or 12.5 mg every 3 or 4 weeks. FDA pregnancy category C.	Onset of action is usually 6-8 wk; may cause nitroid reactions and temporary joint pain after injection. Gluteal injection preferred.
✧ Azathioprine	Imuran*	ORAL: *Adults*—1 mg/kg body weight daily, increasing by 0.5 mg/kg body weight daily after 6-8 wk, then every 4 wk as necessary for maximum dose of 2.5 mg/kg body weight daily. Maintenance: reduce to minimum effective dose in steps of 0.5 mg/kg body weight daily at 1-2 mo intervals. FDA pregnancy category D.	CBC should be performed weekly first month; twice monthly second and third month; monthly thereafter. Liver function tests should be performed every 1-3 mo.
Gold sodium thiomalate	Myochrysine*	INTRAMUSCULAR: *Adults*—10 mg first week; 25 mg weeks 2 and 3; then 25-50 mg once weekly until total dose of 1000 mg has been given. Maintenance: 25 or 50 mg every 2 wk for 2-20 wk, then 25 or 50 mg every 3 or 4 wk. *Children 6-12 yr*—10 mg first week, then 1 mg/kg body weight, up to 50 mg per dose, until desired therapeutic response is reached or until toxicity occurs. FDA pregnancy category C.	Gluteal injection preferred. If therapy has been halted due to mild adverse reactions, initial dose of 5 mg is given; if tolerated, dose is increased by 5-10 mg increments at weekly to monthly intervals until dose of 25-50 mg is reached.
Hydroxychloroquine sulfate	Plaquenil*	ORAL: *Adults*—up to 6.5 mg/kg lean body weight daily, with meals or glass of milk.	If usual initial dose produces side effects, reduce dose for 5-10 days, then gradually increase. Eye examination should be performed initially and after 6 mo.
✧ Methotrexate	Rheumatrex*	ORAL: *Adults*—2.5-5 mg every 12 hr for 3 doses each week, increasing if necessary by 2.5 mg weekly up to 20 mg weekly. Alternatively, ORAL, INTRAMUSCULAR, OR INTRAVENOUS: *Adults*—10 mg once weekly, increasing dosage if necessary up to 25 mg weekly. FDA pregnancy category X.	Oral route is associated with less toxicity. CBC and liver function tests should be performed every 2 wk initially, then every 1-3 mo. Onset of action is 1-2 mo.
Penicillamine	Cuprimine*	ORAL: *Adults*—125-250 mg once daily, increasing if necessary by 125-250 mg daily every 2-3 mo if necessary, up to 1.5 gm daily.	Side effects are common; CBC and urinalysis should be performed every 2 weeks initially, then every 1-3 mo.
Sulfasalazine	Azulfidine, PMS Sulfasalazine,† Salazopyrin†	ORAL: *Adults*—500 mg-1 mg daily for first week; may increase by 500 mg each week, up to maintenance dose of 2 mg daily. May divide into 2 doses. FDA pregnancy category B.	Not currently listed in U.S. product labeling for rheumatoid arthritis. CBC should be performed periodically. Not for persons allergic to sulfa drugs.

*Available in Canada and United States.
†Available in Canada only.

much earlier in the course of rheumatoid arthritis before inflammatory processes have been in place for decades.

AZATHIOPRINE

Mechanism of Action

Azathioprine (Imuran) is an antimetabolite for purines and interferes with the metabolism of DNA and RNA. The exact mechanism of its immunosuppressive activity is not known, but T cell–mediated immunity is affected more than B cell–mediated immunity.

Pharmacokinetics

Azathioprine may be given orally or by injection. It is well absorbed and rapidly converted by the liver to the active metabolites, 6-mercaptopurine and 6-thioinosinic acid, which account for the actual effects of azathioprine. The actual plasma half-life of the drug and its active metabolites is 5 hours. Metabolites are excreted in the bile. The onset of immunosuppressive action is much longer, 4 to 8 weeks. The clinical effects can persist for some time after the drug is discontinued.

Uses

A major use of azathioprine is to prevent organ transplant rejection. The doses administered to prevent rejection begin with 3 to 5 mg/kg body weight/day initially with maintenance doses of 1 to 2 mg/kg body weight/day.

For autoimmune diseases, including rheumatoid arthritis, systemic lupus erythematosus, and myasthenia gravis, the initial dose is about 1 mg/kg body weight a day, generally 50 or 100 mg, as one or two doses. This dose is increased by 0.5 mg/kg body weight daily after 4 weeks. A usual dose for azathioprine is 50 to 200 mg taken as a single dose. A clinical response should be seen in 12 weeks or therapy discontinued. If a satisfactory clinical response is achieved and there are no adverse reactions, therapy may be continued with careful monitoring of the patient.

Adverse Reactions and Contraindications

The most common adverse reactions to azathioprine are nausea, vomiting, diarrhea, and abdominal pain. These are usually just annoying and do not require that therapy be discontinued.

More serious side effects include liver injury and low blood cell counts (CBC). In particular, low platelet counts may lead to bruising and bleeding. If the white blood cell (WBC) count is markedly depressed, the number of infections experienced may increase. In particular, viral infections such as herpes zoster and chickenpox are more common. Jaundice can indicate liver damage. Severe vomiting may indicate mucosal ulcers.

Less common side effects include skin rash, drug fever, loss of hair, and pancreatitis.

Azathioprine should not be used by pregnant or nursing women because of potential effects on the fetus or infant. Azathioprine is contraindicated for patients with chickenpox, herpes zoster, gout, renal function impairment, or hepatic function impairment.

Toxicity

About 28% of patients who take azathioprine have hematologic reactions, including anemia and a decrease in white cell and thrombocyte counts. Long-term administration of azathioprine may increase the risk of developing cancer or leukemia.

Interactions

Allopurinol, an inhibitor of purine metabolism used to treat gout, will greatly increase the activity and toxicity of azathioprine. Live virus vaccines should not be given to patients who take azathioprine because the lowered immune activity will not allow an adequate immune response and the virus may cause illness. Azathioprine should not be administered with other immunosuppressive agents because of the risk of infections and neoplasms.

Azathioprine also has a steroid-sparing effect, which allows a reduction in steroid dose when the two are combined for treating chronic inflammatory diseases.

GLUCOCORTICOIDS

Glucocorticoids dramatically relieve inflammation and the accompanying pain of arthritis and flares of systemic lupus erythematosus. Because of the profound side effects, the use of glucocorticoids is reserved to control severe cases of rheumatoid arthritis. The use of glucocorticoids for immune and inflammatory conditions is described in detail in Chapter 36.

When used in rheumatoid arthritis, a low oral dose of prednisone daily or on alternate days is sometimes used in conjunction with another slower acting drug such as gold, methotrexate, hydroxychloroquine, sulfasalazine, or azathioprine. Prednisone is either gradually decreased as the slower acting drug starts to have an effect, or it may be continued longer at the smallest possible dose.

GOLD COMPOUNDS: GENERAL CHARACTERISTICS

Mechanism of Action

Although gold compounds have both antiinflammatory and immunosuppressive activity, the exact mechanism of action is not known. They appear to decrease the release of enzymes that degrade the joint. Gold compounds are capable of retarding progression of rheumatoid arthritis and even inducing a remission.

Pharmacokinetics

Aurothioglucose and gold sodium thiomalate are administered by weekly intramuscular injection. The onset of action is very slow. Gold is stored in the body, particularly the reticuloendothelial system, and only slowly excreted, over about 6 months, through the kidney and feces.

Auranofin is a gold compound that can be taken orally. Clinical trials indicate that auranofin is as effective as the injectable gold drugs in inducing remission in rheumatoid arthritis. Auranofin is taken twice daily.

Uses

Gold is administered to reduce joint pain and to induce a remission in patients with rheumatoid arthritis.

When given intramuscularly to adults, 10 mg is given the first week, 25 mg the second week, and 50 mg the third week and thereafter until 800 to 1000 mg total has been administered. If there has been no response, the drug is discontinued. If there is a response of decreased joint pain, the injections are continued. When the clinical status stabilizes, the dose can be reduced to 25 to 50 mg every 2 weeks and then to monthly injections. After a year of remission, some doctors will discontinue the drug, others will continue at a reduced dosage. Only 30% to 60% of patients treated with gold respond over a 2- to 3-year course of treatment.

Gold may also be administered to patients with juvenile rheumatoid arthritis. The initial dose is 0.2 mg/kg, 0.5 mg/kg the second week and 1 mg/kg weekly thereafter. No single dose is more than 50 mg.

When administered orally, the adult dose is 6 mg daily as a single or divided dose. If an adequate response is not achieved in 6 months, the dose may be raised to 9 mg daily, but therapy is discontinued if there is still no response after an additional 3 months.

Adverse Reactions and Contraindications

Gold compounds are either well tolerated or produce toxic effects that lead to their discontinuance.

The most common reason for discontinuing successful gold therapy is the appearance of serious side effects such as skin reactions, mouth ulcers, fever, kidney damage, or abnormalities in the blood count. About 40% of patients develop an adverse reaction. These effects can occur at any time during therapy but are more common after a cumulative dose of 400 to 800 mg. Skin reactions and mouth ulcers are the most common side effects. If these are mild, gold therapy may be halted temporarily and then tried again. CBCs and a urinalysis to measure protein should be done before each dose early in gold therapy and continued periodically throughout therapy.

Contraindications for gold therapy include uncontrolled diabetes mellitus, renal disease, hepatic dysfunction, congestive heart failure, hypertension, or blood dyscrasia. Patients who take other immunosuppressive drugs should not receive gold therapy. Because gold crosses the placenta and also appears in breast milk, pregnant and nursing women should not receive gold therapy.

Toxicity

Early symptoms of toxic reactions include a rash, purple blotches, pruritus, mouth lesions, and a metallic taste. Patients should be questioned about these before each injection. Since toxicity can appear even after therapy has been discontinued, the patient should be followed for at least the next 6 months for gold toxicity.

About 20% of patients experience dermatitis or lesions of the mucous membranes, usually in the first 6 months of therapy. The first sign of a skin reaction is often pruritus, and therapy may be temporarily discontinued to avoid severe dermatitis. Sunlight can aggravate skin reactions.

Severe hematologic reactions are rare, but therapy should be discontinued if the white blood cell count falls below 3500/mm^3. Renal damage is manifested by proteinuria. Urinary protein estimates should be done before any gold injection and the injection withheld if protein is found. About 70% of patients with proteinuria have that condition resolve when gold therapy is discontinued. Glucocorticoids should not be used to treat this kidney damage.

Interactions

Penicillamine is a chelating agent and should not be given with gold salts. Drug interactions are not common with gold therapy.

GOLD COMPOUNDS: SPECIFIC DRUGS

Auranofin

Auranofin (Ridaura) is the one gold preparation that is given orally rather than by injection. It is considered less effective than injectable gold for severe cases of rheumatoid arthritis. Gastrointestinal (GI) reactions, including diarrhea, abdominal pain, nausea, and loss of appetite are common early in therapy but usually subside in the first 3 months. Skin reactions occur in about 30% of patients but are generally mild.

Aurothioglucose

Aurothioglucose (Solganal) is a suspension in sesame oil, administered intramuscularly (IM) once a week. It is used for active adult and juvenile rheumatoid arthritis. NSAIDs are usually continued until improvement with gold therapy is seen. Dermatitis is the most common side effect and is worsened by sunlight. Mouth ulcers are also common and may be preceded by a metallic taste in the mouth.

Gold Sodium Thiomalate

The vehicle for gold sodium thiomalate (Myochrysine) may give an anaphylactoid type of reaction with flushing, fainting, dizziness, sweating as well as nausea, vomiting, and weakness.

HYDROXYCHLOROQUINE

Mechanism of Action

Hydroxychloroquine (Plaquenil) is an antimalarial drug. The mechanism of action in treating rheumatic diseases is not clear. It appears to have immunosuppressive effects and may also indirectly inhibit collagen and cartilage breakdown.

Pharmacokinetics

Hydroxychloroquine is readily absorbed after oral administration. The plasma half-life is quite prolonged, up to 30 days, because the drug is deposited in tissues, especially the eye, liver, lungs, and kidney, and only slowly released. Metabolites are excreted in the urine and may be found months or years after the drug is discontinued.

Uses

Hydroxychloroquine, an antimalarial drug, is also effective in treating rheumatic diseases, especially systemic lupus erythematosus and rheumatoid arthritis. A response may not be seen for 3 to 6 months after the start of therapy, and therapy is discontinued after 1 year if no response is seen. About 70% of patients with rheumatoid arthritis experience at least moderate relief of symptoms. Hydroxychloroquine is used for patients with systemic lupus erythematosus to control arthritis, skin rashes, and mouth ulcers.

Chloroquine is also occasionally used, but it has a higher incidence of pigment changes to the eye.

Adverse Reactions, Toxicity, and Contraindications

Hydroxychloroquine can produce GI upset, dry skin, and pruritus. These effects are usually mild. Ophthalmic examination is recommended and therapy should be discontinued if pigment changes are noted. Rarely, emotional changes or muscle weakness are noted.

Hydroxychloroquine is fairly toxic to children; doses of 750 to 1 gram are fatal. However, hydroxychloroquine has been successfully used to treat juvenile rheumatoid arthritis. The drug crosses the placenta and is not recommended for use during pregnancy. Use by nursing mothers is not recommended because of the greater toxicity in children, although no adverse actions have been reported.

Contraindications for hydroxychloroquine include blood dyscrasia, severe neurologic disorders, hepatic function impairment, and a history of retinal or visual field changes.

Interactions

Hydroxychloroquine should not be combined with penicillamine, because the penicillamine plasma concentrations are increased with a higher incidence of adverse reactions.

✣ METHOTREXATE

Mechanism of Action

Methotrexate (Rheumatrex) is a folic acid antagonist. It inhibits DNA, RNA, and protein synthesis and thereby slows rapidly growing cells.

Pharmacokinetics

Methotrexate is variably absorbed and has a half-life of 3 to 10 hours. Most of the drug is excreted unchanged in the urine in the first 24 hours.

Uses

In high doses, 75 to 150 mg per week, methotrexate is used to treat various carcinomas and leukemia. In low doses, 5 to 20 mg per week, methotrexate can be effective in treating psoriasis and rheumatoid arthritis. Improvement is noted in 2 to 6 weeks and plateaus at about 6 months. Although many DMARDs become ineffective after a couple of years, methotrexate remains effective over time. Although methotrexate originally was used only for severe cases of rheumatoid arthritis, this drug is becoming more widely used in preference to other DMARDs because in low doses it has proven to be effective and well tolerated.

Adverse Reactions, Toxicity, and Contraindications

Side effects include nausea, mucositis, GI discomfort, rash, diarrhea, and headaches. Toxic reactions are possible but most are reversible if detected early; these include liver damage, lung disease, bone marrow depression, severe diarrhea, and ulcerative stomatitis. Baseline studies include blood chemistry, renal function, liver function, and chest x-ray films; these are repeated periodically throughout treatment. There have been rare reports of non-Hodgkin's lymphoma and other lymphomas. Contraindications to the use of methotrexate include pregnancy and nursing, alcoholism, blood dyscrasia, immunodeficiency syndromes, or hypersensitivity to the drug.

Interactions

Methotrexate given concurrently with phenylbutazone increases the risk of developing agranulocytosis. Probenecid can inhibit renal excretion of methotrexate and increase its toxicity. Because of immunosuppression, live viral vaccines may have increased adverse effects and may not be effective in producing immunity. Alcohol and drugs with potential hepatotoxicity can increase the risk of damage to the liver.

PENICILLAMINE

Mechanism of Action

Penicillamine (Cuprimine, Depen) is a chelating agent. It has an immunosuppressive action through suppression of T-cell activity, but the mechanism for this effect is unknown.

Pharmacokinetics

Penicillamine is administered orally and has a peak plasma concentration in 2 hours. The drug should be taken on an empty stomach about 1 hour before a meal. It is metabolized extensively with most metabolites excreted in the feces.

The onset of action for relieving symptoms of rheumatoid arthritis may take 2 to 3 months. To minimize side effects, the dosage is kept low, 125 to 250 mg once a day, for at least a month, and then increased stepwise monthly in 125 to 250 gm increments. If there is no remission after 4 months on 1000 to 1500 mg daily, therapy is discontinued. Otherwise therapy is continued. The maximum therapeutic effect is usually seen after 6 to 9 months.

Uses

Penicillamine is used to treat rheumatoid arthritis that has not responded to other drugs. It is also used to treat Wilson's disease, a disease of excessive copper deposition in tissues. As a chelating agent, penicillamine is also used to treat heavy metal toxicity, especially from mercury, lead, copper, and iron, by forming soluble complexes that are readily excreted in the urine. Penicillamine also combines chemically with cystine to prevent the formation of renal cystine calculi and to dissolve existing stones.

Adverse Reactions and Contraindications

Penicillamine has a high incidence of adverse actions. The most common side effects include pruritus, rash, loss of appetite, nausea, vomiting, alteration in taste, and diarrhea. More serious side effects include mouth ulcers, bone marrow depression, leukopenia, and thrombocytopenia. Blood tests should be performed initially, every 2 weeks during the first 6 months of therapy, and monthly thereafter. Possible damage to the kidney should also be monitored with urinary protein excretion, blood urea nitrogen (BUN), and creatinine levels.

Penicillamine can occasionally trigger another autoimmune disease, including lupus, pemphigus, Goodpasture's syndrome, myasthenia gravis, or dermatomyositis. These are usually reversible if penicillamine is discontinued. Penicillamine is contraindicated for individuals with any of these autoimmune diseases.

Contraindications for penicillamine include impaired renal function and pregnancy. Persons allergic to penicillin should not receive penicillamine.

Interactions

Penicillamine should not be given with gold therapy or other immunosuppressants except glucocorticoids. Phenylbutazone can cause serious hematologic and renal toxicity when combined with penicillamine. Iron supplements should be avoided.

SULFASALAZINE

Mechanism of Action

Sulfasalazine (Azulfidine, Salzopyrin, others) is metabolized to a salicylate and acts as an NSAID.

Pharmacokinetics

Sulfasalazine is composed of a sulfa compound and a 5-aminosalicylic acid. In the colon the drug is metabolized by bacteria to the component drugs.

Uses

Sulfasalazine is particularly effective in the treatment of inflammatory bowel disease. The effectiveness of sulfasalazine in treating rheumatoid arthritis is about equal to that of hydroxychloroquine or penicillamine. Sulfasalazine is also effective in treating ankylosing spondylitis.

Adverse Reactions, Toxicity, and Contraindications

Side effects include dizziness and GI disturbances. The more serious side effects include hypersensitivity and photosensitivity. Patients with elevated hepatic enzymes should not take sulfasalazine. CBCs should be done periodically to monitor for agranulocytosis and neutropenia.

Interactions

Sulfasalazine can potentiate the activity of anticoagulants and oral antidiabetic agents by displacing them from protein binding. Methotrexate, phenylbutazone, and sulfinpyrazone can also be potentiated.

NURSING PROCESS OVERVIEW

Rheumatoid Arthritis

Assessment

Obtain a careful history of the presenting problem in addition to vital signs, weight, and subjective and objective data related to the complaint and the overall condition of the patient. Monitor laboratory work, including hematocrit and hemoglobin level, blood counts, tests to confirm the diagnosis or to monitor diseases such as the rheumatoid factor, antinuclear antibody (ANA), complement, erythrocyte sedimentation rate (ESR), and tests to monitor the activity or side effects of drugs the patient is taking. Assess joint function, mobility, and ability to perform activities of daily living.

Nursing Diagnoses

- Risk for stomatitis (with gold compounds)
- Potential complication: hematologic disorders
- Potential anxiety related to chronic disease, changing medical therapies, and use of drugs with high potential for causing side effects

Patient Outcomes

The patient will state improved function and less discomfort. The nurse will minimize and manage blood dyscrasias. The patient will take drugs as ordered but will seek medical assistance as side effects develop.

Planning/Implementation

No drug can cure rheumatoid arthritis. Goals of drug therapy are to provide analgesia, to reduce inflammation and decrease pain, and to maintain or increase joint function. Monitor patient response to the therapeutic regimen, including pain, joint function, subjective and objective data related to the patient's complaints, new signs and symptoms possibly because of the therapy, and laboratory work specific for the drugs in use or the patient's problems. Plan goals so that patient management is directed to a mutually satisfactory outcome. Teach the patient that maintaining ideal weight is less stressful to joints in cases of arthritis; dietary restriction and instruction may be necessary. Refer to occupational therapy, physical therapy, and visiting nurses.

Evaluation

Ascertain that the patient can explain the disease process and the specific drugs being used, is aware of possible side effects of the drugs and what action to take if they should appear, knows how to take ordered drugs correctly, understands the need for frequent follow-up and data that will be obtained at these visits to monitor for effectiveness and side effects, and recognizes the need to avoid self-medication with over-the-counter (OTC) drugs unless approved by the physician.

Therapeutic Rationale: Systemic Lupus Erythematosus

Systemic lupus erythematosus (SLE, or simply lupus) is a chronic, inflammatory multisystem disorder of the immune system that affects about 1 in 2000 persons in the United States. It usually develops in young women; it is nine times more common in women than in men. Persons of African or Hispanic background and those with relatives having SLE are more likely to develop SLE. Lupus varies greatly in severity, from mild cases that require minimal intervention to those with significant damage to the lungs, heart, kidney, and brain. No two cases are exactly alike. SLE is also characterized by exacerbation of activity (flares) with periods of remission that may last weeks to years.

The autoimmune disorder underlying lupus is not well understood. It is characterized by an overproduction of autoantibodies. Tissue damage results from inflammatory response to deposition of immunoglobulins and complement. Early symptoms of lupus are vague, nonspecific, and easily confused with other disorders. Profound fatigue is an almost universal symptom. Other symptoms that are commonly seen can include the following: arthralgia, arthritis, fever >100°F, skin rashes, anemia, kidney involvement, pleurisy, malar rash, photosensitivity, hair loss, Raynaud's phenomenon, seizures, and mouth or nose ulcers. Lupus flares are eruptions of symptoms and often have erratic patterns. Potential life-threatening complications include damage to the kidney, central nervous system, and vascular system.

Use of certain drugs may induce a lupus-like syndrome with a positive ANA test, pleuropericardial inflammation, fever, rash and arthritis. The symptoms subside when the drug is discontinued. Drugs that have definitely been associated with drug-induced lupus include chlorpromazine, hydralazine, isoniazid, methyldopa, and procainamide. Drugs with possible association include beta-blockers, captopril, carbamazepine, cimetidine, diphenylhydantoin, ethosuximide, methimazole, penicillamine, phenazine, quinidine.

Therapeutic Agents: Systemic Lupus Erythematosus

Drug therapy for lupus is directed at controlling symptoms to prevent or control serious complications as a result of organ

TABLE 37-3 Agents for Systemic Lupus Erythematosus

GENERIC NAME	TRADE NAME	ADMINISTRATION/DOSAGE	COMMENTS
✣ Azathioprine	Imuran*	ORAL: *Adults*—1 mg/kg body weight daily, increasing by 0.5 mg/kg body weight daily after 6-8 wk, then every 4 wk as necessary for maximum dose of 2.5 mg/kg body weight daily. Maintenance: reduce to minimum effective dose in steps of 0.5 mg/kg body weight daily at 1-2 mo intervals. FDA pregnancy category D.	CBC should be performed weekly first month; twice monthly second and third month; monthly thereafter. Liver function tests should be performed every 1-3 mo. Can be used with prednisone or another glucocorticoid to reduce dosage needed to control symptoms.
✣ Cyclophosphamide	Cytoxan*	INTRAVENOUS: *For lupus nephritis: Adults*—0.5-1 gm/m² once monthly for 6 mo. FDA pregnancy category D.	Pulse therapy decreases mortality when lupus nephritis develops. Ovulation is inhibited and may be permanently impaired.
Hydroxychloroquine sulfate	Plaquenil*	ORAL: *Adults*—up to 6.5 mg/kg lean body weight daily, with meals or glass of milk.	If usual initial dose produces side effects, reduce dose for 5-10 days, then gradually increase. Eye examination should be performed initially and after 6 mo.
Prednisone	Apo-Prednisone,† Deltasone,* Orasone, others	ORAL: *Adults*—1-10 mg once daily for maintenance or larger doses to control active disease. FDA pregnancy category C.	Side effects are related to dosage and length of therapy.

*Available in Canada and United States.
†Available in Canada only.

damage by the inflammatory processes. The drugs most commonly used include NSAIDs, glucocorticoids, hydroxychloroquine, and azathioprine (Table 37-3). Cyclophosphamide is primarily used to treat lupus nephritis.

Azathioprine

The major use of azathioprine (Imuran) for lupus is for the glucocorticoid sparing effect. Azathioprine potentiates the immunosuppressive action of glucocorticoids and thereby allows a lower dosage of glucocorticoid to have a greater immunosuppressive action. See Table 37-1 and the earlier section on rheumatoid arthritis.

Cyclophosphamide

Cyclophosphamide (Cytoxan, Endoxan) is a cytotoxic drug used to treat a number of cancers. The role of cyclophosphamide in lupus is the immunosuppressive treatment of diffuse proliferative nephritis and other organ inflammation unresponsive to glucocorticoids. Its use is reserved for severe cases because of the many adverse side effects. Cyclophosphamide is administered intravenously once a month (pulse therapy) for 6 months, and the results are evaluated. Cytotoxic drugs to treat cancer are covered in Chapter 49.

Glucocorticoids

Glucocorticoids are used in high doses to treat exacerbations of the lupus and in low doses to control lupus symptoms when other drugs do not work. Glucocorticoids are discussed in detail in Chapter 36.

Hydroxychloroquine

The antimalarials, particularly hydroxychloroquine (Plaquenil), are prescribed for the control of lupus arthritis, skin rashes, and mouth ulcers (see previous section on rheumatoid arthritis).

Nonsteroidal Antiinflammatory Drugs

Salicylates and NSAIDs are commonly prescribed for patients with lupus, especially to control fever and arthralgia (Chapter 30).

NURSING PROCESS OVERVIEW

Systemic Lupus Erythematosus

Assessment

Complete a total assessment. Pay special attention to history of fever, weight loss, fatigue, pain in joints, dyspnea, cough, pleuritic pain, lung sounds, and presence of edema. Assess for rash, purpura, alopecia. Assess vital signs and weight. Monitor CBC, renal function tests, and urinalysis. Assess electrocardiogram (ECG), if available. Question the patient about ability to perform activities of daily living and activity tolerance.

Nursing Diagnoses

- Activity intolerance and/or fatigue related to disease progression
- Fluid volume excess related to renal failure and/or drug side effects
- Anxiety related to variable course of disease

Patient Outcomes

The patient will achieve optimal activity level (describe level appropriate for patient). The patient will describe methods to decrease edema. The patient will state a lessened degree of anxiety.

Planning/Implementation

The course of systemic lupus erythematosus is highly variable and characterized by remissions and exacerbations. Management will depend on the patient's situation. Provide emotional support. Instruct the patient about prescribed drug regimen. Depending on drugs being used and presence of renal dysfunction, instruct the patient about concomitant dietary modifications that may be helpful, such as limiting calories and sodium intake and increasing intake of protein and potassium if the patient is taking glucocorticoids. Work with the patient to modify the daily routine to permit periods of rest, if needed. Emphasize the importance of regular medical follow-up to monitor the progress of disease and effectiveness of therapy.

Evaluation

At present there is no cure for this disease. Ascertain that the patient can explain the disease process and the specific drugs being used and is aware of possible side effects of the drugs and what action to take if they should appear. Determine if the patient understands the need for regular follow-up. If fatigue or activity intolerance are present, evaluate the efforts of the patient to increase strength and incorporate regular periods of rest into daily activities.

Therapeutic Rationale: Multiple Sclerosis

Multiple sclerosis is a crippling autoimmune disease in which the myelin sheath of nerve fibers of the brain and spinal cord is destroyed. Multiple sclerosis affects about 250,000 people in the United States, two thirds of them women. It begins slowly, usually in young adulthood, and continues with periods of flares and remission. The first signs are tingling (paresthesia) in the extremities or on one side of the face. Other signs include muscular weakness, vertigo, and visual disturbances, especially double vision, nystagmus, or partial blindness. Later symptoms include emotional lability, abnormal reflexes, ataxia, and difficulty in urination. Because of the periods of remission and the vagueness of the symptoms, diagnosis of multiple sclerosis is difficult and involves ruling out other diseases.

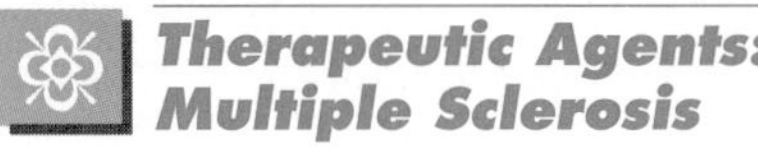

Therapeutic Agents: Multiple Sclerosis

A mouse model for multiple sclerosis has been developed by injecting myelin basic protein to produce an autoimmune disease in susceptible mice, experimental allergic encephalomyelitis (EAE). This model has helped researchers understand the autoimmune events underlying multiple sclerosis. One new drug for multiple sclerosis has emerged from this research, beta-interferon. Otherwise, the major treatment for exacerbations of the disease has been corticotropin and, to a lesser degree, methylprednisolone (Table 37-4).

Corticotropin

Corticotropin (ACTH) is the hormone released by the pituitary to act on the adrenal cortex and increase the natural production of corticosteroids (see Chapter 60). A 2-week course of intramuscular corticotropin injections may improve the recovery from an acute relapse of multiple sclerosis.

✣ Interferon Beta-1b

Mechanism of Action

Interferons (Betaseron) are cytokines that inhibit the proliferation of certain cell types. Interferon beta-1b appears to decrease T-cell proliferation and inhibit interferon gamma synthesis. The drug interferon beta-1b is manufactured by recombinant DNA techniques and differs by a single amino acid from the natural human form.

Pharmacokinetics

Interferon beta-1b is administered by subcutaneous injection every other day. The serum levels are undetectable.

Uses

Interferon beta-1b is indicated for patients who have the relapsing-remitting form of multiple sclerosis. In clinical trials this drug significantly reduced the frequency and intensity of relapses.

Adverse Reactions and Contraindications

Reactions at the injection site are fairly common as are flu-like symptoms of fever, chills, myalgia, malaise, and sweating. Women may experience menstrual disorders. Less common reactions include palpitations, hypertension, tachycardia, and peripheral vascular disorders.

Blood studies should be performed, especially to monitor the neutrophil count and serum levels of bilirubin and alanine amino transferase (ALT). The drug should be discontinued if the absolute neutrophil count is $<750/mm^3$ or if AST (aspartate amino transferase)/ALT levels exceed 10 times the upper limit of normal. Some patients may experience confusion and anxiety. Signs and symptoms of depression should be monitored because a few patients have become suicidal while taking the drug.

Interferon beta-1b is contraindicated for pregnant women because spontaneous abortions have been reported.

Interactions

No drug interactions have been reported with the use of interferon beta-1b.

Methylprednisolone

Methylprednisolone is one of the intermediate acting glucocorticoids. High-dose intravenous administration of methylprednisone improves the recovery from acute exacerbations of multiple sclerosis, although there is no long-term improvement in the disease.

Nursing Process Overview

Multiple Sclerosis

Assessment

Perform a complete assessment. Multiple sclerosis is highly individualized: what is a problem for one patient may not affect another. Monitor vital signs and weight. Auscultate lung sounds. Obtain a history of ability to perform activities of daily living, presence of fatigue, or activity intolerance. Question the patient about changes since the last visit.

TABLE 37-4 Agents for Multiple Sclerosis

GENERIC NAME	TRADE NAME	ADMINISTRATION/DOSAGE	COMMENTS
Corticotropin	Acthar*	INTRAMUSCULAR: *Adults*—80-120 USP U/day for 2 or 3 wk. FDA pregnancy category C.	For acute exacerbations of multiple sclerosis.
✣ Interferon beta-1b	Betaseron	SUBCUTANEOUS: *Adults*—0.25 mg every other day.	For prophylactic treatment of multiple sclerosis when there are recurrent attacks followed by partial or complete remission.
Methylprednisolone sodium succinate	Solu-Medrol*	INTRAMUSCULAR OR INTRAVENOUS: *Adults*—160 mg daily for 1 wk, followed by 64 mg every other day for 1 mo. FDA pregnancy category C.	For acute exacerbations of multiple sclerosis.

*Available in Canada and United States.

Nursing Diagnoses

- Anxiety related to presence of chronic disease, specific symptoms, or inability to maintain usual level of daily activities
- Risk for self-concept disturbance related to loss of usual role responsibilities

Patient Outcomes

The patient will learn strategies to optimize physical abilities (specify). The patient will discuss anxiety. The patient will discuss recent changes in role and feelings about those changes.

Planning/Implementation

At the present time there is no cure for multiple sclerosis. The course is highly variable from person to person. Provide emotional support as needed. Seek assistance as needed from other members of the health care team, including the physical or occupational therapist, home care nurses, and social worker. Teach the patient about the disease itself and about any prescribed medications. Emphasize the importance of regular follow-up to monitor disease process, effectiveness of any medications, or treatments.

Evaluation

Ascertain that the patient can explain the disease process and any drugs being used, is aware of possible drug side effects, and what action to take if they should appear. Verify that the patient can state the importance of regular follow-up visits to monitor progress.

NURSING IMPLICATIONS SUMMARY

DRUGS FOR DIAGNOSIS AND TREATMENT OF MYASTHENIA GRAVIS

Drug Administration

- Assess the patient for signs of myasthenic crisis (inadequately treated myasthenia gravis) such as positive Tensilon test; increased blood pressure and pulse; difficulty chewing, swallowing, and coughing; bladder and bowel incontinence; increasing ptosis; difficulty breathing; and cyanosis. Differentiate symptoms of myasthenic crisis from those of cholinergic crisis (over-treated myasthenia gravis) such as negative Tensilon test; abdominal cramps; diarrhea; fasciculations; nausea, vomiting, and blurred vision. The following may be seen in myasthenic or cholinergic crisis: generalized weakness; increased salivation, tearing, and bronchial secretions; general feeling of apprehension; restlessness; and difficulty breathing. Have a suction machine at the bedside.
- Keep edrophonium, pyridostigmine, atropine, neostigmine, and syringes and a tourniquet at the patient's bedside or in a convenient place on the patient care unit for rapid treatment of a myasthenic or cholinergic crisis.
- Assess the patient's ability to swallow before preparing an ordered oral dose of anticholinesterase. If the ability to swallow is deteriorating, it may be necessary to administer a parenteral dose of medication. Obtain written orders for oral and parenteral doses at the time of admission so time is not lost if the patient can no longer swallow.
- Schedule off-unit diagnostic studies and therapies for the patient with myasthenia gravis so that medication administration is not delayed while the nurse waits for the patient to return. If the patient is not present when a medication is due, take the dose of the medication to the patient.
- Assess blood pressure, pulse, vital capacity, presence and degree of ptosis, muscle strength, and ability to swallow as indicators of adequate drug control.
- When one of these drugs is used as an antidote for tubocurarine or other neuromuscular blockade agents, administer via slow intravenous push. Continue appropriate ventilatory support until the patient is breathing well unassisted. Have atropine at the bedside. If the pulse is less than 80 beats/minute, administer atropine before the neostigmine.
- For constant infusion of anticholinesterases, use a volume control device and microdrip tubing. Monitor respiratory and cardiovascular status. The dose may be titrated to peripheral nerve stimulator response.

Intravenous Edrophonium

- May be given undiluted at a rate of 2 mg (0.2 ml) over 15 to 30 seconds. A physician or nurse anesthetist should be present. Read drug labels carefully: Enlon contains edrophonium, whereas Enlon-Plus contains edrophonium and atropine. The dose may be titrated to peripheral nerve stimulator response.

Intravenous Neostigmine

- Read the drug label: must be for IV use. May be given undiluted at a rate of 0.5 mg or less over 1 minute. A physician or nurse anesthetist should be present. The dose may be titrated to peripheral nerve stimulator response.

Intravenous Pyridostigmine

- May be given undiluted at a rate of 0.5 mg or less over 1 minute. A physician or nurse anesthetist should be present. The dose may be titrated to peripheral nerve stimulator response.

Continued.

NURSING IMPLICATIONS SUMMARY—cont'd

Patient and Family Education

- Teach the patient and family about the signs and symptoms of myasthenia gravis, myasthenic crisis, and overdose with anticholinesterases.
- Teach the patient and family to take medications exactly as ordered. Forgetting, omitting, or doubling a dose of medication may cause the patient's condition to deteriorate.
- No medication, whether prescription or OTC, should ever be taken without the approval of the physician. In addition, give the patient a list of drugs known to be contraindicated for patients with myasthenia gravis (see box on p. 448). Suggest that the patient plan a medication schedule that includes taking doses of anticholinesterases 30 to 60 minutes before meals to increase strength for chewing and swallowing. Take anticholinesterases with milk or a snack to reduce gastric irritation. Use a reliable alarm clock with battery back-up to wake the patient for early morning or nighttime doses of medication.
- Keep careful watch on supplies of drugs on hand, and refill prescriptions before they run out. Reinforce to the patient and family the need to seek medical assistance immediately if the patient's condition seems to be deteriorating. Encourage the patient to wear a medical identification tag or bracelet and to carry a list of the names and doses of medication being taken. Refer the patient and family to local, state, or national myasthenia gravis support groups.
- If intramuscular (IM) forms are prescribed for self-administration, teach injection technique to the patient and family members.

THERAPEUTIC AGENTS FOR RHEUMATOID ARTHRITIS

Azathioprine

Drug Administration

- Assess vital signs. Monitor CBC, WBC differential, and platelet count.
- There may be some risk to personnel who prepare and administer immunosuppressant drugs. Check agency procedures. When preparing doses, use a biologic containment cabinet, and wear disposable gloves and masks. Use careful technique in the handling and administration of these medications. Dispose of vials, syringes, needles, intravenous (IV) equipment, and unused medication in biohazard containers.
- Monitor CBC and differential, platelet count, and liver function tests.
- Assess for signs of hepatitis, including right upper quadrant abdominal pain, jaundice, fever, malaise, nausea, vomiting, and anorexia. Tell the patient to report these signs and symptoms if they develop.

Intravenous Azathioprine

- Reconstitute by adding 10 ml of sterile water for injection to the vial and swirling to dissolve drug. May be further diluted in at least 50 ml of 0.9% sodium chloride injection or 5% dextrose in normal saline. Administer a diluted dose over at least 30 to 60 minutes, but rate may vary from 5 minutes to 8 hours depending on use, volume of fluid, and size and age of patient.

Patient and Family Education

- Review the reasons for using this drug with the patient. See the patient problem boxes on bleeding tendencies (p. 586) and leukopenia (p. 585).
- Emphasize the importance of returning for regular follow-up and not discontinuing the medication without consulting the physician.
- Remind the patient to take doses after meals or at bedtime if the drug causes nausea. If the patient vomits shortly after taking a dose, have the patient contact physician to see if the dose should be repeated.
- Instruct the patient to avoid immunizations unless first discussed with the physician. Others in the patient's house should avoid immunization with oral poliovirus vaccine. If the patient must be in contact with someone who has received the polio vaccine, tell the patient to limit close contact and wear a protective mask that covers the nose and mouth.
- For missed doses, if the ordered dose is once a day, omit the missed dose, and resume the regular dosing schedule the next day. Do not double up for missed dose. If doses are ordered more than once a day, take missed dose as soon as remembered. Contact the physician with questions.
- Teach injection technique if required. Refer the patient to a home nursing care agency for follow-up.

Gold Compounds

Drug Administration

- Assess respiratory rate and auscultate lung sounds. Monitor intake and output, and weight. Monitor CBC and differential, platelet count, BUN level, serum creatinine level, and liver function tests. Monitor urinalysis to detect proteinuria and hematuria. Inspect the skin and mouth for presence of rashes, ulcers, stomatitis, and irritation.
- For IM injection, use large muscle masses. Record and rotate injection sites. Aspirate before administering dose to prevent inadvertent IV administration. Keep the patient supine for at least 15 minutes after dose. Monitor vital signs and blood pressure. Have available drugs, equipment, and personnel to treat an acute allergic reaction when parenteral gold compounds are administered.

NURSING IMPLICATIONS SUMMARY—cont'd

Intramuscular Aurothioglucose

- This drug form is an oil-based suspension (see box on p. 60).

Patient and Family Education

- Review the anticipated benefits and possible side effects of drug therapy with the patient. Instruct the patient to notify the physician if severe or persistent vomiting or diarrhea, rashes, skin irritation, itching, mouth ulcers, oral irritation, stomatitis, metallic taste, unexplained bruising, bleeding of gums, bleeding in stool, nosebleeds, jaundice, right upper quadrant abdominal pain, malaise, fever, sore throat, eye irritation, or visual changes develop. Reinforce the importance of reporting new signs or symptoms to the physician.
- Instruct the patient to take oral compounds with meals or a snack to lessen gastric irritation.
- Review oral hygiene with the patient if stomatitis develops. See the patient problem box on stomatitis (p. 587), and review the patient problem box on photosensitivity (p. 649).
- Explain that weeks to months of therapy may be necessary before full benefit of gold therapy can be seen. Emphasize the importance of continuing other prescribed therapies, including prescribed exercise program, weight reduction, application of heat and cold, and physical therapy.
- For patients receiving the injectable forms: immediately after the injection, dizziness, feeling faint, nausea and vomiting, increased sweating, or weakness may develop, but these symptoms should resolve in a short time. The patient should lie down after injection in anticipation of these effects. If these symptoms worsen, or other symptoms develop within 10 minutes of the injection, notify the physician. Joint pain may occur for 1 or 2 days after each injection but should diminish after several doses.
- Teach injection technique if prescribed for patients self-administering gold preparations at home.
- For missed doses, oral form: if ordered dose is once a day, take the missed dose when remembered, unless not remembered until the next day, then omit missed dose. For missed doses if ordered more than once a day, take missed dose as soon as remembered, unless almost time for the next dose, then omit. Do not double up for missed doses.
- Women of childbearing age may wish to use some form of birth control while on gold therapy; discuss this issue before initiating gold therapy.

Glucocorticoids: Prednisone and Methylprednisolone

- See Chapter 36 for a detailed discussion of these drugs.

Hydroxychloroquine

- See Chapter 48 for a detailed discussion of this drug, also used to treat malaria.

Methotrexate

- See Chapter 49 for a detailed discussion of this drug, used in higher doses to treat cancer.

Penicillamine

Drug Administration

- Monitor weight and blood pressure. Auscultate lung sounds. Inspect for presence of skin rashes and lesions. Monitor CBC and differential, platelet count, serum creatinine level, BUN level, and liver function tests. Monitor urinalysis to detect proteinuria.
- Assess penicillin allergy before administering. Cross-sensitivity between the two drugs is possible although rare.
- Penicillamine is a copper chelating agent and is also used in the treatment of Wilson's disease, a disorder of copper metabolism. Teach patients with Wilson's disease to avoid foods higher in copper including chocolate, nuts, shellfish, mushrooms, liver, molasses, broccoli, and copper-enriched cereals.

Patient and Family Education

- Review the anticipated benefits and possible side effects of drug therapy. Instruct the patient to notify the physician if severe or persistent vomiting or diarrhea, skin rashes, lesions, scaling, dermatitis, hair loss, fever, inflamed mouth, mouth lesions, stomatitis, swelling or edema, bruising, bleeding, nosebleeds, blood in stool, malaise, sore throat, jaundice, or abdominal pain develop. Explain that side effects may develop any time during therapy. Report new signs and symptoms to the physician.
- Review the patient problem box on stomatitis (p. 587).
- Emphasize the importance of taking drugs as ordered. Sporadic or intermittent use (unless prescribed by the physician) may contribute to further allergic reactions.
- Capsules may be opened and contents mixed with 15 to 30 ml of chilled applesauce, other pureed foods, or fruit juice for ease in administering.
- For prevention of cystinuria, tell the patient to take the bedtime dose with at least two 8-ounce glasses of water, and to drink two more 8-ounce glasses of water during the night. Take daytime doses with a full glass of water.
- Teach patients taking oral iron preparations to allow at least 2 hours to elapse between the two drugs.
- Penicillamine increases the body's requirement for pyridoxine. If pyridoxine is also prescribed, emphasize the importance of taking this supplement. See the dietary consideration box on vitamins (p. 215) for dietary sources of pyridoxine.
- Penicillamine may lead to impaired taste. For all patients except those with Wilson's disease, normal taste may be returned with administration of copper each day (e.g., several drops of cupric sulfate solution diluted in fruit juice); check with the physician.

Continued.

NURSING IMPLICATIONS SUMMARY—cont'd

- Women of childbearing age may wish to use some form of birth control while on penicillamine therapy; discuss this issue before initiating therapy.
- Emphasize that weeks to months of therapy may be necessary before full benefit of penicillamine can be seen. Reinforce the importance of continuing other prescribed therapies; that might include a prescribed exercise program, weight reduction, application of heat and cold, and physical therapy.
- For treatment of arthritis, teach the patient to take doses 1 hour before or 2 hours after meals, and 1 hour before or after other medications, food, or milk.
- For treatment of Wilson's disease, take doses on an empty stomach, 30 to 60 minutes before or 2 hours after meals.
- For treatment of lead poisoning, take doses on an empty stomach, 2 hours before or 3 hours after meals.
- Teach patients with Wilson's disease to avoid multivitamin preparations that contain copper. Teach the patient to use distilled or demineralized water for drinking if the patient's water supply contains more than 100 μg of copper per liter.

Sulfasalazine

Patient and Family Education

- Assess the patient for allergy to other sulfonamides, furosemide, thiazide diuretics, salicylates, carbonic anhydrase inhibitors, or sulfonylureas (see Chapter 44).
- Take doses with meals or a snack to lessen gastric irritation.
- Take enteric-coated tablets whole, without chewing or crushing.
- Teach the patient to take doses with a full glass (8 ounces) of water and to maintain a daily fluid intake of at least 2000 to 2500 ml.
- Instruct the patient to avoid driving or operating hazardous equipment if dizzy.
- See the patient problem boxes on photosensitivity (p. 649), leukopenia (p. 585), and bleeding tendencies (p. 586).
- Encourage regular dental care and good dental hygiene (flossing and brushing). Leukopenia and thrombocytopenia may contribute to gum infections and bleeding gums.
- Teach the patient to return to the physician if symptoms, including diarrhea, do not improve in 4 to 6 weeks. Encourage the patient to return for regularly scheduled follow-up.
- This drug may cause the skin of some patients to turn yellow-orange. This discoloration does not need medical attention.

THERAPEUTIC AGENTS FOR SYSTEMIC LUPUS ERYTHEMATOSUS

Cyclophosphamide

- See Chapter 49 for a discussion of this drug, which is also used to treat cancer.

THERAPEUTIC AGENTS FOR MULTIPLE SCLEROSIS

Corticotropin

- See Chapter 60 for a discussion of this drug.

Interferon Beta-1b

Drug Administration

- See the manufacturer's insert for detailed information about this drug.
- Reconstitute with the diluent provided by the manufacturer. Use within 3 hours of reconstituting drug. Administer subcutaneously.

Patient and Family Education

- For home management, teach the patient self-administration, including injection technique and proper handling and disposal of syringes and needles.
- Emphasize the importance of returning for follow-up visits to monitor for drug effectiveness and side effects. Remind the patient not to discontinue medications without consulting the physician.

CRITICAL THINKING

APPLICATION

1. Describe the mechanism by which acetylcholinesterase inhibitors increase activation of the neuromuscular junction.
2. What muscarinic side effects of neostigmine and pyridostigmine would you observe? Which drug would you administer as an antidote for neostigmine?
3. Describe two diagnostic uses of edrophonium.
4. Develop a teaching plan for the patient taking anticholinesterases.
5. What is meant by disease-modifying agents for rheumatic diseases (DMARDs)? Which drugs are classified as DMARDs?
6. Which drugs are commonly used to treat lupus? Which drug is used for lupus nephritis?
7. Which drugs are used as therapeutic agents for multiple sclerosis?

CRITICAL THINKING

1. Autoimmune diseases are chronic diseases for which there are no cures. They are marked by periods of remission, but over time they may become progressively more debilitating. Research one of these diseases and describe some of the challenges in working with a patient not only related to adjusting medications but also to other aspects of care.

SECTION X

Antiinfective Agents

This section discusses drugs that act as selective poisons against certain organisms or types of cells. Chapter 38, *Introduction to the Use of Antiinfective Agents,* introduces the principle of selective toxicity that underlies all the information in the remaining chapters and focuses on the use of selective poisons to treat disease caused by bacteria or closely related microorganisms. Chapters 39 through 44 discuss specific antiinfective agents, grouping drugs into chapters on the basis of similar mechanisms of action or similar uses.

Chapters 45 to 48 consider several types of drugs. Each chapter not only discusses specific drugs but also delineates the differences between the therapy of diseases produced by viruses, fungi, or eucaryotic parasites from the therapy of bacterial disease.

CHAPTER 38

Introduction to the Use of Antiinfective Agents

OBJECTIVES

After studying this chapter, you should be able to do the following:

- *Discuss the principle of selective toxicity.*
- *Describe the difference between bactericidal and bacteriostatic agents.*
- *Discuss the influence of plasmids on antibiotic resistance.*
- *Describe the factors that influence the outcome of antibiotic therapy.*
- *Explain why antibiotics should not be discontinued until the prescribed therapy is complete.*
- *Outline important patient teaching points related to general use of antiinfective agents.*

KEY TERMS

acquired resistance
antimicrobial spectrum
bactericidal drugs
bacteriostatic drugs
eucaryotic cells
inherent resistance
minimum bactericidal concentration (MBC)
minimum inhibitory concentration (MIC)
plasmids
procaryotic cells
selective toxicity
superinfections
therapeutic index (TI)

CHAPTER OVERVIEW

Preceding chapters presented the use of drugs intended to alter processes that occur naturally in the body. For example, cardiotonic drugs alter existing patterns of ion flow in heart cells; the therapeutic goal of increasing contractility of the heart is achieved by this direct action of the drug. Similarly, a direct action on normal physiologic functions can be cited for each drug discussed previously. In contrast, the drugs considered in this section ideally do not directly affect any physiologic process in the patient. The antiinfective agents may be considered selective poisons because the goal of therapy with these drugs is to poison invading pathogenic microorganisms without poisoning the patient.

This introductory chapter presents concepts important in understanding antibiotic therapy. Microbiologic principles that make antibiotic therapy effective are reviewed, general mechanisms by which these drugs act are discussed, and major problems associated with antimicrobial therapy are presented.

Therapeutic Rationale: Infectious Disease

Although the world of microbes was discovered by Anton Van Leeuwenhoek in 1676, the impact of these tiny organisms on human destiny was not appreciated until the last third of the nineteenth century. During this period Louis Pasteur and Robert Koch, working in separate laboratories and on different microorganisms, showed that bacteria could cause human disease. After these discoveries two subsequent developments became almost inevitable.

Microbiologists and physicians began to classify human diseases in terms of the organism that produced the disease. By the early twentieth century, microorganisms that cause cholera, typhoid, bubonic plague, gonorrhea, leprosy, malaria, syphilis, and other diseases were isolated and identified.

This new knowledge put therapy of microbially induced diseases on a more rational basis. The first attempts at controlling diseases caused by microorganisms involved immunization. This approach allowed certain diseases to be prevented, but immunization was not effective for all diseases nor was it effective once the disease was established. Thus chemists sought out agents that could eradicate invading pathogens in a living patient. A leader in this area was Paul Ehrlich, who in 1912 introduced salvarsan, a drug specific for syphilis. Salvarsan and a related drug, neosalvarsan, established the validity of drug therapy for infectious diseases. In 1935 a synthetic agent was discovered that could cure streptococcal infections, and in 1939 development was begun on an extract of culture fluid from the mold *Penicillium*. These discoveries marked the beginnings of the sulfonamides and penicillin. The search for more effective antimicrobial agents has not ceased. As subsequent chapters illustrate, that search has been extraordinarily fruitful.

Antimicrobial agents are possible because bacterial pathogens differ significantly from their human hosts. Bacteria are **procaryotic cells,** which have genetic material that exists free within the cell protoplasm. Human cells are **eucaryotic** and have membrane-bounded nuclei that contain the genetic material. Other distinguishing characteristics exist. For example, procaryotes possess cell walls composed in part of peptidoglycan, a complex molecule that contains amino acids and sugars. Human cells have no cell wall but only a cell membrane. Single-celled eucaryotic organisms such as algae and fungi may possess complex rigid cell walls, but these walls do not contain peptidoglycan.

Procaryotes and eucaryotes also differ in certain internal functions. For example, ribosomes in eucaryotes are larger than those in procaryotes, and the two forms differ in their response to certain chemicals (see Chapters 41 through 43). Likewise, folic acid metabolism may differ. Many procaryotes cannot use folic acid from the environment but must synthesize the vitamin from simpler starting materials (Chapter 44). In contrast, eucaryotes cannot synthesize folic acid but must absorb it from the diet.

The structural and metabolic differences in procaryotes and eucaryotes form the basis for selective toxicity. **Selective toxicity** is the selective poisoning of an invading disease-causing organism by means of an agent that has no effect on the person in whom the disease exists.

No drug is yet available that is a perfectly selective agent; at some dose every antiinfective agent currently available may cause a direct effect on the host. One way to evaluate the degree of selective toxicity that may be achieved with a drug is by means of the therapeutic index (see Chapter 1). The **therapeutic index (TI)** is the ratio of the dose of a certain drug that kills 50% of the test animals to the dose of that drug that is effective in 50% of the animals ($TI = LD_{50}/ED_{50}$). A drug that is relatively nontoxic may be given in very large doses before it kills animals. If the drug is also potent, it may require small doses to achieve the desired clinical effect, which in this case is to cure the infection. Such a drug would have a large TI and would be considered to display good selective toxicity: it attacks the pathogen at doses well below those that are dangerous to the host. In contrast a drug with low TI would not have good selective toxicity. A drug with a TI of 1 would be equally toxic to the bacteria and to the patient.

The TI is derived from studies on laboratory animals. Because correlating animal studies with the clinical effectiveness of a drug is sometimes difficult, other indexes of selective toxicity have been used to indicate clinical experience with a drug. For example, the safety margin of a drug is the percentage increase above the standard therapeutic dose that is required to produce serious toxic reactions in a certain percentage of patients. This evaluation is based entirely on clinical experience.

A drug with a large TI and a wide safety margin may be given to patients in larger than normal doses without causing significant toxicity in most patients. To illustrate this principle, consider the antibiotics gentamicin and penicillin G. Gentamicin must be given in carefully controlled doses because it can damage the kidneys if the concentration in blood becomes too high. Gentamicin has such a low TI and narrow safety margin that increasing the dose by 50% may cause significant toxicity (see Chapter 43). In contrast, penicillin G has a very wide safety margin and a high TI. Direct toxicity with this drug is low, and doses 3 or 4 times the standard dose may be administered with little risk of toxic reactions in most patients (see Chapter 39).

Therapeutic Agents: Antimicrobial Drugs

Most antibiotics achieve selective toxicity by acting on microorganisms in one of the following five ways: inhibit cell wall formation, block protein synthesis, disrupt cell membranes, interfere with nucleic acid synthesis, or prevent synthesis of folic acid. Each mechanism of action exploits a biochemical difference between eucaryotic and procaryotic cells.

In addition to classifying antibiotics by specific mechanisms, they may be broadly described as bacteriostatic or bactericidal. **Bactericidal drugs** directly kill bacterial cells. For example, several antibiotics, by interfering with cell wall synthesis, may cause the bacterial cell to explode because the osmotic forces generated within the cytoplasm can no longer be contained by the defective cell wall. Likewise, antibiotics that disrupt the bacterial cell membrane allow the cytoplasmic contents of the cell to leak out, and the cell dies. **Bacteriostatic drugs** do not directly kill bacteria but rather halt bacterial reproduction. With bacteriostatic drugs, bacteria removed from exposure to the drug can resume growth. The host's immune system must attack, immobilize, and kill the pathogens for therapy with bacteriostatic drugs to achieve a long-term cure. In theory, cures can be effected with bactericidal drugs independent of the immune system, but such cures are not easily achieved. In immunosuppressed patients cures of bacterial infections are much more difficult to achieve than in patients with normal immune function, even with appropriately prescribed bactericidal drugs. These observations suggest that cures of bacterial disease in ordinary persons depend strongly on immunologic factors.

To classify a drug as exclusively bactericidal or bacteriostatic may be misleading. Many antibiotics are bacteriostatic or bactericidal depending on dose, site of infection, and the causative organism. For example, sulfonamides, which prevent folic acid synthesis in sensitive bacteria, might be considered bacteriostatic for a systemic infection, but, because of the high drug concentration in urine, they may be bactericidal in urine. Other examples are cases in which two types of microorganisms differ greatly in sensitivity to a certain antibiotic. For the more sensitive organism, the serum and tissue levels achievable with normal dosage may be sufficient for bactericidal action, whereas the more resistant organism may simply suffer growth inhibition, a bacteriostatic effect, at that same antibiotic concentration.

The **antimicrobial spectrum** is the range of microorganisms against which the drug is effective. Table 38-1 lists common pathogenic microorganisms according to criteria established by microbiologists. A drug effective against only a few of these organisms has a narrow spectrum, such as penicillin G, which is primarily effective against gram-positive bacteria. In contrast a drug that can be used against several groups of organisms has a broad spectrum, such as tetracycline, which is effective against gram-positive and gram-negative bacteria, as well as against *Rickettsia* and *Chlamydia.*

Minimum inhibitory concentration (MIC) and **minimum bactericidal concentration** (MBC) relate to the antimicrobial spectrum. For each antibiotic and microorganism, it is possible to determine in the laboratory the amount of that drug required to halt the growth of the organism and the amount required to kill the organism. The concentrations are the lowest ones at which growth inhibition or cell death can be observed. A consideration of these figures and determination of safe blood levels for an antibiotic help determine an effective therapeutic regimen. For example, a blood concentration above the MBC is desirable, but whether that concentration can be obtained depends on the pharmacologic properties governing drug absorption and elimination and the threshold for toxicity produced by the drug in the host.

TABLE 38-1 Microbial Pathogens of Humans

ORGANISMS	COMMON DISEASES PRODUCED
Viruses	
Influenza	Flu and upper respiratory tract infection
Herpes simplex	Skin, eye, and brain infections
HIV	Immunodeficiency, AIDS
Chlamydia	Psittacosis; eye and genital infections
Rickettsia	Typhus, Q fever, and Rocky Mountain spotted fever
Spirochetes	Syphilis and yaws
Eubacteria, Gram-Negative	
Haemophilus	Meningitis
Escherichia	Urinary tract infections
Proteus	Urinary tract infections
Klebsiella	Urinary tract infections and pneumonia
Pseudomonas	Urinary tract infections and meningitis
Neisseria	Meningitis and gonorrhea
Salmonella	Typhoid and gastroenteritis
Shigella	Dysentery
Eubacteria, Gram-Positive	
Staphylococcus	Soft tissue infections
Streptococcus	Upper respiratory tract infections
Mycobacteria	Tuberculosis, leprosy
Actinomycetes	Organ lesions and abscesses
Fungi	
Candida	Minor skin, mild respiratory, and severe systemic infections
Cryptococcus	
Histoplasma	
Blastomyces	

FACTORS AFFECTING OUTCOME OF ANTIBIOTIC THERAPY

Microbial Resistance to Antibiotics

Not all microorganisms are sensitive to all antibiotics. Resistance to antibiotics may be inherent or acquired. **Inherent resistance** to an antibiotic is a stable genetic trait. For example, *Pseudomonas aeruginosa* is resistant to penicillin G in part because the drug cannot penetrate the cell wall complex of this organism. This property of the bacteria does not change significantly over time or on exposure to penicillin G.

In contrast, **acquired resistance** represents a genetic change that converts a previously drug-sensitive bacteria to a drug-resistant one. *Staphylcoccus aureus* is a good example of the clinical importance of acquired resistance. Strains of this bacteria isolated from clinical infections during the 1940s, before penicillin use became widespread, were almost always penicillin sensitive, whereas today clinically isolated *S. aureus* strains are mainly penicillin resistant. Resistance can also be acquired on a much shorter time scale. An example is the drug ciprofloxacin. When originally introduced, this drug was active against many gram-negative bacteria, including *Pseudomonas aeruginosa,* and against gram-positive bacteria, including methicillin-resistant *Staphylococcus aureus.* Within a year some institutions reported wide-spread resistance to the drug.

One particularly important mechanism for acquiring antibiotic resistance involves **plasmids.** Plasmids are small circular pieces of DNA found separate from the chromosome in some bacteria. Many genes for antibiotic resistance reside on plasmids. Because plasmids may be rapidly passed between bacterial cells, antibiotic resistance can spread rapidly through an entire bacterial population. This mechanism for acquired resistance usually results in serious therapeutic difficulty because resistance to several antibiotics may occur simultaneously.

Microbiologists have recently discovered that plasmids can be shared between distantly related bacteria normally found in the human gastrointestinal tract. This fact leads us to the unsettling realization that if *any* bacteria is resistant to a drug, the gene for that resistance may be acquired by *many* bacteria, given time and exposure to the drug.

The mechanisms by which microorganisms achieve resistance to an antibiotic may be divided into three categories. Destruction of the antibiotic by the microorganism usually involves enzymes that chemically alter and thereby inactivate the drug. Examples of this process include penicillinase, which destroys penicillin and the acetylase, phosphorylase, and adenylating enzymes that inactivate the aminoglycoside antibiotics.

Bacteria may also achieve antibiotic resistance by reducing the uptake of the drug into the bacterial cell. Many antibiotics freely enter and in some cases are concentrated within bacterial cells. Resistance is achieved by blocking this uptake. An example of this type of resistance is with tetracyclines, which can freely enter sensitive bacteria but not resistant strains.

The third mechanism for resistance involves a mutation or an alteration in the target of the antibiotic in the microorganism. For example, erythromycin inhibits protein synthesis by binding to certain sites on the bacterial ribosome. Certain resistant microorganisms form altered ribosomes that do not bind erythromycin and are therefore resistant to its inhibitory action. Some types of streptomycin resistance may occur through similar means. A clinically important example of this type of resistance is methicillin-resistant *S. aureus.*

Identifying Bacteria Causing the Infection

In antibiotic therapy the first step is proper identification of the microorganism causing the disease. In some infections the symptoms are sufficiently clear to allow accurate diagnosis with a physical examination only. In other cases culturing must be done to identify the organism. At some institutions nursing personnel are trained to take specimens for culture, whereas in others laboratory personnel or physicians perform this function. The second step in treatment is the selection of the proper antibiotic, a process that depends on knowledge of the pathogen involved. This decision may be based entirely on clinical experience or may be aided by antibiotic susceptibility testing carried out in the microbiology laboratory on the pathogen isolated from the patient.

Site of Infection

Even when the proper drug has been selected, several factors influence effectiveness of therapy. One is the site of infection. For example, meningitis is difficult to treat partly because many antibiotics do not penetrate the blood-brain barrier very well, making an effective drug concentration difficult to obtain at the infection site. Similarly, many abscesses or soft tissue infections are not easily treated because the areas of infections are poorly perfused, and many drugs do not penetrate well into these areas. Healing is frequently hastened by surgical drainage.

Other Drugs

Other drugs the patient is receiving may influence the outcome of antibiotic therapy. Immunosuppressant drugs, for example, limit antibiotic effectiveness by depressing immune mechanisms that ordinarily assist in clearing the infection. Large doses of glucocorticoids cause significant immunosuppression. The use patterns of antibiotics can also influence resistance. For example, resistance to ciprofloxacin was more likely in settings where ciprofloxacin or its chemical relatives were widely used.

Clinical Status of Patient

The patient's clinical status can alter the outcome of antibiotic therapy. For example, renal function is important because many antibiotics are excreted by the kidney. If renal function is impaired, drugs eliminated through the kidney may accumulate. Likewise, hepatic disease may cause accumulation of drugs that are eliminated primarily by liver mechanisms. Patients with insufficiencies in these organ systems must be watched closely for signs of drug toxicity, which may occur at lower doses than would be expected in normal persons. Resistance to antibiotics is also more frequent in patients with certain chronic diseases such as cystic fibrosis. These patients are likely to have received multiple courses of antibiotic therapy, which also increases the risk of developing antibiotic resistance.

PROBLEMS IN ANTIBIOTIC THERAPY

Side Effects of Antibiotics

Direct Toxicity

Each antibiotic should be considered for its potential toxicity to the patient when it is administered. The signs of direct toxicity are frequently highly characteristic for a given class of drugs. For example, any aminoglycoside antibiotic can cause kidney damage and loss of hearing or equilibrium. When these drugs are given, patients should be observed closely for these toxic signs. Even drugs with a high TI occasionally cause direct toxic reactions. For example, at high enough doses penicillin can have direct effects on the central nervous system. Nurses should be alert to these signs. Direct toxic reactions to antibiotics are often dose dependent and would be expected to be more frequent and serious when high doses of drugs are given or when drug accumulation occurs in patients with renal or hepatic impairment.

Allergic Reactions

Allergies occur frequently with several antibiotics. The penicillins can produce allergic reactions that range from simple rashes to anaphylactic shock. Allergies occur in patients who have previously been exposed to the antibiotic or compounds chemically related to it in the medical setting or in the environment. Environmental exposure may be direct, as in workers in the antibiotic industry, or more subtle. For example, animals intended for immediate slaughter may not be treated with antibiotics also used in humans, but meat occasionally has contained sufficient residues of antibiotics to sensitize some people who consumed it.

Superinfections

Superinfections are infections that arise during antibiotic therapy. By definition, they involve microorganisms resistant to the antibiotic originally used; thus superinfections are often serious and difficult to treat. Such infections are more common with broad-spectrum than narrow-spectrum antibiotics. This observation is based on the fact that broad-spectrum antibiotics eliminate much more of the natural bacterial flora and upset the ecologic controls that normally keep resistant pathogens in check. With tetracyclines, for example, yeasts such as *Candida* are often involved in superinfections.

Misuse of Antibiotics

Viral Infections

One common misconception is that antibiotics can cure any type of infectious disease including those caused by viruses. In fact, no effective drugs exist to treat minor viral infections such as colds or sore throats (Chapter 47). It is not always easy to distinguish these viral infections from bacterial infections that might respond to antibiotics, and patients often request antibiotics for every cold or sore throat they experience.

Early Discontinuation of Antibiotics

Many infections resolve quickly once appropriate antibiotics are administered. Thus it is tempting for patients to discontinue medication much earlier than the physician planned, namely as soon as they feel better. This practice is dangerous for several reasons. Antibiotics with bacteriostatic action inhibit growth of bacteria, but the bacteria remain alive, at least until the immune system can eliminate them. Therefore if therapy is stopped too early, these organisms may again proliferate and relapse may occur. Not only does this prolong recovery, but it may also make the disease more difficult to treat. If we consider that the organisms most resistant to the drugs being used are the ones that probably survive longest, we can appreciate that these resistant organisms may cause the relapse. Therapy may therefore be difficult because some degree of drug resistance has occurred.

One excuse frequently given when patients discontinue antibiotic therapy early is that they wish to have the medication on hand in case they ever need it again. This practice is dangerous not only for the reasons just discussed but also because it assumes that patients can diagnose future illnesses accurately. Self-medication with old unused antibiotic prescriptions may delay proper medical attention and prolong or worsen the patient's disease. Once medication has been started, culture results become unreliable and proper diagnosis may be impossible. Thus patients should be discouraged from saving previously prescribed antibiotics to take them "just until I can get to the doctor."

Instability of Stored Antibiotics

Many drugs require special storage conditions and do not remain active for long when exposed to the warm, humid environment of most bathroom medicine cabinets. Drugs stored for weeks or months under such conditions may be inactive or may convert to forms that are more toxic. For example, tetracyclines tend to be light-sensitive and break down to toxic compounds.

Potential Dangers to Children

Any drug that remains in the household may be a hazard to children. Proper use and disposal of drugs is important to protect children from accidental poisoning. In addition, young children may be much more sensitive to certain antibiotics than adults. Antibiotics should never be given to children without first consulting a physician.

NURSING PROCESS OVERVIEW

Antiinfective Therapy

Assessment

Perform a complete physical assessment. Assess for fever, drainage, elevation of the white blood cell count, and signs of inflammation such as redness, swelling, or tenderness. Monitor vital signs. Assess for symptoms appropriate to the problem being treated: cough, production of phlegm, nasal drainage; difficulty or pain while urinating, frequent urination. Obtain a history of any exposure to infecting organisms and preexisting medical condition. Obtain the ordered cultures.

Nursing Diagnoses

- Altered bowel elimination: diarrhea and cramping related to antiinfective use
- Risk for vaginal superinfection with *Candida*

Patient Outcomes

The patient will complete the course of antiinfective therapy with minimal gastrointestinal (GI) discomfort. The patient will have vaginal superinfection diagnosed early if it occurs and will complete a course of appropriate drug therapy to treat it.

Planning/Implementation

Obtain additional data relevant to the antibiotic prescribed, such as renal function or liver function studies, and assessment of possible ototoxicity. Monitor vital signs, blood count, culture reports, and the patient's subjective and objective signs of infection. Maintain adequate nutritional and fluid intake, and use other therapies appropriate to the problem being treated: warm soaks, debridement of infected areas, and special wound-cleaning procedures. Use agents for patient comfort such as antipyretics for fever or bladder analgesics for bladder discomfort. Assess for side effects and for superinfection.

Evaluation

Before discharge, ascertain that the patient can explain why and how to take the prescribed drug, why it is necessary to continue the course of therapy as prescribed, what side effects may occur and which ones warrant contacting the physician, and what symptoms indicate that the medication is not effective.

NURSING IMPLICATIONS SUMMARY

Antiinfective Agents

Drug Administration

- Assess for history of allergy to antibiotics or antiinfectives before administering dose. Phrase questions appropriately. For example, "Are there any medicines you should not take and why?" may elicit more information than "Are you allergic to any antibiotics?" Have the patient describe previous problems. A gastric upset is probably a side effect; the development of hives is probably an allergic reaction. If there is a question about whether the patient is allergic to a medication, consult the physician before administering the dose.
- Label the patient's health record, chart, medication Kardex, and armband (per agency procedure) if the patient is allergic to any medications. In some hospitals patients with allergies wear a second specially marked or colored identification bracelet indicating allergies.
- Observe all patients receiving antiinfective agents for possible allergic reactions. Monitor vital signs. Have equipment and personnel available to treat acute allergic reactions. Have drugs such as epinephrine, antihistamines, and steroids available to treat allergic reactions.
- Nurses who are allergic to any antiinfective agent should wear gloves when preparing or administering doses of that drug.
- Read the physician's orders and drug labels carefully. Within a class of antiinfectives there may be several drugs with similar names.
- Reconstitute parenteral forms as directed by the label or in the manufacturer's literature. Date and initial the vial if some of the drug will be saved for later use. Do not use undated reconstituted medications. Observe expiration dates.
- For intramuscular (IM) administration, use large muscle masses (see Chapter 5). Aspirate before administering to prevent inadvertent intravenous (IV) administration. Record and rotate injection sites. If the ordered dose is a large volume of medication, divide the dose and administer in two injections.

Patient and Family Education

- Review the anticipated benefits and possible side effects of drug therapy with the patient. Instruct the patient to report the development of any unexpected sign or symptom.
- Encourage patients with a known allergy to any drug to wear a medical identification tag or bracelet indicating allergies.
- Instruct the patient to take antiinfective agents for as long as prescribed (usually 1 week to 10 days) even if he or she begins to feel better. Emphasize the following points: Do not share drugs with other family members. Do not save remaining doses to treat later infections. Do not administer drugs prescribed for adults to children.
- Antiinfectives work best when taken at evenly spaced intervals throughout the day. Discuss with the patient an appropriate dosing schedule based on the prescribed drug frequency.
- Tell pregnant or lactating women not to take any antiinfective agents without consulting the physician.
- Remind the patient to shake suspensions thoroughly before pouring dose. Use the same spoon or same size medicine cup to ensure the same dosage each time.
- Some oral liquids are dispensed in bottles with droppers, although the medicine is to be taken orally; review this with patients.
- Chewable tablets should be chewed and swallowed for best effect.
- Tell the patient to swallow enteric-coated preparations whole, without crushing or chewing. Consult the pharmacist if in doubt.
- Review with the patient any restrictions about taking the drug with meals, milk, or a snack and special storage con-

Continued.

NURSING IMPLICATIONS SUMMARY—cont'd

siderations such as refrigeration. Pharmacists usually label drugs that must be refrigerated.

- If a dose is missed, tell the patient to take it as soon as remembered, unless the time is close to the next dose, in which case the forgotten dose should be omitted. Exact guidelines vary depending on the frequency of doses. Instruct the patient not to double up for missed doses.
- Remind parents to keep drugs out of the reach of children. Pediatric dosage forms are often disguised in pleasant-tasting syrups and diluents, and children may want to take more than ordered doses. Tell parents to give children only drugs and doses prescribed for children.
- Instruct the patient to keep all health care providers informed of all drugs being taken. Review all drugs a patient is taking. If questions about drug incompatibilities arise, consult the physician or pharmacist.
- In the home check drug containers for expiration dates and encourage the patient to discard expired medications. Assess the area where the patient stores medications, and make recommendations if needed.

CRITICAL THINKING

APPLICATION

1. What is the principle of selective toxicity?
2. Why is selective toxicity possible to achieve?
3. How is selective toxicity achieved? How is it measured?
4. What is the difference between a bacteriostatic and a bactericidal drug?
5. What is the antimicrobial spectrum of a drug?
6. Define minimum inhibitory concentration (MIC) and minimum bactericidal concentration (MBC).
7. What is the difference between inherent and acquired resistance?
8. What are the three ways microorganisms resist the action of antibiotics?
9. Name five factors that influence the outcome of antibiotic therapy.
10. What problems may arise during antibiotic therapy?
11. What two dangers are associated with saving leftover antibiotics in the home?

CRITICAL THINKING

1. How would you assess for superinfections?
2. What are some of the common misuses of antibiotics? What should you teach patients to help avoid these problems?
3. What are the dangers associated with premature cessation of antibiotic therapy? What would you teach patients about this problem?

CHAPTER 39

Penicillins, Cephalosporins, and Related Drugs

OBJECTIVES

After studying this chapter, you should be able to do the following:

- *Explain the specific antibacterial effects of penicillins and cephalosporins.*
- *Describe the classes of penicillins.*
- *Explain the mechanism of resistance that bacteria develop to penicillins and cephalosporins.*
- *Describe the most common reaction to penicillins.*
- *Describe the most common reactions to cephalosporins, aztreonam, and imipenem.*
- *Develop a nursing care plan for a patient receiving one of the drugs discussed in this chapter.*

KEY TERMS

beta-lactam antibiotics
beta-lactamases
cephalosporins
methicillin-resistant *Staphylococcus aureus*
penicillin G

CHAPTER OVERVIEW

This chapter introduces the most widely used family of antibiotics in medical practice today, the **beta-lactam antibiotics,** of which penicillins and cephalosporins are the most important representatives. These agents share many properties, but individual drugs also have some important distinguishing characteristics.

Therapeutic Rationale: Bacterial Infections

Infections caused by bacteria take many forms, ranging from mild local infections to life-threatening systemic disease. The large family of beta-lactam antibiotics includes agents that are effective against most commonly encountered pathogens.

Therapeutic Agents: Bacterial Infections

Beta-Lactam Antibiotics

Mechanism of Action and Bacterial Resistance

Penicillins, cephalosporins, and other beta-lactam antibiotics are irreversible inhibitors of a bacterial enzyme called *transpeptidase.* This enzyme cross-links strands of cell wall material called *peptidoglycan.* When cross-linking occurs, peptidoglycan becomes rigid and is an effective cell wall. When cross-linking is blocked by beta-lactam antibiotics, cell wall synthesis continues, but the unreinforced strands formed cannot resist the osmotic forces within the bacterial cell. The bacterium may explode. Since exposed bacteria may be directly killed, beta-lactam antibiotics are classified as *bactericidal drugs.* However, even at doses below those required to kill bacteria, penicillins and cephalosporins are effective in some circumstances. Minimum disruption of the bacterial cell wall by these drugs may make the bacteria more liable to elimination by the immune system of the host.

Beta-lactam antibiotics do not directly destroy existing bacterial cell wall but prevent formation of new, intact cell wall. Thus these drugs are most effective against actively multiplying bacteria. These drugs are highly selective because they attack a process that does not exist in mammalian cells.

Resistance to penicillins and cephalosporins develops in microorganisms. The most common mechanism for resistance involves enzymes called **beta-lactamases.** These enzymes are usually referred to as *penicillinases* or *cephalosporinases,* depending on which type of drug the enzyme is most effective against. These enzymes destroy the penicillin or cephalosporin molecule, rendering the drug inactive. Some organisms possess these enzymes as part of their normal metabolic makeup and therefore are intrinsically resistant to beta-lactam antibiotics. Other organisms may acquire the enzyme and thus be converted from antibiotic sensitivity to resistance. Clinically important examples of acquired penicillin resistance are *Staphylococcus aureus* and *Neisseria gonorrhoeae.* Although 25 years ago both organisms could routinely be considered sensitive to penicillin G, today significant resistance to penicillin G exists for both organisms. In some hospitals, more that 90% of *S. aureus* strains are resistant.

Although resistance to penicillins is most commonly acquired by developing beta-lactamase, other important forms of resistance are known. The most clinically relevant example may be **methicillin-resistant *Staphylococcus aureus* (MRSA).** In this organism, resistance is conferred by altered penicillin targets. Altered targets are also the basis for resistance of *S. pneumoniae* to penicillin, which is an increasingly common clinical problem today.

Pharmacokinetics

Most penicillins and cephalosporins are excreted renally, by a combination of glomerular filtration and active tubular secretion. Exceptions are cefotaxime, cephalothin, and cepapirin, which are metabolized in liver to a significant degree. Both metabolites and unchanged drug are eliminated in urine. Nafcillin, ceftriaxone, and cefoperazone are also exceptions in that they are eliminated primarily in bile.

Penicillins, cephalosporins, and other beta-lactam antibiotics may accumulate in patients with impaired renal function. For this reason, the dosage of many of these drugs may be reduced when renal function is lower than normal. Dosage is adjusted based on creatinine clearance, according to guidelines in the package insert for each individual drug.

Uses

The primary clinical uses of the beta-lactam antibiotics is summarized in Table 39-1 and in the following sections on individual drugs.

Adverse Reactions and Contraindications

Allergies are the most common adverse reaction to penicillins. Many patients experience skin rashes or urticaria, but anaphylaxis is a much more dangerous allergic response. Injections of penicillin are responsible for most anaphylactic episodes, but any form of exposure to penicillin may produce anaphylaxis in sensitive individuals. Cephalosporins are good allergens much like penicillins, and many patients suffer similar allergic reactions. Many patients who are allergic to penicillins are also allergic to cephalosporins and vice versa.

Allergic rashes and drug fevers usually appear after several days of therapy, but the onset of anaphylaxis is nearly always within 10 minutes. A patient beginning therapy with a beta-lactam antibiotic should remain under medical supervision for 30 minutes after the injection so that if anaphylaxis develops, help is immediately available. If anaphylaxis occurs, medical personnel first should administer subcutaneous epinephrine. Anaphylaxis involves profound vasomotor collapse, and laryngeal edema may further complicate resuscitation efforts. Steroids may be required, as well as a tracheostomy and oxygen under positive pressure. All these emergency supplies should be on hand in any clinical setting where antibiotics are administered.

An estimated 3% to 5% of the general population is allergic to penicillin, but 10% of those who have previously received penicillin in a medical setting may be allergic. Patients about to receive penicillin must be asked if they have ever been given penicillin before and if they have ever had a rash or other allergic symptom during drug therapy. This information, although necessary, is somewhat unreliable. Many patients cannot recall what drugs they have received. Other patients may report past allergy to penicillin, yet they do not experience allergic reactions when reexposed. In these cases

TABLE 39-1 Primary Uses of Beta-Lactam Antibiotics

ORGANISM	TYPICAL INFECTIONS	BETA-LACTAM ANTIBIOTICS USED*
Gram-Positive Bacteria		
Streptococcus pneumoniae	Otitis media, sinusitis, pneumonia, meningitis	PENICILLIN G, PENICILLIN V, amoxicillin, ampicillin, imipenem, mezlocillin, piperacillin
Group A streptococci (e.g., *S. pyogenes*)	Pharyngitis, scarlet fever, impetigo, rheumatic fever	PENICILLIN G, PENICILLIN V, amoxicillin, ampicillin, cephalosporins, mezlocillin, piperacillin
Group B streptococci (e.g., *S. agalactiae*)	Neonatal sepsis, postpartum infections, meningitis	AMOXICILLIN, AMOXICILLIN + CLAVULANATE, AMPICILLIN, MEZLOCILLIN, PENICILLIN G, PENICILLIN V, PIPERACILLIN, cephalosporins
Enterococci	Endocarditis, urinary tract infections, nosocomial infections	AMPICILLIN, PENICILLIN G, imipenem, mezlocillin, penicillin V, piperacillin
Staphylococcus aureus nonpenicillinase	Boils, wound infections, skin infections, bone infections, endocarditis, meningitis	FIRST-GENERATION CEPHALOSPORINS, PENICILLIN G, PENICILLIN V, amoxicillin, ampicillin, imipenem
Staphylococcus aureus penicillinase strains	Boils, wound infections, skin infections, bone infections, endocarditis, meningitis	FIRST-GENERATION CEPHALOSPORINS, CLOXACILLIN, DICLOXACILLIN, METHICILLIN, NAFCILLIN, OXACILLIN, imipenem
Gram-Negative Bacteria		
Haemophilus influenzae	Pneumonia, bacteremia, tissue infections, meningitis, otitis media	AMOXICILLIN, AMOXICILLIN + CLAVULANATE, AMPICILLIN, AMPICILLIN + SULBACTAM, CEFUROXIME, THIRD-GENERATION CEPHALOSPORINS (parenteral), aztreonam
Neisseria gonorrhoeae	Gonorrhea, pelvic inflammatory disease	AMOXICILLIN, AMOXICILLIN + CLAVULANATE, AMPICILLIN, AMPICILLIN + SULBACTAM, CEFMETAZOLE, CEFOTETAN, CEFOXITIN, CEFUROXIME, THIRD-GENERATION CEPHALOSPORINS (except cefprozil)
Neisseria meningitidis	Meningitis	PENICILLIN G, amoxicillin, ampicillin, cefotaxime, ceftriaxone, cefuroxime
Escherichia coli	Diarrhea, wound infections, urinary tract infections	CEPHALOSPORINS, LORACARBEF, amoxicillin, ampicillin, aztreonam, imipenem, mezlocillin, piperacillin
Klebsiella pneumoniae	Pneumonia, urinary tract infections	CEPHALOSPORINS (except cefadroxil, cefprozil, cephalexin), aztreonam, imipenem
Serratia, Providencia	Bacteremia, nosocomial infections	CEFOPERAZONE, CEFOTETAN, CEFTAZIDIME, CEFTIZOXIME, ceftriaxone
Pseudomonas aeruginosa	Urinary tract infections, burn infections, wound infections, pneumonia	MEZLOCILLIN, PIPERACILLIN, TICARCILLIN, aztreonam, ceftazidime, imipenem
Bacteroides fragilis	Abscesses, infections at anaerobic sites	AMPICILLIN + SULBACTAM, IMIPENEM, TICARCILLIN + CLAVULANATE, mezlocillin, piperacillin, ticarcillin
Spirochetes		
Treponema pallidum	Syphilis	PENICILLIN G, PENICILLIN V
Borrelia burgdorferi	Lyme disease	CEFOTAXIME, CEFTRIAXONE, PENICILLIN G, PENICILLIN V

*Primary drugs = UPPER CASE; alternative drugs = lower case.

the original reaction may not have been a true penicillin allergy. Ampicillin, for example, may cause a benign macular eruption rather than a urticarial reaction. This toxic rash is not a sign of allergy but may be reported as an allergy by the patient.

In spite of the uncertainties in assessing past allergic responses, a medically documented prior allergic response to a penicillin, a cephalosporin, or penicillamine is the only contraindication to the use of most beta-lactam antibiotics.

The second most common reaction to beta-lactam antibiotics is gastrointestinal (GI) tract distress. Oral penicillin or cephalosporin preparations are the most likely to cause this side effect. Reactions include irritation and inflammation of the upper GI tract, nausea, vomiting, and diarrhea. Severe reactions may include antibiotic-associated pseudomembranous colitis. This condition arises when normal bacterial flora of the bowel are destroyed by an antibiotic, allowing *Clostridium difficile* to flourish. This anaerobic organism releases a toxin that causes the symptoms of pseudomembranous colitis, which include violent watery diarrhea and sloughing of tissue lining the GI tract.

Toxicity

Direct drug toxicity with penicillins is low; massive doses have been given with no ill effects. The tissue most sensitive to direct effects is the central nervous system (CNS). Intrathecal injection (into the subarachnoid space or cerebrospinal fluid) may produce convulsions. Convulsions also occur occasionally in patients given high doses intramuscularly or intravenously, especially if renal impairment exists and the drug accumulates. A relatively high concentration must be achieved in the cerebrospinal fluid before convulsions occur. This complication could occur in older adult patients being treated for serious infections such as streptococcal endocarditis. These patients may receive 25 to 40 million units of penicillin daily to maintain continuous bactericidal drug concentrations. Healthy persons can readily eliminate these large amounts through their kidneys, but older adults may have diminished renal function (see box). Therefore drug accumulation may occur, and penicillin may enter the CNS. The first sign may be loss of consciousness or myoclonic movements. Generalized seizures may follow.

Another group of patients with reduced ability to excrete penicillin are newborn infants. Because of this limitation, neonates receive carefully adjusted penicillin doses based on their body weight and reduced clearance of penicillin.

Interactions

Penicillins and cephalosporins require care in handling and diluting for intramuscular (IM) or intravenous (IV) therapy. Many penicillins require properly buffered solutions for stability, and thus not all are compatible with common IV fluids. Check the package insert or ask the pharmacist before adding penicillins or cephalosporins to any IV fluid.

Beta-lactam antibiotics are also incompatible in solution with aminoglycoside antibiotics. Both drugs are inactivated. When patients must receive both drugs, they are given at least 1 hour apart at separate sites.

Probenecid is sometimes used with penicillins to increase their effective duration of action by slowing active tubular secretion in the kidney. Probenecid may cause toxic reactions that are difficult to distinguish from a penicillin reaction. For example, probenecid may cause chills, fever, rash, GI tract irritation, and anemia. Probenecid also blocks renal excretion of some, but not all, cephalosporins.

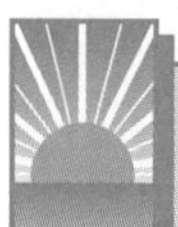

GERIATRIC CONSIDERATION

Penicillins and Cephalosporins

THE PROBLEM

Most beta-lactam antibiotics are excreted primarily through the kidneys, with biliary excretion as an alternative route. If renal function is impaired, excretion may be slowed, and the drug can accumulate. Healthy geriatric patients may have significantly lower renal function than younger adults and perhaps should be considered as renally impaired.

SOLUTIONS

When administering these drugs to older adult patients, it is important to monitor renal function. Adjust doses for renal function as prescribed or as described in the package insert.

Many penicillins and cephalosporins may block excretion of methotrexate since these drugs may compete for elimination by active tubular secretion. If methotrexate accumulates, significant toxicity may result.

Individual penicillins and cephalosporins occasionally have specific interactions with other drugs. These are listed under the individual antibiotics in the following sections.

Narrow-Spectrum Penicillins

Penicillin G, penicillin V

Mechanism of Action and Bacterial Resistance

All beta-lactam antibiotics share the same bactericidal mechanism of action: they inhibit bacterial cell wall biosynthesis. Resistance to **penicillin G** and penicillin V (Table 39-2) is often caused by penicillinases, enzymes that destroy the antibiotic. Examples include *S. aureus* and *N. gonorrhoeae*. Resistance in *S. pneumoniae* is mediated by changes in the penicillin target protein that render them impervious to inhibition by the antibiotic.

Pharmacokinetics

The penicillin molecule must remain intact to retain antibacterial activity. At least one bond in the molecule is sensitive to acid, which explains the lability of penicillin G in the stomach. Approximately 30% of an oral dose is absorbed, the rest being destroyed in the stomach or retained in the intestine and destroyed by bacteria in the large bowel. Because of the incomplete and somewhat variable absorption of penicillin G by this route, oral doses of penicillin G are not recommended.

Attempts to improve the oral absorption of penicillin G led to the development of penicillin V. Penicillin V is more acid stable and thus more efficiently absorbed from the GI tract than penicillin G; however, penicillin V is less potent as an antibacterial agent. Penicillin V should be given 1 hour before or 2 hours after meals, because food can interfere with absorption.

Penicillin G is rapidly and completely absorbed after IM injection, so that serum concentrations reach a peak 20 to 30 minutes after injection (Figure 39-1). This peak concentration persists for only a short time, primarily because the kidney so efficiently removes penicillin from the blood. Within 2 to 3 hours after IM injection, about 60% of the penicillin dose appears in urine. The drug in urine is unchanged and still possesses antibacterial activity. Penicillin enters urine by active secretion in the renal tubule.

Penicillin G is distributed to many tissues, with high concentrations found in blood, liver, kidney, and bile. Very little drug is found in brain or cerebrospinal fluid in healthy persons. If the meninges are inflamed, as in meningitis, penicillin can enter the CNS in significant amounts.

Uses

Penicillin G is a narrow-spectrum antibiotic; the organisms against which it is effective are summarized in Table 39-1. Most of the sensitive organisms are gram-positive bacteria.

TABLE 39-2 Common Dosages of Representative Penicillins

GENERIC NAME	TRADE NAME	ADMINISTRATION/DOSAGE
Narrow-Spectrum Penicillins		
✣ Penicillin G	Pentids	ORAL: *Adults*—200,000-500,000 U every 4-6 hr administered ½ hr before or 2 hr after meals. FDA pregnancy category B. *Children*—25,000-90,000 U/kg body weight daily in 3-6 doses. INTRAMUSCULAR, INTRAVENOUS: *Adults*—1 million-5 million U every 4-6 hr. *Children*—12,500-25,000 U/kg body weight every 6 hr.
Penicillin V	Pen-Vee K V-Cillin-K*	ORAL: *Adults*—125-500 mg every 6-8 hr. FDA pregnancy category B. *Children*—3.75-12.5 mg/kg body weight every 6 hr.
Repository Penicillins		
Benzathine penicillin G	Bicillin* Megacillin†	ORAL: *Adults*—200,000-500,000 U (base) every 4-6 hr. FDA pregnancy category B. *Children*—25,000-90,000 U/kg daily, divided into 3, 4, or 6 doses. INTRAMUSCULAR: *Adults*—1.2 million U every 2-4 wk. *Children*—50,000 U/kg body weight up to 1.2 million U every 1-4 wk.
Procaine penicillin G	Crysticillin Wycillin*	INTRAMUSCULAR: *Adults and children*—600,000-1.2 million U every 12-24 hr. FDA pregnancy category B. *Infants*—50,000 U/kg body weight once daily.
Penicillinase-Resistant Penicillins		
Cloxacillin	Orbenin† Tegopen	ORAL: *Adults*—0.25-0.5 gm every 6 hr. FDA pregnancy category B. *Infants*—6.25-12.5 mg/kg body weight every 6 hr. Administer 1 hr before or 2 hr after meals.
Dicloxacillin	Dycill Dynapen	ORAL: *Adults*—0.125-0.25 gm every 6 hr. FDA pregnancy category B. *Children*—3.125-6.25 mg/kg body weight every 6 hr. Administer 1 hr before or 2 hr after meals.
Methicillin	Staphcillin	INTRAMUSCULAR: *Adults*—1 gm every 4-6 hr. FDA pregnancy category B. *Children*—25 mg/kg body weight every 6 hr. INTRAVENOUS: *Adults*—1 gm every 6 hr. *Children*—same as for IM.
Nafcillin	Nafcil Nallpen Unipen*	ORAL: *Adults*—0.25-1 gm every 4-6 hr. FDA pregnancy category B. *Children*—6.25-12.5 mg/kg body weight every 6 hr. *Neonates*—10 mg/kg body weight every 6-8 hr. INTRAMUSCULAR: *Adults*—500 mg every 4-6 hr. *Children*—25 mg/kg body weight every 12 hr. INTRAVENOUS: *Adults*—0.5-1 gm every 4 hr. *Children*—20-40 mg/kg body weight every 8 hr.
Oxacillin	Bactocill Prostaphlin	ORAL: *Adults*—0.5-1 gm every 4-6 hr. FDA pregnancy category B. *Children*—12.5-25 mg/kg body weight every 6 hr. Administer 1 hr before or 2 hr after meals. INTRAMUSCULAR, INTRAVENOUS: *Adults*—0.25-2 gm every 4-6 hr. *Children*—12.5-25 mg/kg body weight every 6 hr.
Extended-Spectrum Penicillins		
✣ Amoxicillin	Amoxil* Polymox	ORAL: *Adults*—250-500 mg every 8 hr. *Infants and children 8-20 kg*—6.7-13.3 mg/kg body weight every 8 hr.
Amoxicillin + K clavulanate	Augmentin Clavulin†	ORAL: *Adults*—250 mg amoxicillin + 62.5 clavulanate or 500 mg amoxicillin + 125 mg clavulanate every 8 hr. FDA pregnancy category B. *Infants*—amoxicillin 6.7-13.3 mg/kg body weight + 1.7-3.3 mg clavulanate every 8 hr.
Ampicillin	Ampicin† Omnipen Polycillin Principen	ORAL: *Adults*—250-500 mg every 6 hr. FDA pregnancy category B. *Infants*—12.5-25 mg/kg body weight every 6 hr. INTRAMUSCULAR, INTRAVENOUS: *Adults*—same as for oral. *Infants*—25-50 mg/kg body weight every 6 hr.
Ampicillin + sulbactam	Unasyn	INTRAMUSCULAR, INTRAVENOUS: *Adults*—1-2 gm ampicillin and 0.5-1 gm sulbactam every 6 hr. FDA pregnancy category B.
Bacampicillin	Penglobe† Spectrobid	ORAL: *Adults*—400-800 mg every 12 hr (400 mg bacampicillin = 280 mg ampicillin). FDA pregnancy category B. *Children*—12.5-25 mg/kg every 12 hr.
Anti-*Pseudomonas* Penicillins		
Carbenicillin	Geocillin Geopen* Pyopen†	INTRAMUSCULAR, INTRAVENOUS: *Adults*—1-2 gm every 6 hr. Doses increased for life-threatening infections but should not exceed 40 gm daily. FDA pregnancy category B. *Children*—25-75 mg/kg body weight every 6 hr.
Carbenicillin indanyl sodium	Geocillin	ORAL: *Adults*—500-1000 mg (1 or 2 tablets) every 6 hr.

*Available in Canada and United States.
†Available in Canada only.

Continued.

TABLE 39-2 Common Dosages of Representative Penicillins—cont'd

GENERIC NAME	TRADE NAME	ADMINISTRATION/DOSAGE
***Anti-Pseudomonas* Penicillins—cont'd**		
Mezlocillin	Mezlin	INTRAMUSCULAR, INTRAVENOUS: *Adults*—3-4 gm every 4-6 hr. Severe infections may be treated with up to 24 gm daily in equally divided doses. FDA pregnancy category B. *Children*—50 mg/kg body weight every 4 hr.
Piperacillin	Pipracil*	INTRAMUSCULAR, INTRAVENOUS: *Adults*—3-4 gm every 4-6 hr. Up to 24 gm may be given daily for life-threatening infections. FDA pregnancy category B.
Piperacillin + tazobactam	Zosyn Tazocin†	INTRAVENOUS: *Adults*—3-4 gm piperacillin and 0.375 to 0.5 gm tazobactam every 6-8 hr. FDA pregnancy category B.
Ticarcillin	Ticar*	INTRAMUSCULAR: *Adults*—1 gm every 6 hr. FDA pregnancy category B. *Children*—50-75 mg/kg body weight every 6 hr. INTRAVENOUS: *Adults and children*—75 mg/kg body weight every 6 hr.
Ticarcillin + clavulanate	Timentin*	INTRAVENOUS: *Adults*—3 gm ticarcillin and 100 mg of clavulanic acid every 4-6 hr. FDA pregnancy category B. *Children*—50 mg ticarcillin and 1.7 mg clavulanic acid per kg body weight every 4-6 hr.

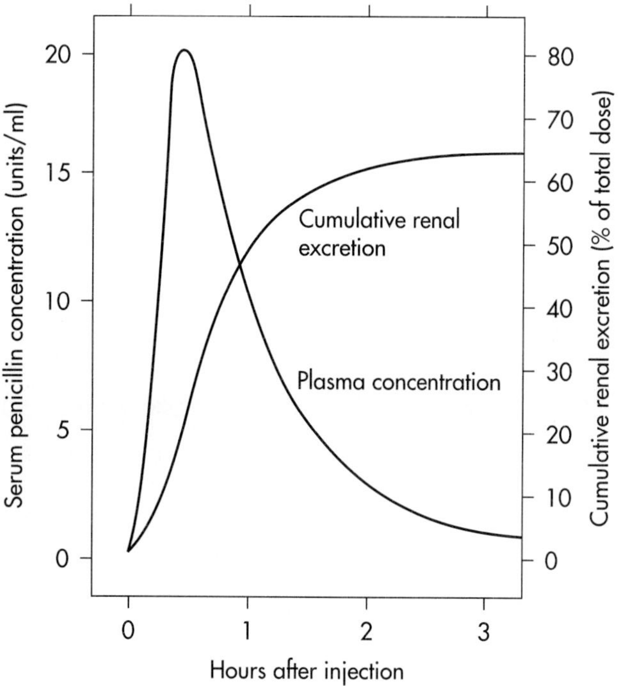

FIGURE 39-1
Serum concentration and urinary excretion of IM dose of penicillin G. Penicillin G is efficiently and rapidly absorbed after IM injections. Peak plasma concentrations of drug appear 20 to 30 minutes after injection. Penicillin G is actively secreted by renal tubules, accounting for rapid elimination half-time of about 20 to 30 minutes. Most of drug dose ends up in urine as unaltered penicillin.

These bacteria are characterized by thick, peptidoglycan-rich cell walls, which react with the Gram stain. Some of these gram-positive organisms such as *S. aureus, Streptococcus* species, and *S. pneumoniae* cause common infections of the upper respiratory tract and soft tissues, as well as more serious infections. Other rare gram-positive organisms, such as the ones that cause anthrax, gas gangrene, tetanus, and diphtheria, are also sensitive to penicillin G.

Among gram-negative organisms, clinically significant sensitivity to penicillin G is seen only with *N. meningitidis* (meningococcus) and *N. gonorrhoeae* (gonococcus). Other common gram-negative organisms normally found in the bowel and those frequently responsible for urinary tract infections are clinically resistant to penicillin G. In the laboratory, some of these gram-negative bacteria can be affected by high doses of penicillin G, but these high drug levels cannot routinely be achieved in patients.

Although penicillin G is not effective against common pathogens in routine urinary tract infections, it is effective against syphilis and gonorrhea. Syphilis, caused by a spirochete, is frequently treated effectively with single-dose penicillin G therapy. Gonorrhea was at one time also treated with a single dose of penicillin G but the organism that causes gonorrhea *(N. gonorrhoeae)* has gradually developed resistance to penicillins. Therefore cephalosporins or other drugs are now preferred.

The uses of penicillin V are restricted to conditions in which oral antibiotic therapy is appropriate. Mild to moderately serious infections caused by penicillin-sensitive organisms may be treated with penicillin V. Penicillin V also may be used in prophylaxis, especially in patients who have had rheumatic fever. In these patients, penicillin V prophylaxis may prevent recurrent streptococcal infections, which could lead to heart or kidney damage.

Adverse Reactions and Contraindications

Rashes and other allergic reactions are the primary side effects with narrow-spectrum penicillins. Because anaphylaxis, although rare, is potentially lethal, a medically documented allergy is a contraindication to the use of these drugs.

Toxicity

Potassium or sodium included in drug formulations may cause difficulties for some patients. For example, 1 million units of penicillin G and penicillin V may contain 1.5 mEq of potassium. Given in high enough doses for long enough periods, potassium intoxication and cardiac arrhythmias may occur. Some preparations of penicillin G contain high concentrations of sodium, which may cause difficulties in patients with preexisting cardiac or renal dysfunction.

Interactions

Active secretion of penicillins involves a specific renal transport system for which several drugs may compete. Physicians may take advantage of this trait by using another actively secreted drug such as probenecid to block penicillin excretion, thereby increasing peak penicillin concentration in the serum and increasing its effective duration.

Potassium supplements should be discontinued when potassium penicillin G or potassium penicillin V is being used to avoid potassium toxicity.

Repository Penicillins

Procaine penicillin G, benzathine penicillin G

Mechanism of Action and Bacterial Resistance

The repository penicillins (see Table 39-2) contain penicillin G as the active ingredient and therefore have the same mechanism of action.

Pharmacokinetics

Repository penicillins were designed for slow absorption from IM injection sites, creating a long duration of action. Once drug is absorbed from depot sites, it is hydrolyzed to release penicillin G, which is the active agent.

Slower absorption of drug means that peak concentrations are lower and take longer to achieve. For example, procaine penicillin G yields peak drug concentrations in serum 3 to 4 hours after injection, and significant serum concentrations may persist for 48 hours. A single dose of 300,000 U of aqueous penicillin G gives peak serum levels of 6 to 8 U/ml within one-half hour of injection, but procaine penicillin G at that same dose produces peak concentrations of only 1 to 2 U/ml. Benzathine penicillin G is absorbed even more slowly; thus peak serum levels occur 8 hours after injection, and useful serum levels persist for at least 2 weeks. An adult dose of 1.2 million U of benzathine penicillin G produces peak serum levels of only 0.1 to 0.3 U/ml.

Uses

Repository penicillins are not appropriate for serious infections when high serum concentrations of drug are required. Rather, these drugs are best used to maintain modest serum levels for relatively long periods. These conditions occur when very sensitive organisms are involved in mild to moderately serious infections or when prophylaxis is required.

Adverse Reactions and Contraindications

Procaine penicillin G is associated with CNS side effects because of the procaine content of the formulation. After injection, procaine may be released in significant amounts into the blood and may produce anxiety, lowered blood pressure, respiratory depression, and convulsions. These CNS reactions to procaine are usually transient, lasting less than 1 hour.

As with any penicillin, allergies can also occur, and documented prior allergies to beta-lactam antibiotics or penicillamine are a contraindication.

Toxicity

Repository penicillins are intended for deep muscular injections. Both preparations are stabilized suspensions of relatively insoluble forms of penicillin and contain up to about 2% weight/volume of emulsifying agents in addition to buffers. Such preparations should never be given by IV routes. Care must be taken on IM injection to prevent the accidental entry of these preparations into blood vessels since occlusion of blood vessels may result.

Penicillinase-Resistant Penicillins

Cloxacillin, dicloxacillin, methicillin, nafcillin, oxacillin

Mechanism of Action and Bacterial Resistance

These drugs retain the same mechanism of action as other penicillins, interfering with cell wall biosynthesis. These drugs were developed to resist the penicillinase produced by *S. aureus,* and thus are useful in many situations in which infections are caused by penicillinase-producing strains of that organism. Cloxacillin, dicloxacillin, and oxacillin are more potent than methicillin but are less potent than penicillin G.

Although these drugs resist penicillinase, other mechanisms of resistance may develop. A good example is methicillin, where resistance to the drug involves developing altered targets that render the bacteria tolerant to the drug. When methicillin resistance occurs, the organism also becomes resistant to all beta-lactam antibiotics and other antibiotics as well. Treatment of MRSA is a difficult clinical problem because of the limited number of effective drugs.

Pharmacokinetics

Methicillin is destroyed by stomach acid and therefore must be given parenterally. The other penicillinase-resistant penicillins are more stable in acid and thus may be used orally. Although nafcillin is sometimes used orally, it is not as well absorbed as oxacillin, cloxacillin, and dicloxacillin. With these latter drugs, oral absorption can be approximately doubled by fasting.

Nafcillin is unique among the penicillins since it is excreted primarily in the bile. All other penicillins are excreted primarily by the kidney.

Uses

Penicillinase-resistant penicillins are primarily used in initial therapy when a penicillinase-producing gram-positive bacteria is suspected. In all other penicillin-sensitive infections penicillin G is preferred because it is more potent than penicillinase-resistant drugs. One of the dangers in too frequent use of penicillinase-resistant penicillins is that the unusual drug-tolerance type of resistance may increase in bacterial populations. This type of resistance then affects all beta-lactam antibiotics and makes the resistant organism quite difficult to eradicate.

Adverse Reactions and Contraindications

As with any oral antibiotics, GI tract disturbances may occur. Methicillin and oxacillin can cause significant blood dyscrasias and interstitial nephritis. These reactions are uncommon with other penicillins.

Toxicity

Allergies may occur and documented prior allergic reactions to beta-lactam antibiotics or penicillamine are a contraindication.

Hepatotoxicity is associated with cloxacillin, dicloxacillin, and oxacillin more than with other penicillins. Hepatotoxicity may be more prevalent in human immunodeficiency virus (HIV)–positive patients.

Interactions

Drug interactions seldom influence the use of these drugs.

Extended-Spectrum Penicillins

Ampicillin, ✣ amoxicillin, bacampicillin

Mechanism of Action and Bacterial Resistance

Amoxicillin, ampicillin, and bacampicillin have the same mechanism of action as other beta-lactam antibiotics, in that they interfere with bacterial cell wall biosynthesis. Resistance to these drugs is commonly mediated by penicillinases.

Pharmacokinetics

Ampicillin may be used orally, but only 35% to 50% of an oral dose is absorbed. Bacampicillin is a prodrug designed to be more rapidly and completely absorbed than ampicillin and to release ampicillin on breakdown in the body. Amoxicillin is more acid stable than ampicillin and therefore better absorbed orally.

Uses

The penicillins discussed previously have narrow antimicrobial spectra, being primarily useful against gram-positive bacteria (see Table 39-1). The development of ampicillin and related drugs broadened the penicillin spectrum to include several common gram-negative pathogens. These drugs penetrate gram-negative cell walls better and are therefore more effective than penicillin G against these organisms. The extended-spectrum penicillins are not resistant to penicillinase and so may not be effective against *S. aureus* strains resistant to penicillin G.

Ampicillin is available in a fixed combination with sulbactam, and amoxicillin is available in fixed combination with clavulanic acid. Sulbactam and clavulanic acid are inhibitors of beta-lactamases. Inclusion of these inhibitors in fixed combinations protects the active drugs from destruction, allowing their use against some organisms that would otherwise be resistant.

Adverse Reactions and Contraindications

All beta-lactam antibiotics have the potential to cause allergic reactions and are avoided in patients with reported penicillin allergies.

Ampicillin commonly causes GI tract complaints and is one of the leading causes of antibiotic-associated colitis. In its worst form, this condition progresses to pseudomembranous colitis, which is associated with destruction of the GI tract lining by a toxin formed by *C. difficile.*

Toxicity

Ampicillin frequently causes a rash that is not allergic in origin and is referred to as a toxic rash. This rash appears 8 to 10 days after the start of therapy. Incidence of rash is greatly increased in patients with mononucleosis.

Interactions

Ampicillin and amoxicillin may reduce effectiveness of oral contraceptives by effects on steroid metabolism. Alternate birth control may be sought during the cycle when the antibiotics are used.

Ampicillin and bacampicillin may increase the incidence of rashes in patients receiving allopurinol.

The interaction of ampicillin and amoxicillin with sulbactam and clavulanic acid produces synergistic antibacterial action, as described above (see discussion of uses).

Anti-*Pseudomonas* Penicillins

Carbenicillin, mezlocillin, piperacillin, ticarcillin

Mechanism of Action and Bacterial Resistance

Like all other penicillins the anti-*Pseudomonas* penicillins interfere with bacterial cell wall synthesis in susceptible bacteria. These drugs are sensitive to penicillinases, including the one produced by *S. aureus.*

Pharmacokinetics

These drugs must be administered parenterally. For carbenicillin, an indanyl ester is available, which allows the drug to be used orally. However, indanyl carbenicillin does not produce high enough serum levels of carbenicillin to make the drug effective for most infections. Therefore it is reserved for use in urinary tract infections because the drug does accumulate to high concentrations in urine after oral dosage.

Uses

One pathogenic organism that is not sensitive to extended-spectrum penicillins is *Pseudomonas aeruginosa.* This gram-negative bacterium is responsible for certain urinary tract infections, bacteremias, and infections in burn patients and is unusually resistant to many antibiotics. Thus the anti-*Pseudomonas* drugs were developed specifically for use against this organism. Anti-*Pseudomonas* penicillins may be used with gentamicin or another anti-*Pseudomonas* aminoglycoside (see Chapter 43) to treat severe *Pseudomonas* infections.

Adverse Reactions and Contraindications

Carbenicillin, piperacillin, and ticarcillin frequently interfere with platelet function. This problem is worse in uremic patients because they have preexisting platelet dysfunction as a result of their renal disease.

Toxicity

Anti-*Pseudomonas* penicillins and especially preparations of ticarcillin contain high concentrations of sodium, which may cause difficulties in patients with preexisting cardiac or renal dysfunction.

Interactions

Gentamicin or other aminoglycosides must never be directly mixed in the syringe or IV bottle with these agents since the drugs inactivate each other.

Cephalosporins

Mechanism of Action and Bacterial Resistance

Cephalosporins (Table 39-3) share the same mechanism as penicillins; both types of drugs inhibit the action of transpeptidase enzymes that cross-link bacterial cell wall peptidoglycan. The drugs are considered bactericidal because the weakened cell wall can rupture, leading to death of the bacteria.

Resistance to cephalosporins occurs most often because bacteria produce beta-lactamases that destroy the antibiotic. The enzymes that attack cephalosporins are often different from those that destroy penicillins. For example, the beta-lactamase of *S. aureus* that confers resistance to many penicillins does not attack cephalosporins.

Pharmacokinetics

Several cephalosporins are currently available for oral use (see Table 39-3). These preparations are well absorbed and produce effective serum concentrations of antibiotic. Absorption of cephalosporins from the GI tract is slowed by food in the stomach, but about the same amount of drug is ultimately absorbed as in a fasting patient.

Most cephalosporins are given parenterally because they are well absorbed from IM sites. The elimination half-times of all these drugs are about twice as long as that of penicillin G and are roughly equivalent to those of ampicillin or the penicillinase-resistant penicillins.

Cephalosporins are distributed in the body in a manner similar to that of penicillins, except that first-generation and most second-generation cephalosporins do not penetrate the CNS well enough to be used in meningitis. Cephalosporins, with the exception of cefoperazone and ceftriaxone, are excreted primarily by the kidney and are highly concentrated in urine, making them useful in treating several common types of urinary tract infections.

Uses

The cephalosporins are divided into three subgroups, referred to as *generations.* Among the first-generation cephalosporins, cephalothin and cefazolin are the most widely used parenteral agents, and cephalexin is the most widely used oral agent, although other members of this class differ little from these three. Second-generation cephalosporins differ from the first-generation drugs by having slightly extended activity against gram-negative bacteria. For example, the second-generation drug cefamandole has better activity than first-generation cephalosporins against *Enterobacter.* Other second-generation cephalosporins are especially active against *Haemophilus.* Third-generation cephalosporins generally have lower activity against gram-positive organisms than first-generation drugs, but some third-generation cephalosporins have significant activity against the gram-negative pathogen *P. aeruginosa.* They are the only cephalosporins to possess such activity. In addition, several third-generation cephalosporins are distributed reliably into the CNS.

The primary usefulness of cephalosporins is based on the differences in the antimicrobial spectra of penicillins and cephalosporins. First-generation cephalosporins resemble ampicillin in their effectiveness against gram-negative bacteria. Unlike ampicillin, cephalosporins resist the action of staphylococcal penicillinase and can be used when the organism is resistant to penicillin G. Cephalosporins are not effective against MRSA. Second- and third-generation cephalosporins are used for specific, serious infections caused by gram-negative bacteria.

Adverse Reactions and Contraindications

Many cephalosporins cause pain at the injection site. When given intravenously, these drugs cause phlebitis or thrombophlebitis and pain along the affected vein. Orally administered cephalosporins may cause gastric irritation, nausea, and vomiting. Superinfections may arise when these relatively broad-spectrum drugs are used, the most common being oral or vaginal candidiasis (yeast infections). Allergies to cephalosporins may take the form of rashes, serum sickness, hemolytic anemia, Stevens-Johnson syndrome, or anaphylaxis.

Cefamandole, cefmetazole, cefoperazone, and cefotetan have been associated with platelet dysfunction. Patients should be observed for signs of unusual bleeding or bruising. The bleeding time or prothrombin time may require monitoring. Patients with bleeding disorders should not receive these drugs.

The only contraindication to the use of cephalosporins is a prior history of serious allergic reaction to penicillamine, a penicillin, or a cephalosporin. Caution should be used if these drugs must be given to patients with hepatic disease or renal impairment, and doses may require reduction. Patients with GI tract disease may be more likely to develop antibiotic-associated pseudomembranous colitis.

Toxicity

Overdoses of cephalosporins may cause seizures. The drugs should be discontinued if seizures occur; specific treatment for controlling seizure activity may be required.

TABLE 39-3 Common Dosages of Representative Cephalosporins

GENERIC NAME	TRADE NAME	ADMINISTRATION/DOSAGE
First Generation		
Cefadroxil	Duricef* Ultracef	ORAL: *Adults*—0.5 gm every 12 hr. FDA pregnancy category B. *Children*—15 mg/kg body weight every 12 hr.
✣ Cefazolin	Ancef* Kefzol*	INTRAMUSCULAR, INTRAVENOUS: *Adults*—250 mg every 8 hr, up to 1.5 gm every 6 hr. FDA pregnancy category B. *Children*—6.25-25 mg/kg body weight total every 6 hr.
Cephalexin	Keflex*	ORAL: *Adults*—250-500 mg every 6 hr. FDA pregnancy category B. *Children*—6.25-25 mg/kg body weight every 6 hr.
Cephalothin	Keflin*	INTRAVENOUS: *Adults*—1-2 gm every 4-6 hr. FDA pregnancy category B. *Children*—20-40 mg/kg body weight every 6 hr.
Cephapirin	Cefadyl*	INTRAMUSCULAR, INTRAVENOUS: *Adults*—500 mg-1 gm every 4-6 hr. FDA pregnancy category B. *Children*—10-20 mg/kg body weight every 6 hr.
Cephradine	Velosef*	ORAL, INTRAMUSCULAR, INTRAVENOUS: *Adults*—1-6 gm total daily dose. FDA pregnancy category B. *Children*—6.25-25 mg/kg body weight every 6 hr.
Second Generation		
Cefactor	Ceclor*	ORAL: *Adults*—250-500 mg every 8 hr. FDA pregnancy category B. *Children*—20-40 mg/kg body weight, not to exceed 1 gm daily.
Cefamandole	Mandol*	INTRAMUSCULAR, INTRAVENOUS: *Adults*—500 mg-2 gm every 4-6 hr. FDA pregnancy category B. *Children*—16.7-33.3 mg/kg body weight every 8 hr.
Cefixime	Suprax*	ORAL: *Adults*—200 mg every 12 hr or 400 mg once daily. FDA pregnancy category B. *Children*—4 mg/kg body weight every 12 hr or 8 mg/kg body weight once daily.
Cefonicid	Monocid	INTRAMUSCULAR, INTRAVENOUS: *Adults*—1-2 gm once daily. No more than 1 gm should be given at single IM site. FDA pregnancy category B.
Cefotetan	Cefotan*	INTRAMUSCULAR, INTRAVENOUS: *Adults*—1-3 gm every 12 hr. FDA pregnancy category B.
Cefoxitin	Mefoxin*	INTRAVENOUS: *Adults*—1-2 gm every 4-8 hr. FDA pregnancy category B. *Children*—20-40 mg/kg body weight every 6 hr.
Cefprozil	Cefzil	ORAL: *Adults*—250-500 mg every 12 hr. FDA pregnancy category B. *Children >6 mo*—7.5-15 mg/kg every 12 hr.
Cefuroxime	Kefurox* Zinacef*	INTRAMUSCULAR, INTRAVENOUS: *Adults*—0.75-1.5 gm every 8 hr. FDA pregnancy category B. *Children >3 mo*—16.7-33.3 mg/kg body weight every 8 hr.
Cefuroxime axetil	Ceftin*	ORAL: *Adults*—250-500 mg every 12 hr. FDA pregnancy category B. *Children*—125 mg every 8-12 hr.
Third Generation		
Cefmetazole	Zefazone	INTRAVENOUS: *Adults*—2 gm (base) every 6-12 hr. FDA pregnancy category B.
Cefoperazone	Cefobid*	INTRAVENOUS: *Adults*—2-4 gm every 8 hr. Daily dose not to exceed 12 gm. FDA pregnancy category B.
✣ Cefotaxime	Claforan*	INTRAVENOUS: *Adults*—1-2 gm every 4-12 hr. More severe infections may require up to 12 gm daily. FDA pregnancy category B. *Children*—50 mg/kg body weight every 8 hr. INTRAMUSCULAR: *Adults*—250 mg as single dose for uncomplicated gonorrhea.
Cefpodoxime	Vantin	ORAL: *Adults*—100-400 mg every 12 hr. FDA pregnancy category B. *Children >6 mo*—5 mg/kg every 12 hr.
Ceftazidime	Fortaz* Tazicef	INTRAMUSCULAR, INTRAVENOUS: *Adults*—0.5-2 gm every 8-12 hr. FDA pregnancy category B. *Children*—30-50 mg/kg body weight every 8-12 hr.
Ceftizoxime	Cefizox*	INTRAVENOUS: *Adults*—1-4 gm every 8-12 hr. FDA pregnancy category B. *Children >6 mo*—50 mg/kg body weight every 6-8 hr. INTRAMUSCULAR: *Adults*—1 or 2 gm (1 gm per site) once, for uncomplicated gonorrhea.
Ceftriaxone	Rocephin*	INTRAMUSCULAR, INTRAVENOUS: *Adults*—1-2 gm every 24 hr. FDA pregnancy category B. *Children*—25-37.5 mg/kg body weight every 12 hr.

*Available in Canada and United States.

Interactions

Interstitial nephritis is sometimes seen with these drugs. There is danger of synergistic nephrotoxicity when a cephalosporin is given with other nephrotoxic agents such as an aminoglycoside antibiotic or the diuretics furosemide or ethacrynic acid. In spite of this risk, third-generation cephalosporins such as ceftazidime or cefoperazone may be given with an aminoglycoside such as amikacin, netilmicin, tobramycin, or gentamicin when synergistic activity is required to treat serious infections caused by *P. aeruginosa*.

Probenecid may prolong the persistance of cephalosporins in the body by blocking renal tubular secretion. Probenecid has no effect on the duration of action of cefoperazone, ceftriaxone, or ceftazidime because these three drugs depend less on active tubular secretion for elimination than do the other cephalosporins.

Cefamandole, cefmetazole, cefoperazone, and cefotetan are a chemically related subset of cephalosporins that may cause excessive bleeding if used with anticoagulants or platelet-aggregation inhibitors such as aspirin. These drugs are also more likely than other cephalosporins to cause a disulfiram reaction if alcohol is ingested while the drugs are being taken.

OTHER BETA-LACTAM ANTIBIOTICS

Aztreonam

Mechanism of Action and Bacterial Resistance

Aztreonam (Table 39-4) acts in a way similar to other beta-lactam antibiotics, interfering with bacterial cell wall synthesis. Unlike most penicillins and cephalosporins, aztreonam inhibits or destroys primarily gram-negative aerobic bacteria. Aztreonam is ineffective for gram-positive or anaerobic bacteria because the drug fails to bind to critical targets in those organisms.

Pharmacokinetics

Aztreonam must be administered parenterally to obtain useful concentrations in plasma. The drug is distributed well to many body tissues and fluids but is relatively low in cerebrospinal fluid. Excretion is primarily via the kidneys, and only minor amounts of drug are eliminated by hepatic mechanisms.

Uses

Aztreonam is given to treat urinary tract infections, septicemia, infections of the lower respiratory tract, intraabdominal or gynecologic infections, and soft tissue infections. These infections are typically caused by gram-negative bacteria, including *Pseudomonas.*

Adverse Reactions and Contraindications

The principal adverse reactions to aztreonam include pain or phlebitis at the injection site in up to 2.4% of patients. GI tract symptoms (including nausea, diarrhea, or vomiting) occur in up to 1.3% of patients. Rash and other symptoms of allergic reactions can occur, as with all beta-lactam antibiotics.

The only contraindication to the use of aztreonam is prior allergic reaction to a beta-lactam antibiotic, but caution should be used when the drug must be given to patients with cirrhosis or renal impairment. Doses may require reduction in these conditions.

Imipenem

Mechanism of Action and Bacterial Resistance

Imipenem (see Table 39-4) is an extremely potent inhibitor of bacterial cell wall synthesis. The mechanism of action resembles that of other beta-lactam antibiotics. Imipenem has a broad antimicrobial spectrum that includes gram-positive, gram-negative, and anaerobic bacteria. Imipenem is effective against penicillinase-producing *S. aureus.*

Resistance to imipenem has begun to appear in MRSA and *P. aeruginosa. Enterococcus faecium* is also resistant to imipenem. In some cases, unusual beta-lactamases are involved in resistance, but other mechanisms of resistance also occur.

Pharmacokinetics

Imipenem is well distributed to many tissues but is low in cerebrospinal fluid. Excretion is through the kidneys. When given alone, imipenem is hydrolyzed in the kidneys and excreted as inactive products. The clinical preparation includes cilastatin, an agent chemically related to imipenem but with little antibacterial activity. Cilastatin inhibits destruction of imipenem in the kidneys and allows active imipenem to accumulate in renal tissue and urine.

Uses

Because imipenem has such a broad antimicrobial spectrum, it is used to treat a variety of infections at many sites. *P. aeruginosa* is usually sensitive, but resistant strains may occur.

Adverse Reactions and Contraindications

Imipenem can cause mild-to-serious allergic reactions, as can other beta-lactam antibiotics. Imipenem can also cause rare CNS reactions, which may include seizures. Pseudomembranous colitis can also occur.

Toxicity

Doses of imipenem greater than 2 gm daily increase the risk of seizures. Imipenem is more likely to cause seizures than are other beta-lactam antibiotics.

Interactions

Imipenem is used in fixed combination with cilastatin to avoid destruction of imipenem in the kidneys, as described above (see discussion of pharmacokinetics).

TABLE 39-4 Clinical Summary of Aztreonam and Imipenem

GENERIC NAME	TRADE NAME	ADMINISTRATION/DOSAGE
Aztreonam	Azactam	INTRAMUSCULAR, INTRAVENOUS: *Adults*—1-8 gm daily, divided into 2-4 equal doses. FDA pregnancy category B.
Imipenem-cilastatin	Primaxin*	INTRAVENOUS: *Adults*—1-4 gm daily, divided into 3 or 4 equal doses. FDA pregnancy category C.

*Available in Canada and United States.

Nursing Process Overview

Penicillins, Cephalosporins, and Related Drugs

Assessment

Assess the patient and monitor for clinical signs of infection. Pay special attention to subjective data suggesting the patient has a history of allergy to penicillins or to related drugs. Monitor renal function.

Nursing Diagnoses

- Possible complication: allergic reaction
- Risk for diarrhea related to drug side effects

Patient Outcomes

Ideally, the patient will not experience an allergic reaction; but if one occurs, the nurse will manage and minimize complications associated with the allergic response. The patient will not experience diarrhea related to drug side effects.

Planning/Implementation

Observe the patient closely for possible allergic response for 20 to 30 minutes after the first dose is administered. Have available drugs and equipment for resuscitation. In preparation for discharge, review with the patient the need to take the prescribed drug for the full course of therapy and to try to space doses evenly throughout the 24-hour day.

Evaluation

Penicillins, cephalosporins, and related drugs seldom cause long-term side effects. Before discharge, ascertain that the patient can judge improvement in the infection and describe possible side effects and situations that warrant consulting the physician.

Nursing Implications Summary

Penicillins, Cephalosporins, and Related Drugs

Drug Administration

- Review the Nursing Implications Summary in Chapter 38 (p. 469).
- Assess for history of allergy before administering these drugs.
- Monitor vital signs and temperature. Inspect for rash.
- Monitor serum creatinine and blood urea nitrogen (BUN) levels, liver function tests, complete blood count (CBC), and differential count. Monitor serum electrolyte level of patients with hypertensive, renal, or cardiovascular disease and in patients receiving drugs high in potassium or sodium.
- For IV administration, consult the manufacturer's literature or Table 39-5 for the approximate rate of IV push administration. Too rapid administration of penicillins has resulted in the occurrence of seizures. Too rapid administration of the cephalosporins contributes to venous irritation and patient discomfort.
- Warn patients that IM injection may be painful. Use large muscle masses. Record and rotate injection sites. See Chapter 5 for a description of IM injection sites.
- See text; penicillins and cephalosporins are incompatible with aminoglycosides.
- Read drug labels and orders carefully. Products containing procaine, benzathine, or a combination of these are never given by IV routes. Occasional patients are sensitive to procaine; symptoms include anxiety, confusion, agitation, fear of impending doom, and convulsions.

Patient and Family Education

- Review the Nursing Implications Summary in Chapter 38 (p. 469).
- The following drugs should be taken on an empty stomach, 1 hour before or 2 hours after meals, with a full (8-ounce) glass of water: ampicillin, liquid bacampicillin, carbenicillin, cloxacillin, dicloxacillin, flucloxacillin, nafcillin, oxacillin, and penicillin G.
- The following drugs may be taken with food or on an empty stomach: amoxicillin, amoxicillin and clavulanate, the tablet form of bacampicillin, penicillin V, pivampicillin, pivmecillinam, and oral cephalosporins.
- Instruct the patient to take amoxicillin suspension straight or mix with formula, milk, fruit juice, ginger ale, or other cold drink. Instruct the patient to take dose immediately after mixing dose.
- Instruct the patient to avoid acidic fruit juices or beverages within 1 hour of taking a dose of penicillin G.
- Cefuroxime axetil should be taken with food or snack and may be crushed and mixed with food to ease taking and to help disguise the taste.
- Liquid forms may be dispensed with a calibrated measuring device or may be in the form of pediatric drops. Review measurement and administration of the dose with the patient and family.
- The penicillins, cephalosporins, and related drugs may cause false-positive reactions with copper sulfate urine glucose tests. Advise the patient to check with the physician before changing insulin or diet. Instruct the patient to monitor blood glucose levels.

NURSING IMPLICATIONS SUMMARY—cont'd

- If chewable tablets are prescribed, encourage the patient to chew or crush the tablets before swallowing them.
- Penicillins, cephalosporins, and related drugs may cause diarrhea. Instruct the patient to notify the physician if diarrhea is severe or persistent. For mild diarrhea, only medicines containing kaolin or attapulgite should be used.
- Warn the patient taking cefamandole, cefmetazole, cefoperazone, or cefotetan to avoid the use of alcohol while taking these drugs and for several days after completing the course of therapy. Ingestion of alcohol may cause a disulfiram-type of reaction (see the patient problem box on alcohol use and disulfiram on p. 635).
- Warn the female patient taking ampicillin, amoxicillin, or penicillin V that oral contraceptives containing estrogen may not work during the course of antiinfective drug therapy. Female patients should use an alternate or additional form of birth control while taking these antiinfectives; advise the patient to consult the physician or pharmacist.

TABLE 39-5 Direct Infusion Rate for Penicillins, Cephalosporins, and Related Drugs

DRUG	RECOMMENDED DILUTION*	RATE OF ADMINISTRATION†
Penicillins		
Ampicillin	500 mg/at least 5 ml diluent	1 dose/10-15 min
Ampicillin + sulbactam	1.5 gm/4 ml diluent, then further diluted in at least 50 ml compatible diluent	1 dose/15-30 min
Carbenicillin	Dilute as directed on vial, then further dilute each gram in at least 5 ml diluent	1 gm/5 min
Methicillin	500 mg reconstituted drug in at least 25 ml diluent	10 ml/min
Mezlocillin	1 gm in at least 10 ml diluent	1 dose/3-5 min
Nafcillin	Desired amount of drug in 15-30 ml diluent	500 mg/5-10 min
Oxacillin	1 gm/10 ml diluent	1 ml/min
Piperacillin	1 gm/5 ml diluent	1 dose/3-5 min
Piperacillin + tazobactam	Dose/5 ml diluent, then further dilute in desired volume	1 dose/30 min
Ticarcillin	1 gm in at least 4 ml diluent, then further diluted to 1 gm/10 ml	1 gm/5 min
Ticarcillin + clavulanate	3.1 gm/13 ml diluent; further dilute in 50-100 ml of fluid	1 dose/30 min
Cephalosporins		
Cefamandole	1 gm/10 ml diluent	1 gm/3-5 min
✚ Cefazolin	1 gm/10 ml diluent	1 gm/5 min
Cefmetazole	Dilute as directed on vial	1 dose/3-5 min
Cefonicid	0.5 gm/2 ml diluent	1 dose/3-5 min
Cefoperazone	1 gm/5 ml diluent	1 dose/3-5 min
✚ Cefotaxime	1 dose/10 ml diluent	1 dose/3-5 min
Cefotetan	1 gm/10 ml diluent	1 dose/3-5 min
Cefoxitin	1 gm/10 ml diluent	1 gm/3-5 min
Ceftazidime	0.5 gm/5 ml	1 dose/3-5 min
Ceftizoxime	1 gm/10 ml diluent	1 dose/3-5 min
Ceftriaxone	250 mg/2.5 ml; further dilute in 50-100 ml of fluid	1 dose/30 min
Cefuroxime	750 mg/9 ml diluent	1 dose/3-5 min
Cephalothin	1 gm/10 ml diluent	1 gm/3-5 min
Cephapirin	1 gm/10 ml diluent	1 gm/5 min
Cephradine	500 mg/5 ml diluent	1 gm/3-5 min
Others		
Aztreonam	1 dose/6-10 ml diluent	1 dose/3-5 min
Imipenem and cilastatin	1 dose/10 ml diluent; further dilute in 100 ml fluid	500 mg/20-30 min 1 gm/40-60 min

*For information about appropriate diluents, preparations for constant infusion, compatibilities with infusion fluids, storage conditions, and other questions, consult the pharmacist and the manufacturer's information. Because the cephalosporins are so irritating to the vein, diluting these drugs more than is indicated in the table is preferable, when possible.

†These rates are for direct IV push unless otherwise noted. When diluted in 50 to 100 ml or more, the rate is determined in part by the total volume.

CRITICAL THINKING

APPLICATION

1. What is the mechanism of action of penicillins and cephalosporins?
2. What is the effect of beta-lactam antibiotics on existing bacterial cell walls?
3. What is the most common mechanism by which bacteria gain resistance to beta-lactam antibiotics?
4. What is the mechanism of excretion for most penicillins and cephalosporins?
5. What is the most common toxic reaction to penicillins and cephalosporins? What should you watch for?
6. What is the purpose of skin tests for penicillin allergies?
7. What is the effect of penicillin on the CNS?
8. Name two groups of patients most at risk for accumulating penicillins given at normal doses.
9. What type of patient would be most at risk from the potassium and sodium contained in many penicillin and cephalosporin preparations? What tests should you monitor?
10. Why is probenecid sometimes administered with penicillin G?
11. Why is penicillin G absorbed erratically from the GI tract?
12. When does the peak concentration of penicillin G appear in the bloodstream after an IM dose of the drug?
13. What is the elimination half-time for penicillin G in normal patients?
14. How does the penetration of penicillin G into the cerebrospinal fluid differ in healthy patients and in those with meningitis?
15. Why do procaine penicillin G and benzathine penicillin G have longer durations of action than penicillin G?
16. What is the danger to patients from accidentally administering the repository penicillins by IV routes?
17. What advantage does penicillin V have over penicillin G?
18. Why is methicillin useful in treating infections caused by penicillinase-producing *S. aureus?*
19. How do bacteria become resistant to methicillin?
20. What is the route of excretion of nafcillin?
21. What advantages do oxacillin, cloxacillin, and dicloxacillin have over methicillin?
22. How does the antimicrobial spectrum of ampicillin and amoxicillin differ from that of penicillin G?
23. What advantage does amoxicillin possess over ampicillin?
24. Why is clavulanic acid or sulbactam included in fixed combination with ampicillin, amoxicillin, or ticarcillin?
25. Infections caused by what pathogen are appropriately treated with carbenicillin or ticarcillin?
26. How does carbenicillin indanyl sodium differ from carbenicillin?
27. Why are first-generation cephalosporins not useful in treating meningitis?
28. What is the most common reaction expected from most cephalosporins when administered by IV routes?
29. How does the antimicrobial spectrum of the cephalosporins differ from that of penicillin G?
30. What is the antimicrobial spectrum of aztreonam?
31. What is the antimicrobial spectrum of imipenem?
32. Why is imipenem given with cilastatin?

CRITICAL THINKING

1. Which would produce a higher serum concentration of antibiotic, 1 million units of penicillin G or 1 million units of procaine penicillin G?
2. Compare and contrast one drug from each generation of cephalosporins. Consider spectrum of activity, route of administration, frequency of dose, and cost.
3. What are the main points of a nursing care plan for patients receiving drugs discussed in this chapter?
4. What teaching points are important for patients receiving one of the antiinfective agents discussed in this chapter?

CHAPTER 40

Quinolones

OBJECTIVES

After studying this chapter, you should be able to do the following:

- *Explain the unique mechanism of action of quinolone antibiotics.*
- *Discuss the side effects that are most common with quinolones.*
- *Explain why quinolones are generally not used in children.*
- *Explain why quinolones may be avoided in patients with a history of seizures.*
- *Develop a nursing care plan for a patient receiving ciprofloxacin.*

KEY TERMS

ciprofloxacin
crystalluria
DNA gyrase
lomefloxacin
norfloxacin
ofloxacin
quinolones

CHAPTER OVERVIEW

This chapter introduces a new group of potent antibiotics that were developed from older agents such as nalidixic acid, which was too weak for use in systemic infections. The newer agents are sometimes referred to as fluoroquinolones because the greater antibacterial potency of the new agents comes from a fluorine substitution on the quinolone ring. This chapter focuses on these newer drugs.

Therapeutic Rationale: Bacterial Infections

Infections caused by bacteria range from mild local infections to life-threatening systemic disease. Infections caused by gram-positive bacteria are associated with many infections of the throat and ears, as well as soft tissue infections and pneumonia. Gram-negative bacteria are likely to be the cause of urinary tract infections. In addition these organisms may cause pneumonia in hospitalized or chronically ill patients. The newer quinolone antibiotics are especially useful against gram-negative pathogenic bacteria.

Therapeutic Agents: Bacterial Infections

Quinolone Antibiotics

Mechanism of Action and Bacterial Resistance

Quinolones interfere with DNA replication in bacteria by inhibiting the proper functioning of **DNA gyrase.** DNA gyrase is the enzyme that allows bacterial DNA to unwind (relax) so that replication may proceed. The quinolones block this action and lead to breaks in the double-stranded DNA. At achievable clinical concentrations, these agents are bactericidal. **Ciprofloxacin, lomefloxacin, norfloxacin,** and **ofloxacin** have broad antibacterial spectra, with activity toward aerobic gram-positive and gram-negative bacteria, including *Pseudomonas aeruginosa.* Cinoxacin and nalidixic acid are older agents with much more restricted spectra, covering many common gram-negative pathogens but not *P. aeruginosa.* Enoxacin also has restricted activity against *P. aeruginosa* and is not as effective as other quinolones against gram-positive bacteria but is active against pathogens causing common urinary tract infections (UTIs) and gonorrhea.

Resistance to these drugs can occur, but plasmid-mediated resistance is not yet significant. One mechanism of resistance may involve blockage of antibiotic transport into the bacterial cell. Mutations of DNA gyrase may also confer resistance.

Pharmacokinetics

Quinolone and related antibiotics (Table 40-1) are generally well absorbed when given orally. Portal circulation carries absorbed drug directly to the liver, where metabolism occurs. Nalidixic acid is the most extensively metabolized drug of this group, with glucuronide and hydroxylated derivatives being formed. The hydroxylated form of nalidixic acid is biologically active and comprises a significant proportion of the active drug in blood or urine. Over 90% of nalidixic acid in blood is bound to serum proteins. Little enters most body tissues. The only organs in which drug concentration exceeds the plasma concentration are the kidneys. Nalidixic acid has the lowest plasma concentration of any drug in this group.

Tissue penetration and persistance in plasma is greater with ciprofloxacin, enoxacin, ofloxacin, lomefloxacin, and norfloxacin than with cinoxacin or nalidixic acid.

Ciprofloxacin, enoxacin, norfloxacin, and cinoxacin are less extensively metabolized than nalidixic acid; about 20% of a dose of these drugs is metabolized in liver. From 30% to 60% of an oral dose of these drugs appears unchanged in urine. Biliary excretion accounts for an additional 20% to 35% of a drug dose. The half-lives of these drugs are 3-6 hours.

Lomefloxacin and ofloxacin rely almost exclusively on renal mechanisms for elimination, with little contribution by hepatic metabolism or biliary excretion. The half-lives of these drugs range up to 8 hours.

Doses of quinolones may require adjustment in patients with renal impairment because the kidneys are the primary

TABLE 40-1 Quinolone and Related Antibiotics

GENERIC NAME	TRADE NAME	ADMINISTRATION/DOSAGE	COMMENTS
Cinoxacin	Cinobac	ORAL: *Adults*—250 mg every 6 hr or 500 mg every 12 hr. FDA pregnancy category C.	For UTIs
✤ Ciprofloxacin	Cipro*	ORAL: *Adults*—500-750 mg every 12 hr. FDA pregnancy category C. INTRAVENOUS: *Adults*—400 mg infused over 1 hr every 12 hr for 7-14 days.	For bone and soft tissue infections, bronchitis, pneumonia, bacterial diarrhea, or UTIs
Enoxacin	Penetrex*	ORAL: *Adults*—200-400 mg every 12 hr. FDA pregnancy category C.	UTIs and gonorrhea
Lomefloxacin	Maxaquin*	ORAL: *Adults*—400 mg once daily for 10-14 days.	For bronchitis or UTIs
Nalidixic acid	NegGram*	ORAL: *Adults*—1 gm 4 times daily for 1-2 wk.	UTIs only; emergence of resistant bacterial strains commonly causes treatment failure
Norfloxacin	Noroxin*	ORAL: *Adults*—For UTIs, 400 mg every 12 hr for 3-21 days. For gonorrhea, 800 mg as single dose. FDA pregnancy category C.	For UTIs and gonorrhea
Ofloxacin	Floxin*	ORAL, INTRAVENOUS: *Adults*—200-400 mg every 12 hr. FDA pregnancy category C.	UTIs, gonorrhea, chlamydial infection, pneumonia, bronchitis, soft tissue infections, prostatitis

*Available in United States and Canada.

organ of excretion of active drug or metabolites. Typically, doses are cut in half and/or the dosing interval is doubled when creatinine clearance falls below about 50% of normal values.

Uses

Nalidixic acid, cinoxacin, and enoxacin are used for urinary tract infections. Enoxacin may also be used for gonorrhea. These three agents are not appropriate for systemic infections or for infections caused by *P. aeruginosa.*

Ciprofloxacin, lomefloxacin, norfloxacin, and ofloxacin are more potent than other members of this family and thus can be used for a variety of bacterial infections. They are especially useful for infections caused by gram-negative organisms, including *P. aeruginosa.* All four agents are used for urinary tract infections. Lomefloxacin may also be used for bronchitis caused by susceptible bacteria, and norfloxacin may be used for gonorrhea. Ofloxacin is used for bronchitis, pelvic chlamydial infections, gonorrhea, gram-negative or streptococcal pneumonia, prostatitis, and skin or soft tissue infections.

Ciprofloxacin has the broadest range among the quinolones. This drug is used for bone and joint infections, skin and soft tissue infections, pneumonia, bronchitis, and gastroenteritis, as well as urinary tract infections.

Penicillinase-producing strains of gram-positive bacteria may be susceptible to quinolones. Methicillin-resistant *Staphylococcus aureus* (MRSA) can be susceptible to quinolones, but resistance of this and other gram-positive bacteria may develop rapidly. Occasionally, streptococcal pneumonia has developed or progressed during therapy with ciprofloxacin or other quinolones. This risk of resistance has limited the application of quinolones to serious infections caused by gram-positive bacteria.

Adverse Reactions and Contraindications

Quinolones have two major side effects. The first involves the central nervous system (CNS). Symptoms range from headache, dizziness, tinnitus, insomnia, shakiness, and changes in vision to seizures. These drugs are used cautiously in patients with preexisting CNS disease such as prior seizure activity because they can exacerbate the problem. The second side effect shared by the quinolones is a tendency to damage cartilage, especially in the young (see box). This reaction has been observed in the young of several animal species and has led to permanent damage and lameness. For this reason, quinolones are not given to children.

In addition to the serious side effects noted above, quinolones, like many other oral antibiotics, can cause mild to moderate gastrointestinal (GI) tract symptoms including nausea, vomiting, or diarrhea.

Allergies to quinolones are uncommon but can be severe. Symptoms include rashes, itching, shortness of breath, serum sickness, or Stevens-Johnson syndrome. Allergy to nalidixic acid or any other quinolone may be a contraindication for receiving any quinolone because cross-allergenicity does exist.

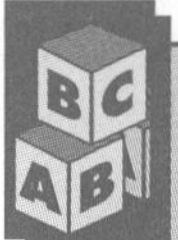

PEDIATRIC CONSIDERATION

Quinolones

THE PROBLEM

Quinolones, including nalidixic acid and cinoxacin, have damaged cartilage in tests in young animals, leading to permanent joint impairment.

SOLUTIONS

- Avoid quinolone use in children
- Remind adults not to share drugs with children, even if symptoms appear to be the same; some drugs should not be used in children

Toxicity

Overdoses may require gastric lavage or induction of emesis. High doses of ciprofloxacin or norfloxacin may cause renal difficulties because both drugs are relatively insoluble, especially in alkaline urine. Most people have slightly acidic urine, but strict vegetarians and persons taking certain drugs (see the following discussion) may have alkaline urine. Under these conditions the drug may crystallize in the urinary tract, causing pain and obstruction. The risk for this complication, called **crystalluria,** can be lessened by acidifying the urine and maintaining an adequate fluid intake.

Interactions

Antacids containing aluminum or magnesium compounds can block absorption of quinolones. Lower plasma and urinary concentrations of antibiotic and loss of antibacterial effectiveness result. To avoid this interaction the antibiotics should be taken 2 hours before the antacids.

Sodium bicarbonate, citrates, carbonic anhydrase inhibitors, and antacids containing calcium may alkalinize urine, which renders ciprofloxacin and norfloxacin less soluble. Avoiding these agents and maintaining an adequate fluid intake lessen the risk of crystalluria developing.

Ciprofloxacin lowers hepatic clearance of the asthma medication theophylline, which can cause theophylline to accumulate. As serum theophylline levels increase, so does the risk of CNS toxicity; nausea, vomiting, tremors, restlessness, agitation, and palpitations may occur. Most case reports of seizure activity in patients receiving ciprofloxacin have involved patients who were also receiving theophylline. Caffeine clearance can also be slowed by some quinolones. Lomefloxacin and ofloxacin are two quinolones that have little or no effect on caffeine or theophylline clearance and thus are not subject to this interaction.

Didanosine, a drug used against human immunodeficiency virus (HIV), reduces absorption of ciprofloxacin and possibly other quinolones because the didanosine preparation contains aluminum. These combinations should be avoided.

Warfarin anticoagulation may be increased by ciprofloxacin or norfloxacin and possibly other quinolones. Prothrombin times should be monitored in patients receiving warfarin and a quinolone to avoid bleeding episodes.

NURSING PROCESS OVERVIEW

Assessment

Assess vital signs and signs and symptoms of presenting problem. Assess for history of allergy to antiinfective drugs and in women assess for pregnancy. Check complete blood count (CBC), liver function tests, and renal function tests. Obtain baseline weight.

Nursing Diagnoses

- Knowledge deficit related to need to increase fluid intake while taking quinolones

Patient Outcomes

The patient's infection will resolve, and the patient will increase fluid intake to 2500 ml/day while taking a quinolone.

Planning/Implementation

Continue to monitor presenting symptoms. Assess for GI tract disturbance, skin changes, and CNS side effects. Encourage fluid intake. Monitor renal function and weight.

Evaluation

Ascertain that the patient states the need to maintain an adequate fluid intake, states major side effects, and describes how to take the prescribed medication correctly.

NURSING IMPLICATIONS SUMMARY

Drug Administration

- See Nursing Implications Summary in Chapter 38 (p. 469).
- Assess for pregnancy or history of allergy before administering drug.
- Assess for CNS side effects such as headache, dizziness, tinnitus, insomnia, shakiness, and changes in vision.
- Monitor CBC and differential, platelet count, blood urea nitrogen (BUN) level, serum creatinine level, and liver function tests.

Patient and Family Education

- See Nursing Implications Summary in Chapter 38 (p. 469).
- Review the anticipated benefits and possible side effects of drug therapy with the patient. Instruct the patient to report any new sign or symptom.
- Reinforce the importance of not giving quinolones to children (see box on p. 487).
- Instruct the patient to take oral doses with a full (8-ounce) glass of water or fluid, and increase daily intake of water by several 8-ounce glasses a day. Instruct the patient to take doses of ciprofloxacin, lomefloxacin, or nalidixic acid on a full or empty stomach. Instruct the patient to take doses of enoxacin, norfloxacin, or ofloxacin on an empty stomach 1 hour before or 2 hours after meals.
- See the patient problem boxes on urinary tract infections (p. 514), photosensitivity (p. 649), and dry mouth (p. 300).
- Note the drug interactions. Instruct the patient to take ciprofloxacin or norfloxacin 2 hours before or 2 hours after antacids containing aluminum or magnesium, or sucralfate. Review the patient's other medications, and counsel as necessary. Remind the patient to inform all health care providers of all drugs being used.
- Caution the patient to avoid driving or operating hazardous equipment if CNS symptoms develop. Advise the patient to report dizziness, tinnitus, and visual changes to the physician.
- If photophobia develops (eyes have increased sensitivity to light), instruct the patient to wear sunglasses and to avoid bright lights or sunlight.
- Inform the diabetic patient taking nalidixic acid that the drug may interfere with urine glucose results. Inform the patient with diabetes not to change diet or insulin dose without consulting the physician. Instruct the patient with diabetes to monitor blood glucose level.

CRITICAL THINKING

APPLICATION

1. What is the mechanism of the antibacterial effect of quinolones?
2. By what routes are quinolones given?
3. What is the major clinical use of nalidixic acid, cinoxacin, enoxacin, and norfloxacin?
4. What are the clinical uses of ciprofloxacin, lomefloxacin, and norfloxacin?
5. What is the major route of excretion of the quinolones?
6. How does the elimination of ofloxacin differ from that of ciprofloxacin?
7. What types of patients are most likely to develop seizures when they receive quinolones?
8. Why are quinolones not used in children?
9. Why is it important to know the renal status of a patient receiving a quinolone antibiotic?
10. What special precaution may be required in an asthmatic patient using theophylline who is given ciprofloxacin?
11. What process should be monitored when warfarin is given with ciprofloxacin?

CRITICAL THINKING

1. Patients taking one of the quinolones should increase their fluid intake to at least 2400 ml/day. Think of specific suggestions to give to patients to help them remember to do this.

CHAPTER 41

Macrolides, Clindamycin, and Miscellaneous Penicillin Substitutes

OBJECTIVES

After studying this chapter, you should be able to do the following:

- *Explain the common indications for erythromycin, azithromycin, and clarithromycin.*
- *Describe common side effects of erythromycin, azithromycin, and clarithromycin.*
- *Develop a nursing care plan for a patient receiving a macrolide.*
- *Explain the common indications for clindamycin, vancomycin, or spectinomycin.*
- *Describe common side effects of clindamycin and vancomycin.*
- *Develop a nursing care plan for a patient receiving clindamycin, vancomycin, or spectinomycin.*

KEY TERMS

azithromycin
clarithromycin
clindamycin
erythromycin
macrolides
penicillin substitutes
pseudomembranous colitis

CHAPTER OVERVIEW

This chapter introduces several antibiotics that are effective against the same gram-positive bacteria covered by narrow-spectrum penicillins. Because of this property, these drugs are sometimes grouped together as **penicillin substitutes.** The mechanisms of action, modes of bacterial resistance, absorption properties, drug distribution and excretion, and the unique toxic reactions these drugs may induce are discussed.

Therapeutic Rationale: Bacterial Infections

Infections caused by bacteria range from mild local infections to life-threatening systemic disease. Infections caused by gram-positive bacteria are associated with many infections of the throat and ears, as well as soft tissue infections and pneumonia. Certain gram-negative bacteria are also associated with specific pneumonias or other respiratory tract infections. The macrolides may be especially useful for these conditions, but the other drugs covered in this chapter are primarily used as substitutes for narrow-spectrum penicillins.

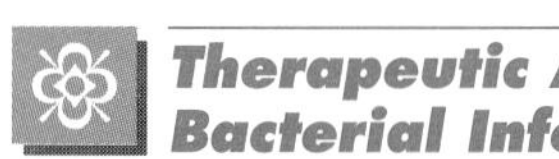

Therapeutic Agents: Bacterial Infections

Macrolides

Azithromycin, clarithromycin, ✤erythromycin

Mechanism of Action and Bacterial Resistance

Macrolides bind to bacterial ribosomes and thus prevent bacterial protein synthesis. At low concentrations this effect is bacteriostatic, but at high concentrations the drugs may be bactericidal. For example, **azithromycin** has been shown to be bactericidal against *Streptococcus pyogenes, Streptococcus pneumoniae,* and *Haemophilus influenzae.*

Bacteria are resistant to **erythromycin** by two mechanisms. Gram-negative bacteria from the bowel, such as *Escherichia coli,* seem to be relatively impermeable to erythromycin and are therefore intrinsically resistant. Cell wall–deficient forms of these bacteria (L-forms) are permeable to erythromycin and are highly sensitive to the drug. In contrast, gram-positive bacteria acquire resistance by chemically altering their ribosomes so that the ribosomes no longer bind erythromycin; thus protein synthesis is not inhibited. This ribosomal alteration is catalyzed by an enzyme that is synthesized from genes carried on a bacterial *plasmid.* Plasmids are discrete circular molecules of deoxyribonucleic acid (DNA) that are separate from the bacterial chromosome (see Chapter 38). These plasmids can be transferred directly from one bacterial cell to another. Therefore resistance to erythromycin may spread rapidly throughout a bacterial population.

The mechanism of resistance to other macrolides such as azithromycin and **clarithromycin** is similar to that of erythromycin, but the spread of resistance has not been fully assessed for these newer drugs.

Pharmacokinetics

Erythromycin is sensitive to acid and therefore may be extensively degraded in the stomach. Thus erythromycin base is formulated with acid-resistant coatings so that the drug will pass intact through the stomach and be dissolved and absorbed in the small intestine. This tactic is based on the knowledge that the pH of the duodenum is near neutrality (see Chapter 1).

Certain chemical forms of erythromycin are used clinically primarily because of their increased resistance to acid and their better oral absorption. These compounds are the stearate, ethylsuccinate, and estolate esters of erythromycin (Table 41-1). Erythromycin stearate and erythromycin ethylsuccinate are absorbed more rapidly and completely from the gastrointestinal (GI) tract than erythromycin base. Free erythromycin apparently is absorbed from the duodenum with these agents after hydrolysis of the esters. With erythromycin estolate, much better absorption of drug is achieved, and serum levels may be four times higher than with other forms of erythromycin. However, with erythromycin estolate, most of the drug in the serum is actually the ester, and controversy exists regarding whether this form of the drug has biologic activity. Many physicians prefer erythromycin estolate because of the high tissue and blood levels and note that many tissues and bacteria can hydrolyze the ester form of the drug to release free erythromycin at the infection site.

Oral bioavailability for the macrolides varies from 30% to 65%, depending on which preparation is used. Food may interfere with the oral absorption of most macrolides. Erythromycin estolate and erythromycin ethylsuccinate are exceptions, being well absorbed even when food is present.

Erythromycin is available as the lactobionate or the gluceptate for intravenous (IV) injection (see Table 41-1). These water-soluble products may be diluted with sterile water for injection but should not be diluted in sterile water containing preservatives. Erythromycin lactobionate and erythromycin gluceptate should be infused slowly into the vein to avoid pain. Intramuscular (IM) administration of erythromycin is avoided because injections are extremely painful.

Erythromycin readily distributes to tissues, where concentrations of drug may persist well beyond when it can be detected in serum. Erythromycin is especially concentrated in the liver and spleen. It enters fluids of the middle ear and pleural fluids but not cerebrospinal fluid unless the meninges are inflamed. The drug does cross the placenta, but fetal blood levels are less than 20% of maternal blood levels. Erythromycin also enters breast milk, in which the concentrations may equal that of maternal serum.

Azithromycin and clarithromycin are more strongly concentrated in tissues than is erythromycin and therefore persist longer in the body. Azithromycin in particular concentrates in the lungs and other organs but like erythromcyin does not accumulate in normal brain tissue.

The liver is the major excretory organ for erythromycin and other macrolides. A large percentage of orally administered drug is concentrated in bile and excreted in feces. Some reabsorption from the intestine occurs in a process called *enterohepatic circulation* (Chapter 1). Another significant proportion of erythromycin is apparently inactivated in the liver. Less than 10% of orally administered erythromycin appears as active drug in urine; with IV dosage, about 15% of the dose appears in urine.

TABLE 41-1 Summary of Macrolides

GENERIC NAME	TRADE NAME	DRUG FORM	ADMINISTRATION/DOSAGE
Azithromycin	Zithromax*	Capsules	ORAL: *Adults and children >16 yr*—500 mg on first day, then 250 mg once daily. For chlamydial infections, 1000 mg as single dose. FDA pregnancy category B.
Clarithromycin	Biaxin	Tablets, oral suspension	ORAL: *Adults and children >12 yr*—250-500 mg every 12 hr. FDA pregnancy category C.
Erythromycin base	ERYC E-Mycin* Erythromid†	Enteric or film-coated tablets or capsules	ORAL: *Adults*—250 mg 4 times/day (15-20 mg/kg body weight/day, not to exceed 4 gm daily.) FDA pregnancy category B. *Children*—7.5-12.5 mg/kg every 6 hr or 15-25 mg/kg every 12 hr.
Erythromycin base	Staticin*	Gel, solution, or swabs	TOPICAL: *Adults and children*—Apply to skin twice daily.
Erythromycin base	Ilotycin*	Ophthalmic ointment	TOPICAL: *Adults and children*—Apply to conjunctiva once daily.
Erythromycin estolate	Ilosone* Novorythro†	Tablets, capsules, and suspension	ORAL: *Adults and children*—Same as for erythromycin base.
Erythromycin ethylsuccinate	E.E.S.*	Oral suspension, chewable tablets, and film-coated tablets	ORAL: *Adults*—400 mg 4 times/day. FDA pregnancy category B. *Children*—Same as for erythromycin base.
Erythromycin ethylsuccinate + sulfisoxazole	Eryzole Pediazole*	Oral suspension	ORAL: *Children*—12.5 mg erythromycin/kg body weight every 6 hr.
Erythromycin gluceptate	Ilotycin*	Powder for reconstitution with sterile preservative-free water	INTRAVENOUS: *Adults*—250-500 mg base every 6 hr. Maximum daily dose 4 gm. FDA pregnancy category B. *Children*—3.75-5 mg/kg every 6 hr.
Erythromycin lactobionate	Erythrocin*	Powder for reconstitution with sterile preservative-free water	INTRAVENOUS: *Adults and children*—Same as for erythromycin gluceptate.
Erythromycin stearate	Erythrocin*	Film-coated tablets and oral suspension	ORAL: *Adults and children*—Same as for erythromycin base.

*Available in Canada and United States.
†Available in Canada only.

Uses

Erythromycin is active against the same gram-positive bacteria that are usually susceptible to penicillin G, but erythromycin is chemically unrelated to penicillins and is not cross-allergenic with them. Therefore it is a useful substitute in patients allergic to penicillins. In addition, since penicillins and erythromycin act by entirely different mechanisms, bacteria that become resistant to one of these drugs are still sensitive to the other. The newer macrolides, azithromycin and clarithromycin, have equal or improved activity over erythromycin toward gram-positive organisms.

Erythromycin is the drug of choice for some infections, including atypical pneumonias such as those caused by *Mycoplasma pneumoniae and Legionella pneumophila* (legionnaires' disease). Azithromycin and clarithromycin have equal or better activity against these organisms and in addition display activity toward other serious pathogens such as *Borrelia burgdorferi* and *Campylobacter pylori.* Erythromycin may be preferred over penicillin G for diphtheria since it eradicates the diphtheria carrier state. Erythromycin also may be useful in relapsing urinary tract infections; the relapse is frequently caused by L-forms of gram-negative organisms such as *E. coli* and *Proteus mirabilis.* These L-forms lack cell walls and are therefore resistant to penicillins. The L-form bacteria remain latent during penicillin therapy, revert to normal, and again produce disease when penicillin therapy is stopped. Since erythromycin penetrates these L-forms and blocks protein synthesis, the infection may be eradicated.

Adverse Reactions and Contraindications

The most common patient complaint with oral erythromycin is some form of GI tract difficulty. Abdominal discomfort and cramping are dose-related reactions to these drugs. Severe pain and nausea may rarely indicate pancreatitis. At normal doses, nausea, vomiting, and diarrhea occur commonly, as with other oral antibiotics. In addition to GI tract side effects, clarithromycin may cause headache or rarely thrombocytopenia with bruising or bleeding. Azithromycin may cause GI tract difficulties or rarely headache, dizziness, allergy, or interstitial nephritis. Fever, rash, and joint pain accompany interstitial nephritis.

Clinical studies suggest that pregnant women have variable absorption of oral erythromycin, and many do not achieve effective serum concentrations of the drug. Erythromycin estolate also causes hepatotoxicity in about 10% of pregnant women. For these reasons erythromycin and especially erythromycin estolate may not be recommended during pregnancy.

Toxicity

Rarely, patients who receive more than 4 gm of erythromycin a day experience hearing loss. Loss of hearing is usually reversible and may appear at any time during therapy.

The most significant toxicity occurs with erythromycin estolate. This drug damages the liver by direct drug toxicity or by an immune reaction. This reaction, called *cholestatic hepatitis*, usually appears 10 to 12 days after therapy is begun but may appear earlier in patients previously exposed to the drug. These patients may experience severe abdominal pain, liver enlargement, fever, and jaundice. When the drug is discontinued, these symptoms rapidly disappear in most patients.

Interactions

Erythromycin is metabolized in the liver and may therefore compete with other drugs for the limited hepatic metabolic capacity. For example, alfentanil, carbamazepine, cyclosporine, warfarin, valproic acid, and theophylline must be eliminated by hepatic mechanisms. When erythromycin is given concurrently, the aforementioned drugs are eliminated more slowly, serum levels rise, and the drugs may accumulate. Because these drugs have dose-related toxicity, erythromycin not only increases serum levels but also increases the risk of serious toxicity. Clarithromycin has also been shown to increase serum concentrations of carbamazepine, theophylline, and terfenadine.

Rarely, erythromycin may cause hepatotoxicity, especially when used at high doses or for long periods. The risk of liver damage is increased if erythromycin is given concurrently with other hepatoxic agents such as acetaminophen (high dose), anabolic steroids, androgens, estrogens, isoniazid, ketoconazole, phenothiazines, rifampin, sulfonamides, or valproic acid.

Macrolides can interact in several ways with other antimicrobial agents. Erythromycin and other macrolides can antagonize the antibacterial effects of lincomycin, clindamycin, or chloramphenicol because they share the same target in bacteria and may displace each other from the target. Erythromycin should not be used concurrently with these antibiotics. Rifabutin, a drug used to treat *Mycobacterium avium-intracellulare* infections, significantly lowers serum concentrations of clarithromycin. Serum concentrations of zidovudine are significantly lowered by clarithromycin; the drugs must be taken at least 4 hours apart to avoid this interaction.

Erythromycin lactobionate or erythromycin gluceptate may be rapidly inactivated if added to fluids below pH 5.5. This sensitivity to extremes of pH makes erythromycin incompatible in solution with a number of other drugs. Before adding erythromycin to any other drug solution, compatibility of the agents should be verified with the pharmacist.

Fewer interactions have been noted with azithromycin than for other macrolides. The major documented interaction involves aluminum and magnesium contained in antacids. These materials lower absorption of azithromycin and should be taken at least 2 hours before the antibiotic.

Lincosamides

Clindamycin and lincomycin

Mechanism of Action and Bacterial Resistance

Clindamycin and lincomycin inhibit the action of bacterial ribosomes in a manner similar to erythromycin. These drugs halt bacterial protein synthesis and may be bacteriostatic or bactericidal, depending on drug concentrations. Bacterial resistance to lincomycin and clindamycin apparently develops in several ways. Some organisms may become impermeable to the drugs. Others alter their ribosomes to prevent binding of lincomycin or clindamycin. With this latter mechanism, organisms may become resistant to lincomyin, erythromycin, or chloramphenicol. In practice, most clinically observed resistance to clindamycin and lincomycin develops slowly and in a gradual, stepwise manner.

Pharmacokinetics

Lincomycin may be administered by oral, IM, or IV routes (Table 41-2). When given orally, peak serum concentrations occur about 4 hours after the dose is administered but only 20% to 30% of the dose is absorbed. Food significantly hinders lincomycin absorption and results in serum levels much lower than those observed in the fasting state. Thus the drug should be administered between meals so that no food is eaten for 1 to 2 hours before and after the drug.

Clindamycin is better absorbed orally than is lincomycin and produces higher blood concentrations, and oral absorption is not significantly impaired by food. Clindamycin palmitate is available as flavored granules to be used in suspension for oral administration. The palmitate is apparently rapidly removed to release active clindamycin.

Clindamycin-2-phosphate may be injected intramuscularly, but clinical reports suggest that local pain after injection may occur. Absorption of drug by this route is good, with serum peaks being achieved 30 to 60 minutes after injection. These drugs are also suitable for IV use. By this route, clindamycin-2-phosphate causes pain and phlebitis. Clindamycin-2-phosphate is inactive as an antibiotic but is rapidly converted to clindamycin in the body.

Clindamycin and lincomycin are well distributed to most body tissues, with the exception of the central nervous system (CNS). Lincomycin does not appear in the cerebrospinal fluid of healthy patients but may enter the CNS when the meninges are inflamed by infection. Clindamycin does not appear in the cerebrospinal fluid even when meningitis is present. Lincomycin and clindamycin appear in the milk of lactating women treated with these drugs.

Clindamycin and lincomycin are extensively biodegraded in the body; the liver is the primary site of biotransformation. Since less than 20% of the total drug administered orally shows up as active antibiotic in urine or feces, these drugs are used at normal dosages in patients with renal insufficiency or failure. Neither lincomycin nor clindamycin is removed by hemodialysis.

TABLE 41-2 Summary of Clindamycin and Miscellaneous Penicillin Substitutes

GENERIC NAME	TRADE NAME	DRUG FORM	ADMINISTRATION/DOSAGE
Clindamycin	Cleocin HCl Dalacin C†	Capsules	ORAL: *Adults*—150-300 mg every 6 hr. *Children*—2-5 mg/kg body weight every 6 hr.
Clindamycin palmitate	Cleocin Pediatric Dalacin C†	Granules in suspension	ORAL: *Children*—8-25 mg/kg body weight/day in 3 or 4 doses for children >10 kg. Smaller children should receive 37.5 mg 3 times daily.
Clindamycin phosphate	Cleocin Phosphate Dalacin C†	Solution with benzyl alcohol, disodium edetate, and hydrochloric acid or sodium hydroxide	INTRAMUSCULAR, INTRAVENOUS: *Adults*—300-600 mg every 6-8 hr to upper limit of 2.4 gm/day (no more than 0.6 gm/injection site intramuscularly). *Children >1 mo*—15-40 mg/kg body weight daily in 3 or 4 doses.
Clindamycin phosphate	Cleocin T	1% topical gel or solution	TOPICAL: *Adults and children*—For acne vulgaris, apply thin film to affected area twice daily.
Lincomycin	Lincocin*	Capsules	ORAL: *Adults*—500 mg 3 or 4 times daily. *Children >1 mo*—30-60 mg/kg body weight/day in 3 or 4 divided doses.
		Solution with 0.9% benzyl alcohol	INTRAMUSCULAR: *Adults*—600 mg once or twice daily. *Children >1 mo*—10 mg/kg body weight once or twice daily. INTRAVENOUS: *Adults*—600 mg to 1 gm 2 or 3 times daily; to upper limit of 8 gm/day. *Children >1 mo*—10 mg/kg body weight once or twice daily.
Spectinomycin	Trobicin*	Powder to be reconstituted with diluent	INTRAMUSCULAR: *Adults*—2-4 gm in single dose.
Vancomycin	Lyphocin Vancocin*	Powder to be reconstituted with sterile water	INTRAVENOUS: *Adults*—500 mg every 6 hr. *Children*—10 mg/kg body weight every 6 hr.
Vancomycin	Vancocin*	Powder, capsules	ORAL: Same as for IV. *Note:* This route is for intestinal infections only.

*Available in Canada and United States.
†Available in Canada only.

Uses

Clindamycin is more effective and less toxic than lincomycin and is much more commonly used. Both drugs have antimicrobial spectra similar to those of penicillin G or erythromycin, being primarily effective against gram-positive organisms. Clindamycin and lincomycin are not as effective as penicillin against *Neisseria gonorrhoeae* or other gram-negative cocci. Clindamycin is effective against several anaerobic organisms, particularly *Bacteroides fragilis.* Infections caused by these organisms are a major indication for clindamycin.

The dangers of severe colitis have largely restricted the use of clindamycin and lincomycin to cases in which patients are allergic to safer drugs or the pathogenic organism is demonstrated by the microbiology laboratory to be sensitive to these agents.

Adverse Reactions and Contraindications

The most serious reaction to lincomycin or clindamycin is colitis. Symptoms range from mild diarrhea to a severe, life-threatening condition called **pseudomembranous colitis.** Any increase in frequency of bowel movements or softness of the stools may be reason to discontinue the drug, especially in older adult patients. Significant diarrhea should prompt discontinuation of the drug and may be relieved by that measure alone. The appearance of blood or mucus in the stool may signal severe colitis.

Pseudomembranous colitis is caused by a toxin produced by *Clostridium difficile.* Overgrowth of this organism in the bowel can result from antibiotic disturbance of the bacterial flora in the bowel. This superinfection and its associated colitis may be treated with vancomycin. Fluid and electrolyte replacement and other supportive therapy also may be required. Agents that slow peristaltic action may worsen the condition or prolong it; thus opiates or diphenoxylate with atropine are not appropriate for use in these patients.

In addition to colitis, clindamycin and lincomycin may produce GI tract irritation ranging from nausea and vomiting to glossitis and stomatitis. These drugs are usually avoided in patients with significant preexisting GI tract disease.

Allergies to clindamycin and lincomycin range from mild rashes to fever and anaphylactic shock. These reactions may occur in anyone but are more common in those with other allergies. The appearance of any allergic response is cause for discontinuing the drug.

Some reports suggest that blood dyscrasias and liver dysfunction occur during lincomycin or clindamycin therapy. Clindamycin doses are often lowered when patients have significant preexisting hepatic disease to avoid clindamycin accumulation.

Toxicity

Direct toxicity of oral doses of these drugs is low, except for the increased risk of GI tract symptoms arising from alteration of bacterial populations in the bowel. In addition, direct infusion of these drugs may affect the cardiovascular system. Lincomycin should be administered in an IV solution no more concentrated than 1 gm/dl at a rate no more rapid than 100 ml/hr to avoid hypotension or cardiac arrest. Clindamycin should be administered in an IV solution no more concentrated than 0.6 gm/dl at a rate no more rapid than 100 ml/20 min.

Interactions

Clindamycin is incompatible in solution with aminophylline, ampicillin, barbiturates, calcium gluconate, magnesium sulfate, and phenytoin. Chloramphenicol and erythromycin antagonize the antibacterial effect of clindamycin and lincomycin.

Since clindamycin and lincomycin have neuromuscular blocking properties, they may enhance the action of various neuromuscular blocking agents and inhalation anesthetics.

Absorption of oral doses of lincomycin may be decreased by food and other agents. The use of kaolin-pectin-antidiarrheal agents given at the time oral lincomycin or clindamycin is ingested markedly lowers the serum concentrations of the antibiotic.

Glycopeptide Antibiotics

Vancomycin

Mechanism of Action and Bacterial Resistance

Vancomycin prevents synthesis of bacterial cell walls by blocking peptidoglycan strand formation. This site of action is different from the sites sensitive to penicillin and other antibiotics interfering with cell wall synthesis.

Resistance to vancomycin is relatively uncommon and has developed slowly. As the drug is used clinically, it is a rapidly bactericidal agent, which may partly explain why the low incidence of bacterial resistance to vancomycin persisted for so many years.

Pharmacokinetics

Vancomycin is a complex glycopeptide that may be positively or negatively charged, depending on pH. Therefore vancomycin does not easily cross biologic membranes and is not significantly absorbed after oral administration (see Table 41-2). Vancomycin is most often administered by intermittent IV infusion but may rarely be given by mouth for intestinal infections. Bactericidal concentrations of drug are not obtained in systemic circulation with oral doses.

Vancomycin is well distributed throughout the body and reaches clinically effective concentrations in various body fluid compartments such as pericardial, synovial, and pleural fluids. It does not penetrate normal cerebrospinal fluid but does enter the CNS when the meninges are inflamed.

Active vancomycin appears in very high concentrations in urine. The kidney is the major excretory organ for vancomyin, and nonrenal elimination is limited. In patients with renal insufficiency, vancomycin may accumulate unless drug doses are reduced to compensate for loss of excretory efficiency. In patients who lack kidney function, vancomycin is usually given only once between dialysis treatments. Vancomycin is not cleared from the body by hemodialysis.

Uses

Vancomycin is most often used in serious or life-threatening staphylococcal or streptococcal infections. Because the drug is chemically unrelated to penicillins and has a different mechanism of action, it acts against organisms that resist penicillins, including methicillin-resistant *Staphylococcus aureus.* Since vancomycin and penicillin are not cross-allergenic, vancomycin is useful in patients allergic to penicillins. Vancomycin also has special utility in treating antibiotic-induced colitis, which arises from a superinfection with *C. difficile* in the bowel.

Adverse Reactions and Contraindications

IV infusion of vancomycin has produced nausea, flushing, and itching. These reactions are more likely when undiluted vancomycin is dripped directly into a running IV line rather than being properly diluted beforehand. The reaction, which is caused by generalized histamine release, is sometimes referred to as "red man syndrome" because of the intense flushing reactions observed.

Toxicity

Vancomycin causes deafness in some patients, especially when serum concentrations exceed 80 μg/ml serum. Patients with impaired renal function and older adult patients are more likely than healthy or younger persons to show drug accumulation (see box) and should be closely watched for ringing in the ears (tinnitus) or hearing loss. Some patients have regained some hearing acuity when vancomycin was stopped. For others, hearing loss may persist.

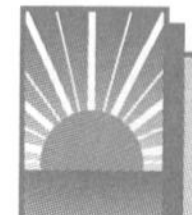

GERIATRIC CONSIDERATION

Vancomycin

THE PROBLEM

Patients over 60 years of age have reduced renal function and therefore excrete vancomycin more slowly than do younger adults. The drug may accumulate because alternative paths of elimination are limited. Older adults also have some hearing loss because of their age.

SOLUTIONS

- Lower doses to avoid accumulation.
- Monitor serum vancomycin concentration.
- Monitor renal function tests.
- Perform baseline auditory function tests; repeat during therapy.

Nephrotoxicity may occur, with symptoms of increased thirst, altered urination, anorexia, or weakness. Blood and protein in urine occasionally have been noted.

If vancomycin inadvertently enters muscle or skin around the IV site, local tissue necrosis may develop.

Interactions

Vancomycin is compatible with many common IV fluids. The major consideration in combining vancomycin with another drug should be to avoid administering another ototoxic or nephrotoxic drug such as an aminoglycoside antibiotic, bumetanide, cisplatin, ethacrynic acid, or furosemide. Combining one of these drugs with vancomycin may result in additive toxic effects. Complete loss of hearing or renal failure is possible.

Aminocyclitol

Spectinomycin

Mechanism of Action and Bacterial Resistance

Spectinomycin inhibits protein synthesis in many bacteria, but the ability of spectinomycin to inhibit *N. gonorrhoeae* is the basis for its clinical usefulness. On this basis, it is classified as a penicillin substitute. Resistance to spectinomycin may occur.

Pharmacokinetics

Spectinomycin is injected intramuscularly to treat gonorrhea (see Table 41-2). Absorption produces high serum concentrations of drug that are maintained long enough after a single injection to eradicate *N. gonorrhoeae* from the infection site. Within 2 days, nearly all the injected drug appears in active form in urine.

Uses

Spectinomycin is used only for gonorrhea. It is not effective for chlamydial infections, which often occur along with gonorrhea.

Adverse Reactions and Contraindications

Single doses of spectinomycin have caused nausea, chills, and dizziness. Patients may report pain at the injection site, urticaria, or fever. Spectinomycin is contraindicated when known allergy to the drug exists.

Toxicity

No significant toxicity is noted with single doses in adults. The preparation is not used in children because benzyl alcohol included as a preservative is toxic in infants.

Interactions

No significant interactions occur with single doses used in adults.

NURSING PROCESS OVERVIEW

Macrolides, Clindamycin, and Miscellaneous Penicillin Substitutes

Assessment

Perform a thorough patient assessment, focusing on the presenting problem. Depending on the antiinfective agent prescribed, obtain baseline hearing acuity. Monitor vital signs, complete blood count (CBC) and white blood cell (WBC) differential.

Nursing Diagnoses

- Potential complication: pseudomembranous colitis
- Potential complication: ototoxicity
- Knowledge deficit related to prevention of sexually transmitted diseases

Patient Outcomes

The patient's infection will resolve without side effects. If pseudomembranous colitis or ototoxicity develop, the nurse will manage and minimize side effects of these problems.

Planning/Implementation

Monitor renal function tests or liver function tests, depending on drug prescribed. Monitor serum drug levels, if available. Teach patients to report the development of side effects. Monitor vital signs and clinical signs of the initial infection.

Evaluation

Before discharge, verify that the patient can explain what drug reactions might be expected and when to notify the physician.

NURSING IMPLICATIONS SUMMARY

Macrolides

Drug Administration

- See Nursing Implications Summary in Chapter 38 (p. 469).
- Assess for history of allergy before administering the drug.
- Assess baseline hearing acuity. Assess for GI tract symptoms and signs of liver dysfunction.
- Monitor intake and output and weight.
- Monitor liver function tests.

Intravenous Erythromycin Lactobionate or Gluceptate

- Dilute each 500 mg with 10 ml of sterile water for injection without preservatives and further dilute as instructed in drug insert. Administer at a rate of 1 gm diluted in 100 ml over 20 to 60 minutes. Monitor vital signs.

Patient and Family Education

- See Nursing Implications Summary in Chapter 38 (p. 469).
- Instruct the patient to report tinnitus or hearing loss, malaise, fever, jaundice, right upper quadrant abdominal pain, and change in the color or consistency of stools.
- Patients should take oral doses of erythromycin with meals or a snack to reduce gastric irritation. Instruct the patient to take doses of azithromycin on an empty stomach 1 hour before or 2 hours after meals. Instruct the patient to take doses of clarithromycin with meals or snack or on an empty stomach.
- Instruct the patient to swallow delayed-release capsules or tablets whole, without chewing or breaking.

Clindamycin and Lincomycin

Drug Administration

- See Nursing Implications Summary in Chapter 38 (p. 469).
- Assess for history of allergy before administering the drug.
- Assess for diarrhea or GI tract distress. Monitor intake and output and weight.
- Monitor CBC and WBC differential, platelet count, liver function tests, and serum electrolyte level.

Intravenous Clindamycin

- IV clindamycin is available premixed, or each 300 mg can be diluted with at least 50 ml of suitable diluent; see drug insert. Administer at a rate of 300 mg or less over at least 10 minutes. Do not administer too rapidly. Monitor vital signs. Supervise ambulation.

Intravenous Lincomycin

- Dilute 1 gm with at least 125 ml of suitable diluent; see drug insert. Administer at a rate of 1 gm or less/hr. Monitor vital signs. Do not administer too rapidly. Supervise ambulation.

Patient and Family Education

- Instruct the patient to report diarrhea to the physician. Warn the patient to not self-medicate for severe diarrhea; for mild diarrhea, the patient may self-medicate with antidiarrheal drugs containing kaolin or attapulgite. These medications should be taken 2 hours before or 3 to 4 hours after lincomycin or clindamycin.
- Instruct the patient to take oral capsules of clindamycin with a full (8-ounce) glass of fluid, with or without meals. Instruct the patient to measure doses of the oral liquid form with the dropper provided by the pharmacist.
- The patient should take oral lincomycin with a full (8-ounce) glass of fluid on an empty stomach 1 hour before or 2 hours after meals or a snack.
- For topical administration of clindamycin, instruct the patient to apply carefully, avoiding the eyes, nose, mouth, or mucous membranes, and to apply over the entire affected area, not just to pimples. Instruct the patient to use the drug regularly for best effect and to use only water-based cosmetics. Instruct the patient to notify the physician if acne does not improve in 6 weeks, if skin irritation develops, or if any GI tract symptoms develop.
- For vaginal cream, review administration technique with the patient. See the patient problem box on vaginal infections (p. 539). Instruct the patient to wear a minipad or sanitary napkin to absorb leaking medication; the patient should not use tampons. Instruct the patient to avoid intercourse during the course of therapy and to avoid latex (rubber) contraceptives during therapy and for 72 hours after completing the course of therapy since clindamycin may weaken the latex, causing it to be ineffective.

Vancomycin

Drug Administration

- See Nursing Implications Summary in Chapter 38 (p. 469).
- Assess for history of allergy before administering the drug.
- Assess baseline hearing acuity.
- Monitor serum creatinine level, blood urea nitrogen (BUN) level, CBC, and WBC differential count. Monitor urinalysis. Monitor serum drug levels, if available.

Intravenous Vancomycin

- Dilute each 500 mg with 10 ml of sterile water for injection. Further dilute with 100 ml of normal saline or 5% dextrose in water (D5W). Administer each diluted dose over 60 minutes. Monitor vital signs. Too rapid IV administration may be associated with hypotension, cardiac arrest, or "red man syndrome" or "red neck syndrome": maculopapular or erythematous rash of the face, head, chest, and arms; fever; chills; fainting; nausea; vomiting; tachycardia; or itching.

NURSING IMPLICATIONS SUMMARY—cont'd

Patient and Family Education

- See Nursing Implications Summary in Chapter 38 (p. 469).
- Instruct the patient to report tinnitus or hearing loss.
- Patients should not take oral doses within 4 hours of taking cholestyramine or colestipol.
- If vancomycin is prescribed to treat diarrhea caused by other antibiotics, avoid antidiarrheal medicine unless first approved by the physician.

Spectinomycin

Drug Administration and Patient and Family Education

- See Nursing Implications Summary in Chapter 38 (p. 469).
- Caution the patient to avoid driving or operating hazardous equipment if dizziness develops; the patient should notify the physician.
- Warn the patient that IM injections may cause burning at the injection site. Use diluent supplied by the manufacturer. Dilute as directed on the vial label.
- If given to treat gonorrhea, warn the patient that the sexual partner may also need treatment to avoid passing the organism back and forth. Also instruct the patient about sexually transmitted diseases as appropriate. Caution the patient that the male sexual partner should wear a condom to prevent transmission of infection.

CRITICAL THINKING

APPLICATION

1. Why are erythromycin, clindamycin, vancomycin, and spectinomycin called penicillin substitutes?
2. What advantages do the esters of erythromycin have over erythromycin base?
3. Which of the erythromycin esters is best absorbed orally and may be taken with meals?
4. Which forms of erythromycin can be used parenterally?
5. What property limits parenteral use of erythromycin?
6. What is the major route of excretion of macrolides?
7. What is the most common adverse reaction to macrolides?
8. What toxic reaction is unique to erythromycin estolate?
9. How does azithromycin differ from erythromycin in distribution in the body and in antibacterial spectrum?
10. Bacterial resistance to clindamycin is associated with resistance to which other antibiotic?
11. What form of clindamycin is appropriate for parenteral use?
12. How is clindamycin eliminated from the body?
13. What is the limiting toxicity to clindamycin? What implications does this have for nursing care?
14. How is antibiotic-associated colitis best treated?
15. Why is bacterial resistance to vancomycin relatively rare?
16. By what route is vancomycin usually administered?
17. What is the major route of excretion of vancomycin?
18. What toxic reactions are most common with vancomycin?
19. Name three clinical uses for vancomycin.
20. What is the primary clinical indication for spectinomycin?
21. What pharmacologic property of spectinomycin makes it a useful replacement of penicillin in treating gonorrhea?

CRITICAL THINKING

1. Develop a nursing care plan for a patient receiving erythromycin, clindamycin, or vancomycin.

CHAPTER 42

Tetracyclines and Chloramphenicol

OBJECTIVES

After studying this chapter, you should be able to do the following:

- *Describe how the antimicrobial spectra of tetracyclines and chloramphenicol differ from those of erythromycin (see Chapter 41) and penicillin G (see Chapter 39).*
- *Name the most common route of administration for tetracyclines and chloramphenicol.*
- *Explain how doxycycline and minocycline differ from other tetracyclines.*
- *Describe common side effects of tetracyclines.*
- *Describe the serious side effects of chloramphenicol.*
- *Develop a nursing care plan for a patient receiving doxycycline or chloramphenicol.*

KEY TERMS

chloramphenicol
chlamydia
rickettsia
spirochete
tetracyclines

CHAPTER OVERVIEW

This chapter introduces antibiotics with very broad antimicrobial spectra: tetracyclines and chloramphenicol. The **tetracyclines** are a large family of chemically related compounds, many of which are clinically useful both in human and in animal medicine.

Chloramphenicol is the only member of its chemical class approved for use in the United States.

Therapeutic Rationale: Microbial Infections

Infections caused by bacteria range from mild local infections to life-threatening systemic disease. Other organisms cause similar diseases. For example, *Chlamydia trachomatis* causes genitourinary tract infections, and various **rickettsia** cause typhus and Rocky Mountain spotted fever. A **spirochete,** *Treponema pallidum,* causes syphilis, and protozoans of the species *Plasmodium* cause malaria. These nonbacterial diseases comprise the primary indications for tetracyclines today.

Therapeutic Agents: Tetracyclines and Chloramphenicol

Tetracyclines

Demeclocycline, doxycycline, minocycline, oxytetracycline, tetracycline

Mechanism of Action and Bacterial Resistance

Tetracyclines block bacterial growth by preventing ribosomes from binding messenger RNA, thereby preventing the initiation of protein synthesis. Members of this drug family are therefore bacteriostatic rather than bactericidal.

For tetracyclines to be effective, they must first be transported into the bacterial cell. Antibiotic uptake is accomplished by an energy-dependent transport system. Resistant bacteria lose the ability to transport tetracyclines into the bacterial cell, and the antibiotic does not come in contact with its intracellular target. Much observed tetracycline resistance involves a *plasmid* (see Chapter 38) that is transmitted from bacterium to bacterium and may therefore spread rapidly throughout bacterial populations. For example, families of patients treated on a long-term basis with low doses of tetracyclines may show a conversion of the normal tetracycline-sensitive bacterial flora to tetracycline-resistant forms. Cross-resistance between the older tetracyclines is complete. The newer tetracyclines minocycline and doxycycline are more lipid soluble than the other drugs and are transported into the bacterial cell by different mechanisms than the older drugs. These drugs may therefore penetrate bacterial cells that do not concentrate the older tetracyclines.

Pharmacokinetics

Tetracyclines are most often administered orally (Table 42-1), usually as a hydrochloride or as a phosphate salt to increase solubility and thereby increase absorption. Tetracyclines are variably absorbed from the gastrointestinal (GI) tract. Absorption is influenced by acid lability, water solubility, and lipid solubility. All tetracyclines except doxycycline and minocycline are acid labile and are partly destroyed by stomach acid. Tetracyclines are not highly water soluble, and this solubility may be further reduced by complex formation with metal ions or with solid material in the intestine. In these insoluble forms, drugs are not absorbed but remain in the intestine and are excreted in feces. Doxycycline and minocycline are exceptions; being highly lipid soluble, both drugs pass freely through GI tract membranes and are much more completely and rapidly absorbed than most other tetracyclines.

Absorption of tetracyclines from intramuscular (IM) sites is poor and often causes local tissue irritation and pain at the injection site. IM use of tetracyclines is therefore limited.

Tetracyclines may be used intravenously in serious infections. Oxytetracycline, doxycycline, and minocycline can be obtained in a form suitable for intravenous (IV) use. These drugs have low water solubility and must be diluted extensively before use by this route. When used intravenously, tetracyclines may cause thrombophlebitis. Improper dilution of the drug or repeated infusion into the same vein increases the likelihood of thrombophlebitis.

Tetracyclines are well distributed in most body tissues and fluids, appearing in liver, spleen, bone marrow, bile, and cerebrospinal fluid even in the absence of inflammation. The drugs pass the placental barrier and enter fetal circulation in appreciable amounts. Tetracyclines also appear in the milk of nursing mothers.

Differences in lipid solubility among the tetracyclines affect their elimination. The more polar or water-soluble drugs are eliminated through the kidneys in greater amounts than are the lipid-soluble tetracyclines doxycycline and minocycline. All tetracyclines enter urine by passive glomerular filtration, but lipid-soluble drugs are more completely reabsorbed from kidney tubules than drugs that are charged at the acid pH of the tubular fluid. This high degree of reabsorption is reflected in the longer elimination half-life for doxycycline and minocycline (12 to 15 hours) than those of less lipid-soluble tetracyclines such as oxytetracycline, tetracycline, or chlortetracycline (6 to 9 hours).

The second major route of elimination is by biliary excretion. Tetracyclines are concentrated in liver and bile and carried into the intestine, where they may be reabsorbed by enterohepatic circulation. The liver is also the site for biotransformation of several tetracyclines. In general, the more lipid-soluble drugs penetrate liver cells and are more extensively biotransformed. In particular, minocycline is extensively biotransformed. The high lipid solubility of doxycycline and its tendency to form insoluble complexes with intestinal solids account for an unusual mode of elimination for this drug. It seems to diffuse directly into the intestine, where the drug is sequestered by complex formation with fecal material. Because of this unusual mechanism for excretion, doxycycline does not accumulate in renal failure.

Uses

Tetracyclines are clinically important because of their wide antibacterial spectrum. Most gram-positive organisms are sensitive to tetracyclines; however, most infections caused by these organisms are best treated by other agents because penicillins, cephalosporins, erythromycin, and clindamycin are equally or more effective against these organisms and are less toxic.

TABLE 42-1 Clinical Summary of Chloramphicol and Tetracyclines

GENERIC NAME	TRADE NAME	ADMINISTRATION/DOSAGE
Chloramphenicol	Chloromycetin Novochlorocap†	ORAL: *Adults and children*—12.5 mg/kg every 6 hr. *Infants up to 2 wk*—6.25 mg/kg every 6 hr. OPHTHALMIC: *Adults and children*—Apply solution or ointment to conjunctiva every 3 hr or more frequently.
Chloramphenicol	Chloromycetin*	OTIC: *Adults and children*—Apply 2 or 3 drops to ear canal every 6-8 hr.
Chloramphenicol palmitate	Chloromycetin	ORAL (suspension): *Children*—As for other oral forms.
Chloramphenicol succinate	Chloromycetin*	INTRAVENOUS: As for oral.
Demeclocycline	Declomycin*	ORAL: *Adults*—150 mg every 6 hr. FDA pregnancy category D. *Children >8 yr*—6-12 mg/kg/day in 2-4 doses.
Doxycycline	Doryx* Vibramycin*	ORAL, INTRAVENOUS: *Adults*—100-200 mg/day. FDA pregnancy category D. *Children >8 yr*—2-4 mg/kg/day in 2 doses.
Minocycline	Minocin*	ORAL, INTRAVENOUS: 200 mg initially, then 400 mg every 12 hr. FDA pregnancy category D. *Children >8 yr*—4 mg/kg initially, then 2 mg/kg every 12 hr.
Oxytetracycline	Terramycin	ORAL: *Adults*—250-500 mg every 6 hr. *Children >8 yr*—6.25-12.5 mg/kg every 6 hr. INTRAMUSCULAR: *Adults*—100 mg every 8 hr. *Children >8 yr*—5-8.3 mg/kg every 8 hr. INTRAVENOUS: *Adults*—250-500 mg every 12 hr. *Children >8 yr*—5-10 mg/kg every 12 hr.
Tetracycline	Achromycin* Sumycin Tetracyn*	ORAL: *Adults*—250-500 mg every 6 hr. *Children >8 yr*—6.25-12.5 mg/kg every 6 hr. INTRAMUSCULAR: *Adults*—100 mg every 8 hr. *Children >8 yr*—5-8.3 mg/kg every 8 hr, not to exceed 250 mg/dose.

*Available in Canada and United States.
†Available in Canada only.

Gram-negative bacterial pathogens cause diseases including urinary tract infections (*Klebsiella* species) and pneumonia *(Haemophilus influenzae)* that may respond to tetracyclines. Gram-negative bacteria found in the bowel (e.g., *Escherichia coli*) may be susceptible to tetracyclines, but resistance does develop. *Serratia, Proteus,* and *Pseudomonas* strains are usually resistant. *Neisseria gonorrhoeae* is sensitive to tetracyclines. Clinically, tetracyclines are used to treat gonorrhea only when penicillin is contraindicated. Tetracyclines are clinically effective for a number of bacterial infections that are relatively rare in the United States including chancroid *(Haemophilus ducreyi),* rabbit fever or tularemia *(Francisella tularensis),* black plague *(Yersinia pestis),* brucellosis (*Brucella* species), and cholera *(Vibrio cholerae).*

Tetracyclines are highly effective for diseases caused by rickettsiae (tick fever, Rocky Mountain spotted fever, typhus, and Q fever), **chlamydia** (parrot fever or psittacosis, trachoma, lymphogranuloma venereum), and *Mycoplasma pneumoniae* (atypical or "walking" pneumonia).

Tetracyclines are useful in treating Lyme disease *(Borrelia burgdorferi),* relapsing fever *(Borrelia recurrentis),* syphilis *(T. pallidum),* and yaws *(T. pertenue),* which are all caused by spirochetes. Tetracyclines may have a useful role in treating amebic dysentery. Minocycline in particular may be useful in nocardial infections.

Tetracyclines are widely used to treat acne. Relatively low doses may be prescribed over long periods of time. Although this treatment is effective for many patients, questions arise as to long-term adverse effects of the drugs and to the contribution this practice makes to the development of tetracycline-resistant bacterial populations.

Pharmaceutic formulations of tetracyclines are quite varied. These antibiotics are available in 50 to 500 mg tablets or capsules, syrups for pediatric use, ophthalmic ointments or drops, and various forms for topical use.

Adverse Reactions and Contraindications

Tetracyclines cause a wide variety of adverse reactions. The most common complaint is GI tract irritation. Many patients suffer nausea, vomiting, or pain with oral tetracyclines. Diarrhea may occur as a result of irritation by unabsorbed tetracycline remaining in the bowel. Diarrhea may also result from changes in the intestinal flora. Occasionally, the effects of these broad-spectrum drugs on intestinal flora are so extensive that overgrowth of drug-resistant bacteria occurs. Staphylococcal enterocolitis may result and may be life threatening, producing bloody diarrhea and extensive damage to the intestinal epithelium. *Candida* infections of the throat, vagina, and bowel also occur occasionally.

Tetracyclines are also commonly associated with central nervous system (CNS) effects, causing dizziness or unsteadiness.

Allergies to tetracyclines are uncommon. Urticaria, morbilliform rashes, and dermatitis occur, as do more serious reactions such as asthma, angioedema, and anaphylaxis.

Tetracyclines are not entirely specific for bacterial ribosomes and may inhibit mammalian protein synthesis to a small degree. This may explain their toxic effect on various tissues. For example, kidney function may be impaired by tetracyclines, and the effects may be worse in a kidney already damaged by disease or by trauma. Renal function should therefore be carefully watched in patients receiving these drugs.

Tetracyclines also delay blood coagulation. The exact mechanism for this reaction is not known, but it may involve binding the calcium that is required in coagulation.

The ability of tetracyclines to bind calcium also leads to their deposition in bones and teeth. In adults, this binding produces little visible effect, but in children under 8 years of age the newly formed permanent teeth may be stained by the drug. This staining is irreversible. Binding of tetracyclines to bones may slow bone growth visibly in fetuses or young children. Infants may also display increased intracranial pressure with bulging fontanelles when given tetracyclines (see box).

All tetracyclines can be degraded to toxic products by exposure to light, but demeclocycline is most effective in producing these reactions. The drug is broken down by the action of ultraviolet light on the skin, and the toxic products released cause an intense sunburn reaction. Since tetracyclines other than demeclocycline can cause this reaction, it is prudent to suggest that patients receiving these drugs limit their exposure to direct sunlight, especially in subtropical or tropical climates.

Outdated tetracycline preparations have been implicated in occasional severe adverse reactions, apparently caused by toxic breakdown products of the drugs. A reaction called the *Fanconi syndrome* has been observed, in which the patient loses amino acids, proteins, and glucose in urine and suffers polyuria and polydipsia, acidosis, nausea, and vomiting. These reactions slowly disappear after the drug is discontinued. In other cases, patients show symptoms reminiscent of systemic lupus erythematosus.

Specific tetracyclines may cause unique adverse reactions. For example, minocycline can damage vestibular function, thereby impairing balance. Minocycline may also discolor skin and mucous membranes. Demeclocycline is the tetracycline most likely to induce nephrogenic diabetes insipidus, with weakness, thirst, and increased urination.

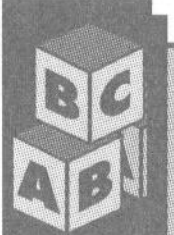

Pediatric Consideration

Tetracyclines

THE PROBLEM

Young children rapidly form bones and teeth, which are composed primarily of calcium phosphates. As this material is deposited, tetracyclines may be so tightly bound to the calcium in bones and teeth that it cannot be released. Fetal bone growth may be slowed. Tetracyclines over time are degraded by light and exposure to chemicals. This process occurs even though the drug is incorporated into the solid matrix of teeth. The degraded tetracyclines appear as brown to gray-colored permanent stains on the teeth.

SOLUTIONS

- Avoid tetracyclines in the last half of pregnancy.
- Avoid tetracyclines in children younger than 8 years.

Toxicity

The liver may be sensitive to tetracyclines. Hepatotoxicity may progress to jaundice, fatty liver, and death unless the drug is discontinued at the first sign of difficulty. Pregnant women are most sensitive to this complication and should rarely, if ever, be given tetracyclines.

Older adult patients who are extremely debilitated or patients recovering from extensive surgery or traumatic injuries may suffer metabolic derangement when given tetracyclines. These patients often show negative nitrogen balance. This reaction may result from tetracycline inhibition of mammalian protein synthesis.

Interactions

Several tetracycline interactions with other drugs result from the ability of tetracyclines to form insoluble complexes with metal ions. For example, oral tetracyclines frequently cause gastric irritation; for this reason, patients may wish to take antacids along with the antibiotic. This practice should be discouraged since common antacids include magnesium and aluminum salts, which complex with tetracyclines and prevent their absorption from the GI tract. Therefore the antacids reduce the antibacterial effect of the antibiotic. Likewise, iron-containing preparations such as vitamin or mineral supplements may prevent tetracycline absorption. Milk and other dairy products are high in calcium and also impair absorption. Sodium bicarbonate taken with a tetracycline tablet may impede tablet dissolution in the stomach and thereby reduce absorption of the drug.

Food in the stomach impairs absorption of oral tetracyclines, with the exception of doxycycline and minocycline. These lipid-soluble tetracyclines are absorbed well even in the presence of food or milk products in the stomach.

Cholestyramine and colestipol bind tetracyclines and impair oral absorption of the antibiotics. As a result, effective blood concentrations may not be achieved with concurrent use of these drugs.

Several tetracyclines, especially doxycycline and minocycline, are metabolized to some degree in the liver. Drugs such as barbiturates, which increase hepatic drug-metabolizing enzymes, shorten the duration of action of doxycycline and minocycline. This action may decrease the antibacterial effectiveness of these agents.

Estrogen-containing contraceptives may be less effective when tetracyclines are used over prolonged periods. Metabolism of the estrogen may be influenced by tetracyclines.

The bacteriostatic mechanism of action of tetracyclines leads to specific interactions. For example, penicillins given with tetracyclines may be less effective than penicillin given alone. Penicillins are bactericidal and act against actively multiplying bacteria. By inhibiting bacterial growth, tetracyclines make the bacteria resistant to the action of penicillins.

Tetracycline nephrotoxicity may become significant and dangerous when these antibiotics are given with other nephrotoxic agents.

Chloramphenicol

Mechanism of Action and Bacterial Resistance

Chloramphenicol inhibits bacterial protein synthesis. The mechanism of action is different from that of tetracyclines in that chloramphenicol inhibits late rather than early steps in ribosomal function. Like tetracyclines, chloramphenicol is bacteriostatic rather than bactericidal.

Bacterial resistance to chloramphenicol nearly always involves destruction of the antibiotic by bacterial enzymes. These enzymes are not always present but may be induced by exposure of potentially resistant bacteria to sublethal doses of chloramphenicol. The genes required for synthesizing this enzyme are usually carried on small DNA molecules called *plasmids,* which may exist separately from the bulk of genetic material in bacteria. Plasmids may be transmitted from bacterium to bacterium, and resistance to chloramphenicol may thereby be transmitted widely throughout bacterial populations.

Pharmacokinetics

Chloramphenicol is nearly completely absorbed from the GI tract after oral administration. The peak serum concentration achieved by an oral dose is about the same as that produced by an equivalent dose given intravenously, although attainment of peak serum concentration is somewhat delayed with oral administration. IM injection produces lower blood levels than oral administration and for this reason is not recommended. Seriously ill patients should receive chloramphenicol intravenously since oral absorption may be impaired in these patients. The succinate form of chloramphenicol is used for IV administration only, whereas the parent drug, chloramphenicol, is used orally.

Chloramphenicol is well distributed throughout body tissues and fluids. Significant and effective concentrations of the drug enter the eye, joint (synovial), and pleural fluids. Unlike many other antibiotics, chloramphenicol enters cerebrospinal fluid relatively easily, even when the meninges are not inflamed. Chloramphenicol also easily crosses the placenta and appears in human milk.

Most of a dose of chloramphenicol is inactivated in the liver. The drug is conjugated with glucuronic acid to form chloramphenicol glucuronide. This inactive drug form may be excreted in the kidneys by tubular secretion, whereas unaltered chloramphenicol is excreted solely by glomerular filtration. The actual concentration of active chloramphenicol in urine is high enough to be antibacterial, but active chloramphenicol in urine is only a small fraction of the total drug excreted via this route.

Uses

Because of dangerous toxic reactions, chloramphenicol is used only in serious infections. Chloramphenicol is the drug of choice for typhoid fever. In addition, life-threatening infections such as bacteremias or meningitis may be treated with chloramphenicol when the pathogen has been tested and has proved sensitive to the drug. The antibacterial spectrum of chloramphenicol is similar to that of tetracyclines and includes gram-negative bacteria (except *Pseudomonas aeruginosa*), rickettsiae, and chlamydia. Chloramphenicol is especially effective against the important anaerobic pathogen *Bacteroides fragilis.*

Adverse Reactions and Contraindications

Chloramphenicol is an effective antibiotic, but its clinical use is limited by its potential for bone marrow toxicity. A reversible form of bone marrow depression causes leukopenia and a reduction of reticulocytes. These symptoms usually resolve quickly when chloramphenicol is discontinued. Patients receiving chloramphenicol should have routine blood tests performed during therapy to detect early signs of this toxic reaction.

Chloramphenicol may also induce irreversible bone marrow depression, which leads to aplastic anemia, a condition with high mortality. This condition is usually characterized by pancytopenia (loss of all forms of blood cells), but in some cases, one or more types of blood cells continue to be formed. Aplastic anemia, although rare, may appear weeks or months after chloramphenicol therapy. This time lag between drug administration and appearance of aplastic anemia complicates accurate calculation of drug-associated risk, especially considering that most patients have received more than one other drug during the interim between chloramphenicol therapy and development of aplastic anemia. Best estimates of incidence suggest that roughly one in 30,000 chloramphenicol-treated patients will develop aplastic anemia. Although this incidence is low, the frequently fatal outcome is sufficient cause to restrict the use of chloramphenicol to the treatment of very serious infections.

Less severe problems also occur with chloramphenicol therapy. Allergies of various types and GI tract irritation may occur. Long-term therapy has been associated with neuritis, which may involve the optic nerve. Blindness has occurred in a few patients. CNS symptoms are also seen in some patients; these include headache, mental confusion, depression, or delirium.

Chloramphenicol crosses the placenta and may concentrate in fetal liver. For this reason, the drug is not given to pregnant women near term.

Toxicity

Patients with reduced liver function are at risk of severe toxic reactions because of drug accumulation. The liver normally converts over 90% of administered chloramphenicol, which is toxic, to a glucuronide, which is nontoxic. Therefore any reduction in the liver's ability to detoxify the drug may cause accumulation of the toxic drug, unless dosages are appropriately reduced. Newborn infants are especially at risk for this complication. Neonates have an immature liver that lacks the enzyme to form glucuronides. When these infants are given a weight-adjusted dosage based on adult doses, many develop *gray syndrome.* Drug accumulation proceeds without symptoms for 3 to 4 days, after which time the infant may develop abdominal distension, emesis, progressive pallid cyanosis, and irregular respiration. In a high percentage of cases, vasomotor collapse and death result. Infants receiving smaller doses are less likely to develop these symptoms. If early signs of the condition are noted by alert health care personnel and the drug is discontinued, most infants recover.

Interactions

Chloramphenicol can inhibit drug-metabolizing enzymes in the liver. This property may lead to dangerous interactions with drugs that have a low therapeutic index and are eliminated by microsomal hepatic enzymes. Drugs in this category include alfentanil, chlorpropamide, phenytoin, tolbutamide, and coumarin anticoagulants. When a patient receiving one of these drugs on a long-term basis is given chloramphenicol, these liver-metabolized drugs tend to accumulate. As a result, the patient's previously well-controlled conditions may escape control. For example, well-controlled diabetic patients may become hypoglycemic, successfully anticoagulated patients may develop spontaneous bleeding, or controlled epileptic patients may develop phenytoin toxicity.

Chloramphenicol competes with erythromycin and clindamycin for binding sites on bacterial ribosomes. As a result, the drugs may be antagonistic with one another and should not be combined.

NURSING PROCESS OVERVIEW

Tetracyclines and Chloramphenicol

Refer to Chapter 38 for general guidelines on the nursing process with antibiotic therapy. The additional material in this chapter relates specifically to the tetracyclines and chloramphenicol.

Assessment

Carry out a thorough patient assessment. Monitor liver and kidney function. Monitor signs of clinical infection.

Nursing Diagnoses

- Potential complication: gastrointestinal distress
- Potential complication: bone marrow depression

Patient Outcomes

The patient's infection will resolve without incident. The nurse will manage and minimize complications.

Planning/Implementation

Monitor renal and liver function. Assess for GI tract distress. Adjust timing of ordered doses to allow for interactions with food or other drugs (especially with tetracycline).

Evaluation

Before discharge, ascertain that the patient can take drugs as ordered and can explain signs and symptoms warranting consultation with the physician.

NURSING IMPLICATIONS SUMMARY

Tetracyclines

Drug Administration

- See Nursing Implications Summary in Chapter 38 (p. 469).
- Assess for allergy to tetracyclines or "caine" drugs (lidocaine, procaine) before administering drug.
- Assess for dizziness and vertigo in patients receiving minocycline. Inspect for bruising, bleeding, or blood in stool.
- Monitor blood urea nitrogen (BUN) level, serum creatinine level, liver function tests, complete blood count (CBC) and differential, and platelet count.
- Palpate the fontanelles of infants every 4 hours; report bulging to the physician.
- Do not administer tetracyclines to children younger than 8 years of age unless absolutely necessary.
- Warn the patient that IM injections are painful.
- Administer IV doses slowly, and well diluted, to lessen the chance of venous irritation and phlebitis. Make certain IV infusion is patent before administering drug to avoid extravasation.

Intravenous Oxytetracycline

- Dilute as directed in drug insert. Administer at a rate of 100 mg or less over at least 5 minutes.

Intravenous Doxycycline

- Check expiration date. Dilute each 100 mg with 10 ml sterile water for injection or normal saline. Further dilute as directed in drug insert with 100 to 1000 ml of compatible fluid. Administer at a rate of 100 mg over 1 to 4 hours.

Intravenous Minocycline

- Dilute as directed in drug insert. Final dilution is in a volume of 500 to 1000 ml. Administer at an appropriate rate for the volume and the age and size of the patient.

Continued.

NURSING IMPLICATIONS SUMMARY—cont'd

Patient and Family Education

- See Nursing Implications Summary in Chapter 38 (p. 469).
- Instruct the patient to take oral doses with a full (8-ounce) glass of water.
- Usually the patient should take oral tetracyclines on an empty stomach 1 hour before or 2 hours after meals. However, if the drug causes stomach upset, the physician may permit it to be taken with meals or a snack. Doxycycline and minocycline may be taken on a full or empty stomach.
- Instruct the patient not to take oral demeclocycline, oxytetracycline, or tetracycline within 1 to 2 hours of having milk, milk products, or formula. Instruct the patient not to take any tetracycline within 1 to 2 hours of any of the following medications: antacids, calcium supplements, choline and magnesium salicylate combinations, magnesium salicylate, magnesium-containing laxatives, or sodium bicarbonate. Review other prescribed medications with the patient to clarify these instructions.
- Instruct the patient not to take iron or vitamin preparations containing iron within 2 to 3 hr of taking a tetracycline.
- Warn the patient that tetracyclines may cause the tongue to become darkened or discolored. This effect is not significant and clears when the drug is stopped.
- Contraceptive pills containing estrogen may not be effective while patients are taking tetracyclines; other forms of birth control should be used. Discuss this effect with the physician or pharmacist.
- This drug may cause photosensitivity (see the patient problem box on photosensitivity, p. 649).
- Demeclocycline may be used to treat the syndrome of inappropriate antidiuretic hormone (SIADH) and, when used for this, functions as a diuretic. This diuretic action is effective in patients with SIADH but is not satisfactory in other patients who may require diuresis.
- When tetracyclines are used in children younger than 8 years of age, discoloration of the teeth may occur. Notify the physician if this happens.
- Instruct the patient to observe expiration dates on all medications but especially tetracyclines. Use of outdated preparations or those that have deteriorated or changed color may cause severe adverse reactions.
- Warn the patient taking minocycline to avoid driving or operating hazardous equipment if vertigo or dizziness occurs and to notify the physician.
- Teach proper injection technique to a patient who will self-administer IM forms.
- Instruct the patient to swallow the capsule form of doxycycline whole, without crushing or breaking.
- Topical tetracyclines: Read the patient instruction leaflet provided by manufacturer. The cream, ointment, and topical liquid forms may stain clothing. Instruct the patient to notify the physician if skin condition does not improve in 4 to 6 weeks or if skin irritation or excessive dryness develops.
- Tetracyclines are also available in eye ointment and eyedrop forms. See Chapter 5 for information about administering these drug forms. Instruct the patient in the appropriate administration technique.

Chloramphenicol

Drug Administration

- See Nursing Implications Summary in Chapter 38 (p. 469).
- Assess for history of allergy before administering the drug.
- Assess visual acuity before beginning therapy and at regular intervals. Assess for GI tract side effects, skin changes, and signs of hematologic side effects.
- Monitor infants for appearance of gray syndrome. Assess for failure to feed, abdominal distension, progressive pallid cyanosis, and irregular respiration. Note that gray syndrome can develop in infants of women who received chloramphenicol during labor or the last few days of pregnancy.
- Monitor serum drug levels, CBC and differential, platelet count, BUN level, serum creatinine level, and liver function tests.

Intravenous Chloramphenicol

- Dilute 1 gm with 10 ml of sterile water or 5% dextrose in water (D5W). Chloramphenicol may be further diluted with 50 to 100 ml of compatible solution; see the drug insert.
- Administer IV push at a rate of 1 gm over at least 1 minute. For infusion, administer a volume of 50 to 100 ml over 30 to 60 minutes.
- Warn the patient that he or she may experience a bitter taste in the mouth after IV administration but that it should resolve after a few minutes.

Patient and Family Education

- See Nursing Implications Summary in Chapter 38 (p. 469).
- Instruct the patient to report unexplained bruising or bleeding, nosebleed, bleeding gums, blood in stools and fever, sore throat, malaise, fatigue, or symptoms of infection. Instruct the patient to report these symptoms even if they develop after the drug has been stopped.
- Instruct the patient to take oral doses with a full (8-ounce) glass of water on an empty stomach 1 hour before or 2 hours after meals for best effect. Caution the patient to avoid driving or operating hazardous equipment if confusion or visual changes occur.
- Warn the diabetic patient that chloramphenicol may cause false results with urine glucose tests. Instruct the diabetic patient to consult the physician before changing diet or diabetes medications and to monitor blood glucose levels.
- Chloramphenicol is also available in eye ointment, eyedrop, topical cream, and eardrop form. See Chapter 5 for information about administering these drug forms. Instruct the patient in the appropriate administration technique.

Critical Thinking

APPLICATION

1. What is the mechanism of action of tetracycline antibiotics?
2. What is the mechanism by which bacteria become resistant to tetracyclines?
3. How does the absorption of minocycline and doxycycline differ from that of other tetracyclines?
4. What factors limit the IM use of tetracyclines?
5. What precautions are necessary for using tetracyclines by IV routes?
6. What are the three main routes of excretion for tetracyclines?
7. Are minocycline and doxycycline eliminated in the same way as other tetracyclines?
8. What are the main toxic reactions common to all tetracycline antibiotics?
9. What toxic reaction is especially associated with demeclocycline?
10. What toxic reaction is especially associated with minocycline?
11. What toxicity is associated with outdated tetracycline preparations?
12. What is the effect of administering tetracyclines with antacids? What is the education implication?
13. Why do tetracyclines interfere with the antimicrobial action of penicillins?
14. Name three groups of organisms against which the tetracyclines are effective.
15. What is the mechanism of action of chloramphenicol?
16. What is the mechanism by which bacteria become resistant to chloramphenicol?
17. Which routes of administration give the most rapid and complete absorption of chloramphenicol?
18. Does chloramphenicol efficiently enter cerebrospinal fluid?
19. What is the primary route of elimination of chloramphenicol?
20. What is the most dangerous toxic reaction associated with chloramphenicol?
21. What is gray syndrome?
22. Name a clinical indication for chloramphenicol.

CRITICAL THINKING

1. What factors influence the oral absorption of tetracycline antibiotics? What are some education implications?
2. Develop a nursing care plan for a patient receiving one of the drugs discussed in this chapter.

CHAPTER 43

Aminoglycosides

OBJECTIVES

After studying this chapter, you should be able to do the following:

- *Explain why aminoglycosides are administered only by parenteral routes.*
- *Describe the toxicity associated with aminoglycoside use.*
- *Explain why aminoglycosides are sometimes used along with penicillins for serious infections.*
- *Develop a nursing care plan for a patient receiving an aminoglycoside.*

KEY TERMS

amikacin
aminoglycosides
gentamicin
streptomycin

CHAPTER OVERVIEW

In this chapter a group of antibiotics with primary usefulness for infections caused by gram-negative aerobic bacteria are introduced. Aminoglycoside antibiotics are composed of three or four amino sugars held together in glycosidic linkage. Great variability in structure is possible in these component sugars, and as a result several antibiotics of this type exist.

Therapeutic Rationale: Bacterial Infections

Diseases caused by aerobic gram-negative bacteria include pneumonias, urinary tract infections, septicemia, and central nervous system (CNS) infections. Because aminoglycosides have serious dose-limiting toxicity, they are used only in serious or life-threatening infections caused by aerobic gram-negative organisms.

Therapeutic Agents: Aminoglycosides

Aminoglycosides

Amikacin, ✤ gentamicin, kanamycin, neomycin, netilmicin, streptomycin, tobramycin

Mechanism of Action and Bacterial Resistance

The **aminoglycosides** inhibit early steps in bacterial protein synthesis by binding to bacterial ribosomes. Under certain conditions, bacterial protein synthesis may continue in the presence of aminoglycosides but with a greatly increased error rate. Defective proteins formed may damage the bacterial cell. Aminoglycosides also have a somewhat delayed effect on bacterial cell membranes. Aminoglycosides are bactericidal, unlike many other antibiotics that inhibit bacterial protein synthesis.

Resistance to aminoglycosides occurs as a result of decreased antibiotic uptake, changes in antibiotic binding to ribosomes, or enzymatic destruction of the aminoglycosides. By far the most common mechanism for resistance involves antibiotic destruction. Many sites for enzymatic attack exist on the amino sugars in aminoglycosides. Bacterial enzymes modify aminoglycosides in several ways. The primary sites of attack are amino and hydroxyl groups on the sugars. Amino groups may be acetylated, and hydroxyl groups may have a phosphate or an adenylate group added. Any of these substitutions inactivates the aminoglycoside. At least 13 separate enzymes catalyzing these reactions have been identified. Aminoglycosides differ in susceptibility to degradation, ranging from kanamycin, which is destroyed by at least six different enzymes, to amikacin, which is sensitive to only two enzymes.

Rarely, bacterial resistance may result from reduced drug uptake. This mechanism has been observed especially with amikacin. An equally rare mechanism of resistance involves lowering drug binding to the ribosome. Occasional streptomycin-resistant strains arise by this mechanism.

Pharmacokinetics

Aminoglycosides are polycationic molecules at physiologic pH. As a result of being charged, these drugs do not readily penetrate mammalian membranes and are not absorbed orally. Therapy with aminoglycosides is therefore by intramuscular (IM) or intravenous (IV) routes and usually involves hospitalized patients suffering from moderate-to-severe infections. Absorption of aminoglycosides from IM injection sites is rapid, and peak serum concentrations occur between 1 and 1½ hours after injection.

Aminoglycosides do not enter the CNS to any significant extent in normal persons. Some drug does appear in cerebrospinal fluid when meningitis is present. Aminoglycosides enter most other body fluids and tissues. These drugs cross the placenta and achieve significant concentrations in fetuses.

Aminoglycosides are excreted by glomerular filtration in the kidney. Active drug is concentrated in urine. Since the kidney is the primary site for elimination of these drugs, any reduction in renal function may lower excretion sufficiently to cause aminoglycoside accumulation. The approximate half-time for elimination of these drugs is 2 to 4 hours, but in renal failure it may be greatly prolonged. Excretion is also lower in neonates, who have immature kidneys, and in older adult patients, whose renal function is diminished simply as a function of age (see box).

Uses

The clinical use of these drugs is limited by their toxic potential. As a general rule the aminoglycosides are reserved for serious infections caused by aerobic gram-negative bacteria or by mycobacteria (see Chapter 45). Individual drugs in this family differ in specific uses as a result of differences in relative toxicity and antibacterial activity. Table 43-1 lists the most important clinical uses of individual aminoglycosides.

Streptomycin is most useful today in combination with other agents to treat infections in which strict bactericidal action is required for most effective therapy. Examples of these infections are bacterial endocarditis and tuberculosis (see Chapter 45).

One difference among aminoglycosides is their different degree of activity against *Pseudomonas aeruginosa.* **Amikacin, gentamicin,** netilmicin, and tobramycin are most effective

GERIATRIC CONSIDERATION

Aminoglycosides

THE PROBLEM

Patients older than 60 years of age have reduced renal function and therefore may excrete aminoglycosides more slowly than younger adults. In older adults aminoglycosides may accumulate because alternative paths of elimination are limited. Older adults also have some hearing loss because of their age and may therefore be more susceptible to drug-induced hearing loss.

SOLUTIONS

- Lower doses to avoid accumulation.
- Monitor serum aminoglycoside concentrations.
- Monitor renal function tests.
- Perform baseline auditory function tests; repeat during therapy.

against this pathogen. Kanamycin usually is not effective. Amikacin differs from other aminoglycosides in being less sensitive to common aminoglycoside-degrading enzymes. Amikacin is therefore active against some bacterial strains that are resistant to other aminoglycosides. Table 43-2 lists common dosages for aminoglycosides used in patients with normal renal function.

Adverse Reactions and Contraindications

Less common adverse reactions include effects on a variety of organ systems. Blood dyscrasias, while rare, may occur with any aminoglycoside. Rare neurotoxicity causes headaches, paresthesias, tremor, confusion, and disorientation. The aminoglycosides are also somewhat irritating and may cause pain at the injection site.

Allergies to aminoglycosides are possible, and a prior allergic reaction to any aminoglycoside is a contraindication to receiving the drugs again.

Because aminoglycosides may be nephrotoxic, renal function must be monitored in patients receiving aminoglycosides (see next section). Serum levels of these drugs are monitored to prevent intoxication.

Aminoglycosides must be used with caution in patients with any condition that impairs transmission at the neuromuscular junction or otherwise weakens muscular function. For this reason, patients with myasthenia gravis, Parkinson's disease, or infant botulism would normally not receive aminoglycosides; if they receive aminoglycosides, they must be watched carefully for excessive muscle weakness during therapy.

Patients with preexisting renal, auditory, or vestibular damage would ordinarily not be given an aminoglycoside if an alternative drug was available. These patients may be more at risk for the dose-related toxicity described in the next section.

Toxicity

The aminoglycosides exert significant toxicity of three major types: ototoxicity, renal toxicity, and neuromuscular blockade. Ototoxicity may cause hearing loss, loss of equilibrium control, or both. Hearing loss in some patients continues even after the drug is discontinued. Loss of equilibrium may be less obvious than hearing loss but can usually be revealed by

TABLE 43-1 Aminoglycoside Antibiotic Use

DRUG	INDICATIONS
Amikacin, gentamicin, netilmicin, tobramycin	Serious infections caused by aerobic gram-negative bacteria, including *Pseudomonas aeruginosa.*
Kanamycin	Serious infections caused by aerobic gram-negative bacteria other than *P. aeruginosa.*
Neomycin	Topical use only.
Streptomycin	Used alone to treat tularemia (rabbit fever) and bubonic or black plague. Used in combination with other antibiotics to treat bacterial endocarditis (with penicillin G), tuberculosis (with isoniazid or other antituberculosis agents), brucellosis (with tetracyclines), and *Listeria* infections (with ampicillin or penicillin G).

TABLE 43-2 Aminoglycoside Antibiotics

GENERIC NAME	TRADE NAME	ADMINISTRATION/DOSAGE
Amikacin	Amikin*	INTRAMUSCULAR, INTRAVENOUS: *Adults and children*—5 mg/kg body weight every 8 hr. Do not exceed 1.5 gm daily. IV doses are given by slow infusion. FDA pregnancy category D. *Neonates*—10 mg/kg initially, then 7.5 mg/kg every 18-24 hr.
✣ Gentamicin	Cidomycin† Garamycin*	INTRAMUSCULAR, INTRAVENOUS: *Adults*—1-1.7 mg/kg every 8 hr. Do not exceed 8 mg/daily. FDA pregnancy category C. *Children*—2.5 mg/kg every 8-24 hr. *Neonates*—2.5 mg/kg every 12-24 hr.
Kanamycin	Kantrex	INTRAMUSCULAR, INTRAVENOUS, INTRAPERITONEAL: *Adults and children*—Not to exceed 15 mg/kg daily, divided into 2 or 3 doses. FDA pregnancy category D.
Neomycin		TOPICAL: *Adults and children*—Commonly used as 0.35% creams and ointments. Also used in numerous combinations with other antibiotics.
Netilmicin	Netromycin*	INTRAMUSCULAR, INTRAVENOUS: *Adults*—1.3-2.2 mg/kg every 8 hr. FDA pregnancy category D. *Children*—2.75-4 mg/kg every 12 hr. *Neonates-6 wk*—2-3.25 mg every 12 hr.
Streptomycin		INTRAMUSCULAR: *Adults*—1-4 gm daily in 1-4 doses. Older adult patients may require less drug. Lower doses are used for long-term treatment of mild tuberculosis. FDA pregnancy category D. *Children*—10-20 mg/kg every 12 hr.
Tobramycin	Nebcin*	INTRAMUSCULAR, INTRAVENOUS: *Adults and infants*—1-1.7 mg/kg every 8 hr. FDA pregnancy category D. *Children*—2-2.5 mg/kg every 8-16 hr.

*Available in Canada and United States.
†Available in Canada only.

appropriate tests. Nausea or dizziness may signal disturbance of equilibrium. Ototoxicity is usually more severe when serum concentrations of aminoglycosides exceed 8 to 10 μg/ml. The total dose administered may also be a factor since some patients treated over long periods may display these symptoms in spite of never having excessively high serum levels of the drug.

Aminoglycosides may damage both tubules and glomeruli in the kidney, especially when high doses are given. This toxic potential can cause a rapid clinical deterioration since renal damage can cause drug accumulation, which in turn causes further damage to the kidney. This cycle of accumulation and increasing renal damage can destroy kidney function. Patients who accumulate the drug because of renal dysfunction are also more prone to ototoxicity.

The third characteristic toxic reaction to aminoglycosides is neuromuscular blockade. This reaction is usually observed in surgical patients when an aminoglycoside is used in peritoneal lavage. Neuromuscular blockade usually is manifested by respiratory paralysis since the muscles of the chest involved in breathing are prevented from functioning. Some of the aminoglycosides produce a competitive neuromuscular blockade, which may be reversed by neostigmine. Others such as kanamycin produce an irreversible blockade, which neostigmine does not affect, although calcium may relieve the blockade in some cases. Patients who have recently received muscle relaxants are more prone to suffer neuromuscular blockade with aminoglycosides. Patients with myasthenia gravis are also more sensitive to this effect.

Interactions

The ototoxicity and nephrotoxicity of aminoglycoside antibiotics may be enhanced by a variety of agents. For example, if a patient who is receiving an aminoglycoside is also given a nephrotoxic drug such as a cephalosporin or methoxyflurane (Penthrane), the risk of kidney damage is increased. Likewise, ototoxic drugs such as ethacrynic acid may enhance ototoxicity in a patient receiving an aminoglycoside antibiotic. All aminoglycosides possess neuromuscular blocking activity. This action has led to enhancement of agents used for neuromuscular blocking action during surgery.

Gentamicin is frequently combined with an anti-*Pseudomonas* penicillin to treat *P. aeruginosa* infections. Although these drugs may be used in the same patient, they should never be physically mixed since penicillins chemically inactivate gentamicin in solution.

Aminoglycosides are many times more effective at the slightly alkaline pH of normal serum (pH 7.4) than at the acidic pH of normal urine (pH 5). Therefore in the treatment of urinary tract infections with these drugs a therapeutic advantage may be gained by alkalinizing urine.

NURSING PROCESS OVERVIEW

Aminoglycosides

Refer to Chapter 38 for general guidelines on the nursing process with antibiotic therapy. The additional material in this chapter relates specifically to the aminoglycosides and polymyxins.

Assessment

Perform a full assessment focusing on the signs and symptoms of infection. Assess renal function, hearing acuity, and vestibular function. Note other medications the patient is receiving.

Nursing Diagnoses

- Potential complication: ototoxicity related to aminoglycoside therapy
- Potential complication: renal damage or failure related to aminoglycoside therapy

Patient Outcomes

The patient's infection will resolve without serious drug side effects. If ototoxicity or renal failure develops, the nurse will manage and minimize these side effects.

Planning/Implementation

Once the decision is made to administer aminoglycosides, gather the proper supplies for proper administration by the parenteral route chosen. Note whether the patient has received any other neuromuscular blocking agents or whether the patient has any other condition such as myasthenia gravis that would predispose the patient to respiratory paralysis. Have available equipment to deal with respiratory paralysis if it occurs. Ensure that the medications are administered at the times prescribed. If samples are being taken for the measurement of blood levels of these drugs, obtain samples as ordered since the timing is critical for proper interpretation of the information.

Evaluation

Monitor vital signs closely, and assess objective and subjective signs and symptoms. Hearing loss caused by aminoglycosides may progress during and after therapy. Continue to evaluate the patient for this symptom and for any loss of control of equilibrium as evidenced by difficulty in walking or by staggering or dizziness.

NURSING IMPLICATIONS SUMMARY

Aminoglycosides

Drug Administration

- See Nursing Implications Summary in Chapter 38 (p. 469).
- Assess for history of allergy before administering drug.
- Review discussion of toxicity observed with these drugs. Assess for changes in hearing and balance and for development of tinnitus and buzzing.
- Monitor intake and output and weight. Assess for increased thirst, nausea, vomiting, loss of appetite, and increase or decrease in frequency of urination.
- Monitor vital signs and auscultate lung sounds.
- Monitor serum creatinine level, blood urea nitrogen (BUN) level, urinalysis, liver function tests, serum electrolyte level, complete blood count (CBC) and WBC differential, and platelet count.
- Monitor serum drug levels. Peak and trough levels may be available. Peak levels indicate serum levels after a dose is given and reflect the highest serum level for that patient at that dose. Trough levels are drawn shortly before a dose is given and reflect the lowest serum level for that patient at that dose. If peak and trough levels are ordered, notify the laboratory of the time a dose will be given so that blood specimens can be obtained at the proper times for drug level calculations.
- Have available neostigmine and calcium chloride in settings where aminoglycosides are used with high-risk patients such as in the operating room, recovery room, and intensive care units.
- Monitor respiratory status. Have available a suction machine at the bedside.
- Use gentamicin without preservatives for intrathecal administration.
- Do not mix aminoglycosides in a syringe with other medications.
- For pediatric doses and dilutions, consult the manufacturer's literature.
- Because of the possibility of hypotension or vertigo, keep siderails up. Supervise ambulation.
- Neomycin may be ordered orally or via enema to inhibit ammonia-forming bacteria in the gastrointestinal (GI) tract of patients with hepatic encephalopathy.
- Streptomycin may cause peripheral neuritis. Assess for burning of face, numbness, and tingling.

Intramuscular Streptomycin

- Dilute as directed on the label of the vial. Use a large muscle mass. This drug is not administered by the IV route. Teach IM administration technique to patients who will self-administer at home.

Intravenous Amikacin

- Dilute 500 mg in 100 to 200 ml of normal saline or 5% dextrose in water (D5W); administer to adults over 30 to 60 minutes. Administer doses to infants over 1 to 2 hours.

Intravenous Gentamicin

- Dilute a single dose in 50 to 200 ml of normal saline or D5W. The concentration should not exceed 0.1% (1 mg/ml). Administer each dose over 30 to 60 minutes in adults or up to 2 hours in children. Prepared dilutions are available.

Intravenous Kanamycin

- Dilute the prescribed dose in normal saline or D5W to a concentration of 500 mg in 100 to 200 ml. Administer over 30 to 60 minutes.

Intravenous Netilmicin

- Dilute a single dose in 50 to 200 ml of diluent; see the drug insert. Administer over 30 minutes to 2 hours.

Intravenous Tobramycin

- Dilute the dose in 50 to 100 ml of D5W or normal saline and administer over 20 to 60 minutes.

Patient and Family Education

- See Nursing Implication Summary in Chapter 38 (p. 469).
- Instruct the patient to report hearing loss, nausea, dizziness or vertigo, decreased urinary output, nausea, vomiting, loss of appetite, and increased thirst.
- Streptomycin is often given in combination with other drugs in long-term therapy for tuberculosis.
- Streptomycin may cause peripheral neuritis. Caution the patient to report changes in vision, burning, numbness, or tingling.
- With topical preparations, systemic side effects are rare but can occur. Factors that influence the likelihood of toxicity include the frequency of application, the size of the area to which the preparation is being applied, whether the skin surface was intact, and the amount and kind of other ototoxic or nephrotoxic drugs the patient might be receiving concomitantly.
- Photosensitivity has been reported with topical preparations (see the patient problem box on photosensitivity, p. 649).

CRITICAL THINKING

APPLICATION

1. What is the mechanism of action of aminoglycoside antibiotics?
2. What is the most common mechanism for bacterial resistance to aminoglycosides?
3. Which routes of administration are appropriate for aminoglycosides?
4. What is the primary route of excretion of aminoglycosides?
5. What effects may aminoglycoside antibiotics have on the ears?
6. What groups of patients might be more prone to aminoglycoside ototoxicity and nephrotoxicity?
7. How do aminoglycosides affect the neuromuscular junction?
8. What special precautions must be taken when gentamicin and carbenicillin are used together?
9. Name three clinical uses of streptomycin.
10. Name one clinical indication for neomycin.
11. How does the clinical indication for the use of kanamycin differ from the indications for gentamicin, tobramycin, netilmicin, and amikacin?

CRITICAL THINKING

1. How do aminoglycoside antibiotics affect the kidneys? How should you assess for these effects?
2. What groups of patients are most likely to develop respiratory paralysis after therapeutic use of aminoglycoside antibiotics? How should you monitor these patients?
3. Develop a nursing care plan for a patient receiving gentamicin.

CHAPTER 44

Sulfonamides, Trimethoprim, and Drugs for Urinary Tract Infections

OBJECTIVES

After studying this chapter, you should be able to do the following:

- *Explain why sulfonamides are especially useful for urinary tract infections.*
- *Explain why trimethoprim is given in fixed combination with a sulfonamide.*
- *Discuss the limited indications for nitrofurantoins.*
- *Develop a nursing care plan for patients receiving drugs discussed in this chapter.*

KEY TERMS

crystalluria
nitrofurantoin
sulfamethoxazole
sulfonamides
trimethoprim
urinary tract infections (UTIs)

CHAPTER OVERVIEW

This chapter focuses on drugs used mainly to treat urinary tract infections (see box, p. 514). Sulfonamides and trimethoprim have antimicrobial mechanisms and pharmacokinetic properties that make these drugs useful in certain systemic infections as well, but nitrofurantoins are used only in urinary tract infections.

Patient Problem

Urinary Tract Infections

THE PROBLEM

Urinary tract infections (UTIs) are more common in females than in males since the urethra is shorter in females. UTIs are also more common in patients wearing urinary retention catheters (Foley catheters) and in patients requiring intermittent catheterization or urinary tract manipulation. Drugs may be prescribed when an infection develops, prophylactically when genitourinary examination or manipulation is planned, or when a history of chronic UTI exists.

SIGNS AND SYMPTOMS

Burning on urination, frequent urination, itching in the area of the urinary meatus, fever, and malaise.

PATIENT AND FAMILY EDUCATION

- Instruct the patient to drink sufficient fluids to ensure a daily urine output of 1500 to 2000 ml. Usually, this means drinking at least 6 to 8 full (8-ounce) glasses of fluid for adults.
- Instruct the female patient to always wipe from front to back after voiding or defecating to avoid accidental contamination of the urinary meatus with bacteria from the anal region.
- Instruct the patient to avoid bubble baths. Some patients, especially female patients, may have to eliminate all baths and shower only.
- Wash soap off the perineal region completely to avoid irritation from the soap. Some patients may have to wash with water only.
- Instruct the patient to void immediately after sexual intercourse.
- Some drugs for UTIs are most effective if urinary pH is changed. This is difficult to do through diet alone, so other drugs may be prescribed by the physician. If sodium bicarbonate or other drugs are prescribed, instruct the patient to take as ordered for best treatment of the UTI.
- Instruct the patient to take drugs for the full prescribed dose (often 7 to 10 days) and not stop when symptoms begin to subside.

FOR PATIENTS WITH URINARY CATHETERS

- Secure catheter well, so there is minimal pulling on the meatal area.
- Wash the catheter insertion area with soap and water, but avoid rough scrubbing. Rinse well.
- Avoid opening the drainage system unless necessary.
- Clean the tubing and bag as directed (unless replacing them with a new device), usually with a dilute bleach solution or as instructed by the discharge nurse.
- In the hospital, use sterile technique to insert catheters. In the home, use clean technique as instructed.
- Maintain a good fluid intake.

Therapeutic Rationale: Urinary Tract Infections

Bacterial infections of the urinary tract are one of the most common complaints seen by physicians. The organisms that cause these infections are mostly gram-negative bacteria, but chlamydia may also cause genitourinary tract infections, as well as infections of the eye. The agents that are covered in this chapter are effective because they act against the organisms most likely to cause **urinary tract infections** (**UTIs**) and because the drugs are concentrated in the urinary tract.

Therapeutic Agents: Urinary Tract Infections

Sulfonamides

Sulfacytine, sulfadiazine, sulfadoxine, sulfamethizole, sulfamethoxazole, sulfapyridine, sulfasalazine, sulfisoxazole

Mechanism of Action and Bacterial Resistance

Sulfonamides are metabolic inhibitors that block bacterial synthesis of folic acid, a vitamin required for the synthesis of amino acids and nucleic acids (Figure 44-1). The metabolically active form of folic acid, tetrahydrofolic acid (THFA), is synthesized in bacteria from simple precursor molecules. Two of the enzymes involved in these conversions have been exploited as targets of antibacterial drugs. Dihydropteroate synthetase, which converts paraaminobenzoic acid (PABA) and other small molecules to dihydropteroate, is the target for sulfonamides. The sulfonamides competitively inhibit this enzyme. The second target in this pathway is dihydrofolic acid reductase, the enzyme that forms THFA (see trimethoprim).

Sulfonamides are selectively toxic to organisms that must form folic acid from PABA and the other precursors. Fortunately, humans are not sensitive to this action because we cannot synthesize folic acid but must absorb it preformed in our diet. Sulfonamides are primarily bacteriostatic against those organisms they affect.

Bacterial resistance to sulfonamides has become widespread and has reduced the clinical usefulness of these drugs. Some bacteria such as pneumococci acquire an altered dihydrofolic acid synthetase, which is less sensitive to sulfonamides. Overproduction of PABA is a common mechanism of resistance for several pathogens, including staphylococci, pneumococci, and gonococci. Since sulfonamides are only competitive inhibitors of PABA incorporation into folic acid, excess PABA overcomes the sulfonamide inhibition.

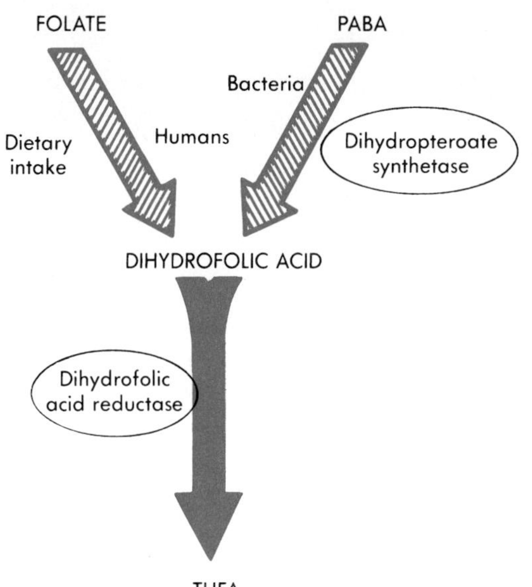

FIGURE 44-1
Synthesis of tetrahydrofolic acid (THFA) in bacteria and humans. THFA is vitamin required for nucleic acid and amino acid synthesis. Many bacteria form this vitamin from paraaminobenzoic acid (PABA) and other small molecules. Two enzymes involved in this synthesis have proved useful in chemotherapy, dihydropteroate synthetase and dihydrofolic acid reductase. Sulfonamides inhibit dihydropteroate synthetase, thereby blocking THFA synthesis in bacteria. Humans are immune from this action because preformed folate and dihydrofolic acid are supplied in diet. Dihydrofolic acid reductase in bacteria is inhibited by trimethoprim.

Pharmacokinetics

Sulfonamide antibacterial agents with a wide variety of pharmacokinetic properties are available (Tables 44-1 to 44-3). For example, sulfasalazine is poorly absorbed from the gastrointestinal (GI) tract but is cleaved within the bowel to release sulfapyridine, which is the active agent. This preparation is useful for ulcerative colitis, as active material is released at the site of infection.

Topical sulfonamides such as mafenide and silver sulfadiazine are used to treat or prevent infections on burned or abraded skin. Systemic absorption is not expected by this route but can occur when the drugs are used on extensive areas of burned skin.

The sulfonamides used to treat systemic infections are well absorbed orally. Distribution of these drugs to body tissues including brain is good. Concentrations of sulfonamides in cerebrospinal and other body fluids may approach those of serum. Sulfonamides also pass the placental barrier and enter fetuses. Elimination of sulfonamides from the body involves both liver and kidneys. The liver converts a portion of the sulfonamide in blood to an acetylated derivative, which is usually bacteriologically inactive. Acetylated as well as free drug are eliminated by the kidneys, primarily by glomerular filtration. Tubular reabsorption is significant for some sulfonamides. Excretion of sulfonamides is favored by alkalinizing urine. This procedure increases the solubility of these drugs in urine and also converts the drugs to a charged form that does not undergo renal tubular reabsorption.

TABLE 44-1 Summary of Sulfonamides: Single-Component Formulations

GENERIC NAME	TRADE NAME	ADMINISTRATION/DOSAGE	CLINICAL USE
Sulfadiazine		ORAL: *Adults*—Single loading dose of 2-4 gm, then 1 gm every 4-6 hr. FDA pregnancy category C. *Children >2 mo*—75 mg/kg body weight to load, then 25 mg/kg every 4 hr.	Used with pyrimethamine for toxoplasmosis and malaria.
Sulfamethizole	Thiosulfil Forte	ORAL: *Adults*—0.5-1 gm every 6-8 hr. FDA pregnancy category C. *Children >2 mo*—7.5-11.25 mg/kg every 6 hr.	UTIs only.
Sulfamethoxazole	Gantanol*	ORAL: *Adults*—Single 2 gm loading dose, then 1 gm 2 or 3 times daily. FDA pregnancy category C. *Children >2 mo*—50-60 mg/kg loading dose, then 25-30 mg/kg twice daily, not to exceed 75 mg/kg daily.	Conjunctivitis, nocardiosis, otitis media, trachoma, and UTIs.
Sulfapyridine	Dagenan†	ORAL: *Adults*—500 mg 4 times daily. Reduce dose as improvement allows.	Dematitis herpetiformis.
Sulfasalazine	Azulfidine Salazopyrin*	ORAL: *Adults*—1 gm every 4-6 hr. FDA pregnancy category B. *Children >2 yr*—10 mg/kg every 4 hr initially, then 7.5 mg/kg every 6 hr.	Ulcerative colitis; sulfapyridine is released from sulfasalazine as active agent in bowel.
Sulfisoxazole	Gantrisin NovoSoxazole†	ORAL: *Adults*—2-4 gm loading dose, then1-2 gm every 6 hr. FDA pregnancy category C. *Children >2 mo*—75 mg/kg loading dose, then 25 mg/kg every 4 hr.	UTIs and systemic infections caused by sensitive organisms and nocardiosis.

*Available in Canada and United States.
†Available in Canada only.

TABLE 44-2 Summary of Sulfonamides: Fixed Combinations for Oral Use

COMPONENTS OF COMBINATION	DRUG FORM	TRADE NAME	DOSAGE	CLINICAL USE
✤ Sulfamethoxazole: 400 mg Trimethoprim: 80 mg	Tablet	Bactrim* Cotrim Roubac† Septra*	*Adults*—2 tablets every 12 hr. For pneumocystis pneumonia, 25 mg/kg sulfamethoxazole and 5 mg/kg trimethoprim every 6 hr. *Children >2 mo*—4-6 mg/kg trimethoprim and 20-30 mg/kg sulfamethoxazole every 12 hr.	UTIs, otitis media, enteritis caused by sensitive *Shigella,* pneumocystis pneumonia.
Sulfadiazine: 410 mg Trimethoprim: 90 mg	Tablet	Coptin†	*Adults*—2 tablets once daily. *Children 3 mo-5 yr*—¼-½ tablet every 12 hr. *Children 5-12 yr*—½-1 tablet every 12 hr.	UTIs.
Sulfadoxine: 500 mg Pyrimethamine: 25 mg	Tablet	Fansidar*	*Adults*—for treatment, 3 tablets as single dose on third day of quinine treatment; or 1 tablet every 7 days for chemoprophylaxis. FDA pregnancy category C. *Children 2 mo-4 yr*—¼ tablet every 7 days for chemoprophylaxis. *Children 5-8 yr*—½ tablet once every 7 days for chemoprophylaxis. *Children 9-14 yr*—¾ tablet once very 7 days for chemoprophylaxis.	Malaria, chloroquine-resistant.
Sulfamethoxazole: 500 mg Phenazopyridine: 100 mg	Tablet	Azo Gantanol	*Adults*—4 tablets to load, then 2 tablets every 12 hr for 2 days.	UTIs only.
Sulfisoxazole: 500 mg Phenazopyridine: 50 mg	Tablet	Azo Gantrisin*	*Adults*—4-6 tablets to load, then 2 tablets every 6 hr for 2 days.	UTIs only.

*Available in Canada and United States.
†Available in Canada only.

TABLE 44-3 Summary of Sulfonamides: Topical Agents

GENERIC NAME	TRADE NAME	APPLICATION FORM	CLINICAL USE	COMMENTS
Malenide acetate	Sulfamylon	Cream: 85 mg mafenide acetate/gm	Treatment of second- and third-degree burns.	Drug is effective against broad spectrum of pathogens, including *Pseudomonas aeruginosa.*
Silver sulfadiazine	Silvadene Flamazine† Thermazene	Cream: 10 mg/gm	Treatment of second- and third-degree burns.	Drug is effective against broad spectrum of pathogens, including *P. aeruginosa* and certain yeasts.
Sulfacetamide	Bleph* Cetamid* Sulamyd*	Solution: 10%, 15%, or 30% Ointment: 10%	Ophthalmic only. For conjunctivitis, corneal ulcer, and trachoma.	Drug allergy may develop in sensitive patients.
Sulfisoxazole diolamine	Gantrisin	Solution: 4% Ointment: 4%	Ophthalmic only. For conjunctivitis, corneal ulcer, and trachoma.	Drug allergy may develop in sensitive patients.

*Available in Canada and United States.
†Available in Canada only.

Uses

Sulfonamides are potentially active against a wide range of gram-positive and gram-negative organisms, as well as *Nocardia, Chlamydia,* and *Actinomyces,* but bacterial resistance has limited use for many bacterial infections requiring systemic therapy. **Sulfamethoxazole** is the most widely used sulfonamide for general infections.

Sulfonamides may be combined with phenazopyridine to treat UTIs (see Table 44-2). The sulfonamide component supplies antibacterial activity and the phenazopyridine, which is excreted in urine, exerts an analgesic effect on the mucosa of the urinary tract. The added phenazopyridine therefore relieves the pain, burning, and itching associated with the UTI.

Sulfonamide preparations are available for vaginal application, but no evidence of effectiveness exists. Moreover, sensitization may be produced.

Adverse Reactions and Contraindications

Sulfonamides induce allergic reactions in a significant proportion of patients receiving the drugs. The most common reactions are skin rashes and itching, but drug fever and other more serious reactions such as Stevens-Johnson syndrome may occur. Anaphylaxis has been reported. Since sulfonamides are chemically related to the thiazide diuretics, acetazolamide, and oral hypoglycemic agents, a patient who becomes allergic to a sulfonamide may also become allergic to one or more of these agents. Photosensitivity to sulfonamides may also be a problem. The redness of the skin may be confused with an allergic reaction, but photosensitivity is localized to skin exposed to sun or sunlamps.

GI tract disturbances also occur with sulfonamides. In addition to nausea, vomiting, and diarrhea, more serious reactions such as pancreatitis, hepatitis, and stomatitis may occur. Central nervous system (CNS) alterations have also been observed, including headache, ataxia, hallucinations, and convulsions.

Deaths from aplastic anemia and other blood dyscrasias, although rare, have been connected with sulfonamide therapy. Sore throat, fever, or pallor may signal a serious blood dyscrasia (see box below).

Patients with preexisting renal or hepatic disease are more prone to develop side effects since these organs remove sulfonamides from the body. Patients with a genetic deficiency of glucose-6-phosphate dehydrogenase (G6PD) have greater risk for hemolytic anemia induced by sulfonamides. The highest frequency of G6PD deficiency is observed among African-Americans and Mediterranean populations; patients from these groups should be watched carefully for signs of anemia. Sulfonamides may worsen the condition of patients with anemias caused by folate deficiency.

Toxicity

Renal toxicity was common with sulfonamides in use before 1960. Most of the renal damage associated with these older agents was produced by drug crystallization in urine or tubular fluid, a condition called **crystalluria.** These drugs precipitated because of their low solubility in normal acidic urine. Newer sulfonamides are more soluble under these conditions, and drug precipitation is seldom a problem. The least soluble sulfonamides in use today are sulfadiazine and the acetylated metabolite of sulfamethoxazole. Patients receiving any sulfonamide should receive sufficient fluids to produce at least 1 L of urine daily. If there is a problem, solubility of sulfonamides in urine may be increased by alkalinizing urine. Sulfamethizole and sulfasalazine produce a yellow-orange coloration in alkaline urine. This coloration, also observable in skin, is not harmful.

Interactions

Sulfonamides are highly bound to serum proteins and may therefore displace other drugs from protein-binding sites. This displacement can occur with oral anticoagulants, sulfonylureas, the anticonvulsant phenytoin, the antiinflammatory agents phenylbutazone and sulfinpyrazone, and the antineoplastic agent methotrexate. In newborns displacement of bilirubin by sulfonamides may place the patient at risk (see box below).

Hemolytic agents such as sulfonylureas, primaquine, procainamide, and quinidine increase the risk of hemolysis with sulfonamides. The urinary antiseptic methenamine is designed to release formaldehyde in acidic urine for antibacterial effect. Sulfonamides can form insoluble complexes with formaldehyde and thus lead to crystalluria.

Dihydrofolate Reductase Inhibitors

Trimethoprim

Mechanism of Action and Bacterial Resistance

Trimethoprim inhibits dihydrofolic acid reductase,thus preventing THFA formation in bacteria. Dihydrofolic acid reductase functions in humans and in bacteria since much of the vitamin in mammalian diets is dihydrofolic acid that must be converted to THFA. Therefore trimethoprim might be expected to be toxic to humans and to bacteria. This is not the case, however, because dihydrofolic acid reductase in humans is relatively resistant to the action of trimethoprim, and the drug may be given at doses that inhibit this enzyme in bacteria but not in humans.

Pharmacokinetics

Trimethoprim is most often used in fixed combination with sulfamethoxazole (see Table 44-2). This combination represents an exploitation of drug properties for therapeutic effect. These drugs are administered in tablets with a 1:5 trimethoprim-sulfamethoxazole ratio. Both drugs are well

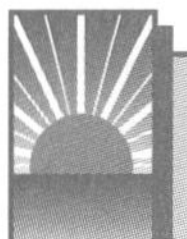

GERIATRIC CONSIDERATION

Sulfonamides

THE PROBLEM

Older adult patients are more likely to suffer severe blood and skin reactions to sulfonamides than younger adults. Diuretics, commonly taken by older adult patients for high blood pressure, compound the risk.

SOLUTIONS

- Monitor blood tests for signs of bone marrow depression.
- Watch for bleeding or reduced platelet counts.
- Inspect carefully for rash or purpura.
- Ascertain if the patient is taking a thiazide diuretic, either alone or as a component of other preparations.

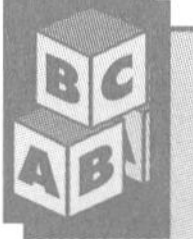

PEDIATRIC CONSIDERATION

Sulfonamides

THE PROBLEM

Sulfonamides displace bilirubin from serum proteins. In neonates, who typically have elevated bilirubin, this displacement may be sufficient to produce kernicterus.

SOLUTIONS

- Avoid sulfonamides in pregnancy near term.
- Avoid sulfonamides in infants younger than 1 month of age.

absorbed from the GI tract. Serum concentrations of the free drug not bound to serum proteins are usually in a 1:20 trimethoprim-sulfamethoxazole ratio. At this concentration ratio, the drugs have maximum antibacterial activity. The combination is synergistic, or more effective in combination than would be expected from the action of either drug alone. Synergy may result because both drugs starve sensitive bacteria for THFA, but the drugs work on two different enzymes in the sequence of reactions leading to THFA. Sequential blockade of this metabolic pathway is much more effective than blockade of a single step by one drug at high concentrations.

Trimethoprim penetrates body tissues better than sulfamethoxazole. Trimethoprim concentrations in breast milk, bile, prostatic fluid, vaginal fluids, liver, spleen, skin, and kidneys may exceed plasma concentrations of the drug. Penetration into other tissues is adequate, including the CNS.

Trimethoprim appears in urine at a concentration approximately 100 times the plasma concentration, with most of the drug in the active form. The urinary concentration of sulfamethoxazole is about 5 times the plasma concentration.

Uses

Trimethoprim has a spectrum of antimicrobial activity similar to that of sulfonamides, with some exceptions. Trimethoprim is more active against the gram-negative bacteria *Proteus* and *Klebsiella.* It is not useful alone against *Chlamydia* or *Nocardia.* Trimethoprim resistance has not yet become widespread. Although trimethoprim is used in the United States most commonly in combination with a sulfonamide, a preparation of trimethoprim alone is available for use in UTIs.

Adverse Reactions and Contraindications

Serious reactions to trimethoprim are rare, but anorexia, diarrhea, headache, nausea, or vomiting sometimes occurs.

Toxicity

Toxicity from trimethoprim is expected only with large overdoses. Treatment may include acidifying the urine to hasten excretion of trimethoprim and giving leucovorin to overcome its antifolate effects.

Trimethoprim may be less toxic than sulfonamides, but when trimethoprim is used in combination with sulfamethoxazole, patients should be observed for all signs of sulfonamide toxicity.

Interactions

Trimethoprim is synergistic with any systemically effective sulfonamides. Sulfamethoxazole was chosen for use in the fixed combination with trimethoprim because the kinetics of elimination of the two drugs are similar, as discussed above.

Trimethoprim should not be combined with methotrexate, pyrimethamine, or trimetrexate because these drugs have potent antifolate activity. The result could be megaloblastic anemia.

Nitrofurantoin

Mechanism of Action and Bacterial Resistance

Nitrofurantoin is activated in bacteria to compounds that attack bacterial proteins. It is effective against some gram-positive and gram-negative organisms, including many common pathogens of the urinary tract. *Pseudomonas* species are, however, usually intrinsically resistant. Development of resistance to nitrofurantoin therapy is not a significant problem.

Pharmacokinetics

Many compounds that are effective antibacterial agents in the laboratory are ineffective when used to treat systemic infections because of their unfavorable pharmacokinetics. One example of such a compound is nitrofurantoin (Table 44-4). This drug, in spite of being well absorbed from the small intestine, never achieves satisfactory blood levels. Low blood levels result from a rapid excretion of the drug by the kidneys. Removal of the drug occurs so quickly that it fails to accumulate in blood. Therefore despite its broad antibacterial spectrum, it is ineffective against systemic infections. Nitrofurantoin is concentrated in the kidneys and achieves bactericidal concentrations in urine. The drug diffuses from renal tubules into renal tissues so that final renal concentrations are much greater than would be expected from the very low blood concentrations of the drug. These properties make nitrofurantoin effective against UTIs.

TABLE 44-4 Nitrofurantoin and Trimethoprim

GENERIC NAME	TRADE NAME	ADMINISTRATION/DOSAGE	COMMENTS
Nitrofurantoin	Furadantin Furalan	ORAL: *Adults*—50-100 mg 4 times daily. *Children >1 mo*—0.75-1.75 mg/kg every 6 hr.	Gastric irritation may be minimized by administering drug with food or milk.
Nitrofurantoin	Macrobid	ORAL (extended release): *Adults*—100 mg every 12 hr for 7 days.	Take with food or milk.
Nitrofurantoin macrocrystals	Macrodantin*	As for nitrofurantoin.	Large crystal size minimizes gastric irritation.
Trimethoprim	Proloprim* Trimpex	ORAL: *Adults*—100 mg every 12 hr. FDA pregnancy category C.	UTIs only, unless combined with sulfonamide.

*Available in Canada and United States.

Uses

Nitrofurantoin is effective against UTIs caused by susceptible strains of *Escherichia coli, Enterobacter* species, enterococci, *Klebsiella* species, *Proteus* species, and staphylococci.

Adverse Reactions and Contraindications

Gastric irritation with anorexia, nausea, and emesis is common with nitrofurantoin. The large crystal form (Macrodantin, see Table 44-4) may be less irritating than the microcrystalline form. Gastric irritation is lessened by taking the drug with milk or food.

Another common side effect with nitrofurantoin is lung injury. Patients receiving nitrofurantoin for long periods should be observed for pneumonitis or pulmonary fibrosis, which may develop gradually or may appear as an acute illness.

Rashes, allergies, and reversible blood dyscrasias have been observed with nitrofurantoin. Hemolytic anemia similar to that seen with sulfonamides may also be seen. Infants under 3 months of age have undeveloped enzyme systems that make them especially susceptible to hemolytic anemia induced by nitrofurantoin. It should be used with care in pregnant patients and never at term. Persons with G6PD deficiency are also at risk for hemolysis.

Nitrofurantoin causes urine to turn brown, but this reaction is harmless. As with any drug that is excreted primarily by the kidneys, nitrofurantoin may accumulate in patients with renal failure. Therefore patients with renal failure are more likely to suffer from significant side effects of nitrofurantoin therapy. Vitamin B deficiency, common in individuals with alcoholism, may also predispose a patient to peripheral neuropathy. Diabetes mellitus, a disease that may cause peripheral neuropathy, may produce added risk of neural complications.

Toxicity

Peripheral neuropathy is one of the most serious toxic effects of nitrofurantoin. If detected early, the condition disappears after discontinuation of the drug. Damage may be permanent if the drug is continued after signs of peripheral neuropathy have developed.

Interactions

To avoid excessive risk of hemolysis, nitrofurantoin should not be used with hemolytic agents. To avoid excessive neurotoxicity, nitrofurantoin should not be combined with neurotoxic medications. If nitrofurantoin is used with probenecid or sulfinpyrazone, the effectiveness of nitrofurantoin may be impaired because these drugs block renal secretion of nitrofurantoin. As a result, lower concentrations of the antibacterial agent are achieved in urine.

NURSING PROCESS OVERVIEW

Sulfonamides, Trimethoprim, and Nitrofurantoin

Refer to Chapter 38 for general guidelines on the nursing process with antibiotic therapy. The additional material in this chapter relates specifically to drugs used mainly to treat urinary tract infections.

Assessment

The drugs described in this chapter are used mainly to treat UTIs. Focus assessment on renal function. Monitor other clinical signs of infection. Include objective data such as blood tests, history of allergies, and mental function.

Nursing Diagnoses

- Potential altered home maintenance management related to the need to increase fluid intake to 1500 ml or more per day
- Potential complication: blood dyscrasias

Patient Outcomes

The patient's infection will resolve without side effects. The patient will increase fluid intake while taking a sulfonamide. The nurse will manage and minimize any blood dyscrasias that develop.

Planning/Implementation

Monitor the progress of treatment for UTIs by assessing clinical signs such as relief of pain and itching and by culturing urine. Ascertain that urine samples are appropriately collected to prevent trivial contamination, which renders the culture results meaningless. Blood tests may be required for patients receiving sulfonamides. Encourage adequate fluid intake to maintain good urine flow. Teach the patient about the signs of blood dyscrasias for those receiving sulfonamides and signs of pulmonary distress and peripheral neuropathy for those receiving nitrofurantoin. These side effects are usually sufficient cause for the physician to discontinue medication.

Evaluation

Ascertain that the patient can explain how to take the prescribed medication and can point out which side effects are sufficient reason to call the physician.

Nursing Implications Summary

Sulfonamides and Trimethoprim

Drug Administration

- Review Nursing Implications Summary in Chapter 38 (p. 469).
- Assess for history of allergy to other sulfonamides, thiazide diuretics, acetazolamide, or oral hypoglycemic agents before administering sulfonamides.
- Inspect for rashes or skin changes and GI tract distress. Monitor temperature.
- Monitor complete blood count (CBC) and differential, platelet count, blood urea nitrogen (BUN) level, serum creatinine level, liver function tests, and urinalysis.
- Topical sulfonamide preparations are used to treat burns (see Table 44-3). Wear sterile gloves when applying medication. The drugs are most effective when the area is cleaned of debris and pus. Dressings are not necessary but may be used. Medicate for pain before redressing the wound. Monitor serum drug and serum electrolyte levels, in addition to blood work noted previously.

Intravenous Trimethoprim and Sulfamethoxazole

- Dilute each 5 ml ampule in 125 ml 5% dextrose in water (D5W). Administer diluted dose over 60 to 90 minutes. Flush tubing well after administration. For patients who must restrict their fluid intake, see the package insert.

Patient and Family Education

- Review Nursing Implications Summary in Chapter 38 (p. 469).
- Review the benefits and possible side effects of drug therapy. Instruct the patient to report fever, sore throat, unexplained bleeding or bruising, malaise, jaundice, rashes, and skin changes.
- Review the patient problem box on urinary tract infections (p. 514). Even if drug is not used to treat UTIs, instruct the patient to increase daily fluid intake to 2500 to 3000 ml/day.
- Inform the patient receiving sulfasalazine that this drug may turn urine or skin a yellow-orange color.
- Instruct the diabetic patient that sulfonamides may produce false-positive results with Benedict's test for urine glucose. Monitor blood glucose.
- Inform the patient taking combination products that contain phenazopyridine that this compound turns urine reddish orange in color and may stain clothing.
- Phenazopyridine dye may produce false results with urine glucose and ketone tests. Inform the diabetic patient about this effect.
- Instruct the diabetic patient not to change insulin dose or diet without discussing this with the physician. Monitor blood glucose level.
- Instruct the patient to take doses with a full (8-ounce) glass of water or other liquid.
- Instruct the patient and family not to give sulfonamide drugs to children younger than 12 years of age unless specifically prescribed for the child by a physician.
- Review the patient problem box on photosensitivity (p. 649) with the patient.
- Caution the patient to avoid driving or operating hazardous equipment until the effects of this medication are known and to report dizziness to the physician.
- Sulfonamides are available for ophthalmic use. See Chapter 5 for a discussion of application of drops and ointment.
- Sulfonamides are available for intravaginal use. Make certain that the patient can apply the ordered dose correctly. (Review the patient problem box on treatment of vaginal infections (p. 539).
- Remind the patient to inform all health care providers of all drugs being used.

Nitrofurantoin

Drug Administration

- See Nursing Implications Summary in Chapter 38 (p. 469).
- Assess for GI tract disturbance, skin changes, and peripheral neuropathy. Assess lung sounds and respiratory rate. Monitor weight.
- Monitor CBC and differential and liver function tests.

Patient and Family Education

- See Nursing Implications Summary in Chapter 38 (p. 469).
- Nitrofurantoin may cause false results with urine glucose tests.
- Instruct the patient to monitor blood glucose. Caution the patient not to change diet or insulin without checking with the physician.
- Review the anticipated benefits and possible side effects of drug therapy with the patient. Instruct the patient to report any new sign or symptom.
- Review the patient problem box on urinary tract infections (p. 514).
- Instruct the patient to take oral doses with meals or a snack to reduce gastric irritation. Warn the patient that oral suspensions may stain teeth. Instruct the patient to dilute doses of suspension with milk, formula, water, or juice before taking.
- Inform the patient that nitrofurantoin may cause urine to turn rusty-yellow to brown.

CRITICAL THINKING

APPLICATION

1. What is the mechanism for the antibacterial effect of sulfonamides?
2. Why are sulfonamides not equally toxic to humans and bacteria?
3. By what routes may sulfonamides be administered?
4. Do sulfonamides enter the cerebrospinal fluid?
5. How are sulfonamides eliminated from the body?
6. What are the major toxic reactions to sulfonamides?
7. Why should patients be cautioned to drink several liters of water each day they receive sulfonamides?
8. What is the mechanism for the antibacterial effect of trimethoprim?
9. Why is trimethoprim not equally toxic to humans and bacteria?
10. Why are trimethoprim and sulfamethoxazole combined to treat UTIs and infections at other sites?
11. Why is nitrofurantoin not effective for systemic infections?
12. By what route is nitrofurantoin administered?
13. What reactions to nitrofurantoin are commonly encountered with short-term therapy?
14. What reactions to nitrofurantoin are associated with long-term therapy?

CRITICAL THINKING

1. What is the purpose of combining sulfonamides with phenazopyridine to treat UTIs? What should you teach patients about this?
2. Develop a nursing plan for a patient receiving one of the drugs discussed in this chapter.

CHAPTER 45

Drugs for Tuberculosis and Other Mycobacterial Infections

OBJECTIVES

After studying this chapter, you should be able to do the following:

- *Explain why therapy of mycobacterial diseases must continue for years.*
- *Describe the use of isoniazid and identify the types of patients most at risk for severe reactions to the drug.*
- *Describe the use of dapsone.*
- *Discuss why drug combinations are commonly used for tuberculosis and leprosy.*
- *Develop a nursing care plan for a patient receiving drug therapy for tuberculosis, leprosy, or* Mycobacterium avium *complex.*

KEY TERMS

dapsone
isoniazid
leprosy
Mycobacterium avium complex (MAC)
rifabutin
rifampin
tuberculosis

CHAPTER OVERVIEW

The acquired immunodeficiency syndrome (AIDS) epidemic has led to a resurgence of interest in mycobacterial diseases. Tuberculosis has once again become a public health problem, especially in urban populations where the incidence of human immunodeficiency virus (HIV) infection and intravenous (IV) drug abuse is high. Other mycobacterial diseases that are insignificant in persons with intact immune systems may add significantly to morbidity and mortality in AIDS patients. For example, patients with AIDS who also have *M. avium* complex face a poor prognosis. In this chapter the clinical features of *Mycobacterium* infections, which make treatment more difficult than that of most other bacterial diseases, are considered. Second, the properties of the drugs used to treat these diseases and the ways they are used are covered.

Therapeutic Rationale: Tuberculosis

Tuberculosis and leprosy are diseases produced by *Mycobacterium* infections. Both diseases have been known since ancient times and are among the earliest examples of diseases that were recognized as infectious. Tuberculosis, or the white plague, was a major cause of death in Europe and the Orient throughout the Middle Ages and until recent times. Leprosy, although less common, was greatly feared because of the disfigurement it caused. This grim picture changed in the early 1940s when the first effective antituberculosis agent, streptomycin, was discovered. Around the same time a sulfone was discovered to be effective in controlling leprosy. With these and more recently discovered agents, both diseases may be treated effectively in many patients.

Tuberculosis is produced by *Mycobacterium tuberculosis* or less commonly by other mycobacteria harbored by cattle or birds. Three features of *M. tuberculosis* are especially important for understanding how disease is produced in humans by these organisms. First, mycobacteria are strict aerobes, which means that they must live in an oxygen-rich environment and may explain why the first site of infection in humans is usually the alveoli in lungs. Second, mycobacteria induce activity of macrophages, causing these cellular immunity factors to phagocytize *M. tuberculosis.* Rather than helping prevent infection, this action actually may enhance survival and spread of the disease-causing organisms because *M. tuberculosis* resists the acids and enzymes that usually destroy bacteria within macrophages. *M. tuberculosis* reproduces within macrophages at a near-normal rate and may be carried by them throughout the body. Third, mycobacteria are slow-growing organisms relative to other bacteria. This slow growth contributes to the difficulty encountered in treating the disease because it is during active growth that an organism is most susceptible to metabolic interference.

Tuberculosis may pass through several phases. The initial or primary infection usually occurs in the lungs as a result of inhaling droplets containing live *M. tuberculosis.* These infective aerosols are generated when a patient with an active infection coughs or sneezes. Once in alveoli, *M. tuberculosis* is phagocytized and begins to multiply. Infected macrophages may remain in the lungs, but many enter the lymphatic system, and a few enter the blood and are carried throughout the body. In response to the increasing number of tubercle bacilli in the lungs, a pneumonia-like condition may develop within a few weeks. This inflammatory response to the infection may continue for a few weeks, but in most people this process is ultimately halted by the delayed immune reaction provoked by the infection. Lesions within the lungs resolve when infective loci become calcified. Living tubercle bacilli no longer appear in sputum at this stage, and the disease is said to be inactive. Living *M. tuberculosis* remain within the body, however, and relapses may occur months or years after the initial infection. When relapse occurs, localized areas again become sites of active multiplication of tubercle bacilli. Local necrosis develops while the cellular immunity factors attempt to isolate the infection. Necrosis may spread as a result of this inflammatory response and may cause large cavities within the lungs or other tissues.

M. tuberculosis, like most bacteria, can acquire resistance to drugs. Development of resistance is common when patients are treated with a single drug. To minimize this complication, multiple drug therapy is used. The rationale for this therapy is simple: when two drugs with different mechanisms of action are administered together, the organism must acquire two independent mutations to become resistant to both drugs. Since mutations are rare, the likelihood of simultaneously acquiring two specific mutations is small. Using three or more drugs lowers the probability of developing resistance even further. The options for treating tuberculosis use three to six drugs initially, with therapy continuing 6 to 24 months (see box, p. 524). Treated patients rapidly cease to be infectious, but chemotherapy must be continued for long periods to eliminate most of the dormant tubercle bacilli.

The properties and uses of antituberculosis agents are considered in the following sections, with the drugs considered in order of their clinical importance.

Therapeutic Agents: Tuberculosis

Primary Drugs for Tuberculosis

Isoniazid

Mechanism of Action and Bacterial Resistance

Isoniazid is a potent inhibitor of mycolic acids involved in cell wall synthesis and also blocks pyridoxine (vitamin B_6) utilization in a number of intracellular enzymes. Isoniazid is bactericidal and affects both intracellular (within macrophages) and extracellular mycobacteria.

Mycobacteria can rapidly acquire resistance to isoniazid. In early trials when isoniazid was used alone to treat active pulmonary tuberculosis, 11% of the patients carried isoniazid-resistant strains at the end of 1 month of therapy. At the end of 3 months, 71% of these patients harbored resistant *Mycobacterium.* Observations such as these have led to the clinical practice of combining isoniazid therapy with one or more drugs.

Isoniazid, at a concentration of 0.2 mg/ml, inhibits the growth of over 90% of *M. tuberculosis* strains. Resistant strains of *M. tuberculosis* may be less pathogenic than sensitive strains. For this reason, isoniazid therapy may be continued even after isoniazid-resistant strains are cultured.

Pharmacokinetics

Isoniazid is well absorbed after oral administration, achieving peak serum levels in 1 to 2 hours. Bactericidal concentrations are found in most tissues, including pleural fluids and caseous exudates surrounding active loci of infection in lungs.

Isoniazid undergoes several metabolic conversions in liver, most resulting in inactive drug, which is excreted primarily by the kidneys. The major metabolite is an acetylated form

TREATMENT REGIMENS FOR TUBERCULOSIS

Patient criteria	Treatment schedule
Option 1 ■ Born in United States ■ Never treated for tuberculosis ■ Low risk of drug-resistant *Mycobacterium*	Isoniazid, rifampin, and pyrazinamide daily for 2 months; then isoniazid and rifampin daily or twice weekly for 4 to 22 months
Option 2 ■ Born in the United States ■ Never treated for tuberculosis ■ Risk of drug-resistant *Mycobacterium*	Isoniazid, rifampin, ethambutol, and pyrazinamide daily for 6 to 24 months
Option 3 ■ Non-HIV patients ■ Isoniazid resistance ≥4% in locality ■ Medications taken under direct observation	Isoniazid, rifampin, pyrazinamide, and streptomycin for 8 weeks; isoniazid and rifampin daily or 2 to 3 times weekly for 16 weeks if organism is susceptible
Option 4 ■ Non-HIV patients ■ Medications taken under direct observation	Isoniazid, rifampin, pyrazinamide, and streptomycin daily for 2 weeks, then twice weekly for 6 weeks; isoniazid and rifampin twice weekly for an additional 16 weeks
Option 5 ■ Non-HIV patients ■ Medications taken under direct observation	Isoniazid, rifampin, pyrazinamide, and streptomycin or ethambutol 3 times weekly for 6 months
Option 6 ■ HIV-infected patients ■ Medications taken under direct observation	Options 3, 4, or 5, but continued for at least 9 months and at least 6 months beyond culture conversion
Option 7 ■ Known drug-resistant *Mycobacterium* ■ Retreatment (received drugs before)	Option 5 plus one or two other drugs to include at least 3 drugs demonstrated effective in culture

of isoniazid. The rate of drug acetylation differs markedly among populations, and two genetically determined types may be distinguished. Rapid acetylators inactivate isoniazid 2 to 3 times as rapidly as slow acetylators. As would be expected, rapid acetylators have lower blood concentrations of active drug than slow acetylators, but both types of patients respond well to standard therapeutic doses given once daily. Increasing the drug dose or frequency of administration in slow acetylators is not wise since these patients tend to be more prone to side effects. Slow acetylators include 45% to 65% of Northern European and African-American or Caucasian populations. Oriental and Eskimo populations contain predominantly rapid acetylators.

Uses

Isoniazid is considered to be the most useful antituberculosis agent. The drug is available as a single agent formulation and in combination with other antituberculosis agents (Table 45-1).

Isoniazid may be used alone for prophylaxis. The drug is prescribed for persons with known exposure to tuberculosis or patients who have recently converted from negative to positive reactions in the skin test for tuberculosis. These people usually have smaller numbers of *Mycobacterium* than would be found in an active, symptomatic case of tuberculosis, and for them the use of isoniazid alone is usually successful.

Adverse Reactions and Contraindications

Isoniazid is relatively nontoxic, but untoward reactions can occur in a small percentage of patients. The most commonly encountered adverse reaction is peripheral neuropathy. Diabetic patients, patients with alcoholism, and malnourished persons are more prone to this complication than the general population. At least some of these reactions are related to low vitamin B_6 levels and may be prevented by taking 5 mg of the vitamin daily. Peripheral neuropathies are more likely to occur in slow acetylators.

TABLE 45-1 Antituberculosis Drugs

GENERIC NAME	TRADE NAME	ADMINISTRATION/DOSAGE	CLINICAL USE
Aminosalicylate sodium	Nemasol† Tubasal	ORAL: *Adults*—5-6 gm every 12 hr. *Children*—50-75 mg/kg every 6 hr, not to exceed 12 gm daily.	Alternate drug. Patients with congestive heart failure may be unable to tolerate sodium load with this drug.
Capreomycin	Capastat*	INTRAMUSCULAR: *Adults*—1 gm daily in single dose. FDA pregnancy category C.	Alternate drug. Patients with hearing impairment, renal function impairment, or muscle weakness may suffer exacerbations of their condition.
Cycloserine	Seromycin	ORAL: *Adults*—250 mg every 12 hr initially, then 250 mg every 6 to 8 hr, up to maximum daily dose of 1 gm. FDA pregnancy category C. *Children*—5-20 mg/kg in divided doses.	Alternate drug. Central nervous system toxicity, including seizures, is more likely in alcoholics or patients with prior seizure disorders.
Ethambutol	Etibi† Myambutol*	ORAL: *Adults*—15-25 mg/kg once daily or 50 mg/kg twice weekly. Single dose should not exceed 2.5 gm. *Children <13 yr*—Should not receive drug.	Primary drug. Patients with reduced renal function require reduced drug doses. Patients with preexisting visual defects may be difficult to evaluate for drug-induced visual changes.
Ethionamide	Trecator SC	ORAL: *Adults*—250 mg every 8-12 hr. *Children*—4-5 mg/kg every 8 hr.	Alternate drug. Patients also receiving cycloserine are at greater risk for seizures.
✚ Isoniazid (INH)	Isotamine† Laniazid Nydrazid	ORAL: *Adults*—300 mg daily maximum. FDA pregnancy category C. *Children*—10-20 mg/kg daily. INTRAMUSCULAR: As for oral.	Primary drug. Older adult patients, alcoholic patients with liver impairment, or patients also receiving rifampin have increased risk of drug-induced hepatitis.
Pyrazinamide	Pyrazinamide* Tebrazid†	ORAL: *Adults*—15-30 mg/kg daily up to 2 gm or 50-70 mg/kg 2 or 3 times weekly. FDA pregnancy category C. *Children*—15-30 mg/kg body weight daily.	Primary drug. Hepatotoxicity; increased blood concentration of uric acid (hyperuricemia).
Rifampin	Rifadin* Rimactane* Rofact†	ORAL: *Adults*—600 mg daily in 1 dose. FDA pregnancy category C. *Children*—10-20 mg/kg up to 600 mg daily. INTRAVENOUS: *Adults*—As for oral.	Primary drug. Patients with prior liver disease and alcoholics are more likely to suffer drug-induced hepatotoxicity. Patients also receiving isoniazid have increased risk of drug-induced hepatitis. Also used as prophylaxis for meningococcal infections.
Rifampin and isoniazid	Rifamate	ORAL: *Adults*—600 mg of rifampin and 300 mg of isoniazid (2 tablets) once daily.	Treatment of pulmonary tuberculosis after dose of separate drugs has been established.
Rifampin, isoniazid, and pyrazinamide	Rifater	ORAL: *Adults*—As for individual components.	Short-course treatment of tuberculosis. This preparation is orphan drug product.
Streptomycin	Streptomycin	INTRAMUSCULAR: *Adults*—1 gm daily for 2-4 mo or longer. Dosage may then be reduced to 1 gm 2 or 3 times weekly. FDA pregnancy category D. *Children and older adult patients*—May require smaller doses.	Primary drug. Patients with renal insufficiency or older adult patients are more prone to accumulate streptomycin and to develop ototoxicity.

*Available in Canada and United States.
†Available in Canada only.

Various other reactions have occasionally been reported with isoniazid, including allergies, blood dyscrasias, gastric distress, and metabolic acidosis.

Toxicity

Hepatotoxicity is the most serious side effect associated with isoniazid. Fatalities resulting from liver failure have occurred even among persons receiving the drug prophylactically. Hepatitis caused by isoniazid is rare among patients younger than 20 years of age and occurs in patients 20 to 34 years of age at a rate of approximately 3 cases per 1000 patients. After age 50, the incidence increases to 23 cases per 1000 patients. Patients also have an increased risk of hepatitis if they are rapid acetylators of isoniazid, if they ingest ethanol daily, or if they also receive the drug rifampin. Liver function should be monitored in all patients receiving isoniazid. Symptoms of hepatitis include anorexia, dark urine, jaundice, nausea, tiredness, or weakness.

Interactions

Isoniazid may enhance metabolism of the antifungal drug ketoconazole and may reduce effectiveness of the agent. In contrast, metabolism of alfentanil, carbamazepine, and phenytoin is inhibited by isoniazid, and serum concentrations of these drugs may increase when isoniazid is given. Isoniazid should never be given with other hepatotoxic drugs because of the greatly increased risk of hepatic failure.

Rifampin

Mechanism of Action and Bacterial Resistance

Rifampin inhibits DNA-dependent RNA polymerase in sensitive organisms. As a result, gene transcription halts, and protein synthesis ceases. Metabolic activity in the bacteria stops, and the bacteria ultimately die or are eliminated by host defenses.

Resistance to rifampin can occur when the drug is used alone against *Mycobacterium*. Resistant strains have an altered DNA-dependent RNA polymerase that is no longer inhibited by the drug. Cross-resistance to other antituberculosis drugs does not occur.

Pharmacokinetics

Rifampin is adequately absorbed orally in the presence or absence of food. Rifampin is a relatively lipid-soluble agent. This property explains why it is found in higher concentrations in body tissues than in serum. Lipid solubility also explains its ability to penetrate white blood cells and to attack *Mycobacterium* living there.

About 40% of a dose of rifampin is excreted in bile, with less in urine. The drug is also deacetylated by the liver to an active metabolite that is excreted via bile into feces.

Uses

Rifampin, originally developed as an antibacterial drug, is now used against *Neisseria meningitidis* and mycobacteria. Rifampin is as potent as isoniazid against mycobacteria and distributes well to many sites where mycobacteria survive. These advantages have made rifampin a primary drug for tuberculosis.

Rifampin is available as a single-ingredient formulation and in fixed combination with other antituberculosis drugs (see Table 45-1).

Adverse Reactions and Contraindications

Rifampin can cause a variety of mild reactions such as gastrointestinal (GI) tract upset and rashes. The drug also turns body fluids such as tears, sweat, saliva, and urine an orange-red color, which might be mistaken for blood. This coloration is harmless.

Liver abnormalities may occur with rifampin. Mild abnormalities in liver function may return to normal without discontinuing the drug, but increases in alkaline phosphatase or the appearance of jaundice signals that the drug should be discontinued.

Intermittent doses of rifampin may cause an immune reaction that is associated with a variety of symptoms. This flu-like syndrome may progress from chills, fever, vomiting, diarrhea, and myalgia to acute renal failure. Deaths have occurred. Since these symptoms occur when therapy is resumed, patients should be advised not to miss doses of rifampin, especially if they are receiving relatively high doses. Some treatment centers have significantly lowered rifampin dosage for intermittent therapeutic programs and have reduced these immune reactions.

Toxicity

Overdoses of rifampin can produce serious reactions including generalized itching, facial edema, and mental changes. Activated charcoal may be used orally as a slurry to remove unabsorbed or recirculated rifampin from the system.

Interactions

Rifampin induces liver enzymes involved in drug and hormone metabolism in humans. This action leads to several drug interactions. Patients receiving coumarin anticoagulants, oral hypoglycemic agents, theophylline, phenytoin, methadone, various antiarrhythmics, verapamil, or digitalis may require adjustment of the dosage of these agents because rifampin induces liver microsomal enzymes that degrade these drugs. Patients receiving oral contraceptives or replacement doses of cortisol may lose the effectiveness of these agents because rifampin accelerates breakdown of the steroids. Patients receiving isoniazid along with rifampin or patients who regularly use alcohol have an increased risk of drug-induced hepatitis.

Pyrazinamide

Mechanism of Action and Bacterial Resistance

Pyrazinamide may be bacteriostatic or bactericidal, depending on the site of infection and the strain of mycobacteria. The mechanism of action or resistance is unknown.

Pharmacokinetics

Pyrazinamide is rapidly and completely absorbed orally. The drug distributes freely to most tissues, including the brain. In the liver, pyrazinamide is converted in part to pyrazinoic acid, which is also active. Renal elimination half-times for these compounds are 10 to 12 hours in normal persons, but 22 to 26 hours when renal function is impaired.

Uses

Pyrazinamide is effective only against mycobacteria and is a primary drug for treatment of tuberculosis (Table 45-1).

Adverse Reactions and Contraindications

Pyrazinamide often causes joint pain, which may arise from hyperuricemia. Rarely, the drug may cause gouty arthritis or jaundice.

There are no contraindications to pyrazinamide, but the drug should be used cautiously in patients with impaired hepatic function or allergies to ethionamide, isoniazid, or niacin.

Toxicity

Doses of 40 to 50 mg/kg daily, if sustained for prolonged periods, may cause hepatotoxicity.

Interactions
Drugs such as allopurinol, colchicine, probenecid, or sulfinpyrazone may be less effective when pyrazinamide is given because pyrazinamide tends to elevate blood levels of uric acid.

Ethambutol
Mechanism of Action and Bacterial Resistance
Ethambutol is most effective against rapidly dividing mycobacteria but the precise antibacterial action is unknown. The drug is bacteriostatic. Resistance to ethambutol develops if the drug is used alone in therapy. Ethambutol does not induce cross-resistance to other antituberculosis agents.

Pharmacokinetics
Ethambutol is well absorbed from the GI tract in the presence or the absence of food. Peak serum concentrations are observed 2 to 4 hours after an oral dose. Ethambutol is less extensively metabolized than isoniazid or rifampin, and up to 50% of the drug excreted in urine is in the unaltered active form. Fecal concentrations of the drug represent unabsorbed material.

Ethambutol has been detected in cerebrospinal fluid after oral therapy, although the levels are below those found in plasma. The drug also concentrates in erythrocytes.

Uses
Ethambutol is a primary antituberculosis drug that is chemically unrelated to other antituberculosis drugs or antibiotics. It is effective only against mycobacteria and no other bacteria, viruses, or fungi. It has become a first-line antituberculosis drug because of its relatively wide spectrum of activity against *Mycobacterium* species and its relatively low toxicity.

Adverse Reactions and Contraindications
Elevated uric acid levels have been reported in patients receiving ethambutol. Gouty arthritis may occur. The drug also causes confusion and headaches, as well as GI tract disturbances.

Other reactions to ethambutol appear rarely. Allergic reactions have occasionally been reported. Peripheral neuritis can occur with higher doses.

Toxicity
A serious adverse reaction to ethambutol is visual disturbance. Some patients report changes in color vision, whereas others suffer a more prominent loss of visual acuity. These signs are cause to terminate ethambutol use. If the drug is discontinued when these visual signs appear, the changes are reversible, although full recovery may take months. These visual changes are caused by optic neuritis and are more common with doses of 25 mg/kg given for 2 months or longer. The drug should not be used in patients with preexisting optic neuritis.

Interactions
Ethambutol has been associated with few significant interactions but should not be used with other neurotoxic drugs.

Streptomycin
Mechanism of Action and Bacterial Resistance
Streptomycin inhibits protein synthesis in sensitive bacteria (see Chapter 43) and in mycobacteria. The drug is highly effective against most types of pathogenic mycobacteria with the exception of *M. avium*. Resistance to streptomycin develops quickly when the drug is used alone.

Pharmacokinetics
Streptomycin is not absorbed orally and must be administered by IM injection for routine clinical use. This property restricts its use to the hospital or to a well-supervised outpatient program.

Streptomycin is well distributed in the body and may be used to treat nonpulmonary tuberculosis. Streptomycin is excreted almost exclusively by renal mechanisms.

Uses
The first antituberculosis drug to be discovered, streptomycin is still a reliable agent for initial therapy in multidrug regimens (see the box on p. 524). It is usually discontinued after the number of infective organisms has been greatly reduced, usually after 2 to 4 months, but other drugs continue.

Adverse Reactions and Contraindications
Streptomycin can produce any reaction seen with other aminoglycoside antibiotics (see Chapter 43). Patients with renal insufficiency, older adult patients, and patients receiving long-term streptomycin therapy are more prone to develop side effects or toxic reactions.

Toxicity
Ototoxicity is the most common reaction in tuberculosis patients. Careful attention to maintaining dosage within safe limits (see Table 45-1) prevents the reaction in most patients.

Interactions
Because streptomycin causes ototoxicity, it should not be combined with other ototoxic drugs such as the diuretic ethacrynic acid. Patients receiving muscle relaxants along with streptomycin may suffer excessive muscle relaxation because streptomycin is a weak neuromuscular blocking agent.

Alternate Drugs for Tuberculosis
Aminosalicylate, capreomycin, cycloserine, ethionamide
Mechanism of Action
Aminosalicylate inhibits folic acid metabolism in mycobacteria. Cycloserine interferes with cell wall biosynthesis. The mechanism of capreomycin and ethionamide are unknown.

Pharmacokinetics
Aminosalicylate, cycloserine, and ethionamide are efficiently absorbed orally, but capreomycin must be given intramuscularly. Distribution is adequate to most tissues, but only cycloserine and ethionamide achieve significant concentrations

in the central nervous system (CNS). Excretion is primarily renal for all four drugs, but hepatic metabolism of ethionamide forms mostly inactive products.

Uses

These drugs are included in multidrug regimens when significant resistance to other drugs is expected.

Adverse Reactions and Contraindications

Most patients receiving aminosalicylate report GI tract irritation, which may be relieved by taking the drug with food or antacids. Allergic symptoms have also been reported, including exfoliative dermatitis and severe organ damage.

Nephrotoxicity is the most common side effect with capreomycin. The characteristic reactions to cycloserine are CNS reactions, including anxiety, confusion, depression, dizziness, irritability, nervousness, mood changes, and thoughts of suicide.

Ethionamide commonly causes anorexia, nausea, vomiting, and a metallic taste in the mouth. The drug also causes orthostatic hypotension. Jaundice, mental changes, or peripheral neuritis are less common.

Toxicity

High doses or prolonged therapy with aminosalicylate may cause crystalluria or changes in thyroid function. High doses of capreomycin increase the risk of ototoxicity or nephrotoxicity. High doses of cycloserine (500 mg or 1 gm daily) increase the risk and severity of CNS reactions. Neurotoxicity from ethionamide may be reduced by giving pyridoxine.

Interactions

Aminobenzoates may block absorption of aminosalicylate. Risk of nephrotoxicity, ototoxicity, and neuromuscular blockade with capreomycin is increased by aminoglycosides or loop diuretics. Use of cycloserine with alcohol or ethionamide increases the risk of seizures.

NURSING PROCESS OVERVIEW

Treatment of Tuberculosis

Assessment

Antituberculosis therapy is used in patients diagnosed with active tuberculosis, those whose tuberculosis skin tests convert from negative to positive, or in some instances in those receiving high doses of adrenocortical steroids. In the latter group of patients the concern is that high doses of steroids will alter the patient's ability to resist infection from tuberculosis or will cause reactivation of earlier tubercular infections. Perform a thorough total assessment, emphasizing subjective complaints, possible history of tuberculosis in the patient and family, and recent activities such as travel or moving that might have influenced exposure to the disease. Tuberculosis can appear in other organs besides the lungs (e.g., tuberculosis meningitis). The focus of the assessment would be different if the patient had a nonpulmonary form of tuberculosis.

Nursing Diagnoses

- Anxiety related to diagnosis and long-term drug therapy
- Potential altered home maintenance management related to lack of knowledge about how to incorporate drug therapy into daily activities

Patient Outcomes

The patient will take medication as ordered, and tuberculosis will resolve. Side effects will be reported early and will be treated, or drug therapy will be modified. The patient will state a decrease in anxiety and will describe the risk, transmission, and course of tuberculosis.

Planning/Implementation

As soon as diagnosis is made, begin patient education. If unsure of the local standards regarding care of tuberculosis patients, contact the local health department or hospital-infection control department. Place hospitalized patients in isolation until no longer infectious. Remember that many tuberculosis patients are diagnosed and treated entirely on an outpatient basis.

Evaluation

Noncompliance is a major cause of treatment failure. Before a patient begins self-management, ascertain that the patient can explain why and how to take the drugs ordered, possible side effects, ways to treat minor side effects such as nausea associated with taking medication, and side effects that require notification of the physician. Verify that the patient can explain when and why to return for evaluation of laboratory work and other patient data. Also check that the patient can demonstrate measures to decrease the possibility of spreading the disease to others. Because exposure to tuberculosis may occur any time the nurse provides care for a patient, nurses should have regular tuberculosis skin tests.

Therapeutic Rationale: Leprosy

Leprosy is currently found primarily in developing countries and is rarely encountered in the United States or Canada. Leprosy is curable with appropriate drug therapy. Patients are usually treated for at least 6 months, and some must be treated for life. Long-term treatment is required because *Mycobacterium leprae,* the causative agent of leprosy, is a slow-growing organism and may remain dormant for long periods in humans.

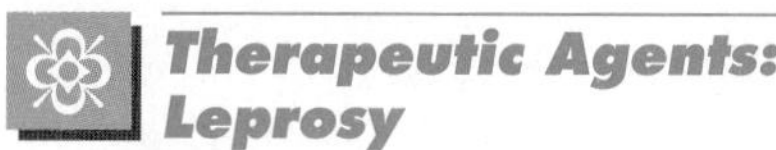

Therapeutic Agents: Leprosy

Primary Drugs for Leprosy

Dapsone

Mechanism of Action and Bacterial Resistance

Dapsone is an antifolate with actions much like sulfonamides. The drug is bacteriostatic, and resistance can develop.

Pharmacokinetics

Dapsone is slowly but nearly completely absorbed orally. The drug distributes well to tissues. Dapsone is metabolized in the liver and excreted in urine. The half-life for elimination of the drug is very long, ranging from 10 to 50 hours.

Uses

Dapsone is the first choice for treating leprosy in the United States. It is also used for dermatitis herpetiformis. Combined with trimethoprim, the drug may be used for prophylaxis of *Pneumocystis carinii* pneumonia in AIDS patients.

Resistance to dapsone appears more frequently today than in previous years; therefore combination therapy has become accepted in the United States. Combining drugs lessens the likelihood that resistance will occur and increases the likelihood that all mycobacteria will be eradicated to achieve a permanent cure. Rifampin or clofazimine is combined with dapsone for the first 6 months to 3 years, after which dapsone alone may be continued for as long as is necessary. A gluten-free diet (see box) may be prescribed for patients with dermatitis herpetiformis. The properties of drugs used to treat leprosy are summarized in Table 45-2.

Adverse Reactions and Contraindications

Dapsone often causes rashes and potentially serious blood dyscrasias such as methemoglobinemia and hemolytic anemia. Symptoms include cyanosis, shortness of breath, bluish coloration to fingernails or lips, anorexia, paleness, or unusual tiredness and weakness. Dapsone is usually avoided if possible in patients with preexisting anemia or glucose-6-phosphate dehydrogenase (G6PD) deficiency, which would increase the risk of hemolytic anemia.

Toxicity

At higher doses, dapsone may cause GI tract disturbances and CNS toxicity, characterized by headache, insomnia, and restlessness. Overdoses can lead to death by methemoglobin accumulation. Treatment may include IV infusion of methylene blue to preserve oxygenation of tissues.

Interactions

Dapsone requires an acidic environment for good oral absorption. Didanosine may block dapsone absorption because preparations of didanosine include strong buffers to reduce gastric acidity. Dapsone should not be combined with other hemolytic agents to avoid unacceptable risk of hemolysis.

Rifampin

Rifampin is used in the recommended combination with dapsone for initial therapy of leprosy in the United States. The properties of rifampin are covered in the section on tuberculosis.

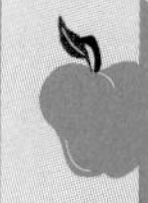

DIETARY CONSIDERATION

Gluten-Free Diet

Gluten, which is found in many grains, is restricted in the management of several health problems, including celiac disease (nontropical sprue) and dermatitis herpetiformis. Food items to avoid on a gluten-free diet include cereal grains such as wheat, barley, oats, rye, bran, graham, millet, wheat germ, bulgur, and malt and products containing these grains. Products made with gluten-containing grains include prepared meats, thickened stew, breaded vegetables, root beer, pasta, macaroni products, gluten stabilizer, brewer's yeast, flour (when the source is not indicated), and pizza.

The following foods are permitted: rice, corn, flours made from soybeans, buckwheat, lima beans, gluten-free wheat starch, cornmeal, and hominy.

- Encourage patients to read food labels carefully.
- Refer patients as needed to the dietitian.

TABLE 45-2 Drugs to Treat Leprosy

GENERIC NAME	TRADE NAME	ADMINISTRATION/DOSAGE	CLINICAL USE
Dapsone	Avlosulfon† Dapsone*	ORAL: *Adults*—100 mg daily for 4 yr to life, with rifampin for first 6-36 mo. FDA pregnancy category C. *Children*—1.4 mg/kg daily.	Primary therapy.
Clofazimine	Lamprene	ORAL: *Adults*—50-100 mg daily for 4 yr to life, with rifampin for first 6-36 mo. FDA pregnancy category C.	Alternate or combination therapy. GI distress; discoloration of the skin is an expected, reversible side effect.

*Available in Canada and United States.
†Available in Canada only.

Alternative Drugs for Leprosy

Clofazimine, ethionamide, thalidomide

The primary drug used to treat leprosy is the sulfone dapsone, but alternatives are now available. Clofazimine has a different mechanism of action from dapsone, and strains of *M. leprae* that acquire resistance to dapsone remain sensitive to clofazimine. The antituberculosis drugs rifampin and more rarely ethionamide have also been used to treat leprosy. Thalidomide is an orphan drug (Chapter 3) that may sometimes be used for leprosy.

NURSING PROCESS OVERVIEW

Treatment of Leprosy

Assessment

In the United States the diagnosis of leprosy is unusual. Perform a thorough total assessment, with special emphasis on subjective and objective deviations from normal.

Nursing Diagnoses

- Anxiety related to diagnosis and long-term drug therapy
- Potential complication: depression related to change in skin color related to drug side effect

Patient Outcomes

The patient will state a decrease in anxiety. The patient will take the drug therapy as ordered. If clofazimine is prescribed, the patient will report the development of depression if it occurs, and symptoms will be managed or drug therapy will be changed.

Planning/Implementation

The diagnosis of leprosy causes a great deal of fear and anxiety in patients. Refer the patient to appropriate agencies for education and support and begin patient and family education. Appropriate agencies include the local health department and the Centers for Disease Control and Prevention in Atlanta. Continue regular total patient assessment, with a focus on identifying possible toxic and side effects of the drugs prescribed.

Evaluation

Therapy for leprosy often continues for years. Before discharging patients, ascertain that they can explain why and how to take the drugs prescribed, possible side effects, side effects that require notification of the physician, and possible ways to treat more common side effects. Any additional measures that may be prescribed related to the stage of the disease as it was diagnosed should be discussed. Report the diagnosis of leprosy to the local health department for family follow-up.

Therapeutic Rationale: Mycobacterium avium Complex

Patients in the latter stages of AIDS are increasingly debilitated from infections not seen in persons with intact immune systems. ***Mycobacterium avium* complex** (MAC) is one of those infections. *Mycobacterium avium* and *Mycobacterium intracellulare* are the causative organisms. This infection will occur in most, if not all, AIDS patients as the disease progresses. MAC causes affected patients to require prolonged nursing care and medical support.

Therapeutic Agents: Mycobacterium avium Complex

Rifabutin

Mechanism of Action and Bacterial Resistance

Rifabutin has a mechanism similar to rifampin against most bacteria, but the mechanism against *M. avium* and *M. intracellulare* has not been established. Cross-resistance can develop with rifampin.

Pharmacokinetics

Rifabutin is a highly lipophilic drug that is adequately absorbed orally and distributes well to tissues, including the brain. Elimination is mostly by hepatic metabolism to inactive products that appear in feces and urine.

Uses

Rifabutin is used only to prevent MAC in patients with advanced HIV disease. The drug is given for life.

Adverse Reactions and Contraindications

Rifabutin commonly causes skin rashes, nausea, and vomiting. The drug also produces a red discoloration of body fluids like urine, tears, sweat, and saliva; this effect is harmless.

Rifabutin is avoided in patients with active tuberculosis because single-drug therapy is likely to cause development of resistance of *M. tuberculosis* to rifampin, one of the primary drugs for treating tuberculosis.

Toxicity

Overdoses of rifabutin may cause uveitis, with loss of vision and pain in the eye.

Interactions

Rifabutin may decrease plasma concentrations of zidovudine, but clinical trials have not consistently shown this effect.

Clarithromycin

Clarithromycin, a macrolide covered in Chapter 41, is active against MAC; because resistance develops easily, clarithromycin is best used in combinations.

NURSING PROCESS OVERVIEW

Treatment of *Mycobacterium avium* Complex

Assessment

Assess vital signs. Assess weight and history of weight loss, persistent fever, diarrhea, and night sweats. Assess hemoglobin and hematocrit and alkaline-25-phosphatase. If the patient has AIDS, obtain a history of AIDS progression. Monitor CD4 cell count and culture reports. Assess the patient for activity level, general sense of well-being, and other subjective symptoms.

Nursing Diagnoses

- Potential complication: septicemia

Patient Outcomes

The patient will report subjective improvement. The nurse will manage and minimize complications of septicemia.

Planning/Implementation

The clinical picture may vary from a patient mildly ill to a patient critically ill. After assessing the patient, determine the priorities for the patient. Emphasize the importance of taking all medications as prescribed. Work with the dietitian to increase nutritional intake. Continue to monitor vital signs, intake and output, and laboratory work. Patients with MAC may be severely debilitated. Work with the health care team to develop a long-range plan to provide comfort and physical care.

Evaluation

The goal is to treat the infection so it resolves. In fact, the patient's general condition may make cure impossible. Provide physical and emotional support to patient and family. Success may be in the form of slowing deterioration and helping the patient and family cope with the symptoms and physical care.

NURSING IMPLICATIONS SUMMARY

General Guidelines: Patient With Tuberculosis or Leprosy

- Provide emotional support for the patient and the family when a diagnosis of tuberculosis or leprosy is made. Both diseases may be associated with patient fears and misunderstandings. Inform the patient and family about the diseases, their spread and control, and about drug therapy.
- Review anticipated benefits and possible side effects associated with drug therapy.
- Emphasize the importance of long-term therapy for best effect, even if the patient feels subjectively better.
- Encourage the patient to return as scheduled for follow-up appointments. Blood work must be monitored to rule out side effects.
- Refer the patient to the local health department for teaching and for follow-up.
- Emphasize the importance of taking drugs on a regular basis. Review guidelines for missed doses, which are to be taken as soon as remembered unless shortly before the next dose. Inform the patient not to double up for missed doses.
- Health care personnel should obtain a routine annual tuberculosis screening test.
- Instruct the patient to inform all health care providers of all drugs being taken.
- Some of these drugs are contraindicated during pregnancy or breastfeeding. Advise female patients to consult with their physicians before getting pregnant, if possible.
- Instruct patients taking combination drugs (e.g., Rifamate, which is a combination of rifampin and isoniazid) about each of the drugs in the combination.

Aminosalicylate

Drug Administration/Patient and Family Education

- See the general guidelines for the patient with tuberculosis or leprosy.
- Instruct the patient to take oral doses with meals or a snack to lessen gastric irritation. Provide positive reinforcement. This drug is difficult to take. A 5 gm dose requires ten 500 mg tablets.
- Instruct the patient to discard discolored tablets and obtain a fresh supply. Aminosalicylates deteriorate rapidly. Caution the patient against storing this drug in the bathroom, in damp areas, or near the kitchen sink. Instruct the patient to observe expiration dates.
- Instruct the patient to prevent crystalluria by maintaining a fluid intake of 2000 to 2500 ml/day.
- Instruct the patient not to take aminosalicylates within 6 hours of doses of rifampin.
- Warn diabetic patients that aminosalicylates may cause false urine glucose results. Do not change diet or insulin dose without consulting the physician. Monitor blood glucose level if possible.

Capreomycin

Drug Administration/Patient and Family Education

- Review the general guidelines for the patient with tuberculosis or leprosy.
- Capreomycin is for intramuscular (IM) administration only. Reconstitute as directed on label. If for home management, instruct the patient in proper administration technique.

Continued.

Nursing Implications Summary—cont'd

- Give cautiously with other drugs known to cause renal impairment or ototoxicity. Examples include aminoglycosides, furosemide, and cisplatin.
- Monitor renal function including blood urea nitrogen (BUN) level and serum creatinine level.
- Assess for ototoxicity including hearing acuity and balance.
- Instruct the patient to avoid driving or operating hazardous equipment if drowsiness or dizziness occurs and to notify the physician if these symptoms occur.

Cycloserine

Drug Administration/Patient and Family Education

- Review the general guidelines for the patient with tuberculosis or leprosy.
- Assess for signs of depression including malaise, lack of interest in personal appearance, insomnia, withdrawal, and weight gain or loss. Review these symptoms with patient and family. Instruct the patient to notify the physician if depression or suicidal thoughts develop.
- Monitor serum drug levels if available.
- Instruct the patient to take doses after meals if GI tract irritation develops.
- Instruct the patient to avoid driving or operating hazardous equipment if drowsiness or dizziness occurs and to notify the physician if these symptoms occur.
- Instruct the patient to avoid alcoholic beverages while taking cycloserine.

Ethambutol

Drug Administration

- See the general guidelines for the patient with tuberculosis or leprosy and the Nursing Implications Summary in Chapter 38 (p. 469).
- Assess for visual changes (blurred vision, loss of vision, red-green color blindness, eye pain) and peripheral neuropathy.
- Monitor complete blood count (CBC), and white blood cell (WBC) differential, and uric acid levels.

Patient and Family Education

- Review the general guidelines for the patient with tuberculosis or leprosy.
- Instruct the patient to take oral doses with meals or a snack to lessen gastric irritation. Inform the patient that taking a single daily dose maintains the serum drug level better than two or more smaller daily doses.
- Instruct the patient to report changes in vision to the physician.
- Instruct the patient to avoid driving or operating hazardous equipment until the effects of this medication are known; it may cause drowsiness or dizziness.

Ethionamide

Drug Administration/Patient and Family Education

- See the general guidelines for the patient with tuberculosis or leprosy and the Nursing Implications Summary in Chapter 38 (p. 469).
- Instruct the patient to take doses with or after meals if gastric irritation develops.
- Assess for peripheral neuropathy including numbness, tingling, paresthesia, and feelings of heaviness of the fingers, arms, and legs.
- Pyridoxine may also be prescribed with this drug. Emphasize the importance of taking both drugs. See the dietary consideration box on vitamins on p. 215.
- Instruct the patient to report changes in vision to the physician.
- Instruct the patient to avoid driving or operating hazardous equipment until the effects of ethionamide are known; it may cause drowsiness or dizziness.
- Assess for depression including malaise, lack of interest in personal appearance, insomnia, withdrawal, and weight gain or loss.

Isoniazid

Drug Administration

- Review Nursing Implications Summary in Chapter 38 (p. 469).
- Assess for peripheral neuropathy including numbness, tingling, paresthesia, and feelings of heaviness of the fingers, arms, and legs; review these symptoms with the patient.
- Monitor CBC and WBC differential, platelet count, liver function tests, and blood glucose level.
- Warn the patient that IM injection may produce pain at the injection site.

Patient and Family Education

- Review the general guidelines for the patient with tuberculosis or leprosy.
- Instruct the patient to report any new sign or symptom.
- Emphasize to the patient the importance of taking pyridoxine if prescribed. Review the dietary consideration box on vitamins (p. 215) for information about dietary sources of pyridoxine.
- Instruct the patient to avoid the use of alcohol while taking isoniazid and to notify the physician if any signs of hepatitis develop: anorexia, nausea, vomiting, excessive fatigue, jaundice, dark urine, malaise.

NURSING IMPLICATIONS SUMMARY—cont'd

- Instruct the patient to take oral doses with meals to avoid gastric irritation.
- See the patient problem box on dry mouth (p. 300).
- Caution the patient to avoid driving or operating hazardous equipment if dizziness, ataxia, tinnitus, or vision changes occur and to notify the physician if these symptoms do occur.
- Ingestion of fish or cheese while taking isoniazid may cause a reaction. Symptoms include headache, flushing, nausea, vomiting, tachycardia, itching skin, and light-headedness. Instruct the patient to limit or avoid cheese or fish and to notify the physician if these symptoms develop.
- Inform diabetic patients that isoniazid may cause false results in urine glucose tests. Instruct the diabetic patient not to change diet or insulin dose without contacting the physician. Monitor blood glucose level if possible.
- Instruct the patient not to take aluminum-containing antacids within 1 hour of taking isoniazid.

Pyrazinamide

Drug Administration/Patient and Family Education

- Review Nursing Implications Summary in Chapter 38 (p. 469) and the general guidelines for the patient with tuberculosis or leprosy.
- Monitor liver function tests and serum uric acid level.
- Warn diabetic patients that pyrazinamide may alter results of urine ketone tests; monitor blood sugar level.

Rifampin

Drug Administration

- See the general guidelines for the patient with tuberculosis or leprosy and the Nursing Implications Summary in Chapter 38 (p. 469).
- Assess CBC and WBC differential, platelet count, and liver function tests.

Intravenous Rifampin

- Dilute 600 mg in 10 ml sterile water for injection and swirl gently to dissolve the drug. Further dilute the solution in 500 ml 5% dextrose in water (D5W). Administer dose over 3 hours.

Patient and Family Education

- Review the general guidelines for the patient with tuberculosis or leprosy.
- Instruct the patient to take rifampin on an empty stomach 1 hour before or 2 hours after meals with a full (8-ounce) glass of water. Instruct the patient to take rifampin with meals if gastric irritation is severe when taken on an empty stomach.
- Instruct the patient not to take rifampin within 6 hours of taking a dose of aminosalicylate.
- Warn the patient that body fluids (tears, sweat, feces, and urine) may turn orange-red while undergoing rifampin therapy. Soft contact lenses may be permanently stained.
- It is especially important not to miss rifampin doses. Encourage the patient to take rifampin regularly, as prescribed, for best results.
- Instruct the patient to avoid driving or operating hazardous equipment if drowsiness, dizziness, or visual changes occur and to notify the physician if these symptoms do occur.
- Instruct the patient to avoid alcoholic beverages while taking rifampin and to report signs of possible hepatitis to the physician: excessive fatigue, anorexia, nausea, vomiting, jaundice, or dark urine.
- Oral contraceptives containing estrogen may not be effective in patients who are also taking rifampin. Instruct the patient to use another means of birth control while taking rifampin and to consult the physician.
- Inform the patient that capsules of rifampin may be opened and the contents may be mixed with applesauce or jelly for ease in taking.
- A suspension can also be made; the patient should consult the pharmacist.

Streptomycin

- Streptomycin is discussed in Chapter 43.

Dapsone

Drug Administration/Patient and Family Education

- See the general guidelines for the patient with tuberculosis or leprosy.
- Assess for skin changes and peripheral neuropathy.
- Monitor CBC and WBC differential, platelet count, BUN level, and serum creatinine level. Monitor urinalysis.
- Instruct the patient to take ordered doses with meals or a snack to lessen gastric irritation.
- Instruct the patient to take once-daily doses in the morning if insomnia occurs.
- Instruct the patient to avoid driving or operating hazardous equipment if dizziness or light-headedness occurs and to notify the physician if these symptoms do occur.
- Patients with dermatitis herpetiformis may be prescribed a gluten-free diet (see the dietary consideration box on gluten-free diet on p. 529).

Clofazimine

Drug Administration/Patient and Family Education

- Instruct the patient to take oral doses with meals or a snack to lessen gastric irritation.

Continued.

NURSING IMPLICATIONS SUMMARY—cont'd

- Warn the patient that clofazimine may cause red-to-brown pigmentation of the skin and eyes. Assess for discoloration. If skin changes produce depression or extreme sadness, notify the physician.
- See the patient problem box on photosensitivity on p. 649.
- Clofazimine may discolor feces, sputum, sweat, tears, and urine. It may also produce black, tarry, or bloody stools; instruct the patient to notify the physician if these symptoms occur.
- Instruct the patient to use lotion or skin cream to treat dry, scaly skin.
- Instruct the patient to avoid driving or operating hazardous equipment if drowsiness or dizziness occurs and to notify the physician if these symptoms occur.

Rifabutin

Drug Administration/Patient and Family Education

- Review the general guidelines for patients with tuberculosis or leprosy.
- Monitor WBC count and platelet count.
- Warn the patient that body fluids (tears, sweat, feces, and urine) may turn orange-red while undergoing rifabutin therapy. Soft contact lenses may be permanently stained.
- Instruct the patient to take doses on an empty stomach unless gastric irritation develops, then take with meals or snack.
- Inform the patient that capsules may be opened and contents mixed with applesauce for ease in swallowing.

CRITICAL THINKING

APPLICATION

1. What properties of mycobacteria make controlling tuberculosis more difficult than many other bacterial diseases?
2. During what phase of tuberculosis is the disease contagious?
3. What is the duration of therapy for tuberculosis?
4. What is the mechanism of action of isoniazid?
5. What is the outcome of using isoniazid alone to treat active tuberculosis?
6. When is isoniazid used alone?
7. How is isoniazid administered?
8. What is the fate of isoniazid in the body?
9. What toxicity is associated with isoniazid? What types of patients are most at risk?
10. What is the mechanism of action of rifampin?
11. How is rifampin administered in tuberculosis therapy?
12. What is the route of administration of pyrazinamide?
13. What side effect is characteristic of pyrazinamide?
14. How is ethambutol administered in tuberculosis therapy?
15. What toxicity is associated with ethambutol?
16. How is streptomycin administered?
17. What toxicity is associated with streptomycin?
18. Why are aminosalicylate, capreomycin, cycloserine, and ethionamide classified as alternate drugs in tuberculosis therapy?
19. What drugs are most useful in treating leprosy?
20. How long must therapy continue for control of leprosy?
21. What drugs are most useful for control of MAC?
22. How long must therapy continue for MAC?

CRITICAL THINKING

1. Why is tuberculosis usually treated by multiple drug therapy? Name the implications for patient assessment and teaching.
2. How would you advise a patient receiving multidrug therapy for tuberculosis who confided that he had omitted his rifampin dose for the last week?
3. Develop a nursing care plan for a patient with tuberculosis, leprosy, or MAC.

CHAPTER 46

Antifungal Agents

OBJECTIVES

After studying this chapter, you should be able to do the following:

- *Explain the mechanism of action of amphotericin B and azole antifungal drugs.*
- *Discuss the dose-limiting toxicity of amphotericin B.*
- *Explain why drugs that are too toxic for systemic use may be used for local fungal infections.*
- *Develop a nursing care plan for the patient receiving one of the parenteral, oral, or topical antifungal agents discussed in this chapter.*

KEY TERMS

azole antifungal agents
dermatophytes
ergosterol
fungi
opportunistic infection
polyene antifungal agents
systemic fungal infections

CHAPTER OVERVIEW

Fungal diseases range from mild infections in localized areas of the skin to grave systemic infections. Diseases of various types may be produced by a wide range of fungi, and to a great extent the seriousness of the infection is determined by the nature of the infective organism and the immune status of the host. In this chapter some of the more common and the more serious fungal diseases are examined, and the drugs used to control these specific infections are considered.

Therapeutic Rationale: Fungal Diseases

Although the **fungi** that cause disease in humans are single-celled organisms, they are eucaryotes (see Chapter 38) and therefore resemble human cells more than bacteria in their biochemical properties. These biochemical similarities to human cells present therapeutic problems. For instance, none of the antibiotics that inhibit bacterial protein synthesis affect that process in fungi because fungal ribosomes resemble those in humans and are sensitive to the same drugs. Therefore selective toxicity cannot be achieved by this mechanism. Moreover, fungal cells do not contain a peptidoglycan cell wall, which renders them resistant to all antibiotics that block peptidoglycan synthesis (e.g., penicillins). For these reasons the antimicrobial agents discussed in previous chapters cannot be used to treat fungal diseases.

Design of new antifungal agents is limited by the small number of known biochemical differences between fungal and mammalian cells. The only systematically exploited difference lies in the outer membranes of the cells. Human cells contain cholesterol in their membranes, whereas those of fungi contain **ergosterol.** This feature of membrane structure is the basis of action of polyene antifungal agents that bind to ergosterol, and the azole antifungal agents that inhibit the synthesis of ergosterol.

Fungal cells possess many antigens, which ultimately provoke host immune responses. Most fungal infections resolve in this way, many times without the host ever being aware of an active disease. This pattern is especially common with fungal diseases spread by breathing in spores from contaminated soil. Examples of diseases of this type are histoplasmosis, blastomycosis, cryptococcosis, coccidioidomycosis, and aspergillosis. Several of these diseases are concentrated in specific geographic areas. For example, coccidioidomycosis is most common, or endemic, in the southernmost portions of California, Nevada, Utah, Arizona, New Mexico, and Texas, whereas histoplasmosis is endemic in the states bordering the Mississippi and Ohio rivers. Blastomycosis is endemic in isolated areas along the Mississippi and Ohio Rivers, around the Great Lakes, along the St. Lawrence River, and in the Carolinas.

Some fungal diseases are spread by contact with soil contaminated with bird droppings. Birds are not necessarily affected by these diseases, but they frequently carry the organisms. Cryptococcosis frequently follows exposure to high concentrations of pigeon droppings. Histoplasmosis is associated with avian excreta such as chicken or starling droppings or bat guano. Although pulmonary forms of these diseases are usually mild and limited by effective development of immunity in the victim, in rare cases the fungus may become disseminated and invade other body tissues. A notorious example is the yeast *Cryptococcus neoformans,* which can cause meningitis, pulmonary disease, and infections at many other sites. The disseminated, or systemic, fungal diseases are most likely to develop in patients with immune systems depressed by disease or drug therapy, especially with glucocorticoids or immunosuppressant antineoplastic agents.

The yeast *Candida* may cause a range of infections from serious systemic disease to annoying mucous membrane infections. Since *Candida* is normally found on the skin and mucous membranes of healthy persons, the growth of *Candida* to cause disease usually represents an **opportunistic infection.** *Candida* infections are therefore most common in persons receiving broad-spectrum antibacterial drugs such as tetracyclines (see Chapter 38) or in persons with suppressed immune systems. *Candida* infections are very common in patients with acquired immunodeficiency syndrome (AIDS).

Therapeutic Agents: Drugs for Systemic Fungal Infections

Systemic fungal infections pertain to the whole body. Table 46-1 summarizes drugs used to treat systemic fungal infections.

Polyenes

✣ Amphotericin B

Mechanism of Action

Amphotericin B is the only polyene antifungal agent used for systemic fungal infections. **Polyene antifungal agents** have a greater affinity for ergosterol than for cholesterol and therefore react with ergosterol from fungal cell membranes. This action destroys the integrity of the cell membrane and the cell dies as its cytoplasmic components are lost. This membrane-disruptive effect is not entirely selective, and some of the cholesterol-containing membranes of mammalian cells are also damaged.

Pharmacokinetics

Amphotericin B must be administered intravenously, although the drug irritates vascular tissue and frequently causes phlebitis. This lipid-soluble agent is administered as a colloidal suspension stabilized with small amounts of the detergent desoxycholate. Amphotericin B must be infused at a concentration of less than 0.1 mg/ml in a 5% dextrose solution. Higher drug concentrations cause precipitation of the drug in the intravenous (IV) solution and endanger the patient.

Amphotericin B has a high affinity for lipids and thus tends to bind to tissues rather than remain in blood. The elimination half-life of the drug is about 12 hours after a single IV dose. During long-term therapy, only a fraction of the daily dose can be recovered in urine or feces. The unrecovered drug is held in tissues and continues to appear in urine for long periods after therapy is halted. The tissue-binding properties and the relative water insolubility of amphotericin B prevent the drug from entering body fluids efficiently. For this reason concentrations of the drug in the cerebrospinal fluid or in ocular fluid may be too low to effectively eliminate infections at those sites. To overcome this problem, amphotericin B may be injected intrathecally (into the cerebrospinal fluid) to treat meningitis.

TABLE 46-1 Drugs to Treat Systemic Fungal Infections

GENERIC NAME	TRADE NAME	ADMINISTRATION/DOSAGE	CLINICAL USE
✤ Amphotericin B	Fungizone*	INTRAVENOUS: *Adults*—0.25-0.7 mg/kg/day infused at 0.1 mg/ml in 5% dextrose over 6 hr. Daily dose should not exceed 50 mg. Total drug course usually <4 gm. FDA pregnancy category B. *Children*—0.25 mg/kg/day infused as for adults.	Disseminated, symptomatic fungal disease caused by *Histoplasma, Blastomyces, Coccidioides, Cryptococcus, Aspergillus, Candida,* and others.
Fluconazole	Diflucan*	ORAL, INTRAVENOUS: *Adults*—100-400 mg once daily. FDA pregnancy category C.	Meningitis caused by *C. neoformans;* systemic, esophageal, or oropharyngeal candidiasis.
Flucytosine	Ancobon Ancotil†	ORAL: *Adults and children*—12.5-37.5 mg/kg every 6 hr. Lower drug doses are required when renal function is impaired. FDA pregnancy category C.	Disseminated fungal infections caused by sensitive *Candida* strains, cryptococcal meningitis, and other infections; usually combined with amphotericin B.
Itraconazole	Sporanox*	ORAL: *Adult*—200 mg daily. FDA pregnancy category C.	Aspergillosis, blastomycosis, and histoplasmosis.
✤ Ketoconazole	Nizoral*	ORAL: *Adults*—200-400 mg once daily. FDA pregnancy category C. *Children >2 yr*—3.3-10 mg/kg once daily.	Disseminated infections caused by *Histoplasma, Paracoccidioides,* and *Candida.* Also used topically (see Table 46-2).
Miconazole	Monistat IV	INTRAVENOUS: *Adults*—0.2-3.6 gm, divided into 3 equal doses, depending on causative organism. FDA pregnancy category C. *Children*—Total daily dose 20-40 mg/kg with no single infusion exceeding 15 mg/kg.	Alternate drug for severe systemic infections caused by susceptible fungi. Also used topically (see Table 46-2).

*Available in Canada and United States.
†Available in Canada only.

Uses

Amphotericin B can be used to treat many different fungal diseases, including those caused by *Histoplasma, Blastomyces, Cryptococcus,* and *Aspergillus* organisms. Amphotericin B may also treat systemic *Candida* and *Coccidioides* infections. Topical use of amphotericin B is not recommended because other topical agents such as ciclopirox, clotrimazole, econazole, and miconazole are more effective.

Adverse Reactions and Contraindications

Most patients start on low doses of amphotericin B, and the dosage is increased as tolerance to ensuing side effects develops. Fever, headache, nausea, and vomiting may occur after the first few injections, but these side effects usually subside as therapy continues. Renal damage progresses with length of therapy and may become irreversible when total doses of amphotericin B approach 4 gm. Anemia also develops with time, as do electrolyte disturbances including acidosis and hypokalemia (low blood potassium).

There are no absolute contraindications to the use of amphotericin B for serious systemic fungal disease, but in patients with renal disease the risk of increased nephrotoxicity is significant.

Toxicity

Amphotericin B therapy must be continued for long periods to attempt to cure disseminated fungal disease. No firm guidelines for therapy exist, although physicians try to limit the total drug dose to less than 4 gm. Even with doses approaching this limit, cures are not always obtained. For many patients therapy must be discontinued early because of toxic effects of the drug.

Amphotericin B has been experimentally infused encapsulated in liposomes (lipid vesicles). Patients whose therapy was ineffective with standard preparations responded to the liposomal form of the drug. This experimental method of administration may also reduce the drug's toxicity. Development of this technique continues.

Interactions

Amphotericin B is incompatible in solution with sodium chloride and with benzyl alcohol. These compounds cause precipitation of the colloidal suspension of amphotericin B used for IV administration.

Because amphotericin B has significant toxicity on its own, it can also cause serious interactions with other agents. Bone marrow depressants and radiation therapy may increase the risk of anemia with amphotericin B. Nephrotoxic drugs increase the risk of renal damage with amphotericin B.

Amphotericin B tends to cause hypokalemia. This action increases the risk of toxicity with digitalis glycosides and with potassium-depleting diuretics. The risk of serious hypokalemia is also increased with corticosteroid use.

Antimetabolite

Flucytosine

Mechanism of Action

Flucytosine is a pyrimidine analogue that is converted to the cytotoxic agent 5-fluorouracil in sensitive fungi. Because this metabolite is not freely formed in humans, a degree of selective toxicity is achieved.

Pharmacokinetics

Flucytosine is a water-soluble drug that is well absorbed from the gastrointestinal (GI) tract and well distributed into body fluids. Drug concentration in cerebrospinal fluid may be 50% to 70% of serum levels, in contrast to amphotericin B, for which cerebrospinal fluid levels are less than 5% of serum levels. The primary organ of excretion for flucytosine is the kidney. More than 90% of an oral dose can be recovered intact in urine, in which concentrations of the drug are high. The elimination half-life is about 6 hours.

Uses

A relatively narrow range of fungi are sensitive to flucytosine, including *Cryptococcus, Candida,* and a few other rarely encountered pathogenic fungi. Intrinsic resistance to flucytosine may exist in a significant number of clinically encountered *Candida* strains, and resistance to the drug may be acquired by *Cryptococcus* during therapy. This pattern of resistance has limited the drug's usefulness.

Adverse Reactions and Contraindications

Flucytosine therapy is usually continued for several weeks to months. Nausea and diarrhea appear in roughly one fourth of patients. Blood dyscrasias such as anemia and thrombocytopenia (unusual bruising or bleeding) and transient liver abnormalities have been reported.

The only absolute contraindication to the use of flucytosine is a documented allergy to the drug, but the drug should be used cautiously in patients with impairment of renal function or with bone marrow depression caused by drugs or disease.

Toxicity

High serum concentrations of flucytosine increase the risk of hematologic toxicity. Hemodialysis may be required to remove the drug from the system, especially in patients with poor renal function.

Interactions

Because of its effects on the bone marrow, flucytosine should not be used with other agents that also depress bone marrow function.

Flucytosine is often combined with amphotericin B for treatment of disseminated fungal disease. The rationale for combining these drugs for serious infections is twofold: the combination allows the dose of amphotericin B to be lowered somewhat, thereby reducing toxicity, and resistance to flucytosine is minimized by combination chemotherapy.

Azole Antifungal Agents

Fluconazole, itraconazole, ✣ ketoconazole, miconazole

Mechanism of Action

Azole antifungals inhibit synthesis of ergosterol. As a result, the function of fungal cell membranes are impaired. Development of invasive hyphae by *Candida* cells may also be retarded, enhancing the ability of the host immune system to eliminate fungal cells.

Pharmacokinetics

Ketoconazole is adequately absorbed orally, but bioavailability depends on sufficient stomach acidity. Ketoconazole is best absorbed on an empty stomach and should not be administered within 2 hours of administration of antacids or H_2 histamine receptor blocking drugs such as cimetidine. Ketoconazole is not well distributed to all tissues and is especially low in cerebrospinal fluid. Elimination is primarily by the liver, which forms inactive metabolites and excretes the drug into bile.

Fluconazole is well absorbed orally, with a bioavailability of about 90%; absorption does not depend on stomach acidity as much as with ketoconazole. Fluconazole is well distributed to most body tissues, including the cerebrospinal fluid. Little hepatic metabolism of fluconazole occurs, and most of the drug is excreted unchanged in urine. The half-life of the drug in patients with normal renal function is 30 hours.

Itraconazole is relatively lipid soluble and is absorbed after oral administration. Food increases absorption of oral doses of this drug. Itraconazole concentrates in tissues such as skin and lung but does not enter the vitreous humor or the cerebrospinal fluid adequately to treat infections at those sites. Itraconazole metabolites are formed in the liver and excreted in urine.

Miconazole must be administered intravenously in systemic infections. The drug enters vitreous humor but poorly penetrates into the cerebrospinal fluid; therefore intrathecal injections must be used for meningitis.

Uses

Azole antifungal agents are used to treat a variety of fungal infections. Fluconazole is indicated for cryptococcal meningitis and for systemic, esophageal, or oropharyngeal candidiasis. Ketoconazole is used against *Histoplasma* and *Paracoccidioides.* It may also be effective in certain patients with disseminated candidiasis and blastomycosis. Itraconazole is indicated for aspergillosis, blastomycosis, and histoplasmosis. Miconazole may be used against systemic coccidioidomycosis, cryptococcosis, and candidiasis but is primarily used as a topical agent. Clotrimazole, econazole, oxiconazole, sulconazole, and terconazole are used topically for a variety of infections including vaginal infections caused by *Candida* (see box, p. 539) and tinea (see Table 46-2).

Adverse Reactions and Contraindications

Ketoconazole is relatively nontoxic for many patients. Nausea and pruritus occur in less than 5% of treated patients.

PATIENT PROBLEM

Vaginal Infections

THE PROBLEM

The dark, moist environment of the vagina is prone to infection by a variety of organisms. Some chronic health problems such as diabetes mellitus increase susceptibility to vaginal infection. Treatment with some groups of drugs such as antibiotics may increase susceptibility to fungal superinfection. Finally, some invading organisms are passed as venereal diseases. Treatment of vaginal infection may be messy and difficult. It is difficult to reach all mucosal surfaces. Also, since the woman is upright during most of the day, medications drain out because of gravity.

SOLUTIONS

- Use prescribed agents for the full course of therapy; do not stop when symptoms disappear.
- Do not wear tampons during therapy. Wear sanitary napkins to prevent staining of clothing.
- Continue therapy through the menstrual period.
- Wash hands carefully before and after using prescribed medications.
- Use once-daily doses of vaginal medication in the evening, before retiring. Insert vaginal suppository, ointment, or cream just before going to bed to allow the medication to remain in the vaginal area as long as possible.
- If douching is prescribed, wash douche equipment carefully after each use and dry it.
- Depending on the infecting agent, it may be necessary to treat the sexual partner also; consult the physician.
- Usually, avoid sexual intercourse during the course of therapy. If not possible, the sexual partner should wear a condom.

TO HELP PREVENT VAGINAL INFECTION

- Wear clean underwear daily, preferably of cotton material. Synthetic fabrics do not allow air to circulate as well, and thus they keep the vaginal area more moist than normal. Avoid pantyhose for the same reason.
- Wipe from front to back after voiding or defecating.
- Do not douche unless prescribed by the physician. Do not douche between doses of vaginal medications.
- Avoid bubble baths and soaps that may irritate vaginal mucosa. Wash the vaginal area gently and rinse soap off well. Some women may need to wash with water only if soap is irritating to the vaginal area.
- Use water-soluble lubricants, if needed, in the vagina. Do not use oil-based products such as petroleum jelly.

Dizziness, nervousness, and headache have been reported less frequently.

Fluconazole may cause side effects in up to 13% of treated patients. GI tract disturbances such as nausea or diarrhea and headaches are the most common complaints. Thrombocytopenia, which produces unusual bleeding or bruising, and hepatotoxicity are more serious rare effects. Rarely, patients may develop dangerous allergic reactions such as Stevens-Johnson syndrome or exfoliative skin disorders.

Miconazole may produce rashes, itching, redness at the injection site, or phlebitis. Reversible platelet dysfunction, anemia, and thrombocytopenia may also occur with systemic administration.

Itraconazole appears to cause less hepatotoxicity than does ketoconazole and alters platelet function less than miconazole. All azole antifungals are capable of inducing allergic reactions.

Toxicity

Hepatotoxicity is an idiosyncratic reaction that occurs in about 1 in 10,000 patients receiving ketoconazole. High doses of ketoconazole may inhibit testosterone and cortisol synthesis. This inhibition may produce gynecomastia (excessive development of mammary glands), which has been noted in about 10% of males receiving ketoconazole.

Interactions

Azole antifungal agents are subject to a wide array of drug interactions. Pharmacokinetic interactions include those that block absorption of the azoles. For example, antacids or H_2 receptor blockers that raise gastric pH lower absorption of ketoconazole and itraconazole because these azoles require strong acidity for absorption. Didanosine also lowers absorption of azoles because didanosine preparations contain buffers to raise gastric pH.

Another potentially serious pharmacokinetic interaction arises because the azole antifungals, and especially ketoconazole and itraconazole, can inhibit hepatic metabolism of a variety of drugs. This action leads to a rise in blood concentrations of drugs like the antihistamines astemizole and terfenadine, cyclosporine, digoxin, phenytoin, warfarin, and the sulfonylurea antidiabetic medications. Increased blood levels of these agents can produce serious or even life-threatening side effects.

A few drugs lower the blood concentrations of the azole antifungal agents and cause failure of therapy. Examples include carbamazepine and the antituberculosis drugs rifampin and isoniazid.

Ketoconazole has been linked to hepatotoxic reactions when given with other hepatotoxic agents or when used in patients suffering from chronic alcohol abuse. Concurrent use of ketoconazole and alcohol has caused a disulfiram-like reaction (facial flushing, tightness in the chest, difficulty breathing).

Sterol Biosynthesis Inhibitor

Terbinafine

Mechanism of Action

Terbinafine inhibits ergosterol biosynthesis by a different mechanism than the azole antifungal agents. Terbinafine disrupts fungal cell membranes and kills affected fungi.

Pharmacokinetics

Terbinafine is well absorbed orally with or without food. The drug is highly lipophilic and therefore distributes well to tissues and especially to skin, hair follicles, and nail beds. Terbinafine is readily metabolized in liver to inactive forms that are eliminated primarily in urine. In spite of relatively effective elimination processes, terbinafine persists in tissues for prolonged periods as a result of its high lipid solubility.

Uses

Terbinafine is used for dermatophytic infections, including those of the scalp and nails.

Adverse Reactions and Contraindications

Terbinafine commonly causes anorexia, diarrhea, nausea, stomach pain, or vomiting. The drug may also change the sensation of taste. Allergies are possible and rarely these may be severe, including life-threatening conditions such as Stevens-Johnson syndrome.

There are no absolute contraindications to the use of terbinafine, but the drug should be used cautiously, if at all, in patients with a history of alcoholism or hepatic impairment. These patients may be at increased risk of terbinafine-induced hepatotoxicity. Patients with renal impairment may require reduced doses of the drug.

Toxicity

Terbinafine rarely may cause hepatitis or toxic epidermal necrolysis.

Interactions

Terbinafine should not be used along with other hepatotoxic drugs. Therefore patients receiving terbinafine should avoid the use of alcohol or high doses of vitamin A or niacin. Other drugs to avoid include steroids, sulfonamides, phenothiazines, or zidovudine.

Terbinafine is metabolized by hepatic cytochrome P-450 systems. Therefore drugs that affect this system can affect clearance of terbinafine. Barbiturates, griseofulvin, phenytoin, and rifampin are examples of drugs that induce P-450, which increases metabolism of terbinafine and lowers blood levels of the drug.

In contrast, cimetidine, clarithromycin, estrogens, erythromycins, azole antifungals, fluoroquinolones, and isoniazid inhibit P-450 and therefore block metabolism of terbinafine. The result is higher concentrations of terbinafine, which may increase risk of toxicity.

Therapeutic Rationale: Topical Fungal Infections

Dermatophytes are fungi whose growth is almost always restricted to the skin of humans. These fungi cause the annoying infections commonly known as *ringworm* and *athlete's foot,* as well as several others. This group of infections is frequently referred to as *tinea.* Many of the drugs used topically are not absorbed extensively through the skin. Therefore more toxic agents may be used than can be used systemically, and selective toxicity is achieved against many dermatophytes.

Therapeutic Agents: Drugs to Treat Topical Fungal Infections

In this section drugs that are used to treat topical fungal infections, or those restricted to skin, mucous membranes, or GI tract, are considered. The properties of specific drugs are listed in Table 46-2. Most of these agents are used strictly locally, being applied at the site of infection. For example, tolnaftate is used to treat simple cases of tinea, but the effectiveness is limited by the accessibility of locally applied drug to the infective fungi. For this reason tinea infections around nails and heavily keratinized skin are hard to eradicate.

Griseofulvin

Griseofulvin is effective against several types of dermatophytic infections, including infections of the scalp. It is used orally rather than topically. The usefulness of this drug as an oral agent depends on its ability to localize in skin after oral absorption. Those skin cells containing high concentrations of griseofulvin are resistant to infection by dermatophytes. Ultimately, all infected cells will be lost through the natural sloughing off of skin cells, and the disease will be cured. This process takes a considerable period of time, and accordingly griseofulvin therapy may need to be continued for several weeks or months, depending on the site and the severity of the infection.

Nystatin

Nystatin is sometimes given orally to treat intestinal fungal infections. This treatment may be considered topical since nystatin is not absorbed orally and is retained in the intestine. Nystatin is also used to treat vaginal infections such as those caused by *Candida.* This treatment is also topical since the drug is administered intravaginally and is not systemically absorbed. Nystatin is too toxic to be used for systemic infections.

TABLE 46-2 Drugs to Treat Topical Fungal Infections

GENERIC NAME	TRADE NAME	ADMINISTRATION/DOSAGE	CAUTIONS
Carbol-fuchsin (Castellani's paint)	Castel Plus	TOPICAL: *Adults and children*—For athlete's foot and ringworm, solution swabbed over affected area 1-3 times daily.	Contact sensitivity may cause reactions; poisonous if ingested.
Ciclopirox olamine	Loprox*	TOPICAL: *Adults*—For tinea infections, including tinea versicolor and cutaneous candidiasis, cream or lotion applied twice daily. FDA pregnancy category B.	Avoid contact with eyes. Do not use occlusive dressing.
Clioquinol (iodochlor-hydroxyquin)	Vioform	TOPICAL: *Adults and children*—For localized dermatophytoses, 3% cream or ointment applied 2 or 3 times daily.	Causes false-positive ferric chloride test for phenylketonuria (PKU); can alter iodine content of blood
Clotrimazole	Canesten† Lotrimin Mycelex Canesten† Gyne-Lotrimin Myclo† Mycelex	TOPICAL: *Adults and children*—For tinea and cutaneous *Candida*, 1% cream, lotion, or solution applied twice daily. FDA pregnancy category B. INTRAVAGINAL: *Adults*—For vulvovaginal candidiasis, tablets or creams containing 100 mg inserted once daily. FDA pregnancy category B. ORAL: *Adults and children >4 yr*—For oropharyngeal candidiasis, 10 mg lozenge dissolved in mouth 5 times daily. FDA pregnancy category C.	Avoid contacting eyes with lotions, creams, and solutions.
Econazole	Ecostatin† Spectazole	TOPICAL: *Adults and children*—For mucocutaneous *Candida* or tinea, 1% cream applied to skin 2 times daily. FDA pregnancy category C.	Avoid eyes; do not use occlusive dressings.
Gentian violet	Genapax	INTRAVAGINAL: *Adults*—For vaginal candidiasis, one tampon (Genapax) inserted once or twice daily for 12 days. FDA pregnancy category C. TOPICAL: *Adult, child*—For candidiasis, apply 1 or 2% solution 2 or 3 times daily for 3 days.	This dye stains skin and clothing.
Griseofulvin	Fulvicin* Grifulvin Grisactin Grisovin†	ORAL: *Adults*—For tinea infections with exception of tinea versicolor, 500 mg microcrystalline form in single or divided dose. Avoid during pregnancy. *Children*—5-10 mg/kg daily.	Headache, GI disturbances, neuritis, allergies, and hepatotoxicity may occur. Warfarin anticoagulant activity blocked. Barbiturates decrease griseofulvin activity.
Haloprogin	Halotex	TOPICAL: *Adults and children*—For tinea and other superficial fungal infections, 1% cream or solution applied twice daily. FDA pregnancy category B.	Local tissue irritation may occur; avoid contact with eyes.
✤ Ketoconazole	Nizoral	TOPICAL: *Adults and children*—For tinea and cutaneous *Candida*, 2% cream applied once daily or shampoo used every 4 days for dandruff. FDA pregnancy category C.	Avoid contact with eyes.
Miconazole nitrate	Micatin Monistat-Derm Monistat*	TOPICAL: *Adults and children*—For dermatophytoses, 2% cream, lotion, or aerosol applied twice daily. INTRAVAGINAL: *Adults*—For vaginal candidiasis, 1% cream, tampon, or suppositories applied once daily.	Local tissue irritation occurs; avoid contact with eyes.
Naftifine	Naftin	TOPICAL: *Adults and children*—For tinea, 1% cream or gel applied to skin twice daily. FDA pregnancy category B.	Local irritation may occur. Avoid contact with eyes or mucous membranes.
Natamycin	Natacyn	OPHTHALMIC: *Adults and children*—For fungal blepharitis, conjunctivitis, or keratitis, 5% ophthalmic suspension, 1 drop every 2-6 hr.	Eye irritation may occur with this chemical relative of amphotericin B.
Nystatin	Mycostatin* Nadostine† Nilstat* Nystex	ORAL: *Adults and children*—For oropharyngeal *Candida* infections, 0.5-1 million U 3 times daily. *Infants*—0.1-0.2 million U 4 times daily.	Nausea, vomiting, or diarrhea may occur. Drug is not absorbed from intestinal tract.
		TOPICAL: *Adults and children*—For *Candida* infections of skin, ointments, creams, and powder (0.1 million U/gm) applied twice daily.	Irritation of skin may occur.
		INTRAVAGINAL: *Adults*—For *Candida* infections of vagina, cream or tablets, 0.1-0.2 million U daily.	Irritation is rare.

*Available in Canada and United States.
†Available in Canada only.

TABLE 46-2 Drugs to Treat Topical Fungal Infections—cont'd

GENERIC NAME	TRADE NAME	ADMINISTRATION/DOSAGE	CAUTIONS
Oxiconazole	Oxistat	TOPICAL: *Adults and children*—For tinea infections, 1% cream or lotion once or twice daily. FDA pregnancy category B.	Rash or burning may occur.
Sulconazole	Exelderm	TOPICAL: *Adults*—For tinea infection, 1% cream or solution applied once or twice daily.	Solution is not appropriate for athlete's foot.
Terbinafine	Lamisil	TOPICAL: *Adults*—For tinea infections, 1% cream applied twice daily.	Rarely causes irritation or sensitization.
Terconazole	Terazol	VAGINAL: *Adults*—For *Candida* vulvovaginal, 5 gm 0.4% cream or 80 mg suppository applied once daily. FDA pregnancy category C.	Vaginal burning may occur.
Tolnaftate	Aftate Tinactin*	TOPICAL: *Adults and children*—For tinea infections, 1% cream, gel, solution, powder, or aerosol applied twice daily.	Rarely causes irritation or sensitization. Avoid eyes.

NURSING PROCESS OVERVIEW

Fungal Infections

Assessment

Fungal infections are relatively common and can occur in patients of any age. Perform a thorough total assessment, focusing on the specific subjective complaints or objective signs that indicate possible fungal infection. Include as part of the history recent use of drugs that may alter the patient's immune response and measures the patient has tried for eradication of the problem. Patients most likely to have fungal infections include those receiving cancer chemotherapy, immunotherapy, antibiotic therapy, or drugs that alter the normal pH of areas such as the vagina; those receiving nutritional support via peripheral or central venous catheters; patients with AIDS; and those taking high doses of adrenocortical steroids.

Nursing Diagnoses

- Potential altered comfort: nausea and vomiting as a side effect of drug therapy
- Potential complication: renal damage and failure

Patient Outcomes

The patient will not experience nausea and vomiting caused by antifungal drug therapy. The nurse will manage and minimize complications related to renal failure.

Planning/Implementation

Teach the patient about the drugs prescribed, the infection, and possible ways to limit the spread of the infection and to prevent its recurrence. Treatment of systemic fungal infections is more serious. Monitor the vital signs and appropriate laboratory work to evaluate possible side effects.

Evaluation

Before discharge, ascertain that the patient can explain why the drug is being used, how it should be used and under what circumstances, what to do if side effects should occur, and which side effects require notification of the physician.

NURSING IMPLICATIONS SUMMARY

Amphotericin B

Drug Administration

- Assess for side effects such as nausea, vomiting, chills, phlebitis, headache, anemia, and electrolyte imbalances.
- Monitor temperature, vital signs, intake and output, and weight. Monitor blood glucose levels.
- Monitor complete blood count (CBC) and differential, platelet count, and serum creatinine, blood urea nitrogen (BUN), and serum electrolyte levels.
- Use an infusion monitoring device to assist in regulating the rate. Too rapid infusion may be associated with cardiac toxicity.
- To prevent side effects, corticosteroids may be administered before or during therapy or may be added to the infusion.
- If ordered, administer antiemetics 30 minutes before starting the infusion to help prevent nausea and vomiting.
- If ordered, administer acetaminophen before or during infusion to treat fever or headache. Codeine or other analgesics may also be used to treat headache.
- Other drugs may be administered to prevent or treat side effects. Heparin may be added to infusions to help prevent thrombophlebitis; IV meperidine may be used to treat rigors (shaking chill); mannitol may be administered before and after amphotericin B to reduce nephrotoxic effects; a potassium-sparing diuretic may be administered to limit hypokalemia; and diphenhydramine may be administered to prevent chills.
- Disagreement exists about the need to cover the tubing and fluid reservoir containing amphotericin B. Follow agency custom; most agencies still cover the bag with a plastic or paper bag.
- Keep siderails up and call bell within easy reach. Do not leave the patient unattended for long periods.
- Use of IV filters is controversial. If an IV filter is used, it must be at least 1 micron in diameter.
- Prepare IV doses as directed in the package insert. Dissolve doses in sterile water with no bacteriostatic agent. Further dilute to the desired volume in 5% dextrose in water (D5W); no other diluent may be used. Do not administer other IV medications via the amphotericin B line without flushing well before and after the dose with D5W. If other IV medications are to be administered during amphotericin B infusion, start and maintain a separate IV access line.
- The diluted drug is a suspension. Gently agitate the bag or bottle regularly during the infusion to promote uniform dilution.
- If the course of therapy is interrupted for more than a few days, it may be necessary to resume therapy with low doses and increase the dose gradually to the desired dose.
- In addition to IV administration, amphotericin B may be administered via intracavitary instillation, intrathecal administration, or bladder irrigation; see the package insert.

Patient and Family Education

- Review anticipated benefits and possible side effects of drug therapy with the patient. The patient may require not only teaching but also continued emotional support since IV therapy is continued for weeks to months. Some patients are suitable candidates for home therapy. Assess the patient and consult the physician. Refer home therapy patients to a community-based nursing care agency.
- Instruct the patient to report any new sign or symptom.
- Provide instruction on dietary sources of sodium, potassium, and iron as indicated.
- Warn the patient to avoid driving or operating hazardous equipment if visual changes occur and to notify the physician if these changes do occur.
- Remind the patient to inform all health care providers of all drugs being used.
- Side effects with topical preparations are uncommon. Instruct the patient not to cover affected areas with an occlusive dressing. Instruct the patient to use topical forms regularly, as prescribed. Intermittent use may cause the fungal infection to return. The cream form may stain skin. Fabric discoloration from lotion or cream can be removed with soap and water. Fabric discoloration from ointment can be removed with cleaning fluid.

Flucytosine

Drug Administration

- Inspect the patient for bruising, bleeding, or other signs and symptoms of blood dyscrasias. Assess for GI tract side effects. Monitor weight.
- Monitor BUN and serum creatinine levels, CBC and differential, platelet count, and liver function tests.
- Check stools for blood and guaiac regularly.

Patient and Family Education

- Review the anticipated benefits and possible side effects of drug therapy with the patient. Instruct the patient to report any new sign or symptom.
- Provide emotional support as needed; weeks to months of therapy may be required for adequate treatment.
- Instruct the patient to take oral doses with meals or a snack over a 15-minute period to lessen gastric irritation.
- Warn the patient to avoid driving or operating hazardous equipment if vertigo or sleepiness occurs and to notify the physician if these symptoms do occur.
- See the patient problem box on photosensitivity (p. 649).

Ketoconazole and Itraconazole

Drug Administration

- Monitor for side effects such as central nervous system (CNS) effects and GI tract distress.
- Monitor liver function tests.
- A potentially fatal drug interaction exists between ketoconazole or itraconazole and astemizole or terfenadine

Continued.

NURSING IMPLICATIONS SUMMARY—cont'd

(see Interactions). Inform all health care providers of all drugs being used.

Patient and Family Education

- Review anticipated benefits and possible side effects of drug therapy with the patient. Instruct the patient to report any new sign or symptom.
- Warn the patient to avoid driving or operating hazardous equipment if dizziness or lethargy develops and to notify the physician if these symptoms occur.
- Instruct the patient not to take H_2 receptor blocking drugs (e.g., cimetidine, ranitidine), omeprazole, or antacids within 2 hours of ketoconazole or itraconazole doses.
- Instruct the patient to avoid alcoholic beverages while taking either ketoconazole or itraconazole.
- If photophobia develops (sensitivity of the eyes to light), instruct the patient to wear sunglasses and avoid bright lights and sunlight.
- For the patient using the oral liquid form: use the calibrated measuring device provided by the pharmacist for measuring doses.
- Absorption of ketoconazole or itraconazole requires an acid pH in the stomach. For patients with achlorhydria, the physician may recommend that the patient dissolve the dose in cola or seltzer water before taking the dose that the patient dissolve each dose in 4 ml of 0.2N HCl solution. Instruct the patient to use a straw to avoid contact with the teeth and to follow the dose with another half glass of water. Consult the pharmacist and physician as needed.

Fluconazole

Drug Administration

- Monitor BUN level, serum creatinine level, and liver function tests.
- Monitor for side effects including exfoliative skin disorders, hepatotoxicity, thrombocytopenia, GI tract distress, and headache.

Intravenous Fluconazole

- Fluconazole is prepacked in a ready-to-use form. Administer at a rate of 200 mg or less over 1 hour.

Patient and Family Education

- Review the anticipated benefits and possible side effects of drug therapy with the patient. Instruct the patient to report any new sign or symptom.
- Instruct the patient to avoid alcoholic beverages while taking fluconazole.
- Review the patient problem box on bleeding tendencies (p. 586).

Miconazole

Drug Administration

- Perform neurologic assessment regularly. Monitor vital signs and weight. Inspect injection site for phlebitis and pruritus.
- Monitor CBC and serum electrolyte level.

Intravenous Miconazole

- Dilute 200 mg in 200 ml of normal saline or D5W. Administer each 200 mg over 2 hours. Monitor vital signs with IV doses and do not administer too rapidly.

Patient and Family Education

- Review the anticipated benefits and possible side effects of drug therapy with the patient. Instruct the patient to report any new sign or symptom. Provide emotional support as needed since therapy may be required for weeks to months.

Terbinafine

Patient and Family Education

- Instruct the patient to take doses with meals or on an empty stomach.
- Emphasize the importance of taking the drug for the full course of therapy, as prescribed, for best effect. Weeks of therapy may be required to treat specific fungal infections.
- Instruct the patient to avoid alcoholic beverages while taking this drug.
- There are many significant drug interactions with terbinafine. Remind the patient to keep all health care providers informed of all drugs being used.
- Instruct the patient to read drug labels and orders carefully and to not confuse terbinafine with terbutaline or terfenadine.

Topical Antifungal Agents

Patient and Family Education

- Instruct the patient that for best effect tropical antifungal agents must be used regularly, as prescribed. Instruct the patient to contact the physician if redness, itching, discharge, or other problems develop while using a prescribed topical antifungal agent.
- With ointments and creams, instruct the patient to apply the dose as directed and gently rub into the area. The patient should not cover the area with a dressing unless instructed to do so by the physician.
- Instruct the patient to shake aerosol powders or solutions well before using, hold the spray opening 6 to 10 inches away from the area to be treated, and spray well. Caution the patient not to inhale powder or solution and to avoid the eyes.
- Instruct the patient to sprinkle powder forms liberally on the affected area such as the toes and feet.

NURSING IMPLICATIONS SUMMARY—cont'd

- When treating toes and feet, the patient should make certain the drug reaches the area between toes and on the bottom of the feet. The patient should sprinkle or spray onto socks or in shoes if directed to do so by the physician.
- For vaginal forms, see the patient problem box on vaginal infections (p. 539). Instruct the patient to insert a medicated tampon (e.g., miconazole) at bedtime and remove it in the morning.
- Azole vaginal forms may cause the latex in condoms, diaphragms, or cervical caps to weaken and break, so these forms of birth control will be unreliable; use an alternate method of birth control. Drugs in this group include butoconazole, clotrimazole, econazole, miconazole, terconazole, and tioconazole.
- Remind women that no medications, even topical ones, should be used during pregnancy or lactation without prior consultation with the physician.
- For tinea cruris (jock itch): Instruct the patient to avoid underwear that is tight or made of material that does not breathe well, wear loose cotton underwear, and change it daily. Instruct the patient to use an absorbent powder or antifungal powder but to not apply powder at the same time as antifungal creams, lotions, or solutions.
- For tinea pedis (athlete's foot): Instruct the patient to carefully dry feet, especially between toes, after bathing or showering. Instruct the patient to avoid wearing socks made of materials that hold moisture and to wear clean cotton socks and change at least daily. Instruct the patient to wear sandals or well-ventilated shoes with air holes and to rotate shoes so they can dry thoroughly between wearings. Instruct the patient to use an absorbent powder or antifungal powder but to not apply powder at the same time as antifungal creams, lotions, or solutions.

Nystatin

Drug Administration/Patient and Family Education

- Side effects are uncommon. Instruct the patient to report any new sign or symptom.
- With nystatin suspension, the drug may be dispensed with a dropper; use this to measure the dose. Place half the dose in one side of the mouth and the other half in the other side. Instruct the patient to hold, swish, and gargle for as long as possible before swallowing.
- With nystatin powder, add the dose (about ⅛ teaspoon) to 4 to 5 ounces of water and stir well. Instruct the patient to take a mouthful of the suspension and to hold, swish, and gargle for as long as possible before swallowing. The patient should repeat the process with another mouthful until the entire dose has been taken.
- Instruct the patient to allow the lozenge form to dissolve slowly in the mouth, which may take 15 to 30 minutes. The patient should swallow the saliva as needed but should not chew or break the lozenge. Warn the patient not to allow children younger than 5 years to have lozenges since they may choke on them.

CRITICAL THINKING

APPLICATION

1. Why are fungi resistant to drugs such as penicillins and tetracyclines?
2. What types of infections are commonly caused by *Candida?* What are signs and symptoms of these infections?
3. What are dermatophytes?
4. What is the mechanism of action for the polyene antifungal agent amphotericin B?
5. By what route is amphotericin B administered? What are nursing care activities associated with administration of amphotericin B?
6. What types of fungal infections are properly treated with amphotericin B?
7. How does the lipid solubility of amphotericin B influence its tissue distribution?
8. What are the characteristic toxic reactions associated with systemic use of amphotericin B?
9. What is the mechanism of action of flucytosine?
10. May flucytosine be used as an oral agent?
11. What is the main route of excretion of flucytosine?
12. What toxic reactions occur with the use of flucytosine?
13. Why are flucytosine and amphotericin B sometimes combined for antifungal therapy?
14. What is the mechanism of action of azole antifungal agents?
15. By what route are azole antifungal agents administered?
16. What side effects may occur with azole antifungal agents? How should you assess for these?
17. What is the mechanism of action of griseofulvin?
18. Is therapy with griseofulvin long or short term?

CRITICAL THINKING

1. A colleague places a filter in the IV line through which a patient is to receive amphotericin B. What should you do?

CHAPTER 47

Antiviral Agents

OBJECTIVES

After studying this chapter, you should be able to do the following:

- *Explain why acyclovir is selectively active against virus-infected cells.*
- *Discuss the basis of anti-HIV activity of zidovudine.*
- *Develop a nursing care plan for a patient receiving an antiviral agent.*
- *Summarize the points that the nurse teach the patient about topical treatment of genital herpes.*

KEY TERMS

acquired immunodeficiency syndrome (AIDS)
host specific
human immunodeficiency virus (HIV)
interferons
retroviruses
viruses

CHAPTER OVERVIEW

Viral diseases are among the most common infections in humans, but the prevention and treatment of these diseases has lagged far behind the ability to control bacterial infections. This chapter discusses the properties of viral diseases that make them difficult to treat and the mechanisms of action of antiviral drugs that have been developed.

Therapeutic Rationale: Viral Diseases

Viruses cause a wide variety of clinical disease, both chronic and acute. Acute illnesses include the common cold, influenza, and various other respiratory tract infections. These illnesses frequently resolve quickly and leave no latent infections or sequelae. Chronic infections are those in which the disease runs a protracted course with long periods of remission interspersed with reappearance of the disease. An example is herpes infections in which active disease alternates with latent periods during which the virus remains dormant.

Many viruses attack specific cell types within the host. For example, several viruses affect only the tissues of the respiratory tract. For these diseases, symptoms develop as the infection spreads from the original site to immediately adjacent cells. The severity of symptoms depends in part on how many host cells are affected. Other viruses have affinity for nervous tissues. For example, herpesvirus resides in nerves during the long latent periods of herpetic diseases. The rabies virus also specifically attacks nervous tissue, traveling along nerves and eventually invading the brain, causing the characteristic symptoms of rabies.

For some viruses the cell specificity is known to arise from interactions with receptors found on only one cell type. For example, **human immunodeficiency virus (HIV)** causes a brief acute illness that may be unnoticed, but chronic infection of lymphoid tissue is established. HIV at this site infects T lymphocytes as they move in and out of the lymphoid tissue. HIV attacks those cells specifically because the virus attaches to the T-lymphocyte cell surface receptor, CD4. This infection has such devastating effects because the cells attacked by HIV are critical for immune function. The progressive destruction of immune function caused by HIV ultimately produces **acquired immunodeficiency syndrome (AIDS)**.

Some viruses have the potential for more generalized invasion of tissues throughout the body by a mechanism called *viremic spread.* Viremic spread is detailed in Table 47-1. Clinical symptoms do not appear in most diseases spread in this manner until very late in the disease, when the secondary viremia occurs. At this stage, most viral infections are self-limiting and resolve even without medical attention. However, certain viruses can attack the brain after the secondary viremia. An example is the poliovirus, which causes relatively mild disease during the respiratory phase and secondary viremic stage but becomes life-threatening when it invades the central nervous system (CNS). Even with polioviruses, invasion of the CNS is rare, and most infections end with the secondary viremia.

With infections caused by bacteria, symptoms occur during the period of most active bacterial reproduction; therefore therapy can begin relatively early in the disease and may include bactericidal agents. With viral diseases, this is not the case. Symptoms occur after most of the virus particles have reproduced, and therapy would be instituted late in the disease. Furthermore, the antiviral drugs currently available inhibit reproduction but do not eradicate latent viruses.

TABLE 47-1 Viremic Spread in Mammalian Body

SITE	SYMPTOMS
Primary Site of Infection	
For example, lung in pox, measles, and mumps; GI tract in polio	First wave of replication produces no symptoms.
Bloodstream	
Viruses free or bound to blood cells	Primary viremia produces no symptoms.
Secondary Sites of Infection	
For example, liver, spleen, bone marrow, or lymphoid tissue	Second wave of replication may produce mild symptoms for some viral diseases.
Bloodstream	
Viruses free or bound to blood cells	Secondary viremia may produce fever, rashes, and other symptoms whose severity depends on number of viruses released.
Central Nervous System	Although this system is rarely involved, infections at this site are serious.

Therapeutic Agents: Vaccines for Viral Diseases

The external surface of viruses contains antigenic substances that promote antibody production. These humoral factors limit the spread of many types of viral disease and allow the body to eliminate the virus. Infected cells are also changed sufficiently in many viral diseases so that these cells are also eliminated.

Many viral diseases are best controlled by inducing antibodies in healthy individuals before exposure to the viral disease. This prophylaxis is successful for many diseases (see Chapter 34) but not for all. The most successful immunization programs are for those viral diseases in which few pathogenic strains exist and with which antigenic properties do not change. The vaccine for poliovirus fits these criteria. The oral vaccine is directed against the three major viral strains; these strains have not shifted in antigenic properties. In contrast, immunization against rhinoviruses, which cause respiratory disease, has not been feasible because there are approximately 100 strains of rhinoviruses and each induces a separate antibody in humans; unfortunately, each antibody protects against only one of the strains.

Influenza viruses illustrate another difficulty in immunizing against viral diseases. With influenza the antigenic properties shift every few years so that those persons who were immunized naturally or artificially against the prevalent strain of the virus are unprotected when the new viral type arises. Therefore influenza immunizations are effective only for a specific viral strain and should not be expected to carry over when new strains appear. Rapid antigenic shift is also a characteristic of HIV.

In addition to the traditional immune responses to viral infection, the body has another mechanism by which it limits the spread of viral diseases. This mechanism is the production of glycoproteins called **interferons** (see Chapter 33). Interferons, released from virus-infected cells, alter the metabolism of uninfected cells to prevent the virus from attacking these new cells. This mechanism prevents the spread of the viral disease to new cells and allows the immune system to eliminate the viruses and infected cells.

Interferons are **host specific** and not virus specific. This property means that interferons induce resistance to several types of viruses at once. Host specificity of interferons determines that only human interferon prevents viral disease in humans. Human interferons are produced as drugs by recombinant DNA technology or are harvested from pooled human leukocytes.

Interferons have a few specific indications for viral diseases. They are also used as anticancer agents because they limit cell proliferation (see Chapter 50).

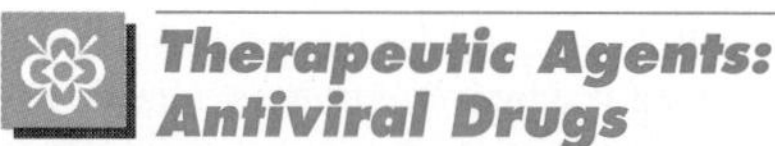

Therapeutic Agents: Antiviral Drugs

Drugs for Systemic Viral Infections

Because viral reproduction is carried out mostly by host cell enzymes and ribosomes, targets for selective toxicity are difficult to identify. Basic research has revealed that some key viral enzymes are required for reproduction inside the host cells. These viral enzymes or processes that occur only in virus-infected cells have been the most successful points for attack with selectively toxic agents.

Development of anti-HIV drugs is proceeding rapidly. A variety of approaches are being explored, including blocking specific absorption of the virus to its target cells, inhibiting virus-specific proteases required for maturation of the virus, and developing new inhibitors of the virus-specific enzyme, reverse transcriptase. The status of these investigational agents changes very quickly. Current information can be obtained by consultation with the AIDS section at the National Institutes of Health or by consulting current publications devoted to AIDS research. Drugs approved as of December 1995 are included in this section. Table 47-2 summarizes specific antiviral drugs used for systemic viral infections.

Acyclovir

Mechanism of Action

Acyclovir is one of the most highly selective of the antiviral agents. The drug is activated by viral thymidine kinase, an enzyme found only in virus-infected cells. The activated form of the drug preferentially and irreversibly inhibits the viral DNA polymerase present in infected cells, effectively halting virus production. Much higher concentrations of acyclovir are required to halt normal human cell metabolism. Therefore effective doses for antiviral activity are relatively nontoxic to normal host cells.

Pharmacokinetics

Acyclovir is used intravenously to treat mucocutaneous herpes simplex in immunocompromised patients and to treat severe genital herpes or herpes simplex encephalitis. Oral administration of acyclovir leads to incomplete absorption, but this route is effective when used for mild-to-moderate genital herpes. Once absorbed, acyclovir is widely distributed to tissues. The topical ointment may be useful in mild herpes infections, but parenteral routes are more effective and usually preferred.

Excretion is by renal mechanisms. Acyclovir may be metabolized by the liver. The drug is eliminated with a half-life of about 2½ hours in patients with normal renal function.

Uses

Acyclovir is used to treat initial lesions or recurrences of genital herpes, mucocutaneous herpes simplex infections in immunocompromised patients, herpes simplex encephalitis, and herpes zoster infections.

Adverse Reactions and Contraindications

Acyclovir generally causes few side effects. Phlebitis at the injection site may occur with intravenous (IV) acyclovir. Rarely, patients receiving parenteral acyclovir may suffer coma, confusion, seizures, or tremors. Light-headedness is common. Oral administration can cause gastrointestinal (GI) tract disturbances.

Acyclovir should not be given at full dose to patients with renal impairment or to dehydrated patients.

Toxicity

Neuropsychiatric reactions and nephrotoxicity are more common with very high doses of acyclovir or in patients who accumulate the drug because of poor renal function. Nephrotoxicity, including crystallization of drug in the renal tubule, can be minimized by giving the drug as a slow infusion rather than as a rapid bolus. Increasing water intake also helps.

Interactions

Because of the potential for nephrotoxicity, acyclovir should not be given with other nephrotoxic agents.

Amantadine

Mechanism of Action

Amantadine blocks early phases of viral replication, but the exact mechanism is unclear. This drug has a narrow antiviral spectrum, being effective only against influenza type A.

TABLE 47-2 Drugs to Treat Systemic Viral Diseases

GENERIC NAME	TRADE NAME	ADMINISTRATION/DOSAGE	COMMENTS
✤ Acyclovir	Zovirax*	ORAL: *Adults*—200 mg 5 times daily. FDA pregnancy category C. INTRAVENOUS: *Adults*—5 mg/kg infused at constant rate over 1 hr, repeated every 8 hr. *Children <12 yr*—250 mg/m^2 infused at constant rate over 1 hr, repeated every 8 hr. TOPICAL: 5% ointment applied directly to initial lesions of genital herpes.	Specific actions on cells infected with herpesvirus.
Amantadine	Symadine Symmetrel*	ORAL: *Adults*—100 mg twice daily. *Older adults*—100 mg once daily. FDA pregnancy category C. *Children*—2.2-4.4 mg/kg every 12 hr, up to 150 mg daily.	Prophylaxis of influenza type A infections in high-risk patients.
Didanosine	Videx*	ORAL: *Adults*—200 mg tablet twice daily, body weight 50-74 kg; 125 mg twice daily, body weight 35-49 kg. FDA pregnancy category B. *Children*—Doses are given every 8-12 hr according to body surface area: up to 0.4 m^2, 25 mg; 0.5-0.7 m^2, 50 mg; 0.8-1.0 m^2, 75 mg; 1.1-1.4 m^2, 100 mg.	Treatment of patients with advanced HIV infection or those intolerant or unresponsive to zidovudine.
Famciclovir	Famvir	ORAL: *Adults*—500 mg every 8 hr for 7 days. FDA pregnancy category B.	For control of herpes zoster infections (shingles) in immunocompetent adults.
Foscarnet	Foscavir	INTRAVENOUS: *Adults*—60 mg/kg 3 times daily for induction; 90-120 mg/kg daily for maintenance therapy.	Treatment of CMV retinitis in patients with AIDS.
Ganciclovir	Cytovene*	ORAL: *Adults*—Maintenance, 1000 mg 3 times daily with food. INTRAVENOUS: *Adults*—5 mg/kg infused over at least 1 hr, every 12 hr for 14-21 days. FDA pregnancy category C.	Treatment of CMV retinitis in immunosuppressed patients, including AIDS patients.
Interferon alfa-2b, recombinant	Intron A*	INTRAMUSCULAR, SUBCUTANEOUS: *Adults*—3 million U 3 times week. FDA pregnancy category C.	For chronic or active hepatitis (non-A, non-B/C).
Interferon alfa-n3	Alferon N	INTRALESIONAL: *Adults*—250,000 U twice weekly for 8 wk. FDA pregnancy category C.	For treatment of external genital warts.
Ribavirin	Virazole*	INHALATION: *Children*—20 mg/ml in Viratek small particle aerosol generator model SPAG-2 12-18 hr/day. FDA pregnancy category X.	Severe pneumonia caused by respiratory syncytial virus (RSV).
Rimantadine	Flumadine	ORAL: *Adults*—100 mg twice daily. FDA pregnancy category C. *Children*—5 mg/kg once daily, not to exceed 150 mg daily.	For prophylaxis or therapy of influenza type A.
Stavudine	Zerit	ORAL: *Adults*—From 15-40 mg every 12-24 hr, individualized based on patient weight and renal function. FDA pregnancy category C.	For advanced HIV infection or AIDS, when other drugs cannot be used or have failed.
Zalcitabine	HIVID*	ORAL: *Adults*—0.75 mg with 200 mg of zidovudine every 8 hr. FDA pregnancy category C.	For advanced HIV infection or AIDS, in combination with zidovudine.
✤ Zidovudine	Retrovir*	ORAL: *Adults*—100 mg every 4 hr around clock. FDA pregnancy category C. *Children 3 mo-12 yr*—90-180 mg/m^2 every 6 hr.	HIV infection (AIDS and AIDS-related complex).

*Available in Canada and United States.

Pharmacokinetics

Amantadine is well absorbed orally and distributes well to tissues. The concentrations in lung tissue may exceed serum concentrations. The concentration of amantadine that reaches the epithelial surfaces of lung tissues is the determining factor in protecting against influenza type A infections. Nearly all elimination of the drug is by renal mechanisms. The half-life for elimination is about 15 hours in patients with normal renal function, 24 to 29 hours in older adults, and 7 to 10 days in renally impaired patients.

Uses

Amantadine is effective at preventing influenzae caused by type A virus. Prophylaxis is usually limited to older adult patients or others in whom influenza is likely to lead to life-threatening complications. If used within 24 hours of the onset of symptoms, amantadine may be helpful in treating influenza type A.

Amantadine has also been used to treat parkinsonism (see Chapter 56).

Adverse Reactions and Contraindications

Amantadine can cause amphetamine-like stimulation of the CNS, lethargy, ataxia, slurred speech, and other symptoms. Because of these CNS effects, the drug should be used cautiously, if at all, in older adult patients (see box) with cerebral arteriosclerosis or in patients with a history of epilepsy.

Anorexia and nausea are common side effects with amantadine. Anticholinergic side effects may also be seen, including constipation, dry mouth, blurred vision, difficulty in urination, and CNS signs.

Side effects are more common when amantadine is used for parkinsonism because the doses of drug are about twice those used for influenza prophylaxis.

Toxicity

Signs of overdose include CNS and cardiopulmonary toxicity. Symptoms may include cardiac arrhythmias, pulmonary edema, toxic psychosis, or convulsions.

Interactions

Alcohol increases the risk of seizure activity with amantadine. Anticholinergics may be dangerously potentiated by the anticholinergic action of amantadine. CNS stimulants increase the risk of CNS irritability or seizures.

Didanosine

Mechanism of Action

Didanosine is a purine analogue that is activated by phosphorylation within cells and in this active form blocks synthesis of HIV DNA by inhibiting the virus-specific enzyme called *reverse transcriptase.* This mechanism of action is similar to that of zidovudine.

Pharmacokinetics

Didanosine has a poor bioavailability in most patients because it is destroyed by stomach acid. Current formulations include buffers to improve absorption by lowering acidity and preserving integrity of the drug. The average plasma half-life of didanosine is between 30 and 80 minutes, but the half-life within cells is longer than 12 hours. Therefore the drug is given every 12 hours. Excretion yields about 20% of a dose present in urine as active drug.

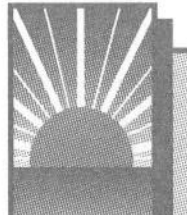

GERIATRIC CONSIDERATION

Amantadine

THE PROBLEM

Older adults are more sensitive to the antimuscarinic side effects of amantadine than are younger adults.

SOLUTIONS

- Cut normal adult dose by half for older adults.
- Watch carefully for antimuscarinic signs such as confusion or difficulty in urination.

Uses

Didanosine is currently used for treating adults or children older than 6 months of age who have advanced HIV disease and who are intolerant to zidovudine or have failed therapy with zidovudine.

Adverse Reactions and Contraindications

Peripheral neuropathy may occur in many patients receiving didanosine. Signs include tingling or aching in the legs or feet. Reflexes may be diminished. Side effects affecting the CNS are also common, including anxiety, headache, irritability, and sleeplessness. Diarrhea, dry mouth, and nausea are common but usually do not require medical attention.

Less frequent side effects include acute pancreatitis, allergies, blood dyscrasias, and cardiac failure (shortness of breath, swelling of feet and legs).

Toxicity

Peripheral neuropathy is more common with higher doses of didanosine or in patients in whom the drug accumulates. High doses were associated with atrophy of the retinal pigment epithelium in three children.

Interactions

The risk for pancreatitis is increased in patients who also have received other drugs causing this reaction (e.g., alcohol, asparaginase, azathioprine, estrogens, furosemide, methyldopa, pentamidine, sulfonamides, sulindac, tetracyclines, thiazides, or valproic acid). Peripheral neuropathy is more likely when patients also receive other neurotoxic drugs (e.g., chloramphenicol, cisplatin, dapsone, ethambutol, ethionamide, hydralazine, isoniazid, lithium, metronidazole, nitrofurantoin, nitrous oxide, phenytoin, stavudine, vincristine, or zalcitabine).

The buffers in didanosine preparations impair absorption of dapsone, itraconazole, and ketoconazole. Fluoroquinolone and tetracycline antibiotics are chelated by components of the buffering system in didanosine, decreasing absorption of the antibiotics.

Famciclovir

Mechanism of Action

Famciclovir is activated only by viral thymidine kinase. Therefore, like acyclovir, famciclovir is converted to an active agent only in virus-infected cells.

Pharmacokinetics

Famciclovir is a pro-drug that is converted to penciclovir in the intestinal wall following oral absorption. Penciclovir is the form that enters cells and is activated by viral thymidine kinase. Oral bioavailability is good. The drug is cleared primarily by the kidneys, but some penciclovir appears in feces.

Uses

Famciclovir is used for herpes zoster infection (shingles) in immunocompetent adults.

Adverse Reactions and Contraindications
Headache is a common complaint, but diarrhea, dizziness, fatigue, nausea, or vomiting may also occur.

Reduced doses of famciclovir may be required in renal impairment.

Toxicity
Little toxicity is noted with famciclovir, presumably because the drug is converted to its cytotoxic form only in virus-infected cells.

Interactions
Probenecid may block renal excretion of penciclovir.

Foscarnet
Mechanism of Action
Foscarnet inhibits viral DNA polymerases and reverse transcriptases. Because foscarnet is a chemical relative of inorganic phosphate, it does not require activation within cells.

Pharmacokinetics
Foscarnet is poorly absorbed orally and must be given by IV injection or infusion. The drug distributes to tissues, including brain tissues, although levels are variable. As an analogue of inorganic phosphate, foscarnet seems to be incorporated into bone. Most of the remainder of the drug is excreted unchanged in urine.

Uses
Foscarnet has shown activity against HIV, herpesviruses, and hepatitis B but is presently indicated only for control of cytomegalovirus (CMV) retinitis in HIV-infected patients.

Adverse Reactions and Contraindications
Renal toxicity is the major concern with foscarnet. Signs of serious renal toxicity may occur in up to 25% of patients receiving the drug. Some protection may be afforded by assuring adequate hydration before administering foscarnet.

Other side effects of foscarnet use include nausea, headache, dizziness, and anemia.

Toxicity
Nephrotoxicity may include acute renal tubular necrosis.

Interactions
Other nephrotoxic drugs should be avoided during therapy with foscarnet.

Ganciclovir
Mechanism of Action
Ganciclovir acts similarly to acyclovir, both drugs being readily activated within virus-infected cells to a form that inhibits virus reproduction. Unlike acyclovir, ganciclovir is also activated to a limited degree by normal cells.

Pharmacokinetics
Ganciclovir is poorly absorbed orally, with a bioavailability of less than 5%. Administration is therefore by IV infusion. The drug distributes widely into tissues, including the eye. Ganciclovir is not biotransformed and is excreted unchanged in urine.

Uses
Ganciclovir is indicated only for treatment of CMV retinitis in immunocompromised patients.

Adverse Reactions and Contraindications
Ganciclovir causes granulocytopenia, marked by sore throat and fever, in about 40% of patients receiving the drug. Ganciclovir also causes thrombocytopenia, marked by bruising and unusual bleeding, in 20% of patients. These reactions are usually reversible. Anemia, allergies, and signs of CNS irritability have also been reported less frequently.

Ganciclovir is used cautiously, if at all, in patients with low neutrophil or platelet counts. Doses must be reduced in renal failure.

Toxicity
Subcutaneous or intramuscular injection leads to severe tissue damage because ganciclovir preparations have a very high pH.

Interactions
Ganciclovir may cause dangerous blood dyscrasias when combined with zidovudine. Other bone marrow depressants may lead to unacceptable side effects with ganciclovir.

Interferons, alfa
Mechanism of Action
Interferons inhibit virus replication in infected cells and in general inhibit cell proliferation.

Pharmacokinetics
Interferons are proteins that must be administered parenterally. Uptake is good from intramuscular or subcutaneous infections.

Uses
Interferon alfa-2b, recombinant, is used to treat non-A, non-B/C hepatitis. Interferon alfa-n3 is used by intralesional injection to treat genital warts, which are induced by papillomavirus.

Adverse Reactions and Contraindications
Adverse reactions are more common when interferon is used systemically to treat hepatitis than when interferon is used locally for genital warts. Possible reactions include anorexia, blood dyscrasias (anemia, leukopenia, thrombocytopenia), diarrhea, fatigue, nausea, or vomiting. A flulike syndrome with fever, chills, and headache is common and may physically stress the patient. Patients with cardiac disease, severe

diabetes, or pulmonary disease may be unable to cope with this stress.

Interferons should be avoided in patients with autoimmune disease because the immune reactions may increase. In contrast, chickenpox or herpes zoster may be worsened. The conditions of patients with CNS disease including psychiatric disorders or seizures may be worsened by interferons.

Interferon alfa-2b should be avoided in patients with impaired thyroid function because thyroid function may be further worsened.

Toxicity
Cardiotoxicity has been reported; however, this condition is rare.

Interactions
Blood dyscrasias may be worsened by other drugs producing the same side effects as the alfa interferons.

Ribavirin
Mechanism of Action
Ribavirin is a synthetic purine nucleoside that interferes with multiple steps leading to synthesis of viral nucleic acids.

Pharmacokinetics
Ribavirin is administered as an aerosol to treat respiratory viruses. In this way, drug levels in the lung are maximized, but systemic absorption is low, which minimizes side effects.

Uses
In the United States, ribavirin is indicated only for therapy of severe respiratory syncytial virus (RSV) in children, but in other parts of the world the drug has been used to treat various viral-induced hemorrhagic fevers.

Adverse Reactions and Contraindications
Skin rashes can occur. Health care workers exposed during administration of the drug can suffer headaches and irritation of the eyes. Oral or IV administration of ribavirin often causes anemia and may cause CNS or GI tract effects.

Toxicity
Little systemic toxicity occurs when ribavirin is given by inhalation.

Interactions
Because ribavirin blocks phosphorylation of nucleosides, it interferes with activation of zidovudine and therefore should not be given to patients receiving zidovudine.

Rimantadine
Mechanism of Action
Rimantadine is thought to interfere with uncoating of the influenza type A virus when it enters mammalian cells. This action prevents viral replication because uncoating is required for release of the viral genome in infected cells.

Pharmacokinetics
Rimantadine is well absorbed orally and extensively metabolized in the liver. Metabolites are eliminated in urine. The half-life of the drug ranges from 13 to 38 hours. In general, older adults or those with liver impairment eliminate the drug more slowly.

Uses
Rimantadine is used only for prophylaxis or treatment of infections caused by influenza type A virus. Treatment is approved only for adults, but prophylaxis may be carried out in adults or children.

Adverse Reactions and Contraindications
Rimantadine causes CNS effects less often than the related drug amantadine, but headache, insomnia, or fatigue are possible. Anorexia, dry mouth, nausea, or vomiting are also possible.

Patients with a history of seizures may be at risk of increased frequency of seizures with rimantadine. Patients with reduced hepatic function require reduced doses of rimantadine to compensate for slower elimination of the drug.

Toxicity
Toxic reactions have not been documented, but CNS toxicity might be expected with very high doses.

Interactions
Acetaminophen and aspirin may reduce peak serum levels of rimantadine by a small amount, and cimetidine may speed clearance of rimantadine; but none of these interactions are thought to be clinically significant for most patients.

Stavudine
Mechanism of Action
Stavudine is an analogue of thymidine, a precursor of DNA. Inside cells, stavudine is activated to a form that inhibits several enzymes including HIV reverse transcriptase and also may cause termination of DNA chains' being synthesized. These actions prevent successful replication of virus.

Pharmacokinetics
Stavudine is well absorbed orally, with or without food. The drug distributes well in the body and enters cells freely. About 40% of the drug administered is excreted unchanged in urine. The remainder is probably metabolized in various tissues.

Uses
Stavudine is used for advanced HIV disease in patients who cannot take the primary drugs or who have failed with established therapy.

Adverse Reactions and Contraindications
Sensory peripheral neuropathy is the most common serious side effect with stavudine. The burning, numbness, or pain in the extremities may resolve if the drug is discontinued.

A variety of other side effects may occur, including allergic reactions, anemia, anorexia, diarrhea, headache, insomnia, pain in muscles and joints, pancreatitis, or weakness.

There are no absolute contraindications to the use of stavudine, but if the drug must be used in patients with peripheral neuropathy or renal function impairment, lower doses may be required.

Toxicity
Neurotoxicity increases with increasing doses. After resolution of neurotoxicity, 50% of normal dose may be used.

Interactions
Stavudine should be avoided in patients also receiving other drugs that cause peripheral neuropathy, such as dapsone, didanosine, ethambutol, ethionamide, isoniazid, metronidazole, vincristine, or zalcitabine.

Zalcitabine
Mechanism of Action
Zalcitabine is an analogue of deoxycytidine, a precursor of DNA. Zalcitabine is activated inside cells to a form that inhibits HIV reverse transcriptase and may terminate DNA chains' being synthesized. These actions prevent successful replication of virus.

Pharmacokinetics
Oral absorption of zalcitabine is high in adults but may be lower in children. The drug distributes well in the body and freely enters cells. Little metabolic degradation occurs, and about 70% of the drug administered is excreted unchanged in urine.

Uses
Zalcitabine is used in advanced HIV disease, in combination with zidovudine.

Adverse Reactions and Contraindications
Peripheral neurotoxicity is the most common serious side effect of zalcitabine. Pancreatitis has caused death in a few patients receiving zalcitabine.

Less serious adverse reactions include abdominal pain, allergic reactions, diarrhea, headache, nausea, pain in muscles and joints, or ulcers in the mouth.

Toxicity
Peripheral neurotoxicity is dose related and therefore is more likely to occur and to be more serious in patients receiving high doses of zalcitabine.

Interactions
Zalcitabine should be avoided if possible in combination with other drugs that cause pancreatitis, such as alcohol, estrogens, furosemide, pentamidine, sulfonamides, tetracyclines, or diuretics. Drugs such as dapsone, didanosine, ethambutol, ethionamide, isoniazid, metronidazole, stavudine, and vincristine may increase the risk of peripheral neuropathy.

Aminoglycosides, amphotericin B, and foscarnet block renal excretion of zalcitabine. The result may be increased zalcitabine toxicity.

✣ Zidovudine
Mechanism of Action
Zidovudine is used in conditions caused by infection with HIV. HIV is a retrovirus that has had several names, including LAV (lymphadenopathy-associated virus) and HTLV-III (human T-cell leukemia/lymphoma virus type III). **Retroviruses** use RNA as their genetic material and must therefore convert RNA into DNA within the host cell for viral replication to take place. This unusual reaction, which does not normally occur in the host cell, is catalyzed by the enzyme, reverse transcriptase. Zidovudine inhibits reverse transcriptase. In addition, some of the drug may be incorporated into viral DNA, in which it causes premature chain termination. Both actions block viral replication. Zidovudine does not cure HIV infection or AIDS but, by slowing replication of HIV, it may delay damage to the immune system and lower the incidence of opportunistic infections in these patients.

Pharmacokinetics
Absorption of zidovudine from the GI tract is rapid and nearly complete, but the drug is quickly metabolized to an inactive glucuronide on first pass through the liver. These factors give zidovudine a half-life of only 1 hour. For this reason, zidovudine is taken every 4 hours around the clock to maintain virustatic concentrations. To be effective, zidovudine must be administered continuously throughout life. The short half-life and toxicity of the drug make this ideal difficult to achieve.

Uses
Zidovudine is the primary drug for HIV infections. It may be used in asymptomatic patients to delay onset of the decline in T-cell counts, as well as in patients with more advanced forms of the disease. Zidovudine has been used in HIV-infected children. The drug has also been used to lower the incidence of transmission of HIV from an infected mother to her fetus.

Adverse Reactions and Contraindications
Nearly all patients suffer toxicity from zidovudine. The most common reactions are granulocytopenia and anemia. Routine blood monitoring is extremely important. Withdrawal from zidovudine may be necessary to allow recovery from drug-induced blood dyscrasias. Neurotoxicity has also been reported but may be difficult to distinguish from the neural effects of HIV infection. Other adverse actions include headache, insomnia, muscle pain, and nausea.

There are no absolute contraindications to the use of zidovudine, but patients with bone marrow depression may be at greater risk of anemia or other blood disorders; these patients should be very carefully monitored. Patients with hepatic impairment may be prone to increased drug toxicity.

Toxicity

A few patients have taken large overdoses of zidovudine, through accidents or in deliberate suicide attempts. Signs of overdose include anemia, ataxia, fatigue, leukopenia, severe nausea, nystagmus, thrombocytopenia, and vomiting. Seizures are rare.

Interactions

Drug interactions may occur with zidovudine and other drugs often used in immunosuppressed patients. Ganciclovir and zidovudine combine to produce severe hematologic toxicity. Other bone marrow depressants may also increase zidovudine toxicity. Ribavirin interferes with activation of zidovudine within the virus-infected cell and thereby blocks the anti-HIV effect of zidovudine.

Clarithromycin lowers the peak of zidovudine in the blood, which may interfere with anti-HIV activity. Probenecid increases the concentration of zidovudine in blood and slows its elimination, which increases the risk of toxicity.

Ophthalmic Antiviral Agents

Ophthalmic antiviral agents are available for use directly in the eye to treat localized viral infections (Table 47-3). The primary disease is keratitis caused by herpes simplex virus. These drugs have mechanisms similar to other antiviral agents but are not as selective and are therefore much more toxic. For this reason the use of these drugs is restricted to topical applications.

Idoxuridine, trifluridine, and vidarabine are potentially mutagenic and carcinogenic. It is not clear how important this potential may be when these agents are used topically since these drugs are not well absorbed from the eye into systemic circulation.

Idoxuridine

Idoxuridine is incorporated into DNA in place of thymidine, thereby preventing normal DNA replication and halting virus formation. Herpes simplex infections of the cornea, conjunctiva, and eyelids tend to recur, and idoxuridine does not prevent reappearance of the infection or scarring and resultant loss of sight in serious cases.

When used topically in the eye, little idoxuridine enters the systemic circulation. The drug can produce local reactions in the eye, the most serious being corneal defects. It may also interfere with corneal epithelial regeneration and healing. Idoxuridine is potentially mutagenic and carcinogenic.

Trifluridine

Trifluridine, like idoxuridine, is activated by viral and host cell thymidine kinase to a form of drug that inhibits DNA polymerase. Trifluridine may be less damaging to the cornea than idoxuridine or vidarabine; nevertheless, conjunctival or corneal burning can occur when the drug is placed in the eye. Swelling of the eyelids (palpebral edema) has also been noted.

Trifluridine is potentially mutagenic and carcinogenic.

Vidarabine

Vidarabine inhibits viral DNA synthesis in a variety of DNA viruses. Vidarabine is activated by host cell enzymes to ara-ATP, a potent and selective inhibitor of viral DNA polymerase. Clinically important selectivity of action is achieved against herpesvirus-infected cells.

Ophthalmic use is not usually associated with serious side effects, but local irritation and sensitivity of the eyes to light may occur. Vidarabine is potentially mutagenic and carcinogenic.

NURSING PROCESS OVERVIEW

Antiviral Agents

Assessment

Use of antiviral agents is limited to patients in whom supportive therapy has not been helpful or who have viruses known to be particularly virulent or frequently fatal. Perform a thorough total assessment. Emphasize the subjective and objective complaints related to the virus. Assess laboratory work, cultures, and other studies that would help monitor the progress of the disease.

Nursing Diagnoses

- Potential complication: blood dyscrasias, renal failure, or pancreatitis related to drug therapy (varies with drug)

TABLE 47-3 Ophthalmic Drugs to Treat Viral Diseases

GENERIC NAME	TRADE NAME	ADMINISTRATION/DOSAGE	COMMENTS
Idoxuridine	Herplex* Stoxil*	OPHTHALMIC: *Adults and children*—0.1% solution, 0.5% ointment used 5 times daily.	Local irritation and pitting defects may occur in cornea. Systemic toxicity is possible but rare.
Trifluridine	Viroptic*	OPHTHALMIC: *Adults and children*—1% solution applied up to 9 times daily.	Local irritation.
Vidarabine	Vira-A*	OPHTHALMIC: *Adults and children*—3% ointment used 5 times daily. FDA pregnancy category C.	Local irritation, superficial punctate keratitis, and allergy.

*Available in Canada and United States.

Patient Outcomes

The nurse will manage and minimize blood dyscrasias, renal failure, or pancreatitis

Planning/Implementation

Monitor appropriate laboratory work, vital signs, and other objective data that help chart the progress of the disease. Monitor for side effects known to occur with the drug used. If the patient will receive antiviral drug therapy after discharge, instruct the patient and family about possible side effects. If the virus is known to be virulent, isolate the patient during the hospitalization phase. For information about specific viruses, consult the infection control department at the local hospital, the local health department, or the Centers for Disease Control and Prevention in Atlanta. Many serious viral illnesses should be reported to the local health department since this information is used for epidemiologic charting of viral spread; examples include polio and rabies. Finally, immunize family members and health care team members if appropriate.

Evaluation

Before discharge, ensure that the patient can explain how to take the drug correctly, identify side effects that may occur, and describe situations that require consultation with the physician.

NURSING IMPLICATIONS SUMMARY

Acyclovir

Drug Administration

- Assess for GI tract symptoms and CNS side effects. Inspect for skin rashes.
- Monitor intake and output and weight.
- Monitor complete blood count (CBC) and differential, platelet count, and blood urea nitrogen (BUN) and serum creatinine levels.
- For best effect in treatment of chickenpox, begin therapy as soon as possible after the rash appears, within 24 hours of onset. For best effect in treatment of recurrent herpes simplex infections, begin therapy as soon as possible after symptoms appear.

Intravenous Administration

- Dilute as directed in the drug insert. Administer dose over 1 hour. Use an infusion control device or microdrip tubing to help regulate infusion rate. Inspect the IV site frequently and question the patient regarding symptoms of phlebitis or irritation. Because excretion is via the kidneys and the drug half-life is about 2½ hours, the patient should be well hydrated during IV infusion to prevent precipitation of the drug in the renal tubules.

Patient and Family Education

- Review the anticipated benefits and possible side effects of drug therapy with the patient.
- Instruct the patient to take oral doses with a full (8-ounce) glass of water. For oral suspension form, instruct the patient to measure doses using the calibrated measuring device supplied by the pharmacist.
- Warn the patient to avoid driving or operating hazardous equipment if dizziness, fatigue, or vertigo develop and to notify the physician if these symptoms do occur.
- For topical application, instruct the patient to use a glove or finger cot to apply ointment to avoid contamination of the finger. Caution the patient to avoid contact with the eyes and to use the drug on a regular basis, as prescribed, for best effect. Instruct the patient to consult the physician if there is no improvement within a week.
- Instruct the patient with genital herpes how to lessen the chance of spreading the virus by avoiding sexual activity when open lesions or scabs are present. Male partners should wear condoms. Acyclovir will not prevent the spread of herpes.
- Instruct the patient to keep areas of infection clean and dry and to wear loose-fitting garments. Caution the patient not to use other creams or ointments on viral lesions unless prescribed by the physician.
- Encourage women with genital herpes to have regular Pap smears to check for cervical cancer.

Amantadine

- See Nursing Implications Summary in Chapter 56 (p. 703).

Didanosine

Drug Administration

- Assess patient for severity of symptoms: fever, night sweats, swollen lymph nodes, weight loss, excessive fatigue, diarrhea, cough, weakness, anorexia, yeast infections (oral or vaginal).
- Assess for peripheral neuropathy including numbness or tingling of fingers and extremities. Assess deep tendon reflexes.
- Assess for pancreatitis including epigastric or left upper quadrant abdominal pain, nausea, vomiting, and fever. Monitor white blood cell (WBC) count, serum lipase, serum triglycerides, serum electrolytes, and serum uric acid.

Patient and Family Education

- Check drug insert for current information. Protocols for treatment and prevention of HIV infection change frequently. Instruct the patient to take doses as ordered, to not increase dose or frequency without talking with the physician, to not omit doses, and to not discontinue therapy if feeling better or symptoms disappear.

Continued.

NURSING IMPLICATIONS SUMMARY—cont'd

- Take oral doses on an empty stomach 2 hours before or 2 hours after eating.
- Instruct the patient taking pediatric oral suspension to measure doses using the calibrated measuring device supplied by the pharmacist.
- Instruct the patient using didanosine for oral solution to pour contents of foil packet into 4 ounces of water and to not mix with fruit juice or any acidic beverage. Instruct the patient to stir for 2 to 3 minutes to dissolve powder, then drink immediately.
- Instruct the patient to chew or crush tablets thoroughly before swallowing or mix with 1 ounce of water until a suspension forms, then swallow the mixture.
- Each tablet contains the drug and a buffer. For patients older than 1 year the prescribed dose should always be 2 tablets. Tablets must be taken together to get enough of the buffer. For children younger than 1 year of age there is enough buffer in 1 tablet.
- Remind the patient to keep all health care providers informed of all drugs being used. Caution the patient not to take any other medication, whether prescription or OTC, without checking with physician first.
- Inform the patient that taking didanosine will not prevent the spread of HIV. If possible, HIV-positive patients should avoid sexual activity or should always use protection to avoid spreading HIV. Men should use latex condoms, and women may wish to carry condoms with them so they will always be available. Using a spermicide may help prevent the spread of HIV. The patient should not use lubricants such as oil-based jelly, cold cream, baby oil, or shortening but can use oil-free lubricants such as K-Y jelly.
- Instruct the patient who injects drugs not to share needles with others.

Foscarnet

Drug Administration

- Check drug insert for current information.
- Monitor intake and output and weight. Monitor serum electrolyte level, CBC, BUN level, and serum creatinine level.
- Assess for nausea.

Intravenous Foscarnet

- Use undiluted solutions in central lines only. For peripheral IV infusion, dilute drug in an equal volume of 5% dextrose in water (D5W) or normal saline for a dilution of 12 mg/ml. Discard any excess drug from the IV bottle; to avoid overdose, only the prescribed dose should be in the IV bottle at the start of the infusion. Administer the dose over at least 1 hour. The dose should not exceed 1 mg/kg/min. Use an infusion pump to deliver accurate dose.

Patient and Family Education

- Instruct the patient to assure adequate hydration before administering the drug to lessen the chance of renal toxicity. Encourage the patient to drink several additional 8-ounce glasses of water each day while taking foscarnet.
- This drug may cause sores to develop on the genitals. Instruct the patient to wash genitals after urinating to decrease the chance of sores forming.
- Encourage the patient with CMV infection of the eyes to have regular ophthalmic examinations to monitor progress.

Famciclovir

Drug Administration/Patient and Family Education

- Instruct the patient to take doses with meals.
- For best effect, begin famciclovir at the first sign of rash or symptoms, within 47 hours of the onset of rash. Instruct the patient to continue therapy for the full course and to not stop when symptoms begin to clear up.
- Instruct the patient to keep the area affected by herpes as clean and dry as possible and to wear loose-fitting clothing.

Ganciclovir

Drug Administration

- See drug insert for preparation guidelines.
- Administer each dose over 1 hour as an infusion. Use microdrip tubing and an infusion monitoring device.
- Monitor CBC and platelet count, liver function tests, and BUN level.
- Monitor intake and output.

Patient and Family Education

- See the patient problem box on bleeding tendencies (p. 586).
- Instruct the patient (men and women) to use measures for contraception during treatment and for at least 90 days after treatment.
- Encourage the patient to have an ophthalmic examination at the start of therapy and at regular intervals to monitor progress. Encourage the patient to report any changes in vision.

Interferons

Drug Administration

- Review the manufacturer's instruction leaflet. If the patient is to administer injections at home, teach proper injection technique as well as proper handling and disposal of contaminated syringes and needles.
- Assess for development of side effects. Be alert to signs of depression including insomnia, weight loss, withdrawal, anorexia, and lack of interest in personal appearance.

NURSING IMPLICATIONS SUMMARY—cont'd

- Monitor pulse and blood pressure. Auscultate lung and heart sounds. Monitor intake, output, and weight.
- Monitor hematocrit or hemoglobin level, platelet count, WBC differential, and liver function tests.

Patient and Family Education

- Review the anticipated benefits and possible side effects of drug therapy with the patient.
- Review the dosing schedule and discuss with the patient what to do if a dose is missed if drugs are to be self-administered. Make certain that the patient can inject the dose correctly.
- Instruct the patient to stay well hydrated to lessen symptoms from hypotension.
- Warn the patient to avoid driving or operating hazardous equipment if fatigue or dizziness develops.
- These drugs often cause a flulike reaction, with fever, chills, and headache. The nurse should consult the physician about appropriate instructions for the patient related to notifying the physician and self-medicating with antipyretics.
- Instruct the patient not to change to other brands of interferon without consulting the physician.
- Instruct the patient to avoid other drugs that may also cause drowsiness or fatigue unless specifically approved by the physician; this includes alcohol, antihistamines, sedatives, sleeping medications, prescription medication for pain, and medications for seizures. Instruct the patient to keep all health care providers informed of all drugs being used.
- Review the patient problem boxes on leukopenia (p. 585) and bleeding tendencies (p. 586).
- Instruct the patient to take doses at night to lessen daytime fatigue.

Ribavirin

Drug Administration/Patient and Family Education

- Review the anticipated benefits and possible side effects of drug therapy with the patient and family. Encourage the patient or family to report new signs or symptoms.
- Auscultate lung sounds and assess respiratory status. Monitor temperature and vital signs.
- Check drug package insert for current information. Do not give simultaneously with other aerosolized medications. Use only the aerosol generator specified by the manufacturer.
- Healthcare workers should avoid contact with the drug if possible since it may cause eye irritation or headaches.

Rimantadine

Drug Administration/Patient and Family Education

- Assess for a history of seizures before administering rimantadine.
- For best results, drug therapy should be started before exposure to influenza type A or as soon as possible after exposure. Instruct the patient to continue therapy as prescribed for the full course, even if feeling better or symptoms improve.
- Instruct the patient to avoid driving or operating hazardous equipment if drowsiness, dizziness, or excessive fatigue develop.

Stavudine

Drug Administration/Patient and Family Education

- Monitor liver function tests, serum amylase, and lipase.
- Assess for peripheral neuropathy: numbness, tingling, or pain of the fingers, hands or feet.
- Instruct the patient to take stavudine as prescribed for the full course of therapy for best results.
- Emphasize to the patient the importance of returning for follow-up visits to monitor progress. Remind the patient to keep all health care providers informed of all medications in use and to check with the physician before taking any other medications.
- Inform the patient that taking stavudine will not prevent the spread of HIV. If possible, HIV-positive patients should avoid sexual activity or should always use protection to avoid spreading HIV. Men should use latex condoms, and women may wish to carry condoms with them so they will always be available. Using a spermicide may help prevent the spread of HIV. Instruct the patient not to use lubricants such as oil-based jelly, cold cream, baby oil, or shortening but to use oil-free lubricants such as K-Y jelly.
- Caution patients who inject drugs not to share needles with others.

Zalcitabine

Drug Administration/Patient and Family Education

- Assess for peripheral neuropathy: numbness, tingling, or pain of the fingers, hands, or feet.
- Monitor liver function tests, serum lipase and amylase, and serum triglycerides.
- Instruct the patient to take zalcitabine as prescribed for the full course of therapy for best results.
- Emphasize to the patient the importance of returning for follow-up visits to monitor progress. Remind the patient to keep all health care providers informed of all medications in use and to check with the physician before taking any other medications.
- Inform the patient that taking zalcitabine will not prevent the spread of HIV. If possible, HIV-positive patients should avoid sexual activity or should always use protection to avoid spreading HIV. Men should use latex condoms, and women may wish to carry condoms with them so they will always be available. Using a spermicide may help prevent the spread of HIV. Instruct the patient not to use lubricants

Continued.

NURSING IMPLICATIONS SUMMARY—cont'd

such as oil-based jelly, cold cream, baby oil, or shortening but to use oil-free lubricants such as K-Y jelly.

- Caution patients who inject drugs not to share needles with others.

Zidovudine

Drug Administration

- Assess for headaches, anxiety, and confusion. Inspect for rashes. Monitor temperature and pulse.
- Monitor CBC, differential, and platelet count.

Intravenous Zidovudine

- Review drug package insert for current information about dilution. Administer the diluted dose evenly over 1 hour.

Patient and Family Education

- Review the anticipated benefits and possible side effects of drug therapy with the patient and family. Encourage the patient to report new signs or symptoms.
- See the patient problem boxes on bleeding tendencies (p. 586) and leukopenia (p. 585).
- Instruct the patient to take zidovudine as prescribed for the full course of therapy for best results.
- Emphasize to the patient the importance of returning for follow-up visits to monitor progress. Remind the patient to keep all health care providers informed of all medications in use and to check with the physician before taking any other medications.
- Inform the patient that taking zidovudine will not prevent the spread of HIV. If possible, HIV-positive patients should avoid sexual activity or should always use protection to avoid spreading HIV. Men should use latex condoms, and women may wish to carry condoms with them so they will always be available. Using a spermicide may help prevent the spread of HIV. Instruct the patient not to use lubricants such as oil-based jelly, cold cream, baby oil, or shortening but to use oil-free lubricants such as K-Y jelly.
- Caution patients who inject drugs not to share needles with others.

Ophthalmic Antiviral Agents

Drug Administration/Patient and Family Education

- Review the technique for administration of eye medications with the patient (see Chapter 5).
- If photophobia develops, instruct the patient to avoid bright lights and to wear sunglasses.
- Caution the patient that vision may be blurry for several minutes after administering eye medications. Instruct the patient to avoid driving or operating hazardous equipment if vision is not clear.
- Encourage the patient to have regular ophthalmic examinations to monitor progress. Remind the patient to use medications as ordered for best effect and to use them for the full course of therapy.
- Instruct the patient to notify the physician if vision worsens or exudate, itching, or other symptoms develop.

CRITICAL THINKING

APPLICATION

1. Are antiviral drugs virucidal or virustatic?
2. Why does HIV specifically attack T lymphocytes?
3. Why is immunization not possible against all viral diseases?
4. What are interferons?
5. How may interferons be used against viruses?
6. What is the mechanism of action of acyclovir?
7. How is acyclovir used to treat viral diseases?
8. What side effects are associated with acyclovir? How should you assess for these?
9. What is the mechanism of action of amantadine and rimantadine?
10. How is amantadine used to treat viral diseases?
11. How are ganciclovir and foscarnet used as antiviral agents?
12. Explain why famciclovir is called a pro-drug.
13. How is ribavirin used to treat viral disease?
14. What is the mechanism of action of zidovudine?
15. How is zidovudine used to treat viral disease? How does the use of didanosine, stavudine, and zalcitabine relate to the use of zidovudine?
16. What side effects are associated with zidovudine? How should you assess for these?
17. Why is zidovudine given every 4 hours around the clock?
18. How does didanosine differ from zidovudine?
19. How are idoxuridine, trifluridine, and vidarabine used as antiviral agents?
20. If you have access to the Internet; try contacting the National Institutes of Health for current information about AIDS. Hint: try http://www.NIH.gov

CRITICAL THINKING

1. You advise your older adult patient to have a flu shot. The patient responds that he had one last year, so why does he need another one this year? What is your response?
2. Patients who are HIV positive are at greater risk for opportunistic infections. These patients may be treated with zidovudine. Does treatment with this drug lessen the risk of infection for these patients?

CHAPTER 48

Drugs to Treat Protozoal and Helminthic Infestations

OBJECTIVES

After studying this chapter, you should be able to do the following:

- *Discuss how the site of infestation may affect the success of drug therapy.*
- *Describe the type of patients in whom specific protozoal or helminthic diseases might be more likely.*
- *Explain hygienic measures that should accompany drug therapy in controlling pinworm infestations.*
- *Develop a nursing care plan for the patient receiving one of the drugs in this chapter.*

KEY TERMS

amebic disease
cestodes
enterobiasis
giardiasis
helminths
malaria
trichomoniasis

CHAPTER OVERVIEW

On a worldwide scale, chronic diseases caused by protozoal or helminthic (worm) infestations are the most common afflictions of humanity. Although these diseases flourish primarily in tropical regions, several are encountered in North America. In this chapter the discussion centers on the treatment of diseases that occur in the continental United States and Canada.

Parasitic diseases are caused by eucaryotic organisms against which selective toxicity is sometimes difficult to achieve. The selection of an effective drug involves matching the tissue distribution of the drug with the sites of infestation of the parasite, as well as choosing an agent that possesses intrinsic activity against the parasite.

For the purposes of discussion, parasitic diseases are divided into the following categories in this chapter: amebic disease, malaria, selected parasitic diseases (cryptosporidiosis, giardiasis, pneumocystosis, toxoplasmosis, trichomoniasis), and diseases caused by helminths.

Therapeutic Rationale: Amebic Disease

Amebic disease is caused by microscopic, single-celled parasitic organisms. *Entamoeba histolytica* is a frequent pathogen of humans, commonly passed from host to host by oral ingestion of fecally contaminated food or water. The organism is ingested as a cyst. Cysts have thick walls and resist desiccation and the action of stomach acids. In the intestine the nonmotile cyst changes to a motile, sexually active form called *trophozoites.* Trophozoites produce active disease as they reproduce and invade tissues.

Amebic disease may be restricted to the intestinal lumen. However, trophozoites invade the intestinal lining in the course of the disease and may penetrate the intestinal wall and create abscesses in other tissues and organs. The liver and lung are most commonly affected in this way.

The choice of drug for treating amebic disease depends on the stage of the disease. For acute colitis that occurs while the disease is limited to the intestinal tract, several drugs are available (Table 48-1). For more extensive intestinal disease or for abscesses in other organs, metronidazole is the safest and most effective agent.

Metronidazole therapy is usually followed by iodoquinol or diloxanide, drugs that more effectively destroy free amebae within the intestinal lumen.

Therapeutic Agents: Amebic Disease

Primary Agents

Iodoquinol

Mechanism of Action

Iodoquinol is an effective amebicidal agent (see Table 48-1). The mechanism of action of idoquinol may relate to the iodine content of the drug.

Pharmacokinetics

Iodoquinol given orally is not significantly absorbed from the intestine. Iodine is increased in the blood, which suggests that some drug is absorbed or that iodine is absorbed after breakdown of the drug in the gut.

Uses

Iodoquinol is used alone for intestinal amebiasis or with metronidazole for serious invasive intestinal amebiasis.

Adverse Reactions and Contraindications

Iodoquinol is relatively nontoxic, but nausea and other gastrointestinal (GI) tract symptoms are not uncommon. Allergic reactions, fevers, and chills may also occur.

Iodoquinol can cause the thyroid gland to enlarge because the drug contains significant iodine. This iodine content also

TABLE 48-1 Drugs to Treat Amebic Infestations

GENERIC NAME	TRADE NAME	ADMINISTRATION/DOSAGE	COMMENTS
✣ Chloroquine	Aralen*	ORAL: *Adults*—For amebic liver abscesses, 250 mg 4 times daily for 2 days, then 250 mg twice daily for up to 3 wk. *Children*—for amebic liver abscesses, 10 mg/kg daily for 3 wk.	Alternate drug used in combinations for amebic liver abscesses.
Diloxanide	Entamide‡ Furamide‡	ORAL: *Adults*—500 mg 3 times daily for 10 days. *Children >2 yr*—6.7 mg/kg 3 times daily. Maximum daily dose 1.5 gm.	Alternate drug for asymptomatic intestinal disease.
Iodoquinol	Diodoquin† Diquinol Yodoxin*	ORAL: *Adults*—650 mg 3 times daily for 20 days. Maximum daily dose 2 gm. *Children*—10-13.3 mg/kg 3 times daily for 20 days. Maximum daily dose 1.95 gm.	Primary drug for asymptomatic intestinal disease.
✣ Metronidazole	Flagyl*	ORAL: *Adults*—For amebiasis, 500-750 mg 3 times daily for 5-10 days. For anaerobic bacterial infections, 7.5 mg/kg 4 times daily. FDA pregnancy category B. *Children*—for amebiasis, 11.6-16.7 mg/kg 3 times daily for 10 days. For anaerobic bacterial infections, 7.5 mg/kg 4 times daily.	Primary drug for intestinal or extraintestinal amebiasis; anaerobic bacteria.

*Available in Canada and United States.
†Available in Canada only.
‡Available in United States only though Centers for Disease Control and Prevention (CDC) in Atlanta.

makes iodoquinol potentially dangerous for patients with hepatic or renal failure.

Toxicity

Prolonged high doses of iodoquinol may produce optic neuritis or atrophy and other signs of neuropathy.

Interactions

No documented drug interactions are clinically important, but iodoquinol does cause persistent interference with thyroid function tests because iodine levels are high in blood.

Metronidazole

Mechanism of Action

Metronidazole is most effective against anaerobic organisms, being reduced in those organisms to a form that directly damages DNA. Metronidazole attacks amebas at intestinal and other tissue sites (see Table 48-1).

Pharmacokinetics

Metronidazole is well absorbed after oral administration. The drug is metabolized by various pathways. Both metabolites and unchanged drug appear in urine. Some patients observe a reddish brown discoloration of urine while taking metronidazole. This harmless discoloration is caused by a colored metabolite of metronidazole.

Uses

Metronidazole is a primary agent for intestinal amebiasis and for tissue abscesses caused by amebae. It has also been used to treat trichomoniasis and giardiasis (see Table 48-3), as well as infections and abscesses caused by anaerobic bacteria.

Adverse Reactions and Contraindications

Metronidazole can produce various GI tract symptoms including a sharp, metallic taste, as well as nausea, diarrhea, vomiting, epigastric pain, and abdominal cramping. Although annoying, these symptoms rarely require stopping the drug.

Metronidazole commonly causes dizziness or headache, but other central nervous system (CNS) effects such as ataxia (incoordination affecting walking), numbness, and paresthesias are uncommon. These latter symptoms may signal that metronidazole should be withdrawn. Metronidazole may also produce discomfort in the pelvic organs. Dysuria, cystitis, and dryness of the vagina may be experienced.

Because of its action on DNA, metronidazole may be mutagenic or carcinogenic in experimental animals. This potential problem precludes routine use of the drug in pregnant women. Metronidazole is also avoided if possible in patients with significant CNS disease or blood dyscrasias because the drug may worsen either condition. Patients with hepatic impairment may accumulate the drug because the liver is the primary organ for elimination of metronidazole; reduced doses may be used.

Toxicity

High doses of metronidazole may cause seizures.

Interactions

Metronidazole causes an alarming reaction when ethyl alcohol is ingested. Patients experience intense flushing, nausea, headaches, and abdominal cramps. This reaction is similar to that experienced by patients taking both disulfiram and ethyl alcohol (Chapter 20).

Metronidazole may potentiate the action of warfarin. Patients receiving both drugs should be observed for signs of bleeding.

Alternate Drugs

Diloxanide

Diloxanide is not available commercially in either Canada or the United States, but it may be obtained from the Centers for Disease Control and Prevention in Atlanta. Diloxanide eliminates *E. histolytica* from the intestine of persons mildly infected and who are passing cysts in their stools (see Table 48-1). The mechanism of action of diloxanide is not known.

Diloxanide is given orally and is well absorbed by that route. Excretion is primarily renal. It is a relatively safe drug, producing few systemic side effects. Flatulence (intestinal gas) is the most frequent side effect. Other GI tract disturbances such as nausea, diarrhea, and esophagitis may rarely occur.

Chloroquine

Chloroquine may be used along with iodoquinol or diloxanide to treat liver abscesses caused by amebic infections. Chloroquine is only an alternate drug for amebic disease (see Table 48-1) but is a primary drug for malaria. Chloroquine is discussed fully under malaria and in Table 48-2.

Therapeutic Rationale: Malaria

Malaria is a serious infectious illness transmitted by the bite of infected mosquitoes. Four species of *Plasmodium* produce human disease: *P. falciparum, P. vivax, P. ovale,* and *P. malariae.*

Plasmodia have complex life cycles. Sporozoites enter human blood, travel directly to the liver and may persist there for prolonged periods. Clinical malaria is produced when merozoites, the plasmodial form produced in liver cells, are released into the blood. Merozoites attack red blood cells and ultimately cause them to rupture, thus producing the fever, chills, and sweating characteristic of malaria. A few gametocytes are also formed. Only gametocytes cause a mosquito to become infectious and capable of transmitting the disease. Thus patients at this stage of the disease can transmit parasites to mosquitoes and thence to other human hosts.

Therapy for malaria depends on the stage of the disease and which plasmodial species is involved. *P. falciparum* and *P. malariae* do not produce persistent tissue forms of the para-

TABLE 48-2 Drugs to Treat Malaria

GENERIC NAME	TRADE NAME	ADMINISTRATION/DOSAGE	COMMENTS
Chloroquine	Aralen*	ORAL: *Adults*—For suppression, 500 mg once every 7 days. For therapy, 1 gm initially, 500 mg 6-8 hr later, then 500 mg once daily for 2 days. *Children*—For suppression, 8.3 mg/kg once every 7 days, not to exceed 500 mg. For therapy, 16.7 mg/kg initially, then 8.3 mg/kg at 6, 24, and 48 hr later. INTRAMUSCULAR: *Adults*—For therapy, 200-250 mg repeated in 6 hr if needed. INTRAMUSCULAR, SUBCUTANEOUS: *Children*—For therapy, 4.4 mg/kg repeated in 6 hr if needed.	Primary drug for therapy or prophylaxis of malaria.
Halofantrine	Halfan‡	ORAL: *Adults*—500 mg, repeated at 6 and 12 hr. Repeat schedule 1 wk later. *Children*—8 mg/kg, repeated at 6 and 12 hr. Repeat schedule 1 wk later.	Therapy for acute malaria caused by chloroquine-resistant *P. falciparum.*
Hydroxychloroquine	Plaquenil*	ORAL: *Adults*—For suppression, 400 mg once every 7 days. For therapy, 800 mg initially, 400 mg 6-8 hr later, then 400 mg once daily for 2 days. *Children*—For suppression, 6.4 mg/kg once every 7 days, not to exceed 400 mg. For therapy, 12.9 mg/kg initially, then 6.4 mg/kg at 6, 24, and 48 hr later, not to exceed 400 mg.	Primary drug for therapy or prophylaxis of malaria.
Mefloquine	Lariam	ORAL: *Adults*—For prophylaxis, 250 mg once a week. For therapy, 1250 mg once. *Children 15-45 kg body weight*—For prophylaxis, one-fourth, one-half, or three-fourths tablet once weekly. For therapy, 16.5 mg/kg as a single dose.	Prophylaxis or therapy of malaria, including disease caused by chloroquine-resistant *P. falciparum.*
Primaquine		ORAL: *Adults*—26.3 mg once daily for 14 days. *Children*—0.68 mg/kg once daily for 14 days.	Primary drug for radical cure of malaria *(P. vivax, P. ovale);* kills gametocytes of *P. falciparum.*
Pyrimethamine	Daraprim*	ORAL: *Adults*—75 mg once with 1.5 gm of sulfadoxine. May be combined with quinine or mefloquine. *Children*—1.25 mg/kg once with 25 mg/kg sulfadoxine.	Therapy for malaria caused by chloroquine-resistant *P. falciparum.*
Quinine		ORAL: *Adults*—600-650 mg every 8 hr for 3-7 days. May be combined with doxycycline, clindamycin, or sulfadoxine/pyrimethamine. *Children*—8.3 mg/kg every 8 hr for 3-7 days. May be combined with clindamycin or sulfadoxine/pyrimethamine.	Therapy for malaria caused by chloroquine-resistant *P. falciparum.*

*Available in Canada and United States.
‡Not commercially available in United States or Canada.

site; therefore therapy that destroys blood forms of the protozoan will be curative. With *P. vivax* and *P. ovale,* therapy must include a drug that destroys the persistent tissue forms of *Plasmodium.*

Chloroquine has been the leading antimalarial drug for decades, but chloroquine-resistant malaria has developed in several regions of the world. Chloroquine-resistant malaria is treated with combinations including quinine, mefloquine, halofantrine, and pyrimethamine with sulfadoxine. Clindamycin, dapsone, doxycycline, and tetracycline have also been included in treatment regimens for chloroquine-resistant disease.

Several of the drugs used to treat malaria may also be used for prophylaxis. Chloroquine, hydroxychloroquine, mefloquine, and pyrimethamine with sulfadoxine are given in once-weekly doses.

Therapeutic Agents: Malaria

Primary Agents

Chloroquine
Hydroxychloroquine

Mechanism of Action

Chloroquine and hydroxychloroquine are both *4-aminoquinolines.* This family of drugs has been the mainstay of antimalarial therapy worldwide since the late 1940s. All effective members of this family can bind tightly to double-stranded DNA, thereby altering the physical properties of DNA. These drugs may also inhibit metabolic processes in *Plasmodium*.

Pharmacokinetics

Chloroquine phosphate and hydroxychloroquine sulfate are satisfactorily absorbed from the GI tract. Chloroquine hydrochloride is available for intramuscular (IM) injection when oral dosage is impossible.

Drugs of the 4-aminoquinoline family are strongly concentrated in the liver, spleen, kidneys, and lungs. More important to the therapeutic usefulness, the drugs are also concentrated in red blood cells. Infected red blood cells may concentrate the drug up to 1000-fold over concentrations in plasma.

The 4-aminoquinolines may be metabolized by hepatic microsomal enzymes; some of the metabolites retain antiplasmodial activity. The drugs and metabolites are eliminated by the kidneys. Renal excretion is enhanced by acidifying urine, which converts the drug to a charged form that is not reabsorbed.

Uses

Chloroquine and hydroxychloroquine are both used for suppressive treatment and treatment of acute malaria caused by *P. falciparum, P. malariae, P. ovale,* and *P. vivax.* Chloroquine-resistant strains of *P. falciparum* require combinations of drugs. Radical cure of *P. ovale* and *P. vivax* requires addition of primaquine to the drug regimen.

Adverse Reactions and Contraindications

At the doses commonly used in therapy, chloroquine and hydroxychloroquine can produce nausea and other GI tract symptoms. These symptoms may be minimized by administering the drugs with meals.

Visual changes may also occur with 4-aminoquinolines; ciliary muscle impairment may be minor, but persistent or more severe changes in vision may signal overdose (see next section).

Chloroquine and hydroxychloroquine are relatively safe drugs if care is taken to avoid overdose, prolonged use, or use in sensitive patients. Patients with glucose-6-phosphate dehydrogenase (G6PD) deficiency are more likely than normal patients to suffer hemolysis when treated with these drugs. Children are also more sensitive to these agents than are adults (see box). Patients with liver disease or retinal damage are also more at risk of severe toxic reactions.

Toxicity

The toxic reactions to 4-aminoquinolines are greatly increased when the drugs are used for prolonged periods such as with long-term malaria prophylaxis. Signs of overdose include cardiovascular signs (arrhythmias, cardiovascular collapse, hypotension), CNS toxicity (drowsiness, excitability, headache, seizures), and visual disturbances (blurred vision). Blurred vision may signal reversible impairment of accommodation, but retinal or corneal changes are not reversible. Patients reporting misty vision, patchy vision, or foggy patches in the visual field may be developing serious eye damage.

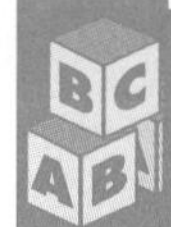

PEDIATRIC CONSIDERATION

Chloroquine and Hydroxychloroquine

THE PROBLEM

Infants and children are more sensitive to 4-aminoquinolines than are adults. Children have died after swallowing as little as 750 mg of chloroquine. Severe reactions and sudden death have been reported with parenteral use.

SOLUTIONS

- Use minimal effective doses in children.
- Do not give these drugs long term to children.
- Carefully observe children receiving these drugs.
- Keep drugs out of easy reach of children.
- Use childproof caps on medication containers.
- Never refer to medication as candy.

Interactions

The 4-aminoquinolines should not be used with penicillamine because they may cause excessive accumulation and toxicity of penicillamine.

Primaquine

Mechanism of Action

Primaquine is an 8-aminoquinoline. The mechanism of action may be different from the related 4-aminoquinolines, but the exact mechanism by which primaquine kills certain forms of plasmodia is unknown (see Table 48-2).

Pharmacokinetics

Primaquine is well absorbed after oral doses. Drug concentrations in plasma peak within 6 hours of the dose, but the drug is extensively metabolized and rapidly cleared from blood.

Uses

Primaquine keeps gametocytes of *P. falciparum* from the blood, thereby preventing the transmission of malaria to the mosquito and thence to human hosts. In addition, primaquine is used to produce a radical cure of *P. vivax* and *P. ovale* infections. By destroying the tissue-bound forms of the pathogen, primaquine prevents relapses.

Adverse Reactions and Contraindications

Primaquine given at normal therapeutic doses produces little toxicity. Abdominal cramps and epigastric distress can occur, but these symptoms can usually be relieved by taking the drug with meals.

Primaquine may damage red blood cells. The drug blocks production of an intracellular reducing agent, NADPH. In normal cells this deficit is made up by glucose metabolism, and the cell continues to function normally, but patients with reduced levels of G6PD cannot use glucose rapidly enough to make up the deficit. Red blood cells in these patients accumulate oxidized products such as methemoglobin, which is not an efficient oxygen carrier. Cyanosis may result. Ultimately, these red blood cells may rupture. Hemolysis can be severe and signals that drug dosage should be reduced or that treatment should be stopped. One sign of hemolysis that may be seen easily is darkening of urine.

Primaquine side effects are more severe in patients lacking G6PD. The lack of G6PD is genetically determined and exists in high proportions of certain populations such as Sardinians, Sephardic Jews, Greeks, and Iranians. African-Americans are less prone to this deficiency than these groups but have a higher incidence than the Caucasian population of the United States. Patients with these increased sensitivities to primaquine may be given lower doses of the drug.

Toxicity

High doses of primaquine cause methemoglobinemia, as well as other signs of blood dyscrasias.

Interactions

Primaquine is not routinely used with other bone marrow suppressants because the risk of leukopenia is too great. Quinacrine is also avoided with primaquine because of excessive toxicity with the combination.

Alternate Drugs

Halofantrine

Halofantrine is not available commercially in North America but is used elsewhere for acute malaria caused by chloroquine-resistant *P. falciparum.*

Halofantrine may interfere with digestion of hemoglobin by the organism. Oral absorption of drug is best when it is taken with a fatty meal. Halofantrine is not excreted renally; drug appears unchanged in feces. GI tract side effects or rashes are the most likely side effects. Cardiovascular toxicity is rare but potentially fatal. For this reason, halofantrine is avoided in patients with a history of cardiac arrhythmias. The drug is also avoided in patients receiving mefloquine because the risk of cardiovascular toxicity is increased.

Mefloquine

Mefloquine is used for prophylaxis or therapy of malaria caused by chloroquine-resistant *P. falciparum* or for malaria caused by *P. malariae, P. ovale,* or *P. vivax.* For radical cure of *P. ovale* or *P. vivax,* primaquine must be added to the regimen. Mefloquine is often considered as an alternate to its chemical relative quinine. Mefloquine, like quinine, acts only against the blood-borne forms of *Plasmodium* (see Table 48-2). The exact mechanism of action is unknown.

Oral absorption of mefloquine is usually in excess of 85%. The drug distributes well to many tissues, including cerebrospinal fluid and brain. Mefloquine is concentrated in red blood cells, which may contribute to the effect against the organisms harbored there.

Mefloquine is metabolized to a variable degree in liver. Elimination is slow, with drug remaining in the body for up to 1 month. This long elimination half-life allows the drug to be given as a single dose to treat malaria.

Mefloquine may cause GI tract distress, including vomiting. At higher doses it may also cause CNS effects such as dizziness, headache, anxiety, confusion, or seizures. Visual disturbances have also been noted. Slowing of the heart rate (bradycardia) is a rare side effect. Mefloquine is not combined with chloroquine to avoid excessive CNS toxicity or with quinidine or quinine to avoid excessive cardiovascular toxicity.

Pyrimethamine

Pyrimethamine in combination with quinine and sulfadoxine is used to treat chloroquine-resistant *P. falciparum.* It is also a primary agent for toxoplasmosis; see p. 567 for a full discussion of pyrimethamine.

Pyrimethamine, as it is normally used in treating chloroquine-resistant malaria, produces few side effects.

Quinine

Quinine may be active against all four forms of *Plasmodium* and is used today primarily for drug-resistant malaria (see Table 48-2). In acute illness when patients require intravenous (IV) medication, the related drug quinidine (Chapter 19) may substitute for quinine, which is too irritating to be given parenterally. Quinine should be combined with pyrimethamine and sulfadoxine for best effect.

Quinine is rapidly absorbed orally. The drug is generally well distributed throughout the body, although it does not enter the cerebrospinal fluid to a significant degree. Quinine is extensively metabolized and excreted in urine. Excretion is enhanced in acidic urine.

Quinine can produce cinchonism (quinine comes from cinchona bark). Symptoms include ringing in the ears (tinnitus), altered hearing acuity, headache, blurred vision, and diarrhea. At the doses used today, these symptoms are usually mild. If the dosage is increased or if the patient is hypersensitive, severe cinchonism can arise. Various blood dyscrasias may occur as well.

Sulfadoxine

Sulfadoxine is a sulfonamide used in combination with pyrimethamine to treat chloroquine-resistant *P. falciparum* malaria (see Table 48-2). For a full description of the properties of sulfadoxine, see Chapter 44.

Therapeutic Rationale: Selected Parasitic Diseases

The diseases covered in this section ordinarily occur in small numbers of patients. The diseases may be related to travel (giardiasis), occur as opportunistic infections mostly in immunosuppressed hosts (cryptosporidiosis, pneumocystosis, toxoplasmosis), or be passed from host to host (trichomoniasis).

Cryptosporidiosis

Cryptosporidia are small protozoans that infect microvilli of host intestinal cells and cause diarrhea in several species of animals and in humans. The most common infections in humans are caused by *Cryptosporidium parvum*. The disease is passed from host to host by ingestion of thick-walled cysts; but within a single host, thin-walled cysts can release sporozoites that are invasive and invade surrounding host cells. This recycling autoinfection is more common in severely immunocompromised patients.

Cryptosporidium has spread as a waterborne infection when the highly chlorine-resistant thick-walled cysts contaminate water supplies. Runoff from feedlots where large numbers of cattle are maintained may pose a risk of contaminating water supplies unless these facilities are kept well away from the watershed area of the water supply. Animals including calves, puppies, kittens, and rodents harbor *Cryptosporidium* and may pass it to humans.

Many patients with acquired immunodeficiency syndrome (AIDS) suffer chronic, debilitating diarrhea in the late stages of their disease; for many of these patients, *C. parvum* infection is a contributing factor to the diarrhea. Patients with intact immune systems generally recover well with only supportive therapy to maintain fluid and electrolyte balance. No effective therapy for *C. parvum* infections exists, although spiramycin has been somewhat helpful for some patients (Table 48-3). New drugs will be required to aid severely immunosuppressed patients.

Giardiasis

Giardiasis is an intestinal infection caused by the protozoan *Giardia lamblia*. This disease, which is passed between human hosts by ingestion of fecally contaminated food, may be asymptomatic in many patients. For others, it may be much more severe, producing diarrhea, GI tract distress, and malabsorption. Quinacrine or metronidazole are primary drugs for giardiasis in adults (see Table 48-3).

Pneumocystosis

Pneumocystis carinii has been recognized as an opportunistic pathogen for several decades, but little is known about the life cycle of this organism. Although the organ-

TABLE 48-3 Drugs to Treat Selected Parasitic Diseases

GENERIC NAME	TRADE NAME	ADMINISTRATION/DOSAGE	COMMENTS
Atovaquone	Mepron*	ORAL: *Adults*—750 mg 2 or 3 times daily, with high-fat meal. FDA pregnancy category C.	Alternate drug for *P. carinii* pneumonia.
Furazolidone	Furoxone	ORAL: *Adults*—100 mg 4 times daily for 7-10 days.	Alternate drug for giardiasis.
✤ Metronidazole	Flagyl*	ORAL: *Adults*—For giardiasis, 2 gm once daily for 3 days. For trichomoniasis, 2 gm once, then 250 mg every 8 hr for 7 days. FDA pregnancy category B. *Children*—For giardiasis, 5 mg/kg 3 times daily for 5-7 days. For trichomoniasis, 5 mg/kg every 8 hr for 7 days.	Primary drug for giardiasis and for trichomoniasis.
Pentamidine	Pentam Pentacarinat†	INTRAVENOUS: *Adults and children*—4 mg/kg infused over 1-2 hr once daily for up to 21 days. FDA pregnancy category C.	Primary drug for pneumocystosis.
Piritrexim		INTRAVENOUS: *Adults*—Up to 170 mg/m^2 of body surface has been used.	Alternate drug for *P. carinii* pneumonia.
Pyrimethamine	Daraprim*	ORAL: *Adults*—50-200 mg daily with 250 mg-1 gm of sulfadiazine for 1-2 days, then 25-100 mg daily with 250 mg-1 gm of sulfadiazine for up to 6 wk. AIDS patients require therapy for life to suppress infection. FDA pregnancy category C. *Children*—1 mg/kg once daily for 1-3 days, then 0.5 mg/kg once daily for 4-6 wk, with sulfonamide.	Primary drug for toxoplasmosis.
Quinacrine	Atabrine*	ORAL: *Adults*—100 mg 3 times daily for 5-7 days. *Children*—2 mg/kg 3 times daily for 5-7 days.	Alternate drug for giardiasis.
Spiramycin	Rovamycine*	ORAL: *Adults*—1 gm 3 times daily for 3-4 wk. *Children*—50-100 mg/kg daily divided into 2 or 3 doses.	Investigational drug for cryptosporidiosis.
Trimetrexate	Neutrexin*	INTRAVENOUS: *Adults*—45 mg/m^2 of body surface once daily for 21 days, with leucovorin 20-40 mg/m^2 every 6 hr continued throughout therapy and for 72 hr after halting trimetrexate. FDA pregnancy category D.	Alternate drug for *P. carinii* pneumonia.

*Available in Canada and United States.
†Available in Canada only.
‡Not commercially available in United States or Canada.

ism is related to fungi, the clinically effective drugs are antiprotozoal agents. *P. carinii* seldom causes disease in healthy humans, but it can produce severe pulmonary disease in patients receiving immunosuppressive drugs or patients with AIDS. Young, malnourished children are also susceptible. As many as half the patients who acquire this disease may die unless treated. Patients receiving immunosuppressive cancer chemotherapy or those receiving immunosuppressive drugs to prevent rejection of a transplanted organ usually respond well to the fixed combination of sulfamethoxazole and trimethoprim for prophylaxis or therapy (Chapter 44).

Sulfamethoxazole and trimethoprim may be used to treat *P. carinii* pneumonia in AIDS, but AIDS patients suffer an unusually high incidence of serious reactions to these drugs. Pentamidine is also effective against *P. carinii* pneumonia but also causes serious toxicity. Alternate therapy for *P. carinii* pneumonia in AIDS patients includes atovaquone, clindamycin with primaquine, dapsone with trimethoprim, and trimetrexate or piritrexim with leucovorin.

Toxoplasmosis

In the United States, toxoplasmosis is primarily acquired from ingestion of the oocyte of *Toxoplasma gondii.* The most common source of infection is cat feces. In adult humans the disease is usually mild and transitory, with symptoms resembling those of mild mononucleosis. Occasionally, the disease may involve the eyes or nervous system in adults, but congenital toxoplasmosis is usually fatal, causing severe damage to eyes, brain, and other organs of the fetus. Because of the dangers this disease poses to fetuses, many obstetricians suggest that pregnant women not handle used cat litter and avoid close contact with cats. Pyrimethamine and sulfadiazine are used in combination to treat this disease (see Table 48-3).

Toxoplasmosis is common in AIDS patients, with encephalitis causing death. Aggressive therapy with pyrimethamine and sulfonamides is usually attempted; for patients who cannot tolerate sulfonamides, other drugs such as clindamycin may be combined with pyrimethamine. Alternate agents include atovaquone or piritrexim.

Trichomoniasis

Vaginal infections caused by *Trichomonas vaginalis* occur commonly. The disease is marked by watery discharge from the vagina and signs of tissue irritation. Trichomonas may be unnoticed in the urinary tract and in the rectum, but these sites can serve as sources of infection.

Vaginal **trichomoniasis** may be treated with local agents applied as gels or douches. Complete cure of the sites outside the vagina and of infections in the male urinary tract may require a systemic agent. Metronidazole is the drug of choice (see Table 48-3).

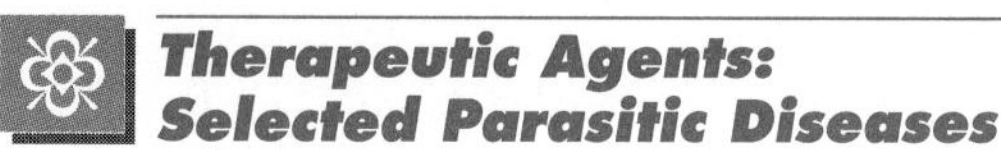

Therapeutic Agents: Selected Parasitic Diseases

Primary Drugs

Metronidazole

Metronidazole has become a primary agent for giardiasis and trichomoniasis (see Table 48-3). A full discussion of the drug appears in the section on amebic disease (p. 561), for which it is also a primary agent.

Pentamidine

Mechanism of Action

The action of pentamidine against *P. carinii* (see Table 48-3) is not completely understood but involves an interference with DNA function.

Pharmacokinetics

Pentamidine is given intravenously for therapy. For prophylaxis of *P. carinii* pneumonia, pentamidine may be aerosolized. When properly administered by this route, the drug is carried into the lungs in droplets small enough to be deposited into the alveoli, where *P. carinii* lodges. Therefore high concentrations are achieved at the site of infection, but because systemic absorption from lungs is low, whole body toxicity is minimized. Unfortunately, *P. carinii* infections at other sites occur because the systemic concentration of drug is low.

Pentamidine is concentrated in renal tissue and is excreted primarily in urine. Complete elimination from the body is slow, with drug appearing in urine as long as 8 weeks after therapy stops.

Uses

Pentamidine is the primary drug for pneumocystis pneumonia in patients who cannot tolerate trimethoprim and sulfamethoxazole.

Adverse Reactions and Contraindications

Patients receiving pentamidine intravenously may suffer acute hypotension, cardiac arrhythmias, and death. Hypoglycemia may be severe. Long-term effects may include hyperglycemia or diabetes mellitus. Nephrotoxicity and blood dyscrasias can also develop. The incidence of side effects can vary, depending on the patient being treated. In general, AIDS patients suffer more of the major and minor reactions to pentamidine than do other patients.

Pentamidine is contraindicated in patients who have had allergic reactions to either parenteral or inhaled pentamidine. Pentamidine worsens the following conditions: bone marrow depression, diabetes mellitus, heart disease, hypoglycemia, or renal impairment.

Toxicity

High doses of pentamidine given rapidly by IV infusion cause dangerous hypotension.

Interactions

Pentamidine worsens the effects of bone marrow depressants or nephrotoxic drugs. The risk of pancreatitis is worsened with didanosine. Foscarnet and pentamidine significantly alter calcium and magnesium levels in blood.

Pyrimethamine

Mechanism of Action

Pyrimethamine inhibits the enzyme dihydrofolate reductase in susceptible organisms, thereby blocking formation of tetrahydrofolic acid (THFA), a cofactor required for several metabolic transformations. The blocked enzyme normally converts dihydrofolic acid (DHA) to THFA. The formation of DHA may be blocked by sulfonamides (Chapter 44). Combining pyrimethamine and a sulfonamide is an example of synergistic effects produced by two drugs acting in the same metabolic pathway. Another example is trimethoprim and sulfamethoxazole (Chapter 44).

Pharmacokinetics

Pyrimethamine is well absorbed orally. The drug concentrates in blood cells and tissues, including liver, where it is metabolized. Metabolites are excreted in urine. Pyrimethamine appears in the milk of nursing mothers.

Uses

Pyrimethamine in combination with sulfadiazine is used to treat or suppress toxoplasmosis. Clindamycin may substitute for sulfadiazine if patients cannot tolerate sulfonamides. Pyrimethamine is an alternate agent for malaria, being used with sulfadoxine and quinine for chloroquine-resistant *P. falciparum* malaria.

Adverse Reactions and Contraindications

Pyrimethamine, as it is normally used in treating chloroquine-resistant malaria, produces few side effects. In higher doses such as those used to treat toxoplasmosis the drug may impair host folic acid metabolism, leading to megaloblastic anemia and various other blood dyscrasias. Treatment with leucovorin (a folinic acid supplement) may be required.

Pyrimethamine is usually avoided if possible in patients with anemia, bone marrow depression, or a history of seizures.

Toxicity

Large doses of pyrimethamine may produce nausea and vomiting. Excitability and signs of CNS overstimulation, including seizures, may occur within 2 hours of the dose. Very high doses may produce respiratory depression or circulatory collapse and death.

Interactions

Pyrimethamine is avoided if possible in persons also receiving other folate antagonists or bone marrow depressants, to avoid excessive actions of these agents.

Quinacrine

Mechanism of Action

Quinacrine has multiple metabolic effects that may account for its usefulness for giardiasis (see Table 48-3).

Pharmacokinetics

Quinacrine is well absorbed from the GI tract, but when given orally, the drug induces vomiting in many patients because it is very bitter tasting. Quinacrine is well distributed throughout the body and seems to bind strongly to tissues. Patients may notice a yellow discoloration of the skin. The reaction is not a sign of jaundice but simply illustrates the distribution of this yellow-colored drug to the skin.

Uses

Quinacrine is a primary drug only for giardiasis. It has been replaced by safer drugs for malaria and for helminthic infestations.

Adverse Reactions and Contraindications

Quinacrine causes few serious side effects when used for short-term treatment. Dizziness and toxic psychosis are occasionally noted. Psoriasis may be exacerbated. The most common reactions to quinacrine are headache, nausea, and vomiting. Quinacrine crosses the placenta and should not be used in pregnant patients. The drug is also avoided if possible in patients with psychosis or psoriasis because these conditions may be worsened.

Toxicity

Use of high doses of quinacrine or prolonged use of the drug may cause aplastic anemia, corneal edema, hepatitis, or retinopathy. Life-threatening overdose is characterized by seizures, hypotension, and arrhythmias followed by cardiovascular collapse.

Interactions

Primaquine toxicity may be worsened because quinacrine may increase primaquine concentrations in blood. This rise in blood levels may result from lowered metabolism of primaquine and displacement of primaquine from tissues.

Alternate Drugs

Atovaquone

Atovaquone is an oral agent used to treat *P. carinii* pneumonia in patients who cannot tolerate trimethoprim and sulfamethoxazole. The agent is also in trials against *T. gondii* in AIDS patients.

Atovaquone is absorbed poorly, and the amount of drug absorbed varies greatly from patient to patient. The half-life of the drug is between 2 and 3 days. There is little biotransformation, with most of the drug being slowly eliminated in feces.

Side effects of atovaquone that were observed in AIDS patients include allergic reactions (fever, skin rash) and GI tract symptoms (diarrhea, nausea, vomiting). Coughing, headache, and insomnia were also reported.

Furazolidone

Furazolidone is a nitrofuran similar in action to those used to treat urinary tract infections (Chapter 44). The drug is used orally to treat infections of the bowel. Like other nitrofurans, it does not reach high serum concentrations.

Furazolidone is metabolized by the liver. One of the breakdown products is a potent inhibitor of monoamine oxidase (MAO). Inhibition of this enzyme lowers elimination of catecholamines, which may cause hypertension. In addition, this action makes drugs such as sympathomimetics (e.g., ephedrine and phenylephrine), MAO inhibitors (e.g., pargyline), or foods rich in tyramine (e.g., cheese, beer, and wine) unsafe for patients receiving furazolidone.

Furazolidone may produce hemolytic reactions, especially in patients who have G6PD deficiency. Allergies and GI tract symptoms may also occur. Patients receiving furazolidone who also drink alcohol may exhibit a disulfiram-like reaction with flushing, difficulty in breathing, and a feeling of constriction in the chest.

Piritrexim

Piritrexim has been in trials for *P. carinii* pneumonia and *T. gondii* in AIDS patients. Piritrexim acts in the same way as pyrimethamine but is a much more potent inhibitor of dihydrofolate reductase and therefore does not require coadministration of a sulfonamide for therapy against these two organisms. Piritrexim does require coadministration of leucovorin, a form of folic acid that rescues mammalian cell from the antifolate effects of piritrexim.

Piritrexim may be given orally or intravenously. The drug distributes well in tissues and has an elimination half-life of 4 hours.

Piritrexim causes mucositis and myelosuppression, side effects that usually limit the dose of drug that can be used. Oral doses of the drug cause nausea and vomiting, which may be reduced somewhat by dividing the daily dose into two equal doses. IV doses of piritrexim cause phlebitis.

Spiramycin

Spiramycin is a macrolide antibiotic related to erythromycin (Chapter 41) and most likely affects bacterial ribosomes in the same way as erythromycin. The mechanism of action on *C. parvum* is unknown.

Oral absorption of spiramycin is often less than 50%. The drug is distributed to many tissues but does not enter the cerebrospinal fluid to any significant degree. Spiramycin is concentrated in bile and excreted almost exclusively by that route. Very little drug appears in urine.

Nausea, vomiting, diarrhea, and indigestion may occur with spiramycin. Fatigue and altered sensation have also been reported.

Sulfamethoxazole and trimethoprim

Sulfamethoxazole and trimethoprim are used together to treat pneumocystosis. For a full description of these drugs, see Chapter 44.

Trimetrexate

Trimetrexate is an alternate drug for *P. carinii* pneumonia. Trimetrexate acts in the same way as pyrimethamine but is a much more potent inhibitor of dihydrofolate reductase and therefore does not require coadministration of a sulfonamide. Trimetrexate does require coadministration of leucovorin, a form of folic acid that rescues mammalian cell from the antifolate effects of trimetrexate.

Trimetrexate is administered intravenously. There is hepatic metabolism of the drug, producing several metabolites including a glucuronide. The drug and metabolites are eliminated by the kidneys.

The most common side effect with trimetrexate is neutropenia, with fever and sore throat. Other blood dyscrasias may also occur, such as thrombocytopenia or anemia; signs include unusual bleeding, bruising, or tiredness. Less common side effects are confusion, itching, and GI tract symptoms.

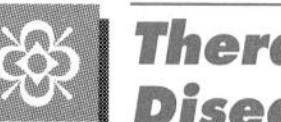

Therapeutic Rationale: Diseases Caused by Helminths

Helminths include flukes, tapeworms, and roundworms that can cause disease. Table 48-4 summarizes antihelminthic agents.

Ascariasis

Ascariasis, also called *roundworm infestation,* is caused by ingesting the eggs of *Ascaris lumbricoides.* This common disease is spread by fecally contaminated food and water. Larvae and adult worms migrate through lungs, liver, gallbladder, or other organs and may cause severe damage. *Ascaris* infestations may be treated effectively with several agents, including albendazole, mebendazole, piperazine, and pyrantel (see Table 48-4).

Enterobiasis

Enterobiasis is pinworm infestation. Pinworms are freely passed between people living close together. Constant reinfection occurs since huge numbers of eggs are passed and they adhere to clothing, towels, and hands. The disease is usually mild, but some patients may suffer pruritus ani, pruritus vulvae, or more serious symptoms.

Since pinworms tend to stay within the intestinal tract, treatment of the disease is relatively simple. Albendazole, mebendazole, and pyrantel are all nearly 100% effective after a single dose. Piperazine is also effective, but therapy continues over a period of several days (see Table 48-4).

Whipworm Infestation

Whipworm infestation is usually asymptomatic, although large numbers of worms in small children may produce diar-

TABLE 48-4 Drugs to Treat Diseases Caused by Helminths

GENERIC NAME	TRADE NAME	ADMINISTRATION/DOSAGE	COMMENTS
Albendazole	Eskazole‡ Zentel‡	ORAL: *Adults and children >2 yr*—For ascariasis, enterobiasis, hookworm, or whipworm, 400 mg once. For threadworms or tapeworms, 400 mg once daily for 3 days. For trichinosis, 400 mg twice daily for 15 days.	Alternate drug for helminthic infestations.
Ivermectin‡		ORAL: *Adults*—up to 200 mg/kg as single dose.	Alternate drug for threadworm infestation.
✤ Mebendazole	Vermox*	ORAL: *Adults and children >2 yr*—For enterobiasis, 100 mg once. Repeat in 2-3 wk. For ascariasis, hookworm, or whipworm, 100 mg in morning and evening for 3 days. Repeat if needed in 2-3 wk. FDA pregnancy category C.	Primary drug for ascariasis, enterobiasis, and hookworm or whipworm infestations.
Niclosamide	Niclocide	ORAL: *Adults*—2 gm as single dose or for up to 7 days, depending on kind of tapeworm. FDA pregnancy category B. *Children 11-34 kg*—1 gm as single dose; may be followed by 500 mg daily for up to 6 days, depending on kind of tapeworm. *Children >34 kg*—1.5 gm as single dose; may be followed by 1 gm daily for up to 6 days.	Primary drug for tapeworm infestation.
Piperazine	Entacyl†	ORAL: *Adults*—Tablet form for ascariasis, 3.5 gm daily for 2 days. For enterobiasis, 65 mg/kg daily for 7 days. *Children*—For ascariasis, 75 mg/kg daily for 2 days. For enterobiasis, as adults.	Alternate drug for ascariasis and enterobiasis.
Praziquantel	Biltricide	ORAL: *Adults and children >4 yr*—20-25 mg/kg 2 or 3 times daily for 1 day. FDA pregnancy category B.	Alternate drug for infections caused by flatworms; primary drug for schistosomiasis.
Pyrantel	Antiminth Combantrin†	ORAL: *Adults and children >2 yr*—For ascariasis or enterobiasis, 11 mg/kg as single dose; repeat in 2-3 wk if needed. Maximum daily dose 1 gm.	Primary drug for ascariasis and enterobiasis.
Thiabendazole	Mintezol	ORAL: *Adults and children >13.6 kg*—25 mg/kg twice daily for 2-7 days, depending on site and type of infection. FDA pregnancy category C.	Primary drug for hookworm or threadworm infestation and trichinosis.

*Available in Canada and United States.
†Available in Canada only.
‡Not commercially available in United States or Canada.

rhea, anemia, and cachexia. Whipworm infestations are effectively treated with mebendazole (see Table 48-4).

Threadworm Infestation

Threadworm infestation, also called *strongyloidiasis*, is more serious than many infestations because the worms may reproduce in humans. Larvae migrate from the intestinal wall into systemic circulation and thence return to the intestine to mature and further increase the numbers of worms in the host. Malabsorption syndrome, diarrhea, and duodenal irritation may occur.

Most drugs used against helminths are ineffective against threadworms since they live within intestinal tissue. Thiabendazole is well distributed to the tissues where this parasite lives and thus eliminates infestation. Ivermectin, a drug developed to treat river blindness and filariasis in tropical regions, is also useful against threadworms (see Table 48-4).

Hookworm Infestation

Hookworm infestation, called *necatoriasis*, occurs in the southern United States. Although two species of hookworms are known, most infestations encountered in the United States are caused by *Necator*. Therefore most patients may be treated with mebendazole or pyrantel. Another type of hookworm from dogs and cats produces a cutaneous lesion called *creeping eruption*, or *cutaneous larva migrans*. Thiabendazole, either topically or orally, may kill the parasites and limit allergic responses, which cause itching, burning, and skin damage (see Table 48-4).

Trichinosis

Trichinosis, or *pork roundworm infestation*, is uncommon today. Ingested cysts from raw or improperly cooked meat develop into adult worms in the intestine. Larvae are released into the circulation and enter muscle to form cysts. Patients suffer GI tract upset, fever, muscle aches, and eosinophilia.

Trichinosis cannot yet be effectively treated. Most patients receive therapy to minimize symptoms rather than produce a cure since most patients survive the disease and carry the quiescent worms encysted in skeletal muscle for the rest of their lives. Thiabendazole, albendazole, and mebendazole have been used in some cases to try to prevent migration of worms to muscles (see Table 48-4).

Tapeworm Infestation

Tapeworms, or **cestodes,** of several types can infest humans. Beef, pork, fish, and dwarf tapeworms are all sensitive to niclosamide. Praziquantel, a drug used primarily in the tropics for schistosomiasis, may also be effective against tapeworms (see Table 48-4). All detected infestations are treated, even though they are mostly asymptomatic. Pork tapeworm infestations may become serious if reflux of eggs from the intestine allows them to reach the stomach and hatch into larvae that invade tissues.

Therapeutic Agents: Diseases Caused by Helminths

Primary Agents

Mebendazole

Mechanism of Action

Mebendazole is an effective broad-spectrum antihelminthic agent that causes microtubules in helminths to disintegrate (see Table 48-4). This action blocks glucose uptake in sensitive helminths. Since these organisms require externally supplied glucose to maintain energy levels, blockade of glucose absorption destroys the worms.

Pharmacokinetics

Mebendazole is used orally for its action against intestinal helminths. Very little drug is absorbed into systemic circulation. The small amount of drug that enters the blood is metabolized by the liver and excreted in urine. If liver function is impaired, the small amount of drug absorbed may accumulate and cause toxicity. Fatty foods favor absorption of mebendazole.

Uses

Mebendazole is an excellent agent against a variety of helminthic diseases, including ascariasis and enterobiasis, as well as infestations caused by hookworm or whipworm (see Table 48-4).

Adverse Reactions and Contraindications

Mebendazole produces few toxic reactions. Abdominal discomfort and diarrhea may result, especially if large masses of worms are expelled.

Toxicity

High doses of mebendazole typically cause GI tract disturbances that last for a few hours. Little systemic toxicity is expected.

Interactions

Few interactions with mebendazole exist, but patients taking mebendazole often have higher than normal liver enzyme (alanine aminotransferase [ALT], aspartate aminotransferase [AST]) and blood urea nitrogen (BUN) levels.

Niclosamide

Mechanism of Action

Niclosamide is effective against tapeworms. These segmented flatworms are killed by a single dose of niclosamide. The dead worm segments are often digested by proteolytic agents in the gut. For this reason a cathartic may be given 1 or 2 hours after the drug has been taken to allow the dead-but-still-intact worm parts to be identified in feces. This purge is required when the tapeworm infestation is caused by the pork tapeworm. With this organism, digestion of the dead worm segments releases living eggs, which can develop in humans and cause more serious, invasive disease. The purge removes the worm segments before they rupture and prevents this complication.

Pharmacokinetics

Niclosamide is not absorbed from the bowel and exerts all of its actions within the lumen of the bowel.

Uses

Niclosamide is a primary drug for a variety of tapeworm infestations that are limited to the intestinal tract. It is not effective for cysticercosis, in which tapeworm larvae live in the intestinal wall.

Adverse Reactions and Contraindications

Niclosamide is almost without side effects because the drug is not absorbed. Some patients have mild GI tract symptoms on the day of therapy. There are no contraindications other than possible history of allergy to the drug.

Toxicity

Niclosamide overdoses are treated with laxatives and enemas to remove the drug. Systemic toxicity is unlikely.

Interactions

Niclosamide interactions with other drugs are unlikely because niclosamide is essentially unabsorbed from the bowel.

Pyrantel

Mechanism of Action

Pyrantel is a depolarizing neuromuscular blocker, similar in action to succinylcholine. Pyrantel causes spastic paralysis and contraction of the muscle in worms (see Table 48-4). The parasites are eliminated from the body by normal peristalsis.

Pharmacokinetics

Pyrantel is not absorbed from the GI tract to any great extent. The small amount absorbed is excreted by the kidneys. Pyrantel produces its desired effects entirely within the lumen of the bowel.

Uses
Pyrantel is effective, when given in short courses, against a variety of worms including roundworms (ascariasis) and pinworms (enterobiasis). Purges are not necessary adjuncts to therapy with this drug.

Adverse Reactions and Contraindications
Since pyrantel is not well absorbed after oral dosage, few systemic effects occur. Headache, muscle twitching, and dizziness may result from CNS effects of this drug. More commonly the drug causes mild GI tract upset and transient changes in liver function tests.

Toxicity
Little toxicity is expected with pyrantel since it is largely contained in the bowel.

Interactions
Piperazine may antagonize the action of pyrantel; they are not used together.

Thiabendazole
Mechanism of Action
Thiabendazole is a potent and specific antihelminthic agent (see Table 48-4). Its exact mechanism of action is unknown, but it is believed to attack a metabolic process essential in helminths but not found in humans.

Pharmacokinetics
Thiabendazole is well absorbed orally, and peak blood levels may be expected within 1 hour of ingestion. Most of the drug is eliminated by hydroxylation and conjugation, these metabolites being the predominant forms of the drug excreted in urine. Very little unchanged drug appears in feces.

Uses
Thiabendazole is used for cutaneous or visceral larva migrans caused by hookworm and other agents, for threadworm infections, and for trichinosis. The drug must be used very soon after infestion of meat infected with *Trichinella spiralis* to lessen subsequent infection in host muscle. Thiabendazole has no effect on larvae encysted in muscle.

Adverse Reactions and Contraindications
Thiabendazole can cause a wide variety of transient, dose-related reactions. The most common effects are anorexia, nausea, vomiting, numbness in the extremities, and dizziness. A few patients experience more severe GI tract symptoms or CNS effects such as drowsiness, headache, or giddiness. Rarely, tinnitus, abnormal sensations in the eyes, or metabolic derangements occur. Although these symptoms may incapacitate a patient, it is rare for the effect to persist beyond 48 hours, and most subside much sooner.

Thiabendazole alters liver function in some patients. Therefore patients with preexisting liver disease should be more carefully observed for progressive liver damage.

Patients frequently report a strong, unpleasant odor to their urine after thiabendazole therapy. The odor is reminiscent of that produced when asparagus is ingested. Patients may be reassured that this odor is caused by a metabolite of thiabendazole and is harmless.

Toxicity
Thiabendazole overdoses can cause significant GI tract and CNS symptoms. There is no specific antidote, but emesis or gastric lavage may help limit reactions.

Interactions
Thiabendazole significantly lowers clearance of theophylline, thereby causing theophylline to accumulate to dangerously high concentrations in blood. Serious CNS toxicity may arise.

Alternate Drugs
Ivermectin
Ivermectin seems to act as an agonist at gamma-aminobutyric acid (GABA) receptors, which interferes with function of the nervous system in threadworms and other parasites (see Table 48-4). The paralyzed worms may die.

Ivermectin is given as a single oral dose that is effective for up to a year. The drug concentrates in the liver and fat tissue in the body. Excretion is primarily in feces, with little drug being found in urine.

Ivermectin may cause dizziness, fever, headache, arthralgia, myalgia, and swollen lymph nodes. Postural hypotension is rare.

Piperazine
Piperazine is effective against *Ascaris* and pinworm infestations (see Table 48-4). The drug apparently blocks the action of acetylcholine on the muscles of these parasites. As a result, the worms are paralyzed and are eliminated from the bowel by normal peristaltic flow. The eliminated worms are alive.

Piperazine is well absorbed after oral administration. A portion of the drug is metabolized to various inactive products. The kidney is the primary route for excretion. Patients with impaired renal or hepatic function may be more sensitive to piperazine than other patients.

Piperazine produces few toxic effects at doses routinely used to treat helminthic infestations. GI tract upset and occasional skin rashes have occurred. Transient neurologic signs ranging from headache and dizziness to ataxia, paresthesias, or convulsions have been seen, but severe reactions are more common with overdoses. The more severe reactions also occur in patients with renal dysfunction, who tend to accumulate the drug, and in patients with seizure disorders, who are more sensitive to the CNS effects of the drug.

Praziquantel
Praziquantel interferes with muscle function in the parasites and can cause local destruction of the integument of these organisms.

Praziquantel is well absorbed after oral administration but undergoes extensive first-pass metabolism in the liver (see Chapter 1). The metabolites that are formed are excreted by the kidneys.

Praziquantel frequently causes mild and transient effects on the CNS. Common signs are headache, dizziness, and malaise. Most patients also report GI tract distress.

NURSING PROCESS OVERVIEW

Protozoal or Helminthic Therapy

Assessment

Perform a baseline assessment of the patient. Include in the patient history questions related to travel within and outside the United States or Canada; recent exposure to new food or water supplies; possible exposure through family members or school or business contacts who have had a similar illness recently; and any previous history of infection with protozoal or helminthic agents. Once drug therapy is ordered, monitor appropriate laboratory work related to potential drug side effects.

Nursing Diagnoses

- Potential knowledge deficit related to transmission of specific protozoal or helminthic infestation

Patient Outcomes

The patient will describe measures to treat and help prevent future infestations.

Planning/Implementation

Monitor the patient's overall condition, with close attention to subjective and objective data related to the infection. It may be appropriate to monitor close family members for the appearance of the infection.

Refer the patient to the local health department for follow-up and for the epidemiologic tracking of health problems.

Evaluation

Many of these drugs do not cause side effects when used for a single infestation and for a short period of time. Before discharge, ascertain that the patient can explain why and how to take the drug, what side effects may occur, what side effects require consultation with the physician, what symptoms indicate unsuccessful treatment or reinfestation, and what other measures to use for assistance in eliminating the protozoa or helminthic agent causing the problem.

NURSING IMPLICATIONS SUMMARY

DRUGS TO TREAT PROTOZOAL AND HELMINTHIC INFESTATIONS

Patient and Family Education

- Encourage the patient to report any unexpected sign or symptom.
- Remind the patient to keep these and all medications out of the reach of children. Many of the medications are available in pleasant-tasting syrups or chewable tablets, which may tempt young children.
- Many of the problems discussed in this chapter require treatment of an entire family. Doses of medication for children may be quite different than adult doses. Emphasize the importance of taking doses as prescribed.
- Remind the patient to keep all health care providers informed of all drugs being used or that have been used in the preceding 6 months.
- Most of these drugs are not recommended for use during pregnancy unless absolutely necessary and should not be used during lactation. Question female patients about possible pregnancy before administering drug.
- Reinforce to the patient the need to continue the course of medication for as long as prescribed and to avoid discontinuing medications without notifying the physician.
- Remind the patient to use medications only as directed. Many of these drugs are dispensed with patient information leaflets; review these with the patient before discharge.
- Review with the patient and family appropriate ways to treat or prevent the problem. Review as appropriate activities such as handwashing, sanitation, and cleaning infected bedding or clothing. Be nonjudgmental and supportive. Obtain information about diseases caused by protozoa and helminths from the local health department or the Centers for Disease Control and Prevention in Atlanta. Refer the patient as appropriate to the local health department for follow-up.
- Suggest that the patient considering international travel contact the Centers for Disease Control and Prevention about health hazards in countries they will be visiting.
- If these are drugs to *prevent* malaria, emphasize the importance of taking the drug on a regular schedule, as prescribed. For example, if ordered once a week, instruct the patient to take doses on the same day each week. The patient should begin therapy at least 2 weeks before exposure to areas where malaria is endemic and for up to 4 weeks after leaving the area.

NURSING IMPLICATIONS SUMMARY—cont'd

- To help avoid exposure to malaria-carrying mosquitoes, advise the patient to sleep under mosquito netting or in an air-conditioned room. Instruct the patient to wear long-sleeved shirts, long pants, and socks, especially when outside. Mosquitoes are out from dusk to dawn. Instruct the patient to use mosquito repellent to exposed skin surfaces during this time and limit outdoor activities. Instruct the patient to use mosquito sprays in living quarters during evening and nighttime hours to kill mosquitoes. These same guidelines apply if patients are trying to avoid exposure to sandflies (which carry kala-azar) or tsetse flies (which carry African sleeping sickness).
- For treatment of *pinworms:* Pinworms are easily passed among household members, so the entire family may be treated. Instruct the patient(s) to take all doses of medication as ordered. Instruct the patient(s) to wear pajamas and underwear to sleep during treatment and to wash all bedding and pajamas after treatment to prevent reinfection.
- For treatment of *hookworms:* Infection with hookworms may cause anemia. If the patient is to take medication to treat anemia, emphasize the importance of taking the iron preparation as prescribed and continuing it for 3 to 6 months after treatment for hookworms.
- For treatment of *tapeworms:* Review with the patient the importance of inspecting meat carefully and cooking it thoroughly.
- For treatment of *threadworms:* Review the importance of cooking vegetables thoroughly before eating to destroy threadworms.

INDIVIDUAL DRUGS

- Any drug not listed below is discussed fully in the text or is similar to others in its class.

Iodoquinol

Drug Administration

- Assess allergy to this drug, chloroxine, clioquinol, iodine, pamaquine, pentaquine, primaquine.
- For treatment of amebiasis, assess signs of dehydration, intake and output, weight, abdominal pain, diarrhea.
- Assess and monitor neurologic function. Assess for visual changes. Inspect for skin changes, rashes, and skin discoloration.

Patient and Family Education

- Review anticipated benefits and possible side effects of drug therapy with the patient.
- Instruct the patient to take doses after meals. Tablets may be crushed and mixed with applesauce or chocolate syrup. Review with the patient how to crush tablets if necessary.
- Because iodoquinol can interfere with thyroid function tests, remind the patient to keep all health care providers informed for at least 6 months after therapy with iodoquinol is completed that this drug has been taken.
- Caution the patient to avoid driving or operating hazardous equipment if visual changes occur and to notify the physician if these changes do occur.

Metronidazole

Drug Administration

- When metronidazole is used for trichomoniasis, assess for vaginal discharge and itching, irritation of bladder, urethra, or vagina.
- When metronidazole is used for amebiasis, assess for signs of dehydration, intake and output, weight, abdominal pain, diarrhea. Monitor stool examination.
- When metronidazole is used for giardiasis, assess diarrhea, characteristics of stool, and abdominal cramping.
- Superinfection can occur. Assess for *Candida* overgrowth in mouth or vagina; assess for diarrhea.

Intravenous Metronidazole

- Review the manufacturer's instructions about reconstitution of IV doses. Do not use syringes with aluminum needles or hubs. Administer prepared dose over at least 1 hour; dose may also be given as a continuous infusion. Instruct the patient to report redness or pain in the extremity. Monitor serum drug levels if available.

Patient and Family Education

- Review anticipated benefits and possible side effects of drug therapy with the patient.
- Instruct the patient to take oral doses with meals or a snack to lessen gastric irritation.
- Instruct the patient to avoid drinking alcohol while taking oral, IV, or vaginal metronidazole. See the patient problem box on disulfiram-like reactions (p. 635).
- See the patient problem boxes on vaginal infections (p. 539) and dry mouth (p. 300).
- For vaginal dryness, suggest that women use a commercially available lubricant designed for vaginal mucosa.
- Warn the patient to avoid driving or operating hazardous equipment if visual changes or dizziness occur and to notify the physician if these symptoms do occur.
- Warn the patient that urine may temporarily turn reddish brown because of the drug.
- Tactfully assess changes in libido. Provide emotional support as appropriate. Remind the patient not to discontinue drug therapy without notifying the physician.
- When metronidazole is used to treat trichomoniasis, the physician may wish to treat the patient and the sexual partner. Also the physician may recommend that the patient use a condom during sexual intercourse until the infection clears.

Continued.

Nursing Implications Summary—cont'd

Diloxanide

Drug Administration/Patient and Family Education

- When diloxanide is used for amebiasis, assess for signs of dehydration, intake and output, weight, abdominal pain, diarrhea. Monitor stool examination.
- Encourage the patient to return for regular follow-up to monitor for drug effectiveness.
- Remind the patient to take drugs as prescribed for the full course of therapy.

4-Aminoquinolines (Chloroquine and Hydroxychloroquine)

Drug Administration

- When 4-aminoquinolines are used for malaria, assess myalgia, fatigue, malaise, chills or history of shaking chills, and lung sounds. Monitor blood smear to confirm malaria.
- Assess for visual changes; signs of depression such as withdrawal, lack of interest in personal appearance, insomnia, or anorexia; and hearing acuity.
- Monitor blood pressure and electrocardiographic (ECG) changes (when patients are receiving long-term therapy), complete blood count (CBC) and differential, platelet count, serum creatinine level, and BUN level.

Patient and Family Education

- Review common side effects. Instruct the patient to report signs of blood dyscrasia including pallor, malaise, sore throat, fever, and unexplained bleeding or bruising.
- Since many CNS side effects have been reported, including personality changes, instruct family members to report any persistent personality changes, apathy, agitation, or irritation.
- Notify the physician if changes in vision or difficulty in reading develop. Caution the patient to avoid driving or operating hazardous equipment if visual changes occur and to notify the physician if these changes do occur. Encourage the patient receiving long-term therapy to have periodic ophthalmic examinations.
- Instruct the patient to notify the physician if hearing loss develops.
- Take doses with milk, meals, or a snack to lessen gastric irritation. Report persistent or severe gastric irritation to the physician.
- These drugs are especially toxic to children. Keep medication out of the reach of children.
- See the general guidelines for information about malaria prophylaxis.
- If used to treat arthritis, lupus, or other chronic problems, instruct the patient that weeks of therapy may be necessary to see improvement. Emphasize the importance of returning to the physician regularly for follow-up.

Primaquine

Drug Administration/Patient and Family Education

- When used for malaria, assess myalgia, fatigue, malaise, chills or history of shaking chills, and lung sounds. Monitor blood smear to confirm malaria.
- Monitor CBC and differential and platelet count.
- Warn the patient to avoid driving or operating hazardous equipment if visual changes occur and to notify the physician if these changes do occur.
- Instruct the patient to take doses with meals or antacids to reduce gastric distress. The patient should notify the physician if gastric distress is severe or persistent.
- Instruct the patient to report any new side effect.

Halofantrine

Drug Administration/Patient and Family Education

- When used for malaria, assess myalgia, fatigue, malaise, chills or history of shaking chills, and lung sounds. Monitor blood smear to confirm malaria.
- Instruct the patient to take doses on an empty stomach.
- See the general guidelines for information about malaria prophylaxis.

Mefloquine

Patient and Family Education

- When mefloquine is used for malaria, assess myalgia, fatigue, malaise, chills or history of shaking chills, and lung sounds. Monitor blood smear to confirm malaria.
- Instruct the patient to take doses with a full (8-ounce) glass of water and with food.
- Caution the patient to avoid driving or operating hazardous equipment if visual changes, vertigo, or light-headedness occur and to notify the physician if these symptoms do occur.
- Take doses of mefloquine at least 12 hours after the last dose of quinidine or quinine if both drugs are prescribed.
- See the general guidelines for information about malaria prophylaxis.

Pyrimethamine

Drug Administration

- When pyrimethamine is used for malaria, assess myalgia, fatigue, malaise, chills or history of shaking chills, and lung sounds. Monitor blood smear to confirm malaria.
- When pyrimethamine is used for toxoplasmosis, assess rash, jaundice, weakness, lung sounds.
- When pyrimethamine is combined with sulfadoxine (Fansidar), assess for allergy to sulfonamides, furosemide, thiazide diuretics, sulfonylureas, and carbonic anhydrase inhibitors.
- Assess and monitor neurologic status; assess for skin changes and visual acuity.

NURSING IMPLICATIONS SUMMARY—cont'd

- Monitor CBC and differential and platelet count.

Patient and Family Education

- Remind the patient to report any new side effects to the physician.
- Warn the patient to avoid driving or operating hazardous equipment if excessive fatigue develops and to notify the physician if this symptom develops.
- See the patient problem box on bleeding tendencies (p. 586).
- Instruct the patient to take oral doses with meals if desired. Tablets may be crushed to make a suspension; consult the pharmacist. Instruct the patient to notify the physician if GI symptoms are severe or persistent. Emphasize to the patient the importance of taking doses at regularly spaced intervals and trying not to forget any doses.
- Pyrimethamine may cause anemia, which is treated with leucovorin (see Chapter 22).

Quinine

Drug Administration

- When quinine is used for malaria, assess myalgia, fatigue, malaise, chills or history of shaking chills, and lung sounds. Monitor blood smear to confirm malaria.
- Assess and monitor neurologic status; assess for cinchonism (see text). Be alert to symptoms of hypoglycemia such as pallor, perspiration, tachycardia, palpitations, nervousness, emotional changes, weakness, trembling, hunger, headache, blurred vision, and incoherent speech. Monitor blood glucose levels.
- Monitor CBC and differential, platelet count, prothrombin time, partial thromboplastin time, and liver function tests.

Intravenous Administration (quinidine gluconate)

- Dilute as directed. Administer a loading dose over 1 to 2 hours, while monitoring for hypotension and widening of the QRS interval. A constant infusion of a lower dose is administered after the loading dose. Keep the patient supine until blood pressure is stable. Keep siderails up. Monitor ECG changes. See Chapter 19.

Patient and Family Education

- Instruct the patient to report any new side effects.
- Warn the patient to avoid driving or operating hazardous equipment if visual changes occur and to notify the physician if these changes do occur.
- Take doses with meals or a snack to reduce gastric irritation. Warn diabetic patients to monitor blood glucose levels carefully.

Sulfadoxine

- See Chapter 44.

Pentamidine

Drug Administration

- For *P. carinii* pneumonia, assess vital signs, lung sounds, cough, dyspnea on exertion, and weight loss. Monitor blood gases and/or pulmonary function tests if available.
- With aerosolized doses, toxicity is less common. Monitor pulse, blood pressure, and respiratory rate. Auscultate lung sounds.
- With systemic administration, assess for signs of hypoglycemia such as pallor, perspiration, tachycardia, palpitations, nervousness, irritability, weakness, trembling, hunger, headache, blurred vision, cycloplegia, incoherent speech, emotional changes, and fatigue. Monitor blood glucose levels.
- Assess for skin changes. Monitor intake and output and weight.
- Monitor serum creatinine and BUN levels, CBC and differential, and serum electrolyte level.
- Warn the patient that IM injections may cause a burning sensation and tenderness at the injection site. Use meticulous technique to avoid abscess formation.

Parenteral Administration

- Review the manufacturer's insert for current guidelines. Keep the patient in a supine position. Monitor blood pressure before administering pentamidine and at 5- to 15-minute intervals. Monitor ECG changes if the patient's condition warrants it. Administer IV doses over 60 minutes. Monitor IV administration sites and instruct the patient to report pain or irritation.
- Have drugs, equipment, and personnel available to treat acute allergic reactions in the setting where pentamidine is administered.

Patient and Family Education

- Instruct the patient to report any unexpected side effects.
- Review the patient problem boxes on bleeding tendencies (p. 586) and leukopenia (p. 585). These problems are more common with the systemic form of pentamidine.
- For *inhalation pentamidine:* If the patient using the inhalation form of pentamidine is also supposed to use an inhalation bronchodilator, instruct the patient to use the bronchodilator first, then wait 5 to 10 minutes before using the pentamidine unless otherwise instructed by the physician. Do not mix any drugs with the pentamidine for inhalation.
- Instruct the patient to avoid smoking while receiving inhalation therapy.
- Inhalation pentamidine may cause a metallic or unpleasant taste in the mouth. Instruct the patient to try sucking on hard candy to relieve this side effect.
- Instruct the patient to report the development of difficulty breathing or swallowing, skin rash, wheezing, nausea and

Continued.

Nursing Implications Summary—cont'd

vomiting, pain in the upper abdomen or chest, chills, cold sweats, headache, shakiness, or unusual fatigue.

Quinacrine

Drug Administration

- When quinacrine is used for giardiasis, assess diarrhea, characteristics of stool, and abdominal cramping.
- Assess and monitor mental status; assess for skin and vision changes. Monitor weight in patients receiving long-term therapy.
- Monitor CBC and differential, platelet count, and liver function tests. Monitor stool examinations for giardiasis.

Patient and Family Education

- Remind the patient to report any new side effects.
- Warn the patient to avoid driving or operating hazardous equipment if dizziness or confusion develops and to notify the physician if these symptoms occur.
- Instruct the patient to notify the physician if GI tract symptoms are severe or persistent.
- Encourage the patient to have regular ophthalmic examinations if recommended by the physician.
- Warn the patient that this drug may cause a yellowish discoloration of the eyes, skin, or urine. This is harmless and will clear when the course of drug therapy is over. Review the drug package insert for information about treating tapeworms.
- Instruct the patient to take doses after meals with a full (8-ounce) glass of water, juice, or tea. Tablets may be crushed and mixed with jam, honey, chocolate syrup, or other sweet foods to mask the bitter taste. Instruct the patient to mix with only a small amount of food and take all the dose as ordered.

Atovaquone

Drug Administration/Patient and Family Education

- For *P. carinii* pneumonia, assess vital signs, lung sounds, cough, dyspnea on exertion, and weight loss. Monitor blood gases and/or pulmonary function tests if available. Monitor CBC and liver function tests.
- For toxoplasmosis, assess rash, jaundice, lung sounds, and weakness.
- Instruct the patient to take doses with a high-fat meal, such as a cheeseburger, milkshake, or ice cream. Crush tablets, if needed, to make them easier to swallow.
- Emphasize the importance of taking all doses, as prescribed, even if feeling better.

Furazolidone

Drug Administration/Patient and Family Education

- Assess for nausea and vomiting. If persistent or severe, notify the physician. For giardiasis, assess diarrhea, abdominal cramping, and characteristics of stool.
- Review information on nitrofurans in Chapter 44.
- Review the patient problem box on disulfiram-like reactions (p. 635). Instruct the patient to avoid alcohol while taking furazolidone and for 4 days after completing therapy.
- Review the dietary consideration box on tyramine (p. 663). Effects of tyramine may persist for up to 2 weeks after finishing the course of furazolidone.
- Instruct diabetic patients to monitor blood glucose levels carefully; furazolidone may cause hypoglycemia.
- Instruct the patient that urine may be dark yellow or brown while taking this drug.
- Doses may be taken with food. For measuring the oral suspension, instruct the patient to use the calibrated measuring device supplied by the pharmacist.
- There are many drug interactions with furazolidone. Remind the patient to keep all health care providers informed of all drugs being taken.

Piritrexim

Drug Administration

- For *P. carinii* pneumonia, assess vital signs, lung sounds, cough, dyspnea on exertion, and weight loss. Monitor blood gases and/or pulmonary function tests if available. Monitor CBC and liver function tests.
- For toxoplasmosis, assess rash, jaundice, lung sounds, and weakness.
- For information about leucovorin, see Chapter 22.
- See the manufacturer's insert for current information.

Spiramycin

Drug Administration/Patient and Family Education

- Assess for side effects noted in the text.
- Review information about erythromycin in Chapter 41.
- Monitor liver function tests. Assess the following for hepatotoxicity: right upper quadrant abdominal pain, jaundice, nausea, vomiting, malaise, and fever.
- Instruct the patient to take oral doses 2 hours before or 3 hours after meals.
- Review the manufacturer's insert for information about IV administration.

Trimetrexate

Drug Administration/Patient and Family Education

- For *P. carinii* pneumonia, assess vital signs, lung sounds, cough, dyspnea on exertion, and weight loss. Monitor blood gases and/or pulmonary function tests if available. Monitor CBC and liver function tests.
- Review the manufacturer's insert for current information.
- See Chapter 22 for information about leucovorin.
- See the patient problem boxes on bleeding tendencies (p. 586) and leukopenia (p. 585).

NURSING IMPLICATIONS SUMMARY—cont'd

Mebendazole

Drug Administration

- For treatment of roundworms (ascariasis): assess lung sounds and cough, fever, anemia, weight loss, vomiting, and abdominal discomfort.
- For treatment of hookworms or threadworms: assess rash or vesicular eruption, cough and lung sounds, abdominal pain, diarrhea, and fever.
- For treatment of tapeworms: assess abdominal discomfort, anemia, and weight loss.
- For treatment of pinworms: assess oral or perianal itching or irritation, especially at night. Monitor laboratory result of cellophane tape swabbing of anal region.
- For treatment of whipworms: assess characteristics of diarrhea and stool, anemia, and weight loss.

Patient and Family Education

- Instruct the patient to report any unexpected signs or symptoms.
- Warn the patient to avoid driving or operating hazardous equipment if visual changes occur and to notify the physician if these changes do occur.
- Instruct the patient to notify the physician if severe or persistent GI tract symptoms occur.
- Tablets may be chewed, swallowed whole, or crushed and mixed with food. Instruct the patient to take doses with high-fat meals.

Niclosamide

Drug Administration

- For treatment of tapeworms: assess abdominal discomfort, anemia, and weight loss.

Patient and Family Education

- Warn the patient to avoid driving or operating hazardous equipment if visual changes occur and to notify the physician if these changes do occur.
- Instruct the patient to report any unexpected finding.
- Instruct the patient to take doses after a light meal to avoid gastric upset.
- Instruct the patient to chew tablets well before swallowing. For small children, crush the tablet and mix with water to form a paste.

Pyrantel

Drug Administration

- For treatment of roundworms (ascariasis): assess lung sounds and cough, fever, anemia, weight loss, vomiting, abdominal discomfort.
- For treatment of pinworms: assess anal or perianal itching or irritation, especially at night. Monitor laboratory result of cellophane tape swabbing of anal region.

Patient and Family Education

- Instruct the patient to notify the physician if new side effects develop.
- To measure doses of the oral suspension, instruct the patient to shake bottle well, then use the calibrated measuring device supplied by the pharmacist.

Thiabendazole

Drug Administration

- For treatment of hookworms or threadworms: assess rash or vesicular eruption, cough and lung sounds, abdominal pain, diarrhea, and fever.
- For treatment of tapeworms: assess abdominal discomfort, anemia, and weight loss.
- For treatment of whipworms: assess characteristics of diarrhea and stool, anemia, and weight loss.
- For treatment of trichinosis: assess rash, periorbital edema, difficulty breathing and lung sounds, abdominal discomfort and diarrhea, photophobia, mental status examination, fever, weakness, headache, edema, and pain in the muscles.
- For cutaneous larva migrans: assess rash or vesicular eruption, cough and lung sounds, abdominal pain, diarrhea, and fever.
- Monitor pulse and blood pressure.
- Monitor CBC and WBC differential, serum creatinine and BUN levels, liver function tests, and blood glucose levels.

Patient and Family Education

- Instruct the patient to report any new side effects.
- Warn diabetic patients to monitor blood glucose levels carefully.
- Warn the patient to avoid driving or operating hazardous equipment if dizziness or visual changes occur and to notify the physician if these symptoms do occur.
- Instruct the patient to take doses after meals or a snack to lessen gastric irritation. Instruct the patient taking the chewable tablets to chew or crush tablets before swallowing them.
- Inform the patient that this drug may cause urine to have a temporary, harmless odor for up to 24 hours.
- For topical preparations, instruct the patient to apply the medicine directly to the infected area and in a large circle around the area, up to 2 to 3 inches in each direction.

Ivermectin

Drug Administration

- For treatment of hookworms or threadworms: assess rash or vesicular erruption, cough and lung sounds, abdominal pain, diarrhea, and fever.

Patient and Family Education

- Caution the patient to avoid driving or operating hazardous equipment if visual changes occur and to notify the physician if these changes occur.

Continued.

Nursing Implications Summary—cont'd

- Review the patient problem box on orthostatic hypotension (p. 157).
- Instruct the patient to notify the physician if any unexpected signs or symptoms develop.

Piperazine

Drug Administration

- For treatment of roundworms (ascariasis): assess lung sounds and cough, fever, anemia, weight loss, vomiting, and abdominal discomfort.
- For treatment of pinworms: assess anal or perianal itching or irritation, especially at night. Monitor laboratory result of cellophane tape swabbing of anal region.

Patient and Family Education

- Instruct the patient to report any unexpected signs or symptoms.
- Instruct the patient to notify the physician if GI tract symptoms are severe or persistent.
- Instruct the patient to take doses after meals or a snack to lessen gastric irritation. Instruct the patient to prepare granules for oral solution by dissolving the contents of 1 packet of granules in 2 ounces of water, milk, or fruit juice. Drink all the liquid to get the full dose.

Praziquantel

Drug Administration

- For treatment of schistosomiasis, assess rash and fever. Monitor stool and urine examination.
- For treatment of tapeworms, assess abdominal discomfort, anemia, and weight loss.

Patient and Family Education

- Warn the patient to avoid driving or operating hazardous equipment if visual changes occur and to notify the physician if these changes occur.
- Instruct the patient not to chew tablets but to swallow them whole. Suggest that the patient take doses during meals to avoid a bitter taste in the mouth.
- Instruct the patient to notify the physician if unexpected signs or symptoms develop.

Critical Thinking

APPLICATION

1. What are the main sites of amebic infection?
2. Why is metronidazole effective for amebic infections outside the intestine but iodoquinol is not?
3. What parasitic diseases other than amebiasis are treated with metronidazole?
4. Why should patients receiving metronidazole avoid ethyl alcohol?
5. Name two sites where plasmodia exist in the human body.
6. How is the use of the 8-aminoquinoline primaquine different from the uses of chloroquine or hydroxychloroquine?
7. What toxicity is associated with primaquine?
8. What drugs may be used for chloroquine-resistant *Plasmodium falciparum* malaria?
9. What type of disease is produced by *Giardia lamblia?*
10. What patients are most at risk from toxoplasmosis?
11. What patient group is most likely to contract pneumocystosis?
12. What two routes are used for pentamidine administration? Why?
13. What is the mechanism of action of mebendazole?
14. How does the tissue distribution of mebendazole affect mebendazole use?
15. What is the tissue distribution of orally administered niclosamide?
16. What is the mechanism of action of pyrantel pamoate?
17. What patient education is most important to help patients with enterobiasis avoid reinfection?
18. What transient effects follow thiabendazole administration?

CRITICAL THINKING

1. How does the tissue distribution of the 4-aminoquinolines increase the usefulness of the drugs in treating malaria?
2. What toxicity is associated with the 4-aminoquinolines? How should you assess for these?
3. What is the rationale for combining trimethoprim with sulfamethoxazole or combining pyrimethamine with sulfadiazine to treat parasitic infections?
4. What toxicity is associated with pyrimethamine? How should you assess for it?

SECTION XI

Drugs Used to Treat Cancer

Drugs that are effective against cancer are a diverse group of agents. Many drugs included in this section are more toxic than agents used for other indications. For this reason nursing care related to drug toxicity is emphasized.

CHAPTER 49 *Cytotoxic Drugs to Treat Cancer* covers agents that are active against cancer primarily because the drugs attack actively dividing cells. The effects of these drugs against cancer are considered in the context of normal cells, which they also affect.

CHAPTER 50 *Tissue-Specific Anticancer Agents* presents agents that often act through receptors. This mechanism localizes the action of the drug to tissues containing those receptors.

CHAPTER 49

Cytotoxic Drugs to Treat Cancer

OBJECTIVES

After studying this chapter, you should be able to do the following:

- *Discuss why most anticancer drugs are toxic toward rapidly growing tissues, both normal and cancerous.*
- *Discuss the side effects common to most anticancer drugs.*
- *Discuss the risks anticancer drugs may pose to health care personnel and how these risks can be minimized.*
- *Discuss the reasons for precautions taken to protect patients who are receiving anticancer drugs from exposure to infectious agents.*
- *Develop nursing care interventions for the patient with depressed white blood cell production, bleeding tendencies, or stomatitis.*
- *Develop a nursing care plan for the patient receiving one or more of the drugs discussed in this chapter.*

KEY TERMS

alkylating agents
alopecia
carcinogenesis
cell cycle
contact inhibition
leukopenia
metastasis
mitosis
oncogenes
stomatitis
thrombocytopenia

CHAPTER OVERVIEW

Cancer occurs when normal cells become transformed by chemicals, viruses, or unknown agents and thereby become resistant to normal regulation of cell division and other cellular processes. In this chapter cell proliferation in normal and cancerous tissues is considered. This presentation forms the basis for understanding the principle of selective toxicity as applied to cancer. Finally, specific cytotoxic agents used in cancer therapy are discussed in conjunction with the rationale behind successful therapeutic regimens.

Therapeutic Rationale: Cancer Chemotherapy

Nature of Cancer

Regulation of Cell Division

The **cell cycle** is the programmed sequence of events that occur during cell division. The cycle is divided into several segments according to the processes that occur during that phase. The first event in the cycle is a rapid increase in RNA synthesis. RNA is formed from the sugar ribose, the purine bases adenine and guanine, and the pyrimidine bases uracil and cytosine. This phase during which RNA synthesis begins is called G_1 (Figure 49-1).

The next phase in the cell cycle is the S phase, during which DNA synthesis occurs. DNA is the nucleic acid that contains the genetic information for the cell. DNA is formed from the same components as RNA, except that thymine is substituted for uracil and deoxyribose is substituted for ribose.

When DNA synthesis is complete, the cell contains twice the amount of DNA found in a nondividing cell. At this point RNA and protein synthesis increase, and the cell enters the G_2 phase. At the end of this phase the cell contains enough material to form two complete cells, and mitosis begins.

In **mitosis** DNA condenses to form chromosomes. As mitosis begins the cell has two copies of each chromosome. To separate these pairs so that one copy of each chromosome goes into each daughter cell, the cell forms microtubules that are organized into the mitotic spindle. Without the mitotic spindle to pull the chromosomes into opposite ends of the cell, reproduction would halt. Once the chromosomes have been successfully segregated into two complete sets, division is completed by closing the cell membrane to divide the mother cell into two daughter cells.

After cell division a cell may immediately reenter the reproductive cycle or it may become temporarily nonreproductive. In this nonreproductive phase, called G_0, the cell only repairs existing DNA and synthesizes only the RNA and protein needed for maintenance of the cell. A cell in the G_0 phase may become altered so that it is no longer capable of dividing, or after some time, it may enter phase G_1 and divide again (Figure 49-1).

Most normal tissues have very few cells actively reproducing at any one time. Most of the cells are either temporarily or permanently incapable of division, but there are exceptions to this rule. For example, bone marrow is the site for formation of blood cells and as a result is constantly undergoing cell division. Lymphoid tissue is the site for formation of lymphocytes and monocytes and therefore has a high rate of cell division. The intestinal lining, testes, ovaries, endometrium, and hair follicles are all additional sites of rapid cell division.

Cell division in cancer is perturbed so that cells seem to divide independent of any external signal. Significant genetic changes are associated with this property, including the expression of **oncogenes.** When these genes are expressed, cells may proliferate indefinitely, as opposed to most normal cells that do not proliferate or do so for a limited time. The altered metabolism of cancer cells reflects this commitment to pro-

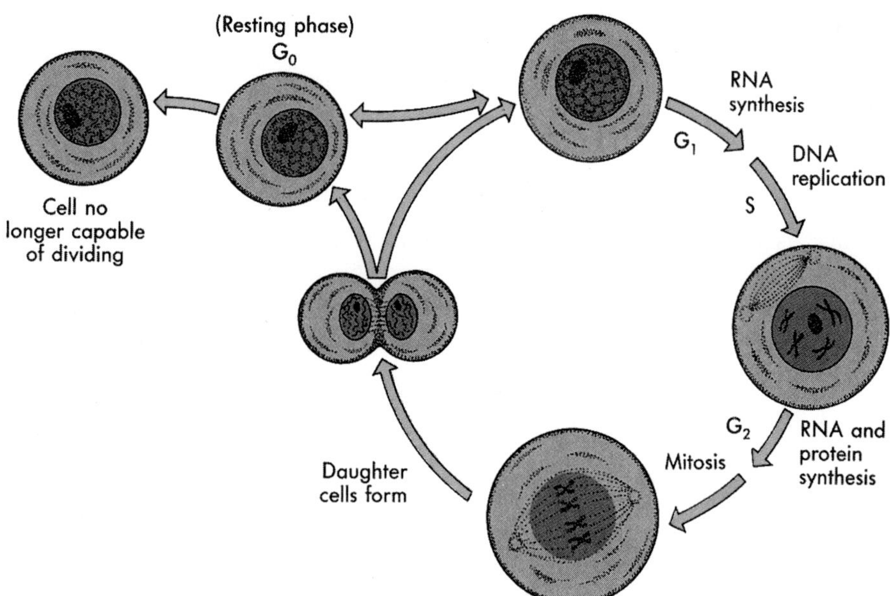

FIGURE 49-1
Proliferative cycle of mammalian cells. In actively dividing cells, metabolic processes required for cell division take place at different times during cycle. DNA synthesis precedes messenger RNA and protein synthesis; these processes must be complete before mitosis, or cell division, can occur. Because of metabolic differences, cells at different phases of cycle have different sensitivities to many drugs used to control cancer.

liferation. DNA and RNA synthesis is increased, along with other metabolic processes necessary for growth and cell division.

Origin of Cancer

Carcinogenesis is the process by which a normal cell is transformed into a cancerous cell. Agents called *carcinogens* may start this transformation by causing mutations or chromosomal translocations. Cells at this stage may divide, die, or lie quiescent. Other factors can influence the fate of the transformed cell. For example, some chemicals can promote division of the altered cell and may cause it to become fully malignant.

Spread of Cancer

Cancer cells lose the normal property of **contact inhibition.** Contact inhibition prevents normal cells from dividing when they are crowded together, but cancer cells continue to divide even when the pressure of the surrounding cell mass is considerable. Uncontrolled proliferation and loss of contact inhibition explain in part how cancer harms the body. In certain tissues, as the cancer proliferates, it forms a solid mass and crowds surrounding normal tissue as the mass, or tumor, grows. In other tissues, such as bone marrow, growth of the neoplastic cells is more diffuse, but ultimately normal tissue is overwhelmed and crowded out by the cancerous tissues.

Cancer cells can metastasize. In this process, cancer cells separate from the original mass and move directly or are carried by blood or lymph to distant sites. There the cells lodge in healthy tissue and begin to divide, thus producing a **metastasis** (secondary tumor). Tumors have been produced in experimental animals with single cancer cells. This property of cancer cells explains why cure of malignancies may require destruction of every cancer cell in the body.

Diseases Called Cancer

The public thinks of cancer as a single disease, but it is a large family of related diseases. Cancers may be categorized according to the tissue of origin (Table 49-1). Within these large categories, many subdivisions are possible. For example, leukemias can arise from any of the various cells within bone marrow. Therefore myelogenous leukemias (arising from myeloid tissue in the marrow), lymphocytic leukemias (arising from cells that form lymphocytes), and other forms of the disease exist.

Some tumors give rise to characteristic disease patterns. For example, Wilms' tumor, Kaposi's sarcoma, and choriocarcinoma all tend to strike a certain age and sex of patient (Table 49-2). Different forms of cancer may also respond differently to chemotherapy. For example, choriocarcinoma is relatively sensitive to chemotherapeutic agents, but Kaposi's sarcoma is not.

TABLE 49-1 Tissue of Origin for Types of Cancer

CANCER	TISSUE OF ORIGIN
Carcinoma	Epithelial cells (e.g., skin and mucous membranes of lung and GI tract)
Leukemia	Blood-forming organ (e.g., bone marrow or lymphoid tissue)
Lymphoma	Lymphoid tissue
Melanoma	Pigmented skin cells
Myeloma	Bone marrow
Sarcoma	Connective tissue (e.g., bone, cartilage, and others)

Controlling Cancer

Host Responses

In theory, one cancer cell left living after therapy can cause recurrence of cancer. In contrast, antibacterial therapy can be successful if bacteria are stopped from growing long enough for the immune system to attack and eliminate the invaders. With cancer the immune system seems much less effective. One reason for this difference is that cancer cells are not easily recognized as foreign by the host immune system. Another factor that seems to lower immune responses to cancer is that as tumors become massive, they produce a specific immune tolerance. Whatever the cause, chemotherapy for most cancers proceeds with little assistance from the host mechanism that so powerfully assists antibacterial agents; thus, therapy for

TABLE 49-2 Selected Neoplastic Diseases

DISEASE	CHARACTERISTICS
Burkitt's lymphoma	Rapidly growing tumor of lymphoid tissue; highly responsive to chemotherapy.
Choriocarcinoma (gestational trophoblastic tumors)	Rapidly growing tumor of embryonic cells; seeded in mother during abortion, childbirth, or after hydatidiform mole; highly responsive to chemotherapy.
Ewing's sarcoma	Rapidly growing tumor most often found in children; responsive to combination of surgery, radiation, and chemotherapy in early stages.
Hodgkin's disease	Tumor of lymph nodes, spleen, and other lymphoid tissue; highly responsive to chemotherapy.
Kaposi's sarcoma	Highly malignant, metastasizing tumor usually noted on skin of extremities. Although characteristic of AIDS patients, tumor is also seen in older men without AIDS.
Lymphocytic leukemia	Cancer of lymphoid tissue causes excess lymphocytes or lymphoblasts in blood; response to therapy is best in acute form of disease.
Myelogenous leukemia	Cancer of myeloid tissue leads to excess granular polymorphonuclear leukocytes in blood; response to therapy not as good as in lymphocytic leukemia.
Wilms' tumor	Rapidly growing tumor of children; highly responsive to combination of surgery, radiation, and chemotherapy.

cancer is often less effective than therapy for bacterial infections. Medical science is just learning how to modulate the immune system (Chapter 35) and there is hope that in the future the immune system can be recruited to combat cancer.

Chemotherapy

Another difficulty in treating neoplastic diseases is that cancer cells offer fewer targets for selective toxicity than do bacterial cells. This similarity in structure and metabolic processes reminds us that cancer cells are derived from host cells. Some differences between normal and cancerous cells can be identified, but they are mostly quantitative rather than qualitative. Specific targets for selective toxicity are discussed with individual drug mechanisms.

Another difficulty with cancer chemotherapy arises because diagnosis cannot be expected until late in the course of the disease. A single transformed cell after 10 cycles of cell division can produce at most 1024 cells, a mass far too small to be noticed. By the time the tumor weighs about 1 gm, it will have gone through about 30 division cycles. A 1 gm tumor is approximately the size of a small grape. In many locations within the body, a tumor this size may easily escape detection, yet in just 10 more cell divisions this tumor could exceed a mass of 1 kg (2.2 lb).

Most tumors do not grow nearly as rapidly as the theoretical example just cited, in which it was assumed that every cell formed immediately reentered the reproductive cycle. Certain cancers are rather slow growing and are described as having a low growth fraction. This description means that most of the tumor cells are temporarily or permanently incapable of division. Other tumors have a very fast growth rate with a high growth fraction.

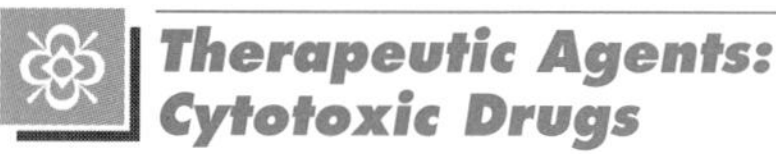

Therapeutic Agents: Cytotoxic Drugs

Agents That Directly Attack DNA

Properties common to this class of drugs are presented below; properties unique to individual drugs are covered with each agent.

Mechanism of Action

The genetic information necessary for cell reproduction resides in DNA. Nucleated cells contain all the genetic information required to form new cells, but information is seldom expressed in normal cells in most tissues because they rarely divide. For this reason, damage to the DNA of many normal cells is undetectable; in contrast, cancer cells with their rapid rates of replication may be killed by damage to the DNA. This rationale explains the use of a large group of anticancer drugs called **alkylating agents.**

Alkylating agents may attack DNA in its double-stranded form, attaching various compounds to one strand or the other. Other agents may form cross-links, or chemical bonds, between the strands. Because the strands must unwind and separate during replication, cross-linking effectively blocks replication.

Pharmacokinetics

Many drugs of this type are rapidly destroyed in the body. A few drugs like cisplatin, mechlorethamine, and melphalan are hydrolyzed or destroyed by nonenzymatic mechanisms in many fluids and tissues. Other drugs like altretamine, bleomycin, busulfan, carmustine, chlorambucil, and lomustine are rapidly metabolized in liver. A few drugs such as bleomycin are degraded by enzymes in many tissues.

Metabolism lowers activity of most of these drugs, but altretamine, chlorambucil, ifosfamide, and lomustine are activated by metabolism or the metabolites retain significant activity.

The duration of action of this class of agents is quite variable. Drugs like mechlorethamine are destroyed within seconds of administration, but the biologic effect may persist for weeks. Other drugs like mitoxantrone bind tightly to DNA and other structures and persist in the body for days to weeks.

Renal excretion is the most common route of elimination with these drugs. Some, such as chlorambucil or lomustine, are eliminated as metabolites; others such as ifosfamide or bleomycin are excreted largely unchanged. The elimination half-lives of these drugs vary from seconds for mechlorethamine to days for mitoxantrone.

Uses

The clinical uses of antineoplastic drugs that directly attack DNA are summarized in Table 49-3.

Adverse Reactions and Contraindications

The specificity of agents that destroy nucleic acid is not great. All cells will undergo attack by these chemicals, although the action is lethal primarily when cells attempt division. Therefore normal tissues with high growth fractions are most sensitive. Clinical symptoms to be expected include bone marrow suppression that produces **leukopenia** (low white cell counts) (see box, p. 585), **thrombocytopenia** (low platelet counts) (see box, p. 586), or other blood dyscrasias; mucocutaneous reactions including **stomatitis** (see box, p. 587) or other signs; and gastrointestinal (GI) toxicity, including acute or delayed nausea and vomiting.

The alkylating agents chemically alter DNA and are thus mutagenic. For this reason this class of agents can induce cancers of various types that may show up years after exposure to the drug. Not every patient will develop a second cancer as a result of chemotherapy, but for patients exposed to alkylating agents the risk is increased many times over the normal low incidence rate.

Some of these drugs have immunosuppressive activity. This action is especially strong with cyclophosphamide but is also observed with chlorambucil, melphalan, and mitoxantrone. Mechlorethamine is weakly immunosuppressive.

Toxicity

As doses increase, the degree of bone marrow suppression increases with these drugs. In addition to these expected effects on bone marrow, which is reflected in lower numbers of var-

TABLE 49-3 Anticancer Drugs That Directly Attack DNA

GENERIC NAME	TRADE NAME	ADMINISTRATION/DOSAGE	COMMENTS/USES
Altretamine	Hexalen Hexastat†	ORAL: *Adults*—260 mg/m² for 14 to 21 consecutive days/month. FDA pregnancy category D.	Used for ovarian carcinomas.
Bleomycin	Blenoxane*	INTRAMUSCULAR, INTRAVENOUS, SUBCUTANEOUS: *Adults and children*—0.25-0.5 U/kg once or twice weekly initially; 1 U daily or 5 U weekly for maintenance.	Palliative therapy for lymphomas, squamous cell carcinomas, and testicular or ovarian carcinomas. Pulmonary toxicity may be fatal.
Busulfan	Myleran*	ORAL: *Adults and children*—60-120 μg/kg daily or 1.8-4.6 mg/m² daily. FDA pregnancy category D.	May prolong survival in chronic myelocytic leukemia.
Carboplatin	Paraplatin*	INTRAVENOUS: *Adults*—300 mg/m² once every 4 wk. FDA pregnancy category D.	Palliative therapy for recurrent ovarian carcinoma.
Carmustine	BiCNU*	INTRAVENOUS: *Adults*—200 mg/m² as single dose, repeated no more often than every 6 wk. FDA pregnancy category D.	Palliative therapy for CNS tumors, lymphomas, and myelomas.
Chlorambucil	Leukeran*	ORAL: *Adults and children*—0.1-0.2 mg/kg daily for treatment; smaller doses for maintenance. FDA pregnancy category D.	Effective against lymphocytic leukemias and lymphomas.
Cisplatin	Platinol*	INTRAVENOUS: *Adults*—Up to 100 mg/m² once every 4 wk after heavy hydration to protect kidneys; doses are lower in combinations. FDA pregnancy category D.	Used to treat testicular cancer and carcinomas in many tissues. Renal damage, ototoxicity, and neurotoxicity may be severe.
Cyclophosphamide	Cytoxan*	ORAL: *Adults*—1-5 mg/kg daily. *Children*—2-8 mg/kg, various schedules. INTRAVENOUS: *Adults*—1.5-3 mg/kg daily. *Children*—2-8 mg/kg on various schedules. FDA pregnancy category D.	Effective for lymphomas, solid tumors, leukemias, myelomas. Hemorrhagic cystitis, leukopenia, or cardiotoxicity may occur.
Dacarbazine	DTIC† DTIC-Dome	INTRAVENOUS: *Adults*—2-4.5 mg/kg for 10 days every month or 150-250 mg/m² for 5 days every 21 days. FDA pregnancy category C.	Used to treat malignant melanoma and lymphomas.
Ifosfamide	IFEX*	INTRAVENOUS: *Adults*—1.2 g/m² daily for 5 days. FDA pregnancy category D.	Used for germ cell testicular tumors.
Lomustine	CeeNU*	ORAL: *Adults*—Up to 130 mg/m² in single dose; repeat in 6 wk. FDA pregnancy category D.	Similar to carmustine in use and properties.
Mechlorethamine	Mustargen*	INTRAVENOUS: *Adults*—0.4 mg/kg total dose in single or several doses. FDA pregnancy category D. INTRACAVITARY: *Adults*—0.2-0.4 mg/kg.	Used to treat Hodgkin's disease and other lymphomas; may be palliative for solid tumors or their effusions.
Melphalan	Alkeran*	ORAL: *Adults*—0.15 mg/kg daily for 2-3 wk or 0.25 mg/kg daily for 5 days. After recovery of bone marrow, 2-4 mg daily. FDA pregnancy category D.	Used to treat multiple myeloma and ovarian carcinomas.
Mitomycin	Mutamycin*	INTRAVENOUS: *Adults*—Up to 20 mg/m² as single dose, repeated no more often than every 6 wk.	Used to treat GI tumors. Renal toxicity may occur.
Mitoxantrone	Novantrone*	INTRAVENOUS: *Adults*—12 mg/m² daily for up to 3 days with other drugs. FDA pregnancy category D.	Used in acute nonlymphocytic leukemia.
Thiotepa	Thiotepa*	INTRAVENOUS: *Adults*—0.3-0.8 mg/kg every 1-4 wk. TOPICAL: *Adults*—30-60 mg in 30-60 ml for application to bladder for bladder carcinoma.	Palliative therapy for lymphomas, carcinomas, and malignant effusions.

*Available in Canada and United States.
†Available in Canada only.

ious cells in the blood, some of these drugs also have dose-related effects on other organs. For example, bleomycin and carmustine cause pulmonary toxicity, whereas cyclophosphamide and mitoxantrone cause cardiotoxicity.

Interactions

All drugs of this class except bleomycin may have significant interactions with bone marrow suppressants or radiation because the combinations can profoundly depress production of blood cells. Live virus vaccines are avoided in patients who receive any of these drugs because generalized viral infections may occur as a result of the immunosuppression these drugs produce. Oral polio vaccines may also be contraindicated for family members of patients who receive these drugs.

Altretamine

Altretamine is similar to alkylating agents, but its exact mechanism is unknown. This highly lipid-soluble drug is rapidly absorbed orally and must be activated by liver metabolism.

In addition to anemia, leukopenia, and thrombocytope-

PATIENT PROBLEM

Leukopenia

THE PROBLEM

Some drugs suppress the bone marrow, resulting in decreased production of white blood cells. With some drugs, this is a common side effect and is anticipated, as with many cancer chemotherapy drugs. With other drugs this side effect is unexpected and occurs only occasionally. Several medical terms may be used to describe this effect: agranulocytosis or granulocytopenia (severe reduction in granulocytes—basophils, eosinophils, and neutrophils) or neutropenia (reduction in neutrophils). The danger to the patient is the increased susceptibility to infection that results from a decreased supply of granulocytes.

SIGNS AND SYMPTOMS

Signs and symptoms include fever, sore throat, rash, malaise, chills, urinary frequency, dysuria, and altered level of consciousness. If the situation is untreated or unrecognized, the patient may develop a serious bacterial infection requiring IV drug therapy and hospitalization. The first line of treatment is to discontinue the drug causing the problem.

NURSING CARE

- Wash hands meticulously before caring for patients with suppressed white blood cell counts.
- Avoid putting patients with granulocytopenia into multibed rooms where other patients have diagnoses of infection. If possible, admit the patient to a private room.
- Use protective isolation only if necessary because this environment isolates the patient from family and friends; rather, screen visitors, and do not permit visits from individuals with obvious colds, bronchitis, chickenpox, herpes simplex or herpes zoster, childhood infectious diseases, or any other infections.
- Avoid the use of rectal thermometers.
- Carefully assess patients who are also receiving steroids because steroids may mask the symptoms of infection.
- Monitor the complete blood count (CBC), white blood cell differential, and hematocrit, hemoglobin, and platelet counts.

PATIENT AND FAMILY EDUCATION

- Notify the physician if symptoms develop.
- Monitor and record the body temperature (if the patient is able).
- If a period of bone marrow suppression is anticipated with each course or dose of drug, find out when the nadir of bone marrow suppression will occur. The nadir is the period of greatest bone marrow suppression or the period of lowest white blood count.
- If a period of suppressed white blood cell production is anticipated, as with cancer chemotherapy drugs, avoid contact with persons with colds or infections during periods of greatest susceptibility.
- Wash hands carefully after using the bathroom and after contact with other persons. Ask family members and friends to wash hands carefully before coming in contact with the patient.
- Instruct patients to avoid touching their eyes or the inside of the nose unless they have just washed their hands.
- Instruct patients to avoid immunizations.
- Do not bring cut flowers or fresh fruits and vegetables (unless washed carefully) to patients.

nia, side effects such as neurotoxicity that affects both the central and peripheral nervous systems are common. Patients may express anxiety or show awkwardness, confusion, dizziness, depression, numbness in limbs, or weakness. Seizures are less common.

Nausea and vomiting occur commonly with altretamine. This reaction usually appears several days after the start of therapy.

In addition to the expected interactions with bone marrow depressants and live virus vaccines, altretamine also interacts with monoamine oxidase (MAO) inhibitors. Severe orthostatic hypotension can result from this combination.

Bleomycin

Bleomycin is a mixture of glycopeptide antibiotics derived from cultures of *Streptomyces.* Bleomycin produces breaks in DNA strands and may also inhibit enzymes that normally repair damaged DNA.

Most tissues rapidly inactivate bleomycin, but skin and lungs are exceptions; therefore the drug tends to concentrate at those sites and produce toxic reactions. Tumors tend not to inactivate bleomycin, so the drug is also concentrated there.

Bleomycin often produces skin and mucous membrane changes, fever, chills, anorexia, and vomiting. Pulmonary reactions occur in 10% to 40% of treated patients, and 1% may die. Lung toxicity begins as pneumonitis and progresses to pulmonary fibrosis.

Bleomycin usually does not suppress the bone marrow and therefore need not be avoided in patients who receive bone marrow suppressants or live virus vaccines. Bleomycin makes lung tissues more susceptible to damage by oxygen. As a result, general anesthetics may provoke a rapid deterioration in pulmonary function.

Busulfan

Busulfan is an alkylsulfonate capable of cross-linking DNA. For reasons that are unclear, busulfan possesses a degree of selectivity that is unique among this class of drugs. Busulfan is a myelosuppressant at doses that do not significantly lower the levels of other blood cells, although platelets may be re-

PATIENT PROBLEM

Bleeding Tendencies

May be caused by anticoagulant therapy or low platelet count (thrombocytopenia)

THE PROBLEM

The platelet level is low, so the patient bleeds easily, or the patient is receiving anticoagulant therapy.

SIGNS AND SYMPTOMS

Bruising; petechiae (minute, pinhead size hemorrhagic spots on the skin; seen only with reduced platelets); bleeding such as bleeding gums or nose bleeds (epistaxis); change in the color of urine which might indicate bleeding in the kidney; anal bleeding; and bleeding in stools.

PATIENT AND FAMILY EDUCATION

- Notify the physician if unexplained or excessive bleeding or bruising develops.
- Avoid using a razor with a blade; use an electric shaver.
- If gums are bleeding, stop flossing teeth until gums no longer bleed. Use a soft-bristle toothbrush. If brushing causes bleeding, stop brushing and use a water-spraying oral-care device if available.
- Permit only experienced professionals to draw blood from your veins.
- Do not go barefoot because foot injuries may be associated with excessive bruising or bleeding.
- Do not permit intramuscular injections if you are receiving anticoagulants or know your platelet count is below 60,000.
- Avoid getting constipated; drink plenty of fluids, stay active within the guidelines, drink fruit juices, and eat fruit and fiber. Do not use enemas unless told to do so by the physician.
- If you develop a headache or stiff neck, notify the physician.
- Wear a medical identification tag or bracelet identifying the medications you are receiving or that you have a low platelet count.
- Avoid using aspirin and OTC medications unless approved by the physician.

SPECIFICALLY FOR PATIENTS WITH LOW PLATELET COUNTS

- Keep track of platelet counts by maintaining close contact with the physician. When the platelet count is below 10,000 to 15,000, stop flossing teeth and use water-spraying oral care devices on low only. When the platelet count drops to 5000 to 10,000, stop brushing teeth, and clean the mouth with a swab or 4 x 4 gauze pad using a mild mouthwash or saline solution. Avoid mouthwashes containing alcohol and lemon-glycerin swabs.
- Consider limiting activities. The following is one regimen prepared by the American Cancer Society:
  For platelet counts of 50,000 to 100,000, continue with moderate activity including walking, swimming, and usual activities of daily living.
  For platelet counts below 50,000, only mild activities are permitted such as walking, light housework, or yardwork.

ADDITIONAL GUIDELINES FOR THE NURSE

- Check stools for occult blood, and monitor urinalysis.
- Inspect venipuncture sites for hematoma; apply pressure for at least 10 minutes after venipuncture to limit hematoma formation at venipuncture sites.
- Handle patients gently. Avoid restraints; if used, pad and inspect under restraints every 2 hours. Keep siderails padded.

duced. Because of this selectivity, busulfan is used in chronic myelocytic leukemia.

Busulfan is well absorbed orally and is used by this route in chronic intermittent therapy. The drug is highly reactive in blood and tissues and is rapidly broken down in the body to a variety of products that are excreted by the kidneys and other routes.

Busulfan may cause leukopenia, usually beginning 10 days after therapy. Hemorrhage may result if the drug is not discontinued. With long-term therapy, many body systems may show signs of toxicity. Busulfan may destroy large numbers of granulocytes during therapy. These dying cells release chemicals that may be converted to uric acid, excessively elevating blood levels of uric acid. To avoid the toxicity produced by uric acid, allopurinol may be given during busulfan therapy.

In addition to the expected interactions with bone marrow depressants and live virus vaccines, busulfan interacts with probenecid and sulfinpyrazone. This interaction is based on the high levels of uric acid that may be released by busulfan. Allopurinol may be needed to avoid nephrotoxicity.

Carboplatin and cisplatin

Cisplatin (CPDD) and carboplatin are platinum-containing complexes that act like alkylating agents. These drugs cross-link DNA and are not specific for cell cycle. Both drugs must be given by intravenous injection and are hydrolysed in solution; cisplatin is rapidly inactivated by this mechanism. The effects of single doses last for weeks.

Cisplatin is a relatively toxic drug that almost always causes severe nausea and vomiting. The drug is also toxic to the renal tubule and may cause serious damage with high doses or too frequent administration. Cisplatin causes hearing loss in the upper frequency ranges and ringing in the ears (tinnitus). Ototoxicity tends to progress with repeated doses. Myelosuppression manifested by lowered leukocyte and platelet counts persists for 3 weeks or longer after a single injection of cisplatin.

PATIENT PROBLEM

Stomatitis

THE PROBLEM

Mucosal cells lining the GI tract are sensitive to some drugs, especially many of the cytotoxic drugs used in cancer chemotherapy and gold preparations in rheumatoid arthritis. As the mucosal cells are destroyed, there may be pain and inflammation along the entire GI tract, which is called *stomatitis*.

SIGNS AND SYMPTOMS

Included are inflamed oral mucous membranes, oral ulcers, areas of irritation in the mouth, pain on chewing and swallowing, anal discomfort, and pain on defecation.

PATIENT AND FAMILY EDUCATION

- If possible, have teeth professionally cleaned and dental caries repaired before the start of drug therapy.
- If chewing and swallowing are painful, switch to a liquid diet, including milkshakes and ice cream. If discomfort is severe, try to maintain an intake of clear fluids of at least 2000 ml (approximately eight 8-ounce glasses) per day to prevent dehydration.
- Try chilling food before eating it.
- If tooth brushing is irritating, try using swabs to clean the mouth. Avoid flossing when stomatitis is severe. Use water-spraying oral care devices on low setting only. Rinse the mouth after each meal with a mild solution of baking soda and water; baking soda, salt and water; or hydrogen peroxide and water.
- Try painting the inside of the mouth with substrate of magnesia up to four times per day. Allow the milk of magnesia to settle to the bottom of the bottle. Pour off the liquid portion at the top of the bottle, and paint the mouth with the white pasty portion remaining.
- If a special mouthwash has been prescribed, use it as ordered. Many mouthwashes are effective only when used regularly throughout the day. OTC mouthwashes may be irritating because many contain alcohol; avoid them unless the physician has prescribed them.
- Avoid spicy foods and foods with hard crusts or edges.
- Try keeping a humidifier running to keep the room air moist.
- Wear dentures or bridgework only while eating, and remove them at other times to decrease irritation.
- Keep the lips moist with a lip balm or moisturizer.
- For anal irritation, avoid suppositories, enemas, rectal thermometers. Try sitting in a tub of warm water several times daily. After bowel movements, clean the anal area completely; some patients find a babywipe to be cooling for this purpose.
- If vaginal irritation is a problem, keep the vaginal area clean and dry; wipe from front to back; avoid soaps in the vaginal area; and pat dry. Avoid douching or using tampons. Notify the physician if vaginal discharge develops or a change in the color, consistency, odor, or amount occurs. To decrease irritation during intercourse, use a commercially available, water-soluble lubricant; avoid hand lotion or petroleum jelly.

ADDITIONAL NURSING CARE MEASURES

- Assess the mouth of patients at high risk for stomatitis at least once each shift. In addition, inspect for development of oral fungal infections (thrush).
- Monitor intake and output.
- Some physicians suggest that patients suck on ice or iced pops during IV administration of drugs known to cause stomatitis. The local vasoconstriction caused by the cold may decrease the severity of stomatitis.

In addition to anemia, leukopenia, neutropenia, and thrombocytopenia, carboplatin causes pain at the site of injection. Extreme tiredness or weakness is also common. Nausea and vomiting usually start in 6 to 12 hours after a dose and last for 24 hours. About 65% of treated patients experience vomiting. Carboplatin causes less renal toxicity than does cisplatin.

Peripheral neuropathies may occur with either drug. Loss of taste has also been reported. Anaphylactoid reactions may occur when cisplatin or carboplatin are given to patients who have previously received these platinum-containing agents.

In addition to the expected interactions with bone marrow depressants and live virus vaccines, carboplatin may show additive nephrotoxicity with cisplatin.

Carmustine and lomustine

Carmustine (BCNU) is a rapidly acting alkylating agent that affects numerous enzymes and nucleic acids. Lomustine (CCNU) is chemically related to carmustine and similarly alkylates DNA and has widespread metabolic effects. One advantage carmustine and lomustine have over many other alkylating agents is that they penetrate the blood-brain barrier very well.

Carmustine is given by intravenous (IV) infusion. The drug is rapidly degraded so that only metabolites are detectable in blood or in tissues a few minutes after the dose is administered. Metabolites are excreted in urine for several days after therapy. These metabolites of carmustine may be active. Lomustine is used orally and is well absorbed by that route. Once absorbed, it is metabolized and excreted similarly to carmustine.

Carmustine and lomustine cause delayed bone marrow suppression. After a single dose of drug, bone marrow function may reach its lowest point 4 to 6 weeks after therapy. For this reason, doses must be given no more frequently than every 6 weeks or at more widely spaced intervals if the bone marrow does not promptly recover.

Pulmonary fibrosis may be an insidious side effect with these drugs. Shortness of breath or cough should be investigated quickly for cause. Nausea and vomiting are dose-related toxic reactions to carmustine and lomustine. Carmustine is highly irritating and may cause hyperpigmentation if it touches the skin. Pain during infusion is common. Patient discomfort can be reduced by slowing the rate of infusion of the drug and by properly diluting it before use.

Carmustine may decompose in solution. The drug in the dry form in the unopened vial may also decompose at temperatures above 80°F (or 27°C). Clear colorless solutions may be used within 8 hours (or stored for short periods in the cold). Lomustine capsules are stable when stored at room temperature in sealed containers.

Chlorambucil

Chlorambucil is chemically related to mechlorethamine and is cytotoxic by the same mechanism. Chlorambucil is distinguished by being the slowest acting and the least toxic of the nitrogen mustard alkylating agents. In addition to its cell cycle nonspecific cytotoxicity, chlorambucil displays a somewhat selective lympholytic action.

Chlorambucil is administered orally. Large doses (20 mg or more) may produce nausea and vomiting, but more common doses are well tolerated and reliably absorbed. The drug is rapidly metabolized by the liver, and the major metabolite is active.

Chlorambucil commonly suppresses the bone marrow, although at normal doses the effects are usually mild and reversible. Chlorambucil can produce central nervous system (CNS) stimulation, GI irritation, pulmonary fibrosis, liver toxicity, and skin reactions at high doses, but these responses are not commonly seen with normal clinical doses. Chlorambucil is often very well tolerated when used at low doses for maintenance therapy.

In addition to the expected interactions with bone marrow depressants and live virus vaccines, chlorambucil interacts with probenecid and sulfinpyrazone because of changes in uric acid production. Uric acid in the blood can reach dangerous levels after chlorambucil treatment. Allopurinol may be needed to avoid nephrotoxicity.

Cyclophosphamide

Cyclophosphamide is a noncytotoxic form of nitrogen mustard that must be activated by liver microsomal enzymes. Several metabolites of cyclophosphamide are formed in the liver, and at least one of these metabolites is a potent alkylating agent with activity similar to that of nitrogen mustard. Because the drug as administered is not active, it does not possess the strong vesicant activity (direct blistering and damage of tissues) seen with other nitrogen mustards.

Cyclophosphamide may be used either orally or parenterally, which is a distinct advantage over most alkylating agents. Oral absorption is good; the absorbed drug passes through portal circulation directly to the liver where the drug is activated.

Cyclophosphamide produces all the expected side effects of nonspecific alkylating agents. Bone marrow suppression occurs and is frequently used to guide the physician in adjusting doses. In most patients the bone marrow begins to recover 7 to 10 days after the drug is discontinued.

GI toxicity with cyclophosphamide is common and usually consists of nausea and vomiting although more severe reactions can occur. Hair loss **(alopecia)** occurs with cyclophosphamide therapy much more commonly than with other drugs of this class. Most patients report regrowth of hair after therapy.

Immunosuppression is an expected side effect. Cyclophosphamide suppresses gonadal tissue, and the effects may be irreversible. Complete suppression of the menstrual cycles and of sperm formation have been reported.

Cyclophosphamide and its metabolites are excreted predominantly through the kidneys. The accumulation of these cytotoxic compounds in the bladder can produce hemorrhagic cystitis. Bladder fibrosis and carcinoma occur more often in patients who receive long-term therapy with cyclophosphamide.

High-dose or long-term therapy is associated with increased risk of cardiotoxicity, pneumonitis, renal toxicity, and uric acid accumulation.

In addition to the expected interactions with bone marrow depressants and live virus vaccines, cyclophosphamide may produce excessive uric acid levels; this latter action may cause interactions with probenecid or sulfinpyrazone. Immunosuppressants contribute to the risk of infection with cyclophosphamide. Cocaine toxicity is worsened because cyclophosphamide inhibits the cholinesterase that normally terminates the action of cocaine. Cytarabine increases the risk of cardiotoxicity with cyclophosphamide.

Dacarbazine

Dacarbazine apparently acts as an alkylating agent and is cell cycle nonspecific. The drug must be given intravenously. It is secreted by renal tubules, with about half the dose excreted by this route; the remaining drug appears in blood as a metabolite.

Dacarbazine causes delayed bone marrow toxicity (16 to 20 days after therapy). Most patients report nausea and vomiting within a few hours after therapy. Tolerance to this symptom develops. Dacarbazine can cause severe pain and tissue damage if it seeps from the vein into surrounding tissues.

Dacarbazine causes the expected interactions with bone marrow depressants and live virus vaccines.

Ifosfamide

Ifosfamide is metabolically activated to a form that acts as an alkylating agent. The drug must be given by IV infusion. Unchanged drug as well as active and inactive metabolites are excreted by the kidneys.

In addition to leukopenia and thrombocytopenia, ifosfamide also causes dose-related CNS effects and hemorrhagic cystitis. Nausea and vomiting are also common side effects, as is alopecia.

Ifosfamide causes the expected interactions with bone marrow depressants and live virus vaccines.

Mechlorethamine

Mechlorethamine (nitrogen mustard) is a potent alkylating agent that may attack DNA at one site or may cause cross-linking. Mechlorethamine is so highly unstable that it must be administered intravenously immediately after the solution is prepared. The drug is so highly reactive that it is destroyed within minutes of its injection. No active drug appears in urine or is excreted by any other route.

Mechlorethamine may induce various malignancies. The drug is also an immunosuppressant and predisposes the patient to infections.

Mechlorethamine is an extremely toxic agent with a very narrow margin of safety. Significant toxicity is to be expected in every treated patient. Bone marrow suppression usually appears within a day and its function is lowest 1 to 3 weeks later. Platelet counts may decrease sufficiently to cause bleeding gums and subcutaneous hemorrhages. Nausea and vomiting are common acute toxic reactions.

Germinal tissue may be severely damaged by mechlorethamine. Men may have complete arrest of spermatogenesis. Women may have menstrual irregularities. Fetuses of treated mothers are damaged by mechlorethamine.

Mechlorethamine is a potent vesicant. Patients and medical personnel must be rigorously protected from improper contact with the drug. Because of its instability the drug must be dissolved immediately before use and injected directly into a free-flowing IV line. This procedure avoids the danger of extravasation (leakage into tissues around the vein), which produces extreme pain and tissue destruction.

In addition to the expected interactions with bone marrow depressants and live virus vaccines, mechlorethamine may cause excessive uric acid levels, which leads to interactions with probenecid or sulfinpyrazone.

Melphalan

Melphalan (L-PAM, or phenylalanine mustard) is a derivative of nitrogen mustard that acts as an alkylating agent. Melphalan is adequately absorbed orally in most patients. The drug persists in blood longer than most alkylating agents; it is detectable for up to 6 hours after a single dose.

Melphalan produces bone marrow suppression. Dosages are usually adjusted to produce mild leukopenia but no further damage. High doses can produce severe bone marrow depression, bleeding, and nausea and vomiting.

In addition to the expected interactions with bone marrow depressants and live virus vaccines, melphalan may raise uric acid levels, which leads to interactions with probenecid or sulfinpyrazone.

Mitomycin

Mitomycin is an antibiotic derived from cultures of *Streptomyces.* The drug is activated by enzymes in the body, so it becomes capable of alkylating DNA. Like other alkylating agents, mitomycin is nonspecific for cell cycle. Mitomycin must be given intravenously because it is not absorbed orally and is highly irritating to skin and muscle. The drug does not distribute to the brain.

Mitomycin produces severe and progressive myelosuppression. Leukopenia and thrombocytopenia occur within 3 to 8 weeks and may persist for up to 10 weeks or longer after therapy. Mitomycin should not be readministered until platelet and white blood cell counts show the bone marrow has recovered. Mitomycin also frequently causes nausea and vomiting, skin rashes, and alopecia. A few patients may also suffer renal failure with hemolysis, liver toxicity, and lung damage. Mitomycin also causes local necrosis if allowed to escape into cutaneous tissues during IV injection.

Mitomycin causes the expected interactions with bone marrow depressants and live virus vaccines.

Mitoxantrone

Mitoxantrone reacts with DNA probably by tight binding to the nucleic acid. The drug is not specific for a particular phase of the cell cycle. Mitoxantrone is available for IV use only. The drug is metabolized in the liver and excreted to some degree in bile. The small amount of drug or its metabolic products in urine add a blue-green color to urine for 24 hours after each dose.

Mitoxantrone is an extremely potent myelosuppressant, which limits its clinical utility. Up to two thirds of treated patients experience some signs of infection. Most patients also suffer GI irritation or distress. Approximately one third of patients experience cough or dyspnea. Cardiovascular toxicity is a risk, especially as the total dose exceeds 140 to 160 mg/kg.

In addition to the expected interactions with bone marrow depressants and live virus vaccines, mitoxantrone may raise uric acid levels, which leads to interactions with probenecid or sulfinpyrazone.

Thiotepa

Thiotepa, also known as triethylenethiophosphoramide, is a nonspecific alkylating agent. Because it is so nonselective, the drug is applied directly to the tumor when possible. This therapy allows high doses to be achieved at the tumor site, with lower doses escaping into systemic circulation. Because toxicity is dose related, such a treatment regimen minimizes systemic toxicity.

Thiotepa is primarily toxic to bone marrow. Because the drug produces its effects slowly, care must be taken not to excessively damage the bone marrow by too high a dose in the early stages of therapy. White blood cell (WBC) counts may be used as an index of toxicity. The drug may also produce nausea and anorexia. Thiotepa is relatively nonirritating and can be administered rapidly through IV lines.

In addition to the expected interactions with bone marrow depressants and live virus vaccines, mitoxantrone may raise uric acid levels, which leads to interactions with probenecid or sulfinpyrazone.

Agents That Block DNA Synthesis (S-Phase Inhibitors)

Properties common to this class of drugs are presented below; properties unique to individual drugs are covered with each agent.

Mechanism of Action

The uncontrolled proliferation of cancerous cells is frequently expressed as rapid cell division or as a high growth fraction. This property distinguishes cancers from most normal tissues, in which a very low growth fraction is the rule. Because only cells in the S phase of the cell cycle synthesize DNA, they are most sensitive to agents that block DNA synthesis.

Drugs may block DNA synthesis in several ways. Some of the drugs in this section are specific enzyme inhibitors and prevent the action of an enzyme that is required for DNA synthesis. Other drugs that are chemically very similar to the natural purines and pyrimidines used to form DNA may be incorporated into DNA but make the DNA unstable and nonfunctional.

A cell that is not forming DNA will not be damaged by a drug that inhibits DNA synthesis. For this reason nonproliferating cells or cells in resting phase are relatively insensitive to these drugs. These drugs are called *cycle-specific* or *phase-specific agents* because they affect primarily cells in S phase.

The property of phase specificity explains why S-phase inhibitors must be given on a repeating schedule. In a single treatment, only the growing fraction of cells in the tumor will be affected. A recovery period with no drug given allows normal tissues with high growth fractions such as bone marrow to return to normal function. During this recovery period, many cells in the cancerous tissue will move from G_0 phase into the reproductive cycle. Other cells that were not in S phase during treatment continue to proliferate, and the tumor continues to grow. Repeated widely spaced doses of the drug give the maximum opportunity for the drug to catch the dividing cells in S phase when they will be sensitive.

Pharmacokinetics

Many S-phase inhibitors must be activated before they exhibit anticancer activity. Some are activated in liver, but others are activated in cells of many types.

Uses

The clinical uses of cycle-specific anticancer drugs are summarized in Table 49-4.

Adverse Reactions and Contraindications

Because the specificity of S-phase inhibitors is toward any active DNA synthesis, many normal cells will be sensitive. At highest risk of toxicity are tissues with a high growth fraction. Bone marrow depression and suppression of lymphocyte formation are characteristic side effects of these drugs. Lowered lymphocyte formation reduces the ability of the patient to fight infection (immunosuppression), which may reduce the patient's chance for survival. GI mucosa also has a high growth fraction and is a target of serious toxic reactions to the drugs of this family. Nausea, vomiting, or stomatitis are observed.

Toxicity

Bone marrow suppression is frequently a dose-related side effect. Therefore very high doses may have profound effects on the bone marrow.

Interactions

S-phase inhibitors all may produce serious interactions with bone marrow suppressants or radiation because the combinations significantly depress production of blood cells. The immunosuppression these drugs produce also puts patients at risk of generalized viral infections if they are given a live virus vaccine during or shortly after receiving an S-phase inhibitor. Oral polio vaccines for family members may also put these patients at risk.

In addition to these expected interactions, a wide variety of other interactions are also possible; these are noted with the individual drugs in the section below.

Cladribine

Cladribine is an analogue of adenosine, a normal component of DNA. The drug is activated in cells and accumulates in monocytes and lymphocytes where it impairs DNA repair. Although the primary action is this antimetabolite activity, cladribine is unlike other antimetabolites in affecting not only S-phase cells but also cells in other phases of the cell cycle. Cladribine is used by IV injection for a single course of therapy. The effect on lymphocytes is noted within a week, but the antileukemic effect may take up to 4 months to become evident.

In addition to the expected effects of anemia, neutropenia, and thrombocytopenia, cladribine also causes skin rashes, fever, infections, nausea, anorexia, vomiting, headache, and excessive tiredness in significant numbers of patients.

Cladribine causes the expected interactions with bone marrow depressants and live virus vaccines. In addition, cladribine elevates uric acid concentrations and may change the dosage of probenecid or sulfinpyrazone needed to control hyperuricemia.

Cytarabine

Cytarabine is a chemical analogue of cytidine, a normal component of DNA. Cytarabine interferes with the function of the enzyme DNA polymerase, which inserts cytidine into DNA but cannot insert cytarabine; therefore cytarabine slows or stops DNA synthesis. Cytarabine is rapidly inactivated by enzymes that deaminate the molecule. Blood and liver enzymes apparently contribute to this process.

Cytarabine must be injected, either subcutaneously, intrathecally, or intravenously. Subcutaneous injections are used only to maintain remissions and are given once or twice a week. Cytarabine does not easily pass into the cerebrospinal fluid. If it is administered intrathecally, it may persist in cere-

TABLE 49-4 Anticancer Drugs That Block DNA Synthesis

GENERIC NAME	TRADE NAME	ADMINISTRATION/DOSAGE‡	COMMENTS/USES
Cladribine	Leustatin*	INTRAVENOUS: *Adults*—0.1 mg/kg daily for 7 days. FDA pregnancy category D.	Used for hairy cell leukemia.
Cytarabine	Cytosar*	INTRAVENOUS: *Adults and children*—100 mg/m² daily for 5-10 days. SUBCUTANEOUS: *Adults and children*—1 mg/kg once or twice per week. FDA pregnancy category D.	Used to induce and maintain remission in leukemia patients.
Floxuridine	FUDR	INTRAARTERIAL: *Adults*—0.1-0.6 mg/kg over 24 hr. FDA pregnancy category D.	Palliative for solid tumors not treatable by other means.
Fludarabine	Fludara*	INTRAVENOUS: *Adults*—25 mg/m² daily for 5 days; repeat monthly. FDA pregnancy category D.	Used for chronic lymphocytic leukemia.
Fluorouracil, or 5-FU	Adrucil*	INTRAVENOUS: *Adults*—7-12 mg/kg for 4 days as initial therapy. Less frequent dosing is used for maintenance therapy. FDA pregnancy category D.	Palliative for solid tumors incurable by surgery or other means. Topical fluorouracil is used to treat multiple actinic (solar) keratoses.
	Efudex Fluoroplex*	TOPICAL: *Adults*—Used as 1%, 2%, or 5% solution or cream.	
Hydroxyurea	Hydrea*	ORAL: *Adults*—Doses range from 20-30 mg/kg daily up to 80 mg/kg every 3 days.	Used to treat melanoma, myelocytic leukemia, and carcinomas.
Mercaptopurine	Purinethol*	ORAL: *Adults and children >5 yr*—2.5 mg/kg/day initially. May continue for weeks if toxicity does not supervene. FDA pregnancy category D.	Produces remissions in leukemias.
✚ Methotrexate	Folex Mexate	ORAL: *Adults and children*—From 2.5 mg daily to 40 mg/m² once weekly, depending on disease. INTRAMUSCULAR: *Adults and children*—15-30 mg daily for 5 days, or 3.3 mg/m² in combinations. INTRAVENOUS: *Adults*—0.4-2.5 mg/kg every 14 days. INTRATHECAL: *Adults and children*—0.2-0.5 mg/kg up to 15 mg total. FDA pregnancy category X.	Methotrexate can cure choriocarcinoma; maintains remissions in lymphocytic leukemia; is palliative for lymphomas and carcinomas.
Procarbazine	Matulane Natulan†	ORAL: *Adults*—2-4 mg/kg daily for 1 wk; then 4-6 mg/kg daily until bone marrow toxicity occurs. On recovery of marrow, doses are 50-100 mg daily. *Children*—50 mg daily.	Palliative for Hodgkin's lymphoma.
Thioguanine	Lanvis†	ORAL: *Adults*—2 mg/kg daily initially. May continue for weeks if toxicity does not supervene.	Used for myelocytic leukemia.

*Available in Canada and United States.
†Available in Canada only.
‡The doses listed are representative. Very different doses and schedules may be indicated in specific diseases or protocols.

brospinal fluid for several hours because that fluid has little of the deaminating enzyme that inactivates cytarabine.

Cytarabine is a potent bone marrow suppressant, acting on that tissue by the same mechanism effective in cancer cells. Bone marrow depression is most profound 1 to 3 weeks after the drug is stopped. Recovery of marrow function takes at least 1 month for most patients and longer for those receiving the drug for extended periods. Cytarabine may also cause significant GI toxicity. Some patients may suffer perforation or necrosis of the bowel. CNS toxicity is reported in up to 10% of treated patients.

Cytarabine causes the expected interactions with bone marrow depressants and live virus vaccines. The drug may also have additive effects with other immunosuppressants, which can increase the risk of infections. In addition, cytarabine elevates uric acid concentrations and may change the dosage of probenecid or sulfinpyrazone needed to control hyperuricemia. Cytarabine with cyclophosphamide increases the risk of cardiotoxicity.

Floxuridine and fluorouracil

Fluorouracil and floxuridine are synthetic pyrimidine bases that may be converted in the body to an active agent (floxuridine monophosphate). This active form of fluorouracil resembles the pyrimidine that is directly incorporated into RNA or that is converted to the pyrimidine, thymidylate. Thymidylate is used exclusively for DNA synthesis.

Fluorouracil and floxuridine disrupt these pathways in at least two ways. First, the activated drug may enter RNA, creating a defective form of that nucleic acid that does not allow normal protein synthesis. Second, thymidylate synthase, the enzyme required to form thymidylate for DNA synthesis, is inhibited. With thymidylate synthase blocked, DNA synthesis halts.

Oral absorption of fluorouracil is erratic, and the drug is commonly given intravenously. For most patients, best results seem to be produced by giving loading doses intravenously for 4 consecutive days and then tapering to weekly maintenance doses.

Fluorouracil is extensively metabolized by the liver and other tissues. Less than 15% of the drug dose appears as active drug in the urine. Fluorouracil is cleared from the blood within 3 hours of an IV injection, but the effects persist longer.

The route of administration of floxuridine determines its metabolic fate and its effectiveness. Floxuridine given intravenously by rapid injection is broken down to fluorouracil and thence to the normal breakdown products of fluorouracil. When floxuridine is given slowly by intraarterial infusion, metabolism to fluorouracil is minimized, and most of the drug is converted to floxuridine monophosphate. The intraarterial route requires a lower dose yet is more effective than IV administration.

Fluorouracil and floxuridine are highly toxic to the GI tract. Inflammation of the membranes of the mouth and pharynx may be an early sign of such toxicity. Nausea, vomiting, and diarrhea almost always occur, and if the drug is not discontinued, duodenal ulcers may occur and the bowel may perforate. Patients with preexisting poor nutritional status are at much greater risk with these drugs.

Blood dyscrasias also occur with fluorouracil and floxuridine and may limit therapy. Leukopenia continues for 1 or 2 weeks after therapy is stopped. Various skin reactions and alopecia also occur but usually do not cause the drug to be discontinued.

Both fluorouracil and floxuridine cause the expected interactions with bone marrow depressants and live virus vaccines.

Fludarabine

Fludarabine is an analogue of adenine, but it resists inactivation by adenosine deaminase. The drug is activated to the triphosphate inside cells. The drug is given by IV injection and is rapidly altered in the blood to a form better able to enter cells.

In addition to the expected side effects of anemia, leukopenia, and thrombocytopenia, fludarabine also causes diarrhea, nausea, pain, pneumonia, skin rash, vomiting, and excessive tiredness.

Interactions with fludarabine include those expected with bone marrow depressants and live virus vaccines. In addition, fludarabine elevates uric acid concentrations and may change the dosage of probenecid or sulfinpyrazone needed to control hyperuricemia. The use of fludarabine with pentostatin increases the risk of potentially fatal pulmonary damage.

Hydroxyurea

Hydroxyurea inhibits the enzyme that converts ribonucleotide precursors of RNA to deoxyribonucleotides, which form DNA; thus, DNA synthesis is inhibited.

Hydroxyurea is well absorbed when given orally and distributes well to many tissues including the brain. The drug is excreted by the kidneys.

Hydroxyurea produces bone marrow suppression as the most common side effect. This reaction is reversible. GI disturbances, renal impairment, and skin reactions are reported less often.

Interactions with hydroxyurea include those expected with bone marrow depressants and live virus vaccines. Hydroxyurea may also elevate uric acid concentrations and change the dosage of probenecid or sulfinpyrazone needed to control hyperuricemia.

Mercaptopurine and thioguanine

Mercaptopurine (6-Mercaptopurine or 6-MP) resembles adenine and guanine and blocks several points in the synthesis of these nucleic acid precursors. Thioguanine (TG or 6-TG) blocks two reactions, which are also sensitive to mercaptopurine. As a result of the blockade of purine synthesis, DNA synthesis is blocked by either drug; therefore both mercaptopurine and thioguanine are S-phase specific inhibitors.

Mercaptopurine is adequately absorbed orally. Part of the dose is excreted renally, but significant metabolic degradation also occurs. The properties of thioguanine are similar to those of mercaptopurine.

Bone marrow suppression may occur with mercaptopurine or thioguanine. Anemia may contribute to weakness and to fatigue. Immunosuppression contributes to increased risk of infection in treated patients.

Mercaptopurine toxicity may be greatly increased by concomitant treatment with allopurinol. Allopurinol blocks uric acid synthesis and is frequently used to prevent toxic accumulation of that substance after extensive tumor cell destruction by chemotherapy, but allopurinol also inhibits the metabolism of mercaptopurine. Therefore when the drugs are combined, more mercaptopurine persists in blood and in tissues for longer periods, and greater toxicity results. Thioguanine metabolism is not significantly affected by allopurinol.

Both mercaptopurine and thioguanine have significant interactions with bone marrow suppressants and live virus vaccines. Mercaptopurine also interacts with immunosuppressants and hepatotoxic medications.

✣ Methotrexate

Methotrexate is commonly described as a folic acid antagonist because it prevents the regeneration of the metabolically active form of folic acid, tetrahydrofolate (THF). Without THF, cells cannot carry out carbon-transfer reactions, and normal metabolism is blocked at several points. One of these blockades prevents the formation of thymidylic acid, and another arrests adenine and guanine nucleotide synthesis in an early state. Without these precursors, DNA synthesis halts. Methotrexate is therefore specific for the S phase of the cell cycle.

Methotrexate may be administered by oral, intramuscular (IM), IV, intraarterial, or intrathecal routes. For many patients, the oral route is satisfactory because effective serum concentrations are reached within 1 hour. Parenteral administration results in a slightly faster absorption rate. The intrathecal route is required to treat patients with leukemias that have penetrated the CNS. Methotrexate does not pass from the blood into cerebrospinal fluid in useful amounts.

Methotrexate is well distributed in the body and may accumulate in some tissues. Liver cells seem especially able to bind the drug for long periods. It also persists in the kidneys. These tissue sites of drug accumulation normally account for a small fraction of the total dose of methotrexate. Most of the drug is excreted directly in urine. Little degradation of methotrexate occurs, and the excreted drug is unchanged.

Methotrexate produces toxicity typical for drugs of this class. The rapidly dividing tissues of the GI mucosal lining are severely damaged. Stomatitis and diarrhea are common signs of toxicity that call for discontinuation of the drug. If therapy continues after these symptoms arise, severe GI damage, including perforation, can result.

Bone marrow function is also compromised with methotrexate. The result, as with other drugs of this class, is leukopenia. Other blood changes may occur and may ultimately produce uncontrolled bleeding (see box). Methotrexate is an immunosuppressant and may damage the body's ability to fight infection.

The effectiveness and toxicity of methotrexate may be affected by a variety of other drugs. Bone marrow suppressants and live virus vaccines produce the expected interactions. In addition, salicylates (e.g., aspirin) tend to increase methotrexate toxicity by displacing methotrexate from plasma proteins. The increase in free plasma methotrexate frequently produces toxicity.

Acyclovir may increase the risk of CNS effects when methotrexate is excreted intrathecally. Alcohol or other hepatotoxic drugs increase the risk of liver damage. Asparaginase may block the action of methotrexate. Nonsteroidal antiinflammatory agents may increase bone marrow effects of methotrexate.

Methotrexate produces cytotoxicity by blocking regeneration of THF. It is thus possible to prevent the action of the drug by supplying the body with THF. This use has been exploited for treating methotrexate overdose. Tumors such as osteosarcoma are treated with massive doses of methotrexate. Under ordinary circumstances, these doses would destroy the bone marrow and would be lethal, but if the patient receives IV leucovorin (citrovorum factor), an agent containing THF and other forms of folic acid, the bone marrow can be protected. This type of therapy is called *leucovorin rescue.*

Procarbazine

Procarbazine has multiple effects on cellular enzyme systems and nucleic acids. It apparently oxidizes nucleic acids. In addition, nucleic acid synthesis is inhibited.

Procarbazine is well absorbed after oral administration. The drug rapidly equilibrates between plasma and cerebrospinal fluid. Procarbazine is converted to an active metabolite by the liver and is excreted primarily by the kidneys.

Procarbazine frequently produces bone marrow depression and immune suppression. CNS stimulation and pneumonitis are also common. Menstrual periods are typically suppressed. Nausea and vomiting are common, as is excessive tiredness.

Procarbazine causes the expected interactions with bone marrow suppressants and live virus vaccines. The drug also causes many other reactions because it inhibits monoamine oxidase. Patients should therefore not receive both procarbazine and drugs that elevate biogenic amine levels (e.g., sympathomimetics, tricyclic antidepressants, phenothiazines, and tyramine-containing food).

Ethyl alcohol can produce a disulfiram-like reaction with procarbazine. Procarbazine can also produce significant interactions with anesthetics, agents with anticholinergic effects, antidiabetic agents, MAO inhibitors, CNS depressants, dextromethorphan, fluoxetine, levodopa, meperidine, methyldopa, and methylphenidate.

Agents That Block RNA or Protein Synthesis

Properties common to this class of drugs are presented below; properties unique to individual drugs are covered with each agent.

Mechanism of Action

The rapid proliferation of cancer cells can be inhibited by agents that block RNA formation or interfere with the use of RNA as a template for protein synthesis. Many of these drugs have this action because they bind very tightly to DNA and prevent reading of genes. These agents are not highly specific for cancer cells but rather interfere with RNA and protein synthesis in any rapidly dividing tissue. The exception to this rule is asparaginase, a drug with some selectivity for cancer cells.

Pharmacokinetics

The pharmacokinetics of these drugs is varied. Many persist for some time inside cells. The effects of the drugs persist for days to weeks.

Uses

The clinical uses of these drugs are summarized in Table 49-5.

Adverse Reactions and Contraindications

These inhibitors of RNA and protein synthesis attack all rapidly dividing tissues and therefore produce the expected

TABLE 49-5 Anticancer Drugs That Block RNA and Protein Synthesis

GENERIC NAME	TRADE NAME	ADMINISTRATION/DOSAGE‡	COMMENTS/USES
Asparaginase	Elspar Kidrolase†	INTRAMUSCULAR: *Children*—6000 IU/m^2 with other drugs. INTRAVENOUS: *Adults and children*—200 IU/kg daily for 28 days. FDA pregnancy category C.	Induces remissions in acute lymphocytic leukemia in children.
Dactinomycin	Cosmegen*	INTRAVENOUS: *Adults*—0.5 mg/m^2 once weekly for 3 wk. FDA pregnancy category C. *Children*—0.015 mg/kg or 0.45 mg/m^2 for 5 days.	Used to treat choriocarcinoma, Wilms' tumor, sarcomas, and carcinomas
Daunorubicin	Cerubidine*	INTRAVENOUS: *Adults*—45 mg/m^2 daily for 3 days. Lifetime dose should not exceed 550 mg/m^2. FDA pregnancy category D. *Older adults:* 30 mg/m^2 daily for 3 days. *Children*—25 mg/m^2 once weekly, with vincristine and prednisone.	Used primarily for leukemias. Heart toxicity occurs especially when total doses approach 500 mg/m^2.
Doxorubicin	Adriamycin*	INTRAVENOUS: *Adults*—60-75 mg/m^2 as single injection repeated no more often than every 3 wk. Lifetime dose should not exceed 550 mg/m^2. *Children*—30 mg/m^2 daily for 3 days; repeat every 4 wk.	Effective against leukemias, lymphomas, sarcomas, and carcinomas. Heart toxicity occurs especially when total doses approach 500 mg/m^2.
Epirubicin	Pharmorubicin†	INTRAVENOUS: *Adults*—75-90 mg/m^2; repeat every 3 wk.	Used for carcinomas and lymphomas.
Idarubicin	Idamycin*	INTRAVENOUS: *Adults*—12 mg/m^2 daily for 3 days. FDA pregnancy category D.	Used for acute myelocytic leukemia.
Plicamycin	Mithracin	INTRAVENOUS: *Adults*—0.025-0.050 mg/kg every other day for 8 doses. FDA pregnancy category X.	Used to treat embryonal cell carcinoma and metastatic bone tumors associated with hypercalcemia.

*Available in Canada and United States.
†Available in Canada only.
‡The doses listed are representative. Very different doses and schedules may be indicated in specific diseases or protocols.

array of side effects: bone marrow suppression leading to lower production of various blood cells; damage to the epithelial layer of the gastrointestinal tract producing symptoms ranging from nausea to stomatitis; and damage to the hair follicles causing hair loss. The exception is asparaginase, a drug whose different mechanism for inhibiting protein synthesis leads to a different array of side effects.

Toxicity

Bone marrow suppression tends to be a dose-dependent side effect. Therefore high doses cause more profound suppression in more patients.

Interactions

Inhibitors of RNA and protein synthesis, with the exception of asparaginase, may produce serious interactions with bone marrow suppressants or radiation because the combinations significantly depress production of blood cells. The immunosuppression these drugs produce also put patients at risk of generalized viral infections if they are given a live virus vaccine during or shortly after receiving one of these agents. Oral polio vaccines for family members may also put these patients at risk.

Treatment with an inhibitor of RNA and protein synthesis often causes an elevation in uric acid in the blood. For this reason, dosages of drugs like probenecid or sulfinpyrazone may need to be changed to prevent hyperuricemia or gout.

In addition to these expected interactions, a wide variety of other interactions are also possible; these are noted with the individual drugs in the section that follows.

Asparaginase

Asparaginase is an enzyme that converts the amino acid asparagine to aspartic acid. The therapeutic effect of this agent arises because many types of cancer cells cannot form asparagine fast enough to support their growth. The enzyme destroys circulating asparagine, starving the cancer cells for asparagine. Normal cells are spared because they can form asparagine internally.

To be most effective, asparagine starvation should occur in the G_1 phase of the cell cycle. If asparagine levels are kept low during that period, the asparagine-dependent cancer cell will be unable to carry out protein synthesis and, ultimately, RNA and DNA synthesis will cease. If asparagine starvation occurs later in the cell cycle after many critical proteins and nucleic acids have been formed, the cell may not die.

Asparaginase is a protein and must therefore be administered by parenteral routes. The drug persists in blood for extended periods and is slowly eliminated. It does not enter cerebrospinal fluid in useful amounts and is not excreted in urine.

Asparaginase produces a wide range of toxic reactions. Because the drug is a protein, it is an effective antigen and may provoke severe allergic reactions. Renal and hepatic function may be impaired, and some patients have bleeding episodes because the drug suppresses various clotting factors. Hyperglycemia has also been observed. Many patients show signs of CNS toxicity, including depression, lowered consciousness, and coma. Asparaginase toxicity is increased by vincristine or prednisone. Nevertheless, these drugs are cautiously used together in certain combination treatment regimens. The anticancer effects of methotrexate may be diminished by asparaginase.

In addition to the interactions noted above, asparaginase has the expected interactions with probenecid, sulfinpyrazone, and live virus vaccines.

Dactinomycin

Dactinomycin (actinomycin D) is an antibiotic derived from *Streptomyces.* The drug binds strongly to double-stranded DNA and prevents the DNA from serving as a template for RNA synthesis. The cell, unable to form messenger RNA, is thus unable to synthesize proteins or complete cell division.

Dactinomycin is not well absorbed orally. The drug is also extremely corrosive to soft tissues and must therefore be given only by the IV route. Dactinomycin is rapidly cleared from blood, entering the liver and other tissues. The drug does not cross the blood-brain barrier in effective amounts. Excretion of dactinomycin is mainly into bile, with smaller amounts of unchanged drug also appearing in urine.

Dactinomycin is very toxic and must be administered with great care. The highly corrosive nature of the compound makes it imperative that IV injection be given properly, with no leakage of drug into tissues that surround the vein. Such extravasation can cause extensive tissue damage.

Dactinomycin causes significant hematologic changes, which may include aplastic anemia. These blood changes are most pronounced several days after therapy. GI toxicity is severe with dactinomycin. Patients may experience extreme nausea and vomiting within hours of drug administration. Phenothiazine antiemetics may be required to control vomiting. Dactinomycin also irritates the lining of the entire GI tract. Patients commonly report lip inflammation (cheilitis), difficulty in swallowing (dysphagia), mouth sores (ulcerative stomatitis), inflammation of the pharynx (pharyngitis), abdominal pain, and anal inflammation (proctitis).

Dactinomycin also severely damages hair follicles causing alopecia. The drug may cause reddening of the skin (erythema) and signs of inflammation, especially in an area also receiving irradiation.

Dactinomycin has the expected interactions with bone marrow suppressants, probenecid, sulfinpyrazone, and live virus vaccines.

Daunorubicin, doxorubicin, epirubicin, and idarubicin

These drugs bind strongly to double-stranded DNA and thus stop the formation of RNA. Cells are most markedly affected during S and G_2 phases of the cell cycle.

Doxorubicin has a wide range of antitumor activity, including leukemias, lymphomas, sarcomas, genitourinary carcinomas, squamous cell carcinomas of the head and neck, and lung cancer. Daunorubicin has been used primarily in patients with leukemias. Idarubicin, which has very similar properties to doxorubicin and daunorubicin, is used primarily for patients with acute myelocytic leukemia. A related compound, epirubicin (Pharmorubicin), has been used in Canada for patients with carcinoma of the breast.

These drugs are not well absorbed orally, are highly irritating to skin and soft tissues, and must therefore be given intravenously. The drugs enter any tissues and organs, but rapid and extensive metabolism occurs in the liver. Active and inactive metabolites are formed. Most drug elimination occurs through the liver. These drugs do not readily enter the CNS.

Doxorubicin causes delayed leukopenia and other blood changes. Damage to bone marrow limits the amount of drug that may be used and the frequency of administration. Ordinarily, 21 days will be required for the bone marrow to recover. Toxicity to the heart also limits the total amount of drug that can be administered. Total doses of more than 550 mg/m^2 may produce irreversible toxicity to the heart, including ECG changes and congestive heart failure. Preexisting heart disease, prior irradiation to the region of the heart, or prior use of the cardiotoxic drugs cyclophosphamide, mitomycin, or dactinomycin may greatly increase the likelihood for heart damage with these drugs.

Because these drugs are metabolized and eliminated by the liver, patients with impaired liver function may have drug accumulation and increased toxicity unless doses are appropriately reduced. Some metabolites of doxorubicin and daunorubicin appear in urine of all treated patients and produce a harmless red coloration of urine. These drugs can cause severe tissue necrosis if allowed to escape from the vein during drug administration. Damage to veins may occur if the same vein is used repeatedly. Alopecia and GI irritation also occur commonly.

These drugs have the expected interactions with bone marrow suppressants, probenecid, sulfinpyrazone, and live virus vaccines.

Plicamycin

Plicamycin binds DNA, thereby preventing RNA synthesis. Plicamycin also blocks parathyroid hormone activity on osteoclasts, thereby lowering the release of calcium into the blood. This ability to lower blood calcium levels may be useful in patients with hypercalcemia as a result of metastatic cancer of the bone. Plicamycin must be given intravenously, because oral absorption is poor. It damages skin and muscle tissues.

Plicamycin produces anorexia, nausea, vomiting, skin changes, liver damage, kidney damage, and lowered blood concentrations of calcium, potassium, and phosphorus. Plicamycin also produces an unusual syndrome involving episodes of bleeding from various sites. Nosebleed (epistaxis) frequently signals the onset of this syndrome. The condition may stabilize after a few episodes or may progress to extensive hemorrhage, usually within the GI tract, and death.

The tendency of plicamycin to cause bleeding establishes the cause of several important interactions. Risk of hemorrhage is increased when plicamycin is used with anticoagulants, antiinflammatory drugs, dipyridamole, heparin, sulfinpyrazone, or valproic acid. Hepatotoxic or nephrotoxic medications may be more toxic in the presence of plicamycin. Plicamycin also produces the expected reactions with bone marrow suppressants and live virus vaccines.

Agents That Prevent or Arrest Mitosis

Properties common to this class of drugs are presented here; properties unique to individual drugs are covered with each agent.

Mechanism of Action

To segregate chromosomes, a dividing cell must form a mitotic spindle composed of microtubules. Microtubules normally function as part of the cytoplasmic transport systems in cells and are required for certain types of cell movement. The major component of microtubules is the protein tubulin.

The structure of microtubules can be disrupted by substances that bind to tubulin and cause it to be released from microtubules. Breakdown of microtubular structure may not be lethal to a cell unless it is in the process of forming the mitotic spindle. Cells exposed at this stage of division are arrested at that point, and reproduction cannot proceed. Ultimately, these cells die. Substances that act in this way are frequently referred to as *mitotic poisons.*

Another class of drugs inhibits an enzyme called topoisomerase II, preventing normal DNA replication. Etoposide and teniposide act by this mechanism to block the entry of a cell into mitosis.

Pharmacokinetics

Most of the compounds in this class have relatively long half-lives that range from a few hours to longer than 2 days. Most of the compounds are biotransformed by the liver and excreted in bile, but renal mechanisms may also operate.

Uses

The clinical properties of mitotic poisons and related compounds used to treat cancer are summarized in Table 49-6.

Adverse Reactions and Contraindications

The effects of these drugs are most pronounced on actively dividing cells; therefore side effects can be expected to be related to normal rapidly dividing tissues. Bone marrow suppression with altered production of blood cells is a common feature with these drugs, resulting in immunosuppression. Alopecia is especially common with this group of drugs. Gastrointestinal symptoms, including nausea and vomiting, also occur.

TABLE 49-6 Anticancer Drugs That Prevent or Block Mitosis

GENERIC NAME	TRADE NAME	ADMINISTRATION/DOSAGE‡	COMMENTS/USES
Etoposide VP-16	VePesid*	ORAL: *Adults*—100 mg/m^2 daily for 5 days. Repeat every 3-4 wk. INTRAVENOUS: *Adults*—50-100 mg/m^2 daily for 3-5 days. Repeat at 3-4 wk. FDA pregnancy category D.	Used for refractory testicular tumors and small-cell lung carcinoma.
Paclitaxel	Taxol*	INTRAVENOUS: *Adults*—135 mg/m^2 as 24 hr infusion; repeat every 21 days. FDA pregnancy category D.	Used for ovarian carcinoma.
Teniposide	Vumon†	INTRAVENOUS: *Adults*—Up to 180 mg/m^2, various schedules. *Children*—Up to 250 mg/m^2 once weekly for 6-8 wk.	Used in lymphomas, acute lymphocytic leukemia, and neuroblastoma.
Vinblastine (VLB)	Velban Velbe† Velsar	INTRAVENOUS: *Adults*—Doses must start at 0.1 mg/kg weekly and increase gradually. Range is usually 0.15-0.2 mg/kg weekly. *Children*—2.5 mg/m^2 weekly, increased gradually to maximum dose allowed by bone marrow toxicity.	Palliative for lymphomas, carcinomas, and sarcomas.
Vincristine (VCR)	Oncovin* Vincasar Vincrex	INTRAVENOUS: *Adults*—Up to 1.4 mg/m^2 as single dose. *Children*—Up to 2 mg/m^2 as single dose. FDA pregnancy category D.	Used in acute leukemia, lymphomas, sarcomas, and Wilms' tumor.
Vindesine	Eldisine†	INTRAVENOUS: *Adults*—3 mg/m^2 every 7-10 days, for 8 doses.	Indicated for acute lymphocytic leukemia.
Vinorelbine	Navelbine	INTRAVENOUS: *Adults*—30 mg/m^2 over 6-10 minutes once weekly. FDA pregnancy category D.	Used for non–small-cell lung carcinoma.

*Available in Canada and United States.
†Available in Canada only.
‡Doses listed are representative. Very different doses and schedules may be indicated in specific diseases or protocols.

Toxicity
Each drug in this category has specific dose-limiting toxicity. For example, for vincristine it is neurotoxicity but for vinblastine it is bone marrow suppression.

Interactions
All drugs of this class increase the risk of severe generalized viral disease if the patient receives a live virus vaccine. Bone marrow suppressants also cause excessive depression of the bone marrow if used with most of these agents. Specific interactions are noted with each individual drug below.

Etoposide and teniposide
Etoposide (VP-16) and teniposide (VM-26) are podophyllotoxin derivatives. Podophyllotoxins are microtubule or spindle poisons that are naturally found in the American mandrake or mayapple plant. These drugs prevent the entry of cells into mitosis rather than arresting cells in metaphase. The exact mechanism of action is unknown but may involve inhibition of topoisomerase II.

Although about 50% of a dose may be absorbed orally, etoposide is administered primarily intravenously. The drug is highly protein bound and is slowly eliminated by the kidney, mostly as unchanged drug. Etoposide is lipid soluble but is poorly distributed to the CNS.

Etoposide produces bone marrow suppression with anemia and thrombocytopenia. Anorexia, nausea, vomiting, and alopecia also occur. Interactions with bone marrow depressants and live virus vaccines are those expected for the drug class.

Paclitaxel
Paclitaxel is a new drug that alters microtubule function inside cells and prevents normal cell division. Paclitaxel must be used intravenously. It is eliminated by liver and renal mechanisms, but the exact kinetics are not understood. The half-life ranges from 5 to 17 hours.

Adverse reactions of paclitaxel include the expected effects on bone marrow, with anemia, leukopenia, neutropenia, and thrombocytopenia. Diarrhea, nausea, and vomiting also occur commonly, as does hair loss.

Adverse reactions unique to paclitaxel include pain in muscles and joints. The drug also causes peripheral neuropathy that may produce numbness or tingling in the limbs. Interactions with paclitaxel are those expected with bone marrow depressants and live virus vaccines.

Vinblastine, vincristine, vindesine, and vinorelbine
Vinblastine, vincristine, vindesine, and vinorelbine are all vinca alkaloids with similar mechanisms of action. These drugs interfere with microtubule assembly, preventing the formation of a functional mitotic spindle, ultimately arresting the cell in mitosis.

These drugs must be administered intravenously. They do not cross the blood-brain barrier well enough to combat CNS spread of leukemia but are well distributed to other tissues. They are rapidly cleared from blood and concentrated in the liver. The drugs are excreted primarily in bile, with little drug appearing in urine. Biliary obstruction or liver impairment can dangerously impede elimination of these agents.

Vincristine doses are usually limited by the peripheral neuropathy it produces. Many symptoms of nerve dysfunction may be observed, but loss of the Achilles tendon reflex is viewed as the first sign of neuropathy. Vinblastine produces neurologic toxicity similar to that produced by vincristine. Mental depression and headache may accompany signs of peripheral neuritis or other peripheral neurologic disorders.

These drugs may be extremely irritating if they are allowed to escape from the vein into surrounding tissues during administration. Severe pain is produced, and necrosis may develop in the exposed tissue.

Vincristine produces alopecia in approximately 20% of treated patients. Many patients complain of constipation and abdominal pain, but these symptoms can usually be relieved with enemas and laxatives. Unlike other members of this class, vincristine usually does not produce significant bone marrow depression.

Vinblastine produces significant bone marrow suppression, primarily leukopenia. Leukopenia normally progresses to a low point 4 to 10 days after the dosage, but recovery usually occurs within 7 to 14 days. Nausea and vomiting are frequent. Stomatitis, diarrhea, or constipation can also occur.

Alopecia is common but often reverses even while the drug therapy is continued.

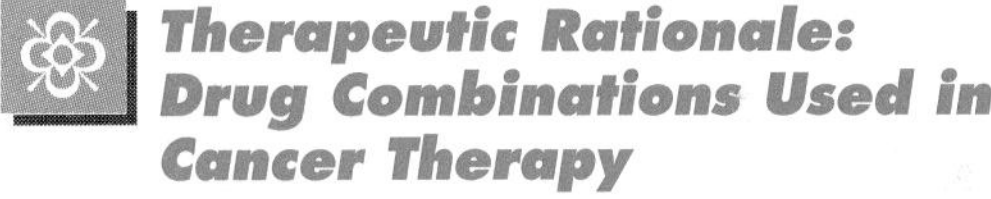

Therapeutic Rationale: Drug Combinations Used in Cancer Therapy

Combinations of Anticancer Drugs
Few of the anticancer drugs discussed in this chapter are used alone. Experience has demonstrated that combinations of these drugs are much more effective than single agents. Several reasons for this increased success exist. First, combinations of drugs acting by different mechanisms are less likely to cause drug resistance. Like microbial cells, cancer cells can adapt and become drug resistant. This process occurs easily if only a single drug is used. If several are used, the cancer cell has greater difficulty in developing simultaneous resistance.

Second, drug combinations allow the physician to select agents that produce different patterns of toxicity and thereby reduce the damage directed at any one organ system. Most of the drugs discussed produce bone marrow suppression. Combining these suppressive drugs with drugs such as bleomycin or vincristine, which do not damage the bone marrow, allows more anticancer effect to be achieved with no added damage to the bone marrow.

Third, combining anticancer agents that act at different stages of the cell cycle allows for more tumor cells to be killed than would occur with the use of only one drug. For example, a drug like procarbazine is specific for the S phase of the cell cycle. Therefore tumor cells that pass into that phase while exposed to procarbazine die, but cells in resting phase survive. If an alkylating agent is added to the treatment regimen, we can expect a percentage of the cells that survive procarbazine treatment to be killed by the second drug. Adding a third drug with yet a different mechanism of action such as vincristine further reduces the number of surviving cancer cells.

Finally, if it is possible to add a tissue-specific drug to the regimen, even more anticancer effect may be gained (Chapter 50). An established and effective treatment regimen such as has just been described exists for Hodgkin's disease. The regimen includes the alkylating agent mechlorethamine (Mustargen), the mitotic poison vincristine (Oncovin), the DNA synthesis inhibitor procarbazine (Matulane), and the lympholytic agent prednisone. This particular regimen is abbreviated MOPP. Many other established combination therapies exist for various types of cancer (Table 49-7).

Drugs Used in Supportive Therapy of Cancer Patients

Cancer patients require many drugs during the course of their disease. The drugs previously discussed attack the cancer directly. In addition to these agents, cancer patients frequently require other drugs to relieve symptoms of the disease or to ameliorate the side effects of the highly toxic antineoplastic drugs. A brief summary of drugs used in supportive care of cancer patients follows.

TABLE 49-7 Combination Chemotherapeutic Regimens

REGIMEN	DRUGS INCLUDED	DISEASE
ABVD	Doxorubicin (Adriamycin) Bleomycin (Blenoxane) Vinblastine (Velban) Dacarbazine (DTIC-Dome)	Hodgkin's disease
CHOP	Cyclophosphamide (Cytoxan) Doxorubicin (Adriamycin) Vincristine (Oncovin) Prednisone	Non-Hodgkin's lymphomas
CMF	Cyclophosphamide (Cytoxan) Methotrexate Fluorouracil	Breast carcinoma
CVP	Cyclophosphamide (Cytoxan) Vincristine (Oncovin) Prednisone	Non-Hodgkin's lymphomas
MOPP	Mechlorethamine (Mustargen) Vincristine (Oncovin) Procarbazine (Matulane) Prednisone	Hodgkin's disease
POMP	Prednisone Vincristine (Oncovin) Methotrexate Mercaptopurine (Purinethol)	Acute lymphocytic leukemia

Allopurinol

Allopurinol may be needed when large tumor masses are quickly destroyed by chemotherapy, releasing many breakdown products, including uric acid. Uric acid can severely damage kidney cells if it is allowed to increase unchecked. Allopurinol inhibits the formation of uric acid and therefore can prevent this complication. Allopurinol is also used to treat gout (Chapter 30).

Analgesics

Because pain associated with advanced cancer can be severe, hospitals and hospices specializing in care for dying cancer patients have a policy of liberal use of narcotic analgesics (Chapter 31). Frequent dosing and high doses may be needed to control pain. Fear of addiction should not prevent adequate pain control in terminal cancer.

Antiemetics

Many drugs used to attack cancer cells also attack the GI mucosa. Nausea or vomiting are therefore common side effects of chemotherapy. Some anticancer drugs cause such severe vomiting that it must be treated to prevent electrolyte imbalance. In other cases, it is transient and less severe. Nevertheless, control of nausea and vomiting can improve a patient's sense of well-being and aid in maintaining good nutrition.

Many antiemetic agents are available (Chapter 25). The severe nausea and vomiting encountered in cancer patients who receive cytotoxic drugs often requires the strong antiemetic action of phenothiazines. Patients may also be sedated to control nausea.

Control of Direct Drug Toxicity

Ifosfamide and cyclophosphamide produce toxic metabolites including acrolein that cause bladder damage (hemorrhagic cystitis). Mesna binds these toxic metabolites and protects the bladder from injury. A new drug, dexrazoxane, may prevent some of the heart damage caused by doxorubicin by binding toxic free radicals.

Control of Hypercalcemia

Hypercalcemia can be a dangerous side effect of cancer chemotherapy, especially when tumor metastases exist in bone. Several agents are available to protect patients from this complication. Etidronate, pamidronate, and gallium nitrate block overproduction of calcium (Chapter 62). Plicamycin helps with this symptom and in addition has anticancer activity as described previously.

Isotopes

The use of radioactive isotopes is generally considered palliative therapy for cancer. These agents have their effect by virtue of the ionizing radiation they release. Sodium phosphate P^{32}

(^{32}P) enters forming DNA, so it tends to be concentrated where that process is highest. Clinically, the use of this drug is to attempt to control proliferation of blood cells in polycythemia vera or in myelocytic leukemia. Gold 198 (^{198}Au) is used to control ascites. Ascites occurs when tumor cells are widely disseminated in the abdominal cavity, and large amounts of fluid accumulate. This condition differs from edema because ascitic fluid is free within the abdominal cavity and is not trapped in tissues. Pleural effusions may also be relieved by radioactive gold. The use of sodium I 131 (^{131}I), a radioactive isotope of iodine, to destroy overactive thyroid tissue is discussed in Chapter 61.

NURSING PROCESS OVERVIEW

Antineoplastic Chemotherapy

Assessment

Patients requiring chemotherapy may be of any age. Perform a thorough total assessment. Include as areas of focus probable drugs that will be used and their known side effects. Obtain a detailed health history, especially if the patient has previously received chemotherapy. Previous response to chemotherapy will be a guide to anticipating response to a repeated dose of chemotherapeutic drugs. Assess laboratory work, including the hematocrit, hemoglobin, and blood count; liver function and renal function studies; and bone, liver, and other scans.

Nursing Diagnoses

- Altered comfort: nausea and vomiting as drug side effect
- Self-concept disturbance related to alopecia as side effect of drug therapy
- Fatigue

Patient Outcomes

The patient will not experience nausea and vomiting or will experience minimal nausea and vomiting. The patient will discuss feelings about alopecia. The patient will establish priorities for daily and weekly activities to lessen fatigue.

Planning/Implementation

Continue to monitor vital signs, body weight, and progress of anticipated side effects. When a side effect occurs with regularity, begin preventive or prophylactic measures as soon as possible. Monitor fluid intake and output. Monitor appropriate laboratory work, and institute nursing interventions based on that information. If medications are being administered via constant infusion, use an infusion control device. Ensure that IV infusion lines are patent, and avoid extravasation. Investigate thoroughly any new signs or symptoms.

Evaluation

There are a few drugs used by the patient in the home for cancer treatment. For many patients cancer chemotherapy is administered in the hospital or in the physician's office because many of these drugs must be administered intravenously. Before discharge, ascertain that the patient can explain how to take medications correctly, side effects that may occur, how to treat side effects, side effects that require notification of the physician, and any measures to be used to prevent complications caused by side effects. Because the nadir or most profound bone marrow suppression often occurs days to weeks after the drug is administered, the patient should know when to anticipate the side effects and what actions to take to deal with them. Teach all patients which situations require immediate notification of the physician.

NURSING IMPLICATIONS SUMMARY

General Guidelines: Patient Receiving Cancer Chemotherapy

Drug Administration

- See the patient problem boxes on stomatitis (p. 587), bleeding tendencies (p. 586), constipation (p. 304), and leukopenia (decreased white blood cell count) (p. 585).
- Many patients receiving cancer chemotherapy develop anemia, which may be due in part to anorexia, poor nutrition, and bone marrow depression. The anemia may be caused by the drugs or by the cancer.
- See the manufacturer's literature for current information about preparation and administration of IV drugs.

Nursing Measures to Decrease Anemia

- Assess for malaise, fatigability, and pale skin color. Monitor hematocrit and hemoglobin counts, and check stools for occult blood.
- Obtain a dietary history. Teach the patient about diet and counsel as appropriate. Iron-rich foods may be unappealing if anorexia or nausea is present; see the dietary consideration box (p. 285).
- Encourage frequent, small feedings. See interventions under anorexia.
- Suggest that patients eat their largest meal in the morning, before increasing fatigue makes them too tired to eat late in the day.

Continued.

NURSING IMPLICATIONS SUMMARY—cont'd

- Encourage the use of iron preparations, if prescribed, although they may have limited value until chemotherapy is completed. Fluoxymesterone (Halotestin), an androgen, or other drugs, may also be prescribed to reverse anemia.

Nursing Measures to Decrease Anorexia

- Anorexia may arise from drug therapy or may be caused by the underlying disease.
- Assess dietary intake; monitor weight.
- Avoid foods having a strong odor. Cool or cold foods may be more appealing than hot foods. Red meat may be less appealing than fish or chicken.
- Encourage small frequent feedings. Instruct caregivers to fix small portions in an attractive manner.
- If the patient craves a specific food item, it is usually permissible for the patient to have it. The alternative may be a completely skipped meal.
- If food preparation is tiring to patients, suggest that they prepare and freeze small portions of food on days they feel better so that when not feeling well, it is necessary only to thaw and eat the food. Encourage interested friends and family members to prepare individual servings for the patient also. Encourage snacking and nibbling during the day. Encourage the patient to keep available in the refrigerator high-protein beverages or snacks that may be appealing such as milk shakes, eggnogs, frozen yogurt, and ice cream. Obtain recipes for high protein snacks from dietitians, the American Cancer Society, or the oncologist's office. Some patients may wish to purchase commercially prepared high-protein supplements that can be consumed as a drink or frozen and eaten as ice cream.
- Although a microwave oven is not a necessity, the patient may find it helpful to have one to quickly heat food. Explore this possibility with the patient and family and community resources.
- Some patients may find that a small glass of sherry or wine before dinner will stimulate their appetite. Consult the physician and the patient.

Nursing Measures to Decrease Diarrhea

- Certain drugs used for cancer chemotherapy cause diarrhea. This symptom may appear within 24 to 48 hours of receiving the drug or may be delayed for 5 to 10 days.
- Instruct the patient to switch to a clear-liquid diet or a low-residue diet high in protein and calories. The goal is to maintain a fluid intake of at least 2000 to 2500 ml per day. Caution the patient to avoid foods known to be irritating to the GI tract such as fruit, fruit juices, spicy foods, raw vegetables, corn, and coffee.
- Review possible clear-liquid food the patient may like such as broth, gelatin, tea, iced pops, soft drinks, and water. The patient may be able to tolerate chicken noodle soup. Although electrolyte-containing drinks such as Gatorade are not required, they may provide a pleasant-tasting alternative less irritating than fruit juice.
- Instruct the patient to notify the physician if diarrhea is severe or persists longer than 2 to 4 days.
- Teach the patient that diarrhea can lead to electrolyte imbalance. When possible, monitor serum electrolyte level. In severe cases the patient may need to be admitted to the hospital for IV replacement of fluids and electrolytes.
- Instruct the patient not to use enemas, rectal suppositories, or rectal thermometers.
- If anal irritation occurs, suggest that the patient shower or sit in a warm tub of water several times per day. Wash the anal area with mild soap and water, and pat the area dry gently after each loose bowel movement.
- Some patients may find it easier or more comfortable to wash the area with prepackaged towelettes such as those used to clean infants during diaper changes or with preparations such as Tucks.

Nursing Measures to Decrease Nausea and Vomiting

- Nausea and vomiting may occur within hours of receiving a dose of chemotherapy or may be delayed for 5 to 10 days.
- Monitor response to chemotherapy. Record on the care plan actions that seem to contribute to or lessen the incidence of nausea and vomiting.
- Administer antiemetics, sedatives, and other drugs as ordered to decrease nausea. They are usually more effective if administered ahead of chemotherapy or at least before severe nausea and vomiting occur, rather than afterward.
- Consider the following interventions: Reschedule chemotherapy time in relation to meal times, either closer to or further from usual mealtimes. Limit oral intake to clear liquids on the day of or the evening before chemotherapy. Keep the environment odor free; do not wear perfume. Have the patient avoid spicy, fatty, or greasy foods the day of or before chemotherapy.
- Instruct the patient and family in relaxation techniques, hypnotism, guided imagery, or distraction techniques if they are interested.
- Instruct the patient to report severe or persistent vomiting occurring at home to the physician, because dehydration and electrolyte imbalance may develop.

Nursing Measures to Decrease Alopecia

- Alopecia (hair loss) occurs when sensitive cells in the hair follicle are damaged by chemotherapy or radiation.
- Before starting chemotherapy, inform patients about the possibility of alopecia. Some patients may wish to invest in a wig resembling their own hair color and style before hair loss begins. In some communities the American Cancer Society has a "wig bank" from which cancer patients can borrow wigs during periods of alopecia. Explore this possibility. In addition, some insurance companies may reimburse patients for the cost of wigs.

NURSING IMPLICATIONS SUMMARY—cont'd

- Point out that alopecia may involve eyebrows, eyelashes, nasal hair, and pubic hair, although hair loss may be patchy rather than total in these areas.
- Some drugs typically cause complete baldness, including cyclophosphamide, daunorubicin, doxorubicin, vinblastine, and vincristine. Some drugs cause a moderate degree of alopecia, including busulfan, etoposide, floxuridine, methotrexate, and mitomycin. Finally, some drugs cause only mild alopecia or sporadic thinning of hair. These drugs include bleomycin, carmustine, fluorouracil, hydroxyurea, and melphalan.
- Reassure the patient that in most cases hair will grow back after the course of chemotherapy is finished. Some patients will begin to have hair growth before the course of chemotherapy is completed; this is variable from person to person. Usually, new hair is the same color and texture as the hair that was lost, but occasionally it is different.
- During alopecia, instruct the patient to wash hair infrequently, every 2 to 4 days. Use a mild shampoo but not necessarily "baby shampoo," which may be a little harsh. The patient's barber or hairdresser may be able to recommend a specific product. Use a cream rinse or conditioner. If the scalp is dry, apply a thin layer of baby oil, mineral oil, or A and D ointment. Brush and comb hair gently. Do not use dyes, tints, rinses, or any unnecessary chemicals on remaining hair.
- Suggest that patients use satin pillow covers.
- Avoid direct exposure to the sun either by wearing a hat or by using a maximum-protection sunscreen when out of doors (SPF 15 or greater). During cold weather, wear a hat when out of doors.
- Sometimes, the patient's head may be cooled with cold compresses prior to IV chemotherapy. This approach is used to cause vasoconstriction to the area, with the hope that less of the medication will reach the scalp, so alopecia will be less severe. Inform patients that hair loss will probably occur even with the use of cold compresses.

Nursing Measures to Decrease Extravasation

- Many cytotoxic agents are highly irritating to normal tissues. When these drugs are administered intravenously, great care must be taken to prevent them from escaping into tissues surrounding the injection site. Pain, tissue damage, and necrosis can result.
- Assess for signs of extravasation when administering IV chemotherapy such as redness or swelling at the insertion site, decreased infusion rate, inability to obtain return of blood, pain, or resistance during injection of medication.
- Signs of extravasation may not be evident at the time a drug is administered, or may be subtle. The patient may note simply that the infusion feels different than previously. If extravasation of a vesicant has occurred, and ulceration is going to develop, it may take several weeks for the full damage to appear.
- Try to avoid extravasation of any IV drugs, but be especially alert when the following drugs are administered because of tissue necrosis and sloughing that may occur: dactinomycin, mitomycin, carmustine, cisplatin, dacarbazine, daunorubicin, plicamycin, streptozocin, mitoxantrone, vincristine, and vinblastine.
- In the ideal situation, perform a fresh venipuncture for administering chemotherapy. Otherwise, ascertain that the infusion line to be used is patent.
- Use a forearm infusion site rather than the dorsum of the hand for infusion of drugs that may cause necrosis and sloughing if extravasation occurs. Extravasation in the forearm may be less severe than in the dorsum of the hand, where muscles and tendons that control hand movement and function may be affected. Remain with the patient during the infusion.
- If extravasation occurs, discontinue the infusion but leave the needle or catheter in place. Attempt to aspirate any drug that can be retrieved. Follow agency procedures for managing the situation. A typical procedure would be to administer a corticosteroid subcutaneously in the area of extravasation or via the infusion catheter that is still in place, cover the area with a topical steroid, then cover with an occlusive dressing. Finally, apply ice compresses for 15 minutes four times a day, and keep the extremity elevated for 48 hours. Notify the physician. Use a fresh venipuncture site for infusion of any remaining chemotherapy drug.
- Medical orders for treatment of extravasation should be written before infusion is begun. These orders should be readily available to all persons who administer chemotherapy. Keep drugs ordered for treatment of extravasation readily available.

Safe Handling of Chemotherapeutic Drugs

- Avoid direct contact with chemotherapeutic agents, because the nurse may be exposed to drug toxicity through repeated skin or aerosolization contact.
- Prepare IV medications with a laminar airflow hood. Wash hands before and after handling chemotherapy drugs.
- Wear disposable gloves and long-sleeved gown during drug preparation. Wear gloves during drug administration.
- Use correct technique to avoid skin contact with prepared dosages. Use Luer-Lok fittings whenever possible to avoid inadvertent separation of syringe and needle. Establish and follow procedures for disposal of drug containers, contaminated gloves, syringes, and IV tubing.
- After drawing up dosages into the syringe, discard the needle, and attach a new sterile needle to avoid skin contact with any traces of medication that might be on the outside of the first needle.
- Check ordered doses carefully. Several drugs have similar names.

Continued.

NURSING IMPLICATIONS SUMMARY—cont'd

- Consult the manufacturer's literature for information about dilution and rate of administration.
- These drugs are highly toxic. Many agencies limit the number of persons who can administer these drugs to a few nurses who have had experience and additional training in their use.
- Allergic reactions have been reported with many of these drugs. Question patients about drug allergy before administering the drug. Have drugs, equipment, and personnel available to treat an acute allergic reaction in the setting in which these drugs are administered. Assess patients frequently during IV administration. Do not leave patients unattended for prolonged periods during treatment.
- Monitor laboratory work on an ongoing basis including complete blood cell count (CBC) and differential, platelet count, blood urea nitrogen (BUN) and serum creatinine serum uric acid level, and liver function tests.
- These drugs are contraindicated during pregnancy. Counsel about contraceptive measures as appropriate. Menstrual irregularities are common in women receiving chemotherapy. Instruct women to keep a record of menstrual periods and to consult a physician immediately if pregnancy is suspected.
- Chemotherapy may cause diminished production or viability of sperm. Male patients may wish to arrange for deposit of sperm in a sperm bank before beginning chemotherapy.

Nursing Measures to Reduce Uric Acid Levels

- Elevation of uric acid levels often accompanies administration of chemotherapy to patients with leukemia or some lymphomas. This is caused by the release of large quantities of breakdown products in these rapidly dividing forms of cancer. For this reason, chemotherapy orders may routinely be accompanied by orders for allopurinol. Monitor the uric acid levels. Keep the patient well hydrated (see Chapter 30).

Patient and Family Education

- Review with the patient and family the anticipated benefits and possible side effects of drug therapy. Provide support to these patients who may be facing a difficult diagnosis and anticipating serious drug side effects.
- Encourage the patient to notify the physician if any new side effects develop.
- Encourage the patient to return for follow-up visits as directed. Point out that many side effects may not become evident for 2 to 3 weeks after the final dose of therapy.
- Remind the patient to inform all health care providers of all medications being taken. This is especially important because bone marrow suppression, stomatitis, and other side effects may not appear until days to weeks after the drug has been administered.
- Remind the patient not to use over-the-counter (OTC) preparations without first consulting the physician. Emphasize the importance of keeping these and all drugs out of the reach of children.
- Warn the patient not to receive immunizations while taking cytotoxic drugs unless first approved by the physician. Instruct persons living with the patient to avoid oral polio vaccine while the patient is receiving chemotherapy. Also have the patient avoid contact with others who have recently had oral polio vaccine; if contact is necessary, have the patient wear a mask over the nose and mouth. Before starting chemotherapy, some physicians recommend that patients receive flu shots or update immunizations; consult the physician.
- Inform the patient that ridges in the fingernails may appear during chemotherapy; these reflect the effect of the drugs on the dividing cells of the nails.
- For information about the drugs, drug protocols, protocols to treat extravasation, oral gargles, mouthwashes, dietary supplements, snack recipes, patient teaching aids, and other information for patients, families, and health care providers, contact the chemotherapy department of local medical centers; the American Cancer Society; the Office of Cancer Communications at the National Cancer Institute, Bethesda, MD 20892, Telephone 1-800-4-CANCER [Spanish-speaking staff members are also available]; the Department of Health and Human Services; or local oncologists' offices. Refer patients as appropriate to the local visiting nurse agencies or hospice.
- Unless additional teaching points are listed, points on patient and family education about the drugs discussed in this chapter are the same.
- Teach the patient to take prescribed medications as ordered, even if not feeling well. Before discharge, review what to do if the patient vomits shortly after taking oral doses.

Altretamine

Drug Administration/Patient and Family Education

- See the general guidelines for information about anemia, leukopenia, thrombocytopenia (bleeding tendencies), nausea and vomiting, and diarrhea.
- Assess for CNS effects, including clumsiness, confusion, dizziness, weakness, and numbness in the arms and legs.
- Assess for depression: depressed mood, lack of interest in personal appearance, insomnia, weight gain or loss.
- Monitor the CBC, white blood cell (WBC) differential, and platelet count.
- Take doses after meals.

Bleomycin

Drug Administration

- The physician may order a test dose of medication to be given before the full dose to test for idiosyncratic reaction. See the manufacturer's literature.

NURSING IMPLICATIONS SUMMARY—cont'd

- See the general guidelines for information about nausea and vomiting, alopecia, and stomatitis.
- Assess for dyspnea and cough, and auscultate lung sounds. Tell the patient to report cough, shortness of breath or difficulty breathing, which may develop for up to a month after the last dose of medication. Encourage patients to stop smoking.
- Assess for skin changes; monitor blood pressure and pulse.
- Monitor CBC and differential, platelet count, BUN, serum creatinine, and urinalysis. Monitor pulmonary function tests if ordered.

Busulfan

Drug Administration

- See the general guidelines for information about thrombocytopenia (bleeding tendencies), depressed WBC count, anemia, elevated uric acid levels, nausea and vomiting, and alopecia.
- Auscultate lung sounds, and assess for dyspnea and cough. Monitor weight and blood pressure. Assess for skin changes.
- Monitor CBC and differential, platelet count, serum uric acid, and liver function tests.

Carboplatin and Cisplatin

Drug Administration

- See the general guidelines for information about depressed WBC count, thrombocytopenia (bleeding tendencies), anemia, nausea and vomiting, and with carboplatin, alopecia.
- Assess hearing acuity, and assess for tinnitus. Refer appropriate patients for audiograms; consult the physician.
- Assess for metallic taste in the mouth. Because this may affect nutritional intake, monitor weight.
- Monitor blood pressure and pulse; auscultate lung sounds.
- Monitor CBC and differential, platelet count, liver function tests, BUN and serum creatinine levels, serum electrolyte level, and uric acid levels.
- To limit the severe nausea and vomiting that frequently accompany cisplatin administration, the regimen may include administration of antiemetics, sedative, steroids, and other drugs. In addition, to limit renal toxicity, the drug is often infused with large fluid volumes, such as 250 ml/hr for 4 hours, or with mannitol. Monitor intake and output hourly for the first 6 to 8 hours, then every 12 to 24 hours.

Carmustine (BCNU) and Lomustine (CCNU)

Drug Administration

- See the general guidelines for information about depressed WBC count, thrombocytopenia (bleeding tendencies), anemia, stomatitis, alopecia, and nausea and vomiting.
- Assess for dyspnea and cough; auscultate lung sounds. Encourage the patient to stop smoking. Monitor weight. Inspect for skin changes and edema.
- Monitor CBC and differential, platelet count, liver function tests, serum uric acid, BUN and serum creatinine level. Monitor pulmonary function tests, if available.
- Wear gloves when preparing or administering these drugs; hyperpigmentation may occur if the drug touches the skin.
- Teach the patient taking lomustine to take doses on an empty stomach. In addition, when the prescription is filled, the correct dose may be a combination of different kinds of capsules. Take all the capsules in one container, as ordered. If there are questions, consult the pharmacist or physician.

Chlorambucil

Drug Administration

- See the general guidelines for information about nausea and vomiting, depressed WBC count, thrombocytopenia (bleeding tendencies), and high uric acid levels.
- Auscultate lung sounds, and assess for dyspnea and cough. Inspect for jaundice, skin changes, and rash.
- Monitor uric acid levels, liver function tests, CBC and differential, and platelet count.

Cyclophosphamide

Drug Administration

- See the general guidelines for information about depressed WBC count, thrombocytopenia (bleeding tendencies), anemia, nausea and vomiting, diarrhea, oral ulcers, high uric acid levels, and alopecia.
- Auscultate lung sounds; assess for cough and dyspnea. Assess pulse and blood pressure. Monitor weight.
- Monitor CBC and differential, platelet count, liver function tests, serum electrolyte levels, uric acid levels, BUN and serum creatinine, urinary specific gravity, and urinalysis.

Patient and Family Education

- See the general guidelines.
- Tell the patient to take doses in the morning on an empty stomach, unless otherwise instructed by the physician.
- Teach the patient to force fluids, up to eight 8-ounce glasses of water daily and to notify the physician if there is blood in urine.
- Warn the patient to avoid driving or operating hazardous equipment if blurred vision, confusion, or lethargy occurs; notify the physician.

Dacarbazine

Drug Administration

- See the general guidelines for information about depressed WBC count, thrombocytopenia (bleeding tendencies), anemia, nausea and vomiting, alopecia, stomatitis (rare), and extravasation.
- Assess for skin changes.

Continued.

Nursing Implications Summary—cont'd

- Monitor the CBC and differential, platelet count, liver function tests, BUN and serum creatinine level, and serum uric acid.
- Monitor the infusion carefully to avoid extravasation.

Patient and Family Education

- See the general guidelines.
- Warn the patient to avoid driving or operating hazardous equipment if blurred vision, confusion, or lethargy occurs; notify the physician.

Mechlorethamine

Drug Administration

- See the general guidelines for information about anemia, depressed WBC count, thrombocytopenia (bleeding tendencies), nausea and vomiting, elevated uric acid level, amenorrhea, and azoospermia. Alopecia is a rare side effect.
- Assess neurologic function: tinnitus, loss of hearing, numbness or tingling of fingers, toes, face. Emphasize the importance of audiometric testing, if prescribed.
- With IV administration, if extravasation occurs, discontinue the infusion and aspirate any remaining drug. Promptly infiltrate the area with sterile isotonic sodium thiosulfate injection, then apply cold compresses for 6 to 12 hours.
- If the drug comes in contact with the skin, wash immediately with copious amounts of water for 15 minutes, then rinse with a 2% sodium thiosulfate solution. If the drug comes in contact with the eye, irrigate immediately with 0.9% sodium chloride or balanced salt ophthalmic solution, then promptly consult an ophthalmologist.
- Prepare the drug just before administration.
- For *topical* administration: wear protective gloves. Assess for rashes. Shower or wash the area before applying the solution or ointment. Make certain the skin surfaces are dry. Apply to the prescribed areas, but apply lightly to the axillary, perineal, inguinal, and inframammary areas to avoid irritation. Do not shower again until before the next dose. Topical preparations may cause the skin to darken, but this should disappear when the drug is stopped.

Patient and Family Education

- See the general guidelines.
- Warn the patient to avoid driving or operating hazardous equipment if drowsiness, vertigo, weakness, or other neurologic symptoms develop; consult the physician.

Melphalan

Drug Administration

- See the general guidelines for information about depressed WBC count, thrombocytopenia (bleeding tendencies), nausea and vomiting, diarrhea, and stomatitis; alopecia is uncommon.
- Monitor pulmonary function; auscultate lung sounds. Assess for dyspnea and cough. Inspect for skin changes.
- Monitor CBC, differential and platelet count, BUN, serum creatinine, and serum uric acid.

Mitomycin

Drug Administration

- See the general guidelines for information about depressed WBC count, thrombocytopenia (bleeding tendencies), anemia, anorexia, nausea and vomiting, and alopecia.
- Auscultate lung sounds, and assess for dyspnea and cough. Monitor intake and output and weight.
- Monitor CBC and differential, platelet count, serum creatinine level, and BUN level.

Mitoxantrone

Drug Administration

- See the general guidelines for information about depressed WBC count, thrombocytopenia (bleeding tendencies), nausea and vomiting, diarrhea, stomatitis, and alopecia.
- Monitor intake and output and weight. Auscultate lung sounds. Inspect for edema. Monitor vital signs.
- Monitor the CBC and differential, platelet count, serum uric acid, and liver function tests.
- Tell the patient that urine may be bluish green and sclera may be blue for a day or two after therapy. This effect is not significant and will disappear.

Thiotepa

Drug Administration

- See the general guidelines for information about depressed WBC count, thrombocytopenia (bleeding tendencies), anemia, nausea and vomiting, alopecia, elevated uric acid, and stomatitis.
- Assess for skin changes. Auscultate lung sounds. Instruct the patient to report wheezing or the development of other respiratory symptoms. Assess for urinary tract problems such as urgency, frequency, and change in urine color.
- Monitor CBC and differential, platelet count, BUN and serum creatinine, liver function tests, serum uric acid, and urinalysis.

Cladribine

Drug Administration/Patient and Family Education

- See general guidelines for information about anemia, leukopenia, thrombocytopenia (bleeding tendencies), anorexia, nausea and vomiting, and elevated uric acid.
- Assess for fever, skin rash, edema in lower extremities.
- Monitor CBC, WBC differrential, platelet count, CD4 and CD8 T lymphocyte counts, and serum uric acid.

Cytarabine

Drug Administration

- See the general guidelines for information about depressed WBC count, thrombocytopenia (bleeding tendencies),

NURSING IMPLICATIONS SUMMARY—cont'd

anemia, anorexia, nausea and vomiting, diarrhea, elevated uric acid levels, and alopecia.

- Auscultate lung sounds, and assess for dyspnea and cough. Monitor pulse and blood pressure. Assess for skin changes, and inspect for edema.
- Assess for changes in vision, and instruct patients to report changes in vision.
- Use brands and diluents that do not contain benzyl alcohol as a preservative for intrathecal administration or for pediatric administration. Intrathecal administration may be associated with CNS side effects. Keep side rails up. Anticipate CNS effects.
- Monitor CBC and differential, platelet count, liver function tests, and serum uric acid level.

Floxuridine and Fluorouracil

Drug Administration

- See the general guidelines for information about depressed WBC count, thrombocytopenia (bleeding tendencies), anemia, nausea and vomiting, diarrhea, alopecia or thinning of hair, and stomatitis.
- Assess for ataxia, and assess mental status. Inspect for skin changes.
- Monitor CBC and differential, platelet count, and liver function tests.

Fludaribine

Drug Administration/Patient and Family Education

- See the general guidelines for information about anemia, leukopenia, thrombocytopenia (bleeding tendencies), nausea and vomiting, stomatitis, alopecia (rare), and elevated uric acid.
- Auscultate lung sounds. Assess for cough, shortness of breath. Assess lower extremities for swelling. Assess for CNS effects, including agitation, confusion, blurred vision, loss of hearing, numbness or tingling in fingers or toes.
- Monitor the CBC, WBC differential, platelet count, and serum uric acid level.

Hydroxyurea

Drug Administration

- See the general guidelines for information about depressed WBC count, thrombocytopenia (bleeding tendencies), anorexia, diarrhea, stomatitis, nausea and vomiting, and elevated uric acid levels.
- The contents of the capsule may be opened and emptied into water. The powder floating on the top of the water is inert filler.
- Assess neurologic and mental status. Monitor weight, and inspect for skin changes and edema.
- Monitor CBC and differential, platelet count, serum creatinine, BUN, and uric acid levels.

Mercaptopurine and Thioguanine

Drug Administration

- See the general guidelines for information about depressed WBC count, thrombocytopenia (bleeding tendencies), anemia, anorexia, diarrhea, nausea and vomiting, stomatitis, and elevated uric acid levels.
- Assess for skin changes.
- Monitor CBC and differential, platelet count, serum uric acid, serum creatinine, and BUN levels, urinalysis, and liver function tests.
- Instruct patients taking mercaptopurine to avoid alcoholic beverages because they may contribute to increased toxicity.

Methotrexate

Drug Administration

- See the general guidelines for information about depressed WBC count, thrombocytopenia (bleeding tendencies), anemia, nausea and vomiting, stomatitis, diarrhea, alopecia, and elevated uric acid levels.
- Monitor weight; inspect for skin changes and edema.
- Intrathecal administration is associated with CNS changes. Monitor mental status. Keep side rails up; supervise ambulation.
- Monitor CBC and differential, platelet count, urinalysis, liver function tests, and serum uric acid, serum creatinine, BUN, and blood glucose levels.
- See also the discussion of leucovorin rescue in Chapter 22.

Patient and Family Education

- See the general guidelines.
- Warn patients to avoid driving or operating hazardous equipment if blurred vision, drowsiness, dizziness, or ataxia develops; notify the physician.
- Instruct the patient to avoid other medications that contain aspirin or other salicylates or NSAIDs because these drugs in combination with methotrexate may contribute to toxicity.
- Review the patient problem box on photosensitivity (p. 649).
- Instruct the patient to avoid alcoholic beverages, which may increase liver toxicity.

Procarbazine

Drug Administration

- See the general guidelines for information about depressed WBC count, thrombocytopenia (bleeding tendencies), anemia, nausea and vomiting, anorexia, diarrhea, and alopecia.
- Assess mental status, and monitor neurologic status. Anticipate CNS side effects. Keep siderails up, supervise ambulation, and keep a night light on.
- Monitor pulse and blood pressure. See the patient problem box on orthostatic hypotension (p. 157).

Continued.

NURSING IMPLICATIONS SUMMARY—cont'd

- Auscultate lung sounds. Assess for cough and dyspnea. Inspect for skin changes.
- Monitor CBC and differential, platelet count, blood glucose level, and urinalysis.

Patient and Family Education
- See the general guidelines.
- Warn the patient to avoid the use of alcohol; see the patient problem box on disulfiram-like reactions (p. 635). Warn the patient to avoid foods containing tyramine (see the dietary consideration box on tyramine, p. 663). Warn the patient to limit intake of caffeine-containing foods such as chocolate, coffee, tea, or cola drinks. These dietary limitations should continue for at least 2 weeks after the last dose of procabazine.
- Tell diabetic patients to monitor blood glucose levels carefully; an adjustment in diet or insulin dose may be necessary.
- Warn the patient to avoid driving or operating hazardous equipment if disorientation, dizziness, or unsteadiness develops; notify the physician.
- Encourage the patient to wear a medical identification tag or bracelet if taking procabazine.

Asparaginase
Drug Administration
- See the general guidelines for information about depressed WBC count, bleeding tendencies, anorexia, elevated uric acid, and nausea and vomiting.
- Assess neurologic and mental status. Monitor blood pressure and pulse. Monitor weight. Assess for skin changes and edema. Check stools for guaiac or occult blood.
- Monitor CBC and differential, prothrombin time, partial prothrombin times, liver function tests, and serum creatinine, BUN, blood glucose, and serum amylase levels.

Dactinomycin
Drug Administration
- See the general guidelines for information about depressed WBC count, thrombocytopenia (bleeding tendencies), anemia, nausea and vomiting, stomatitis, diarrhea, alopecia, and extravasation.
- Monitor weight, blood pressure, pulse, and intake and output. Assess for edema. Auscultate lung sounds. Inspect for skin changes.
- Monitor CBC and differential and platelet count.

Daunorubicin, Doxorubicin, Epirubicin, and Idarubicin
Drug Administration
- See the general guidelines for information about depressed WBC count, thrombocytopenia (bleeding tendencies), anemia, elevated uric acid levels, alopecia, nausea and vomiting, stomatitis, diarrhea, and extravasation.
- Monitor pulse and blood pressure. Assess for signs of congestive heart failure such as weight gain, edema of dependent areas, dyspnea, and jugular venous distention. Auscultate lung sounds, and monitor respiratory rate. Monitor serial electrocardiogram (ECGs), and results of echocardiographs and radionuclide determination of ejection fraction.
- Monitor CBC and differential, platelet count, lactate dehydrogenase (LDH) and liver function tests, serum creatinine, and serum uric acid level.
- Inform the patient that urine may be reddish in color for 1 to 2 days after each dose.

Plicamycin (Mithramycin)
Drug Administration
- See the general guidelines for information about depressed WBC count, thrombocytopenia (bleeding tendencies), anorexia, diarrhea, nausea and vomiting, stomatitis, and extravasation.
- Monitor mental status. Warn the patient to avoid driving or operating hazardous equipment if drowsiness, dizziness, fatigue, or lethargy develops; notify the physician.
- Monitor CBC and differential, platelet count, serum creatinine, BUN, and serum electrolyte levels, and urinalysis.
- Assess for hypercalcemia and hypocalcemia. See Table 17-1 for a description of common electrolyte abnormalities. Some physicians recommend a low-calcium, low–vitamin D diet for patients taking this drug.
- Avoid medications containing aspirin, salicylates, or acetaminophen.

Etoposide and Teniposide
Drug Administration
- See the general guidelines for information about depressed WBC count, thrombocytopenia (bleeding tendencies), anemia, anorexia, stomatitis, nausea and vomiting, and alopecia.
- Monitor pulse, blood pressure, and weight. Auscultate lung sounds; assess for dyspnea. Monitor ECGs at regular intervals. See the patient problem box on orthostatic hypotension (p. 157). Assess for skin changes.
- Monitor CBC and differential and platelet count.

Paclitaxel
Drug Administration/Patient and Family Education
- See the general guidelines for information about anemia, leukopenia, thrombocytopenia (bleeding tendencies), extravasation, stomatitis (rare), nausea and vomiting, diarrhea, and alopecia.
- Monitor vital signs. Assess for CNS effects: numbness, burning or tingling of hands or feet. Assess for hypersen-

NURSING IMPLICATIONS SUMMARY—cont'd

sitivity reaction: flushing of face, skin rash or itching, shortness of breath. Monitor ECG.
- Monitor the CBC, WBC differential, and platelet count.

Vinblastine

Drug Administration

- See the general guidelines for information about depressed WBC count, thrombocytopenia (bleeding tendencies), anemia, nausea and vomiting, anorexia, diarrhea, stomatitis, elevated uric acid, alopecia, and extravasation.
- Assess neurologic and mental status. Warn the patient to avoid driving or operating hazardous equipment if dizziness or numbness develops; notify the physician.
- Assess for peripheral neuropathy including tingling or numbness of extremities. Assess for skin changes. See the patient problem box on photosensitivity (p. 649).
- Monitor CBC and differential, platelet count, and serum uric acid.

Vincristine

Drug Administration

- See the general guidelines for information about anemia, extravasation, constipation, nausea and vomiting, stomatitis, alopecia, and elevated serum uric acid level.
- Assess neurologic and mental status. Assess for peripheral neuropathy including depressed deep tendon reflexes, changes in gait, tingling of extremities (paresthesias), and other changes in the neurologic assessment.
- Monitor intake and output, blood pressure, pulse, and respiratory rate. Auscultate lung and bowel sounds. Monitor reflexes and gait.
- Monitor CBC, serum electrolyte and uric acid levels.

CRITICAL THINKING

APPLICATION

1. What are the phases of the cell cycle, and what events take place during each phase?
2. What is carcinogenesis?
3. What properties of cancer cells allow them to spread through the body?
4. How does the growth fraction of most normal tissues differ from that of most tumors?
5. On what property of cancer cells does most cancer chemotherapy depend?
6. What is the mechanism of action of alkylating agents used as anticancer medications?
7. What type of toxicity is most common with the use of alkylating agents?
8. Which of the alkylating agents is not a strong vesicant as administered because it must be activated by liver microsomal enzymes?
9. Which drugs that directly damage the structure of DNA do not produce bone marrow suppression?
10. What is the mechanism of action of anticancer agents that block purine and pyrimidine formation or utilization?
11. Why are inhibitors of purine and pyrimidine formation or utilization considered phase-specific agents?
12. Which anticancer drug inhibits DNA synthesis by preventing regeneration of tetrahydrofolate (THF)?
13. What is the basis of the anticancer effect of drugs that block RNA or protein synthesis?
14. What properties of asparaginase make it unique among anticancer drugs?
15. Which anticancer drugs that inhibit RNA formation have special toxicity toward the heart?
16. What is the basis of the anticancer effects of drugs that disrupt microtubule formation?
17. What toxicity is characteristic of mitotic poisons? How should you assess for these effects?
18. Which of the mitotic poisons is least associated with bone marrow suppression?
19. What is the rationale behind combination chemotherapy in the treatment of cancer?
20. Why is allopurinol frequently used in cancer treatment programs?
21. What principle governs the use of analgesics in treating cancer patients?
22. Why are antiemetics frequently used as adjuncts to cancer chemotherapy?
23. Why are drugs to lower blood calcium levels often required in cancer patients?

CRITICAL THINKING

1. What normal cells are especially vulnerable to attack by alkylating agents? How should you assess for these effects?
2. What type of toxicity is most common with drugs that inhibit DNA synthesis? How should you assess for these effects?
3. What toxicity is most common with anticancer drugs that inhibit RNA or protein synthesis? How should you assess for these effects?

CHAPTER 50

Tissue-Specific Anticancer Agents

OBJECTIVES

After studying this chapter, you should be able to do the following:

- *Discuss why hormones such as estrogens, androgens, or progestins may have anticancer activity.*
- *Explain the anticancer activity of glucocorticoids.*
- *Name the target organ for mitotane, trilostane, or streptozocin.*
- *Develop a nursing care plan for the patient receiving one or more of the drugs discussed in this chapter.*

KEY TERMS

antiandrogens
antiestrogen

CHAPTER OVERVIEW

Most of the anticancer drugs discussed in the previous chapter are not tissue specific in their cytotoxic action. For example, although chlorambucil is clinically useful because it attacks lymphoid tissue, it also attacks other tissues, especially at higher doses. In this chapter we discuss anticancer agents that are effective not because of general cytotoxicity but because they interact with specific receptors on or in specific types of cells.

Therapeutic Rationale: Tissue-Specific Anticancer Agents

Most of the tissue-specific anticancer agents are derivatives of hormones and interact with those cells bearing specific receptors for the hormone. For example, glucocorticoids suppress lymphoid tissue because that tissue contains specific receptors for glucocorticoids. This action may be helpful in controlling cancers arising from lymphoid tissue.

The sex steroids (androgens, estrogens, and progestins) are also used in cancer chemotherapy. These steroid hormones enter sensitive cells and, complexed with specific receptor proteins, are transported to the cell nucleus. Within the nucleus they alter RNA and protein synthesis, thereby changing the function of the cell. The use of these agents in cancer chemotherapy depends on a knowledge of the hormone dependence of certain tissues. For example, the prostate gland depends on androgens; without these hormones the gland shrinks and loses function. Estrogens, hormones that produce feminization, antagonize the action of androgens on the prostate. Carcinoma of the prostate gland seems to retain a degree of this hormonal control, and tumor regression can frequently be produced by suppressing androgens and supplying excess estrogens.

Similar results can be achieved in many breast carcinomas in women by treating them with estrogens, antiestrogens, or androgens. To a certain extent, hormonal therapy of tumors of the reproductive tissues is empiric. The rationale behind all forms of this therapy is that (1) reproductive tissues proliferate in response to the proper balance of male and female hormones and (2) tumors of reproductive tissues tend to retain some dependence on hormones. Tumors in postmenopausal women respond to hormone therapy better than do those in premenopausal women.

Therapeutic Agents: Tissue-Specific Anticancer Agents

The clinical properties of these tissue-specific anticancer agents are summarized in Table 50-1.

Steroids and Related Agents

Androgens

Mechanism of Action

Androgens interact with certain reproductive tissues, altering RNA and protein synthesis. This action is independent of the cell cycle. For estrogen-dependent tissues, androgens frequently interfere with estrogen function. Androgens can therefore cause involution of these tissues. This action forms the basis for the use of androgen to control some forms of breast cancer in postmenopausal women. Results of this form of therapy usually do not become evident until after 8 weeks of treatment or longer.

Pharmacokinetics

Androgens are in general not well absorbed orally, although a few synthetic androgens are exceptions (see Table 50-1). When given by injection, these oil-soluble substances are slowly absorbed from intramuscular (IM) sites. Androgens are metabolized by the liver. Patients with impaired renal function may have difficulty eliminating the amounts of androgen used therapeutically and may suffer excessive toxicity.

Uses

Testolactone is used almost exclusively for breast carcinoma (see Table 50-1). Other androgens, used primarily in replacement therapy, may occasionally be used to treat specific cancers. These drugs include fluoxymesterone, methyltestosterone, testosterone enanthate, and testosterone propionate (Chapter 66).

Adverse Reactions and Contraindications

An advantage of testolactone is that it does not cause as much virilization in women as other androgens. Side effects are minimal; peripheral neuropathy with numbness or tingling in the face or extremeties, anorexia, diarrhea, nausea, or vomiting is possible. Water retention with swelling of feet and ankles may also occur.

Toxicity

Gastrointestinal (GI) tract symptoms may be more severe with high doses. Hypercalcemia may arise from rapid destruction of tumors; testolactone may need to be withdrawn and the patient may need support with large fluid volumes.

Interactions

Anticoagulant effects may be increased; dosage adjustment may be required.

Antiandrogens: flutamide and LH-RH analogues

Mechanism of Action

Flutamide blocks uptake of androgens into cells or blocks binding of androgens in cell nuclei. Leuprolide, buserelin, and goserelin are synthetic analogues of luteinizing hormone–releasing factor (LH-RH) that on continuous administration suppress secretion of gonadotropin-releasing hormone. The result is lower synthesis and release of testosterone. These three agents are able to produce the same low levels of male sex steroids produced by surgical castration. Because of their actions, these agents are called **antiandrogens.**

Pharmacokinetics

Leuprolide, buserelin, and goserelin are peptides and therefore cannot withstand the acidic environment of the stomach. These drugs are absorbed from subcutaneous sites. Flutamide is absorbed orally but undergoes extensive metabolism in the liver. These agents tend to increase testosterone levels during the first week of therapy, but full suppression of testosterone occurs by 2 to 4 weeks.

Uses

Flutamide and one of the LH-RH analogues are used in combination for metastatic carcinoma of the prostate, a tumor that often depends on androgens for its growth.

TABLE 50-1 Drugs Used to Control Cancer of Specific Tissues

GENERIC NAME	TRADE NAME	ADMINISTRATION/DOSAGE	COMMENTS/USES
Steroids and Related Agents			
Androgens			
Testolactone	Teslac	ORAL: *Adults*—250 mg 4 times daily. FDA pregnancy category C.	Palliation for carcinomas of breast in postmenopausal women.
Antiandrogens			
Buserelin	Suprefact†	SUBCUTANEOUS: *Adults*—0.5 mg 3 times daily for 7 days; then 0.2 mg daily for maintenance.	Analogue of LH-RH lowers follicle-stimulating hormone and luteinizing hormone, thus lowering androgens to castration levels; for prostatic carcinoma.
Flutamide	Euflex† Eulexin	ORAL: *Adults*—250 mg every 8 hr. FDA pregnancy category D.	Blocks androgen actions on cells; use with leuprolide for prostatic carcinoma.
Goserelin	Zoladex*	SUBCUTANEOUS (IMPLANT): *Adults*—3.6 mg base every 28 days.	For prostatic carcinoma; action similar to that of buserelin.
Leuprolide	Lupron*	SUBCUTANEOUS: *Adults*—1 mg daily. INTRAMUSCULAR: *Adults*—7.5 mg once a month. FDA pregnancy category X.	Suppresses secretion of androgens like buserelin; used with flutamide for prostatic carcinoma.
Estrogens			
Chlorotrianisene	TACE	ORAL: *Adults*—12-25 mg daily.	Long-acting; for prostatic carcinoma.
Diethylstilbestrol	Stilphostrol Honvol†	INTRAVENOUS: *Adults*—0.5-1 gm/250 ml for 5 days. Maintenance, 250-500 mg once or twice weekly. ORAL: *Adults*—50-200 mg 3 times daily. FDA pregnancy category X.	Palliative for prostatic carcinoma.
Estramustine	Emcyt*	ORAL: *Adults*—14 mg/kg daily in 3 or 4 doses.	For prostatic carcinoma.
Antiestrogens			
Tamoxifen	Nolvadex* Tamofen†	ORAL: *Adults*—10 or 20 mg twice daily. FDA pregnancy category D.	Palliative for advanced carcinoma of breast.
Progestins			
Medroxyprogesterone	Depo-Provera*	INTRAMUSCULAR: *Adults*—400-1000 mg in weekly injections. FDA pregnancy category X.	Palliative for advanced endometrial or renal carcinomas.
Megestrol	Megace*	ORAL: *Adults*—40-320 mg daily in divided doses. FDA pregnancy category X.	Palliative for advanced endometrial or breast carcinomas.
Adrenal Antagonists			
Mitotane	Lysodren*	ORAL: *Adults*—2 gm 4 times daily; maximum 16 gm/day. FDA pregnancy category C.	Used to control adrenal cortical carcinoma.
Trilostane	Modrastane	ORAL: *Adults*—30 mg 4 times daily; increase slowly to 90 mg 4 times daily. FDA pregnancy category X.	Suppresses steroid production from adrenals and tumors.
Beta-Cell Antagonist			
Streptozocin	Zanosar*	INTRAVENOUS: *Adults*—500 mg/m^2 daily for 5 days every 6 wk. FDA pregnancy category C.	Used for pancreatic tumors.
Interferons			
Interferon alfa-2a, recombinant	Roferon-A*	INTRAMUSCULAR, SUBCUTANEOUS: *Adults*—up to 36 million U daily. FDA pregnancy category C.	Used for hairy cell leukemia, Kaposi's sarcoma, other tumors.
Interferon alfa-2b, recombinant	Intron-A*	INTRAMUSCULAR, SUBCUTANEOUS: *Adults*—up to 30 million U/m^2 3 times weekly. FDA pregnancy category C.	Used for hairy cell leukemia, Kaposi's sarcoma, other tumors.
Interferon alfa-n1 recombinant	Wellferon†	INTRAMUSCULAR, SUBCUTANEOUS: *Adults*—up to 3 million U daily for 16-24 wk. FDA pregnancy category C.	Used for hairy cell leukemia, carcinomas, melanoma, lymphomas.

*Available in Canada and United States.
†Available in Canada only.

Adverse Reactions and Contraindications

When given together, flutamide and an LH-RH analogue reduce testosterone levels to those expected in castrated males. Many of the side effects are the result of low testosterone levels. Hot flashes are very common. Most patients report reduced libido or impotence. Gynecomastia occurs in about 9% of patients.

In addition to symptoms arising from testosterone suppression, flutamide also often causes diarrhea. Less commonly anorexia, edema, gynecomastia, and peripheral neuropathy may arise.

Buserelin and goserelin may cause an initial flare of the disease, with pain and swelling, difficult urination, and possibly weakness. Approximately 10% of patients on goserelin experience disease flare, but only about 1% of patients on buserelin have this reaction. Hot flashes and decreased sexual desire are common with both drugs. Anorexia, breast tenderness, edema, nausea, and vomiting are also possible. In addition, goserelin may cause cardiovascular effects including arrhythmias, strokes, or infarctions. Goserelin may also be associated with chronic obstructive pulmonary disease or congestive heart failure.

Leuprolide causes all the side effects associated with low testosterone levels mentioned above. In addition, it may be associated with cardiac arrhythmias or other cardiac symptoms, especially in men. In women the drug suppresses menstrual cycles. Both men and women may show blurred vision, dizziness, edema, headache, insomnia, nausea, numbness in hands or feet, or vomiting.

Toxicity

Most of the side effects of flutamide and LH-RH analogues are related to the very low levels of testosterone they induce. For this reason, higher doses may not produce side effects that are significantly worse than with regular doses.

Interactions

The combination of flutamide with one of the LH-RH analogues produces a desired interaction in that flutamide prevents the full activity of androgens and the LH-RH analogues lower the production of androgens. The end result is an almost complete abolition of androgen action.

Estrogens

Mechanism of Action

Estrogens can interact with certain reproductive tissues, altering RNA and protein synthesis. This action is independent of the cell cycle. For androgen-dependent tissues, estrogens frequently interfere with androgen function. Estrogens can therefore cause involution of these tissues. This action forms the basis for the use of estrogens to control prostatic carcinoma. Some carcinomas of the breast also respond to exogenous estrogen therapy, especially in postmenopausal women.

Estramustine phosphate sodium combines estradiol with a nitrogen mustard. The rationale for the combination is that the drug will be most concentrated in estrogen-sensitive tissues, including tumors. In those tissues the anticancer effects of the estradiol and the nitrogen mustard may be focused. The toxicity of the drug is largely caused by the estrogen component because release of the active nitrogen mustard into blood is low.

Pharmacokinetics

Natural steroid estrogens are not absorbed orally, but several of the synthetic, nonsteroidal estrogens may be given successfully by this route (see Table 50-1). Estrogens are also available for IM or intravenous (IV) injection. Estrogens are metabolized by the liver. Patients with marked liver impairment may accumulate these compounds.

Estramustine is concentrated in the prostate gland because the drug binds to specific receptors. This concentration of the drug contributes to the tissue-specific action.

Uses

Of the many estrogen preparations available, three are recommended primarily for use in prostatic carcinoma (see Table 50-1). Many of the estrogens discussed in Chapter 64 may also be used in palliative therapy for prostatic carcinoma or carcinoma of the female breast. Estramustine is indicated only for prostatic carcinoma because of the cytotoxic component in the preparation.

Adverse Reactions and Contraindications

Estrogens increase the risks of thromboembolytic disease. Estrogens also increase salt and water retention, alter mood in some patients, decrease glucose tolerance, elevate calcium levels, produce nausea and vomiting, and cause breast tenderness and abdominal cramps. Of these reactions, thromboembolytic disease, hypercalcemia, and edema are the most threatening for cancer patients.

Toxicity

When estrogens are used at high doses in men with prostatic or breast carcinoma, the risk of heart attack, pulmonary embolism, and thrombophlebitis is increased.

Interactions

None of the estrogens should be used with other potentially hepatotoxic drugs because the risk of hepatotoxicity is increased. Cardiovascular side effects are more likely to occur in patients who smoke.

Antiestrogen: tamoxifen

Mechanism of Action

Tamoxifen is an **antiestrogen** that blocks estrogen binding at receptor sites in cells. This action prevents estrogens from supporting the growth of estrogen-dependent cells. Tamoxifen is therefore most useful in palliating symptoms of breast carcinoma in which estrogen dependence of the tumor has been established.

Pharmacokinetics

Tamoxifen is administered orally. The drug is extensively metabolized. Tamoxifen and its metabolites enter the blood slowly, with peak concentrations occurring 4 to 7 hours after an oral dose. However, the drug persists in blood for days as a result of its entry into enterohepatic circulation. Most of the drug is slowly eliminated from the body in feces. The kidney contributes little to the excretion of this drug. The full anticancer effect of tamoxifen takes months to develop.

Uses
Tamoxifen is indicated for breast carcinoma. Tamoxifen is more likely to benefit women whose tumors contain estrogen receptors.

Adverse Reactions and Contraindications
Tamoxifen may produce cancer and birth defects in animals. It is not known whether tamoxifen produces these effects in humans. The drug seems less toxic than the estrogens and androgens used in anticancer therapy. It may occasionally alter platelet or white blood cell (WBC) counts, but the changes observed are mild and usually innocuous. The most frequent reactions are nausea, vomiting, and hot flashes. Fewer patients report vaginal bleeding or menstrual irregularities. These reactions do not usually require discontinuance of the drug.

Patients who begin tamoxifen therapy sometimes report an increase in pain at the tumor site and within metastases in bone. Tumor metastases within soft tissue may temporarily increase in size, and the surrounding tissue may become inflamed. This reaction, sometimes referred to as *disease flare,* may occur even when therapy is effective.

Toxicity
Side effects may become more severe with higher doses of the drug.

Interactions
Interactions are generally of minor importance. Antacids or histamine H_2 receptor blockers may disrupt the enteric coating on tamoxifen tablets, leading to loss of some tamoxifen activity. Estrogens may antagonize the effect of tamoxifen.

Progestins
Mechanism of Action
Progestins normally establish secretory function in the estrogen-primed endometrium (Chapter 64). When used as anticancer agents, progestins may be effective by blocking tissue reponses to other steroid hormones such as estrogens, androgens, or glucocorticoids.

Pharmacokinetics
Progestins are available in various forms suitable for oral or IM administration. The drugs are metabolized primarily in the liver; derivatives of progestins appear in urine.

Uses
The use of progestins as antineoplastic agents has been limited primarily to palliative therapy in endometrial carcinoma, but renal and breast carcinomas may also be susceptible (see Table 50-1).

Adverse Reactions and Contraindications
Progestins usually produce few reactions. Patients should be observed for signs of thromboembolytic disease or sudden changes in vision. Fluid retention and disruption of normal menstrual cycles may also occur. Progestins that are injected may cause pain and tissue changes at the injection site.

Toxicity
High doses of progestins are associated with greater risk of thromboembolism.

Interactions
Drugs such as carbamazepine, phenobarbital, phenytoin, rifabutin, or rifampin induce liver enzymes that metabolize progestins. As a result, these drugs may interfere with the action of progestins.

Glucocorticoids: prednisone
Glucocorticoids are steroid hormones that regulate RNA and protein synthesis in various cells. This action is independent of cell cycle. Prednisone is the glucocorticoid most commonly used as an anticancer agent, although several of these agents are used for symptomatic relief. Prednisone is an effective anticancer agent because it causes regression of lymphoid tissue (Chapter 36). Prednisone is therefore effective against lymphoid tumors and lymphoblastic leukemias, especially in children.

Prednisone is effectively absorbed orally and is metabolized to the active form of the drug, prednisolone. Liver disease may impair this process and thus interfere with the effectiveness of prednisone.

Prednisone may produce all the well-known signs of glucocorticoid excess if given long enough at high doses. These symptoms are outlined in Chapter 36.

Adrenal Antagonists
Mitotane
Mechanism of Action
Mitotane is a derivative of the insecticide DDT. Toxicity studies with DDT showed specific effects on the adrenal cortex. Mitotane causes specific atrophy of the zona fasciculata and reticularis, the two inner layers of the adrenal cortex where the glucocorticoid cortisol is formed. Mitotane is not cell cycle specific and is not a general cytotoxic agent.

Pharmacokinetics
Mitotane is satisfactorily absorbed when given orally. The drug is metabolized by the liver before excretion. If liver function is impaired, the drug may accumulate, and toxic reactions may increase.

Uses
Because of its unusual tissue selectivity, mitotane is used to treat adrenal cortical carcinoma.

Adverse Reactions and Contraindications
Mitotane causes anorexia, nausea, and vomiting in almost every patient. Nearly half those treated experience lethargy or dizziness as a result of adrenal insufficiency. Dermatitis occurs in 20% of patients. Less frequent but serious reactions include abnormalities of the eye, changes in blood pressure, and hemorrhagic cystitis.

Toxicity
Higher doses are associated with more severe side effects.

Interactions
Central nervous system (CNS) depressants are usually avoided when patients receive mitotane to prevent excessive depression of CNS function.

Trilostane
Mechanism of Action
Trilostane is a competitive inhibitor of enzymes involved in adrenal steroid synthesis. It blocks cortisol synthesis in the zona fasciculata, aldosterone synthesis in the zona glomerulosa, and androstenedione synthesis in the zona reticularis (Chapter 60).

Pharmacokinetics
Trilostane is absorbed after oral administration and is biotransformed by the liver.

Uses
The primary use of trilostane is in Cushing's syndrome, but the drug can also be used in various carcinomas, including breast carcinoma.

Adverse Reactions and Contraindications
Trilostane produces signs of adrenocortical insufficiency, which may include darkening of the skin, fatigue, loss of appetite, and vomiting. These symptoms require medical attention. Diarrhea and stomach pains are also common but are usually not severe.

Toxicity
High doses may produce excessive adrenal suppression.

Interactions
Trilostane should not be used with mitotane to avoid profound adrenal suppression.

Pancreatic Beta-Cell Antagonist
Streptozocin
Mechanism of Action
Streptozocin is a specific toxin for the beta-cells of the pancreatic islets. Although streptozocin resembles alkylating agents, cells other than pancreatic beta-cells are relatively insensitive to the drug.

Pharmacokinetics
Streptozocin is unstable and must be given intravenously. It is biotransformed by the liver. Both metabolites and unchanged drug are excreted in urine.

Uses
Because of its strong tissue specificity, streptozocin is primarily used to treat insulin-secreting islet cell tumors of the pancreas.

Adverse Reactions and Contraindications
Streptozocin can destroy beta-cells. Therefore insulin production may cease. The drug is also toxic to the kidneys. Streptozocin does not ordinarily affect blood-forming cells, so blood dyscrasias are rarely encountered. Nausea and vomiting occur often.

Toxicity
Renal toxicity is dose related. At high doses renal function can be fatally compromised.

Interactions
Streptozocin should not be combined with other nephrotoxic drugs. Live virus vaccines may cause a generalized disease if used in a patient receiving streptozocin. Phenytoin may interfere with the action of streptozocin in pancreatic cells.

Interferons
Interferon alfa-2a, alfa-2b, alfa-n1, and alfa-n3
Mechanism of Action
Natural interferons are produced mainly by leukocytes and serve as part of the body's defense system. Interferons modulate the function of macrophages and lymphocytes and generally impede proliferation. Recombinant interferons share these properties. Recombinant interferons are produced by genetic engineering, which uses microorganisms to produce human proteins. Nonrecombinant interferons are produced from cultures of human cells after stimulating interferon production with *Sendai* virus. The anticancer activity of the interferons is not completely understood.

Pharmacokinetics
As proteins, these interferons cannot be administered orally. Absorption is adequate from IM or subcutaneous sites, producing peak serum concentration in 4 to 7 hours. These proteins are completely metabolized in the kidney and other tissues.

Uses
The recombinant interferons, interferon alfa-2a and interferon alfa-2b, are used in hairy cell leukemia, genital warts, and Kaposi's sarcoma in AIDS patients. In addition, these drugs are being investigated for their activity in various lymphomas, leukemias, and solid tumors. Interferons alfa-n1 and alfa-n3 in general have the same uses, but not all interferons have been approved for all indications listed.

Adverse Reactions and Contraindications
A flulike syndrome develops in most patients but resolves within 2 to 4 weeks, even when the drug is continued. Signs of neurotoxicity may involve the CNS (depression, nervousness,

and insomnia) or the periphery (numbness or tingling in extremities). Loss of appetite builds during treatment with alfa-interferons and may persist for some time after therapy ends. Diarrhea, nausea, vomiting, skin rash, and unusual tiredness are common side effects when interferons are used as anticancer agents.

Toxicity

The flulike syndrome is not dose related, but neurotoxicity, GI tract toxicity, and cardiovascular toxicity are worse at higher doses.

Interactions

Interactions are usually unimportant with interferons, but the action of CNS depressants or bone marrow depressants may be enhanced by interferons.

NURSING PROCESS OVERVIEW

Tissue-Specific Anticancer Agents

Assessment

Perform a complete physical assessment. Monitor vital signs and blood pressure. Obtain a history of the problem being treated.

Nursing Diagnoses

- Activity intolerance related to excessive fatigue caused by interferons
- Pain at tumor site(s) related to drug therapy

Patient Outcomes

The patient will identify measures to reduce activity tolerance and/or set priorities for activities that must be completed each day. The patient will state relief of pain at tumor sites.

Planning/Implementation

The drugs in this chapter vary widely. Monitor vital signs. Monitor the patient receiving interferons for severe and continuing flulike symptoms. Monitor the patient receiving steroid drugs for weight gain, skin changes, and depression. Instruct the patient needing to administer drugs via injection form how to administer the prescribed drugs and dispose of contaminated needles and syringes. Encourage the patient to return for regular follow-up to monitor for drug effectiveness and the development of side effects. See the general guidelines in the Nursing Implications Summary in Chapter 49 for additional suggestions.

Evaluation

Continue to monitor for expected effects and side effects. Before discharge, verify that the patient can administer the prescribed drugs as needed. Verify that the patient can list side effects and symptoms that would indicate a need to call the physician.

NURSING IMPLICATIONS SUMMARY

STEROIDS AND RELATED AGENTS

Androgens

- Androgens are discussed in Chapter 66.

Flutamide and LH-RH Analogues

Drug Administration

- See the general guidelines in Chapter 49 (p. 599) for information about anorexia, nausea and vomiting, and diarrhea.
- Consult the manufacturer's literature for current information.
- Assess for tingling of face, fingers, and toes. Assess for numbness and tingling of hands or feet, difficulty urinating, or weakness in legs.
- Monitor pulse, blood pressure, and weight. Inspect for edema. Monitor intake and output. Auscultate lung sounds.
- Allergic reactions have been reported. Ensure that the patient remains in the health care setting for at least 15 minutes after doses. Have drugs, equipment, and personnel available to treat an acute allergic reaction.
- Monitor hematocrit, hemoglobin, serum creatinine, blood urea nitrogen (BUN), and liver function tests.

Patient and Family Education

- Review the anticipated benefits and possible side effects of drug therapy with the patient.
- When flutamide and an LH-RH analogue are prescribed, emphasize the importance of taking both medications for best effect.
- Assess tactfully for impotence and decreased libido since the patient may not wish to discuss them. Provide emotional support as appropriate. Remind the patient not to discontinue medications without consulting the physician. Reinforce to the patient the importance of taking medications as prescribed for best effect.
- Warn the patient that hot flashes may occur as a side effect to the LH-RH analogue; provide support as possible.
- Warn the patient to avoid driving or operating hazardous equipment if dizziness, blurred vision, lethargy, or memory disorders occur and to notify the physician.
- Warn the patient to notify the physician if severe or persistent bone pain develops.
- Buserelin (an LH-RH analogue) is also available as a nasal spray; review with the patient the instruction sheet provided.

NURSING IMPLICATIONS SUMMARY—cont'd

- Goserelin is a subcutaneous implant inserted by the physician.
- Leuprolide is administered via IM injection. Review the instruction leaflet with the patient and instruct the patient in injection technique. This drug is also used to treat endometriosis; see Chapter 64.

Estrogens

- Estrogens are discussed in Chapter 64.

Tamoxifen

Drug Administration

- See the general guidelines in Chapter 49 (p. 599) for information about depressed WBC count, thrombocytopenia, nausea and vomiting, and anorexia.
- Assess for depression including withdrawal, change in affect, lack of interest in personal appearance, insomnia, and anorexia.
- Assess mental status and neurologic function.
- Assess for hypercalcemia; see Table 17-1 for a description of common electrolyte abnormalities.
- Monitor weight; assess for edema. Assess visual acuity.

Patient and Family Education

- Review the anticipated benefits and possible side effects of drug therapy with the patient.
- Warn the patient to avoid driving or operating hazardous equipment if confusion, dizziness, lassitude, or light-headedness develops and to notify the physician.
- Instruct the patient to increase fluid intake to 2500 to 3000 ml/day to foster calcium excretion and to help prevent constipation.
- Instruct the patient taking the enteric-coated form and an antacid to allow at least 2 hours to elapse between doses of antacid and tamoxifen.
- Warn the patient that hot flashes are common; provide support as appropriate.
- This drug may cause transient local disease flare, resulting in a temporary increase in bone pain or increase in size of any existing lesions. A flare is temporary; but if it is severe or persistent, instruct the patient to notify the physician.
- Instruct a female patient to use birth control measures, although not birth control pills containing estrogen.

Glucocorticoids and Progestins

- Glucocorticoids are discussed in Chapter 36.
- Progestins are discussed in Chapter 64.

ADRENAL ANTAGONISTS

Mitotane

Drug Administration

- See the general guidelines in Chapter 49 (p. 599) for information about anemia, anorexia, diarrhea, nausea, and vomiting.
- Assess for depression including anorexia, insomnia, lack of interest in personal appearance, and withdrawal.
- Monitor blood pressure and pulse. Inspect for skin changes.
- Monitor the 8 AM plasma cortisol levels or 24-hour urinary 17-hydroxycorticosteroids.

Patient and Family Education

- Review the anticipated benefits and possible side effects of drug therapy with the patient.
- Warn the patient to avoid driving or operating hazardous equipment if confusion, somnolence, dizziness, fatigue, or other CNS side effects develop and to notify the physician.
- Warn the patient to avoid the use of alcohol or other CNS depressants, including antihistamines, sedatives, sleeping medications, narcotics or prescription drugs for pain, muscle relaxants, and other drugs, unless first discussed with the physician.
- Instruct the patient to wear a medical identification tag or bracelet listing medications in use. In the event of trauma or other injury, it is necessary to administer glucocorticoids.
- Instruct the patient to contact the physician if sickness or infection develops or an injury occurs since glucocorticoids may be necessary.

Trilostane

Drug Administration

- See the general guidelines in Chapter 49 (p. 599) for information about nausea and vomiting and diarrhea.
- Assess for electrolyte abnormalities, including hypercalcemia and hyperkalemia. See Table 17-1 for a description of common electrolyte abnormalities.
- Assess for signs of possible adrenocortical insufficiency such as darkening of the skin, fatigue, loss of appetite, vomiting, depression, and hypotension. Monitor serum cortisol level. Monitor blood pressure.
- Inspect for skin changes.
- Monitor 8 AM plasma cortisol level, serum electrolyte level, 24-hour urinary 17-hydroxycorticosteroid levels, and liver function tests.

Patient and Family Education

- Review the anticipated benefits and possible side effects of drug therapy with the patient.
- Instruct the patient taking trilostane to wear a medical identification tag or bracelet listing medications in use. In the event of trauma or other injury, it would be necessary to administer glucocorticoids. Instruct the patient to keep all health care providers informed of medications in use.
- Instruct the patient to contact the physician if sickness, infection, or injury occurs since glucocorticoids may be necessary.

Continued.

Nursing Implications Summary—cont'd

- Emphasize the importance of regular follow-up to monitor for side effects and drug effectiveness.

PANCREATIC BETA-CELL ANTAGONIST

Streptozocin

Drug Administration

- See the general guidelines in Chapter 49 (p. 599) for information about anemia, extravasation, and nausea and vomiting. See the patient problem boxes on leukopenia (p. 585) and bleeding tendencies (thrombocytopenia) (p. 586).
- Monitor intake and output and weight.
- Monitor complete blood count (CBC), differential, platelet count, serum creatinine level, BUN level, serum electrolyte level, liver function tests, and blood glucose level.

Patient and Family Education

- Review the anticipated benefits and possible side effects of drug therapy with the patient.
- Encourage the patient to increase fluid intake to 2500 ml/day.
- Inform a diabetic patient that streptozocin may alter glucose levels. Instruct the patient to monitor blood glucose, and adjust diet or insulin as necessary.

INTERFERONS

Drug Administration

- Assess for numbness or tingling of fingers, toes or face. Flulike symptoms are common following doses. Assess for aching muscles, fever and chills, headache, joint pain, back pain.
- Assess for nausea, vomiting, and diarrhea. Monitor weight.
- Monitor vital signs and blood pressure. Monitor periodic electrocardiographic (ECG) changes.
- Monitor CBC, WBC differential, platelet count, and liver function tests.

Patient and Family Education

- Teach injection technique if the patient is to self-administer at home. See the patient instruction leaflet supplied by manufacturer.
- Encourage the patient to increase daily intake of fluids if directed by the physician.
- Instruct the patient not to change brands of interferon unless directed to do so by the physician.
- Instruct the patient to avoid other drugs that may depress the CNS while taking interferons. Drugs to avoid include alcohol, antihistamines, prescription drugs for pain, tranquilizers, sleeping pills, sedatives, muscle relaxants, and barbiturates. Instruct the patient to keep all health care providers informed of all drugs being used, including over-the-counter drugs.
- Caution the patient to avoid driving or operating hazardous equipment if drowsiness, unusual fatigue, or confusion develop.
- This drug may cause flulike symptoms. Some physicians recommend that the patient take a dose of acetaminophen before receiving interferons and afterward if the patient develops a fever. Check with the physician and review instructions with the patient.
- See the patient problem boxes on leukopenia (p. 585), bleeding tendencies (thrombocytopenia) (p. 586), stomatitis (p. 587), and dry mouth (p. 300). See the general guidelines in Chapter 49 (p. 599) for information about alopecia, which may affect some patients.

CRITICAL THINKING

APPLICATION

1. What is the basis for the anticancer effects of androgens?
2. Why is testolactone the preferred androgen for use in cancer chemotherapy?
3. Why is suppression of androgen action useful for cancer chemotherapy?
4. What is the mechanism of action of flutamide?
5. Buserelin, goserelin, and leuprolide are analogues of what natural peptide?
6. What is the effect of continuous administration of LH-RH analogues?
7. Why are flutamide and an LH-RH analogue used in combination?
8. What is the cause of most side effects seen with the combination of flutamide and an LH-RH analogue?
9. What is the basis for the anticancer effects of estrogens?
10. Why is estramustine used only for cancer and not for estrogen replacement?
11. What is the mechanism of action of tamoxifen?
12. What is the basis for the anticancer effects of glucocorticoids?
13. Mitotane and trilostane are effective against what specific type of cancer?
14. Streptozocin is a specific toxin for what kind of cells?
15. What is the role of natural interferons?

CRITICAL THINKING

1. What side effects of progestins are especially dangerous? How would you assess for these?
2. What side effects are most dangerous with streptozocin? How would you assess for these?
3. A patient receiving an interferon for hairy cell leukemia confides to you that he is experiencing tingling in his hands and feet. Is this important information? Why? What should you do?

Section XII

Drugs for the Psychoneurologic System

This section presents drugs that affect behavior. Chapter 51 includes drugs used to treat insomnia and anxiety. Benzodiazepines are the major class of drugs used because of their favorable therapeutic index and low abuse potential. Barbiturates are less commonly used today, but they remain an important example of how chemical structure determines drug disposition and tolerance. Other sedative-hypnotic, antianxiety drugs are not presented in detail. A major emphasis is the dependency potential of the drugs and their cross-tolerance. Alcohol is presented in detail because of these factors. The importance of alcohol as a source of drug interactions and abuse is noted.

Chapter 52 presents antipsychotic drugs, with emphasis on the antagonism of the central neurotransmitters dopamine, norepinephrine, and acetylcholine in explaining the various effects of these drugs. Chapter 53 presents the major classes of antidepressant drugs: the tricyclic and heterocyclic antidepressants, the selective serotonin reuptake inhibitors and the monoamine oxidase inhibitors, and lithium. The role of these drugs in improving the neurotransmitter functions of norepinephrine and serotonin in the central nervous system is emphasized. Chapter 54 concentrates on the therapeutic roles of central nervous system stimulants in treating narcolepsy, hyperactivity, and obesity and in improving deficient respiratory drive. The abuse of amphetamine, cocaine, and caffeine is also presented.

CHAPTER 51

Sedative-Hypnotic Agents, Antianxiety Agents, and Alcohol

OBJECTIVES

After studying this chapter, you should be able to do the following:

- *Discuss central nervous system depression, drug dependence and central nervous system depression, and the stages of sleep.*
- *Differentiate among sedatives, hypnotics, and antianxiety agents.*
- *Develop a nursing care plan for patients receiving benzodiazepines, barbiturates, or miscellaneous hypnotics or antianxiety agents.*
- *Describe the effects of alcohol ingestion on the body.*
- *Develop a teaching plan for the patient receiving disulfiram or a drug that may produce a disulfiram-like reaction when alcohol is ingested.*

KEY TERMS

anxiety
barbiturates
benzodiazepines
cross-tolerance
delirium tremens
drug addiction
drug dependency
fetal alcohol syndrome
hypnotic
insomnia
rapid eye movement (REM) sleep
reticular activating system
sedative

CHAPTER OVERVIEW

Sedative-hypnotic drugs and antianxiety drugs are considered together because they are not different so much in their clinical action as in their historic origin. The term *sedative-hypnotic* is reserved for older drug classes, primarily barbiturates. Barbiturates are a class of chemically related drugs developed in the early 1900s, effective as sedatives and as hypnotics. A small dose to calm an anxious patient is called a **sedative.** A larger dose sufficient to induce sleep is a **hypnotic.**

After the 1950s, drugs were developed specifically as hypnotics. Other drugs were developed as sedatives to treat anxiety. The benzodiazepines are the drug class most used today to treat anxiety. These drugs are referred to as *antianxiety drugs.* The older term was *minor tranquilizer.*

An additional drug appropriate to this chapter is alcohol because it has the pharmacologic actions characteristic of a sedative-hypnotic or an antianxiety drug. The social use of alcohol is mainly as a self-prescribed antianxiety agent. Alcohol, when recognized as a drug, is viewed as a major source of drug abuse and dependence.

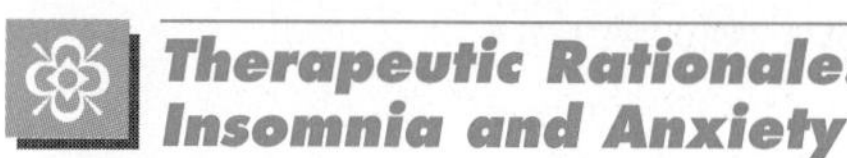

Therapeutic Rationale: Insomnia and Anxiety

Effects Produced by Depression of the Central Nervous System

Reticular Activating System

The effects of a single dose of a sedative-hypnotic drug, an antianxiety drug, or alcohol are very similar. All these drugs act pharmacologically as general depressants of the central nervous system (CNS), since they depress the reticular activating system of the brainstem. The **reticular activating system** refers to neural pathways in which incoming signals from the senses (sight, sound, smell, touch, taste, and balance) and viscera are collected, processed, and passed on to the higher brain centers (Figure 51-1). Higher brain centers also have neural pathways to the reticular activating system to modulate activity. This system determines the level of awareness of the environment and therefore governs reactions to it.

Stages of Depression

Depression of the reticular activating system by a general CNS depressant accounts for the behavioral changes seen in a person who has taken one of these drugs. The degree of depression depends on the amount of drug taken. At a low dose, sedation is produced, characterized by decreased physical and mental responses to stimuli. With an increased dose, disinhibition is the next level of depression reached. Disinhibition falsely appears as a stimulated state of awareness. This is because neurons inhibiting arousal become depressed. The result of disinhibition may be euphoria, excitement, drunkenness, loss of self-control, and impaired judgment. Relief of anxiety produced by a general CNS depressant results from sedation or disinhibition. Loss of motor coordination (ataxia) and involuntary eye movements (nystagmus) are frequently seen at this level of depression and are clues when drug use is suspected. Pain can intensify disinhibition and can result in paradoxical excitement in postoperative patients who are given a sedative-hypnotic or an antianxiety drug. Increasing the drug dose further produces sleep (hypnosis). Anesthesia, the loss of feeling or sensation, is achieved at high doses of a general CNS depressant drug.

The effect of a single dose of a sedative-hypnotic drug, an antianxiety drug, or alcohol therefore depends on the dose taken. In practice, not much distinction can be made in the sedative vs. hypnotic dose for drugs used primarily as hypnotics. Similarly, drugs most popular as sedative or antianxiety drugs are those that produce minimal sleepiness at an effective dose.

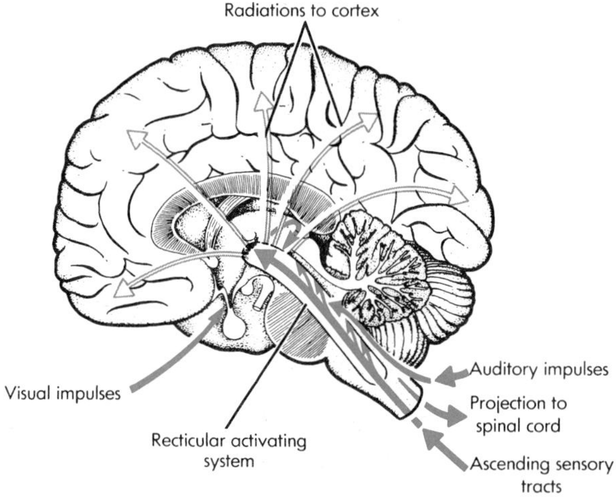

FIGURE 51-1
Awareness is a function of reticular activating system. Diagram illustrates reticular activating system as integration network. General CNS depressants act on reticular activating system, although mechanisms are not understood.

Drug Dependence

Origin

Continued administration of a general CNS depressant drug can cause drug dependence. Drug dependence means that the body has adjusted to the continual CNS depression so that it now requires the presence of the drug to function. If administration is discontinued abruptly, the body experiences withdrawal symptoms. The symptoms of withdrawal from a general CNS depressant drug reflect CNS hyperactivity. Mild withdrawal symptoms include agitation, tremulousness, and insomnia, whereas the major withdrawal symptom is convulsions, a life-threatening emergency. The symptoms disappear when the drug is retaken.

Doses That Produce Dependence

It is not possible to state simply what dose produces drug dependence because great variation exists among individuals. In broad terms, general CNS depressant drugs can produce drug dependence when taken at twice their prescribed doses for 2 to 8 weeks. The dependence potential varies among the drug classes somewhat, as is discussed more fully for each class. A thought-provoking observation is that each new sedative-hypnotic and antianxiety drug has been introduced with the conviction that it was not addicting, but no general CNS depressant drug has turned out to be nonaddictive. The benzodiazepines, a class of drugs accounting for at least 15% of all prescriptions written in the United States, have only recently been widely recognized as capable of producing drug dependence. Now major questions are being raised about drug dependence with benzodiazepines.

Development of Drug Abuse

The time required for drug dependence to develop depends on the drug dose. Long-term use of low doses does not necessarily lead to drug dependence. Many people take low doses of barbiturates to control epilepsy and do not experience withdrawal symptoms if their medication is changed. Moderate alcohol consumption, even on a daily basis, does not necessarily lead to alcohol dependence. However, tolerance does develop to the sedative and euphoric effects of general CNS depressants. People abuse a drug when their reaction to this tolerance is to increase the amount of drug taken. As the drug dose increases, a point is reached at which failure to take the drug produces withdrawal symptoms. At this point, drug use may be continued as much to avoid withdrawal symptoms as to produce drug effects. This stage is referred to as **drug dependency** or **drug addiction.** The individual's life may become centered around the drug, and personal, family, and social interactions become less important.

Drug addiction cannot be explained merely by drug tolerance and physical dependence. In general, physical dependence can be overcome by decreasing the drug intake by 10% of the initial dose daily for 10 days. This gradual reduction prevents withdrawal symptoms from becoming severe. However, many patients revert to drug abuse after they have been withdrawn from drug dependence. Drug addiction therefore involves social and psychologic factors that underlie drug abuse.

Cross-Tolerance

Tolerance to any sedative-hypnotic drug, antianxiety drug, or alcohol results in tolerance to any other of these general CNS depressants. This property is called **cross-tolerance** and is a major factor in drug abuse. The most common pattern of drug abuse is alcohol in combination with one or more sedative-hypnotic or antianxiety drugs. This combination works in an addictive fashion. One way an individual can avoid taking more of the same drug to overcome tolerance is by adding a second drug, usually alcohol. This can be lethal. Although someone drinking enough to die from alcohol alone is relatively uncommon, this becomes possible when another drug such as a sedative-hypnotic or an antianxiety drug is added. Moreover, because of cross-tolerance, a dose that would not lead to drug dependence by itself contributes to drug dependence when added to a second depressant.

Sleep and Hypnotic Drugs

Stages of Sleep

What determines sleep is not well understood. Current sleep research makes use of the brain wave patterns and eye movements recorded during sleep, as shown in Figure 51-2. Four stages of sleep are defined by brain wave patterns. Stage 1 represents the lightest level of sleep, accompanied by muscle relaxation and slowing of the heart rate (bradycardia). Stage 4 represents the deepest level of sleep, accompanied by marked muscle relaxation and bradycardia. During most of the sleep cycle the eye movements are not noticed under closed eyelids. However, during about 20% of the average adult sleep time the eyeballs move rapidly back and forth under the closed eyelids. This is called **rapid eye movement (REM) sleep** and is superimposed on stage 1 or stage 2 sleep. The body is physiologically active during REM sleep so that the heart rate is increased, breathing is irregular, stomach acid is secreted, and the clitoris or penis becomes erect. Muscles lose their tone during REM sleep, however, so that only the mind and autonomic nervous system are active during this stage. Since dreaming occurs exclusively during REM sleep, this time is also called *dreaming sleep.* Many authorities believe that during REM sleep is when we integrate emotionally meaningful experiences.

Sleep Cycles

As indicated in Figure 51-2, an individual normally cycles from stage 1 through stage 4 back to stage 1 about every 90 minutes. Deep sleep (stages 3 and 4) occupies more of the early sleep cycles, whereas dreaming occupies more of the late sleep cycles. Children spend more total time in deep sleep than adults, whereas the older adult may spend little time in deep sleep. With increasing age, it becomes more common to

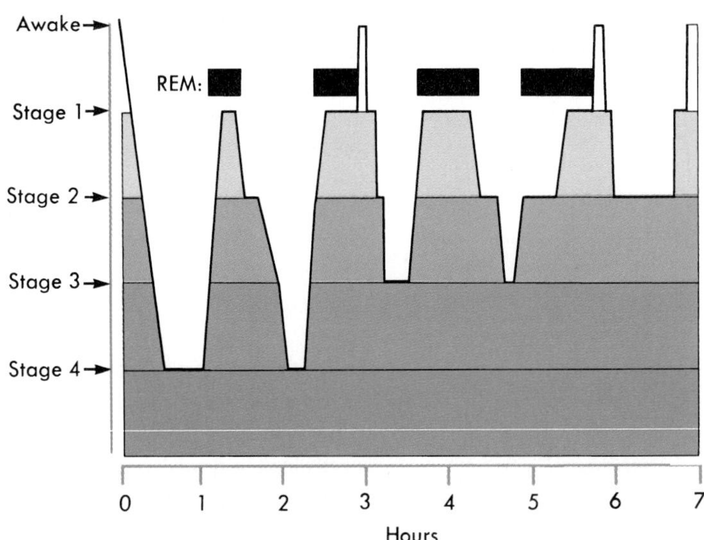

FIGURE 51-2
Normal sleep pattern. Sleep is cyclical. Deep sleep is more frequent during early than later cycles. Dreaming occurs during REM sleep and is associated with stage 1 and stage 2 sleep. Pattern shown is characteristic for adults. Children and older adults often awaken more frequently. Most hypnotics depress REM sleep.

awaken at the end of a sleep cycle, particularly the early morning cycles.

Insomnia

Insomnia, the inability to sleep, is the most common sleep complaint and can be characterized as either difficulty in getting to sleep or in waking up and being unable to get back to sleep. Insomnia is not a disease but a symptom of physical or mental distress. Several conditions in which insomnia is prominent are listed in Table 51-1.

Action of Hypnotic Drugs

Hypnotic drugs are taken to fall asleep faster or to sleep longer. Studies in sleep laboratories show that most hypnotic drugs suppress REM sleep. When the drug is discontinued, even after a single dose, there is a rebound in REM sleep with vivid dreams and increased awakening. Furthermore, after 3 weeks of continuous therapy, most hypnotic drugs are no longer effective in decreasing the time needed to fall asleep or the duration of sleep. Nevertheless, if the patient now discontinues the drug, worse insomnia and associated anxiety will be experienced because of the REM rebound. This reaction may lead the uninstructed patient to continue the drug, perhaps at an increased dose, to regain the hypnotic effect. This is the beginning of drug abuse with hypnotic drugs. Since hypnotic drugs can make insomnia worse rather than better, the cause of insomnia rather than the insomnia should be discovered and treated. Alcohol and antianxiety drugs can interfere with sleep patterns in a similar fashion if taken in large enough doses.

Anxiety and Drug Therapy

Anxiety

Anxiety means different things to different people. Many symptoms are associated with anxiety. These are listed in Table 51-2. An anxious individual will have some, but not all, of these physical symptoms. **Anxiety** may be generalized, in which the individual is unaware of a specific cause of anxiety and may even deny anxiety, or it may be anticipatory, in which the individual is well aware of its origin.

Specific types of anxiety states have also been identified. Phobic disorders are characterized by irrational fear of objects, activities, or situations and by the compelling desire to avoid them. Obsessive-compulsive disorder is characterized by persistent obsessive ideas, thoughts, or images or by compulsive behavior. Posttraumatic stress disorder follows a unique and psychologically traumatic experience.

Action of Antianxiety Drugs

The pharmacologic action of sedatives or antianxiety agents may be to decrease the general level of arousal by inhibiting the reticular activating system of the brainstem. This is not a cure for anxiety, although the response is blunted. Rather, authorities agree that drug therapy for anxiety should be limited to a few weeks, and psychotherapy or behavior modification therapy deals directly with the origin of the patient's anxiety. In part, this recommendation is based on tolerance to these drugs developing after a few weeks so that effective therapy requires larger doses, the first step in drug abuse. Patients taking sedative or antianxiety drugs should be told that drug therapy offers only limited relief.

Information about the regulation of anxiety is becoming more sophisticated. Current research suggests that reduction of anxiety can be achieved without sedation. In addition to the reticular activating system, two other integrating systems control anxiety, the limbic system and the hypothalamus. Although the reticular activating system allows information to enter the brain, the limbic system adds emotion and mediates a sequence of outgoing messages. The hypothalamus integrates the neuroendocrine response to stress, controlling the output of several hormones (see Chapter 58). The goal of current drug research is to identify drugs that affect anxiety without producing sedation. These drugs may act selectively in the limbic system.

TABLE 51-1 Conditions Characterized by Insomnia

CONDITION	CHARACTERISTIC TYPE OF INSOMNIA
Depression	Early morning insomnia is common
Chronic alcoholism	REM sleep and deep sleep are reduced.
Hyperthyroidism	Deep sleep is reduced.
Heart failure	Insomnia is an early complaint.
Pregnancy	Insomnia is common during the last trimester.
Renal insufficiency	
Many neurologic disorders	

TABLE 51-2 Symptoms of Anxiety

APPEARANCE	COMPLAINTS
Excessively alert Easily startled Constantly in motion or inhibited in motion	Cardiorespiratory: heart palpitations, fast heart rate, and breathlessness Gastrointestinal: abdominal cramps, nausea, vomiting, and diarrhea
Excessive and disjointed speech	
Eyes constantly scanning, "fussy" dress	Musculoskeletal: tension headaches, chest pain or tightness, and backache
Tremors, restlessness	General: fatigue, weakness, and insomnia
Dilated pupils	

Therapeutic Agents for Insomnia and Anxiety: Benzodiazepines

Drugs prescribed for insomnia and anxiety are presented in three sections. The first section discusses **benzodiazepines,** the most popular drug class today for treating insomnia and anxiety. The second section presents barbiturates, an older class of drugs used as CNS depressants, from sedation to anesthesia. The third section discusses miscellaneous drugs occasionally prescribed for insomnia or anxiety.

Benzodiazepines: General Characteristics

Mechanism of Action

Specific receptors for the benzodiazepines have been identified in the cerebral cortex and limbic system. Since the limbic system is a major integrating system governing emotional behavior associated with self-preservation, the presence of receptors for benzodiazepines in this system may account for their antianxiety action. Benzodiazepines increase the action of the inhibitory neurotransmitter, gamma-aminobutyric acid (GABA). Benzodiazepines and barbiturates help GABA open a chloride channel in the postsynaptic membrane of many neurons, which reduces the neuron's excitability.

Pharmacokinetics

The benzodiazepines are readily absorbed after oral administration. Only lorazepam is rapidly and completely absorbed after intramuscular (IM) injection. Chlordiazepoxide and diazepam may be administered by IV or IM routes, but chlordiazepoxide is not reliably absorbed after IM administration. Benzodiazepines are highly lipid soluble and therefore are widely distributed in body tissues. They are also highly bound to plasma protein, usually greater than 80%. No drug interactions have been described for protein binding. Protein binding, however, is reduced in patients with cirrhosis and renal insufficiency and in newborns, and these patients often have impaired metabolism of benzodiazepines as well, making a reduction in dosage important.

The benzodiazepines are metabolized by the liver. Several benzodiazepines have active metabolites. *N*-desmethylated metabolites are active and have a longer duration of action than the parent compound. Lorazepam, oxazepam, temazepam, and triazolam do not have active metabolites to prolong their duration of action. These drugs are preferred for older adult patients and for patients with liver disease. Alprazolam is metabolized to weakly active compounds that are eliminated rapidly. The anticonvulsant clonazepam has only weakly active metabolites.

Uses

Benzodiazepines were introduced clinically in the 1960s as antianxiety drugs. By the early 1970s, diazepam (Valium) was the most widely prescribed drug in the United States. The popularity of the benzodiazepines is due in part to their high therapeutic index. Overdoses of 1000 times the therapeutic dose have been reported not to result in death. At therapeutic doses, side effects beyond drowsiness and ataxia are uncommon. No drug interactions are prominent beyond the addictive effect with other CNS depressant drugs.

Benzodiazepines have anxiety reducing (anxiolytic), sedative-hypnotic, muscle relaxing, and anticonvulsant actions. All benzodiazepines are Schedule IV drugs.

Estazolam (ProSom), flurazepam (Dalmane), lorazepam (Ativan), quazepam (Doral), temazepam (Resotril), and triazolam (Halcion) are prescribed primarily as hypnotics. Clonazepam (Klonopin), clorazepate (Tranxene), and diazepam (Valium) have use as anticonvulsants. Diazepam (Valium) is prescribed as a muscle relaxant. Alprazolam (Xanax), chlordiazepoxide (Librium), clorazepate (Tranxene), diazepam (Valium), halazepam (Paxipam), lorazepam (Ativan), oxazepam (Serax), and prazepam (Centrax) are widely prescribed as antianxiety drugs.

Adverse Reactions and Contraindications

Side effects common with benzodiazepines include daytime sedation, ataxia, dizziness, and headaches. Tolerance commonly develops quickly to these side effects. The older adult is more likely to experience these side effects to a disabling degree. Moreover, they do not readily metabolize benzodiazepines, so the drug persists two to three times longer. For these reasons the drug dose is reduced for older adult patients and for patients who have impaired liver function. However, older adult patients are at risk for falling and injuring themselves while taking these drugs for sleep or anxiety. Less common side effects of benzodiazepines include blurred or double vision, hypotension, tremor, amnesia, slurred speech, urinary incontinence, and constipation.

Patients older than 50 years of age with a history of psychosis are the most likely to develop paradoxical excitement or aggression. Benzodiazepines may worsen glaucoma. Benzodiazepines are contraindicated for women in labor and for nursing mothers because of adverse depression of the infant. An increased incidence of cleft lip has been reported among infants whose mothers took diazepam (Valium) during early pregnancy. In general, benzodiazepines are associated with an increased incidence of congenital abnormalities in children whose mothers used the drugs during pregnancy. Benzodiazepines are distributed into breast milk. Infants do not readily metabolize these drugs and can become lethargic, so benzodiazepines are not recommended for nursing mothers.

Acute Toxicity

An acute overdose of benzodiazepines alone is seldom fatal. Patients frequently regain consciousness and normal vital signs with a large concentration of drug still in their bodies. A benzodiazepine antagonist, flumazenil (Mazicon) is available to reverse symptoms of benzodiazepine overdose.

Abuse Potential and Withdrawal

Benzodiazepines are schedule IV drugs since their abuse potential is considered low. Daily use of 30 mg of diazepam in the absence of alcohol or other depressant drugs for 3 months seldom produces dependence. Although tolerance to sedation and ataxia develops rapidly, tolerance to the antianxiety effect develops slowly. If dependence develops, the appearance of withdrawal symptoms after discontinuance will take several days for those benzodiazepines with active metabolites. An acute phase of chronic withdrawal symptoms, consisting of depression, insomnia, nightmares, agitation, and psychologic distress, can persist for 6 weeks. Withdrawal begins during the first week after discontinuance of the drug, with symptoms of agitation, nausea and vomiting, nervousness, sweating, and muscular cramps. Seizures are seldom seen unless high doses have been abused; but if seizures do occur, it is at the end of the first week. To lessen withdrawal symptoms, the dosage of benzodiazepines should be tapered gradually over 2 to 16 weeks, adjusted for the specific drug and starting dose.

Interactions

Like the barbiturates, the sedative effect of the benzodiazepines is increased by other drug classes including alcohol and other general CNS depressants, tricyclic antidepressants, opiate analgesics, antipsychotics, and antihistamines. Unlike barbiturates, benzodiazepines have only slight effects on the liver microsomal enzymes.

Specific Benzodiazepines

Alprazolam

Alprazolam (Xanax) is indicated for the short-term relief of anxiety and may be effective in relieving anxiety associated with depression. Another use is to treat panic disorders. Alprazolam has a potential dependence liability with patients unable to give up use of the drug. Rebound panic, seizures, and delirium have been reported when the drug is rapidly discontinued.

Alprazolam is rapidly absorbed and is effective for about 12 hours. Although the drug is eliminated somewhat more slowly in older than in young adults, the metabolites are only weakly active. Steady-state plasma levels are reached in 2 to 5 days with regular administration.

Bromazepam

Bromazepam (Lectopam) is prescribed as an antianxiety agent. It is available in Canada but not in the United States. Bromazepam has a short-to-intermediate half-life and does not tend to accumulate with multiple doses. The dose for older adult patients should be half the usual adult dose.

Chlordiazepoxide

Chlordiazepoxide (Librium) is prescribed as an antianxiety drug, as a preanesthetic medication for sedation, and to treat symptoms of alcohol withdrawal. Chlordiazepoxide is absorbed better orally than intramuscularly; care must be used with intravenous (IV) injections. Chlordiazepoxide is metabolized by the liver to an active metabolite to give a persistent effect.

Clonazepam

Clonazepam (Klonopin) is mainly used as an anticonvulsant (see Chapter 55). It also treats panic attacks.

Clorazepate

Clorazepate (Tranxene) is prescribed for anxiety, panic attacks, the symptomatic relief of acute alcohol withdrawal, and as adjunctive therapy in the management of partial seizures. Clorazepate is not absorbed orally until converted by stomach acid to an active metabolite. Any condition or medication such as antacids or cimetidine that reduce stomach acidity markedly interferes with clorazepate absorption. The metabolite persists in the body.

Diazepam

Diazepam (Valium) has many clinical uses in addition to treating anxiety and panic attacks. It relieves muscle spasticity in patients with cerebral palsy or other conditions and stops continued convulsions (status epilepticus). Diazepam is also used in the hospital as a preanesthetic medication for sedation. Alcohol withdrawal symptoms may be treated with diazepam.

Diazepam is well absorbed orally and is effective within 1 hour. Absorption from IM injection is erratic, and pain occurs at the injection site, so this route is seldom used. IV injection must be given slowly and carefully into a large vein to minimize irritation and swelling at the injection site, with possible phlebitis or thrombosis.

Estazolam

Estazolam (ProSom) is a new benzodiazepine prescribed for insomnia. It has a fast onset of action and is effective for 6 to 8 hours.

✣ Flurazepam

Flurazepam (Dalmane) is prescribed as a hypnotic only. It suppresses stage 4 sleep but does not markedly depress REM sleep. Flurazepam is effective for more than 2 weeks. Also, it does not produce rebound insomnia when it is discontinued, probably because of the long half-life of its active metabolites. The persistence of active metabolites accounts for decreased mental alertness during the day, particularly after repeated use of flurazepam by older adult patients and by patients with decreased liver function.

Halazepam

Halazepam (Paxipam) an antianxiety drug, is well absorbed orally and is metabolized to an active metabolite with a long half-life. Cumulation of the drug and its metabolite occurs with repeated doses, particularly in older adult patients or in patients with impaired liver function.

Ketazolam

Ketazolam (Loftran) is an antianxiety agent. It is available in Canada but not in the United States. Ketazolam has a long half-life and accumulates with multiple dosing.

Lorazepam
Lorazepam (Ativan) is effective as a hypnotic and an antianxiety drug. It is well absorbed orally and intramuscularly. Parenteral lorazepam is sometimes given as a preanesthetic medication in adults. Lorazepam produces sedation, relieves anxiety, and decreases ability to recall events that day. The drug does not have active metabolites and therefore has a relatively short duration of action, about 15 hours.

Midazolam
Midazolam (Versed) is used as an IV anesthetic and is discussed in Chapter 68.

Nitrazepam
Nitrazepam (Mogadon) is a hypnotic. It is available in Canada but not in the United States. Nitrazepam has a short-to-intermediate half-life and has minimal accumulation with multiple dosing.

Oxazepam
Oxazepam (Serax) is effective as an antianxiety drug, especially in anxiety associated with depression, tension, agitation, and irritability in older adult patients. Oxazepam also reduces the anxiety associated with alcohol withdrawal.

Absorption is slow. The metabolites are not active; thus drug effects are not likely to be cumulative and do not persist for more than 24 hours.

Prazepam
Prazepam (Centrax), an antianxiety drug, is slowly absorbed orally. The metabolites are active; thus cumulative effects are seen with repeated administration.

Quazepam
Quazepam (Doral) is a new benzodiazepine used to treat insomnia. Its characteristics are much like flurazepam.

Temazepam
Temazepam (Restoril) is a hypnotic. Temazepam is slowly absorbed, and onset of sleep is not improved. The number of awakenings is decreased, however, and overall duration and quality of sleep improve. As with flurazepam, stage 4 sleep is suppressed, but REM sleep is not. Unlike flurazepam, temazepam does not have active metabolites, and cumulation is not generally a problem.

Triazolam
Triazolam (Halcion) is a hypnotic, an antianxiety agent, and an anticonvulsant. It may have muscle relaxant effects as well. Triazolam is rapidly absorbed. Its metabolites are not active and are rapidly eliminated. Triazolam and alprazolam are closely related chemically.

The safety of triazolam has been questioned. However, the Food and Drug Administration (FDA) determined that the incidence of severe side effects is not greater for triazolam than for flurazepam and temazepam, two other popular hypnotics, when compared at equivalent doses. Side effects include anxiety, restlessness, amnesia, aggression, and paranoia.

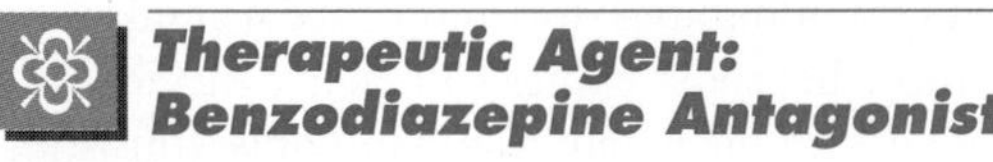

Therapeutic Agent: Benzodiazepine Antagonist

Flumazenil
Flumazenil (Mazicon) is the first benzodiazepine antagonist to be released for clinical use (Table 51-3). Flumazenil binds to the benzodiazepine receptor competitively and thereby inhibits the action of benzodiazepines.

Two major clinical uses are anticipated for flumazenil. First, flumazenil is a diagnostic tool to confirm or exclude benzodiazepine intoxication. Flumazenil, administered intravenously, will reverse benzodiazepine intoxication in 5 minutes. Once benzodiazepine intoxication is confirmed, flumazenil can be given repeatedly to reverse the depression of the respiratory drive caused by benzodiazepine intoxication so that the need for endotracheal intubation and artificial ventilation is avoided or decreased. Second, flumazenil is used to reverse the sedative effects of benzodiazepines given during surgical procedures to induce conscious sedation or general anesthesia. Flumazenil is also being tested as an agent to induce remission of functional CNS impairment, especially that of hepatic encephalopathy.

Flumazenil is generally well tolerated. Surgical patients are more likely to experience nausea and vomiting. Patients being treated for an overdose of benzodiazepines may experience agitation, restlessness, discomfort, and anxiety.

Therapeutic Agents for Insomnia and Anxiety: Barbiturates

Barbiturates: General Characteristics

Mechanism of Action
Barbiturates depress the reticular activating system, probably by promoting the inhibitory synaptic action of the neurotransmitter GABA.

Pharmacokinetics
The **barbiturates** are classified according to their duration of action and have been traditionally divided into four classes: ultrashort-acting, short-acting, intermediate-acting, and long-acting. Although traditional, this classification was derived from animal data and is somewhat arbitrary in the clinical setting, where the variables of dose and patient expectations can modify the degree and duration of effectiveness. In particular the contrast between short-acting and intermediate-acting sedative-hypnotics is not as striking in clinical practice as in drug tables (Table 51-4).

The ultrashort-acting barbiturates are administered intravenously, but other barbiturates are usually given orally and are well absorbed. Differences in onset and duration of action among barbiturates depend on their lipid solubility and protein binding. These properties are determined by the chemical structure. The ultrashort-acting barbiturates are

TABLE 51-3 Sedative-Hypnotic and Antianxiety Drugs: Benzodiazepines and Benzodiazepine Antagonist

GENERIC NAME	TRADE NAME	ADMINISTRATION/DOSAGE	COMMENTS
Benzodiazepines			
Alprazolam	Xanax*	ORAL: *Adults*—0.25-0.5 mg 3 times daily. Maximum daily dose: 4 mg. FDA pregnancy category D. *Older adults*—0.25 mg 2 or 3 times daily.	Used to treat anxiety. Metabolites are only weakly active. Schedule IV substance.
Bromazepam	Lectopam†	ORAL: *Adults*—6-30 mg daily in divided doses.	Used to treat anxiety.
Chlordiazepoxide	Libritabs Librium* Novopoxide† Various others	ORAL: *Adults*—For anxiety, 15-100 mg divided in 3-4 doses or in 1 dose at bedtime. *Older adults*—5 mg 2-4 times daily. *Children*—0.5 mg/kg body weight daily in 3-4 doses. May be given intramuscularly. INTRAVENOUS: *Adults*—For alcohol withdrawal, 50-100 mg slowly over at least 1 min, then 25-50 mg every 6-8 hr, with the total dose not more than 300 mg.	Used to treat anxiety and alcohol withdrawal. Half-life is 24-48 hr. Metabolites are active. Hydrochloride salt is used for injection. Schedule IV substance.
Clonazepam	Klonopin Rivotril†	ORAL: *Adults*—Initially, 0.5 mg 3 times daily. Increase in increments of 0.5 mg-1 mg every 3 days if necessary.	Primarily used as anticonvulsant. Use to treat panic disorders is under investigation. Schedule IV substance.
Clorazepate	Tranxene* Novo-Clopate†	ORAL: *Adults*—13-60 mg divided into 2-4 doses or at bedtime. *Older adults*—6.5-15 mg daily.	Used to treat anxiety. Half-life is 30-200 hr. Metabolites are active. Schedule IV substance.
Diazepam	Apo-Diazepam† Valium* Various others	ORAL: *Adults*—4-40 mg divided into 2-4 doses or single dose of 2.5-10 mg at bedtime. *Older adults*—2-2.5 mg once to twice daily. *Children*—0.12-0.8 mg/kg daily in 3-4 doses. INTRAVENOUS: Administer no more than 5 mg/min. For severe anxiety, severe muscle spasm, status epilepticus, or recurrent seizures: *Adults*—5-10 mg initially, repeated in 3-4 hr if needed. *Children*—0.04-0.2 mg/kg initially, repeat in 3-4 hr if necessary. For basal sedation for cardioversion or endoscopic procedures: *Adults*—10-20 mg as required. For acute alcohol withdrawal symptoms: *Adults*—5-20 mg, then 5-10 mg in 3-4 hr if necessary.	Used to treat anxiety, severe muscle spasm, status epilepticus, and acute alcohol withdrawal symptoms and to provide sedation. Half-life is 48-200 hr. Metabolites are active. Schedule IV substance.
Estazolam	ProSom	ORAL: *Adults*—1 mg at bedtime; some patients may require 2 mg. FDA pregnancy category X. Small or debilitated patients, 0.5 mg.	Used to treat insomnia. New drug.
✤ Flurazepam	Apo-Flurazepam† Dalmane* Novoflupam† Somnol† Various others	ORAL: *Adults*—As hypnotic, 15-30 mg at bedtime. *Older adults*—15 mg. Onset 20-45 min. Duration: 7-8 hr.	Used as hypnotic only. Active metabolite is formed with half-life of 47-100 hr, so repeated use leads to cumulation of this metabolite, which may impair daytime activity. Schedule IV substance.
Halazepam	Paxipam	ORAL: *Adults*—20-40 mg 3 or 4 times daily. FDA pregnancy category D. *Older adults*—Reduce dose to 20 mg 1 or 2 times daily.	Used to treat anxiety. Active metabolite with long half-life. Schedule IV substance.
Ketazolam	Loftran†	ORAL: *Adults*—15 mg 1-2 times daily.	Used to treat anxiety.
✤ Lorazepam	Ativan* Nu-Loraz† Various others	ORAL: *Adults*—For anxiety, 1-2 mg 2-3 times daily, may increase dose to 10 mg maximum daily; as hypnotic, 2-4 mg at bedtime. FDA pregnancy category D. *Older adults*—½ adult dose.	Used to treat anxiety and insomnia. Repeated use for insomnia can cause rebound insomnia. Half-life is 15 hr, so little cumulation occurs. Metabolites are inactive. Schedule IV substance.
Nitrazepam	Mogadon†	ORAL: *Adults*—5-10 mg at bedtime. *Children* (anticonvulsant)—0.3 mg-1 mg/kg body weight in 3 divided doses. May increase gradually if needed and tolerated.	Used as sedative in adults and as anticonvulsant in children.

*Available in Canada and United States.
†Available in Canada only.

Continued.

TABLE 51-3 Sedative-Hypnotic and Antianxiety Drugs: Benzodiazepines and Benzodiazepine Antagonist—cont'd

GENERIC NAME	TRADE NAME	ADMINISTRATION/DOSAGE	COMMENTS
Benzodiazepines—cont'd			
Oxazepam	Apo-Oxazepam† Serax* Novoxapam†	ORAL: *Adults*—For anxiety, 30-120 mg daily in 3-4 doses. *Older adults*—30 mg in 3 divided doses, increased if necessary to 45-60 mg.	Used to treat anxiety. Half-life is 3-21 hr, so little cumulation occurs. Metabolites are inactive. Schedule IV substance.
Prazepam	Centrax	ORAL: *Adults*—20 mg in single dose, increased to 40-60 mg daily in divided doses or once at bedtime. *Older adults*—10-15 mg.	Used to treat anxiety. Half-life is 30-200 hr. Metabolites are active. Schedule IV substance.
Quazepam	Doral	ORAL: *Adults*—Initially, 15 mg. Reduce to 7.5 mg as needed.	Used to treat insomnia. Metabolites have long half life. Schedule IV substance.
Temazepam	Restoril*	ORAL: *Adults*—30 mg at bedtime. FDA pregnancy category X. *Older adults*—reduce dose to 15 mg.	Used as hypnotic only. Slowly absorbed. Metabolites are not active. Schedule IV substance.
Triazolam	Apo-Triazo† Halcion* Novo-Triolam†	ORAL: *Adults*—0.25-0.5 mg at bedtime. FDA pregnancy category X. *Older adults*—Reduce dose to 0.25 mg.	Used as hypnotic. May also be used as antianxiety drug and anticonvulsant. Metabolites are not active. Schedule IV substance.
Benzodiazepine Antagonist			
Flumazenil	Mazicon	Reversal of conscious sedation or in general anesthesia: INTRAVENOUS: *Adults*—0.2 mg administered over 15 sec initially. Wait 45 sec for response. Further doses of 0.2 mg may be repeated at 60 sec intervals if needed, to a cumulative dose of 1 mg per treatment. Treatment may be repeated at 20 min intervals, with no more than 3 mg given in 1 hr. Management of suspected benzodiazepine overdose: INTRAVENOUS: *Adults*—0.2 mg is administered over 30 sec initially. If desired level of consciousness is not seen after waiting 30 sec, further dose of 0.3 mg is administered over another 30 sec. Further doses of 0.5 mg may be administered over 30 sec at 1 min intervals up to cumulative dose of 3 mg. In event of resedation, treatment may be repeated at 20 min intervals, with no more than 1 mg administered at one time and not more than 3 mg given in 1 hr.	New benzodiazepine antagonist for reversal of benzodiazepine-induced sedation.

lipid soluble; on IV administration the concentration of ultrashort-acting barbiturates reaching the brain is large because the brain has a high blood flow and the barbiturates readily cross the blood-brain barrier and depress the reticular activating system. The action is quickly terminated, however, because the barbiturates are redistributed into organs with a lesser blood flow, so the concentration reaching the brain quickly drops. Ultrashort-acting barbiturates may persist in body fat because of their high lipid solubility and in muscle, reflecting their high degree of protein binding.

Barbiturates are released slowly from muscle and fat into the blood for eventual metabolism by the liver and excretion by the kidney. The persistence of low concentrations of barbiturates in the body is believed to account for the "hangovers" after the therapeutic effect has worn off. Short- and intermediate-acting barbiturates are redistributed less rapidly into body fat and muscle, thus acting longer. The long-acting barbiturate phenobarbital binds even less to protein and is much less lipid soluble than the ultrashort-acting barbiturates. Although ultrashort-, short-, and intermediate-acting barbiturates must be metabolized by the liver to water-soluble metabolites for excretion by the kidney, 30% to 50% of a dose of phenobarbital is excreted unchanged in urine.

Uses

Barbiturates have been used for the short-term treatment of insomnia or for sedation to relieve anxiety, tension, and apprehension. However, benzodiazepines have largely replaced barbiturates for these uses.

The ultrashort-acting barbiturates methohexital and thiopental are used as general anesthetics. Amobarbital, butabarbital, pentobarbital, phenobarbital, and secobarbital

TABLE 51-4 Sedative-Hypnotic and Antianxiety Drugs: Barbiturates

GENERIC NAME	TRADE NAME	ADMINISTRATION/DOSAGE	COMMENTS
Amobarbital‡	Amytal*	ORAL: *Adults*—As sedative, 50-300 mg daily in divided doses; as hypnotic, 65-200 mg at bedtime. *Children*—As sedative, 6 mg/kg body weight in 3 divided doses. INTRAMUSCULAR, INTRAVENOUS: *Adults*—65-200 mg as hypnotic dose; 30-50 mg as sedative dose. *Children*—2-3 mg/kg body weight as hypnotic dose; 3-5 mg/kg body weight as sedative dose. FDA pregnancy category D.	Intermediate-acting barbiturate that acts similarly to short-acting barbiturate in humans. Used for daytime sedation, preanesthetic sedation, and hypnosis. Precautions are same as for secobarbital. Schedule II substance.
Aprobarbital	Alurate	ORAL: *Adults*—40-160 mg at bedtime. FDA pregnancy category D.	Intermediate-acting barbiturate. Used as hypnotic. Reduce doses for older adult patients. Schedule III substance. Not available in Canada.
Butabarbital	Butisol Sarisol No. 2	ORAL: *Adults*—As sedative, 50-120 mg/day in 3 or 4 divided doses; as hypnotic, 50-100 mg at bedtime. FDA pregnancy category D. *Children*—As sedative, 6 mg/kg in 3 divided doses daily.	Intermediate-acting barbiturate used for sedation or for insomnia when need is to prolong sleep rather than to induce sleep. Schedule III substance.
Pentobarbital‡	Nembutal* Novopentobarb†	ORAL: *Adults*—As sedative, 30 mg 3 or 4 times daily or 100 mg in timed-release form in morning; as hypnotic, 100 mg at bedtime. FDA pregnancy category D. *Children*—As sedative, 6 mg/kg in 3 divided doses daily. RECTAL: *Adults*—120-200 mg as required for sedation or hypnosis. *Children*—As sedative, 30-120 mg/day. INTRAMUSCULAR: *Adults*—As hypnotic, 150-200 mg. INTRAVENOUS: *Adults*—As hypnotic, 100 mg. After 1 min, can administer small increments, but no more than 500 mg total. *Children*—As hypnotic 50 mg initially.	Short-acting barbiturate used principally for insomnia and preanesthetic sedation and occasionally for daytime sedation. Precautions are same as for secobarbital. Schedule II substance.
Phenobarbital‡	Luminal* Solfoton	ORAL: *Adults*—As sedative, 30-120 mg daily in 2 or 3 divided doses; as hypnotic, 100-320 mg at bedtime. FDA pregnancy category D. *Children*—As sedative, 6 mg/kg daily in 4 divided doses. INTRAMUSCULAR, INTRAVENOUS: *Adults*—As sedative 30-120 mg; as hypnotic 100-320 mg, with no more than 100 mg (2 ml of 5% solution)/min intravenously. Full effect lasts 15 min. RECTAL: *Children*—As sedative, 6 mg/kg divided in 3 doses.	Long-acting barbiturate used principally as sedative. (For use as anticonvulsant, see Chapter 55.) Not readily addictive. Schedule IV substance.
Secobarbital	Seconal* Novosecobarb†	ORAL: *Adults*—As sedative, 30-50 mg; as hypnotic, 100-200 mg at bedtime; for preoperative sedation, 200-300 mg 1-2 hr before surgery. FDA pregnancy category D. *Children*—As sedative, 6 mg/kg in 3 divided doses; for preoperative sedation, 50-100 mg. RECTAL: *Adults*—120-200 mg as required for sedation or hypnosis. *Children*—15-120 mg. INTRAMUSCULAR: *Adults*—As hypnotic, 100-200 mg. *Children*—As hypnotic, 3-5 mg/kg, up to 100 mg. INTRAVENOUS: *Adults*—As hypnotic, 50-250 mg, inject only 50 mg in 15 sec.	Short-acting barbiturate used principally for insomnia and as preanesthetic sedative. Not indicated for repeated use because tolerance develops, rebound insomnia becomes marked, and addiction potential is high. Schedule II substance.

*Available in Canada and United States.
†Available in Canada only.
‡Also available as the sodium salt. Only the sodium salt is suitable for administration as a solution by the rectal, intramuscular, or intravenous route.

are used for preoperative medication. Phenobarbital, mephobarbital, and methabarbital are used in treating epilepsy and convulsions (see Chapter 55).

Adverse Reactions and Contraindications

Side effects are generally mild. Some individuals experience confusion or irritability. Rarely, regular use can cause agranulocytosis, thrombocytopenia purpura, or megaloblastic anemia. Allergic reactions are also a rare reaction but may include angioedema, morbilliform rash, erythema multiforme, or Stevens-Johnson syndrome.

As discussed for hypnotics in general, barbiturates are not effective as hypnotics after 2 weeks of use. Also, even a single dose suppresses REM sleep and leads to REM rebound when the barbiturate is discontinued. Mild withdrawal symptoms from short-term use of barbiturates include nightmares, daytime agitation, and a "shaky" feeling.

An acute overdose of barbiturates causes depression of the medullary centers controlling respiration and the cardiovascular system. The symptoms are a fast heart rate (tachycardia) and a fall in blood pressure (hypotension) that leads to shock. Reflexes disappear, and respiration is markedly depressed. The patient becomes comatose, and death may result from respiratory and cardiovascular collapse. No specific antagonist exists for barbiturates; thus treatment of barbiturate poisoning supports respiration and maintains blood oxygen levels.

Toxicity

Metabolic tolerance. Administration of barbiturates for a few days activates the liver to synthesize more of the drug-metabolizing enzymes. This activation is called *enzyme induction.* Since these enzymes are located in the microsomal fraction of broken cell preparations, these drug-metabolizing enzymes usually are referred to as the *liver microsomal enzyme system.* After induction of the microsomal enzymes, the barbiturates are more rapidly metabolized, decreasing average blood levels after a given dose. This is a classic example of *metabolic tolerance.* Since many other drugs are also metabolized by the same microsomal enzymes, barbiturates can induce tolerance of other drugs. Examples are the coumarins (anticoagulants) and the anticonvulsant phenytoin (Dilantin).

Pharmacodynamic tolerance. In addition to drug-induced tolerance, pharmacodynamic tolerance also develops with repeated administration of the barbiturates. This is the tolerance described previously for all general CNS depressants in which the nervous system adapts to the presence of the depressant. However, the medullary centers controlling respiration and the cardiovascular system do not adapt to general CNS depressants since they are not affected at the usual doses taken. The lethal dose for barbiturates therefore does not increase with drug dependence; this accounts for the accidental death of individuals dependent on high doses of barbiturates since these doses can be lethal. The lethal dose for barbiturates in nontolerant individuals is about 15 times the hypnotic dose.

Abuse Potential and Withdrawal

Barbiturates are a class of widely abused drugs (see box). As with other abused classes of drugs, individual drugs with the most rapid onset are the most abused. This is because the euphoric feeling or "rush" depends on a rapid rate of altering perception. Among the barbiturates, secobarbital, pentobarbital, and amobarbital are schedule II drugs (drugs having a high potential for abuse). Butabarbital is a schedule III drug (lesser abuse potential), whereas phenobarbital and mephobarbital are schedule IV (low abuse potential) drugs (see Chapter 3). With the schedule II barbiturates, a daily consumption of 400 mg leads to severe drug dependence in about 6 weeks. With larger doses, the time decreases.

Severe withdrawal symptoms begin within 24 hours after the drug is discontinued in an individual with severe drug dependence. Grand mal convulsions and delirium are common symptoms; elevated temperature, coma, and death are less common. Because of the danger associated with barbiturate withdrawal, gradual withdrawal is used to detoxify a dependent person. Withdrawal is achieved by reducing the dose of the barbiturate to zero over 10 to 20 days. Sometimes the long-acting barbiturate phenobarbital is substituted for a short-acting barbiturate for once-a-day administration. Phenobarbital (30 mg) is substituted for 100 mg of secobarbital, pentobarbital, or amobarbital.

Interactions

The depressant effect of barbiturates is not only additive with the other general CNS depressants but is also potentiated by

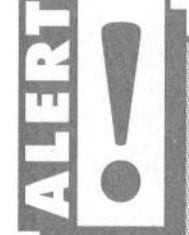

DRUG ABUSE ALERT

Barbiturates

BACKGROUND

Barbiturates are abused to bring about a sense of euphoria and a lessening of anxiety. They can be taken orally or injected.

PHARMACOLOGY

Barbiturates are sedative-hypnotics. Slurred speech, staggering gait, poor judgment, and uncertain reflexes are symptoms of barbiturate use.

HEALTH HAZARDS

There is only a fourfold margin between a sedative dose and an overdose of barbiturates. This margin is decreased by the ingestion of alcohol or another CNS depressant. A barbiturate overdose causes shallow respiration, cold and clammy skin, dilated pupils, and a weak and rapid pulse. In addition to the dangers of overdose, repeated use of barbiturates leads to dependence. Withdrawal symptoms include anxiety, insomnia, tremors, delirium, and convulsions.

antipsychotics and narcotic analgesics. These interactions are important to remember for the patient scheduled to undergo surgery. If secobarbital or pentobarbital is prescribed as the night-before sleeping pill, it should be given at least 8 hours before any of the major tranquilizers, narcotic analgesics, or general anesthetics are administered to avoid undue depression of the medullary control of respiration and the cardiovascular system.

Specific Barbiturates

Thiopental and Methohexital

Thiopental (Pentothal), and methohexital (Brevital) are ultrashort-acting barbiturates administered intravenously for the induction or maintenance of anesthesia. These barbiturates are discussed with the general anesthetics in Chapter 68.

Amobarbital, Aprobarbital, Pentobarbital, and Secobarbital

Amobarbital (Amytal), aprobarbital (Alurate), pentobarbital (Nembutal), and secobarbital (Seconal) are used most frequently as hypnotic drugs. The combination of secobarbital and amobarbital is sold under the name Tuinal as a hypnotic. Although these barbiturates are effective hypnotics for a few days, they lose their effectiveness by the second week of use. Since barbiturates depress REM sleep, REM rebound occurs when they are discontinued. This REM rebound can lead to insomnia. Also drug dependence can develop with the usual hypnotic doses within 2 months, although this does not lead to severe withdrawal symptoms unless the dose has been raised above 400 mg daily.

Butabarbital

Butabarbital (Butisol) is an intermediate-acting barbiturate prescribed for daytime sedation and less commonly for inducing sleep at night. It frequently is combined in sedative doses with other drugs used to treat conditions with psychogenic overtones such as allergies, ulcers, and inflammatory bowel disease.

Phenobarbital

Phenobarbital (Luminal) is the longest acting and most widely used of the barbiturates. Phenobarbital and mephobarbital (Mebaral) control some kinds of epilepsy (see Chapter 55). Phenobarbital is infrequently abused because it is slower in onset of action, and it does not give a rush. Peak blood levels occur 6 to 18 hours after an oral dose, and the half-life is 3 to 4 days.

Phenobarbital is the barbiturate that most readily induces the liver microsomal enzyme system, thereby enhancing its own metabolism and those of many other drugs. Phenobarbital treatment enhances the degradation of bilirubin and is used in infants and children to lower elevated plasma bilirubin levels.

Phenobarbital may be substituted for other barbiturates or nonbenzodiazepine hypnotics when decreasing drug levels for withdrawal. Its longer action allows once-a-day therapy.

Therapeutic Agents: Other Hypnotic and Antianxiety Drugs

The miscellaneous hypnotic and antianxiety drugs listed in Table 51-5 are more similar to the barbiturates than the benzodiazepines in that they are generally shorter acting, which makes them more readily abused. Discontinuance produces withdrawal symptoms resembling those described for the barbiturates. The degree of dependence is sometimes determined by giving 200 mg of pentobarbital every 2 hours until signs of intoxication appear. The patient is then detoxified with divided doses (4 to 6 doses/day) of pentobarbital, and the total daily dose is decreased by 100 mg/day. This approach is possible because pentobarbital is cross-tolerant with these other drugs. Alternatively, the abused drug is decreased daily over a 10- to 20-day period, or phenobarbital is administered in decreasing daily doses.

In addition to these drugs, several antihistamines have a pronounced sedative effect, for which they are sometimes used (see Chapter 28).

Buspirone

Buspirone (BuSpar) is one of the new antianxiety drugs that are not benzodiazepines. Buspirone does not cause the CNS depression characteristic of barbiturates and benzodiazepines. A lag time of 1 to 2 weeks is usual before a decrease in anxiety is noted. Little sedation or mental impairment is noted. However, at higher doses patients may experience sedation or a bad mood. Side effects are uncommon but include headaches, dizziness, nervousness, and light-headedness. Buspirone reportedly has little abuse potential. It is metabolized and excreted in urine.

✣ Chloral Hydrate

Chloral hydrate (Noctec) is the oldest of the currently used hypnotic drugs, introduced in the nineteenth century. Although it is not effective for more than 2 weeks, it does not suppress REM sleep and therefore does not cause REM rebound. Chloral hydrate and its active metabolite, trichlorethanol, have a half-life of only 8 hours, so no persistent effect occurs as does with flurazepam.

Chloral hydrate has an unpleasant taste and odor, which can be masked by taking the drug in capsules, as a chilled elixir or syrup, or as a suppository. The drug produces fewer side effects (particularly paradoxical excitement) among children or older adults than other hypnotics, but it causes gastric irritation in some patients and displaces the coumarin anticoagulants from plasma protein. Drug dependence is produced by long-term use; an acute overdose can result in coma, with the patient having pinpoint pupils. In folklore, chloral hydrate added to an alcoholic beverage produces a "knockout" drink, the Mickey Finn, resulting from the additive effect of the two general CNS depressants.

Ethchlorvynol

Ethchlorvynol (Placidyl) was introduced in the 1950s as a hypnotic. The most frequent patient complaint is an after-

TABLE 51-5 Miscellaneous Sedative-Hypnotic and Antianxiety Drugs

GENERIC NAME	TRADE NAME	ADMINISTRATION/DOSAGE	COMMENTS
Buspirone	BuSpar	ORAL: *Adults*—Initially, 5 mg 3 times daily. May increase by 5 mg daily every 2-3 days until desired response is obtained. Maximum daily dose: 60 mg. FDA pregnancy category B.	New antianxiety drug that causes less sedation. Does not react with alcohol or antidepressants.
✤ Chloral hydrate	Aquachloral Supprettes Novo-Chlorhydrate†	ORAL, RECTAL: *Adults*—As sedative, 250 mg 3 times daily after meals; as hypnotic, 500 mg-1 gm 15-30 min before bedtime. FDA pregnancy category C. *Children*—As sedative, 25 mg/kg body weight in 3-4 doses daily; as hypnotic, 50 mg/kg as bedtime dose, not to exceed 500 mg.	Generally safe hypnotic. Unpleasant taste and odor can be masked by chilling drug or using capsule form. Schedule IV substance.
Ethchlorvynol	Placidyl*	ORAL: *Adults only*—As hypnotic, 500 mg-1 gm at bedtime. FDA pregnancy category C.	Physical and psychologic dependence may occur. Schedule IV substance.
Hydroxyzine hydrochloride, Hydroxyzine pamoate	Atarax* Vistaril Various others	ORAL: *Adults*—For anxiety, 75-500 mg daily in 4 divided doses. For allergic skin reactions: ORAL: *Adults*—25 mg 3 or 4 times daily. *Children <6 yr*—50 mg daily in 3 or 4 divided doses. *Adults*—For anxiety: 50-100 mg every 4-6 hr.	Antihistamine that has antiemetic and antianxiety properties. Used in treating allergic skin rashes and motion sickness and as preanesthetic medication. Usual doses of barbiturates or narcotics must be cut by 50% if given concurrently.
Meprobamate	Equanil* Meprospan* Miltown* Various others	ORAL: *Adults*—For anxiety, 1.2-1.6 gm daily in 3 or 4 divided doses. *Children >6 yr*—For anxiety, 25 mg/kg daily in 2 or 3 divided doses.	Physical and psychologic dependence may occur. Schedule IV substance.
Zolpidem tartrate	Ambien	ORAL: *Adults*—10 mg at bedtime. *Older adults*—5 mg at bedtime. FDA pregnancy category B.	New hypnotic drug with short half-life and negligible hangover side effects. Schedule IV drug.

*Available in Canada and United States.
†Available in Canada only.

taste. Occasionally patients show exaggerated depression, with deep sleep and muscular weakness. Some individuals have an idiosyncratic response of CNS stimulation that may be mild or hysteric. Ethchlorvynol is a schedule IV drug with a duration of action similar to that of the short-acting barbiturates.

Hydroxyzine

Hydroxyzine (Atarax, Vistaril), an antihistamine with sedative properties, is used as an antianxiety agent when it is desirable to have the antiemetic and antihistaminic properties for motion sickness or allergic skin reactions. Hydroxyzine is also used as a preanesthetic medication.

Meprobamate

Meprobamate (Equanil, Miltown) was introduced in the 1950s as the first widely prescribed antianxiety drug. Although physical dependence readily develops with abuse, meprobamate is a Schedule IV drug. Withdrawal symptoms range from insomnia and anxiety to hallucinations and grand mal seizures. Meprobamate is sometimes used as a centrally acting skeletal muscle relaxant, although its effectiveness in this role is questionable.

Zolpidem

Zolpidem (Ambien) is a new nonbenzodiazepine hypnotic. However, like barbiturates and benzodiazepines, zolpidem depresses the reticular activating system, probably by promoting the inhibitory synaptic action of the neurotransmitter GABA. It has short half-life and therefore does not accumulate to cause drowsiness or dizziness the next day. Older adult patients should receive half the normal adult dose.

Therapeutic Rationale: Alcohol and Alcoholism

Alcohol: General Characteristics

Alcohol is a widely used and abused drug. In this section the important actions of alcohol and its interactions with other drugs are reviewed.

Mechanism of Action

As a general CNS depressant, alcohol causes all the behavioral changes described in the overview: sedation, disinhibition, sleep, and anesthesia. As summarized in Table 51-6, the amount of alcohol in the blood, which can be predicted from the amount consumed, produces characteristic behavioral ef-

TABLE 51-6 Alcohol Intake and Its Behavioral Effects

ALCOHOL CONTENT (oz)	BEVERAGE INTAKE IN 1 HR*	BLOOD ALCOHOL LEVEL (mg/dl) IN 150-LB MAN	BEHAVIORAL EFFECTS
½	1 oz 100-proof spirits 1 glass wine 1 can beer	0.025	No noticeable effect
1	2 oz 100-proof spirits 2 glasses wine 2 cans beer	0.050	Lower alertness, impaired judgment, good feeling, and less inhibition
2	4 oz 100-proof spirits 4 glasses wine 4 cans beer	0.100	Slow reaction time, impaired motor function, and less cautious; should not drive; may activate vomiting reflex
3	6 oz 100-proof spirits 6 glasses wine 6 cans beer	0.150	Large increase in reaction times
4	8 oz 100-proof spirits 8 glasses wine 8 cans beer	0.200	Marked depression of sensory and motor abilities
5	10 oz 100-proof spirits 10 glasses wine 10 cans beer	0.250	Severe depression of sensory and motor abilities
6	12 oz 100-proof spirits 12 glasses wine 12 cans beer	0.300	Stuporous and unconscious of surroundings
7	14 oz 100-proof spirits 14 glasses wine 14 cans beer	0.350	Unconscious
8	16 oz 100-proof spirits 16 glasses wine 16 cans beer	0.400	Lethal dose in 50% of the population
12	24 oz 100-proof spirits 24 glasses wine 24 cans beer	0.600	Lethal dose in 95% of the population

*Since only ¼ to ⅓ oz of alcohol is metabolized each hour, alcohol rapidly accumulates.

fects. Alcohol also enhances the sedative-hypnotic effects of other drug classes, including all the general CNS depressants discussed in this chapter and other drug classes with sedative side effects including the antihistamines, the phenothiazines, the narcotic analgesics, the tricyclic antidepressants, and the monoamine oxidase inhibitors. This enhancement of CNS depression means that irreversible coma or death can occur when alcohol is taken concurrently with other drugs, a fact not widely enough appreciated in our society.

Acute ingestion of alcohol has effects in addition to those attributed to its general CNS depression. Rising levels of alcohol may activate the vomiting center. Alcohol acts centrally to produce vasodilation and a feeling of warmth. This vasodilation can produce a marked hypotensive response in persons taking guanethidine or nitroglycerin.

Pharmacokinetics

Alcohol is absorbed more readily from the small intestine than from the stomach. Absorption of alcohol therefore is decreased by food, which dilutes the alcohol and keeps it in the stomach longer. Alcohol in concentrations of 10% or less will stimulate gastric secretions, thereby aiding digestion, but larger concentrations inhibit gastric secretions and damage the cells lining the stomach. This irritation may make some people nauseated the day after heavy drinking and accounts for the inflammation of the stomach (gastritis) and ulcers frequently seen in alcoholics. Aspirin is another drug that readily damages the stomach lining. The combination of aspirin and alcohol can produce bleeding in the stomach.

More than 90% of ingested alcohol is oxidized by the liver, with the remainder being excreted in the breath and urine. The oxidation of alcohol to carbon dioxide and water means that alcohol is a source of calories. Alcoholics may get most of their calories from alcohol but may be malnourished because alcoholic beverages lack vitamins, minerals, and protein. Two enzyme systems in the liver transform alcohol. The major enzyme for alcohol metabolism is alcohol dehydrogenase, which is also the enzyme that limits the rate of alcohol metabolism. In the average adult, the liver alcohol dehydrogenase can metabolize only about 10 ml of alcohol in 1 hour. This means that no matter how much someone has drunk, only 10 ml of alcohol can be metabolized in 1 hour, and alcohol readily accumulates in the body when this amount is exceeded. Neither coffee, fresh air, nor exercise will speed up alcohol metabolism to help someone "sober up."

The product of alcohol metabolism by alcohol dehydrogenase is acetaldehyde, a highly toxic compound. Ordinarily, acetaldehyde does not accumulate because it is metabolized further by aldehyde dehydrogenase. Disulfiram (Antabuse) and other drugs can inhibit this enzyme so that acetaldehyde accumulates and produces unpleasant symptoms, which include headache, nausea, and vomiting.

The liver microsomal enzyme system described for the barbiturates also can degrade alcohol but ordinarily with a very limited capacity. As with phenobarbital, alcohol can induce this enzyme system so that the liver can metabolize not only more alcohol but more of other drugs as well, and this is one source of drug interactions. Alcoholics are able to metabolize twice as much alcohol as those who do not have chronic alcoholism.

An elevated value of serum gamma-glutamyl transpeptidase (GGTP) in the absence of other elevated enzymes is a good predictor of long-term alcohol or drug consumption. This enzyme is induced in the liver by alcohol and drugs and secreted into the circulation. An elevated GGTP is often the first biochemical sign of alcoholism and may occur before overt clinical signs and symptoms develop.

Acute Toxicity

Unless a large amount of concentrated alcohol has been rapidly swallowed on an empty stomach or ingested with another CNS depressant drug, an acute overdose of alcohol commonly causes an individual to pass out before lethal doses can be drunk. However, note that a pint of 100-proof liquor is a lethal dose in 50% of the population (LD_{50}) for a small man (see Table 51-6). With rapid drinking of straight liquor, someone can drink enough to die. The greatest danger of acute alcohol intoxication to nonalcoholic individuals is that they may involve themselves or others in traffic accidents (30,000 alcohol-related traffic deaths per year) or that they may fall and injure themselves.

A hangover is common on recovery from an acute alcohol intoxication and includes such symptoms as an upset stomach, thirst, fatigue, headache, depression, anxiety, and generally feeling out of sorts. Many of these symptoms are caused by congeners, the natural by-products of fermentation and aging. Vodka, which is a mixture of pure alcohol and water and contains a few congeners, also produces few hangover symptoms compared to wines and aged spirits, which have higher congener contents.

TABLE 51-7 Degenerative Changes Common With Chronic Alcohol Consumption

SYSTEM	COMMENTS
Brain	Lack of vitamin B_1 (thiamine) common to alcoholic persons produces *Wernicke's disease:* brain lesions manifested as inability to learn or recall. *Korsakoff's psychosis* describes alcoholic persons who are confused and disoriented as to time or place. Wernicke's disease and Korsakoff's psychosis are considered variations of same brain disease. Replacement of vitamin B_1 helps reverse symptoms in early stages but will not restore lost function later.
Liver	Chronic drinking produces fatty liver because in presence of alcohol, fatty acids are stored in liver rather than being metabolized. About 75% of alcoholic persons show some cirrhosis after 10 years. In cirrhosis, fibrous tissue replaces liver cells. Severe cases result in liver failure and death. Hepatitis (inflammation of liver) is also common among alcoholic persons.
Stomach and GI tract	Alcohol causes gastritis, which leads to ulcers and blood loss. Nonspecific diarrhea is common. Inflammation of pancreas (pancreatitis) is common.
Heart	Some alcoholic individuals develop enlarged heart that functions poorly (cardiomyopathy).
Blood	Because of blood loss and lack of folic acid, alcoholic persons can have both iron deficiency (microcytic) anemia and folate deficiency (macrocytic) anemia. Liver disease may result in clotting factor deficiency. White blood cells and platelets are decreased.
Metabolic	Alcoholic persons are often hypoglycemic because alcohol inhibits glucose production by liver. Since alcohol is converted to substrate for carbohydrate and fat metabolism, high levels of lipids, lactic acid, uric acid, and ketone bodies may appear in blood. Plasma magnesium, plasma phosphate, and plasma albumin concentration are low.
Skin	Vasodilation caused by alcohol eventually produces permanent rosy nose and cheeks. Skin ulcers are common.

Chronic Toxicity

Long-term drinking can produce characteristic degenerative changes in the body, as listed in Table 51-7. These changes are seen after about 10 years of drinking 150 ml of alcohol daily. In addition to these degenerative changes, some alcoholic persons may have blackout spells, periods in which they are awake and functioning but of which they have no memory. Heavy drinking during pregnancy is associated with a 63% incidence of neurologic abnormalities in the offspring. **Fetal alcohol syndrome** is now recognized in the offspring of alcoholic mothers, a syndrome characterized by a flat face with widely spaced, small eyes and mental retardation.

Withdrawal

Long-term drinking also leads to withdrawal symptoms when the person stops drinking. The severity of the withdrawal symptoms depends on the individual's drinking history, but the symptoms are most common when a long-term drinker stays intoxicated for 2 or more weeks and then stops drinking. The first symptoms, which appear within a few hours, are tremors and anxiety. As the first stage progresses, bradycardia occurs, the blood pressure increases, and there is heavy sweating, loss of appetite, nausea and vomiting, and insomnia. The second stage of withdrawal is characterized by hallucinations, usually visual, but sometimes involving hearing or feeling things. The patient is still oriented and only mildly confused despite these hallucinations.

About 10% of untreated patients have seizures within the first 48 hours of withdrawal. **Delirium tremens** is a stage of withdrawal that occurs in about 10% of untreated alcoholic

PATIENT PROBLEM
Alcohol Use and Disulfiram

THE PROBLEM

Disulfiram is prescribed to patients who want to avoid drinking alcohol again. When a patient is taking disulfiram and alcohol is consumed, a serious physiologic reaction occurs. Other drugs also are associated with *disulfiram-like reactions* in combination with alcohol. Examples are furazolidone, metronidazole, chlorpropamide, and the antibiotic moxalactam.

SIGNS AND SYMPTOMS

The combination of alcohol and disulfiram produces flushing, throbbing in the head and neck, throbbing headache, respiratory difficulty, nausea, copious vomiting, sweating, thirst, chest pain, rapid breathing, tachycardia, fainting, weakness, vertigo, blurred vision, and confusion. Severe reactions can cause death.

PATIENT AND FAMILY EDUCATION

- Review the signs and symptoms of disulfiram-like reactions. Instruct the patient to seek medical help for a severe reaction.
- Review sources of alcohol. Obvious sources include ingestion of beer, liquor, or wine. Other dietary sources include sauces that may contain wine, cooking sherry, or liquors; wine vinegars; and some liquid medications such as cough syrups and elixirs. In patients sensitive to this reaction, topical contact with after-shave lotion or colognes, alcohol-containing liniments, or after-bath lotions may produce symptoms. Avoid inhalation of the vapors of any chemical that may contain alcohol such as shellac, varnish, or paint.
- Read the labels on food items and medicines. If in doubt about a drug, consult the pharmacist.
- Wear a medical identification tag or bracelet indicating that disulfiram is being taken.
- Avoid alcohol-containing products for up to 2 weeks after stopping disulfiram or a drug associated with disulfiram-like reactions.

persons 2 to 7 days after the start of withdrawal. Delirium tremens lasts about 2 days, during which time the person is completely disoriented, is extremely agitated, sweats, and has a fever and a changing pulse and blood pressure. The person usually has no memory of this condition.

Withdrawal Treatment

A patient undergoing alcohol withdrawal may be treated with one of the long half-life benzodiazepines, most commonly diazepam or chlordiazepoxide, but occasionally clorazepate or flurazepam. Older alcoholics or those with severe liver disease may be treated with a short half-life benzodiazepine, oxazepam, lorazepam or temazepam. This treatment is effective because alcohol is cross-tolerant with the benzodiazepines.

TABLE 51-8 Drug Interactions With Disulfiram

SYSTEM	COMMENTS
Phenytoin (Dilantin), coumarins (oral anticoagulants)	Potentiated by disulfiram, which inhibits their degradation by liver microsomal enzymes
Benzodiazepines	Potentiated by disulfiram, which inhibits their plasma clearance
Benzodiazepines and ascorbic acid (vitamin C)	Decreased alcohol-disulfiram reaction by protecting acetaldehyde-oxidizing enzymes
Tricyclic antidepressants	Increased alcohol-disulfiram reaction by inhibiting acetaldehyde-oxidizing enzymes
Isoniazid, metronidazole	Can cause neuropsychiatric symptoms by unknown mechanism in presence of disulfiram

Additional therapy during withdrawal is designed to restore normal metabolic parameters and overcome the thiamin, vitamin B_{12}, and folic acid deficiencies. This supportive therapy relieves neurologic symptoms related to hypoglycemia, ketosis, and vitamin deficiency.

Disulfiram (Antabuse) is prescribed for the detoxified patient who wishes to avoid drinking again (see box). Disulfiram blocks the oxidation of acetaldehyde. The accumulation of acetaldehyde causes unpleasant reactions, which include flushing, throbbing in the head and neck, throbbing headache, respiratory difficulty, nausea, copious vomiting, sweating, thirst, chest pain, rapid breathing, tachycardia, fainting, weakness, vertigo, blurred vision, and confusion. These effects can be elicited by alcohol for 1 to 2 weeks after disulfiram is discontinued. The reaction lasts from 30 minutes to 1 to 3 hours. Severe reactions can cause death from cardiovascular collapse or respiratory failure. Because of the severity of the reactions, only well-informed, motivated patients are considered for disulfiram therapy, which is at best a supportive treatment when supplemented by psychiatric therapy. Patients whose drinking problem is lack of moderation after the first drink is taken are considered the best candidates for disulfiram therapy. By itself, disulfiram produces transient effects such as drowsiness, fatigue, impotence, headache, acne, and a metallic or garliclike aftertaste. These effects usually disappear within 2 weeks. Drug interactions with disulfiram are listed in Table 51-8.

Interactions

Alcohol is a major source of drug interactions because it is so widely consumed. Alcohol particularly influences other CNS depressants, drug metabolism, gastric mucosal integrity, blood glucose levels, and vasodilation. Table 51-9 summarizes drug interactions with alcohol. The importance of alcohol as a source of drug interactions can be appreciated by considering the estimate that 5% of adults in the United States are alcoholic and that 30% to 60% of hospitalized individuals are alcoholic.

TABLE 51-9 Sources of Drug Interactions With Alcohol

EFFECT	INTERACTING DRUGS	COMMENTS
Increased CNS depression	Barbiturates Meprobamate Hypnotics Antihistamines Narcotic analgesics Monoamine oxidase inhibitors Tricyclic antidepressants Benzodiazepines Chlorpromazine and other sedating phenothiazines	Any drug causing sedation or drowsiness is potentiated by alcohol. Most of these drugs carry warnings not to drive or operate dangerous equipment and stating that situation worsens if alcohol is ingested. Alcohol can cause coma or death by respiratory depression when combined with CNS depressants even when the dose of either drug is not lethal by itself.
Increased liver metabolism	Barbiturates Phenytoin Tolbutamide Warfarin	When taken over long period, alcohol induces liver microsomal enzyme system for drug degradation. This speeds up metabolism of drugs metabolized by these enzymes so that effective therapeutic dose must be increased. Alternatively, if alcoholic person receiving one of these drugs becomes detoxified, drug dose may need to be lowered.
Gastric and mucosal irritation	Aspirin Nicotine	Aspirin and alcohol act synergistically to irritate stomach and to cause bleeding. Alcoholic smokers have up to a 15-fold greater incidence of oral cancer.
Hypoglycemia	Insulin	Alcohol acts to lower blood glucose levels independently of insulin and may cause marked hypoglycemia when taken with insulin.
Disulfiram-like reaction	Disulfiram Sulfonylureas (oral hypoglycemic agents) Nitroglycerin	Disulfiram inhibits degradation of acetaldehyde, which then accumulates and causes hypotension, GI distress, and headache.
Vasodilation	Guanethidine Nitroglycerin	Alcohol acts centrally to produce vasodilation, which can potentiate action of these drugs.

NURSING PROCESS OVERVIEW

Sedative-Hypnotic and Antianxiety Drugs

Assessment

Perform a systematic assessment, with attention to vital signs, level of consciousness, and emotional affect. Investigate fully any subjective complaints and other health problems.

Nursing Diagnoses

- Potential complication: drug dependence or addiction
- Risk for depressed level of consciousness

Patient Outcomes

The patient will use sedatives or hypnotics for a short period of time, with no accompanying side effects. The patient will state relief of insomnia or anxiety. Other outcomes are appropriate for other uses of these drugs.

Planning/Implementation

The common denominator of the drugs discussed in this chapter is that they produce CNS depression. Assess level of consciousness, affect, vital signs, and blood pressure. Work with the patient to identify nonmedicinal treatments that may help. For example, patients being treated with sedative-hypnotics to produce sleep may be aided by bedtime remedies such as warm milk, relaxing in a warm bath, or reading briefly. Monitor the ability of hospitalized patients to ambulate safely, and keep siderails up at night. If these drugs are being used by IV routes, have appropriate equipment for resuscitation and a suction machine available.

Evaluation

The success of these drugs depends on the original purpose for which they were being used. Before discharge, verify that the patient can explain how to take the prescribed medication correctly, what symptoms may indicate too high a dose of medication, what to do if the medication is no longer effective, and when to return to the physician for follow-up. Determine that the patient can list other drugs to avoid such as alcohol or other antianxiety drugs. Use judgment in indicating to the patient that continued prolonged use of these drugs or use in increasing amounts can lead to drug dependence or addiction.

NURSING IMPLICATIONS SUMMARY

General Guidelines: Use of Antianxiety Agents and Sedative-Hypnotics

Drug Administration

- In the institutional setting, keep siderails up after administering antianxiety and sedative-hypnotic agents. Supervise ambulation and smoking. Keep a night light on.
- Use "sleeping pills" judiciously. Do not deprive patients of needed medication, but use medications as an adjunct to nursing measures such as a backrub, repositioning, a small snack, or a glass of warm milk.
- Tactfully assess side effects. Some drugs cause changes in libido or sexual activity. Provide emotional support as appropriate. Consult with the physician about changes in drug or dosage.
- Be alert in the outpatient setting to patients who return for prescription refills on an increasingly frequent basis; this may indicate improper use or abuse or lack of knowledge about the hazards of continued use of the drugs. Evaluate patients carefully for possible depression and suicidal tendencies.

Patient and Family Education

- Remind the patient to take these drugs only as directed and not to increase the dose or frequency without consulting the physician. Stress the importance of returning for regular follow-up visits if these drugs are used for long-term treatment.
- Warn the patient to avoid driving or operating hazardous equipment if drowsiness, dizziness, unsteadiness, or clumsiness develops. Supervise the play of children.
- Warn the patient to avoid ingestion of alcohol. Instruct the patient to avoid the use of other drugs that may depress the CNS, unless they are specifically prescribed by the physician. Examples include antiemetics, narcotic analgesics, and antihistamines.
- For insomnia, instruct the patient to take doses 30 minutes before bedtime.
- Instruct the patient that the frequently encountered hangover effect in the morning after use of a sedative-hypnotic is a side effect of the medication and not a sign that the patient needs a larger dose of medication the next evening.
- Caution the patient taking anticonvulsant medication that drowsiness may continue for several days to weeks but should gradually diminish. Emphasize the importance of taking the drug as ordered, and not discontinuing the drug without consultation with the physician. Encourage the patient with a history of seizures to wear a medical identification tag or bracelet.
- Instruct the patient to inform all health care providers of all drugs being used, even occasional sleeping pills.
- Instruct the patient to keep these and all drugs out of the reach of children, to use childproof caps in settings where there are small children, and to keep drugs in clearly labeled containers.
- Remind the patient not to share drugs with friends or relatives.
- Refer the patient who is having continuing problems with insomnia or anxiety to appropriate resources for counseling or evaluation.
- After long-term use, the patient may have difficulty discontinuing the medication abruptly. Instruct the patient to consult the physician before discontinuing medications.

Benzodiazepines

Drug Administration

- See the general guidelines.
- Monitor blood pressure and pulse, intake and output, and weight. Monitor the respiratory rate and auscultate breath sounds. Inspect for skin changes.
- Monitor complete blood count (CBC) and platelets, liver function tests, blood urea nitrogen (BUN), and serum creatinine levels.
- Instruct a patient taking flurazepam that several weeks of therapy may be needed to see the full effects of therapy.

Intravenous Benzodiazeplnes

- Have a suction machine and equipment for intubation and ventilatory support available. Too rapid administration may cause apnea, hypotension, or respiratory or cardiac arrest. Monitor respiratory rate and blood pressure. Do not leave the patient unattended unless the individual is sufficiently alert to handle secretions and to call for assistance.
- Keep siderails up.
- Have the patient rest in bed for 2 to 8 hours after IV doses. Monitor vital signs, mental status, and balance.

Intravenous Diazepam

- Administer diazepam undiluted, at a rate of 5 mg (1 ml) or less over 1 minute in adults. Administer the dose over 3 minutes in children and infants. Do not mix with any other drugs.

Intravenous Chlordiazepoxide

- Dilute each 100 mg of chlordiazepoxide with at least 5 ml 0.9% sodium chloride injection or sterile water for injection; do not use the diluent provided for IM injection for IV administration. Administer 100 mg diluted over at least 1 minute.

Intravenous Lorazepam

- Dilute lorazepam just before administering with an equal volume of compatible IV fluid such as 0.9% sodium chloride or 5% dextrose in water (D5W). Administer at a rate of 2 mg or less over 1 minute.

Intravenous Midazolam

- Midazolam may be diluted with normal saline, D5W, or

Continued.

lactated Ringer's solution. Rate of administration is often determined by the patient's response (e.g., 1 mg/4 ml, administered over at least 2 minutes until speech is slurred). For conscious sedation, evaluate carefully to avoid overmedication; wait 2 minutes between increments. Because of the risk of respiratory depression, use this drug only in settings where personnel are trained in the use of the drug and trained in the ability to intubate and provide ventilatory support. Have oxygen, a suction machine, and resuscitation equipment nearby. Monitor vital signs. Use lower doses in older adults or debilitated patients.

Patient and Family Education

- See the general guidelines.
- Instruct the patient to report any new side effects.
- See the patient problem boxes on dry mouth (p. 300) and photosensitivity (p. 649).
- Instruct the patient to take doses with meals or a snack to lessen gastric irritation.

Flumazenil

Drug Administration

- Consult the manufacturer's literature for current guidelines.
- Monitor vital signs, blood pressure, and level of consciousness. Have a suction machine at the bedside. Keep siderails up. Do not leave the patient unattended.
- Administration of this drug to patients who have used benzodiazepines on a long-term basis may precipitate withdrawal symptoms.
- Keep the patient and family informed of the patient's condition.

Barbiturates

Drug Administration

- See the general guidelines.
- Monitor blood pressure and pulse, intake and output, and weight. Monitor the respiratory rate and auscultate breath sounds. Inspect for skin changes.
- Monitor CBC, platelet count, and liver function tests.
- With IV administration, monitor vital signs and respiratory rate. Have a suction machine and equipment for intubation and ventilatory assistance available. The patient should rest in bed until the condition is stable.
- Phenobarbital is also discussed in Chapter 55.

Intravenous Amobarbital

- Dilute each 125 mg of amobarbital with at least 1.25 ml sterile water for injection to make a 10% solution. Administer each 100 mg or less over 1 minute in adults and each 60 mg or less over 1 minute in infants or children. Too rapid injection may cause symptoms of overdose.

Intravenous Pentobarbital

- Pentobarbital may be administered undiluted or may be diluted in sterile water, normal saline for injection, or Ringer's injection. Add 1 ml (50 mg) of pentobarbital or 9 ml diluent to make a dilution of 5 mg/ml. Administer at a rate of 50 mg or less over 1 minute.

Intravenous Secobarbital

- Secobarbital may be administered undiluted or diluted with sterile water for injection, 0.9% sodium chloride injection, or Ringer's injection. Reconstitute powder form by adding 5 ml diluent to 250 mg of drug to make a 5% solution. Administer at a rate of 50 mg or less over 1 minute.

Patient and Family Education

- See the general guidelines.
- Instruct the patient to report any new side effects.
- Instruct the patient to take doses with meals or a snack to lessen gastric irritation.

Miscellaneous Agents

- See the general guidelines.
- Monitor blood pressure and pulse and intake and output.
- When used in the doses ordered, side effects are rare.
- For buspirone: One to 2 weeks of therapy may be required to see full effect of therapy.
- For chloral hydrate: Take capsule form with a full (8-ounce) glass of water, fruit juice, or ginger ale to decrease gastric irritation. For chloral hydrate syrup: Dilute dose in up to 4 ounces (120 ml) of clear liquid such as water, apple juice, or ginger ale to improve taste and decrease gastric irritation. Oral chloral hydrate may be dissolved in olive oil or cottonseed oil to administer as a retention enema if needed; consult pharmacist.
- For ethchlorvynol: Take doses with snack or milk to lessen dizziness caused by rapid absorption.

Disulfiram

Drug Administration/Patient and Family Education

- See the patient problem box on disulfiram-like reactions (p. 635), and review the side effects discussed in the text.
- Treatment with disulfiram is not a cure for alcoholism and should be used only with other forms of supportive therapy. Assess the patient carefully before administering this drug.
- Treatment of severe disulfiram reaction may require hospitalization. Instruct the patient's family regarding the effects of concomitant alcohol consumption and disulfiram use.
- Caution patient to avoid driving or operating hazardous equipment if drowsiness develops after disulfiram administration. The physician may suggest administering dose at bedtime to lessen daytime drowsiness.
- Do not administer disulfiram until patient has been alcohol free at least 12 hours and the blood alcohol level is 0.
- The effects of disulfiram may persist for up to 2 weeks after disulfiram therapy is discontinued.

CRITICAL THINKING

APPLICATION

1. Define sedative, hypnotic, and antianxiety drugs.
2. What is the reticular activating system and how is it affected by general CNS depressants?
3. Describe the stages of CNS depression.
4. What is drug dependence?
5. What are withdrawal symptoms? What symptoms would you observe?
6. What is cross-tolerance? What precautions in medications would you observe?
7. Name the stages of sleep and describe which stages are affected by hypnotics.
8. What is anxiety? What symptoms would you observe?
9. What major advantage do benzodiazepines have over barbiturates?
10. Describe the uses of benzodiazepines. For what conditions are these drugs used?
11. Describe the four categories of barbiturates and list which drugs belong in each category.
12. Describe withdrawal symptoms from barbiturates. What symptoms might you observe?
13. Differentiate between metabolic tolerance and pharmacodynamic tolerance.
14. What are the uses of barbiturates?
15. Are hypnotics more similar to barbiturates or to benzodiazepines?
16. What drug interactions are seen with alcohol?
17. What factors affect alcohol absorption?
18. Describe alcohol metabolism. How does disulfiram interfere with alcohol metabolism?
19. What are the side effects of alcohol ingestion with disulfiram?
20. What physiologic changes are associated with long-term drinking?
21. How is alcohol withdrawal treated? What interventions might you take?

CRITICAL THINKING

1. What drug interactions are seen with benzodiazepines? What steps in patient education would you take?
2. What are some of the resources in your community for patients who express an interest in stopping alcohol consumption?
3. As a home health nurse, what would you assess in the home to provide information about the level of alcohol consumption of your patients?

CHAPTER 52

Antipsychotic Drugs

OBJECTIVES

After studying this chapter, you should be able to do the following:

- *Outline the kinds of psychoses discussed.*
- *Distinguish among the five chemical classes of antipsychotic drugs and the three subgroups of the phenothiazines.*
- *Discuss the role of the neurotransmitters dopamine, norepinephrine, and acetylcholine in the actions of the antipsychotics.*
- *Describe the signs and symptoms of extrapyramidal reactions to antipsychotic drugs.*
- *Develop a nursing care plan for a patient receiving one of the antipsychotic drugs discussed.*
- *Develop a care plan for a patient receiving a drug that may cause photosensitivity.*

KEY TERMS

acute dystonia
akathisia
antipsychotic drugs
functional psychosis
neuroleptic
organic psychosis
phenothiazines
pseudoparkinsonism
psychosis
schizophrenia
sedation and postural hypotension
tardive dyskinesia
toxic psychosis

CHAPTER OVERVIEW

One of the remarkable advances in pharmacology in recent decades has been the discovery and application of drugs effective in treating the major mental illnesses: schizophrenia and depression. This chapter discusses the antipsychotic or antischizophrenic drugs, also called *neuroleptic* drugs. **Neuroleptic** refers to the ability of these drugs to cause a general quiescence and a state of psychic indifference to the surroundings.

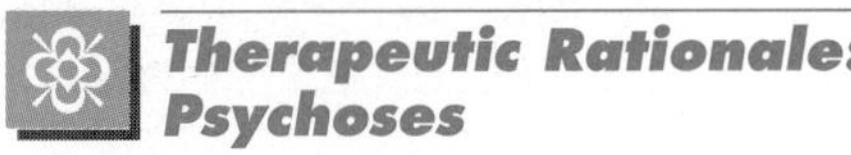

Therapeutic Rationale: Psychoses

A **psychosis** is a major emotional disorder with an impairment of mental function great enough to prevent the individual from participating in everyday life. The hallmark of a psychosis is the loss of contact with reality. There is no one symptom of a psychosis. Symptoms may include agitation, hostility, combativeness, hyperactivity, delusions, hallucinations, disordered thought and perception, emotional and social withdrawal, paranoid symptoms, and personal neglect. **Antipsychotic drugs** specifically reduce at least some of these symptoms so that patients can think and function more coherently.

Psychoses account for most of the hospitalizations for mental illness, disabling as many Americans as heart disease and cancer combined.

Functional Psychoses

A **functional psychosis** may be an isolated "breakdown" caused by a major traumatic event. This psychosis is usually amenable to treatment with an antipsychotic drug. The acute manic phase of manic-depressive illness is treated with an antipsychotic drug or lithium (see Chapter 53).

Schizophrenia

Schizophrenia is a chronic mental illness with psychotic episodes. Before the advent of the antipsychotic drugs in the 1950s, schizophrenia accounted for most of the patient population in mental hospitals. Today, with continued advances in antipsychotic drug therapy, patients with schizophrenia do not usually require the degree of supervision found in mental hospitals. The current trend is to provide acute initial care in the psychiatric intensive care unit followed by minimum care in community facilities. Antipsychotic drugs do not cure schizophrenia. Treatment is lifelong, although patients may not require medication for several weeks or months during a disease remission.

Organic Psychoses

An **organic psychosis** results from damage to the brain by infectious diseases, deficiency diseases, lead poisoning, tumors, and injury through trauma or interrupted blood supply such as in cerebrovascular accidents (stroke). Organic psychoses are not treated with antipsychotic drugs as successfully as functional psychoses.

Toxic Psychoses

A **toxic psychosis** can arise during withdrawal from alcohol or other drugs. Some toxic psychoses are treated with diazepam, an antianxiety drug, rather than with antipsychotic drugs. Amphetamine can cause a toxic psychosis because it releases dopamine in the central nervous system (CNS), and therefore the blockade of dopamine receptors by antipsychotic drugs provides specific therapy for an amphetamine-induced psychosis.

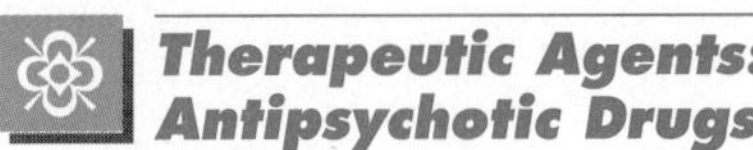

Therapeutic Agents: Antipsychotic Drugs

Antipsychotic Drugs: General Characteristics

Chemical Classes

There are five chemical classes of antipsychotic drugs: phenothiazines, thioxanthenes, butyrophenones, dibenzoxazepines, and dihydroindolones. The latter three classes contribute only four drugs to present clinical use. Ten phenothiazine and two thioxanthene compounds are currently in clinical use as antipsychotic drugs.

The largest antipsychotic drug class is the **phenothiazines.** Chlorpromazine was the first phenothiazine introduced in the United States and is still the most widely used drug in this class. Chlorpromazine originally was licensed as an antiemetic drug, later as a drug to potentiate anesthesia, and finally as an antipsychotic drug. The other major antipsychotic drugs, the thioxanthenes, have a three-ringed main structure that differs by only one atom from that of the phenothiazines. The remaining three drug classes, the butyrophenones, the dibenzoxazepines, and the dihydroindolones are chemically different from the phenothiazines and from each other. However, the three classes behave the same pharmacologically with respect to potency and side effects (Table 52-1).

Subgroups of phenothiazines. The phenothiazines are subdivided into three subgroups based on chemical differences in side groups on the three-ringed main structure. These subgroups are the aliphatic, the piperidine, and the piperazine phenothiazines. The three subgroups differ in potency and in the incidence of key side effects, as summarized in Table 52-2.

Mechanism of Action

Antipsychotic drugs as dopamine receptor antagonists. Four effects of antipsychotic drugs have been linked to the blockade of dopamine receptors in various parts of the brain. The antipsychotic effect arises from receptor blockade in the limbic system and the antiemetic effect from receptor blockade in the chemoreceptor trigger zone. These effects are used therapeutically. Extrapyramidal effects arise from blockade in the corpus striatum of neurons from the basal ganglia and endocrine effects from blockade in the pituitary gland. These two effects are undesired actions of antipsychotic drugs.

Antipsychotic drugs as adrenergic and cholinergic receptor antagonists. The phenothiazines and thioxanthenes block receptors for norepinephrine and dopamine. At one time the antipsychotic action was believed to be the blockade of CNS norepinephrine receptors. The finding that the butyrophenone haloperidol blocked only dopamine and not norepinephrine receptors, however, solidified the data implicating the major role of dopamine rather than norepinephrine in psychotic disorders.

TABLE 52-1 Antipsychotic Drugs

GENERIC NAME	TRADE NAME	ADMINISTRATION/DOSAGE	COMMENTS
Butyrophenone			
✣ Haloperidol	Apo-Haloperidol† Haldol Novo-Peridol† Paridol† PMS-Haloperidol†	Acute psychotic management: ORAL: *Adults and children >12 yr*—1-15 mg in divided doses initially, which can be increased gradually up to 100 mg to bring symptoms under control. Dosage is then gradually reduced. Maintenance dose, usually 2-8 mg daily. FDA pregnancy category C. *Older adult patients and children <12 yr*—0.5-1.5 mg daily initially. Dosage increased by 0.5 mg increments if necessary. Usual maintenance dose, 2-4 mg daily. INTRAMUSCULAR: *Adults and children >12 yr*—2-5 mg every 4-8 hr or every hour if acute state requires. Acute symptoms are usually under control in 72 hr, and 15 mg daily is usually sufficient. Chronic schizophrenia: ORAL: *Adults and children >12 yr*—6-16 mg in divided doses, gradually increased to achieve control. Doses as high as 100 mg may be necessary to achieve control. Doses then are gradually reduced to achieve maintenance of control, usually 15-20 mg daily. *Older adult patients*—0.5-1.5 mg initially, increased very gradually. Maintenance dosage, usually 2-8 mg daily. Mental retardation with hyperkinesia: ORAL: (given after IM treatment as for acute psychoses): *Adults and children >12 yr*—80-120 mg daily, gradually reduced to maintenance dose of about 60 mg daily. *Older adult patients and children <12 yr*—1.5-6 mg daily in divided doses; gradually increase dosage up to 15 mg daily for control, then reduce dosage for maintenance. Gilles de la Tourette's syndrome: Initial dosages to achieve control are same as for chronic schizophrenia. Maintenance dosages: *Adults and children >12 yr*—9 mg daily; *Children <12 yr*—1.5 mg daily.	Management of psychotic disorders. Likely to produce extrapyramidal reactions in patients prone to neurologic reactions. In severe cases of hyperkinetic, retarded patients, large doses may bring improvement in social behavior and concentration. Drug of choice for treatment of Gilles de la Tourette's syndrome. Spectrum of side effects is similar to that of piperazine phenothiazines: low incidence of sedation and autonomic effects but high incidence of extrapyramidal reactions.
Dibenzoxazepines			
Clozapine	Clozaril	ORAL: *Adults*—Initially, 25 mg 1-2 times a day, increasing in increments of 25-60 mg/day, as tolerated, to achieve dose of 300-450 mg/day by end of 2 weeks. Subsequent dosage increments should not exceed 100 mg 1 or 2 times/week.	Atypical antipsychotic, indicated only in management of severely ill schizophrenic patients failing to respond to other drugs. Monitor for agranulocytosis and seizures.
Loxapine succinate	Loxitane Loxapac†	ORAL: *Patients >16 yr*—10-25 mg twice daily initially, with dosage increased rapidly over 7-10 days to achieve control. Dosage reduced for maintenance to 60-100 mg daily; maximum, 250 mg daily. FDA pregnancy category C. *Older adult patients*—⅓-½ dose just listed.	Effective for schizophrenia and acute psychoses.
Dihydroindolone			
Molindone hydrochloride	Moban	ORAL: *Adults*—15-40 mg daily initially, with increased dosage to control symptoms, up to 225 mg daily. Dosage should then be reduced for maintenance. *Older adult patients*—⅓-½ adult dose.	Effective for schizophrenia and acute psychoses.

*Available in Canada and United States.
†Available in Canada only.

TABLE 52-1 Antipsychotic Drugs—cont'd

GENERIC NAME	TRADE NAME	ADMINISTRATION/DOSAGE	COMMENTS
Phenothiazines			
Aliphatic			
✣ Chlorpromazine hydrochloride	Thorazine Chlorpromanyl† Largactil† Thor-Prom Novo-Chlorpromazine† Various others	Psychiatric outpatients: ORAL: *Adults*—12-40 yr, average dose 400-800 mg daily, >40 yr, limit of 300 mg daily is suggested. Acutely psychotic hospitalized patients: INTRAMUSCULAR: *Adults*—25-100 mg every 1-4 hr until symptoms are controlled. *Older adult or debilitated patients*—10 mg every 6-8 hr to control acute symptoms. *Children*—0.5 mg/kg body weight every 6-8 hr, gradually increasing dose to maximum of 40 mg for children <5 yr and 75 mg for those between 5-12 yr. INTRAVENOUS: Not recommended because it is highly irritating. Drug must be diluted to at least 1 mg/ml and no more than 1 mg/min given. ORAL: *Adults*—200-600 mg daily in divided doses, increased every 2-3 days by 100 mg, up to 2 gm if needed. *Older adult or debilitated patients*—⅓-½ adult dose with 20-25 mg increments. *Children*—0.5 mg/kg every 4-6 hr. To control nausea and vomiting: ORAL: 10-25 mg every 4-6 hr. INTRAMUSCULAR: 25 mg initially, then 25-50 mg every 3-4 hr to stop vomiting.	Control of initial acute psychotic episodes is achieved with high doses, which are then tapered to lowest maintenance dose when patient's condition stabilizes. Best tolerated by patients <40 years of age and those hospitalized less than 10 years. Sedation is pronounced at start of therapy, which may be desired for highly agitated patients. Incidence of hypotension, ophthalmic changes, and dyskinesias is high in older adult patients. Antiadrenergic and anticholinergic side effects usually diminish after first week. Not for seizure-prone patients. Severe nausea and vomiting can be controlled by low doses.
		Other uses: ORAL: *Adults*—25-50 mg 3 or 4 times daily. INTRAMUSCULAR: 25 mg every 3 or 4 hr.	Other uses include intractable hiccups, tetanus, and acute intermittent porphyria.
Methotrimeprazine hydrochloride	Nozinan Oral Drops† Nozinan Liquid†	ORAL: *Adults*—For psychotic disorders or presurgical sedation: 6-25 mg/day in 3 divided doses with meals. Severe psychosis: 50-75 mg/day in divided doses with meals. *Children*—0.25 mg/kg body weight/day in 2 or 3 divided doses with meals. Increase gradually as needed, but no more than 40 mg/day in children under 12 yr old.	Used as antipsychotic, analgesic, antianxiety agent, and sedative. For moderate-to-severe pain of bedridden patients; obstetric pain and sedation; anxiety before surgery; and adjunctive therapy in general anesthesia to increase effects of anesthetics.
Methotrimeprazine maleate	Nozinan†	ORAL: *Adults, children*—Same doses as for hydrochloride.	
Methotrimeprazine	Levoprome* Nozinan†	INTRAMUSCULAR: *Adults*—Acute pain: 10-20 mg at 4 to 6 hr intervals; Obstetric pain: 15-20 mg, repeat if needed; postoperative pain: 2.5-7.5 mg immediately after surgery, repeated every 3-4 hr as needed.	For pain relief.
Promazine hydrochloride	Primazine Prozine-50 Sparine*	Severly agitated patients: INTRAMUSCULAR: *Adults*—50-150 mg initially; if no calming effect in 30 min, additonal doses may be given to total of 300 mg. ORAL: *Adults*—10-200 mg every 4-6 hr (may also be given IM).	When IM route is used, take precautions for postural hypotension. Syrup is available for oral administration; dilute concentrate in fruit juice or chocolate flavored drinks.
Triflupromazine hydrochloride	Vesprin	ORAL, INTRAMUSCULAR: *Children >12 yr*—10-25 mg every 4-6 hr.	Total daily dose for adults should not exceed 1000 mg.
		Psychotic disorders: ORAL: *Adults*—50-150 mg daily. *Older adult patients*—20-30 mg orally daily. *Children >2½ yr*—0.5 mg/kg body weight, up to 150 mg maximum.	Management of psychotic disorders. Control of nausea and vomiting.

TABLE 52-1 Antipsychotic Drugs—cont'd

GENERIC NAME	TRADE NAME	ADMINISTRATION/DOSAGE	COMMENTS
Phenothiazines—cont'd			
Aliphatic—cont'd			
		INTRAMUSCULAR: *Adults*—50-150 mg daily. *Older adult patients*—10-75 mg daily. *Children >2½ yr*—0.2-0.25 mg/kg up to 10 mg maximum. All daily doses for children should be divided. Nausea and vomiting: INTRAVENOUS: *Adults*—1 mg up to 3 mg. INTRAMUSCULAR: *Adults*—5-15 mg every 4 hr up to 60 mg daily. ORAL: *Adults*—20-30 mg total daily. ORAL, INTRAMUSCULAR: *Children >2½ yr*—0.2 mg/kg, to 10 mg in 3 doses daily.	
Piperazine‡			
Acetophenazine maleate	Tindal	ORAL: *Adults*—60 mg daily in divided doses that can be increased in 20-mg increments. Optimum level is usually 80-120 mg. Occasionally, severe symptoms require 400-600 mg. *Older adult patients*—⅓-½ adult dose. *Children*—0.8-1.6 mg/kg body weight in divided doses. Maximum, 80 mg daily.	Management of psychotic disorders.
Fluphenazine decanoate	Prolixin Decanoate Modecate†	INTRAMUSCULAR, SUBCUTANEOUS: *Adults <50 yr*—12.5 mg initially, then 25 mg every 2 weeks. Increase by 12.5 mg amounts if needed. Treatment rarely requires more than 100 mg every 2-6 weeks.	Long-acting depot forms last at least 2 weeks. Dosage should be stabilized in hospital because severe episodes of parkinsonism can appear. Not recommended for older adult patients or patients who have had difficulty with extrapyramidal reactions.
Fluphenazine enanthate	Prolixin Moditen Enanthate†	INTRAMUSCULAR, SUBCUTANEOUS: *Adults*—25 mg; repeat or increase every 1-3 weeks as needed and tolerated.	
Fluphenazine hydrochloride	Moditen† Permitil Prolixin	ORAL: *Adults*—2.5-10 mg initially, reduced to 1-5 mg daily for maintenance. *Older adult patients*—⅓-½ adult dose. INTRAMUSCULAR: *Adults*—1.25 mg increased gradually to 2.5-10 mg daily in 3-4 doses. *Older adult patients*—⅓-½ adult dose.	Most potent of phenothiazines used for management of psychotic disorders.
Perphenazine	Apo-Perphenazine† Phenazine† Trilafon*	ORAL: *Adults*—16-64 mg daily in divided doses. *Older adult patients*—⅓-½ adult dose. *Children >12 yr*—6-12 mg daily. INTRAMUSCULAR: *Adults*—5-10 mg initially, then 5 mg every 6 hr with 15 mg maximum daily in ambulatory and 30 mg daily in hospitalized patients. *Older adult patients*—⅓-½ adult dose. *Children >12 yr*—lowest adult dose.	For acute psychotic disorders. Lower doses needed when used as antiemetic.
✣ Prochlorperazine	Compazine	Psychiatric disorders: ORAL: *Adults*—5-10 mg 3 to 4 times daily.	More widely used to control severe nausea and vomiting than for psychiatric treatment. Hypotension is seen when given intravenously for surgery.
Prochlorperazine edisylate	Compazine Edisylate	Raise dosage every 2-3 days as required. From 50-75 mg daily is common range for mild cases and 100-150 mg for severe cases.	
✣ Prochlorperazine maleate	Compazine Maleate PMS-Prochlorperazine† Prorazin† Stemetil†	*Older adult patients*—⅓-½ adult dose. *Children >2 yr*—2.5 mg 2-3 times daily up to total dose of 20-25 mg. Same dosage used rectally. INTRAMUSCULAR: *Adults*—10-20 mg in buttock; repeat every 2-4 hr up to 80 mg total. *Older adult patients*—⅓-½ adult dose. *Children >2 yr*—0.13 mg/kg body weight initial dose only, then switch to oral.	

‡The piperazine phenothiazines are less sedative in effect and have fewer autonomic side effects than other phenothiazine classes. Extrapyramidal reactions are more common, particularly in large doses in patients over age 40. Piperazine phenothiazines are less likely to produce allergic reactions and do not change ECG tracings.

TABLE 52-1 Antipsychotic Drugs—cont'd

GENERIC NAME	TRADE NAME	ADMINISTRATION/DOSAGE	COMMENTS
Phenothiazines—cont'd *Piperazine‡—cont'd*		Nausea and vomiting: ORAL: *Adults*—5-10 mg 3 or 4 times daily. *Children 20-29 lb*—2.5 mg 1-2 times daily; *children 30-39 lb*—2.5 mg 2-3 times daily; *children 40-85 lb*—2.5 mg 3 times daily or 5 mg 2 times daily. INTRAMUSCULAR: *Adults*—5-10 mg every 3-4 hr. *Children*—0.06 mg/lb. RECTAL: *Adults*—25 mg twice daily. *Children*—Same as oral dosage.	
Thiopropazate hydrochloride	Dartal†	ORAL: *Adults*—10 mg 3 times/day, adjusting gradually by 10 mg every 3 or 4 days as needed and tolerated. Maintenance dose, 10-20 mg 2-4 times/day. Reduce dosage for older adult, emaciated, or debilitated patients.	To treat psychotic disorders.
Thioproperazine mesylate	Majeptil†	ORAL: *Adults*—Initially, 5 mg/day, adjusted gradually by 5 mg every 2 or 3 days as needed and tolerated. Usual effective dose is 30-40 mg/day.	To treat psychotic disorders.
Trifluoperazine	Stelazine Terfluzine† Various others	ORAL: *Adults*—2-4 mg daily in divided doses (outpatient), 4-10 mg daily (hospitalized). *Older adult or debilitated patients*—⅓-½ adult dosage. *Children >6 yr*—1 mg 1-2 times daily, gradually raised to maximum of 15 mg. INTRAMUSCULAR: *Adults*—1-2 mg every 4-6 hr, maximum 10 mg daily. *Older adult or debilitated patients*—⅓-½ adult dose. *Children >6 yr*—same as oral dosage.	Management of psychotic disorders.
Piperidine			
Mesoridazine besylate	Serentil†	ORAL: *Adults*—150 mg daily initially. Increased by 50 mg increments until symptoms are controlled. *Older adult patients*—⅓-½ adult dose. INTRAMUSCULAR: *Adults and children >12 yr*—25-175 mg daily in divided doses (irritating).	Management of psychotic disorders. Metabolite of thioridazine with antiemetic activity and no reported retinopathy.
Pericyazine	Neuleptil†	ORAL: *Adults*—Initially, 5-20 mg in morning and 10-40 mg in evening as needed and tolerated. Maintenance: 2.5-15 mg in morning and 5-30 mg in evening.	To treat psychotic disorders.
Pipotiazine palmitate	Piportil L_4†	INTRAMUSCULAR: *Adults*—Initially, 50-100 mg, dosage increased in increments of 25 mg every 2 or 3 wk as needed and tolerated, usually up to maintenance dose of 75-150 mg every 4 wk.	To treat psychotic disorders.
Thioridazine hydrochloride	Apo-Thioridazine† Mellaril* Novo-Ridazine†	Psychotic disorders: ORAL: *Adults*—50-100 mg 3 times daily, increasing up to 800 mg. *Older adult patients*—⅓-½ adult dose. *Children >2 yr*—1 mg/kg body weight in divided doses. Depressive neurosis, alcohol withdrawal syndrome, intractable pain, and senility: 10-50 mg 2-4 times daily.	Management of psychotic disorders. Little antiemetic activity. Safe for patients with epilepsy. Possibly effective in alcohol withdrawal syndrome, intractable pain, and senility. Pronounced sedative and hypotensive side effects initially. One of least likely of antipsychotic drugs to cause extrapyramidal reactions because of pronounced anticholinergic action. Photosensitivity has not been reported. Doses over 800 mg daily have produced serious pigmentary retinopathy.

TABLE 52-1 Antipsychotic Drugs—cont'd

GENERIC NAME	TRADE NAME	ADMINISTRATION/DOSAGE	COMMENTS
Thioxanthenes§			
Chlorprothixene	Taractan Tarasan†	ORAL: *Adults and children >12 yr*—75-200 mg daily in divided doses. Gradually increase if necessary, with total optimum dose usually <600 mg daily. *Older adult patients*—½ adult dose. INTRAMUSCULAR: *Adults and children >12 yr*—75-200 mg daily in divided doses. *Older adult patients*—½ adult dose.	Management of psychotic disorders. Incidence of side effects same as for aliphatic phenothiazines including high sedation, autonomic effects, and low extrapyramidal effects.
Flupenthixol† decanoate	Fluanxol Depot†	INTRAMUSCULAR: *Adults*—initially, 20-40 mg every 4-10 days. May increase in 20 mg increments.	
Flupenthixol hydrochloride	Fluanxol†	ORAL: *Adults*—1 mg 3 times daily initially, increasing by 1 mg every 2-3 days as needed. Maintenance dosages: 3-6 mg, up to 12 mg maximum daily in divided doses. Older adult patients should be given lower dose.	Management of psychotic disorders.
Thiothixene	Navane*	ORAL: *Adults and children >12 yr*—6-10 mg daily in divided doses. Gradually increase, with usual optimal dose 20-30 mg daily, rarely as high as 60 mg daily. *Older adult patients*—⅓-½ adult dose. INTRAMUSCULAR: *Adults and children >12 yr*—4 mg 2-4 times daily; gradually increase if necessary to maximum of 30 mg. *Older adult patients*—⅓-½ adult dose.	Management of psychotic disorders. Incidence of side effects same as for piperazine phenothiazines, including low incidence of sedation and autonomic effects, and high incidence of extrapyramidal effects.

§Chemically related to the phenothiazines.

CNS effects and adrenergic receptor blockade. Norepinephrine is a neurotransmitter associated with specific neurons in the CNS, just as it is associated with the postganglionic neurons of the sympathetic nervous system. Neurons containing norepinephrine in the reticular activating system of the brain are associated with alertness. The sedative effect of the phenothiazines and the thioxanthenes may result from their blockade of these receptors for norepinephrine. The blockade of norepinephrine receptors in the vasomotor center inhibits peripheral sympathetic tone and causes orthostatic hypotension

Pharmacokinetics

The antipsychotic drugs are administered orally in tablet or syrup form. The syrup form is preferred for patients who hide or do not swallow pills. Many antipsychotic drugs are also available in injectable form. Only fluphenazine is available in two different depot forms for intramuscular (IM) injection, which require administration only every 3 to 6 weeks. Normally, antipsychotic drugs are given in divided daily doses initially and in daily doses when the patient's condition has stabilized. Peak plasma levels of the drug are reached 2 to 3 hours after oral administration. Up to 90% of the drug may be bound to plasma proteins. The drugs are metabolized in the liver and excreted in urine and feces. Excretion is slow, however, and metabolites may be found in urine as long as 6 months after the drug is discontinued. Apparently some metabolites are active. Improvement can last as long as 3 months after medication is halted; whether this reflects remission or presence of persistent active metabolites is unclear.

Uses

Dopamine theory of psychosis. Current ideas on the neurochemical origin of psychotic behavior come from an understanding of the action of the antipsychotic drugs. These drugs block receptors in the CNS for the neurotransmitter dopamine. The hypothesis is that too much of this neurotransmitter in the limbic system produces psychotic symptoms. The limbic system is that area of the brain that regulates emotional behavior. Blocking the receptors for dopamine in the limbic system reverses psychotic symptoms.

Antipsychotic effects may not be seen for 7 to 10 days after the start of therapy, and 4 to 6 weeks are needed to see the full effect of a given dosage regimen. Dosages must be adjusted for individual patients.

Emesis and dopamine. Dopamine is the neurotransmitter, located in the medullary chemoreceptor trigger zone, involved in vomiting (emesis). Antipsychotic drugs are effective in preventing vomiting by blocking these dopamine receptors.

Several antipsychotic drugs are prescribed to control vomiting. Chlorpromazine, triflupromazine, perphenazine, and prochlorperazine in particular are widely used as antiemetics. Chlorpromazine is also prescribed for intractable hiccups. Because of the numerous side effects of these drugs, their use

TABLE 52-2 Antipsychotic Drugs: Drug Class, Potency, and Major Side Effects

DRUG	EQUIPOTENT DOSE	RELATIVE INCIDENTS OF SIDE EFFECTS: SEDATIVE EFFECT	ORTHOSTATIC HYPOTENSION	ANTICHOLINERGIC EFFECTS	EXTRAPYRAMIDAL SYMPTOMS
Phenothiazines					
Aliphatic					
✣ Chlorpromazine	100	High	Moderate	Moderate/high	Moderate
Methotrimeprazine	75	High	High	Moderate	Low/moderate
Promazine	200	Moderate	Moderate	High	Moderate
Triflupromazine	25	High	Moderate	Moderate/high	Moderate/high
Piperidine					
Mesoridazine	50	High	Moderate	Moderate	Low
Pericyazine	10	High	Moderate	High	Moderate
Pipotiazine	100	Low	Low	Low	Low
Thioridazine	100	High	Moderate	Moderate/high	Low
Piperazine					
Acetophenazine	20	Moderate	Low	Low	High
Fluphenazine	2	Low/moderate	Low	Low	High
Perphenazine	8	Low/moderate	Low	Low	High
Prochlorperazine	10	Moderate	Low	Low	High
Thiopropazate	20	Low	Low	Low	High
Thioproperazine	10	Low	Low	Low	High
Trifluoperazine	4	Moderate	Low	Low	High
Thioxanthenes					
Chlorprothixene	100	High	Moderate/high	Moderate/high	Low/moderate
Thiothixene	4	Low	Low/moderate	Low	Moderate/high
Butyrophenone					
✣ Haloperidol	2	Low	Low	Low	High
Dibenzoxazepine					
Clozapine	75	High	Moderate/high	Moderate/high	Low
Lozapine	10	Moderate	Low/moderate	Low/moderate	Moderate/high
Dihydroindolone					
Molindone	10	Moderate	Low/moderate	Moderate	Moderate

as antiemetics is restricted to management of postoperative nausea and vomiting, radiation and chemotherapy sickness, nausea and vomiting caused by toxins, and intractable vomiting. Antipsychotic drugs commonly used as antiemetic drugs are listed in Chapter 25.

Antiemetic dosage is much smaller than for the antipsychotic dosage. The antiemetic effect is seen within 1 hour of administration.

Adverse Reactions, Contraindications, and Toxicity

Extrapyramidal reactions and dopamine deficiency. The most important side effects of the antipsychotic drugs are the extrapyramidal reactions described in Table 52-3. Extrapyramidal reactions are most frequent with the piperazine phenothiazines and least frequent with the aliphatic phenothiazines. Extrapyramidal reactions arise from the blockade of dopamine receptors in certain nuclei of the basal ganglia of the brain. This area of the brain is responsible for coordination of movement. A common extrapyramidal reaction is drug-induced parkinsonism. In parkinsonism, degeneration of dopamine neurons going to the basal ganglia occurs, resulting in a local deficiency of dopamine (see Chapter 56). Blockade of dopamine receptors in this area of the brain produces the same symptoms as dopamine deficiency.

Four extrapyramidal syndromes are associated with antipsychotic drugs: acute dystonia, akathisia, pseudoparkinsonism, and tardive dyskinesia. It is important to recognize these bizarre reactions as side effects of drug therapy that require palliative medication or reduction or discontinuance of therapy. Do not treat these reactions as manifestations of the psychotic disease being treated and do not raise the drug dosage.

Acute dystonia is a spasm of muscles of the tongue, face, neck, or back and may mimic seizures. Dystonia is usually seen in the first 5 days of antipsychotic therapy. It may be treated with an antihistaminic or anticholinergic antiparkinsonian drug (see Chapter 56). Injection of one of these drugs

PATIENT PROBLEM

Neuroleptic Malignant Syndrome

THE PROBLEM

Neuroleptic malignant syndrome (NMS), a potentially fatal syndrome, may occur at any time during therapy with neuroleptics. While rare, NMS is more commonly seen at the start of therapy, after patients are switched from one drug to another, after a dosage increase, or when a combination of drugs is used.

SIGNS AND SYMPTOMS

The patient may have convulsions, difficult or fast breathing, tachycardia or irregular pulse rate, fever, high or low blood pressure, increased sweating, loss of bladder control, skeletal muscle rigidity, pale skin, excessive weakness or fatigue, and an altered level of consciousness. There may be severe extrapyramidal side effects such as difficulty swallowing, excessive salivation, oculogyric crisis, and dyskinesia. The white blood cell count may be elevated in the range of 9500 to 26,000 cells/mm^3, and elevated liver function tests and creatine phosphokinase (CPK) level.

TREATMENT

The patient will require intensive care. Monitor vital signs, notify the physician, discontinue neuroleptic therapy. Monitor ECG changes. Administer antipyretics and use a cooling blanket to lower temperature. Monitor electrolytes and administer IV fluids. Drug treatment for NMS includes dantrolene and/or bromocriptine (experimental).

PATIENT AND FAMILY EDUCATION

NMS is rare. Instruct the patient and family to notify the physician of any sudden change in the patient's condition or of any unexpected sign or symptom.

usually dramatically relieves the dystonia. Dystonia reactions are most common in patients under 25 years of age and rarely persist after treatment of the acute reaction. Some of the classic reactions seen in dystonia include neck twisting (torticollis), upward gaze paralysis (oculogyric crisis), stereotyped motions of the jaw, and a spasm in which the head and feet create a horseshoe (∩) configuration (opisthotonos).

Akathisia is a motor restlessness and may be mistaken for psychotic restlessness or agitation. Akathisia commonly appears after the first few days of therapy, and if not recognized, the antipsychotic drug dosage may again be mistakenly increased to relieve the agitation. Patients experiencing akathisia have difficulty sitting still and may pace about, fidget, or constantly move their legs. Anticholinergic drugs or a muscle relaxant such as diazepam may treat these symptoms. If these treatments are not effective, a different antipsychotic drug may have to be tried. Tolerance does not quickly develop to akathisia, but akathisia disappears when the drug is discontinued.

Pseudoparkinsonism is marked by motor retardation and rigidity. Patients find it difficult to initiate movements or to carry them out. The face resembles a mask because emotions do not register on it. The patient has a shuffling gait and hypersalivates. Tremor is seen in the hands and legs. These parkinsonian symptoms commonly appear after a week of therapy and are treated with antiparkinsonian drugs. Tolerance does not develop to the parkinsonian symptoms. If they cannot be controlled with drug therapy, the antipsychotic drug must be changed.

Tardive dyskinesia is associated with long-term, high-dose antipsychotic therapy. It is most common in older adult women and in patients who have had a stroke. Tardive dyskinesia is the worst of the extrapyramidal reactions since it cannot be readily treated, is persistent, and may not altogether

TABLE 52-3 Side Effects of Antipsychotic Drugs

TYPE OF EFFECT	SIGNS AND SYMPTOMS	COMMENTS
Adrenergic blockade (CNS)	Sedation	Usually transient
	Postural (orthostatic) hypotension	
Cholinergic blockade	Atropine-like effects: dry mouth, blurred vision, constipation, and delayed micturition	Usually transient
Endocrine—dopamine blockade	Men: erection problems	Usually transient
	Women: menstrual irregularities and unexpected lactation	
Extrapyramidal—dopamine blockade	Acute dystonia: neck twisting, facial grimacing, abnormal eye movements, and involuntary muscle movements	Most common during first few days of therapy; usually disappears after brief treatment with antiparkinsonian drugs
	Akathisia: restlessness, difficulty in sitting still, and strong urge to move about	Most common during first few days of therapy; control with antiparkinsonian drugs or diazepam
	Parkinsonism: motor retardation, masklike face, tremor, rigidity, salivation, and shuffling gait	Most common after first week of therapy; control with antiparkinsonian drugs
	Tardive dyskinesia: protrusion of tongue, puffing of cheeks, chewing movements, involuntary movements of extremities, and involuntary movements of trunk	Most common when dosage is lowered after prolonged therapy; older adult female patients at greatest risk; may not be reversible
Allergic reactions	Photosensitivity	Common
	Cholestatic hepatitis	Rare
	Agranulocytosis	Rare

disappear when the drug therapy is discontinued. It usually appears some months after therapy has been started when the drug dosage is reduced or discontinued. Tardive dyskinesia may represent the development of receptors that are supersensitive to dopamine after prolonged blockade by the antipsychotic drugs. Thus removing the antipsychotic drug worsens the condition since dopamine then has ready access to these supersensitive receptors. Antiparkinsonian drugs also worsen the condition since they either increase dopamine or block the acetylcholine opposing the dopamine. Some common symptoms of tardive dyskinesia are protrusion of the tongue (fly-catcher sign), puffing of the cheeks or the tongue in a cheek (bonbon sign), chewing movements, and involuntary movements of the extremities and trunk. Recent recognition that tardive dyskinesia is a common reaction in up to 50% of patients treated for a long time with high doses of antipsychotic drugs has prompted reevaluation of long-term therapy with these drugs. The current choice is to use as low a dose as possible and to put the patient on a "drug holiday" during periods of remission.

Sedation and postural hypotension are most often seen early in treatment with the aliphatic phenothiazines, the class of phenothiazines with the most prominent adrenergic blocking activity. These side effects are most likely to be prominent in older adults or debilitated patients. If sedation and hypotension are not severe, the dosage can be reduced and then gradually increased to produce tolerance to these effects, or another drug can be tried. Antipsychotic drugs are not addicting.

Anticholinergic actions. All the antipsychotic drugs have some anticholinergic action. The atropine like effects of dry mouth, blurred vision, delayed micturition, and constipation are common side effects. However, a central anticholinergic action is beneficial in controlling some extrapyramidal reactions. Extrapyramidal reactions such as parkinsonian symptoms are believed to reflect a relative lack of dopamine and a relative abundance of acetylcholine in neuronal areas controlling movement coordination (see Chapter 56). Since antipsychotic drugs produce extrapyramidal reactions by blocking the action of dopamine, those drugs that also have substantial ability to block the action of acetylcholine have less tendency to cause extrapyramidal reactions.

Electrocardiographic changes. The aliphatic phenothiazines are also the most likely to produce nonspecific changes in the T wave of the electrocardiogram (ECG). This change has no particular meaning but is undesirable in a patient with concurrent heart disease who is being monitored for ECG changes.

Seizure potential. Antipsychotic drugs must be used with caution in patients with epilepsy since the drugs can precipitate convulsions. Since antipsychotic drugs lower the convulsive threshold, the drugs are unsuitable to treat drug withdrawal that is likely to produce seizures such as withdrawal from alcohol, barbiturates, and other sedative-hypnotic drugs.

Endocrine disturbances. Dopamine inhibits the release of the hormone prolactin by the pituitary gland. Blockade of dopamine leads to hypersecretion of prolactin and secondarily to endocrine disturbances of the reproductive system by mechanisms not yet understood. Women may experience delayed ovulation and menstruation, lack of menstruation (amenorrhea), milk production (galactorrhea), or weight gain. Men may experience impotence, decreased libido, retrograde ejaculation, or moderate breast growth (gynecomastia).

Allergic reactions. Photosensitivity and cholestatic hepatitis occasionally develop during therapy. Photosensitivity is fairly common and represents an allergic reaction to a metabolite produced not by the body but by reaction with sunlight (see box). The long half-life of the antipsychotic drugs and their metabolites has been discussed. These metabolites accumulate in the skin, where exposure to sun causes chemical changes that can cause skin allergies. Patients taking antipsychotic drugs should not sunbathe since they risk a painful skin rash. Some patients develop slate-blue patches on their skin. This is an accumulation of drug metabolites, not an allergy, and is not dangerous.

Cholestatic hepatitis can develop with antipsychotic therapy. Jaundice develops when the bile duct becomes blocked by an allergic inflammation caused by metabolites excreted in the bile. It is commonly seen in the first month of therapy with one of the aliphatic phenothiazines. It is normally mild and self-limiting; but if jaundice is detected, the drug should

PATIENT PROBLEM

Photosensitivity

THE PROBLEM

Some drugs can cause the skin to become especially sensitive to the effects of ultraviolet rays, so patients become sunburned with minimal exposure to the sun.

SIGNS AND SYMPTOMS

Sunburn develops after relatively brief exposure to the sun or other sources of ultraviolet light. Blisters, red skin, pain, or discomfort over skin surfaces may also occur.

PATIENT AND FAMILY EDUCATION

- Avoid sunbathing or tanning at tanning salons.
- Limit outdoor activities during the middle part of the day (10 AM to 2 PM) as much as possible.
- If outside, wear a wide-brimmed hat, long-sleeved shirt or jacket, long pants, and socks or other foot covering.
- Use a maximum strength sunblock on exposed skin surfaces (SPF 15 or higher). Apply liberally to exposed skin surfaces, and repeat application every 1 to 2 hours. If you suspect that the sunblocking agent is causing skin irritation or rashes, try another agent or a product labeled hypoallergenic, which may be less irritating.
- If you experience moderate-to-severe sunburn, notify the physician.

be stopped and an antipsychotic drug from a different chemical class used.

Blood dyscrasias. A blood dyscrasia, the depression of the synthesis of one of the blood elements, occasionally occurs with antipsychotic therapy. Depression of leukocytes is common with antipsychotic therapy but is usually transient and not serious. Agranulocytosis, however, in which leukocytes are no longer produced, is serious and is often fatal. Agranulocytosis is most common within 3 months of the start of therapy. Therefore blood counts should be done early in the therapy. Any sign of fever or sore throat indicates the possible onset of agranulocytosis and should be checked immediately.

Interactions

Antipsychotic drugs potentiate the action of CNS depressant drugs, including sedative-hypnotic drugs, narcotic analgesics, and anesthetic agents. The potentiation of sedative-hypnotic drugs, including alcohol, is an important drug interaction. The effects of an alcoholic drink or a sleeping pill are greatly exaggerated in patients taking an antipsychotic drug. A toxic overdose of the alcohol or sedative-hypnotic drug therefore becomes possible at a lower dose.

Clinical use is made of the potentiation of narcotic-analgesic drugs by antipsychotic drugs. The chronic pain of terminal cancer patients can be relieved by receiving lower doses of a narcotic-analgesic drug when an antipsychotic drug is also given. This greatly slows the development of tolerance to the narcotics. The antipsychotic drug has the further advantage of controlling the emesis produced by radiation therapy or chemotherapy.

Finally, droperidol, a drug related to the antipsychotic drug haloperidol, is widely used with a narcotic to produce a state of quiescence and indifference to stimuli, which allows bronchoscopy, x-ray studies, burn dressing, and cytoscopy to be performed. Nitrous oxide can be added to this neuroleptic-narcotic combination to produce general anesthesia for surgery, called neuroleptanesthesia. The anesthesia results from the synergistic effect of the drugs with nitrous oxide since nitrous oxide alone is not potent enough to produce surgical anesthesia (see Chapter 68).

NURSING PROCESS OVERVIEW

Antipsychotic Drugs

Assessment

Perform a complete assessment, with a focus on the behavioral component. Assess the patient's emotional affect, ability to interact with others, and ability to initiate appropriate conversation. Assess for abnormal thought processes such as hallucinations or delusions and observe any unusual mannerisms or conversely the lack of any objective activity. Evaluate judgment, decision making, and overall thought processes. Obtain baseline vital signs and weight. Assess for abnormal movements using the abnormal involuntary movement scale (AIMS). Assess serum drug levels if available.

Nursing Diagnoses

- Altered bowel elimination: constipation related to drug side effects
- Potential impaired physical mobility related to extrapyramidal side effects (EPS) of antipsychotic therapy

Patient Outcomes

The patient will not experience constipation related to drug side effects. If EPS develop, the nurse will manage and minimize the severity and effect of these side effects.

Planning/Implementation

Patients requiring antipsychotic drug therapy also require psychiatric care, at least during initial drug therapy. Observe the patient closely for changes in overall affect and behavior. Monitor vital signs, level of consciousness, blood pressure, and signs of drug toxicity. Serious side effects include extrapyramidal reactions or acute dystonia. Continue to monitor serum drug levels and to assess for involuntary movements.

Evaluation

Most patients require continued use of these medications, with brief drug-free periods, for the rest of their lives. Before discharge, verify that the patient or family can explain how to take the medication correctly, what symptoms or side effects should be reported immediately to the physician, what situations indicating overdosage or underdosage should be reported to the physician, and what symptoms of disease exacerbation should be reported to the physician. If other medications are used to treat the underlying condition or side effects of the antipsychotic drugs, ascertain that the patient or family can explain the necessary information about these drugs (see Table 52-3).

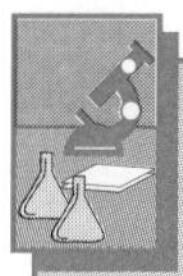

RESEARCH HIGHLIGHT

Noncompliance With Medication Regimens in Severely and Persistently Mentally Ill Schizophrenic Patients

—*JS Mulaik: Issues Mental Health Nurs 13(3):219, 1992.*

PURPOSE

Relapse requiring rehospitalization of schizophrenic patients is a major problem for the patients, the family, and the health care team. Noncompliance (taking significantly less than the prescribed amount of medication over time) with medication regimens is one of many causes of relapse. This study was designed to explore the reasons for noncompliance.

SAMPLE

A convenience sample of eleven "triads" was used. Each triad was composed of a patient, the patient's caretaker or family member, and the primary nurse assigned to the patient. All the patients had a diagnosis of schizophrenia, a history of several admissions, and two or more documented episodes of medication noncompliance. Characteristics of the patients included seven men and four women, with ages from 19 to 58 years; one patient was employed. Family members included six mothers, one grandmother, one daughter, one wife, one sister, and one father.

METHODOLOGY

A structured interview was used to interview the 11 patients, 11 caretaker/family members, and 5 nurses, for a total of 33 interviews (some nurses care for more than one of the patients). Questions on the interview form were developed based on the Health Belief Model.

FINDINGS

Patients reported various reasons for not taking medicines, including "I don't need medicine," and "I'm tired of taking medicine." One half the patients felt they did not need the full dose of medication. There were few side effects; one patient each reported the following: sleepiness, dizziness, impotence, weight gain, and heartburn.

Families and nurses agreed about potential problems patients faced in going home, namely potential for patient violence, refusal to take medication, and problems with drug or alcohol use. Other findings included patients' low self-esteem, lack of knowledge about their medications, inability to identify early symptoms of relapse, and families' stress from patients' abusive, unpredictable behavior.

IMPLICATIONS

Schizophrenic patients and their families require continued support from the health care team. Knowledge of the disease and medications must be provided and reviewed frequently. Patients, families, and the health care team must work together to problem solve when noncompliance is an issue. In this study, drug side effects were not a major reason for noncompliance, but the sample in this study was small. Nurses must continue to assess patients thoroughly for causes of noncompliance when it exists.

NURSING IMPLICATIONS SUMMARY

General Guidelines: Care of Patient Receiving Antipsychotic Drugs

Drug Administration

- Review the common side effects listed in Tables 52-2 and 52-3 since the effects will be frequently encountered. Assess the patient on a regular, ongoing basis for these side effects. Assess thoughtfully: what may appear to be increased agitation may be akathisia, or what may resemble anxiety may be early parkinsonian side effects. Review the box on neuroleptic malignant syndrome (p. 648).
- Monitor blood pressure every 4 hours until stable; this may require several days to 2 weeks. Some physicians prefer that blood pressure be monitored with the patient in lying, sitting, and standing positions.
- Side effects may make the patient unsteady when ambulating. Supervise ambulation and assist when appropriate.
- Monitor fluid intake and output until the patient is stabilized. Weigh the patient weekly. Monitor blood glucose levels.
- Contact dermatitis caused by the phenothiazines has been reported. Avoid getting the drugs on the skin and wash hands carefully after preparing these drugs. If working with these drugs frequently, wear gloves.
- Supervise the patient carefully to ascertain that medication is swallowed and is not hidden in the mouth to be discarded or stored for later use. Some antipsychotic drugs are available in syrup, injection, or depot injection forms to ensure that the patient receives the prescribed dose. On an outpatient basis, it may be necessary for a responsible family member to supervise medication taking.
- Concentrated oral forms of most antipsychotic drugs are available for institutional use. Dilute the dose in 60 to 120 ml in one of the diluents suggested by the manufacturer.

Continued.

Nursing Implications Summary—cont'd

- Monitor the patient with a history of seizures carefully since antipsychotics may alter the seizure threshold.
- For IM injection, choose a large muscle mass. Aspirate the needle before injecting to avoid inadvertent intravenous (IV) administration. Warn the patient that the drug may cause a burning sensation while being injected. Record and rotate injection sites.
- IM injections of nondepot forms of phenothiazines may cause marked hypotension. Keep the patient supine for 30 minutes to 1 hour after the injection, monitor blood pressure, and supervise ambulation. For rare severe reactions, levarterenol and phenylephrine are the vasoconstrictors of choice; do not use epinephrine.
- Read orders and labels carefully. Some drugs are available in an aqueous form and an oil-based depot form. Administer oil-based depot forms intramuscularly, never intravenously.
- When antipsychotics are used as antiemetics, the doses are usually lower. Side effects are milder and include sedation, hypotension, and dry mouth. However, any side effect listed can occur in a patient who is extremely sensitive to the drug. When antipsychotic drugs are given as antiemetics with narcotic analgesics, they may potentiate CNS depressive effects of the analgesics, including hypotension and sedation.
- The care of the mentally ill is complex and involves the use of many treatment modalities. See texts and articles appropriate to the care of psychiatric patients.

Patient and Family Education

- Review the anticipated benefits and possible side effects of drug therapy with the patient and family. Review extrapyramidal side effects listed in Table 52-3. Since there is no effective treatment for tardive dyskinesia, its appearance should be reported immediately. Fine vermicular (wormlike) movements of the tongue may be the first sign of this side effect. Instruct the patient and family to report any new signs or symptoms.
- See the patient problem boxes on dry mouth (p. 300), constipation (p. 304), photosensitivity (p. 649), and orthostatic hypotension (p. 157).
- Inform the patient that several weeks of therapy may be necessary before full benefit can be seen. Encourage the patient to return for follow-up visits to monitor for drug effectiveness and development of side effects.
- Instruct the patient to take oral doses of loxapine, molindone, phenothiazines, or thioxanthenes, with food or a full (8-ounce) glass of water or milk.
- Liquid doses of molindone may be taken undiluted or further diluted in milk, water, fruit juice, or carbonated beverages.
- Instruct the patient to dilute thiothixene oral solution just prior to taking dose with a full glass of water, milk, tomato or fruit juice, soup, or carbonated beverages.
- Instruct the patient not to take oral doses of loxapine, molindone, thioxanthenes, or phenothiazines within 2 hours of taking doses of antacids or medicine for diarrhea.
- Instruct the patient to swallow extended-release forms whole and not to crush or chew.
- Review with the patient how to measure the correct dose if the drug is dispensed with a dropper. Teach correct administration technique if suppositories or injections are ordered.
- Warn the patient to avoid driving or operating hazardous equipment if vision changes or sedation occurs and to notify the physician if these symptoms do occur.
- Instruct the patient to report signs of agranulocytosis including sore throat, fever, and malaise. Instruct the patient to report signs of liver dysfunction including jaundice, malaise, fever, and right upper quadrant abdominal pain.
- These drugs may interfere with the body's ability to regulate temperature. Warn the patient to avoid prolonged exposure to extremes of temperature, to allow for frequent cooling off periods when exercising or in hot environments, and to dress warmly for exposure to the cold.
- Review possible endocrine side effects with patient and family. Assess carefully and tactfully for these side effects. Provide emotional support as appropriate. If endocrine side effects are intolerable, consult the physician for possible drug or dosage change.
- Phenothiazines may cause the eyes to be more sensitive to light. Instruct the patient to wear sunglasses that block ultraviolet light, even on cloudy days.
- For missed doses, if the drug is ordered once a day, advise the patient to take the missed dose as soon as remembered on the day it was due; otherwise, omit the missed dose and resume the regular dosage schedule the next day. If drug is ordered more than once a day, advise the patient to take the missed dose as soon as remembered, if within an hour of when scheduled; otherwise omit the missed dose and resume regular dosing schedule. The patient should not double up for missed doses and should check with the physician if there are questions.
- Instruct the patient to monitor weight (if appropriate to ability and resources). If weight gain is a problem, counsel about low-calorie diets. Refer to a dietitian as needed.
- Caution the patient to inform all health care providers of all drugs being taken. Warn the patient to avoid over-the-counter drugs unless first approved by the physician.
- Caution the patient to avoid alcoholic beverages while taking antipsychotics.
- Warn a diabetic patient that antipsychotics may alter blood glucose levels. Instruct the patient to monitor blood glucose levels carefully and to consult the physician about changes in dietary or drug treatment for diabetes.
- Instruct the patient not to discontinue therapy abruptly or without consultation with the physician. Instruct the patient to keep these and all drugs out of the reach of children.

NURSING IMPLICATIONS SUMMARY—cont'd

- The drugs may produce false-positive pregnancy results. Female patients who suspect they are pregnant should consult the physician. Female patients may desire to use contraceptive measures while taking these drugs; counsel as appropriate. As always, pregnant or lactating women should avoid all drugs unless first approved by the physician.
- If additional drugs are prescribed to treat side effects of antipsychotic agents, review their use and side effects with the patient and family.

Chlorpromazine

Drug Administration

- See the general guidelines.

Intravenous Administration

- For direct IV push, dilute chlorpromazine in 0.9% sodium chloride to make a dilution of 1 mg/ml. Administer at a rate of 0.5 mg/min. For infusion, further dilute and infuse slowly. Monitor blood pressure. Keep siderails up. Supervise ambulation after dose.

Droperidol

Drug Administration

- Droperidol is used as an antiemetic, a preoperative medication, or during anesthesia; see Chapter 68.
- For IV administration droperidol may be given undiluted or may be further diluted. Administer undiluted drug at a rate of 10 mg or less per 1 minute. Monitor blood pressure. Keep siderails up. Supervise ambulation. Titrate diluted doses to patient response.

Flupenthixol

Drug Administration

- Read orders and labels carefully. The decanoate form is a depot, in which the drug is suspended in sesame oil. Use a 21-gauge needle. See information on administering oil-based suspensions in Chapter 5.

Fluphenazine

Drug Administration

- Read orders and labels carefully. The decanoate and enanthate forms are depots, with the drug suspended in sesame oil. Use a dry needle and syringe. A wet needle or syringe causes the drug to turn cloudy. Use a 21-gauge needle. See information on administering oil-based suspensions in Chapter 5.

Haloperidol

Drug Administration

- Read orders and labels carefully. The decanoate form is a depot, with the drug suspended in sesame oil. Use a 21-gauge needle. See information on administering oil-based suspensions in Chapter 5.
- Oral doses are best taken alone but may be mixed with water immediately before taking dose. Do not mix with or take with tea or coffee.

Perphenazine

Drug Administration

Intravenous Administration

- Read label carefully. Use only single-dose 5 mg ampules for IV use. Dilute each 5 mg (1 ml) with 9 ml of normal saline for injection. Administer at a rate of 0.5 mg (1 ml)/1 min. Monitor blood pressure. Keep siderails up. Supervise ambulation.

Prochlorperazine

Drug Administration

Intravenous Administration

- Dilute each 5 mg (1 ml) with 9 ml of normal saline for injection. Administer at a rate of 5 mg or less over 1 minute. Prochlorperazine may also be further diluted and given as an infusion.

Promazine

Drug Administration

Intravenous Administration

- Dilute to 25 mg or less per milliliter with 0.9% sodium chloride injection. Administer at a rate of 25 mg or less over 1 min. Monitor blood pressure. Keep siderails up. Supervise ambulation.

Triflupromazine

Drug Administration

Intravenous Administration

- Dilute 10 mg with 9 ml of normal saline for injection. Administer at a rate of 1 mg (1 ml)/2 min. Monitor blood pressure. Keep siderails up. Supervise ambulation.

CRITICAL THINKING

APPLICATION

1. What is the major chemical class of antipsychotic drugs? List the three subclasses.
2. What are the four actions of antipsychotic drugs attributable to blockade of dopaminergic receptors? What symptoms might you see as a result of this blockade?
3. What are two actions of antipsychotic drugs attributable to blockade of receptors for norepinephrine? What symptoms might you see that may be caused by this blockade?
4. What are two actions of antipsychotic drugs attributable to blockade of cholinergic receptors? What symptoms might you see that may be caused by this blockade?
5. List the four types of extrapyramidal reactions, the key features of each type, and when each type is likely to occur during antipsychotic drug therapy. How can you recognize these reactions?
6. Describe allergic reactions attributed to antipsychotic drugs.
7. For which types of psychoses are antipsychotic drugs generally effective?
8. Name the two clinical uses of antipsychotic drugs other than the treatment of psychoses.

CRITICAL THINKING

1. What would you tell a patient taking an antipsychotic drug (and his or her family) about photosensitivity? What points would you emphasize?
2. Describe the potential side effects of antipsychotic therapy and how you would monitor for these in a care plan.

CHAPTER 53

Antidepressant Drugs

OBJECTIVES

After studying this chapter, you should be able to do the following:

- *Briefly describe reactive depression, endogenous depression, and manic-depressive (bipolar) disorder.*
- *Develop a nursing care plan for patients receiving a tricyclic antidepressant, a heterocyclic antidepressant, a selective serotonin reuptake inhibitor, a monoamine oxidase inhibitor, or lithium.*
- *Describe the toxic symptoms of lithium and the corresponding blood level.*
- *Develop a teaching plan for a patient on a tyramine-restricted diet.*

CHAPTER OVERVIEW

Drugs covered in this chapter are used for severe disturbances of mood, from depression to manic-depressive disorders. Antidepressants, monoamine-oxidase inhibitors, and lithium are presented.

KEY TERMS

depression
endogenous depression
heterocyclic antidepressants
lithium
manic-depressive disorder
monoamine oxidase (MAO) inhibitors
reactive depression
sedative and anticholinergic side effects
selective serotonin reuptake inhibitors (SSRIs)
tricyclic antidepressants

Therapeutic Rationale: Depressive Disorders

Depression

Depression is a disorder of mood (affect) that occurs in an estimated 15% to 30% of all adults at some time during their lives. Depression is not a single entity; rather it is a syndrome that can include various symptoms, as outlined in Table 53-1. Depression becomes a medical problem when normal functioning is significantly hampered. Three major categories of depression are recognized: reactive depression, endogenous depression, and manic-depressive disorder.

Reactive Depression, Endogenous Depression, and Manic-Depressive Disorder

Reactive depression is experienced after some significant loss in life. This depression is usually acute for a couple of weeks and resolves within 3 months. Therapy for reactive depression is to provide emotional support. One subclass of the benzodiazepines, the antianxiety drugs, may be prescribed to relieve anxiety or insomnia if required. An antidepressant drug typically is not needed.

Endogenous depression is depression with no apparent cause. Current views are that endogenous depression is a neurochemical disorder that can be treated with appropriate drug therapy. This concept arose from the observation in the 1950s that reserpine caused depression in patients treated for hypertension. Reserpine depleted the neurotransmitter norepinephrine. About the same time, iproniazid, a drug then used to treat tuberculosis, was found to relieve depression in patients, inhibiting the degradation of norepinephrine by inhibiting the enzyme monoamine oxidase (MAO). These two observations suggested that a deficiency in the brain neurotransmitter norepinephrine is associated with depression. Current evidence favors a biogenic amine theory of depression, in which a deficiency in brain norepinephrine or in another amine neurotransmitter, serotonin, is associated with depression. The two drug classes currently used to treat depression, tricyclic antidepressants and MAO inhibitors, have pharmacologic mechanisms that restore norepinephrine and serotonin in the brain.

Manic-depressive disorder is the third type of depression. The classic manic-depressive patient has a manic period characterized by excessive euphoria, overactivity, a flow of ideas, extreme self-confidence, and little need for sleep, alternating with a period of depression. Lithium is the specific drug treatment for mania.

TABLE 53-1 Symptoms Characteristic of Depression

PARAMETER	CHANGE
General mood	Low for a week or more
Behavior	Appetite or weight change Sleep change; early morning awakening is most common insomnia; some patients may sleep more than usual, although level of activity is exaggerated or depressed Loss of energy Loss of interest in activities and/or sex Feelings of guilt or self-reproach Inability to concentrate Thoughts of suicide

Depression as a Side Effect

In addition to these three classes, depression can also be the side effect of some drugs, especially the antihypertensive drugs reserpine, methyldopa, guanethidine, and propranolol. Alcohol and antianxiety drugs often unmask depression by alleviating the anxiety that frequently accompanies depression. Steroids, particularly glucocorticoids and oral contraceptives, can cause depression. Drug-induced depression mimics endogenous depression but is treated by removing the drug or lowering the dose.

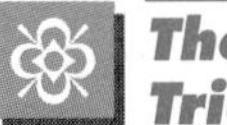

Therapeutic Agents: Tricyclic Antidepressants

Tricyclic Antidepressants: General Characteristics

Mechanism of Action

The **tricyclic antidepressants** (Table 53-2) block the reuptake of norepinephrine or serotonin into the presynaptic neurons, as depicted in Figure 53-1. This causes an increase in the synaptic concentration of these neurotransmitters, which is an early effect of the drug. However, clinically no antidepressant response is seen for 2 weeks. Recent research suggests that the tricyclic antidepressants also alter the sensitivity of brain tissue to the action of norepinephrine and serotonin. Since this effect takes 2 weeks to be established, it more closely correlates with the onset of the clinical antidepressant action.

Pharmacokinetics

The tricyclic antidepressants usually are administered orally, although amitriptyline and imipramine are available in injectable forms. Metabolites of the tricyclic antidepressants are active so that an active form of the drug persists despite the drug being well absorbed and readily metabolized by the intestine and liver. The rate of tricyclic metabolism decreases with age, and people older than 55 years of age generally are started at half the regular adult dose.

Uses

Tricyclic antidepressants elevate mood, counteracting the extreme sadness characteristic of major depression. Physical activity and activities of daily living are increased, overcoming the sense of despair and lack of interest in living. Appetite and sleep patterns are improved.

TABLE 53-2 Antidepressant Drugs

GENERIC NAME	TRADE NAME	ADMINISTRATION/DOSAGE	COMMENTS
Tricyclic Antidepressants			
✣ Amitriptyline hydrochloride	Elavil* Endep Levate† Novotriptyn†	ORAL: *Adults*—Begin with 50 mg at bedtime; increase dosage by 25-50 mg if necessary to 150 mg. Alternately, start with 25 mg 3 times daily and increase to 50 mg 3 times daily. Total dosage should not exceed 300 mg daily. Maintenance doses are usually 50-100 mg at bedtime. These are outpatient dosages; inpatient dosages may be twice as much. FDA pregnancy category C. *Adolescents and older adults*—10 mg 3 times daily plus 20 mg at bedtime (50 mg total) is usually sufficient. INTRAMUSCULAR: 20-30 mg 4 times daily.	Bedtime administration is preferred to lessen discomfort of sedation and anticholinergic effects prominent with this drug.
Clomipramine	Anafranil*	ORAL: *Adults*—Initially 25 mg 3 times/day; then up to 200 mg for outpatients, 300 mg for inpatients. *Older adults*—20-30 mg daily in divided doses. FDA pregnancy category C.	Used for obsessive-compulsive disorders, for blocking panic attacks, and to treat cataplexy associated with narcolepsy.
Desipramine hydrochloride	Norpramin* Pertofrane†	ORAL: *Adults*—Begin with 25 mg 3 times daily; increase gradually to total of 200 mg daily, rarely 300 mg daily; maintenance dosages usually 50-200 mg taken at bedtime. *Adolescents and older adults*—25-50 mg daily; increase to 100 mg in divided doses if necessary. FDA pregnancy category C.	Sedation and anticholinergic effects are not prominent. Metabolite of imipramine.
Doxepin hydrochloride	Novo-Doxepin† Sinequan*	ORAL : *Adults*—75 mg, increased to 150 mg in divided doses or at bedtime; maintenance dose usually 25-150 mg daily (maximum 300 mg daily).	Bedtime administration is preferred to lessen discomfort of sedation and anticholinergic effects prominent with this drug. Doxepin is reported to have much less effect on heart when compared to other tricyclic antidepressants.
Imipramine hydrochloride, Imipramine pamoate	Apo-Imipramine† Novopramine† Tipramine Tofranil* Tofranil-PM	ORAL: *Adults*—75 mg daily in divided doses or at bedtime. Dose may be increased up to 200 mg daily if required. These are outpatient doses; inpatient doses are one third higher. *Adolescents and older adults*—30-40 mg daily, increased to maximum of 100 mg/day. *Children >6 yr*—25 mg, 1 hr before bedtime; if no response in 1 wk, increase to 50 mg; *Children >12 yr*—May receive up to 75 mg.	Imipramine is prototype tricyclic antidepressant. Sedative and anticholinergic effects are moderate. Can be taken at bedtime.
Nortriptyline hydrochloride	Aventyl* Pamelor	ORAL: *Adults*—Initially 40 mg in divided doses or at bedtime; maximum dose 100-150 mg daily. *Adolescents and children*—30-50 mg daily in divided doses. FDA pregnancy category C.	Metabolite of amitriptyline. Sedative effect is moderate; anticholinergic effect is mild. Can be taken at bedtime.
Protriptyline hydrochloride	Triptil† Vivactil	ORAL: *Adults*—15-40 mg daily divided in 3-4 doses; maximum dose 60 mg daily. Increments are added to morning dose. *Adolescents and older adults*—15 mg daily in 3 doses. No more than 20 mg total.	This is only tricyclic antidepressant that has little sedative action and can cause insomnia if given at bedtime. Preferred for patient who has been immobile and sleepy.
Trimipramine maleate	Apo-Trimip† Novo-Tripramine† Rhotrimine† Surmontil	ORAL: *Adults*—75 mg daily increased to 150 mg in divided doses or at bedtime. These are outpatient dosages; inpatient dosages 100 mg daily increased to 200 mg daily with a maximum of 300 mg daily. FDA pregnancy category C. *Adolescents and older adults*—50 mg daily, increased to no more than 100 mg daily as required.	Sedation is high, but anticholinergic effect is moderate.

*Available in Canada and United States.
+Available in Canada only.

Continued.

TABLE 53-2 Antidepressant Drugs—cont'd

GENERIC NAME	TRADE NAME	ADMINISTRATION/DOSAGE	COMMENTS
Heterocyclic Antidepressants			
Amoxapine	Asendin*	ORAL: *Adults*—75 mg initially; increase to 200 mg daily in divided doses. If no improvement in 3 wk, increase dosage 50 mg daily every other week to maximum of 400 mg for outpatients, 600 mg for inpatients. FDA pregnancy category C.	Related to tricyclic antidepressants. Low incidence of anticholinergic, sedative, and cardiovascular effects. May be taken at bedtime to lessen daytime sedation or to treat insomnia.
Bupropion	Wellbutrin	ORAL: *Adults*—Initially 100 mg 2 times/day; increase dosage gradually after 3 days of therapy, to 100 mg 3 times/day as needed and tolerated.	New antidepressant. Seizures may occur at high doses.
Maprotiline	Ludiomil*	ORAL: *Adults*—75 mg, increased to 150 mg daily in divided doses. If no improvement in 3 wk, increase dosage 50 mg daily every other week to maximum of 300 mg. FDA pregnancy category B. *Older adults and adolescents*—⅓ adult dose.	Low incidence of anticholinergic, sedative, and cardiovascular effects. May be taken at bedtime to lessen daytime sedation or to treat insomnia.
Trazodone	Desyrel* Trazon Trialodine	ORAL: *Adults*—75 mg initially; increase by 50 mg daily every 3 or 4 days to 300 mg if necessary. If no improvement in 3 wk, increase dosage 50 mg daily every other week to maximum of 300 mg. FDA pregnancy category C.	Sedation may be noted. Low incidence of anticholinergic and cardiovascular effects. May be taken at bedtime to lessen daytime sedation or to treat insomnia.
Selective Serotonin Reuptake Inhibitors			
✣ Fluoxetine	Prozac*	ORAL: *Adults*—20 mg as single morning dose; may increase dose by 20 mg daily if needed, with second dose at noon. FDA pregnancy category B.	For mild-to-moderate depression; being evaluated for eating disorders (obesity, bulimia), obsessive-compulsive disorders.
Fluvoxamine	Luvox*	ORAL: *Adults*—50 mg at bedtime; increase by 50 mg every 4-7 days if needed. Maximum daily dose is 300 mg. Divide 100 mg or larger doses into 2 doses.	For obsessive-compulsive disorder or for mild-to-moderate depression.
Paroxetine hydrochloride	Paxil*	ORAL: *Adults*—20 mg as single morning dose; may increase weekly by 10 mg/day, up to 50 mg daily. *Older adults*—10 mg daily, increased if necessary. Maximum daily dose is 40 mg. FDA pregnancy category B.	For mild-to-moderate depression.
Sertraline hydrochloride	Zoloft*	ORAL: *Adults*—50 mg daily as morning or evening dose; may increase by 50 mg at weekly intervals if needed. Maximum daily dose is 200 mg.	For mild-to-moderate depression.
Monoamine Oxidase (MAO) Inhibitors			
Isocarboxazid	Marplan*	ORAL: *Adults*—20-30 mg daily in divided doses; maintenance dose usually 10-20 mg daily.	Patient should be instructed in food and drug interactions with MAO inhibitors.
Phenelzine sulfate	Nardil*	ORAL: *Adults*—45-75 mg daily in 3 doses or 1 mg/kg body weight in divided doses. Daily dosage should not exceed 90 mg.	Patient should be instructed in food and drug interactions with MAO inhibitors.
Tranylcypromine sulfate	Parnate*	ORAL: *Adults*—20-40 mg daily in 2 doses for 2 wk. Dosage is reduced after response is obtained. Usually maintenance dose is below 30 mg. Higher doses are not advised for outpatients.	Patient should be instructed in food and drug interactions with MAO inhibitors. Has some psychomotor stimulant activity characteristic of amphetamine.
Lithium			
Lithium carbonate	Eskalith Lithane* Lithizine† Lithonate Lithotabs	ORAL: *Adults*—Initially 0.6-2.1 gm daily divided into 3 doses. Increase or decrease dose by 0.3 gm/day to obtain blood level of 0.8-1.5 mEq/L. FDA pregnancy category D.	Blood should not be drawn for determination of lithium levels earlier than 8 hr after last dose. Levels above 2 mEq/L are toxic. Patients should be instructed not to make up missed dose of lithium.
Lithium citrate	Cibalith-Si	Maintenance dose usually 0.9-1.2 gm daily in divided doses.	

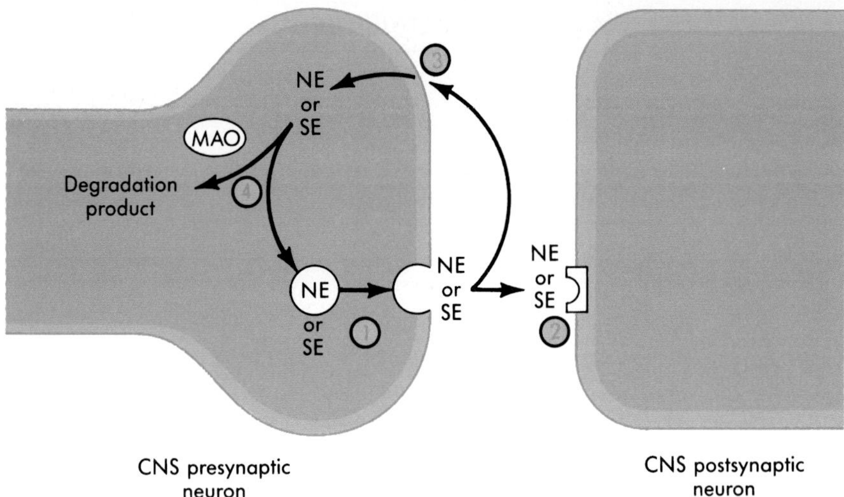

FIGURE 53-1

Depression results from amine concentration too low to activate sufficient receptors; mania results from overabundance of amine acting at receptor. Biogenic amine theory of depression is applied to actions of antidepressant drugs, tricyclic antidepressants and MAO inhibitors, and to action of lithium, used to treat mania (opposite of depression). *1,* Lithium inhibits release of norepinephrine and serotonin. *2,* Tricyclic antidepressants and MAO inhibitors increase receptor sensitivity to norepinephrine and serotonin. *3,* Tricyclic antidepressants block reuptake of norepinephrine and serotonin. Lithium enhances reuptake of norepinephrine and serotonin. Selective serotonin reuptake inhibitors block reuptake of serotonin. *4,* MAO inhibitors prevent degradation of norepinephrine and serotonin.

Adverse Reactions and Contraindications

The major side effects of the tricyclic antidepressants are an atropine-like (anticholinergic) effect and sedation. The relative incidence of these side effects among the tricyclics is listed in Table 53-3. Because of these side effects, the drug is usually given before bedtime so that the patient is asleep when the side effects are at their peak. The more sedating tricyclics, amitriptyline and doxepin, are particularly effective in relieving the insomnia of depression when given as a bedtime dose. These drugs do not interfere with the normal sleep pattern described in Chapter 51.

Sedative and anticholinergic side effects are apparent with the first dose of a tricyclic antidepressant, although little lifting of the depression is seen before 2 weeks of therapy. Thus the dose is started at about a third the expected therapeutic dose to allow the patient to develop tolerance to the side effects. The dose is increased to the expected therapeutic dose over the first week. After 2 weeks of drug therapy, the dosage is reviewed in light of side effects and therapeutic response. The final dosage is individualized for the patient. Therapy is discontinued if no response occurs after 1 month. If the patient's depression is relieved, the duration of therapy depends on the severity of the depression being treated. Mild depression might be treated for 2 to 3 months, whereas severe depression might be treated for 1 to 2 years. The drug therapy is then gradually withdrawn. Reappearance of depression is a sign for reinstitution of drug therapy. The spectrum of therapy for depression ranges from a few weeks to a lifetime, depending on the severity and recurrence of depression.

Anticholinergic side effects include dry mouth, blurred vision, and constipation. Some patients may experience temporary confusion or speech blockage. Patients with glaucoma or those disposed toward glaucoma must have this condition checked when taking tricyclic antidepressants because the anticholinergic effect may worsen this condition. Anticholinergic action also may adversely affect patients, particularly older adult patients, with urinary retention or obstruction.

Cardiac effects. Tricyclic antidepressants have three separate pharmacologic actions on the heart: anticholinergic, adrenolytic, and a quinidine-like action. Therefore the final cardiac effect is complex and depends on dosage. The anticholinergic action increases the heart rate. The adrenolytic action prevents the reuptake of norepinephrine into neurons, an action that tends to deplete norepinephrine stores in peripheral neurons. The most common adrenolytic side effect is orthostatic (postural) hypotension. This decrease in blood pressure affects the heart by lowering the workload. The quinidine-like side effects are seen at high concentrations of the tricyclic antidepressants. This decreases heart rate, myocardial contractility, and coronary blood flow. For these reasons, tricyclic antidepressants are contraindicated for patients with a recent myocardial infarction and present special concern for the patient with cardiac disease. Patients who have hyperthyroidism and are at risk for developing cardiac arrhythmias have this risk potentiated by the tricyclic antidepressants. Doxepin is a tricyclic antidepressant that has minimum cardiac effects.

TABLE 53-3 Incidence of Side Effects of Antidepressant Drugs

	SIDE EFFECT						
		CNS		CARDIOVASCULAR		OTHER	
DRUG	ANTI-CHOLINERGIC	DROWSINESS	INSOMNIA AGITATION	ORTHOSTATIC HYPOTENSION	CARDIAC ARRHYTHMIAS	GASTROINTESTINAL DISTRESS	WEIGHT GAIN (>6 kg)
Tricyclic Antidepressants							
✣ Amitriptyline	++++	++++	0	++++	+++	0	++++
Desipramine	+	+	+	++	++	0	+
Doxepin	+++	++++	0	++	++	0	+++
Imipramine	+++	+++	+	++++	+++	+	+++
Nortriptyline	+	+	0	++	++	0	+
Protriptyline	++	+	+	++	++	0	0
Trimipramine	+	++++	0	++	++	0	+++
Heterocyclic Antidepressants							
Amoxapine	++	++	++	++	+++	0	+
Bupropion	0	0	++	0	+	+	0
Maprotiline	++	++++	0	0	+	0	++
Trazodone	0	++++	0	+	+	+	+
SSRIs	0	0	++	0	0	+++	0
MAOIs	+	+	++	++	0	+	++

Modified from *Clinical practice guideline: depression in primary care,* US Department of Health and Human Services, Agency for Health Care Policy and Research, Pub No 93-0552, April 1993.
MAOI, Monoamine oxidase inhibitor (isocarboxazid, phenelzine, tranylcypromine); *SSRI,* selective serotonin reuptake inhibitor (fluoxetine, fluvoxamine, paroxetine, sertraline).

Toxicity

Tricyclic antidepressants are not addicting, and their abuse potential appears limited. A major problem is their acute toxicity when depressed patients overdose on a tricyclic antidepressant drug in a suicide attempt. Doses of 1 gm of the sedating tricyclics are toxic, and doses of 2 gm are often fatal. Those doses represent only a 5- and 10-fold margin, respectively, over the therapeutic dose.

Overdose. The toxic effects of tricyclic antidepressant overdose are anticholinergic poisoning. The early symptoms are confusion, inability to concentrate, and perhaps visual hallucinations. More severe signs include delirium, seizures, and coma. Respiration may be depressed. The patient may have a low body temperature early but an elevated body temperature later. The pupils are dilated, the eyeballs are restless, the reflexes are hyperactive, and motor coordination is compromised. Depending on the cardiac status of the patient and the degree of overdose, the overall cardiac effect may range from quickening of the heart rate (tachycardia) to slowing of the heart rate (bradycardia) to various arrhythmias related to an atrioventricular block. Especially serious is the slowing of conduction in the atrioventricular node by the quinidine-like action, which can result in heart block. Sudden death from cardiac arrhythmias may occur several days after an overdose.

Physostigmine (Antilirium), a peripherally and centrally active anticholinesterase agent, reverses the anticholinergic toxic symptoms of tricyclic overdose. Two mg of physostigmine is administered every 1 to 2 hours as necessary. This drug must be administered frequently because it is short acting, whereas tricyclics are long acting.

Tricyclic antidepressants do not decrease the suicide potential among depressed patients during the early weeks of therapy. Depressed patients with suicidal thoughts are best hospitalized to begin drug therapy rather than being given quantities of drugs that may be used in a suicide attempt. Patients who have attempted or threatened suicide frequently are treated initially with electroconvulsive shock therapy. Since tricyclic antidepressants can increase the seizure potential, they are not administered concurrently with electroconvulsive shock therapy.

Interactions

The tricyclic antidepressants can potentiate central nervous system (CNS) depression, anticholinergic effects, and sympathomimetic effects of a number of drug classes including antihistamines, phenothiazines, thioxanthenes, and sympathomimetics. Cimetidine and methylphenidate can inhibit the metabolism of tricyclic antidepressants, potentially leading to an overdose. Metrizamide may increase the risk of seizures, while antithyroid agents increase the risk of agranulocytosis.

The interaction of guanethidine and a tricyclic antidepressant is classic; the tricyclic antidepressant inhibits the uptake of guanethidine by the neurons so that guanethidine cannot reach its site of action and is therefore ineffective in lowering blood pressure. Clonidine and guanadrel are also blocked by the tricyclic antidepressants and may become ineffective antihypertensives.

MAO inhibitors and antiarrhythmics have potentially fatal drug interactions with the tricyclic antidepressants and should not be administered concurrently.

Specific Tricyclic Antidepressants

✣ Amitriptyline

Amitriptyline (Elavil) is associated with a high incidence of sedation and anticholinergic effects. These properties are more pronounced than with other tricyclic antidepressants and can cause confusion in the older adult patient. Weight gain sometimes occurs. Amitriptyline has a plasma half-life of 1 to 2 days and is metabolized to nortriptyline, an active tricyclic antidepressant.

Clomipramine

Clomipramine (Anafranil) treats obsessive-compulsive disorder and blocks panic attacks. This drug has a low incidence of sedation but a moderate incidence of anticholinergic and cardiac effects.

Desipramine

Desipramine (Norpramin, Pertofrane) has a low incidence of sedation and anticholinergic effects. It is a metabolite of imipramine and has a plasma half-life of ½ day to 3 days.

Doxepin

Doxepin (Sinequan) has a high incidence of sedative and anticholinergic side effects. Doxepin does not have the quinidine-like cardiac effect to the degree characteristic of the other tricyclic drugs and therefore is indicated when cardiac function must be considered.

Imipramine

Imipramine (Tofranil) has a moderate degree of sedative and anticholinergic side effects. It is metabolized to desipramine, which is also an active tricyclic antidepressant. Imipramine has a plasma half-life of ½ day to 1 day. Imipramine is used to treat enuresis (bed-wetting) in older children or adults.

Nortriptyline

Nortriptyline (Aventyl, Pamelor) is moderately sedating and has minimum anticholinergic side effects. It is a metabolite of amitriptyline.

Protriptyline

Protriptyline (Vivactil) is the one tricyclic antidepressant with minimum sedating effect and is therefore most useful in depressed patients who seem physically immobilized by their depression or who sleep excessively. The plasma half-life of protriptyline is 4 to 9 days.

Trimipramine

Trimipramine (Surmontil) is a tricyclic antidepressant with a high incidence of sedation and a moderate incidence of anticholinergic effects.

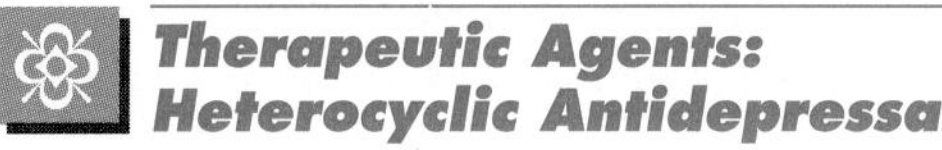

Therapeutic Agents: Heterocyclic Antidepressants

Antidepressant drugs have been introduced that are neither tricyclics nor MAO inhibitors. These **heterocyclic antidepressants** are regarded as alternatives to tricyclic antidepressants, although their action on norepinephrine and serotonin uptake is not necessarily similar to that of the tricyclics. The new antidepressant drugs have, to a varying degree, a lesser incidence of anticholinergic side effects, less cardiotoxicity, and a faster onset of action than the tricyclics.

Amoxapine

Amoxapine (Asendin) inhibits amine uptake and is a more potent inhibitor of norepinephrine than of serotonin uptake. Chemically related to the tricyclic antidepressants, amoxapine is also a chemical metabolite of the antipsychotic drug loxapine and, as with the antipsychotic drugs, blocks dopamine receptors. Overall, amoxapine treats major depression and relieves anxiety and agitation associated with depression.

Amoxapine has minimum anticholinergic and sedative effects and a lesser incidence of cardiac effects than the tricyclics. Drug interactions are similar to those of the tricyclics.

Bupropion

Bupropion (Wellbutrin) is a new antidepressant that only weakly blocks norepinephrine and serotonin. Bupropion differs from tricyclic antidepressants in having a stimulant rather than a sedative effect. Patients may experience restlessness, agitation, anxiety, and insomnia. Cardiac effects are uncommon.

Maprotiline

Maprotiline (Ludiomil) is a tetracyclic antidepressant that inhibits norepinephrine but not serotonin uptake. Drug interactions and side effects are similar to those of the tricyclic antidepressants. Incidence of drowsiness, anticholinergic effects, and cardiac effects is less than with amitriptyline or doxepin.

Trazodone

Trazodone (Desyrel) is chemically unrelated to other antidepressant drugs. It inhibits serotonin uptake but also inhibits alpha-adrenergic receptors. Drowsiness is a side effect, but minimum anticholinergic and cardiac effects occur. Like the tricyclic drugs, trazodone can cause orthostatic hypotension, but taking the drug with food lessens the effect. Rarely, males experience priapism, which may require surgery. Dilute (1:100,000) epinephrine should be administered quickly into the corpus cavernosa to minimize permanent damage.

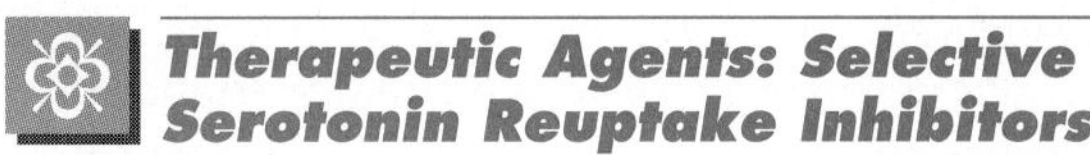

Therapeutic Agents: Selective Serotonin Reuptake Inhibitors

The newest category of antidepressant drugs is the selective serotonin reuptake inhibitors. This drug class has a greater pharmacologic specificity, fewer side effects and minimal potential for fatal overdose compared to the tricyclic antidepressants. Expect to see new drugs from this category.

Selective Serotonin Reuptake Inhibitors: General Characteristics

Mechanism of Action

The **selective serotonin reuptake inhibitors (SSRIs)** block the neuronal reuptake of serotonin but have little effect on the uptake of norepinephrine or dopamine (see Figure 53-1). In addition to having an antidepressant effect, this activity may also lessen obsessive-compulsive disorder and eating disorders.

Pharmacokinetics

The SSRIs are taken orally once a day. They are well absorbed. They bind to plasma protein and may displace other drugs. The SSRIs are metabolized by the liver and metabolites are also pharmacologically active. Metabolites are excreted in the urine.

Uses

The approved use of SSRIs is the treatment of depression, especially mild to moderate depression. The antidepressant effect is usually seen faster than with the tricyclic antidepressants but may still take up to 4 weeks. The SSRIs are also being tested for their efficacy in treating obsessive-compulsive disorders and eating disorders, including obesity and bulimia.

Adverse Reactions and Contraindications

The side effects of the SSRIs are less pronounced than with the tricyclic antidepressants because of the lack of anticholinergic effects or cardiac conduction disturbances characteristic of the tricyclic antidepressants. Overdoses of the SSRIs are not fatal, so they are safer than the tricyclic antidepressants. Side effects of SSRIs include nausea, nervousness, and insomnia. Less frequently reported side effects include headaches, tremor, anxiety, drowsiness, dry mouth, sweating, and diarrhea. Sexual dysfunction may include lack of orgasm in women and ejaculatory delay in men.

Individuals with severe liver or kidney disease may have impaired ability to metabolize and excrete SSRIs, and dosages should be reduced and monitored. Because these drugs are excreted in breast milk and are poorly metabolized by infants, they are not recommended for nursing mothers. SSRIs should be used with caution for patients with seizure disorders.

Interactions

The SSRIs are bound to plasma protein and may displace other drugs, especially oral anticoagulants and phenytoin. The CNS depression of other drugs can be potentiated by the SSRIs. Tryptophan and MAO inhibitors should not be taken concurrently with SSRIs because these also affect serotonin levels.

Specific Selective Serotonin Reuptake Inhibitors

✣ Fluoxetine

Fluoxetine (Prozac) is the first widely used SSRI in the United States. It is well tolerated and effective in treating mild and moderate depression. There has been concern that patients receiving fluoxetine are at increased risk for developing serious suicidal thoughts, but the data does not support this concern.

Fluvoxamine

Fluvoxamine (Luvox) is an SSRI newly released for treating obsessive-compulsive disorders and depression.

Paroxetine and Sertraline

Paroxetine (Paxil) and sertraline (Zoloft) are SSRIs newly released for the treatment of mild to moderate depression.

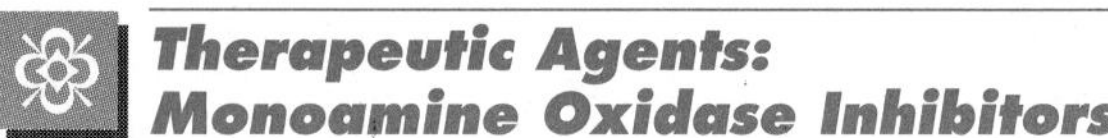

Therapeutic Agents: Monoamine Oxidase Inhibitors

MAO inhibitors are less commonly used because of the poor safety profile that requires strict adherence to dietary limitations and potential for drug interactions. However, they may be the only drugs effective for atypical depression.

Monoamine Oxidase Inhibitors: General Characteristics

Mechanism of Action

The **monoamine oxidase (MAO) inhibitors** were in use before the tricyclic antidepressants were discovered. MAO inhibitors irreversibly inhibit the enzyme MAO. According to the biogenic amine hypothesis of depression, MAO inhibitors are effective because they prevent the degradation of norepinephrine and serotonin so that the concentration of these CNS neurotransmitters is increased (see Figure 53-1).

Pharmacokinetics

MAO inhibitors are well absorbed orally. They are metabolized in the liver to inactive forms and excreted in urine. Despite this, the onset of action requires 2 to 3 weeks. MAO inhibitors act by irreversible inhibition; removal of enough enzyme to produce clinical effectiveness takes time. Similarly, the effect persists for 2 to 3 weeks after MAO inhibitors have been discontinued, reflecting the time to synthesize adequate MAO.

Uses

MAO inhibitors are not as effective as the tricyclic antidepressants in treating common endogenous depression, but they are more effective in treating depressions exhibited as phobias.

Adverse Reactions and Contraindications

Sedation and anticholinergic effects are common side effects associated with MAO inhibitors, but these drugs usually are administered in divided doses during the day because of their tendency to cause insomnia if given in the evening. Orthostatic hypotension is sometimes a side effect. At one time, MAO inhibitors were used as antihypertensive drugs. As with the tricyclic antidepressants, MAO inhibitors are not addicting.

Toxicity

After ingestion of an overdose of an MAO inhibitor, symptoms appear within 12 hours and reflect increased adrenergic activity such as restlessness, anxiety, and insomnia, progressing to include tachycardia and sometimes convulsions. Dizziness and hypotension may occur, whereas some patients have severe headaches and develop high blood pressure. Some patients develop a high fever, which should be reduced with a sponge bath and external cooling. Treatment is supportive to maintain respiration and circulation. Because the effect of the MAO inhibitor is persistent, patients must be watched for at least a week.

Interactions

Several clinically significant problems arise from the interaction of MAO inhibitors with other drugs and certain foods containing tyramine. A hypertensive crisis may be precipitated when a food containing tyramine or a sympathomimetic drug is ingested (see box). Sympathomimetic drugs and tyramine are normally degraded rapidly by MAO of the liver. When MAO is inhibited, tyramine remains undegraded and triggers the release of accumulated norepinephrine, which in turn causes a hypertensive episode. The earliest symptom of such a hypertensive response may be a severe headache. The necessity of avoiding these substances to avert a life-threatening hypertensive crisis is the major limitation of MAO inhibitors. Phentolamine, the alpha-receptor antagonist, may be given to lower blood pressure during a hypertensive crisis.

DIETARY CONSIDERATION

MAO Inhibitors and Tyramine

Patients taking MAO inhibitors may experience a hypertensive crisis if they ingest foods containing a large amount of tyramine. Food high in tyramine include:

- avocados
- bananas
- beer
- bologna
- canned figs
- chocolate
- cheese (except cottage cheese)
- cheese-containing food (e.g., pizza or macaroni and cheese)
- liver
- meat extracts (e.g., Marmite and Bovril)
- offal
- papaya products, including meat tenderizers
- paté
- pickled and kippered herring
- pepperoni
- pods or broad beans (fava beans)
- raisins
- raw yeast or yeast extracts
- salami
- sausage
- sour cream
- soy sauce
- wine and chianti
- yogurt

Specific Monoamine Oxidase Inhibitors

Isocarboxazid

Isocarboxazid (Marplan) is not considered as effective as other MAO inhibitors but is prescribed for depressed patients who are unresponsive to tricyclic antidepressants and electroconvulsive shock therapy.

Phenelzine

Phenelzine (Nardil) is the safest MAO inhibitor. Patients with a high level of anxiety who do not respond to a tricyclic antidepressant may respond to phenelzine. Doses must be individualized since wide variability exists in its metabolism.

Tranylcypromine

Tranylcypromine (Parnate) can have a stimulatory action similar to amphetamine, and the antidepressant activity is seen more rapidly than with other MAO inhibitors.

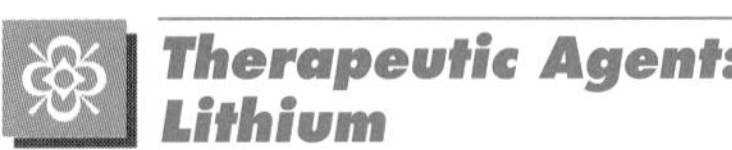

Therapeutic Agent: Lithium

Lithium: General Characteristics

Mechanism of Action

Lithium affects cellular transport mechanisms, second messenger pathways, the dynamics of neurotransmitter processing. Lithium alters both the presynaptic and postsynaptic events affecting serotonin, with a net effect of enhancing central serotonin function. The net effect of lithium is to decrease noradrenergic transmission.

Pharmacokinetics

Lithium is administered orally as the carbonate or citrate salt. Since lithium is an element, related in the atomic table to sodium and potassium, it is not metabolized but is excreted by mechanisms similar to those for sodium and potassium. Of the lithium filtered in the kidney, 80% is reabsorbed in the proximal tubule, and 20% is excreted in urine. The half-life of lithium in the plasma is 24 hours and is increased to 36 hours in older adult patients, so the relative dose of lithium must be decreased to avoid the cumulation to toxic doses. Other factors that decrease lithium excretion include sodium deficiency, extreme exercise, diarrhea, and postpartum status. Factors that increase lithium excretion include high sodium intake and pregnancy.

Uses

Lithium is the drug of choice for treating the manic phase of a manic-depressive disorder. Lithium does not cause CNS depression, excitation, or euphoria. It does stabilize mood, preventing the marked mood swings characteristic of the manic-depressive disorder.

If the patient is severely manic, an antipsychotic drug or electroconvulsive shock therapy may be used initially to subdue behavior. Lithium therapy alone usually reverses mild-to-moderate manic symptoms in 1 to 3 weeks. The duration of lithium therapy depends on the individual. Patients with occasional manic periods may be treated only during those periods.

Continuous lithium therapy is indicated for patients in whom lithium reduces the frequency and intensity of their manic-depressive disorder. Evidence shows that lithium may be effective in treating the depression of the manic-depressive disorder and even endogenous depression. However, lithium is approved only for treating acute mania and as prophylaxis for recurrent mania. In research studies, lithium is being tested for its effectiveness in treating various psychiatric and neurologic brain disorders.

Adverse Reactions and Contraindications

Lithium therapy is contraindicated in early pregnancy because an increased incidence of congenital malformations in infants of treated mothers has been noted. Secretion of the thyroid hormone thyroxine is inhibited by lithium, and a few patients develop an enlarged thyroid gland and may become hypothyroid. A few patients receiving lithium therapy develop nephrogenic diabetes insipidus (see Chapter 59), which is reversed when the lithium dose is lowered or discontinued. Paradoxically, administration of a thiazide diuretic may reverse polyuria. A more serious consequence is permanent renal damage (initially without symptoms), which may develop with long-term lithium therapy. The incidence of this damage remains to be evaluated.

Toxicity

The therapeutic index for lithium is relatively small, and at the start of treatment, patients are tested at least weekly to ensure that the plasma level is in the therapeutic range. The therapeutic range is 0.6 to 1.2 mEq/L but as low as 0.2 mEq/L in older adult patients. Common side effects early in therapy include mild nausea, dry mouth, increased thirst, increased urination (polyuria), and fine tremor of the hands. Toxic symptoms begin to appear at 1.5 to 2 mEq/L and by 4 mEq/L may be fatal. The toxic symptoms are listed in Table 53-4.

Acute lithium toxicity is treated by hastening lithium excretion while maintaining fluid and electrolyte balance. Lithium excretion is increased by administration of an osmotic diuretic such as urea or mannitol. The drugs aminophylline and acetazolamide increase lithium excretion, and one may be given concurrently with the osmotic diuresis. Peritoneal dialysis, or preferably hemodialysis, may be used for severe toxicity or when renal failure occurs.

Interactions

Several drug interactions occur with lithium. Lithium potentiates haloperidol, tricyclic antidepressants, phenothiazines, benzodiazepines, and neuromuscular blocking drugs. Lithium is potentiated by methyldopa, sodium-depleting diuretics, and the phenothiazines.

TABLE 53-4 Toxic Symptoms of Lithium

BLOOD LEVEL (mEq/L)	SYMPTOMS
Below 1.5	Fine tremor of hands Dry mouth Increased thirst Increased urination Nausea
1.5-2	Vomiting Diarrhea Muscle weakness Incoordination (ataxia) Dizziness Confusion Slurred speech
2-2.5	Persistent nausea and vomiting Blurred vision Muscle twitching (fasciculations) Hyperactive deep tendon reflexes
2.5-3	Myoclonic twitches or movements of an entire limb Choreoathetoid movements Urinary and fecal incontinence
Above 3	Seizures Cardiac arrhythmias Hypotension Peripheral vascular collapse Death

NURSING PROCESS OVERVIEW

Antidepressants

Assessment

Antidepressants are used for patients with pronounced, prolonged depression or manic-depressive disease. Perform a thorough physiologic assessment and assess mental status, focusing on objective signs of depression. Monitor vital signs, weight, and blood pressure.

Nursing Diagnoses

- Potential body image disturbance related to weight gain as drug side effect
- Risk for self-harm
- Altered bowel elimination: constipation

Patient Outcomes

The patient will not harm himself or herself. The patient will have no constipation or will carry out dietary or other measures to reduce the incidence of constipation. The patient will discuss feelings about self. The patient will assume responsibility for managing weight.

Planning/Implementation

Monitor fluid intake and output, weight, and blood pressure. Review serum drug levels if available. Assess the patient's level of consciousness, with attention to excessive sedation. Assess for possible suicidal tendencies. Monitor for side effects of the drugs such as the dry mouth and constipation that may occur with tricyclic antidepressants.

Evaluation

Before discharging a patient for self-management, ascertain that the patient or family can explain what drug is being taken, how to take it correctly, the side effects that may occur and those that should be reported immediately to the physician, dietary restrictions associated with the medication being used, and ways in which the success of the drug will be monitored. Verify that patients can explain why follow-up is necessary and when to return for it.

NURSING IMPLICATIONS SUMMARY

General Guidelines: Antidepressants

Drug Administration

- The risk of suicide may exist in seriously depressed patients and may persist for several weeks after they begin antidepressant therapy. Some patients who were not suicidal may become so during initial therapy with antidepressants. Assess patients carefully.
- Monitor vital signs and weight.
- As mood improves, appetite may improve. In addition, some antidepressants contribute to weight gain. If weight gain is significant, counsel patients about weight reduction diets and increased exercise. Provide emotional support as needed. Consult the physician about possible changes in dose or drug.
- Many antidepressants alter the seizure threshold. In patients with a history of seizures, pad siderails, and supervise carefully until effects of the medications can be evaluated.

Patient and Family Education

- Inform the patient and family that several weeks of therapy may be necessary before full effects of a drug regimen can be evaluated. Some side effects may lessen with continued drug use.
- Common side effects are noted in this text, but encourage the patient to consult the physician when any new side effects develop.
- Inform the patient that antidepressants must be taken as ordered, on a regular basis, even if he or she begins to feel better. Instruct the patient to consult the physician before changing the prescribed drug regimen or discontinuing medications.
- Warn the patient to inform all health care providers of all drugs being taken.
- Instruct the patient to avoid over-the-counter drugs unless first approved by the physician.
- Instruct the patient to avoid alcohol unless approved in moderation by the physician.
- Warn the patient to avoid driving or operating hazardous equipment if drowsiness occurs.
- Encourage the patient and family to stay in touch with the physician and to seek assistance from appropriate health care personnel including physicians, psychologists, nurses, and therapists.
- Remind the patient to keep these and all drugs out of the reach of children.

Tricyclic and Heterocyclic Antidepressants

Drug Administration

- See the general guidelines for antidepressants.
- Monitor vital signs and blood pressure.
- Assess for skin changes. Auscultate bowel sounds and keep a record of stools.
- Monitor complete blood count (CBC) and platelet count.
- Concentrated solutions are available for some of the antidepressants; consult the manufacturer's literature for appropriate diluents.
- For amoxapine, see the patient problem box on neuroleptic malignant syndrome (p. 648), and assess for tardive dyskinesia (Table 52-3).
- Supervise the patient carefully to ascertain that the medication is swallowed and not hidden in the mouth to be discarded or stored for later use.
- Imipramine may be used in the treatment of enuresis in children older than 6 years of age. The most frequent side effects are nervousness, sleep disorders, and gastrointestinal (GI) tract upset, although any side effects listed may occur. Treatment is continued for as short a period as possible to obtain relief, then the dose is tapered. The drug should be taken about 1 hour before bedtime, although early night bed-wetters may have a better response if part of the dose is given in the afternoon and part at bedtime; check with the physician. The treatment of enuresis can be complex. Provide emotional support as needed.

Patient and Family Education

- Review the general guidelines for antidepressants with the patient.

Continued.

NURSING IMPLICATIONS SUMMARY—cont'd

- See the patient problem boxes on orthostatic hypotension (p. 157), dry mouth (p. 300), constipation (p. 304), and photosensitivity (p. 649).
- If sedation is a problem, suggest that the patient take daily doses at bedtime.
- Instruct the patient to take doses with meals or a snack to lessen gastric irritation.
- Advise a diabetic patient to monitor blood glucose levels since antidepressants may alter them. A change in diet or insulin dose may be necessary.
- Patient instructions for missed doses: If usually taken at bedtime, but missed, do not take the dose the next morning; check with physician. For missed doses if taken more than once a day, take missed dose as soon as remembered, unless almost time for the next dose, then omit missed dose and resume regular dosage schedule. Do not double up for missed doses.

Selective Serotonin Reuptake Inhibitors

Drug Administration

- See the general guidelines for antidepressants.

Patient and Family Education

- Review the general guidelines for antidepressants with the patient.
- Take doses with food or snack to lessen gastric irritation.
- For a patient taking fluoxetine: Stop drug and notify physician if rash or hives develop.
- Avoid driving or operating hazardous equipment if dizziness, drowsiness, or light-headedness develops.
- See the patient problem box on dry mouth (p. 300).

Monoamine Oxidase Inhibitors

Drug Administration

- See the general guidelines for antidepressants.
- Monitor vital signs and blood pressure.
- Auscultate bowel sounds and keep a record of stools.
- Monitor CBC and platelet count.
- Supervise the patient carefully to ascertain that the medication is swallowed and not hidden in the mouth to be discarded or stored.

Patient and Family Education

- Review the general guidelines for antidepressants with the patient.
- See the patient problem boxes on orthostatic hypotension (p. 157), dry mouth (p. 300), and constipation (p. 304).
- Review dietary restrictions with the patient and family. See the dietary consideration box on MAO inhibitors and tyramine (p. 663).
- Instruct the patient to avoid excessive caffeine intake, although small amounts are acceptable.
- Tell a diabetic patient to monitor blood glucose levels since antidepressants may alter them. A change in diet or insulin dose may be necessary.
- Review drug interactions with the patient.

Lithium

Drug Administration

- See the general guidelines for antidepressants.
- Monitor vital signs. Inspect for edema.
- Assess for symptoms of toxicity (see Table 53-4) .
- Monitor serum drug levels.
- If urinary output is excessive, assess for diabetes insipidus (dilute, high-volume urine with a specific gravity of 1.000 to 1.003).
- Supervise the patient carefully to ascertain that the medication is swallowed and not hidden in the mouth to be discarded or stored.

Patient and Family Education

- Review the general guidelines for antidepressants with the patient.
- Emphasize the importance of returning for follow-up care to have serum drug levels monitored.
- Review the signs and symptoms of lithium toxicity, and teach the patient to report them. Provide emotional support as needed for side effects such as fine hand tremor, polyuria, and metallic taste in the mouth. Remind the patient not to discontinue medications without consulting the physician.
- Inform the patient to take lithium at same time daily. Take doses with meals or a snack to lessen gastric irritation.
- Instruct the patient to maintain a fluid intake of 2.5 to 3 L/day. Instruct the patient to drink limited amounts of coffee, tea, or colas to prevent marked diuresis.
- Instruct the patient to dilute syrup form in fruit juice or other flavored beverage before taking dose.
- See the patient problem box on dry mouth (p. 300). Instruct the patient to notify the physician if fever or severe or persistent diarrhea or vomiting occurs since any of these may contribute to electrolyte disturbance, which may contribute to lithium toxicity.

CRITICAL THINKING

APPLICATION

1. What is the biogenic amine theory of depression?
2. How are the actions of the tricyclic and heterocyclic antidepressants, MAO inhibitors, and lithium consistent with the biogenic amine theory of depression?
3. How can drugs cause depression? How would you determine drug-induced depression?
4. What are the major side effects of the tricyclic antidepressants?
5. How do the heterocyclic antidepressants compare with tricyclic antidepressants?
6. What are the common side effects of MAO inhibitors?
7. What are the symptoms of lithium toxicity?

CRITICAL THINKING

1. Describe the acute toxicity of the tricyclic antidepressants. What are the symptoms?
2. What are the major drug interactions of the tricyclic antidepressants? How should you educate patients?
3. What are the major drug interactions of the heterocyclic antidepressants? How should you educate patients?
4. How can a hypertensive crisis be precipitated in a patient taking an MAO inhibitor? What would you teach a patient to help avoid a hypertensive crisis?

CHAPTER 54

Central Nervous System Stimulants

OBJECTIVES

After studying this chapter, you should be able to do the following:

- *Name the appropriate clinical uses of central nervous system stimulants.*
- *Discuss the side effects of these agents.*
- *Develop a nursing care plan for the patient receiving a central nervous system stimulant.*

KEY TERMS

amphetamines
analeptics
anorexiants
attention-deficit hyperactivity disorder
narcolepsy

CHAPTER OVERVIEW

The central nervous system (CNS) regulates its level of activity by maintaining excitatory and inhibitory systems. Therefore excessive stimulation of the CNS may be produced by excessive activity of excitatory neurons or by blockade of inhibitory neurons. Many types of chemicals at some dose produce a degree of CNS stimulation by one of these mechanisms. Few of these compounds have legitimate pharmacologic uses. CNS stimulants currently are medically accepted only for the treatment of narcolepsy, attention-deficit hyperactivity disorder in children, and obesity. The drugs also are used occasionally as agents to reverse respiratory depression, although they are not recommended for these purposes. This chapter examines the mechanism of action of CNS stimulants used in clinical conditions. The properties that make them drugs of abuse are discussed fully in Chapter 8.

Therapeutic Rationale: Narcolepsy and Attention-Deficit Hyperactivity Disorder

Narcolepsy is a condition in which patients unexpectedly fall asleep during normal activity such as while typing, driving a car, or talking. During an attack, patients experience paralysis of voluntary muscles similar to that experienced while dreaming and may abruptly collapse and fall. Patients with this sleep disorder should be advised to avoid operating cars or dangerous machinery.

The treatment of narcolepsy usually includes the use of CNS stimulants during active daytime periods. These agents have alerting effects and reduce the sleeping episodes. Although drug therapy may be beneficial for many narcoleptic patients, most also require other therapy such as scheduled daytime naps. Psychologic counseling may help patients to reconcile their living patterns with the constraints imposed by the disease.

Children with **attention-deficit hyperactivity disorder** display a variety of symptoms that impair their ability to learn or to maintain appropriate social interactions. These children are excessively active, impulsive, and irritable. Their attention span is very short, and their activity is purposeless. Learning disabilities of various types are frequent in these children. Many children with attention-deficit hyperactivity disorder have abnormal electroencephalographic (EEG) patterns and poorer coordination than normal children of the same age. Intelligence is not impaired. Because of the wide range of symptoms produced, this syndrome has been called by many names, including *minimal brain dysfunction, minimal brain damage, hyperkinesis, attention-deficit disorder with hyperkinesis,* and *hyperkinetic syndrome with learning disorder.*

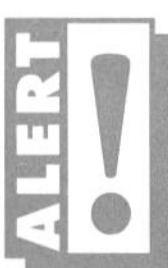

DRUG ABUSE ALERT

Methylphenidate

THE PROBLEM

Methylphenidate rarely causes toxic psychosis but may cause psychologic drug dependence. Both effects are observed after long-term use of doses in excess of therapeutic doses. The primary patient is obviously most at risk of developing dependence, but health care personnel must also be alert to the problem among caregivers. For example, adult guardians of children receiving methylphenidate may divert the drug from the child and use it themselves.

SOLUTIONS

- Confirm that doses are not being extemporaneously increased by the patient or caregiver.
- Advise the patient to seek medical advice if drug seems to become less effective after several weeks.
- See that dosage reduction is gradual so that withdrawal symptoms are minimized

Children with attention-deficit hyperactivity disorder may require drug therapy to reduce hyperactive behavior and to lengthen their attention span. The drugs most effective in controlling this disorder are, paradoxically, CNS stimulants. These agents, which increase agitation and activity in adults, have a calming effect on these children. Although amphetamines have been used for this disorder, an equally effective drug with fewer peripheral side effects is methylphenidate (see box). Pemoline may be used but in general is less effective than amphetamines or methylphenidate.

Controversy surrounds the diagnosis and treatment of children with attention-deficit hyperactivity disorder. Many authorities believe the syndrome is diagnosed more frequently than it exists and suggest that thousands of children may be receiving CNS stimulants unnecessarily. This problem remains to be resolved.

Therapeutic Agents: Narcolepsy and Attention-Deficit Hyperactivity Disorder

Central Nervous System Stimulants

Amphetamine, dextroamphetamine, methamphetamine

Mechanism of Action

Amphetamines increase the release and effectiveness of catecholamine neurotransmitters in the brain and in peripheral nerves by several mechanisms. These drugs seem to increase release of neurotransmitters during normal nervous system activity. In addition, amphetamines block specific reuptake of catecholamine neurotransmitters into presynaptic neurons. Because this reuptake system is normally a major mechanism for terminating the action of neurotransmitters, blockade of the reuptake system produces prolonged and enhanced stimulation of postsynaptic nerves. Norepinephrine and dopamine are thought to be the catecholamines whose actions are most enhanced by amphetamines.

Amphetamines may affect many sites within the brain, but the clinically observed actions of amphetamines probably are related to activity in two particular regions. One is the reticular activating system, which regulates sensory input to the brain and thus controls the level of arousal. Amphetamines stimulate the reticular activating system, creating increased alertness and sensitivity to stimuli.

The second area of the brain affected by amphetamines is in the medial forebrain bundle. This reward, or pleasure, center can be activated by amphetamines. The result to the user is a perception of pleasure unrelated to external stimuli. This stimulation of the pleasure center is thought to be the source of the addictive potential of amphetamines.

Pharmacokinetics

Amphetamines for medical uses are given orally. These drugs are well absorbed from the gastrointestinal (GI) tract and produce peak serum concentrations within 2 to 3 hours after ingestion. The half-lives of the various amphetamines in blood range from 4 to 30 hours. These compounds easily penetrate the blood-brain barrier to produce their CNS effects. Amphetamines are excreted primarily by the kidneys. The rate of excretion is highly dependent on urinary pH. Excretion can be greatly enhanced by acidifying urine.

Uses

Amphetamines may control narcolepsy or attention-deficit hyperactivity disorder, but the high abuse potential of these drugs limits their usefulness (see Chapter 8). Uses for individual amphetamines are shown in Table 54-1.

Adverse Reactions and Contraindications

Generic amphetamine is a mixture of two forms of amphetamine called *d* (dextro) and *l* (levo). The *d* form stimulates the CNS more effectively than does the *l* form. Conversely, the *l* form stimulates the cardiovascular system slightly more effectively than does the *d* form. Amphetamine, a mixture of *d* and *l* forms, causes both CNS and cardiovascular side effects, so patients may experience irritability, nervousness, restlessness, and irregular heartbeat. Dextroamphetamine, the *d* form of amphetamine, is more selective for the CNS and produces primarily CNS side effects.

Children receiving amphetamines may suffer growth retardation. This effect can be minimized by giving holidays during which drug therapy is suspended.

Amphetamines should be used with caution in patients with cardiovascular disease, glaucoma, hyperthyroidism, or psychoses because these conditions may be worsened by amphetamines.

TABLE 54-1 CNS Stimulants for Narcolepsy and Attention-Deficit Hyperactivity Disorder

GENERIC NAME	TRADE NAME	ADMINISTRATION/DOSAGE	COMMENTS
Amphetamine sulfate (also called racemic or *dl*-amphetamine sulfate)		For narcolepsy: ORAL: *Adults*—5-20 mg 1-3 times daily. FDA pregnancy category C. *Children >6 yr*—2.5 mg twice daily; gradually increase to adult dose if needed.	Schedule II substance (U.S.). Dosage is adjusted according to patient's needs and tolerance to side effects.
		For attention-deficit hyperactivity disorder: ORAL: *Children 3-6 yr*—2.5 mg daily; increase by 2.5 mg increments weekly to achieve desired effect; *Children >6 yr*—initially 5 mg daily; increase by 5 mg increments weekly to achieve desired effect.	Dosage should be minimum required for control of symptoms.
Dextroamphetamine sulfate	Dexedrine* Dextrostat	For narcolepsy: ORAL: *Adults*—5-60 mg once daily (extended-release capsules) or in divided doses (tablets). FDA pregnancy category C.	Schedule II substance (U.S.). Class G (Canada).
		For attention-deficit hyperactivity disorder: ORAL: *Children 3-6 yr*—2.5 mg daily; increase by 2.5 mg increments weekly to achieve desired effect; *Children ≥6 yr*—initially 5 mg daily; increase by 5 mg increments weekly to achieve desired effect.	Dosage should be minimum required for control of symptoms.
Methamphetamine hydrochloride	Desoxyn	For attention-deficit hyperactivity disorder: ORAL: *Children ≥6 yr*—5 mg once or twice daily; increase by 5 mg at weekly intervals; or 20-25 mg (extended-release tablets) once daily.	Schedule II substance (U.S.). Dosage should be minimum required for control of symptoms.
✣ Methylphenidate hydrochloride	Ritalin*	For attention-deficit hyperactivity disorder: ORAL: *Children ≥6 yr*—5 mg before breakfast and lunch; increase by 5 or 10 mg weekly; maximum daily dose 60 mg. Extended-release tablets: 20 mg every 8 hr. For narcolepsy: ORAL: *Adults*—5-20 mg 2 or 3 times daily before meals; extended-release tablets: 20 mg every 8 hr.	Schedule II substance (U.S.). Class C (Canada). Drug of choice for most children with attention-deficit hyperactivity disorder.
Pemoline	Cylert*	For attention-deficit hyperactivity disorder: ORAL: *Children ≥6 yr*—37.5 mg daily in single dose; increase weekly by 18.75 mg until response is obtained. Do not exceed 112.5 mg daily.	Schedule IV substance (U.S.). Clinical effects develop over 3-4 wk.

*Available in Canada and United States.

Toxicity

Most CNS toxicity of amphetamines is an extension of effects observed at therapeutic doses. At high doses, amphetamines cause restless behavior, tremor, irritability, talkativeness, insomnia, and mood changes. Excessive aggressiveness, confusion, panic, and increased libido also may occur. More rarely, patients suffer a syndrome resembling schizophrenia, with hallucinations or delirium. Long-term intoxication with amphetamines causes this schizophrenia-like reaction, sometimes called *toxic psychosis.*

The sympathomimetic effects of amphetamines can cause various cardiovascular reactions. Patients report headache, chilliness, and palpitations. Pallor or facial flushing may be present. Angina and various cardiac arrhythmias may arise. Hypertension or hypotension may be observed at various stages during intoxication. Severely intoxicated patients may die in circulatory collapse.

Symptoms of withdrawal seen after prolonged use of high doses include nausea, stomach cramps, vomiting, depression, trembling, and unusual tiredness or weakness.

Interactions

Amphetamines block metabolism of tricyclic antidepressants, causing these drugs to accumulate unless dosage is reduced. Sympathomimetic drugs can increase the effects of amphetamines. Monoamine oxidase (MAO) inhibitors also increase catecholamine levels and potentiate effects of amphetamines; these drugs should not be given within 14 days of one another. Use of amphetamines with beta-adrenergic blockers may cause hypertension and slow heart rate as a result of unopposed alpha-adrenergic activity. Use of amphetamines with meperidine may lead to hypotension, respiratory depression, and vascular collapse. Digitalis glycosides or thyroid hormones may increase the risk of cardiac arrhythmias or coronary insufficiency with amphetamines.

✣ Methylphenidate

Mechanism of Action

Methylphenidate is a mild CNS stimulant. Its exact biochemical mechanism of action is unknown but may involve blockade of dopamine uptake in specific regions of the brain.

Pharmacokinetics

Methylphenidate is well absorbed orally and is usually taken by adults 30 to 45 minutes before meals. Orally administered methylphenidate is extensively metabolized during the first pass through the liver. Metabolites of methylphenidate do not stimulate the CNS or sympathetic peripheral neurons. The drug is excreted in urine mostly as these inactive metabolites.

Uses

Methylphenidate may be useful in narcolepsy as a result of its mild CNS stimulatory effects on the cortex and other portions of the brain. Methylphenidate is very commonly used for attention-deficit hyperactivity disorder, where the CNS effects of the drug have a calming effect.

Adverse Reactions and Contraindications

Methylphenidate often causes nervousness and insomnia. Insomnia may be minimized by not taking the drug in the evening. Nervousness may be controlled by reducing overall drug dosage. Anorexia, nausea, and abdominal pain may occur with methylphenidate. Cardiovascular effects like those produced by amphetamines are also seen and include hypertension and tachycardia.

Methylphenidate causes a temporary slowing of growth in prepubertal children. Most children overcome the deficit and ultimately gain normal stature. Slow growth can be minimized by giving the child a drug-free period during therapy.

Methylphenidate is avoided in patients with severe anxiety, depression, motor tics, or glaucoma because these conditions may be worsened by the drug.

Toxicity

Very high doses cause dangerous CNS effects (agitation, confusion, delirium, seizures, and coma) and cardiovascular effects (arrhythmias, hypertension). Symptoms of withdrawal seen after prolonged use of high doses include bizarre behavior, depression, and unusual tiredness or weakness.

Interactions

Methylphenidate, like the amphetamines, can interact with many other medications. Since methylphenidate causes its effects by release of catecholamines such as norepinephrine, the effects may be greatly increased by MAO inhibitors, sympathomimetic agents, or vasopressors. Pimozide should be avoided in patients receiving methylphenidate because methylphenidate can cause tics.

Pemoline

Mechanism of Action

Pemoline stimulates the CNS in a manner similar to that of amphetamines and methylphenidate but lacks the strong sympathomimetic effects of many of those stimulants. The exact biochemical mechanism for the action of pemoline is unknown.

Pharmacokinetics

Pemoline is well absorbed orally, producing peak serum levels 2 to 4 hours after dosage. The serum half-life for the drug is about 12 hours. Therefore the drug may be given once daily. The kidneys excrete most of the administered pemoline, as unchanged drug and as metabolites.

Although the blood levels reach a plateau within a few days after therapy is begun, the therapeutic effects of pemoline are not immediately evident in hyperkinetic children. Dosage is gradually increased over 2 to 4 weeks after therapy is started. Significant clinical response may not be seen until the third or fourth week.

Uses

Pemoline is only indicated for attention-deficit hyperactivity disorder.

Adverse Reactions and Contraindications

Pemoline, when used in properly selected children at recommended doses, seldom causes serious side effects. CNS signs such as irritability, mild depression, dizziness, headache, and hallucinations are rare. Insomnia often is reported but is a transient reaction in most patients. Pemoline causes anorexia, stomachache, and nausea, which may slow normal weight gain. Children do not seem to suffer permanent growth retardation, but careful records of the child's growth should be maintained to allow assessment during therapy.

Pemoline is avoided in patients with hepatic function impairment because the drug may further impair the liver.

Toxicity

High doses of pemoline cause CNS effects (agitation, confusion, convulsions, hallucinations, restlessness) and cardiovascular effects (severe headache, hypertension, tachycardia). Symptoms of withdrawal seen after prolonged use of high doses include bizarre behavior, depression, and unusual tiredness or weakness.

Interactions

Although pemoline could cause additive stimulation if used with other CNS stimulants, most interactions with pemoline are of limited clinical significance.

Therapeutic Rationale: Obesity

Obesity is a complex problem with psychologic as well as medical components. Persons seeking to lose weight must develop appropriate eating habits and an exercise plan adjusted to their age and physical limitations. For those persons who find it difficult to limit food intake on their own, drugs may be used for short-term suppression of appetite. As a group these drugs are referred to as **anorexiants** or *appetite suppressants* (Table 54-2).

Therapeutic Agents: Obesity

Anorexiants

Benzphetamine, diethylpropion, fenfluramine, mazindol, phendimetrazine, phentermine, phenylpropanolamine

Mechanism of Action

Many CNS stimulants suppress appetite by effects on the hypothalamus in the brain, even while stimulating other CNS functions. Amphetamines were the original CNS stimulants used to control obesity but because of undesirable side effects, including the risk of addiction, they are no longer used in obesity. Currently used anorexiants are listed in Table 54-2.

Fenfluramine is unlike the other anorexiant drugs since it depresses the CNS while suppressing the appetite.

Tolerance develops to all appetite-suppressing drugs in clinical use. Drugs to suppress appetite may help a patient during the initial stages of a weight-reduction program, but these agents are not the key to a successful long-term program.

Pharmacokinetics

Anorexiants are well absorbed orally and have a duration of anorexiant effect ranging from 4 hours (diethylpropion, fenfluramine, phendimetrazine, phentermine) to 15 hours (mazindol). Diethylpropion and phentermine are available in extended release forms that have a duration of action of 12 to 14 hours.

Uses

The anorexiants are for short-term use in a medically supervised program of weight reduction. Diethylpropion, unlike other anorexiants, produces little cardiovascular stimulation and thus may be used in patients with some types of cardiovascular disease.

Phenylpropanolamine mildly suppresses appetite and is included in various nonprescription appetite suppressants, alone or with other agents. Phenylpropanolamine also is often used in nonprescription nasal decongestants (see Chapter 7).

Adverse Reactions and Contraindications

Some anorexiants resemble amphetamines in activity and reactions but produce these reactions less frequently and less severely (Table 54-3); these include benzphetamine and mazindol.

Anorexiants commonly cause irritability and insomnia. Sympathetic nervous system effects include dry mouth, blurred vision, heart palpitations, and hypertension. Because of these sympathetic nervous system effects, these drugs are avoided in patients with hypertension or glaucoma. Most are also avoided in patients with cardiovascular disease, the exception being diethylpropion.

Many of the available effective appetite suppressants have high abuse potential, and many patients experience some level of dependence on these medications (see Table 54-3 and the box on p. 674). For this reason appetite suppressants are avoided in patients with a history of drug or alcohol abuse.

Fenfluramine may produce dangerous mental imbalances, although with this drug the danger is depression rather than stimulation of the CNS. Fenfluramine should be avoided in patients with a previous history of depression or suicidal tendencies.

The anorexiants have not been proved safe during pregnancy; benzphetamine is rated as FDA pregnancy category X. None of these drugs are intended for use in children.

Toxicity

Overdoses with anorexiants can produce dangerous cardiovascular and CNS effects. Symptoms of overdose include GI tract effects (abdominal cramping, diarrhea, nausea, vomiting), CNS effects (aggressiveness, convulsions, coma, hallucinations, hostility, panic, restlessness, tremors), and cardiovascular effects that can be fatal (arrhythmias, fluctuating blood pressure, cardiovascular collapse).

TABLE 54-2 Appetite Suppressants

GENERIC NAME	TRADE NAME	ADMINISTRATION/DOSAGE	COMMENTS
Benzphetamine	Didrex	ORAL: *Adults*—25-50 mg once daily; may increase as needed up to 3 doses daily. FDA pregnancy category X.	Schedule III substance. (U.S.).
Diethylpropion	Tenuate* Tepanil	ORAL: *Adults*—25 mg 1 hr before morning, noon, and evening meals and at midevening if needed. Timed-release formulations (75 mg) are taken once daily. FDA pregnancy category B.	Safest anorexiant for use in patients with mild cardiovascular disease. Schedule IV substance (U.S.). Class G (Canada).
Fenfluramine	Ponderal† Pondimin*	ORAL: *Adults*—20 mg 3 times daily before meals. Dosage may be doubled if required. Extended-release capsules: 60 mg once daily. FDA pregnancy category C.	Only anorexiant that depresses CNS activity; sedation and depression may occur. Schedule IV substance. (U.S.).
Mazindol	Mazanor Sanorex*	ORAL: *Adults*—1 mg daily at breakfast; may increase to 1 mg 3 times daily with meals.	May be used in patients with arteriosclerosis or hyperthyroidism. Schedule IV substance (U.S.).
Phendimetrazine	Anorex Bontril Melfiat Plegine	ORAL: *Adults*—35 mg 2 or 3 times daily taken before meals. Sustained-release: 105 mg taken once in morning.	Schedule III substance. (U.S.).
Phentermine	Adipex Fastin* Zantryl	ORAL: *Adults*—Single dose of 15-37.5 mg may be taken 2 hr after breakfast.	Schedule IV substance (U.S.) Class G (Canada).
Phenylpropanolamine	Acutrim Dexatrim Prolamine	ORAL: *Adults*—25 mg 3 times daily before meals or 50-75 mg of sustained-action formulation once daily at midmorning.	These diet preparations should not be used with cold or allergy medications. Nonprescription drug.

*Available in Canada and United States.
†Available in Canada only.

TABLE 54-3 Systemic Effects of Appetite Suppressants

GENERIC NAME	MOOD	MOTOR ACTIVITY	HEART RATE	BLOOD PRESSURE	ABUSE POTENTIAL
Benzphetamine	Elevated	May increase	May increase	May increase	High
Diethylpropion	May be elevated	May increase	Unchanged	Unchanged	Relatively low
Fenfluramine	Depressed	Depressed	Usually no change	May increase	Relatively low
Mazindol	May be elevated	May increase	Increased	Usually no change	Relatively low
Phendimetrazine	Highly elevated	Increased	Usually no change	Usually no change	High
Phentermine	Usually no change	May increase	Increased	Increased	Relatively low
Phenylpropanolamine	Usually no change	Usually no change	May increase	May increase	Low

Symptoms of withdrawal seen after prolonged use of high doses include GI tract difficulties, insomnia, depression, trembling, and unusual tiredness or weakness.

Interactions

Anorexiants can interact with many other medications. For example, sympathomimetic drugs may have a much greater effect in patients receiving appetite suppressants, because the appetite-suppressing drugs tend to increase the effectiveness of catecholamines. This precaution should be mentioned to patients, and they should be warned to avoid cold remedies, allergy medications, and nasal decongestants that include sympathomimetic agents. For the same reasons, MAO inhibitors should not be used within 14 days of taking an anorexiant.

Thyroid hormones or any drug producing CNS stimulation are avoided with all anorexiants except fenfluramine; fenfluramine is avoided in combination with CNS depressants because of its own CNS depressive effects.

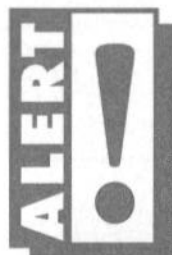

Drug Abuse Alert

Appetite Suppressants

THE PROBLEM

Many patients experience some level of dependence on the CNS stimulants used as appetite suppressants. Patients may seek them from several physicians rather than follow the advice of a single physician who may limit the use of the drugs to 2 to 3 months. Many appetite suppressants also carry the risk of causing psychotic reactions, as a result of either overdosage or prolonged use.

SOLUTIONS

- Warn the patient that the anorectic effect will wear off in 6 to 12 weeks
- Warn the patient not to increase dosage to prolong the anorectic effect
- Observe for signs of dependence
- Offer counseling about healthy dietary limitations and good eating practices

Therapeutic Rationale: Respiratory Depression

Certain CNS stimulants have generalized effects on the brainstem and spinal cord, as well as on higher centers in the brain. These drugs may increase responsiveness to external stimuli and stimulate respiration. As a group, these drugs are referred to as **analeptics** (Table 54-4).

Analeptics have been used to stimulate respiration, but the use of these drugs has become less common because modern techniques of respiratory therapy allow a patient to be adequately ventilated even when the natural reflex is absent. Respiratory paralysis caused by overdoses of narcotic agents is treated with specific narcotic antagonists and not with analeptics.

Therapeutic Agents: Respiratory Depression

Methylxanthines

Caffeine, aminophylline, ✣ theophylline

Mechanism of Action

Methylxanthines block destruction of cyclic adenosine monophosphate (AMP), the compound that mediates the effects of beta-adrenergic stimulation (see Chapter 10). As a result, these compounds affect many body systems, including the CNS.

Caffeine may stimulate any level of the CNS, depending on dose. Caffeine stimulates the medullary centers controlling respiration, vasomotor tone, and vagal tone only at relatively high doses. Very high doses of caffeine may stimulate the spinal cord and produce convulsions. Theophylline also acts as a CNS stimulant but exerts more action on the heart than does caffeine.

Pharmacokinetics

Methylxanthines are well absorbed orally and may be given by nasogastric tube for neonatal apnea. Parenteral solutions are also used for this indication. Metabolism and clearance of methylxanthines may be much lower in neonates than in adults; for this reason blood levels of these drugs may need to be monitored. Clearance of methylxanthines is also lower in patients with liver disease; these patients may also need lower doses.

Uses

Methylxanthines such as aminophylline and theophylline are most often used as bronchodilators (see Chapter 27). These drugs and caffeine are no longer approved as respiratory stimulants in newborn infants.

Adverse Reactions and Contraindications

Two properties of analeptic drugs make them especially hard to control. First, they are nonspecific CNS stimulants and may produce unwanted effects in addition to respiratory

TABLE 54-4 CNS Stimulants for Respiratory Stimulation

GENERIC NAME	TRADE NAME	ADMINISTRATION/DOSAGE	COMMENTS
Aminophylline		ORAL, NASOGASTRIC TUBE: 5 mg/kg initial dose; then 2 mg/kg daily, divided into 2 or 3 doses.	Most commonly used to treat asthma but also used to treat neonatal apnea.
Caffeine (citrated caffeine)		ORAL, NASOGASTRIC TUBE: 10 mg/kg body weight initially; then 2.5 mg/kg daily.	Used in neonatal apnea.
Doxapram	Dopram*	INTRAVENOUS: *Adults*—0.5-2 mg/kg body weight intermittently as needed. For chronic obstructive pulmonary disease: 1-2 mg/min infusion for 2 hr.	Rapidly acting drug whose action is over within 12 min. Do not use in newborn infants because of benzyl alcohol content.
✣ Theophylline		ORAL, NASOGASTRIC TUBE: 5 mg/kg body weight initial dose; then 2 mg/kg daily divided into 2 or 3 doses.	Most commonly used to treat asthma but also used to treat neonatal apnea.

*Available in Canada and United States.

stimulation. Second, all these drugs at a high enough dose or in a predisposed patient may produce convulsions.

Toxicity

High doses of methylxanthines may cause arrhythmias or convulsions.

Interactions

The interactions that may occur with these drugs are presented in Chapters 8 and 27.

Analeptic

Doxapram

Mechanism of Action

Doxapram stimulates respiration in two ways. At low doses the drug stimulates carotid chemoreceptors. This action increases sensitivity to carbon dioxide and thereby increases the impulse to breathe. At slightly higher doses, doxapram stimulates CNS medullary centers controlling respiration. The result is that patients breathe more deeply and may breathe slightly more rapidly.

Pharmacokinetics

Doxapram is administered intravenously. The drug is very rapid acting, with effects observed within 1 minute after injection. The duration of respiratory stimulation is usually 5 to 12 minutes. Doxapram may be given repeatedly or by infusion to sustain a patient throughout a period of respiratory depression, but total doses should normally not exceed 300 mg.

Uses

Doxapram is indicated only for postanesthesia respiratory depression or acute respiratory insufficiency in chronic obstructive pulmonary disease.

Adverse Reactions and Contraindications

Doxapram can produce a variety of reactions. Dizziness, apprehension, and disorientation may be reported. Restless, involuntary muscle activity, and increased reflexes are frequently observed. Patients may report a feeling of warmth with flushing, sweating, and increased body temperature. Blood pressure is elevated. Chest pains and cardiac arrhythmias may occur.

The drug should be avoided in patients with stroke, head injury, coronary artery disease, heart failure, hypertension, epilepsy, airway obstruction, or pulmonary disease. All these conditions may be worsened by doxapram.

Toxicity

If the drug is injected too rapidly, hemolysis may occur. Extreme agitation, hallucinations, or convulsions usually occur only with overdose, but certain patients may be more susceptible to these reactions.

Interactions

Since doxapram increases blood pressure, this drug should not be used in combination with other drugs tending to elevate blood pressure, such as sympathomimetics and MAO inhibitors. Adverse interactions can also occur between doxapram and the inhalation anesthetics that sensitize the heart to catecholamines (e.g., halothane and enflurane). A delay of 10 minutes or more between the cessation of anesthesia with these drugs and the administration of doxapram is suggested to lessen the possibility of excessive cardiac toxicity.

NURSING PROCESS OVERVIEW

Assessment

Perform a complete assessment, with a focus on the problem under treatment. Assess vital signs and blood pressure. For children with attention-deficit hyperactivity disorder, assess weight, height, typical behavior, attention span, and history of any problems in school. For narcolepsy, assess weight, difficulty with activities of daily living, driving, working, or school. For obesity, assess weight and exercise patterns and obtain diet history. For respiratory stimulation, auscultate lung sounds. Assess mental status.

Nursing Diagnoses

- Risk for growth retardation in children
- Altered comfort: nausea and GI tract discomfort
- Risk for hypertension
- Risk for toxic psychosis related to drug therapy

Patient Outcomes

For attention-deficit hyperactivity disorder: The patient will demonstrate less hyperactive behavior, with an increased attention span, improvement in school work, and normal growth patterns. The nurse will manage and minimize growth retardation.

For narcolepsy: The patient will remain awake and alert for longer periods and will be awake for required job or school activities.

For obesity: The patient will lose weight and on the long term will learn behavioral changes to sustain weight loss.

For respiratory stimulation: The patient will breathe spontaneously at a normal rate.

Planning/Implementation

The problems addressed by the drugs in this chapter are varied. Work with the patient and family to set reasonable goals of therapy. Monitor the patient for side effects, ranging from insomnia and weight loss to hypertension and changes in affect. Encourage the patient to return for regular follow-up to monitor progress and to monitor for side effects. Refer the patient to local support groups. For respiratory stimulation, keep a suction machine available, monitor serum drug levels, and assess mental status.

Evaluation

Before discharge, ascertain that the patient knows how to administer prescribed drugs, side effects that should be reported to the physician, what to do about missed doses, and when to return for follow-up. If the patient should keep a weight, height, or blood pressure record at home, check to see that the patient can do this, and has the necessary equipment at home.

NURSING IMPLICATIONS SUMMARY

General Guidelines: Patient Receiving Drugs for Narcolepsy, Attention-Deficit Hyperactivity Disorder, or Appetite Suppression

Drug Administration

- Assess for CNS side effects; if severe, notify the physician.
- In the hospital, pad siderails and keep them up. Have a suction machine nearby.
- Monitor vital signs and blood pressure. Assess mental status.
- Monitor behavior. Assess for restlessness, irritability, confusion, insomnia, and mood changes.
- Assess for GI tract symptoms including vomiting, diarrhea, and abdominal cramps.

Patient and Family Education

- Review the anticipated benefits and possible side effects of drug therapy. Tell the patient to report any new symptoms.
- Instruct the patient to take these drugs only as directed and not to change dose or frequency without consulting the physician. Point out that these drugs are habit forming.
- Remind the patient to inform all health care providers of all drugs being taken. Warn the patient to avoid ingesting drugs or foods that also contribute to cardiovascular side effects such as caffeine and caffeine-containing beverages or over-the-counter (OTC) cold preparations containing phenylpropanolamine.
- Instruct the patient to avoid OTC drugs unless first approved by the physician.
- After long-term use, these drugs should not be discontinued abruptly.
- None of these drugs is appropriate to treat general fatigue.
- Insruct the patient to take the last dose of the day at least 6 hours before bedtime for regular dosage forms, and at least 14 hours before bedtime for extended-release forms to help prevent insomnia. Take the last dose of methylphenidate before 6 PM each day. Insomnia may lessen with continued use of a drug, but may be better treated by eliminating the final dose of medication during the day; consult the physician.
- For missed doses, if the dose is taken once a day, instruct the patient to take the dose as soon as remembered, unless later than the time indicated in the previous guideline, otherwise omit missed dose and resume usual dosing schedule the next day. If two or more doses per day are prescribed, instruct the patient to take the missed dose if remembered within 1 hour of when scheduled, otherwise omit the missed dose and resume the usual dosing schedule. The patient should not double up for missed doses.
- See the patient problem boxes on dry mouth (p. 300) and constipation (p. 304).
- Warn the diabetic patient to monitor blood glucose levels since these drugs may alter blood glucose, necessitating a change in diet or insulin.
- Warn the patient to avoid driving or operating hazardous equipment if dizziness, nervousness, agitation, or other CNS effects are severe and to consult the physician if these symptoms become severe.
- Except when specifically prescribed for attention-deficit hyperactivity disorder, CNS stimulants should not be used in children. Instruct the patient to keep these and all drugs out of their reach.
- These drugs should not be used during pregnancy unless specifically prescribed by the obstetrician. Counsel the patient about contraceptives as needed.
- Instruct the patient to avoid alcoholic beverages unless approved by the physician.

Drugs to Treat Narcolepsy and Attention-Deficit Hyperactivity Disorder

Drug Administration/Patient and Family Education

- See the general guidelines.
- Weigh the patient 2 or 3 times a week until the effects of the drug can be evaluated. Although not being given for the purpose of weight reduction, most of these drugs will suppress the appetite.
- Instruct parents to keep careful weight and height records of children.
- Reinforce to the patient that several weeks of therapy may be necessary until full effect of the drug therapy can be evaluated.
- Refer the patient and family for appropriate teaching and counseling for narcolepsy and attention-deficit hyperactivity disorder.
- Instruct the patient taking drugs for attention-deficit hyperactivity disorder and the parents that drug-free periods may be prescribed periodically to assess whether medication is still needed and to allow for growth if the prescribed drug has caused growth retardation.
- Review dosage schedule with the patient. Some patients require daily dosage, while others may require medication during school or work, but can be drug free on the weekends or during summer for children.

NURSING IMPLICATIONS SUMMARY—cont'd

- For best effect, instruct the patient to take doses of methylphenidate on an empty stomach, 30 to 45 minutes before a meal or snack.

Drugs to Suppress Appetite

Drug Administration/Patient and Family Education

- See the general guidelines.
- Refer the patient for appropriate counseling and instruction on weight-reduction diets. Encourage a regular exercise program.
- Inform the patient that weight reduction will be greatest during the first few weeks of therapy but will slow after that.
- Phenylpropanolamine is also discussed in Chapter 29.
- Assess for signs of depression when fenfluramine is used: withdrawal, lack of interest in personal appearance, insomnia, and change in affect.
- Instruct the patient to take the last dose of the day of mazindol 1 mg tablets 4 to 6 hours before bedtime or the 2 mg dose 10 to 14 hours before bedtime.

CNS Stimulants for Respiration

Drug Administration

- Anticipate that seizures may occur. Have a suction machine at the bedside. Keep siderails up and use padding. Do not leave the patient unattended.
- Have oxygen and resuscitation equipment available.
- Monitor pulse, blood pressure, and respirations. Monitor electrocardiographic (ECG) tracing.
- Monitor temperature.
- See the manufacturer's literature for specific guidelines about administration of doxapram.
- Theophylline and aminophylline are discussed in Chapter 27.
- CNS stimulants are rarely used outside of the intensive care setting to stimulate respiration.
- Keep the family informed of the patient's condition.

CRITICAL THINKING

APPLICATION

1. What is narcolepsy?
2. How is narcolepsy treated?
3. What are potential hazards of untreated narcolepsy? As a community health nurse, what would you assess in the home environment of a patient with narcolepsy?
4. What is attention-deficit hyperactivity disorder? What are some possible signs and symptoms of this problem?
5. How is attention-deficit hyperactivity disorder treated?
6. What is the mechanism of action of amphetamines in the CNS?
7. What two brain areas are especially affected by amphetamines?
8. What is the route of administration of amphetamines used in clinical medicine?
9. What side effects are common with amphetamines? How should you assess for these? What signs may signal overdose?
10. Can you explain why MAO inhibitors may potentiate effects of amphetamines, leading to serious overstimulation of various systems?
11. What are the clinical uses of methylphenidate?
12. What toxicity is associated with use of methylphenidate?
13. The chart for a 10-year-old child receiving methylphenidate includes a note instructing that the child's height should be carefully measured and recorded at each visit. Why is that information especially relevant for this child?
14. How does the action of pemoline differ from that of methylphenidate?
15. How does the duration of action of pemoline differ from that of methylphenidate?
16. How long does it take for full therapeutic effects of pemoline to develop?
17. Why are CNS stimulants used to treat obesity?
18. Which appetite suppressant produces CNS depression?
19. Which appetite suppressant is most often found in OTC obesity medications?
20. What toxic reactions may develop during therapy with the nonamphetamine appetite suppressants?
21. Which methylxanthines are sometimes used to stimulate respiration?
22. What reactions are observed when methylxanthines are used to stimulate respiration?
23. How is doxapram administered, and what is its duration of action?
24. What toxicity is observed with doxapram?

CRITICAL THINKING

1. Should parents keep the school health nurse informed about drug treatment for children with attention-deficit hyperactivity disorder? Why? What are the responsibilities of the school health nurse with children with this diagnosis who are taking medication?
2. If appetite suppressants contribute to weight loss, why not use them with all obese patients?

SECTION XIII

Drugs for the Neurologic System

Section XIII discusses anticonvulsants and drugs to control involuntary muscle movements. Chapter 55, *Anticonvulsants,* reviews the classification of seizures. The anticonvulsants are presented by drug class, but they also are referenced for their role in controlling specific seizure patterns. Chapter 56, *Drugs for Parkinson's Disease and Alzheimer's Disease,* and Chapter 57, *Centrally Acting Skeletal Muscle Relaxants,* cover drugs used to treat disorders of central motor control. Chapter 56 presents the drug classes used to treat parkinsonism and discusses step therapy to control the symptoms of parkinsonism and the role of these drugs in treating drug-induced parkinsonian symptoms. Chapter 57 discusses drugs that control spasticity and drugs that act centrally to relieve local muscle spasms.

CHAPTER 55

Anticonvulsants

OBJECTIVES

After studying this chapter, you should be able to do the following:

- *Define epilepsy and describe the characteristics of simple and complex partial (focal) seizures and generalized seizures, characterizing the major syndromes: tonic-clonic seizures, absence seizures, infantile spasms, myoclonus epilepsy, psychomotor epilepsy, focal motor seizures, and status epilepticus.*
- *Discuss the principles of drug therapy for epilepsy.*
- *Develop a nursing care plan for patients receiving valproate, carbamazepine, phenytoin, ethosuximide, or phenobarbital.*
- *Explain the use of diazepam or lorazepam for the control of status epilepticus.*
- *Develop a teaching plan for a patient receiving drug therapy for control of seizures.*

KEY TERMS

absence epilepsy
aura
automatism
epilepsy
focal seizures
generalized seizures
infantile spasms
myoclonus epilepsy
partial seizures
psychomotor epilepsy
status epilepticus
tonic-clonic epilepsy

CHAPTER OVERVIEW

Anticonvulsants are used to control seizures. The objective of drug therapy is to control seizures as completely as possible without causing intolerable side effects. Therapy is individualized for the drug or drug combinations used and for their doses.

Therapeutic Rationale: Epilepsy

Epilepsy is a neurologic disorder characterized by a recurrent pattern of abnormal neuronal discharges within the brain, resulting in a sudden loss or disturbance of consciousness, sometimes in association with motor activity, sensory phenomena, or inappropriate behavior. The seizure may be preceded by an **aura.** An aura is a sensation peculiar for that patient; it can be a visual disturbance or a certain dizziness or numbness that warns the patient of an impending seizure.

Between 1% and 2% of the population is estimated to have epilepsy. The cause of epilepsy may be unknown (idiopathic) or may be traced to a known brain lesion. In general, epilepsy appearing in childhood or adolescence is likely to be idiopathic, whereas epilepsy appearing in adulthood is likely to relate to a definable cause such as a head injury, cerebrovascular accident (stroke), or brain tumor.

An appropriate choice of drugs, taken on a long-term basis, can control the seizures of epilepsy in about 80% of patients. The choice of drugs depends on a careful diagnosis of the seizure pattern, which ideally is made from the observation of a seizure and the recording of the brain wave pattern with an electroencephalogram (EEG) during the seizure. The diagnosis is critical to the selection of a drug or drugs because different seizure patterns are controlled by different drugs. Other causes of seizures must be ruled out because seizures may be as a result of an organic disorder such as a brain tumor, poisoning, fever, hypoglycemia, and hypocalcemia. Overdose of certain drugs such as local anesthetics and ketamine causes seizures. Abrupt withdrawal of some drugs such as the barbiturates and most other sedative-hypnotic drugs, including alcohol, can precipitate seizures.

CLASSIFICATION OF EPILEPSY

Epilepsy is described most frequently by the classification published by the International League Against Epilepsy. This classification is presented in the accompanying box. It describes the seizure pattern by the area of the brain involved.

The two major categories of epilepsy are partial seizures and generalized seizures. These are pictured in Figure 55-1. **Partial seizures** arise from a focal lesion on one side of the brain. The location of the lesion determines the type of seizure observed—motor, cognitive, behavioral, or sensory. Consciousness is usually not lost, but patients may not remember seizure episodes when cognitive or behavioral function is involved. Focal and psychomotor seizures are examples of partial seizures that are discussed more fully. **Generalized seizures** result from the discharge of cells over both sides of the brain. Tonic-clonic seizures, absence seizures, infantile spasms, and myoclonic seizures are examples of generalized seizures. The patient loses consciousness during generalized seizures.

INTERNATIONAL CLASSIFICATION OF SEIZURES

I. Partial seizures
   A. Simple partial seizures
      1. Motor: most common in older children and adults; consciousness is not lost
      2. Somatosensory or special sensory: odor, taste most common
      3. Autonomic
      4. Psychic
   B. Complex partial seizures
      1. Simple partial onset followed by impairment of consciousness
      2. Impairment of consciousness at onset
   C. Partial seizures evolving to secondarily generalized seizures
      1. Simple partial seizures evolving to generalized seizures
      2. Complex partial seizures evolving to generalized seizures
      3. Simple partial seizures evolving to complex partial seizures evolving to generalized seizures

II. Generalized seizures (convulsive or nonconvulsive)
   A. Absence seizures
      1. Typical absence seizures (petit mal seizures)
      2. Atypical absence seizures
   B. Myoclonic seizures
   C. Clonic seizures
   D. Tonic seizures
   E. Tonic-clonic seizures (grand mal)
   F. Atonic seizures

III. Unclassified epileptic seizures

Modified from Commission on Classification and Terminology of the International League Against Epilepsy: Proposal for revised classification of epilepsies and epileptic syndromes, *Epilepsia* 30:389-399, 1989.

PARTIAL SEIZURES

Simple Partial Seizures

A simple partial seizure begins with a specific symptom that reflects the particular part of the brain in which the seizure originates. The seizure may be visual, such as flashes of light, or tactile, such as a feeling of numbness or tingling. The patient does not lose consciousness; the patient is aware but not in control of what is happening. A **focal** motor seizure can involve just a finite motion such as turning of the head. Motor seizures of the jacksonian type begin with clonic seizures of a few muscles on half of the face or in one extremity; the seizures then progresses (march) to include more body musculature (e.g., finger, hand, and arm).

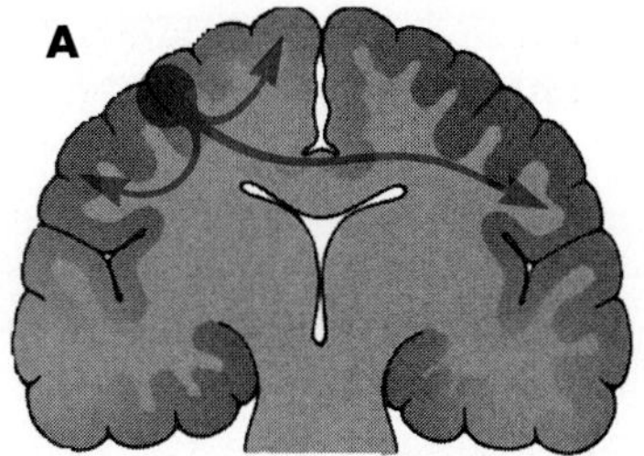

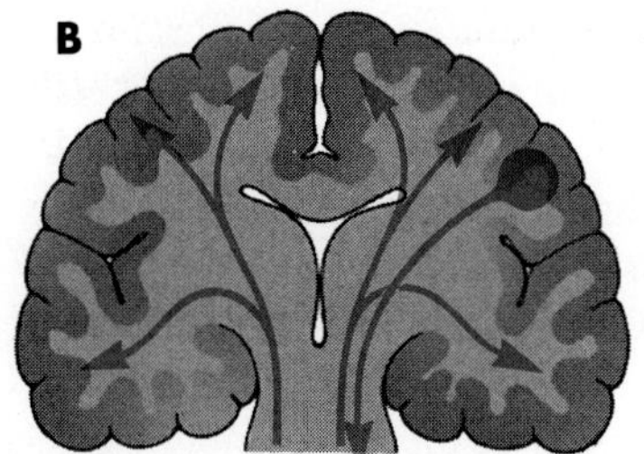

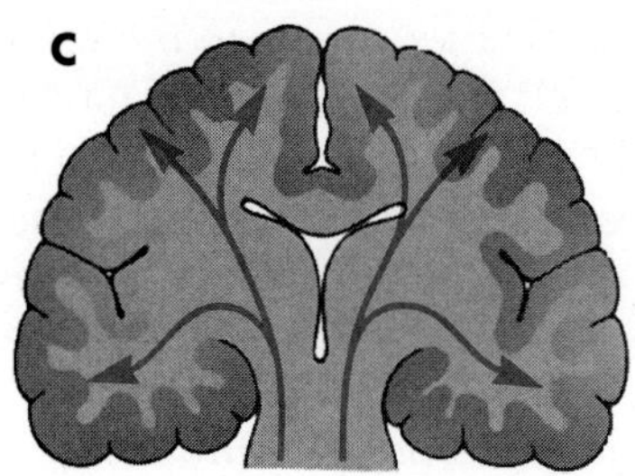

FIGURE 55-1
Schematic representation of how seizures spread. **A,** Focal seizure with spread to adjacent areas, giving rise to partial seizures. **B,** Focal seizure that gives rise to generalized seizure. **C,** Primary generalized seizure.

Psychomotor Epilepsy

Psychomotor epilepsy is a complex partial seizure with complex symptoms that include an aura, automatism, and motor seizures, independently or in combination. These seizures usually last about 5 minutes. The patient remembers the aura but not the automatism or motor seizure. The **automatism** may consist of chewing or swallowing motions, temperamental changes, confusion, feelings of unreality, or unexplained bizarre behavior. A detailed neurologic examination may be required to differentiate psychomotor epilepsy from psychotic mental illness.

GENERALIZED SEIZURES

Tonic-Clonic Epilepsy

Tonic-clonic epilepsy (formerly called grand mal) involves the contraction of all skeletal muscles. Before the seizure begins, the patient may experience an aura. The patient then suddenly loses consciousness and may utter a cry as the diaphragm contracts and expels air from the lungs. The seizure consists of sustained (tonic) contractions or intermittent (clonic) contractions of the muscles. The patient may become incontinent. When the contractions cease, the patient regains consciousness. Usually, the patient is confused and drowsy and lapses into prolonged sleep (postictal depression).

Atonic Seizures

An atonic (drop) seizure is characterized by a sudden loss of tone in postural muscles. Consciousness is impaired. In severe cases the patient may suddenly collapse to the floor.

Absence Epilepsy

Absence epilepsy (formerly petit mal) occurs mainly in children 4 to 12 years of age. The child suddenly loses consciousness for a few seconds, although body tone is seldom lost and consciousness is regained with no confusion. The appearance is one of inattention or daydreaming and may be accompanied by slight blinking or hand movements. Attacks usually occur several times a day. The EEG shows a 3-second spike wave pattern. Absence epilepsy does not generally continue into adulthood, but many patients with absence epilepsy subsequently develop other types of epilepsy, particularly tonic-clonic epilepsy. Thus many physicians treat children prophylactically for tonic-clonic epilepsy in addition to treating absence epilepsy. Some evidence suggests that this prophylactic treatment reduces the incidence of subsequent tonic-clonic epilepsy.

Infantile Spasms

Infantile spasms (West syndrome) denote a major generalized seizure that occurs in the first year of life. The seizure consists of a sudden, transient, repetitive contraction of the limbs and trunk. A sudden shocklike jerk is accompanied by a sharp cry. The legs are extended, and the arms are brought forward in front of the head. These spasms may occur hundreds of times a day and are believed to originate from a congenital malformation or neonatal injury and to reflect an immature nervous system. If the seizures persist after 1 year of age, the seizure pattern changes, usually to a petit mal seizure, a myoclonic seizure, or a head drop seizure in which consciousness is lost for 10 to 15 minutes, accompanied by a loss of muscle tone in the neck.

Myoclonus Epilepsy

Myoclonus epilepsy is a generalized seizure pattern that develops as a result of anoxic brain damage (intentional myoclonus) or as a genetic disorder (progressive myoclonic epilepsy). Intentional myoclonus is a neurologic symptom consisting of sudden involuntary contractions of skeletal muscles, which are aggravated by purposeful activity (hence the term *intentional*) and by visual, auditory, tactile, and emotional activity. Progressive myoclonic epilepsy is a particular form of intentional myoclonus that appears in childhood and becomes progressively worse. When untreated, the genetic disease leads to death after 15 to 20 years.

Status Epilepticus

Status epilepticus refers to seizures that last 30 minutes or longer or that are repeated for 30 minutes or longer and during which consciousness is not regained. Status epilepticus of the generalized tonic-clonic type is a medical emergency. In about 80% of patients, seizures are a result of a disease, frequently associated with a low blood concentration of calcium or glucose, or a result of withdrawal from drugs such as the barbiturates or other sedative-hypnotics. The immediate goals are to establish an airway, to stop the seizures, and then to identify their cause.

Therapeutic Agents: Drug Therapy for Seizures

Molecular Mechanisms

The basis of seizures is a regional imbalance of inhibitory and excitatory neuronal inputs and alterations of membrane stability. Three general molecular mechanisms have been identified for antiepileptic drugs. These mechanisms have not been correlated with specific types of seizures.

The $GABA_A$ receptor mediates the inhibitory activity of gamma-aminobutyric acid (GABA), a major inhibitory neurotransmitter of the brain. Drugs that enhance this activity have an anticonvulsant effect. Such drugs include benzodiazepines, barbiturates, and valproate.

The amino acid glutamate is a major excitatory neurotransmitter of the brain, regulating ion channels. One of these receptor-gated calcium ion channels is identified by stimulation with the agent *N*-methyl-D-aspartate (NMDA). Drugs that inhibit NMDA receptors or activity are anticonvulsants. A newly released drug, lamotrigine, decreases glutamate release.

Neuronal membrane excitability is largely determined by voltage-dependent calcium, potassium, and sodium channels. The antiepileptic drugs carbamazepine and phenytoin modulate sodium channels to decrease cellular excitability.

The understanding of the molecular mechanisms described above is still incomplete and rapidly evolving. The classic route for identifying new antiepileptic drugs has relied on the use of mouse and rat animal models for screening. The identification of new drugs has been slow.

Therapeutic Principles

Several drugs are available for control of epileptic seizures. The drug choice depends on diagnosis of the seizure patterns and on the tolerance and response of the patient to the drug prescribed. Drugs most frequently effective for various seizure patterns are listed in Table 55-1.

One of the first-line drugs for the seizure pattern diagnosed is started in small doses to allow the patient to develop a tolerance to the drowsiness and motor incoordination (ataxia) associated with most of the anticonvulsant drugs. The dose is increased until the seizures are stopped or until toxic effects of the drug appear. If the drug is ineffective or only partly effective in controlling seizures, another first line drug is tried. A second drug is added only if three antiepileptic drugs have failed to control seizures with an acceptable level of side effects.

Because the most common cause of drug failure is the failure of the patient to take the prescribed drugs, the plasma concentration of drug may be determined before deciding

TABLE 55-1 Drug Choice by Seizure Type

SEIZURE TYPE	FIRST-CHOICE DRUGS	SECOND-CHOICE DRUGS	REFRACTORY CASES
Partial (includes secondarily generalized tonic-clonic)	Carbamazepine Phenytoin Valproate	Clorazepate Felbamate Gabapentin Lamotrigine Phenobarbital Primidone	Acetazolamide Ethotoin Mephenytoin Methsuximide Phenacemide
Generalized			
Absence	Ethosuximide Valproate	Clonazepam	Acetazolamide Clorazepate Methsuximide Phensuximide Paramethadione Trimethadione
Tonic-clonic	Carbamazepine Phenytoin Valproate	Phenobarbital Primidione	Acetazolamide Ethotoin Mephenytoin Mephobarbital
Myoclonic, atonic	Valproate	Clonazepam Felbamate	Carbamazepine Clorazepate Ethosuximide Methsuximide Phenobarbital Phenytoin

that the drug is ineffective. Patients must be warned not to discontinue medication when the seizures are under control or when the side effects are disturbing. The sudden discontinuance of medication greatly increases the incidence of seizures. Blood and urine analyses often are routinely carried out because many anticonvulsant drugs infrequently produce blood dyscrasias or renal damage.

Many patients with epilepsy require drug therapy throughout their lives to control seizures. However, some patients can discontinue medication. These patients are those reaching adulthood after childhood treatment for absence epilepsy and those patients who have had several seizure-free years. If the EEG of such a patient appears normal, medication can be gradually discontinued. Seizures recur in 25% to 50% of such patients.

Therapy and Pregnancy

Pregnancy influences the epilepsy itself as well as the metabolism of many anticonvulsant drugs. In general the plasma concentration of anticonvulsant drugs decreases in pregnancy, so that the concentrations need to be monitored closely. Infants of mothers with epilepsy as a whole are at increase risk for prematurity, low birth weight, low Apgar scores, hypoxia, hemorrhage, and congenital malformations. However, the risk of seizures to the fetus is regarded as greater than the risk of anticonvulsant drugs.

A pattern of congenital abnormalities, the fetal antiepileptic drug syndrome, is characterized by prenatal and postnatal growth deficiencies, microencephaly, developmental delay, short nose, hypoplastic fingernails and distal phalanges, and congenital heart defects. Originally described for phenytoin, this syndrome has also been linked with phenobarbital, carbamazepine, and valproate. The highest rate of this syndrome is associated with phenobarbital; and intermediate rate with phenytoin, and the lowest rate with carbamazepine. Both valproate and carbamazepine also increase the risk of spina bifida or neural tube defect. Pregnancies during which the mother takes trimethadione (Tridione) are associated with an 80% incidence of spontaneous abortions or birth defects. If possible, women taking trimethadione should be switched to ethosuximide (Zarontin) before becoming pregnant.

The effectiveness of oral contraceptives may be impaired for women taking phenytoin, phenobarbital, primidone, carbamazepine, and possibly ethosuximide. A high estrogen formulation may be necessary for effective contraception.

FIRST-LINE ANTICONVULSANTS

A summary of first-line anticonvulsant drugs is presented in Table 55-2.

✣ Carbamazepine

Mechanism of Action

Carbamazepine (Tegretol) is chemically related to the tricyclic antidepressants. It limits seizure propagation at the level of synaptic transmission by reducing excitatory sodium currents.

Pharmacokinetics

The plasma half-life is 12 hours, so the drug must be given in divided doses. Carbamazepine is metabolized by the liver, and one of the metabolites has anticonvulsant activity. Absorption from the gastrointestinal (GI) tract is slow; however, this can be improved if the drug is taken at meals.

Uses

Carbamazepine is particularly effective in controlling simple or complex partial seizures, including psychomotor seizures. It is also effective for generalized tonic-clonic seizures. A positive side effect is the increased alertness and improvement of mood in patients. Carbamazepine is also used for the relief of pain caused by trigeminal neuralgia or glossopharyngeal neuralgia. However, carbamazepine is not an analgesic. Other uses include the treatment of alcohol withdrawal, bipolar depression, and excited psychosis.

Adverse Reactions, Contraindications, and Toxicity

Carbamazepine has relatively low behavioral and toxicologic toxicity. The most frequent side effects are drowsiness, dizziness, ataxia, visual disturbances (particularly double vision), and GI upset. Carbamazepine infrequently causes rashes, liver damage, and bone marrow depression, which require its discontinuance. Blood counts should be made frequently in the early course of treatment and occasionally thereafter. Serious adverse effects are rare.

Interactions

Drug interactions encountered include decreased plasma concentration in the presence of other anticonvulsants, because the other agents induce drug-metabolizing enzymes in the liver. Drugs that tend to lower the plasma concentration of carbamazepine by increasing its metabolism include ethotoin, mephenytoin, phenytoin, ethosuximide, methsuximide, phensuximide, clonazepam, primidone, barbiturates, valproate, tricyclic antidepressants, phenothiazines, haloperidol, loxapine, maprotiline, molindone, pimozide, thioxanthines. Other drugs increase the plasma concentration of carbamazepine by inhibiting its degradation. Drugs potentiating the action of carbamazepine by increasing its plasma concentration include cimetidine, propoxyphene, clarithromycin, danazol, diltiazem, verapamil, erythromycin, troleandomycin, and isoniazid.

Carbamazepine can lower the effectiveness of several drugs by increasing their metabolism. Drugs so affected include estrogen, quinidine, glucocorticoids, monoamine oxidase inhibitors, and oral anticoagulants. Prolonged use of carbamazepine with acetaminophen can lead to liver damage.

Ethosuximide

Mechanism of Action

Ethosuximide (Zarontin) is one of the succinimides. These drugs elevate the seizure threshold in cortex and basal ganglia. This reduces synaptic response to low-frequency, repet-

TABLE 55-2 Anticonvulsant Drugs

GENERIC NAME	TRADE NAME	ADMINISTRATION/DOSAGE	COMMENTS
First-Line Anticonvulsants			
✣ Carbamazepine	Apo-Carbamazepine† Epitol Tegretol*	ORAL: *Adults*—100 mg 4 times daily first week; increase by 100 or 200 mg/day at weekly intervals to control seizures. Maintenance: 800-1200 mg daily. *Children 6-12 yr*—50 mg daily, increase by up to 100 mg daily at weekly intervals to control seizures. Maintenance: 400-800 mg daily. *Children to 6 yr*—10-20 mg per kg body weight daily in 2-3 divided doses, increasing by up to 100 mg/day at weekly intervals to control seizures. Maintenance: 250-350 mg daily.	First-line drug because of relative lack of serious side effects and low behavioral and psychologic toxicity. Controls partial seizures with simple or complex symptoms; generalized tonic-clonic seizures; mixed seizure patterns; other partial or generalized seizures. Also indicated for treatment of trigeminal neuralgia and glossopharyngeal neuralgia. Extended-release form available.
Ethosuximide	Zarontin*	ORAL: *Adults and children >6 yr*—15-30 mg/kg body weight daily or initially 250 mg 2 times daily; with dose being increased by 250 mg daily at 4-7 day intervals to control seizures. Maximum daily dose: 1.5 gm. *Children <6 yr*—15-40 mg/kg body weight or initially 250 mg once a day, with dose being increased by 250 mg daily at 4-7 day intervals to control seizures. Maximum daily dose: 1 gm.	First-line drug for simple absence seizures.
✣ Phenytoin	Dilantin*	ORAL: *Adults*—125 mg 3 times/day initially; adjust at 7-10 day intervals to control seizures. *Children*—5 mg/kg body weight daily divided into 2 or 3 doses initially; adjust as needed to control seizures. Maximum daily dose: 300 mg. *Older adults*—3 mg/kg body weight daily in divided doses, adjusted according to patient response. FDA pregnancy category C. INTRAVENOUS: *Adults*—For status epilepticus: 15-20 mg/kg body weight administered at rate not to exceed 50 mg/min. Maintenance: 100 mg every 6-8 hr.	First-line drug for tonic-clonic seizures and simple or complex partial seizures. Used for prophylaxis and treatment of seizures during and following neurosurgery. May be used for sustained control of status epilepticus after diazepam treatment. Used for correction of atrial and ventricular arrhythmias induced by digitalis.
Valproic acid Divalproex sodium	Depakene* Depakote Epival†	ORAL: *Adults*—Monotherapy: 5-15 mg/kg body weight daily; increase at weekly intervals by 5-10 mg/kg body weight daily to control seizures. Polytherapy: 10-30 mg/kg body weight daily; increase at weekly intervals by 5-10 mg/kg body weight daily to contol seizures. If dose exceeds 250 mg daily, divide into 2 or more doses to lessen gastric irritation. *Children 1-12 yr*—Monotherapy: 15-45 mg/kg body weight daily; increase by 5-10 mg/kg body weight weekly to control seizures. Polytherapy: 30-100 mg/kg body weight daily. FDA pregnancy category D.	First-line drug for simple and complex absence seizures. Also effective for partial seizures, tonic-clonic seizures, and myoclonic seizures. Monotherapy is preferred because there are complex drug interactions affecting plasma levels of valproate and many other anticonvulsants.
Alternative or Adjunct Anticonvulsants			
Clonazepam	Klonopin Rivotril†	ORAL: *Adults*—0.5 mg 3 times daily; increase by 0.5-1 mg every 3 days until seizures are controlled or side effects prevent further increase. Maximum daily dose: 20 mg. *Infants and children to 10 yr (or 30 mg/kg body weight)*—0.01-0.03 mg/kg body weight initially divided into 2 or 3 doses; increase by 0.25-0.5 mg every third day until seizures are controlled or maintenance dose of 0.1-0.2 mg/kg body weight is reached.	Treatment for Lennox-Gastaut syndrome; akinetic seizures, myoclonic seizures, absence seizure pattern; adjunctive therapy for simple partial seizure pattern, complex partial seizure patterns. Long-term use by children may impair physical or mental development, which may not be apparent for many years.

*Available in Canada and United States.
†Available in Canada only.

Continued.

TABLE 55-2 Anticonvulsant Drugs—cont'd

GENERIC NAME	TRADE NAME	ADMINISTRATION/DOSAGE	COMMENTS
Alternative or Adjunct Anticonvulsants—cont'd			
Clorazepate	Generic: Apo-Clorazepate† Novo-Clopate† Tranxene*	ORAL: *Adults and children >12 yr—7.5* mg 3 times/day initially; increase by no more than 7.5 mg at weekly intervals, not to exceed 90 mg daily. *Children 9-12 yr—7.5* mg 2 times/day initially; increase by no more than 7.5 mg at weekly intervals, not to exceed 60 mg daily.	Adjunctive therapy for refractory partial or generalized seizures.
Felbamate	Felbatol	ORAL: *Adults*—1200 mg/day divided into 3 or 4 doses initially; increase gradually to no more than 3600 mg daily. *Children 2-14 yr old*—15 mg/kg body weight divided into 3 or 4 doses daily initially; increase gradually to no more than 3600 mg daily. FDA pregnancy category C.	Adjunctive therapy for children with Lennox-Gastaut syndrome not responsive to other treatment; monotherapy for partial seizures refractory to other drugs. Reports of aplastic anemia and liver failure limit use.
Gabapentin	Neurotin	ORAL: *Adults*—300 mg on day 1; 600 mg divided into 2 doses on day 2; 900 mg divided into 3 doses on day 3; then increase as needed to control seizures. Range: 900-3600 mg daily. FDA pregnancy category C.	Adjunct therapy for treatment of partial seizures. Reduce dose for patients with reduced renal function (creatinine < 60 mg/ml).
Lamotrigine	Lamictal	ORAL: *Adults* taking valproate—25 mg every other day for 2 wk; then 25 mg daily for 2 weeks. If needed and tolerated, may increase to 150 mg divided into 2 doses daily.	Adjunct therapy for partial seizures in adults. For patients receiving enzyme-inducing anticonvulsant medications but not valproate, double dose given with valproate.
Phenobarbital	Generic; Solfoton	ORAL: *Adults*—60-250 mg daily as single dose or in divided doses. *Children*—1-6 mg/kg body weight daily as single or divided dose. FDA pregnancy category D.	Alternative agent for treatment of tonic-clonic seizure pattern and simple partial seizure pattern.
Primidone	Apo-Primidone† Mysoline* PMS Primidone† Sertan†	ORAL: *Adults and children >8 yr*—100-125 mg once a day at bedtime for first 3 days; twice a day for days 4-6; three times a day for days 7-9; thereafter adjust as needed; not to exceed 2000 mg daily. *Children up to 8 yr*—50 mg at bedtime days 1-3; 50 mg twice a day for days 3-6; 100 mg twice a day for days 7-9; thereafter 125-250 mg 3 times a day or 10-25 mg/kg body weight daily.	Adjunct or alternate therapy for generalized tonic-clonic, nocturnal myoclonic, complex partial, and simple partial seizures.
Miscellaneous Anticonvulsants			
Acetazolamide	Diamox*	ORAL: *Adults*—4-30 mg/kg body weight daily in up to 4 divided doses (usually 375 mg to 1 gm daily)	Adjunct therapy for other anticonvulsants.
Ethotoin	Peganone	ORAL: *Adults*—500 mg-1gm on first day divided into 4-6 doses; increase over several days, up to 3 gm daily. *Children*—up to 750 mg daily.	Alternative therapy for tonic-clonic and simple or complex partial seizures.
Mephenytoin	Mesantoin*	ORAL: *Adults—50-100 mg once a day, increase by 50-100 mg daily at weekly intervals to control seizures. Maximum daily dose: 1.2 gm.* *Children*—25-50 mg/day; increase by 25-50 mg daily at weekly intervals to control seizures. Maximum daily dose: 400 mg.	Alternative therapy for simple partial seizures in patients not responsive to other agents.
Methsuximide	Celontin*	ORAL: *Adults*—300 mg once a day; increase by 300 mg daily at weekly intervals to control seizures. Maximum dose: 1.2 gm.	Alternative therapy for absence seizures refractory to other agents.
Paramethadione	Paradione	ORAL: *Adults*—300 mg 3 or 4 times daily; increase by 300 mg daily at weekly intervals to control seizures. Maximum dose: 2.4 gm. *Children up to 2 yr*—100 mg 3 times/day. *Children 2-6 yr*—200 mg 3 times/day. *Children ≥6 yr*—300 mg 3 times/day. FDA pregnancy category D.	Alternative therapy for absence seizures refractory to other medications.

TABLE 55-2 Anticonvulsant Drugs—cont'd

GENERIC NAME	TRADE NAME	ADMINISTRATION/DOSAGE	COMMENTS
Miscellaneous Anticonvulsants—cont'd			
Phensuximide	Milontin	ORAL: *Adults*—500 mg 2 or 3 times a day; increase by 500 mg/day at weekly intervals until seizures are controlled. Maximum daily dose: 3 gm.	Alternative therapy for absence seizures refractory to other medications.
Trimethadione	Tridione	ORAL: *Adults*—300 mg 3 or 4 times daily; increase by 300 mg daily at weekly intervals to control seizures. Maximum dose: 2.4 gm. *Children up to 2 yr*—100 mg 3 times/day. *Children 2-6 yr*—200 mg 3 times day. *Children ≥6 yr*—300 mg 3 times/day.	Alternative therapy for absence seizures refractory to other medications.
Anticonvulsants for Status Epilepticus			
Diazepam	D-val Valium*	INTRAVENOUS: *Adults*—5-10 mg initially; repeat at 10-15 min intervals as needed, up to total dose of 30 mg. Repeat in 2-4 hr if necessary. *Children ≥5 yr*—1 mg every 2-5 min up to total dose of 10 mg. Repeat in 2-4 hr if necessary. *Infants >30 days and children up to 5 yr*—0.2-0.5 mg every 2-5 min up to total dose of 5 mg. Repeat in 2-4 hr if necessary. Administer over 3 min to infants and children.	For status epilepticus and severe recurrent convulsive seizures.
✣ Lorazepam	Ativan*	INTRAVENOUS: *Adults*—0.05 mg/kg body weight, up to 4 mg, administered slowly. Repeat twice at 10-15 min if seizures continue or recur, but no more than 8 mg total in 12 hr period.	For status epilepticus and severe recurrent convulsive seizures.

itive stimulation. Related drugs are phensuximide (Milontin), which is sometimes effective in treating psychomotor epilepsy, and methsuximide (Celontin).

Pharmacokinetics

GI absorption is rapid. The plasma half-life is about 30 hours in children and 60 hours in adults. The effective serum concentration is 40 to 80 μg/ml, but serum concentrations of up to 160 μg/ml can be tolerated without excessive toxicity.

Uses

Ethosuximide is a drug of choice for typical absent seizures.

Adverse Reactions and Contraindications

Side effects include dizziness, drowsiness, and GI irritation. Blood counts are performed routinely because of the occasional occurrence of agranulocytosis. The tendency to cause blood dyscrasia may show up in dental problems: increased mouth infection and gingival bleeding. Contraindications for ethosuximide include blood dyscrasias, intermittent porphyria, and hepatic or renal disease. Ethosuximide is excreted in breast milk.

Interactions

Ethosuximide enhances the central nervous system (CNS) depressive effects of other drugs. Use with haloperidol can cause changes in the pattern or frequency of seizures, and the dose of either drug may need to be changed.

✣ Phenytoin

Mechanism of Action

Phenytoin acts to stabilize membranes and raise the threshold for depolarization.

Pharmacokinetics

Since phenytoin has a plasma half-life of 24 hours, it takes 4 days to reach steady plasma levels when initiating therapy. To decrease this time, the initial dose is sometimes given as a loading dose at three times the usual daily dose. At serum concentrations much above therapeutic concentrations, the capacity of the liver to metabolize phenytoin is saturated so that plasma concentrations decrease very slowly. Phenytoin is irregularly absorbed from the intestine. Because absorption depends on formulation, it is best to stay with a particular brand of phenytoin.

Phenytoin should not be given intramuscularly or subcutaneously because it is highly irritating and can precipitate in the tissue. The sodium salt can be administered intravenously, but too-rapid administration can produce severe hypotension and cardiac arrest.

Uses

Phenytoin (Dilantin), formerly called diphenylhydantoin, is a drug of choice in controlling tonic-clonic seizures and partial seizures in adults. Sodium phenytoin is administered intravenously to control status epilepticus alone or after IV diazepam has controlled the seizures. IV sodium phenytoin is also used to control some cardiac arrhythmias (see Chapter 18).

Adverse Reactions and Contraindications

Effective serum concentrations are 10 to 20 μg/ml, and side effects are seen at higher serum concentrations. At greater than 20 μg/ml, involuntary movement of the eyeballs (nystagmus) appears; at greater than 30 μg/ml, ataxia and slurred speech arise. Tremors and nervousness or drowsiness and fatigue may be side effects of higher serum concentrations. However, an acute overdose of phenytoin is seldom fatal. Persistence of these side effects requires reducing the dose or switching to another drug, usually phenobarbital.

About 20% of patients taking phenytoin experience overgrowth of the gums (gingival hyperplasia), which is particularly severe in children. Occasionally, folic acid or vitamin D deficiency can be produced, because phenytoin interferes with the normal metabolism of these compounds. Phenytoin can also cause an allergic rash that can be mistaken for measles or infectious mononucleosis. Phenytoin also worsens acne, which is especially bothersome to teenagers and can increase growth of body hair (hirsutism), which is undesirable in women. There is a higher incidence of congenital malformations in infants of mothers taking phenytoin. These infants are also at risk for hemorrhage and coagulation deficiencies at birth, which can be corrected with vitamin K.

Interactions

Important drugs interactions are noted with phenytoin. Phenobarbital can increase the metabolism of phenytoin in some individuals by inducing liver microsomal enzymes, but in others phenobarbital decreases the rate of drug metabolism of phenytoin by competing with the enzymes for degradation. The oral anticoagulant dicumarol and the anticonvulsant carbamazepine decrease the metabolism of phenytoin by competing with the enzymes for degradation. The anticonvulsant valproic acid displaces bound phenytoin from protein to increase the free concentration of phenytoin while decreasing its total concentration, because more free phenytoin is available for metabolism. Phenytoin enhances the rate of estrogen metabolism, which can decrease the effectiveness of some birth control pills.

Valproate: Valproic Acid and Divalproex Sodium

Mechanism of Action

Valproic acid (Depakene) is an analogue of the inhibitory central neurotransmitter, GABA, which inhibits neuronal activity. One mechanism by which valproic acid may act is to increase the concentration of this inhibitory neurotransmitter. Divalproex sodium (Depakote Epival) is a combination of the acid and salt forms of valproic acid.

Pharmacokinetics

Divalproex sodium is a combination of valproic acid and sodium valproate with an enteric covering to delay absorption for 1 to 4 hours after ingestion. In the GI tract the complex dissolves into valproate. The plasma half life of the active drug is variable, from 6 to 16 hours. Patients with hepatic impairment, older adults, and children younger than 18 months have a long life for valproate.

At low serum concentrations valproate is highly protein bound. At serum concentrations above 50 μg/ml, binding sites become saturated and the fraction of free drug increases, dramatically increasing the incidence of side effects and toxicity. Valproate is metabolized by the liver and some metabolites are active or toxic. Children metabolize the drug more rapidly than adults. Infants and older adults metabolize the drug more slowly than other age groups. The drug and its metabolites are excreted in the urine as glucuronides.

Uses

Valproate is a first-line drug for the treatment of many generalized seizures, including simple and complex absence seizures, myoclonic seizures, and tonic-clonic seizures. Valproate is also a first-line drug for many partial seizures. Clinical studies have shown that valproate is effective in treating manic depression.

Adverse Reactions, Toxicity, and Contraindications

The most frequent side effect seen with valproic acid is GI distress. Sedation is marked at the beginning of treatment unless doses are gradually raised. Occasionally a hand tremor occurs with higher doses. Overdose has produced coma but with uneventful recovery.

Valproate may raise ammonia concentrations in the blood, but this is not associated with any clinical manifestations. Occasionally patients taking valproate may show confusion.

The most serious toxic effect valproate is liver failure. This usually appears in the first 6 months of treatment. Children under 2 years of age or children receiving other anticonvulsants with valproate are at greatest risk for liver failure. Nonspecific symptoms include loss of seizure control, malaise, weakness, lethargy, loss of appetite, vomiting, edema, and a Reye's-like syndrome. The incidence of liver failure is rare but potentially fatal.

Valproate is contraindicated for patients with liver disease because of the potential for liver failure. Valproate also interferes with platelet aggregation. This effect is not a problem for most people, but patients with coagulation disorders or taking anticoagulants should be carefully monitored.

Interactions

Drug interactions with valproic acid include its decreased plasma concentration in the presence of other anticonvulsants that induce liver microsomal enzymes including phenobarbital, primidone, phenytoin, and carbamazepine. Phenytoin also can raise the concentration of free-plasma valproic acid by displacing the fraction bound to plasma proteins.

Drugs that alter coagulation, including oral anticoagulants, heparin, platelet aggregation inhibitors, or thrombolytic agents have an increased risk for bleeding when taking valproate.

Valproate potentiates the CNS depressant effect of other drugs, especially alcohol and CNS depressants.

ALTERNATIVE OR ADJUNCT ANTICONVULSANT DRUGS

Clonazepam

Mechanism of Action

Clonazepam (Klonopin, Rivotril) is a benzodiazepine. These drugs enhance presynaptic inhibition by the inhibitory neurotransmitter, GABA, an action that suppresses the spread of seizures.

Pharmacokinetics

Clonazepam is well absorbed with peak plasma concentrations occurring 1 to 4 hours after administration. The plasma half-life of clonazepam is 20 to 40 hours. Clonazepam is metabolized in the liver to a compound that probably has little anticonvulsant activity.

Uses

Clonazepam is effective in controlling generalized absence seizures, myoclonic seizures, and infantile spasms. Tolerance often develops to clonazepam, and seizures recur in about a third of patients. For this reason, clonazepam is not a first-line drug for epilepsy.

Adverse Reactions and Contraindications

Neurologic side effects are commonly seen during therapy with clonazepam and include drowsiness, ataxia, and personality changes. Children may become hyperactive, irritable, aggressive, violent, or disobedient. Slurred speech, tremors, abnormal eye movements, dizziness, and confusion also may be noticed. These effects are dose related and may subside with time or on lowering the dose. Increased salivation and bronchial secretions sometimes occur and create respiratory problems in children.

Interactions

Clonazepam does not alter the activity of other anticonvulsant drugs. This allows clonazepam to be added to anticonvulsant therapy as a second drug more readily than other agents. However, clonazepam enhances CNS depression, especially with barbiturates. When clonazepam is given with primidone, behavioral disorders may be seen. Cimetidine, oral contraceptives, and disulfiram can increase the plasma concentration of clonazepam.

Clorazepate

Mechanism of Action

Clorazepate (Gen-Xene, Tranxene) is a benzodiazepine. These drugs enhance presynaptic inhibition by the inhibitory neurotransmitter, GABA, an action that suppresses the spread of seizures.

Pharmacokinetics

Clorazepate is rapidly absorbed, but it is inactive until it is metabolized in the stomach or plasma to desmethyldiazepam. This metabolite has a long plasma half-life.

Uses

Clorazepate is mainly used as adjunct therapy in patients with partial or generalized seizures. Tolerance frequently develops to its anticonvulsant activity.

Adverse Reactions and Contraindications

Adverse reactions include drowsiness, ataxia, and sedation. Occasionally, behavioral and personality changes may be noted, especially when given with primidone.

It should be noted that children who are taking chlorazepate may exhibit hyperactivity.

Interactions

Clorazepate enhances the CNS depression of CNS depressant drugs. Cimetidine may slow the metabolism of desmethyldiazepam, resulting in higher plasma concentrations of the active drug, increasing adverse actions.

Felbamate

Mechanism of Action

Felbamate (Felbatol) is chemically related to meprobamate, an anxiolytic agent. Felbamate appears to inhibit indirectly the NMDA receptor and thereby limit excitatory CNS responses.

Pharmacokinetics

Felbamate is well absorbed and has a half-life of 16 to 19 hours. The drug is excreted in the urine unchanged (50%) or as metabolites.

Uses

Felbamate is effective as monotherapy or adjunctive therapy for partial seizures with or without secondary generalization of seizures.

It is also effective as adjunctive therapy in the treatment of partial and generalized seizures associated with the Lennox-Gastaut syndrome. This rare and severe seizure syndrome in children is characterized by frequent absence-like seizures and mental retardation.

However, felbamate is only recommended for the most severe and refractory patients. A high incidence of aplastic anemia and liver failure has been reported in patients taking felbamate.

Adverse Reactions, Toxicity, and Contraindications

Potential side effects associated with felbamate include nausea, headache, weight loss, and insomnia. Toxic side effects have emerged to limit the use of felbamate. Aplastic anemia appears in an estimated 1 of 2000 patients on felbamate for more than a few weeks.

In addition, a few cases of acute liver failure have been reported for patients taking felbamate. Patients with liver function abnormalities should not be put on felbamate. Markers of liver function (ALT, AST, and bilirubin) should be monitored weekly for patients on felbamate.

Interactions

Felbamate decreases the plasma levels of carbamazepine, but it also increases phenytoin and valproic acid levels. Carbamazepine and valproic acid both decrease plasma levels of felbamate.

Gabapentin

Mechanism of Action

Gabapentin (Neurontin) is an analog of the inhibitory CNS neurotransmitter, GABA. However, gabapentin does not interact with GABA receptors, and therefore its mechanism of action is not clear.

Pharmacokinetics

Gabapentin is rapidly absorbed and has a plasma half-life of 5 to 6 hours. About 80% to 100% of the drug is excreted unchanged in the urine. Doses must be adjusted proportionally when renal function as determined by creatinine clearance falls below 60 ml/minutes.

Uses

Gabapentin is effective as adjunctive therapy in refractory partial seizures in adults.

Adverse Reactions and Contraindications

Adverse reactions of gabapentin include somnolence, dizziness, ataxia, fatigue, diplopia, blurred vision, amnesia, nystagmus, and tremor. These are not usually pronounced. Weight increase and depression have also been reported. No toxicity has been reported. Because the drug is excreted unchanged in the urine, patients with reduced renal function require smaller doses.

Interactions

No significant drug interactions have been described with the use of gabapentin.

Lamotrigine

Mechanism of Action

Lamotrigine (Lamictal) inhibits voltage-dependent sodium currents and inhibits the release of the excitatory neurotransmitter, glutamate.

Pharmacokinetics

Lamotrigine is well absorbed. The plasma half-life in adults is about 25 hours. Lamotrigine is extensively metabolized by the liver to glucuronide that are excreted in the urine.

Uses

Lamotrigine is effective as adjunctive therapy in adults with partial seizures. This is a new drug and additional uses may be added with further clinical testing.

Adverse Reactions and Contraindications

Adverse reactions include nausea, headache, diplopia, blurred vision, dizziness, ataxia, somnolence, and rash.

Interactions

Enzyme-inducing drugs such as phenytoin and phenobarbital that enhance liver metabolism decrease the plasma concentration of lamotrigine. Valproic acid markedly retards the metabolism of lamotrigine and increases the plasma concentration.

Phenobarbital

Phenobarbital (Solfoton) has been widely used for 60 years and is an alternative drug for treating patients with partial and generalized seizures. It is also used to treat withdrawal from barbiturates or alcohol. Phenobarbital is cross-tolerant with alcohol and other barbiturates but requires only once-a-day administration because of its long plasma half-life of 4 days. Because of this long plasma half-life, 14 days are required to reach constant serum concentrations.

The main side effects of the barbiturates are sedation and drowsiness at the beginning of treatment, but tolerance usually develops to these effects. In elderly patients and in children a paradoxical excitement may be seen that impairs learning ability. Phenobarbital increases the incidence of congenital malformations in the fetus but not to the degree associated with phenytoin and trimethadione. Phenobarbital induces liver microsomal enzymes and thus can speed its own metabolism and that of other drugs. Sudden rather than gradual withdrawal of the drug can precipitate convulsions. Barbiturates are contraindicated for patients with the metabolic disorder porphyria and for patients who are depressed and might consider suicide.

Primidone

Primidone (Mysoline) is a deoxybarbiturate that is metabolized to phenobarbital and phenylethylmalonamide. Primidone can therefore substitute for phenobarbital to treat partial and generalized seizures. It is not used for the treatment of absence seizures. Primidone has a greater incidence of adverse and toxic effects than does phenobarbital.

MISCELLANEOUS ANTICONVULSANT DRUGS

Acetazolamide

Acetazolamide (Diamox) is used alone or with other drugs in treating absence epilepsy. Mechanism of action is inhibition of the enzyme carbonic anhydrase in the brain, which results in an altered ratio of intracellular to extracellular sodium. Acetazolamide is also a weak diuretic (see Chapter 14). Side effects include loss of appetite, drowsiness, confusion, and tingling. The usefulness of acetazolamide is limited by the frequent development of tolerance to its anticonvulsant action. Acetazolamide may be useful for intermittent use by women whose seizure frequency increases during menstruation.

Adrenocorticotropic Hormone

Adrenocorticotropic hormone (ACTH) is the treatment of choice for infantile spasms. If daily administration for 20 days is effective, the course of treatment is repeated after 2 to 4 weeks or glucocorticoids (usually prednisone) are given. ACTH stimulates the adrenal cortex to synthesize glucocorticoids (see Chapter 60). The effectiveness of ACTH in treating infantile spasms is related to this endocrine action.

Ethotoin and Mephenytoin

Ethotoin (Peganone) and mephenytoin (Mesantoin) are chemically related to phenytoin. Mephenytoin is associated with a high incidence of agranulocytosis and aplastic anemia. Ethotoin is not widely used, although it does not seem to cause gingival hyperplasia, hirsutism, or ataxia.

Methsuximide and Phensuximide

Methsuximide (Celontin) and phensuximide (Milontin) are succinimides. Ethosuximide, listed earlier, is the only widely used drug of this group. Phensuximide is not as effective as ethosuximide for childhood absence seizures. Methsuximide is adjunct therapy for refractor partial complex seizures.

Trimethadione

Trimethadione (Tridione) was the first drug effective in controlling absence epilepsy, but it is now a third-choice drug for absence seizures because of the high incidence of serious side effects.

Trimethadione can produce serious allergic dermatitis, kidney and liver damage, agranulocytosis, and aplastic anemia. Blood counts and urinalyses are done routinely with trimethadione therapy. In adults the drug frequently produces an intolerance to light (photophobia). The incidence of spontaneous abortions or congenital anomalies in infants of mothers taking trimethadione is 80%.

The other anticonvulsant of the oxazolindinedione class, paramethadione (Paradione), is no longer used because of its toxicity.

ANTICONVULSANTS FOR TREATMENT OF STATUS EPILEPTICUS

Diazepam

Diazepam (Valium) administered intravenously (IV) is a drug of choice for terminating the tonic-clonic seizures of status epilepticus and sometimes is used to terminate the seizures of eclampsia. Oral diazepam occasionally is used with other anticonvulsants to control myoclonic and absences seizures. Main side effects are drowsiness, dizziness, and ataxia. Respiratory depression must be watched during IV administration. Overall, diazepam is a safe drug. The major use of diazepam is as an antianxiety drug (see Chapter 51).

✣ Lorazepam

Lorazepam (Ativan) is as effective as diazepam for the initial treatment of status epilepticus. Because lorazepam has a longer duration of action, phenytoin or phenobarbital may then be added for sustained control of seizures. As with diazepam, respiratory depression must be monitored during IV administration.

NURSING PROCESS OVERVIEW

Anticonvulsants

Assessment

Most patients using anticonvulsant drugs have had a seizure, and drug treatment is needed on a long-term basis. Obtain a baseline assessment, with special emphasis on areas known to be affected by the drugs to be used. For example, because phenytoin can cause gingival hyperplasia, assess mouth, teeth, and gums at the start of and periodically during therapy.

Nursing Diagnoses

- Risk for gingival hyperplasia
- Altered comfort: nausea and gastrointestinal distress associated with drug ingestion

Patient Outcomes

The patient will demonstrate good oral hygiene and will state the importance of regular dental care. The patient will not experience nausea or GI distress related to medication regimen.

Planning/Implementation

Drug dosages are adjusted until seizures are controlled or toxic effects are noted. Monitor the general condition of the patient with an emphasis on known drug side effects. Monitor serum levels of the prescribed drugs if available. If the patient continues to have seizures, observe type, duration, and characteristics of the seizure, and continue nursing measures to prevent injury such as padding siderails or supervising ambulation. Refer the patient to health department, social services, or vocational rehabilitation, if appropriate.

Evaluation

Long-term drug therapy often produces side effects. The health care team then must decide which side effects cannot be permitted and which can be treated or tolerated. Evaluate the patient regularly through observation, reassess known problem areas (e.g., the mouth with phenytoin therapy), and make appropriate referrals.

Before discharge, verify that the patient or family can name the drugs being taken and how to take them correctly, including dose, time of day, and correct preparation; can explain side effects that may occur, which of these need to be reported immediately, how to treat or prevent those that are more likely to occur; and can explain what to do if a dose is missed. Determine that the patient can state the importance of wearing a medical identification tag or bracelet.

NURSING IMPLICATIONS SUMMARY

General Guidelines: Anticonvulsant Therapy

Drug Administration

- For seizures, assess frequency, characteristics, previous treatment, alterations in activities of daily living related to seizure activity.
- Monitor serum drug levels if available.
- Assess for side effects. Tactfully question the patient about compliance with therapy.

Patient and Family Education

- Review with the patient the anticipated benefits and possible side effects of drug therapy.
- Provide emotional support as the patient begins anticonvulsant therapy. Drug side effects are common in the first several months of therapy but often diminish with time. Several months of treatment with a drug or regimen may be needed to determine adequate dosage.
- Reinforce to patients the importance of continuing prescribed medications even if they have been seizure-free for an extended period. Stress the need to take drugs as ordered and to avoid abruptly discontinuing prescribed medications because this may precipitate seizures. Recent evidence suggests that anticonvulsants can be discontinued in some patients who have been seizure-free for a long period. This decision must be made on an individual basis in consultation with the physician.
- Counsel the patient to learn from the physician what actions to take in the event of a missed dose of drug. A typical guideline is this one: Take missed dose as soon as remembered, unless almost time for the next dose, then omit missed dose and resume regular dosing schedule. Do not double up for missed doses. Contact the physician for guidelines about what to do if two or more consecutive doses are missed.
- Females of childbearing age may wish to use contraceptives while taking these drugs. If females wish to conceive, counsel them to keep physicians informed so that they can be given current information about drug effects during pregnancy. In addition, remind the patient to inform her gynecologist of the anticonvulsant being used. Oral contraceptives are not effective when some of these drugs are taken.
- Encourage patients to wear a medical identification tag or bracelet indicating they have a history of seizures. In addition, suggest that they carry a card listing current drugs and dosages in their wallets.
- Remind the patient to inform all health care providers of all medications being taken. Tell the patient not to use over-the-counter (OTC) preparations unless approved by the physician. There are many drug interactions with many of these medications.
- Warn the patient to avoid driving or operating hazardous equipment if drowsiness or visual difficulties develop. Teach the patient that visual disturbances are common with many of these drugs; the patient should report the development of double vision, blurred vision, nystagmus.
- Refer the patient as needed to local or national agencies, including the local visiting nurse agency, vocational rehabilitation, or the Epilepsy Foundation of America.
- Instruct the patient to avoid drinking alcoholic beverages unless permitted in small amounts by the physician.
- Tell the patient not to switch brands of anticonvulsant because bioavailability may differ between brands; consult the pharmacist and the physician for specific information.
- Teach the patient using a suspension form to shake the bottle well before pouring each dose. Failure to adequately resuspend the medication may result in inadequate doses when the bottle is nearly full and excessive doses when the bottle is less than half full, because the drug may settle to the bottom of the bottle.
- Review the procedure for the prescribed drug form with the patient. Usually, swallow capsules whole, without breaking them open. Chewable tablets should be chewed well and not swallowed whole. Enteric-coated forms should be swallowed whole, without crushing or chewing. If in doubt, consult the manufacturer's literature and the pharmacist.

Carbamazepine

Drug Administration

- See the general guidelines.
- This drug may be used to treat tic douloureux (trigeminal neuralgia). For this, assess characteristics of pain, aggravating factors, previous treatments.
- Monitor blood pressure and weight. Assess for visual changes, double vision. Assess for possible water intoxication (syndrome of inappropriate antidiuretic hormone, SIADH): weakness, nausea, vomiting, confusion, hostility, stupor, increased seizure frequency.
- Monitor complete blood cell count (CBC) and differential, platelet count, serum electrolytes, and liver function tests.
- Carbamazepine is usually effective at a serum concentration of 6 to 12 μg/ml.

Patient and Family Education

- See the general guidelines.
- See the patient problem boxes on photosensitivity (p. 649), constipation (p. 304), dry mouth (p. 300), bleeding tendencies (p. 586), and leukopenia (p. 585).
- Tell the patient using this medication for trigeminal neuralgia that it is not an analgesic and should not be used for any condition other than that prescribed.
- Tell the diabetic patient that this drug may alter urine glucose results. Monitor blood glucose levels.

NURSING IMPLICATIONS SUMMARY—cont'd

Succinimides (Ethosuximide, Methsuximide, Phensuximide)

Drug Administration

- See the general guidelines.
- Monitor CBC and differential, platelet count, liver function tests, blood urea nitrogen (BUN) and serum creatinine, and urinalysis.
- Ethosuximide and methsuximide are usually effective at a serum concentration of 40 to 100 μg/ml.

Patient and Family Education

- See the general guidelines.
- Encourage the patient to take doses with meals or a snack to lessen gastric irritation.
- Tell the patient taking phensuximide that urine may turn red, pink, or red-brown during therapy with this drug; this effect is harmless.
- Tell the patient taking methsuximide not to take capsules that appear to have melted or are only partly filled.

Hydantoins (Ethotoin, Mephenytoin, Phenytoin)

Drug Administration

- See the general guidelines.
- Assess gait, nausea and vomiting, nystagmus, dizziness, and GI symptoms.
- Therapeutic serum drug level of phenytoin is 10 to 20 μg/ml.
- Monitor complete blood cell count (CBC) and differential, platelet count, liver function tests, and blood glucose level.
- Remember that even if used as an anticonvulsant, phenytoin also has cardiovascular effects (see Chapter 19).

Intravenous Phenytoin

- Prepare dose with diluent supplied by the manufacturer. Slightly yellow-colored solutions may be used, but discard solutions that are not clear. Do not mix with other drugs or many IV solutions, because precipitation may occur. Flush tubing before and after administration with 0.9% sodium chloride. Administer at a rate of 50 mg or less/min. Monitor blood pressure, and if possible, have patient connected to ECG monitor to monitor cardiac rhythm during and immediately after IV administration. Recent studies have involved dilutions in large volumes of normal saline solution or lactated Ringer's injection (e.g., 100 mg phenytoin in 50 ml normal saline solution) to administer phenytoin as an infusion. Use an in-line filter. Consult the manufacturer's literature for current recommendations.

Patient and Family Education

- See general guidelines.
- Review common signs of overdose including ataxia, slurred speech, and nystagmus. Tell the family to report these or any unusual side effects.
- Provide emotional support. Acne or hirsutism may be difficult for some patients. Refer patients to a dermatologist as appropriate.
- Encourage the patient to have regular dental checkups and to have a thorough dental care program that includes flossing, brushing, and rinsing. Even with meticulous oral care, gingival hyperplasia develops in some patients taking phenytoin or mephenytoin. Provide emotional support.
- Instruct the patient to take oral doses with meals or a snack to lessen gastric irritation.
- Instruct the patient to report signs of folic acid deficiency including fatigability, weakness, fainting, and headache.
- Encourage ingestion of foods high in vitamin D (see the dietary consideration box on vitamins, p. 215).
- Advise the diabetic patient to monitor blood glucose levels, because an adjustment in diet or insulin dose may be necessary.
- Tell the patient that these drugs may produce a harmless brownish or pinkish discoloration of urine.
- Instruct the patient not to take doses of these anticonvulsants within 2 to 3 hours of taking antacids or drugs for diarrhea.

Valproic Acid and Divalproex Sodium

Drug Administration

- See the general guidelines.
- Monitor CBC and differential, platelet count, serum ammonia concentration, BUN and serum creatinine, and liver function tests.
- Valproic acid is usually effective at a serum concentration of 50 to 150 μg/ml.

Patient and Family Education

- See the general guidelines.
- See the patient problem box on constipation (p. 304).
- Instruct the patient to take oral doses with meals or a snack to lessen gastric irritation.
- Instruct the patient to take the delayed-release tablet form whole without chewing or breaking the tablet. Instruct the patient taking the delayed-release capsule form to swallow the capsule whole or to pour the contents on a small amount of food such as applesauce or pudding and swallow this food without chewing. Instruct the patient taking the syrup form that the syrup may be mixed with a small amount of food or liquid. Instruct the patient taking the

Continued.

NURSING IMPLICATIONS SUMMARY—cont'd

capsule form to swallow the capsule whole without chewing or crushing.

- Tell diabetic patients that this drug may alter urine tests for ketones, giving false-positive results. Monitor blood glucose levels.

Felbamate

Drug Administration/Patient and Family Education

- See the general guidelines.
- Monitor the CBC and white blood cell (WBC) differential, and platelet count, liver function tests, and serum iron concentration.
- Encourage the patient to take doses with meal or snack to lessen gastric irritation.

Gabapentin

Drug Administration/Patient and Family Education

- See the general guidelines.
- See the patient problem box on leukopenia (p. 585).
- Gabapentin may be taken with food or on an empty stomach. However, instruct patients to follow specific guidelines given by the physician.
- Instruct patients taking doses three times a day not to allow more than 12 hours to elapse between any two doses.

Lamotrigine

Drug Administration/Patient and Family Education

- See the general guidelines.
- See the patient problem boxes on bleeding tendencies (p. 586) and leukopenia (p. 585).
- Instruct the patient to report the development of skin rash immediately.
- Tell the patient that doses may be taken with meals or on an empty stomach.

Long-Acting Barbiturates (Phenobarbital and Primidone)

Drug Administration/Patient and Family Education

- See the general guidelines.
- Barbiturates are discussed in Chapter 51.
- Phenobarbital is usually effective at a serum concentration of 10 to 40 μg/ml. Primidone is usually effective at a serum concentration of 5 to 12 μg/ml.
- Review with families signs of intoxication or overdose including slurred speech, ataxia, and vertigo. If these develop, notify the physician.

Intravenous Phenobarbital

- Dilute sterile powder slowly as directed on the package insert. Drug is also available in solution that must be diluted. Administer diluted dose at a rate of 1 gr (60 to 65 mg) over 1 minute. Monitor vital signs and respiration. Have a suction machine at the bedside and equipment for intubation and ventilatory support available. Do not leave the patient unattended until the patient is stable and alert.

Intramuscular Phenobarbital

- Observe for respiratory depression 30 to 60 minutes after injection. Monitor blood pressure. Supervise ambulation. Keep siderails up.

Dione Anticonvulsants (Paramethadione, Trimethadione)

Drug Administration

- See the general guidelines.
- Monitor CBC and differential, platelet count, liver function tests, serum creatinine and BUN levels, and urinalysis.

Patient and Family Education

- See the general guidelines.
- Tell the patient to report skin rashes or changes immediately. Because side effects are common, encourage patients to stay in close contact with the physician.

Other Drug Groups

- Benzodiazepines are discussed in Chapter 51.
- Acetazolamide is discussed in Chapter 14.
- ACTH is discussed in Chapter 60.

CRITICAL THINKING

APPLICATION

1. Define epilepsy and list some of the known causes. What other conditions can precipitate seizures?
2. Describe tonic-clonic, absence myoclonic, psychomotor, and focal seizures and infantile spasms. List the drug of choice for treating each type of epilepsy.
3. What is status epilepticus and how is it treated?
4. What considerations need to be made in beginning drug administration to control epilepsy?
5. What are the adverse effects and drug interactions of phenytoin?
6. What are the adverse effects of ethosuximide?
7. What are some of the special concerns regarding pregnancy and epilepsy?
8. Which benzodiazepines are used as anticonvulsants? For which seizure types are they effective?
9. What are the uses and side effects of carbamazepine?
10. Why is valproic acid a valuable anticonvulsant?
11. Describe the uses of the newest anticonvulsant drugs, felbamate, gabapentin, and lamotrigine.

CRITICAL THINKING

1. What are some of the factors to monitor when a second anticonvulsant drug is added to the therapy?
2. How would you counsel a patient who has been seizure free for several years and wishes to discontinue medication?

CHAPTER 56

Drugs for Parkinson's Disease and Alzheimer's Disease

OBJECTIVES

After studying this chapter, you should be able to do the following:

- *List three classic symptoms of Parkinson's disease, and explain the role of acetylcholine and dopamine in Parkinson's disease.*
- *Develop a nursing care plan for patients receiving anticholinergic drugs, amantadine, bromocriptine, levodopa or carbidopa-levodopa, pergolide, or selegiline to treat Parkinson's disease.*
- *Describe the rationale for administering tacrine to patients with Alzheimer's disease.*

CHAPTER OVERVIEW

This chapter covers drug therapy for Parkinson's disease and Alzheimer's disease. Parkinson's disease is a progressive neurologic disorder of the extrapyramidal system caused by the degeneration of the dopaminergic neurons. This degeneration results in motor abnormalities. Alzheimer's disease is a progressive dementia characterized by the loss of short-term and long-term memory.

KEY TERMS

akinesia
Alzheimer's disease
bradykinesia
dyskinesia
on-off phenomenon
Parkinson's disease
rigidity

Therapeutic Rationale: Parkinson's Disease

Parkinson's disease is a movement disorder characterized by rigidity, akinesia, and tremor. **Rigidity** means that muscle tone is greatly increased but reflex activity is not. When a limb is passively forced through flexor or extensor movements, the muscular resistance alternately increases and decreases to give a cogwheel effect. **Akinesia** (no motion) refers to the difficulty the patient has in initiating any movement. The face has a masklike, fixed expression devoid of emotion. Early in the course of Parkinson's disease, the difficulty in initiating movement is not as marked and is termed **bradykinesia** (slow motion). The tremor of Parkinson's disease is seen mostly in the limbs at rest and decreases with movement of the limbs.

Role of Acetylcholine and Dopamine

Insight into the neurochemical defect in Parkinson's disease exemplifies our growing knowledge of the role of neurotransmitters in controlling given functions within the central nervous system (CNS). For many years, anticholinergic drugs such as atropine had been used to decrease the tremor characteristics of Parkinson's disease; acetylcholine therefore seemed important in accounting for some symptoms. When the antipsychotic drugs (major tranquilizers) were introduced in the 1950s, symptoms indistinguishable from those of Parkinson's disease began to appear in patients treated with these drugs. It is now known that this is because these drugs block receptors for the CNS neurotransmitter dopamine.

Subsequently, patients with Parkinson's disease were shown to have degeneration of crucial dopaminergic neurons projecting to certain basal ganglia of the extrapyramidal system in the brain. This system is responsible for maintaining motor coordination at the CNS level.

The current understanding of Parkinson's disease is that it represents a deficiency in the neurotransmitter dopamine in certain basal ganglia. Dopamine from these neuronal tracts is believed to exert an inhibitory influence on cholinergic neurons of the extrapyramidal system controlling muscle tone. When dopamine is lacking, muscle tone increases because of the unopposed action of acetylcholine, resulting in muscular rigidity, inhibition of spontaneous movements, and tremor. The lack of dopamine is a result of a progressive degeneration of specific dopaminergic neurons. This degeneration can be caused by encephalitis, carbon-monoxide poisoning, manganese poisoning, cerebrovascular accident (stroke), or, more commonly, unknown causes. This degeneration cannot be arrested. Drugs alleviate the symptoms for only a few years.

The current rationale for the pharmacologic treatment of Parkinson's disease is to diminish the severity of motor symptoms by blocking the excessive action of acetylcholine or by replenishing the dopamine to return the balance of excitatory acetylcholine action and inhibitory dopamine action toward normal.

Drug-Induced Parkinson's Disease

Certain drugs also can cause symptoms of Parkinson's disease. Reserpine (Serpasil), which depletes neuronal stores of dopamine and norepinephrine, and the antipsychotic drugs, which block dopamine receptors, are the usual causes of drug-induced Parkinson's disease. Since symptoms depend on the presence of the drug, lowering the dosage or discontinuing the drug eliminates the symptoms.

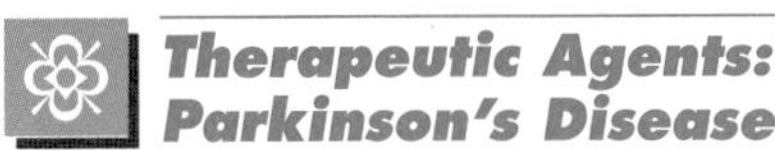

Therapeutic Agents: Parkinson's Disease

Antidyskinetic Drugs: General Characteristics

Mechanism of Action

Antidyskinetic drugs (Table 56-1) are anticholinergic agents that cross the blood-brain barrier and block central muscarinic cholinergic receptors.

Pharmacokinetics

These agents are given orally. The dosage is started low and increased gradually until the tremor and rigidity decrease or the side effects become prominent. When the drug is discontinued, the dosage should be decreased gradually to lessen a rebound appearance of the parkinsonian symptoms.

Uses

Anticholinergic drugs are administered early in the course of Parkinson's disease to lessen rigidity, bradykinesia, and tremor. Atropine and scopolamine, the classic anticholinergic drugs, were used to treat symptoms of Parkinson's disease for many years. Anticholinergic drugs used today are synthetic drugs that are centrally active and produce fewer peripheral side effects. These drugs include biperiden (Akineton), benztropine (Cogentin), ethopropazine (Parsidol), procyclidine (Kemadrin), and trihexyphenidyl (Tremin and others). The antihistamine diphenhydramine (Benadryl) is also used in the treatment of Parkinson's disease for its anticholinergic properties.

An antidyskinetic is also the drug of choice for treatment of extrapyramidal reactions (akathisia, acute dystonia, and parkinsonism) caused by the antipsychotic drugs. Tardive dyskinesia is not reversed by anticholinergic drugs. These extrapyramidal reactions are described in Chapter 52.

Adverse Reactions, Toxicity, and Contraindications

Common side effects of the anticholinergic drugs are dry mouth, constipation, urinary retention, and blurred vision. Common mental effects include impairment of recent memory, confusion, insomnia, and restlessness. Mental effects can become serious, with the development of agitation, disorientation, delirium, paranoid reactions, or hallucinations. Mental problems are more common with elderly patients who have preexisting mental disturbances. Patients who have prior

TABLE 56-1 Drugs to Treat Parkinsonism

GENERIC NAME	TRADE NAME	ADMINISTRATION/DOSAGE	COMMENTS
Anticholinergics			
Benztropine mesylate	Cogentin*	ORAL: *Adults*—0.5-1 mg at bedtime initially; increase gradually to 4-6 mg if required. FDA pregnancy category C. For drug-induced extrapyramidal reactions: ORAL, INTRAMUSCULAR, INTRAVENOUS: *Adults*—1-4 mg 1 or 2 times daily. For acute dystonic reaction: ORAL, INTRAVENOUS: *Adults*—2 mg intravenously, then 1-2 mg orally twice daily.	To treat Parkinson's disease and drug-induced extrapyramidal reactions. Particularly effective in reversing acute dystonic reaction to antipsychotic drug.
Biperiden hydrochloride	Akineton*	ORAL: *Adults*—2 mg 3 times daily; may increase dose up to 20 mg daily if required. FDA pregnancy category C. For drug-induced extrapyramidal reactions: ORAL: *Adults*—2 mg 1-3 times daily. INTRAMUSCULAR: *Adults*—2 mg repeated as often as every 30 min but no more than 4 doses in 24 hr. *Children*—0.04 mg/kg body weight as often as every 30 min but no more than 4 doses in 24 hr.	To treat Parkinson's disease and drug-induced extrapyramidal reactions.
Ethopropazine hydrochloride	Parsidol Parsitan†	ORAL: *Adults*—50 mg 1 or 2 times daily initially. Mild-to-moderate cases require 100-400 mg daily. Severe cases may require 500-600 mg daily. FDA pregnancy category C.	To treat Parkinson's disease. Phenothiazine with only anticholinergic effects and devoid of antidopaminergic effects.
Procyclidine hydrochloride	Kemadrin* Procyclid†	ORAL: *Adults*—5 mg twice daily, up to 20-30 mg daily if required. FDA pregnancy category C. For drug-induced extrapyramidal reactions: ORAL: *Adults*—2-2.5 mg 3 times daily; increase to 10-20 mg daily if required.	To treat Parkinson's disease and drug-induced extrapyramidal reactions.
Trihexyphenidyl hydrochloride	Artane* Trihexy†	ORAL: *Adults*—2 mg 2 or 3 times daily. Increased to 15-20 mg daily (usually) or 40 to 50 mg daily (rarely) to control symptoms. FDA pregnancy category C. For drug-induced parkinsonism: ORAL: *Adults*—1 mg initially. Subsequent doses increased if symptoms do not decrease. Usual daily dose, 5-15 mg.	To treat Parkinson's disease and drug-induced extrapyramidal reactions.
Antihistamines			
✣ Diphenhydramine hydrochloride	Benadryl*	ORAL: *Adults*—25 mg 3 times daily; increase to 50 mg 4 times daily if required. For drug-induced extrapyramidal reactions: INTRAMUSCULAR, INTRAVENOUS: *Adults*—10-50 mg; maximum, 400 mg daily. *Children*— 5 mg/kg body weight intramuscularly daily; maximum 300 mg in 24 hr.	To treat Parkinson's disease and drug-induced extrapyramidal reactions. Marked sedative effects.
Drugs Affecting Amount of Dopamine in Brain			
✣ Amantadine	Symadine Symmetrel*	ORAL: *Adults*—100 mg daily after breakfast for 5-7 days. Additional 100 mg may be added after lunch.	Antiviral agent that augments release of dopamine. Side effects are similar to those of anticholinergic drugs.
Bromocriptine	Parlodel	ORAL: *Adults*—Initially 1.25 mg twice daily; increase every other week or monthly by 1.25-2.5 mg until benefits are achieved or adverse effects become intolerable.	Dopamine agonist. May be added to levodopa or carbidopa-levodopa therapy; occasionally replaces levodopa therapy.

*Available in Canada and United States.
†Available in Canada only.

TABLE 56-1 Drugs to Treat Parkinsonism—cont'd

GENERIC NAME	TRADE NAME	ADMINISTRATION/DOSAGE	COMMENTS
Drugs Affecting Amount of Dopamine in Brain—cont'd			
Carbidopa-levodopa	Sinemet	ORAL: *Adults*—Initial daily dose should be ¼ daily dose of levodopa. Sinemet should be administered 8 hr after last levodopa dose and given in 3 or 4 doses daily. Patients not previously receiving levodopa are started with 10:100 mg (carbidopa : levodopa) 3 times daily; dosage is gradually increased as required.	Carbidopa inhibits degradation of dopamine outside CNS. Levodopa-carbidopa ratio is 10 : 1.
✣ Levodopa	Dopar Larodopa*	ORAL: *Adults*—Initially 300-1000 mg daily in 3-7 doses during waking hours with food. Increase dosage 100-500 mg every 2-3 days or more until desired control is achieved. Usually requires 4-6 gm and 6-8 wk to achieve control. After several months to 1 year, dosage may be lowered.	Levodopa is chemical precursor of dopamine.
Pergolide mesylate	Permax	ORAL: *Adults*—Initially 0.05 mg daily for first 2 days; increase by 0.1-0.15 mg daily at 3-day intervals for 12 days until antiparkinson effect is optimum or maximum of 5 mg daily is reached. Can be administered in 3 divided doses daily.	Pergolide has dopaminergic activity.
Selegiline hydrochloride	Eldepryl	ORAL: *Adults*—10 mg/day.	Inhibits degradation of dopamine by inhibiting monoamine oxidase B. May slow progress of Parkinson's disease. Also used as adjunct for patients who exhibit deterioration in response to carbidopa-levodopa therapy.

histories of glaucoma, particularly narrow-angle glaucoma, or some type of urinary or intestinal obstruction or tachycardia are not good candidates, because anticholinergic drugs can aggravate any of these conditions. Characteristic actions of anticholinergic drugs are discussed in Chapter 11.

Interactions

The antidyskinetics increase the sedative effect of alcohol and other CNS depressant drugs. They also have additive anticholinergic action with other drugs.

Specific Antidyskinetic Drugs

Benztropine

Benztropin (Cogentin) may be administered orally or by intravenous (IV) or intramuscular (IM) injection. When administered orally, the onset of action is 1 to 2 hours. The drug is active in a few minutes after injected. The duration of action is about 24 hours. Benztropin has slight antihistaminic and local anesthetic effects. It increases the efficacy of levodopa if administered concurrently.

Biperiden

Biperiden (Akineton) may be administered orally or by intramuscular or intravenous injection. The duration of action after IV injection is variable, from 1 to 8 hours. Biperiden has a slight effect on the cardiovascular and respiratory system.

✣ Diphenhydramine

Diphenhydramine (Benadryl) is an antihistamine with anticholinergic properties. It can be administered orally or by IM or IV injection. This drug can also be administered to children.

Ethopropazine

Ethopropazine (Parsidol) is administered orally and has a duration of action of about 4 hours. Like benztropine, ethopropazine has slight antihistaminic and local anesthetic effect. It is also a phenothiazine derivative, and at high doses may cause changes in vision, jaundice, hematologic changes, and abnormalities in an electrocardiogram.

Procyclidine

Procyclidine (Kemadrin) is administered orally and has a duration of action of about 4 hours. It has a direct antispasmodic effect on smooth muscle. The action of procyclidine is more pronounced in reducing rigidity than in reducing tremor. Procyclidine enhances the effect of levodopa when administered concurrently.

Trihexyphenidyl

Trihexyphenidyl (Artan) is administered orally. The onset of action is 1 hour and the duration of action 6 to 12 hours. For patients stabilized on the drug, an extended-release capsule formulation (Artan Sequels) is available for twice-a-day administration. Trihexyphenidyl has a direct antispasmodic effect on smooth muscle. Although small doses have a sedative effect, high doses can produce excitement. Trihexyphenidyl enhances the effect of levodopa when administered concurrently.

DRUGS AFFECTING AMOUNT OF DOPAMINE IN BRAIN

Several drugs are used in the treatment of Parkinson's disease to maintain or increase the level of dopamine in the brain. Amantadine and selegiline may be used early in the disease, but most of these agents are reserved for use after disability has begun. The reason is that these drugs are only effective for a few years. They treat only the symptoms of the disease but do not alter its course. However, there are some studies that indicate that selegiline may slow the progression of Parkinson's disease. This drug is now frequently started when the diagnosis is made. The drugs in this section are listed in Table 56-1.

✣ Amantadine

Amantadine (Symmetrel) is an antiviral agent that also has been found effective in reducing the severity of symptoms of Parkinson's disease when used alone or with an anticholinergic drug. Amantadine promotes the release and inhibits the reuptake of dopamine from the central neurons, an action unrelated to its antiviral action.

Amantadine is often used in the early stages of the disease to control parkinsonian symptoms. It has the advantages of being effective when administered as a single daily dose and of having few side effects. Side effects seen include dizziness, nervousness, inability to concentrate, ataxia, slurred speech, insomnia, lethargy, blurred vision, dry mouth, gastrointestinal upset, and rash. Amantadine may also be used with anticholinergic drugs or with levodopa, because it enhances the effectiveness of these other drugs and allows a reduction of their dosage.

Bromocriptine

Bromocriptine (Parlodel) mimics the action of dopamine in the brain. It is an alternative to levodopa when levodopa is contraindicated, is not well tolerated, or does not produce a response. Bromocriptine has a duration of action similar to that of levodopa and may be added to levodopa or carbidopa-levodopa therapy for patients who show symptoms of fluctuating doses such as dystonia and muscle cramps. Doses of bromocriptine must be individualized. Transient dizziness and nausea are common. Hypotension, abdominal pain, blurred vision, double vision, and vasospasm of the fingers and toes in response to cold also occasionally occur.

Carbidopa-Levodopa

Carbidopa (Atamet, Sinemet) inhibits the conversion of levodopa to dopamine. Because carbidopa cannot enter the CNS, only peripheral conversion is inhibited. This means that levodopa is converted to dopamine only in the brain, so the presence of carbidopa lowers the dose of levodopa required by 75%. Because the emetic effects of levodopa reflect peripheral dopamine concentrations, the incidence of nausea and vomiting is reduced greatly with carbidopa-levodopa combination. Carbidopa is available only in a fixed-ratio combination with levodopa.

✣ Levodopa

Mechanism of Action

Levodopa (Dopar and Larodopa) is the chemical precursor of dopamine, and unlike dopamine, it readily crosses the blood-brain barrier. It is converted to dopamine by the enzyme dopa decarboxylase.

Pharmacokinetics

About 95% of a dose of levodopa is converted to dopamine in the periphery rather than in the brain, and the high plasma concentration of dopamine is responsible for the nausea and cardiac effects occurring with this therapy. For these reasons, levodopa is almost always given in combination with carbidopa (see previous entry).

Levodopa is taken orally, and the peak effect is seen 1 to 2 hours later. Dosage is adjusted up or down gradually every 2 to 3 days to lessen the incidence of nausea and to avoid precipitating side effects.

Uses

Levodopa is prescribed when the drugs used in the early stages of Parkinson's disease—anticholinergics, amantadine, or selegiline—no longer control symptoms. Levodopa therapy does not stop the progression of Parkinson's disease but relieves the symptoms and dramatically improves ability to function.

Adverse Reactions, Toxicity, and Contraindications

Dopamine is the neurotransmitter for the chemoreceptor trigger zone of the medulla and thus produces nausea, vomiting, and anorexia. To create tolerance to this emetic action, levodopa therapy must be initiated by starting with low doses that are gradually increased. A snack high in protein also helps to prevent nausea. Antiemetics from the phenothiazine class should not be used because they block the therapeutic action of dopamine. Trimethobenzamide (Tigan) may be taken early in the morning to control nausea.

Additional effects typically noted after the start of levodopa therapy include increased alertness, sense of well-being, and increased libido. These effects are attributed to behavioral roles of dopamine in the brain. Further mental changes may occur with prolonged therapy. Euphoria, restlessness, anxiety, irritability, hyperactivity, insomnia, and vivid dreams frequently occur. Patients occasionally may become paranoid and may experience psychotic episodes or become depressed, with or without suicidal tendencies. These mental changes are usually reversed by lowering the dosage.

Another side effect sometimes seen at the start of levodopa therapy is orthostatic hypotension. The mechanism is not known but is believed to be a CNS effect rather than a peripheral effect. This hypotension tends to decrease with time. An increase in heart rate and force of contraction may also be apparent at the start of therapy. These cardiac actions are caused by the direct action of dopamine on the heart. Cardiac arrhythmias may develop and must be controlled by appropriate medication.

Additional side effects of levodopa therapy may be gastrointestinal (GI) effects, including bleeding, difficulty in swallowing, and a burning sensation of the tongue. Respiratory effects such as cough, hoarseness, and disturbed breathing may appear. Because of these side effects, levodopa therapy is used cautiously for patients with a history of heart disease, asthma, emphysema, or peptic ulcer. Problems in urination from incontinence to retention may arise.

Blurred vision or dilated pupils may be caused by levodopa. Levodopa therapy is not considered for patients with narrow-angle glaucoma and only with careful monitoring for patients with chronic (wide-angle) glaucoma. Hepatic, hematopoietic, cardiovascular, and renal function tests are performed periodically on patients receiving long-term levodopa therapy. This is because many laboratory test values are high in patients receiving levodopa therapy, and only careful monitoring can determine whether or not a real problem exists. Hematocrit and white blood cell counts may be lowered by levodopa therapy, but therapy is discontinued only when abnormally low counts are found. Therapy is not initiated in patients with blood disorders.

After prolonged therapy with levodopa, abnormal involuntary movements (**dyskinesia**) alternating with a sudden lapse in symptom control (the **on-off phenomenon**) may appear. Dyskinesia usually comprises abnormal involuntary movements of the mouth, tongue, face, or neck. Dyskinesia usually appears 1 to 2 hours after the latest dose of levodopa and represents a mild levodopa toxicity. "End-of-dose" akinesia also may occur. This means that the akinesia appears just before a new dose is to be taken and usually can be avoided by increasing frequency of administration.

Interactions

Drugs that reduce the effectiveness of levodopa include the antipsychotic drugs, the rauwolfia alkaloids, phenytoin, papaverine, methyldopa, metoclopramide, and pyridoxine. A hypertensive crisis may be precipitated with levodopa and monoamine oxidase inhibitors are given concurrently.

Pergolide

Pergolide (Permax) has direct dopaminergic action. It is more potent than bromocriptine and has a longer half-life. Overall effectiveness of pergolide with carbidopa-levodopa therapy is similar to bromocriptine. Side effects are similar to those of bromocriptine. The most common reactions are hallucinations, nausea, dry mouth, light-headedness, and dyskinesia.

Selegiline

Selegiline (formerly deprenyl) (Eldepryl) inhibits the enzyme monoamine oxidase B, which degrades dopamine in the brain. Because dopamine is not rapidly degraded in the presence of selegiline, the duration of action and dose of levodopa is reduced. Early morning stiffness and end-of-dose symptoms are decreased.

There are some indications that selegiline may slow the progression of Parkinson's disease. It is often administered in the early stages of the disease as a preventive measure, although early symptoms are in general not well controlled by selegiline alone. In advanced cases of the disease, selegiline lessens the wearing off effects of levodopa or carbidopa-levodopa therapy.

Selegiline should not be administered with meperidine and other opioids or with monoamine oxidase inhibitors or serotonin uptake inhibitors.

NURSING PROCESS OVERVIEW

Drugs to Treat Parkinson's Disease

Assessment

Perform a baseline patient assessment, including vital signs, joint movement, amount of tremor, affect and objective signs of the disease, and ability to ambulate and to perform activities of daily living. Because this is often a disease of the elderly, obtain a baseline view of other known health problems such as hypertension, diabetes, and cardiovascular or renal disease.

Nursing Diagnoses

- Altered bowel elimination: constipation caused by drug side effects
- Risk for urinary retention
- Risk for body image disturbance related to dyskinesia or other drug side effects

Patient Outcomes

The patient will describe methods to prevent constipation. The patient will recognize urinary retention and contact the health care team if it develops. The patient will share feelings about body image changes.

Planning/Implementation

Include the patient in the discussion of the goals of therapy. Monitor for subjective and objective improvement and for drug side effects. Improvement in symptoms should outweigh the discomfort of side effects. Some patients find the side effects from a drug are worse than if the disease is untreated, at least at some stages in its progression. Before discharge, refer the patient to social service, vocational rehabilitation, visiting nurse, and other agencies, if appropriate.

Evaluation

Before discharge and at regular intervals during therapy, ensure that the patient can explain prescribed drugs and doses; how to take the drugs correctly; the expected goals of therapy; and drug side effects, how to treat them, and when to notify the physician. Verify that the patient can explain any necessary dietary or vitamin restrictions.

Therapeutic Rationale: Alzheimer's Disease

Alzheimer's disease is a disease of progressive mental degeneration. The onset is gradual and generally progressive with a dementia characterized by impairment of short-term and long-term memory. At death, brains of those with Alzheimer's disease show abnormal plaques in the affected areas and a shrunken brain. It is a disease primarily of older adults, although some genetic forms have been identified with early onset. The genetic basis of certain proteins associated with Alzheimer's plaques, especially beta-amyloid and apolipoprotein E alleles, is being studied. In addition, many individuals with Down's syndrome (trisomy 21) develop Alzheimer's by the time they are 40 years old.

Therapeutic Agents: Alzheimer's Disease

Pharmacologic treatment for Alzheimer's disease is lacking because the cause of the disease is still unknown. Ergoloid mesylates (Chapter 15) are vasodilators widely used to treat dementia syndromes, although their efficacy remains controversial. Cholinergic drugs have been tried because acetylcholine appears to be the primary neurotransmitter affected by the disease process. Tacrine is an acetylcholinesterase inhibitor specifically approved for the management of Alzheimer's disease. Symptoms associated with Alzheimer's disease include depression, psychotic behavior, and anxiety. These symptoms are treated with appropriate drugs.

Tacrine

Mechanism of Action

Tacrine (Cognex) (Table 56-2) is a centrally acting acetylcholinesterase inhibitor that also blocks potassium channels and inhibits the reuptake of norepinephrine, serotonin, and dopamine.

Pharmacokinetics

Tacrine is rapidly absorbed. It is extensively removed by first-pass metabolism in the liver. The major metabolite has central cholinergic activity.

Uses

The major indication for tacrine is for symptomatic treatment of mild to moderate dementia in Alzheimer's disease. Efficacy is limited.

Adverse Reactions, Toxicity, and Contraindications

The side effects of tacrine include ataxia, loss of appetite, nausea, vomiting, and diarrhea.

Hepatotoxicity limits the use of tacrine. Up to 50% of patients develop elevated levels of liver enzymes. When dose is reduced or the drug discontinued, liver function studies commonly return to normal within 6 weeks.

Interactions

Tacrine interferes with the cytochrome P-450 system, leading to elevated levels of theophylline. Cimetidine can increase the plasma concentrations of tacrine. Because tacrine increases gastric acid secretion, it can increase the gastric irritation and potential for bleeding of nonsteroidal antiinflammatory drugs (NSAIDs). Smoking decreases the plasma level of tacrine by two thirds.

TABLE 56-2 Drug Therapy for Alzheimer's Disease

GENERIC NAME	TRADE NAME*	ADMINISTRATION/DOSAGE	COMMENTS
Tacrine	Cognex	ORAL: *Adults*—10 mg 4 times/day initially. If drug is tolerated and transaminase levels do not increase, may increase dose to 20 mg 4 times/day and at 6 wk intervals up to 40 mg 4 times/day.	Dose must be stopped if transaminase serum value exceeds 5 times normal. May start again if transaminase levels did not exceed 10 times normal and they return to normal.

NURSING IMPLICATIONS SUMMARY

General Guidelines: Patient Receiving Drugs for Parkinson's Disease

- Assess severity of symptoms, including muscle control and movement, ability to perform activities of daily living, dysphagia, posture, and gait.

Patient and Family Education

- Review the anticipated benefits and possible side effects of drug therapy.
- Teach the patient and family that several weeks to months of therapy may be needed in some cases to obtain full benefit of drug therapy. Provide emotional support.
- Parkinson's disease is primarily a problem of the older adults. However, if a premenopausal female develops Parkinson's disease, counsel as needed about contraceptives. These drugs should not be used during pregnancy without consulting the physician.
- Point out to the family that confusion is often a drug side effect in the elderly patient and should not be attributed to Parkinson's disease until fully evaluated.
- Warn the patient not to discontinue these drugs suddenly. A patient should inform all health care providers of all drugs being taken. Over-the-counter medications should be avoided unless approved by the physician.
- Counsel the patient to avoid the use of alcohol unless permitted in small amounts by the physician.

Other Drug Groups

- Anticholinergic drugs are discussed in Chapters 11 and 23.
- See the patient problem boxes on dry mouth (p. 300), constipation (p. 304), and orthostatic hypotension (p. 157).
- Antihistamines are discussed in Chapter 28.
- Phenothiazines are discussed in Chapter 52.

Amantadine

Drug Administration

- Assess mental status regularly. Be alert to signs of increasing depression including lethargy, apathy, decreased appetite, and loss of interest in personal appearance. Be alert to suicidal tendencies.
- Monitor intake and output, daily weight, blood pressure, and pulse. Auscultate lung sounds. Inspect for edema and skin changes.
- Assess for urinary retention. Suggest patients void before taking drug doses.
- Monitor complete blood cell count (CBC) and differential.

Patient and Family Education

- See the general guidelines.
- See the patient problem boxes on orthostatic hypotension (p. 157), dry mouth (p. 300), and constipation (p. 304).
- Warn the patient to avoid driving or operating hazardous equipment if drowsiness or dizziness develops; notify the physician.
- Capsules may be opened and contents mixed with a small amount of food or fluid for ease in taking dose, although a liquid preparation is also available.
- Tell the patient that livedo reticularis (bluish or purplish mottling of the skin) may appear during the first year of therapy and may take several weeks to subside when therapy is discontinued.

Bromocriptine

- Bromocriptine is discussed in Chapter 65.

Carbidopa-Levodopa Combination

Drug Administration/Patient and Family Education

- No specific side effects have been attributed to carbidopa.
- Review with the patient the information about levodopa.

Levodopa

Drug Administration

- Monitor neuromuscular, neurologic, and mental status regularly.
- Monitor blood pressure and pulse, intake and output, and weight.
- Check stools for presence of occult blood. Inspect for skin changes.
- Monitor CBC and differential, platelet count, blood urea nitrogen (BUN) and serum creatinine, and liver function tests.

Patient and Family Education

- See the general guidelines.
- See the patient problem boxes on constipation (p. 304), orthostatic hypotension (p. 157), and dry mouth (p. 300).
- Warn the male patient that priapism has been reported and to notify the physician if it develops.
- Tell the patient that sweat may be darker in color while this drug is taken, and urine may be dark, especially if left standing.
- Instruct the patient to take doses shortly after meals or snack to reduce gastric irritation (15 minutes after).
- Instruct the patient to swallow carbidopa/levodopa extended-release tablets whole, without chewing or crushing. The tablets may be broken in half if approved by the physician. If the patient has difficulty swallowing levodopa capsules or tablets, consult the pharmacist about preparing a liquid form.
- Tell the diabetic patient to monitor blood glucose levels carefully because tests for urinary glucose and ketone levels may be inaccurate.
- There are many side effects of levodopa therapy. Encourage the patient and family to report any new or unexpected findings.
- Pyridoxine (vitamin B_6) may reduce the effectiveness of levodopa. Instruct the patient not to take any vitamin preparations without consulting the physician. Limit in-

Continued.

Nursing Implications Summary—cont'd

take of foods high in pyridoxine; see the dietary consideration box on vitamins (p. 215).

- An on-off phenomenon has been reported with this drug. After long use, some patients report the loss of ability to move. This effect may last for a few minutes to several hours. The patient can then move as before. This problem may occur repeatedly. If it develops, notify the physician.

Pergolide

Drug Administration

- See the general guidelines.
- Assess for common side effects including hallucinations, nausea, dry mouth, light-headedness, and dyskinesia. Monitor weight. See the patient problem box on dry mouth (p. 300).
- Encourage the patient to take doses with meals to lessen gastric irritation.
- Assess the patient for worsening symptoms if pergolide and levodopa are administered concurrently.
- Monitor the blood pressure. Dosages are increased slowly to lessen the degree of hypotension.
- Monitor the patient with a history of cardiac arrhythmias carefully when beginning pergolide therapy; increases in atrial premature contractions and sinus tachycardia have been reported.

Selegiline

Drug Administration

- See the patient problem boxes on orthostatic hypotension (p. 157) and dry mouth (p. 300). Assess for confusion, dizziness, and insomnia.
- Instruct the patient to avoid driving or operating hazardous equipment if dizziness or syncope develops.
- Monitor the blood pressure.
- In doses of 10 mg or less, there are no dietary restrictions with this drug. In higher dosages, the patient should avoid foods high in tyramine. See the dietary consideration box on MAO inhibitors and tyramine (p. 663).

Tacrine for Alzheimer's Disease

Drug Administration/Patient and Family Education

- Assess mental and cognitive status. Monitor vital signs and BP.
- Teach the patient to take doses on an empty stomach, 1 hour before or 2 hours after meals.
- Emphasize the importance of returning for regular follow-up. Blood work must be monitored frequently and regularly for best effect of this drug.
- Tell the patient to avoid driving or operating hazardous equipment if dizziness, clumsiness, or unsteadiness develops.
- Remind the patient to keep all health care providers informed of all drugs being used. Do not take any drugs without first checking with the physician. Do not discontinue tacrine without first discussing it with the physician.
- For missed doses, take as soon as remembered, unless within 2 hours of the next dose; then omit. Do not double up missed doses.
- Avoid smoking while taking tacrine.

Critical Thinking

APPLICATION

1. Describe the physical characteristics seen in Parkinson's disease.
2. What is the neurochemical defect in Parkinson's disease? How do some drugs mimic this defect?
3. Why are anticholinergic drugs, antihistaminic drugs, and amantadine effective in treating symptoms of Parkinson's disease? What are major side effects of these drug classes?
4. What is the rationale for administering levodopa to treat the symptoms of Parkinson's disease? What role does carbidopa play?
5. What are the side effects of levodopa?
6. What is the rationale for administering tacrine to patients with Alzheimer's disease?

CRITICAL THINKING

1. Prepare a care plan for the patient with Parkinson's disease who is about to begin levodopa therapy.
2. What would you tell the family of a patient with Alzheimer's disease to expect from therapy with tacrine? How would tacrine help the depressed patient with Alzheimer's disease?

CHAPTER 57

Centrally Acting Skeletal Muscle Relaxants

OBJECTIVES

After studying this chapter, you should be able to do the following:

- *Develop a nursing care plan for the patient receiving a centrally acting skeletal muscle relaxant such as diazepam, baclofen, or dantrolene.*
- *Develop a nursing care plan for the patient receiving drug therapy for muscle spasms.*

KEY TERMS

muscle spasms
spasticity

CHAPTER OVERVIEW

This chapter discusses drug therapy for spasticity and muscle spasms. Spasticity is a common symptom of upper motor neuron lesions. Muscle spasm is an involuntary contraction of a muscle or group of muscles. This condition can be alleviated with appropriate drug therapy.

Therapeutic Rationale: Spasticity

Spasticity results from the loss of inhibitory tone in the polysynaptic pathways of the spinal cord so that fine control of motor activity is lost.

Because the inhibitory tone is controlled largely by neural pathways from the brain, spasticity is seen in patients in whom these inhibitory pathways have been disrupted through spinal cord injury, strokes, multiple sclerosis, or cerebral palsy. The patient with spasticity demonstrates exaggerated reflexes (spinal spasticity) or inappropriate posture (cerebral spasticity).

Therapeutic Agents: Spasticity

Drugs for the treatment of spasticity are presented in Table 57-1. Three drugs found to be effective in relieving some cases of spasticity are diazepam (Valium), baclofen (Lioresal), and dantrolene (Dantrium). Diazepam and baclofen are believed to act within the spinal cord to restore some inhibitory tone, but dantrolene is unique in acting within the muscle.

Diazepam

Diazepam (Valium) is a benzodiazepine commonly prescribed as an antianxiety drug (see Chapter 51). Although its

TABLE 57-1 Centrally Acting Skeletal Muscle Relaxants

GENERIC NAME	TRADE NAME	ADMINISTRATION/DOSAGE	COMMENTS
✤ Baclofen	Lioresal*	ORAL: *Adults*—Begin with 5 mg 3 times daily. Increase by 5 mg 3 times daily every 3 days as required; maximum, 80 mg.	Diminishes reflex responses by decreasing transmission in spinal cord.
✤ Dantrolene	Dantrium*	ORAL: *Adults*—25 mg 1 or 2 times daily. Increase to 25 mg 3-4 times daily, then 50-100 mg 4 times daily as required. Increments are adjusted every 4-7 days.	Acts peripherally to inhibit calcium release within muscle.
Diazepam	Valium*	ORAL: *Adults*—2-10 mg 4 times daily. *Children*—0.12 to 0.8 mg/kg body weight daily in 3 or 4 doses. INTRAVENOUS: *Adults*—2-10 mg injected no faster than 5 mg (1 ml)/min. Do not mix or dilute with other solutions, drugs, or IV fluids. *Children*—0.04-0.2 mg/kg body weight; maximum, 0.6 mg/kg in 8 hr.	Benzodiazepine also used to treat spasticity or muscle spasm.
Drugs for Muscle Spasms			
Carisoprodol	Rela Soma* Various others	ORAL: *Adults*—350 mg 4 times daily.	Related to meprobamate. May cause drowsiness.
Chlorphenesin	Maolate	ORAL: *Adults*—800 mg 3 times daily. Can decrease to 400 mg 4 times daily as improvement is noted.	May cause drowsiness and dizziness.
Chlorzoxazone	Paraflex Parafon Forte DSC	ORAL: *Adults*—250-750 mg 3 or 4 times daily. *Children*—20 mg/kg body weight in 3 or 4 divided doses.	May cause drowsiness. Watch for signs of liver damage (rare).
Cyclobenzaprine	Flexeril*	ORAL: *Adults*—10 mg 3 times daily up to maximum total dose of 60 mg.	Related to tricyclic antidepressants. Does not cause drug dependence but may cause changes in liver.
Diazepam	Valium*	Same as for diazepam to treat spasticity.	
Metaxalone	Skelaxin*	ORAL: *Adults*—800 mg 3 or 4 times daily.	Monitor patient for development of liver toxicity.
Methocarbamol	Delaxin Robamol Robaxin* Various others	ORAL: *Adults*—1.5-2 gm 4 times daily for 2-3 days. Decrease to 1 gm 4 times daily for maintenance. INTRAMUSCULAR: *Adults*—500 mg every 8 hr, alternating between gluteal muscles. INTRAVENOUS: *Adults*—1-3 gm daily for maximum of 3 days. Inject no faster than 300 mg (3 ml)/min.	Not recommended for patients with epilepsy. Do not administer parenterally to patients with impaired renal function because drug vehicle may worsen kidney function.
Orphenadrine	Flexon Neocyten Norflex* Tega-Flex Various others	ORAL: *Adults*—100 mg twice daily. INTRAMUSCULAR, INTRAVENOUS: *Adults*—60 mg twice daily.	Anticholinergic effects are common side effects. Not for patients with glaucoma, myasthenia gravis, tachycardia, or urinary retention.

*Available in Canada and United States.

action as an antianxiety drug results from depression of the reticular activating system, diazepam also enhances inhibitory descending pathways in the spinal cord governing muscular activity, apparently by enhancing the activity of the inhibitory neurotransmitter gamma-aminobutyric acid (GABA). Diazepam is effective in relieving spasticity associated with spinal cord injury, multiple sclerosis, and cerebral injury and in treating muscle spasms. Relatively high doses are required to relieve muscle hyperactivity, and drowsiness and ataxia may be prominent side effects.

Baclofen

Baclofen (Lioresal) is an analogue of the inhibitory neurotransmitter GABA, and although the effect elicited is that desired of a GABA agonist, this mechanism of action cannot be demonstrated in the laboratory. Baclofen is most effective in relieving spasticity caused by spinal cord injury and is less effective in relieving spasticity from brain damage. Side effects include drowsiness, ataxia, and occasional gastrointestinal (GI) upset.

Dantrolene

Dantrolene (Dantrium) is not a centrally acting skeletal muscle relaxant but instead affects the muscle directly by interfering with the intracellular release of calcium necessary to initiate contraction. At therapeutic doses, this effect is limited to skeletal muscle and is not seen in the heart or smooth muscle. Dantrolene causes muscular weakness and can worsen the overall condition if the patient already has marginal strength. Dantrolene is most useful for the patient whose spasticity causes pain, discomfort, or limits functional rehabilitation. In addition to the spasticity caused by spinal cord injury, dantrolene relieves spasticity of stroke, cerebral palsy, or multiple sclerosis, for which the other drugs have limited effectiveness.

The major limitation to the use of dantrolene is liver damage. Baseline liver function studies are done before therapy starts, and regular liver function studies are performed throughout therapy. Dantrolene is discontinued if no relief of spasticity is achieved in 6 weeks.

Therapeutic Rationale: Muscle Spasms and Treatment

Muscle spasms are local muscle contractions initiated by muscle or tendon injury and inflammation. Muscle spasms occur in sprains, bursitis, arthritis, and lower back pain. The primary treatment includes analgesics, antiinflammatory drugs, immobilization of the affected part (if possible), and physical therapy. If relief is not achieved through these means, a centrally acting skeletal muscle relaxant may be added. Although the mechanism postulated for the centrally acting skeletal muscle relaxants is depression of the polysynaptic pathways in the spinal cord modulating muscle tone, drugs used as centrally acting skeletal muscle relaxants are related to various antianxiety drugs. Since anxiety worsens a muscle spasm, treatment of the accompanying anxiety may be the more important mechanism of action.

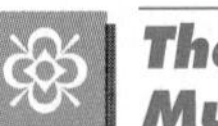

Therapeutic Agents: Muscle Spasms

Centrally acting skeletal muscle relaxants commonly prescribed to treat muscle spasms are listed in Table 57-1. They are used as part of an overall program for the relief of muscle spasms, a program that includes rest and physical therapy.

Centrally acting skeletal muscle relaxants include carisoprodol (Rela and Soma), chlorphenesin (Maolate), chlorzoxazone (Paraflex), cyclobenzaprine (Flexeril), diazepam (Valium), metaxalone (Skelaxin), methocarbamol (Robaxin and others), and orphenadrine (Norflex and others). With the exception of cyclobenzaprine, these drugs are similar to sedative-hypnotic or antianxiety drugs with respect to side effects, drug interactions, and drug dependence (see Chapter 51); thus short-term rather than long-term therapy is the rule. Cyclobenzaprine is related to the tricyclic antidepressants and does not cause drug dependence or alter sleep patterns.

Drowsiness and dizziness are common side effects of all the centrally acting skeletal muscle relaxants, and they should not be combined with alcohol or other drugs that depress the central nervous system (CNS).

Carisoprodol

Carisoprodol (Rela, Soma, others) has a rapid onset of action and the effect lasts 4 to 6 hours. It is chemically related to meprobamate and meprobamate is the principal metabolite. Carisoprodol is contraindicated for patients with acute intermittent porphyria and for nursing mothers.

Chlorphenesin

Chlorphenesin (Maolate) has an onset of action under an hour and a 3- to 4-hour duration of action. Use for more than 8 weeks is not recommended. Chlorphenesin is contraindicated during pregnancy for nursing mothers. Patients with liver impairment should be given chlorphenesin with caution. Rare but serious reactions include drug fever and blood dyscrasias.

Chlorzoxazone

Chlorzoxazone (Paraflex) has an onset of action under an hour and a 3- to 4-hour duration of action. Rarely hypersensitivity reactions occur and include agranulocytosis and angioedema. Hepatotoxicity is another rare but serious hazard.

Cyclobenzaprine

Cyclobenzaprine (Flexeril) is related to the tricyclic antidepressants (see Chapter 53). Drowsiness, dry mouth, and dizziness are the most common side effects. Cyclobenzaprine is contraindicated for patients with hyperthyroidism, arrhythmias, heart block, conduction disturbances, congestive heart failure, or recent myocardial infarction. Monoamine oxidase inhibitors should not be given concurrently.

Metaxalone

Metaxalone (Skelaxin) is active in about an hour. Rarely it is associated with hemolytic anemia or hepatotoxicity. This drug is contraindicated for patients with a history of these conditions.

Methocarbamol

Methocarbamol (Robaxin and others) is effective within 30 minutes when given orally. It is also available for intravenous (IV) or intramuscular (IM) administration. Intravenous administration is used in the treatment of tetanus. When administered intravenously, methocarbamol may cause convulsions, fainting, slow heartbeat, muscle weakness, nystagmus, and facial flushing, especially if administered rapidly. Blurred or double vision are occasional side effects of methocarbamol.

Orphenadrine

Orphenadrine (Norflex and others) is an analogue of diphenhydramine, an antihistamine, and has anticholinergic properties that include blurred vision, dry mouth and skin, and excitation. Orphenadrine is contraindicated for patients with closed-angle glaucoma or myasthenia gravis. Caution should be used for older adult patients or those with tachycardia, cardiac failure, or urinary retention.

NURSING PROCESS OVERVIEW

Centrally Acting Skeletal Muscle Relaxants

Assessment

Perform a general assessment with an additional focus on spasticity, including degree of spasticity, aggravating factors, associated pain, and degree to which spasticity interferes with the activities of daily living or the activities that could increase independence. If dantrolene is used, monitor baseline liver function studies.

Nursing Diagnoses

- Fatigue related to drug side effects (specify drug)

Patient Outcomes

The patient will discuss the causes of fatigue. The patient will establish priorities for daily activities. If appropriate to the patient's situation, the patient will incorporate exercises or other anxiety-reducing activities into the daily schedule.

Planning/Implementation

During dosage adjustment, monitor the patient for drug effectiveness and side effects. Weeks of therapy may be needed before a lessening of spasticity occurs. These drugs may be used with other therapies, including traction, physical therapy, exercises, bed rest, and application of heat.

Evaluation

Evaluate the continuing degree of spasticity. Since not all side effects are undesirable, decisions related to them should be individualized. For example, a patient who is drowsy when receiving short-term diazepam therapy may be better able to tolerate enforced bed rest because of the drowsiness. Before discharge, verify that the patient can explain what drugs to take and how to take them correctly; side effects that may occur and which of them require notification of the physician; how to perform additional therapies such as application of heat and exercises; and when to return for additional help.

NURSING IMPLICATIONS SUMMARY

Diazepam

- For information on diazepam, see Chapter 51.

Baclofen

Drug Administration

- Assess mental status, and monitor regularly.
- Monitor blood pressure every 4 hours until stable. Be alert to hypotension when assisting patients to ambulate, especially if they have been immobilized or mostly sedentary before starting drug therapy.
- Monitor intake and output and weight. Monitor respiratory rate, auscultate lung sounds, and assess for dyspnea. Inspect for skin changes and edema.
- Monitor complete blood cell count (CBC) and urinalysis.
- Tactfully question the patient regarding impotence. Provide emotional support. Remind the patient not to discontinue medications without consulting the physician.

Patient and Family Education

- Teach the patient that several days to weeks of therapy may be necessary before improvement is seen. If improvement is not seen in 6 to 8 weeks, the drug is usually withdrawn. However, teach the patient not to stop the medication without consulting with the physician. Depending on the dose and period of time the patient has been using the medication it may be necessary to withdraw the drug slowly.
- See the patient problem boxes on constipation (p. 304) and dry mouth (p. 300).
- Warn the patient to avoid driving or operating hazardous equipment if drowsiness develops.
- Caution the diabetic patient to monitor blood glucose levels carefully because an adjustment in diet or insulin may be needed.
- Warn the patient to avoid the use of alcohol unless permitted in small amounts by the physician.
- Remind the patient to inform all health care providers of all drugs being taken.
- Take dose with meals or a snack to lessen gastric irritation.

Dantrolene

Drug Administration

- Assess mental status and monitor regularly. Watch for signs of depression, including withdrawal, lack of interest in personal appearance, insomnia, anorexia, and weight loss.
- Monitor blood pressure and pulse. When drug is used for treatment of malignant hyperthermia, attach patient to cardiac monitor.
- Be alert to hypotension when assisting the patient to ambulate, especially if the patient has been immobilized or primarily sedentary before receiving drug therapy.
- Check stools for occult blood.
- Monitor intake and output. Monitor urinalysis, or check urine for blood.
- Tactfully assess men regarding difficulty in achieving erection. Provide emotional support. Caution the patient not to discontinue medications without consulting the physician.
- Auscultate lung sounds, watch for pleural effusion.
- Inspect skin for abnormal hair growth or rash.
- Monitor CBC and liver function tests.

Intravenous Dantrolene

- Dilute each 20 mg with 60 ml sterile water for injection that does not contain a bacteriostatic agent. Shake solution until clear. Administer as rapid intravenous IV push. Once reconstituted and diluted, solution must be protected from light and used within 6 hours.

Patient and Family Education

- Review the anticipated benefits and possible side effects of drug therapy. Tell the patient to notify the physician of any unexpected findings.
- See the patient problem box on constipation (p. 304).
- Reassure the patient that several days to weeks of therapy may be necessary before improvement is seen. If improvement is not seen in 6 to 8 weeks, drug is usually withdrawn.
- Warn the patient to avoid driving or operating hazardous equipment if dizziness or drowsiness develops.
- Warn the patient to avoid the use of alcohol unless permitted in small amounts by the physician.
- Remind the patient to inform all health care providers of all medications being taken.
- Instruct the patients who develop malignant hyperthermia to wear a medical identification tag or bracelet.

Drugs for Muscle Spasms

Drug Administration

- Assess for CNS side effects including dizziness, ataxia, and vertigo.
- Warn the patient that IM injections may cause a burning sensation at the injection site.
- Consult the manufacturer's literature for information about IV administration.
- For IV administration, keep the patient supine. Keep siderails up. Monitor vital signs. Keep the patient recumbent until blood pressure is stable. Supervise ambulation.
- Monitor CBC and differential and liver function tests.
- These drugs may cause allergic reactions. Check the patient frequently when beginning therapy. Have drugs and equipment available to treat acute allergic reactions in settings where these drugs are administered.

Continued.

NURSING IMPLICATIONS SUMMARY—cont'd

Patient and Family Education

- Review the anticipated benefits and possible side effects of drug therapy.
- If necessary, chlorzoxazone, metaxalone, or methocarbamol tablets may be crushed and mixed with a little food or liquid to make them easier to swallow.
- Warn the patient to avoid driving or operating hazardous equipment if drowsiness, dizziness, or visual changes develop.
- See the patient problem boxes on orthostatic hypotension (p. 157), dry mouth (p. 300), and constipation (p. 304).
- Remind the patient to use medications only as directed and to inform all health care providers of all medications being taken.
- Warn the patient to avoid alcohol unless permitted in small amounts by the physician.
- Instruct the patient to take oral doses with meals or snack to lessen gastric irritation.
- Teach the patient to take the final dose of the day at bedtime.
- Warn the patient taking chlorzoxazone that urine may turn orange or purple-red while the drug is taken.
- Warn the patient taking methocarbamol that urine may turn black, brown, or green while the drug is taken.
- Warn the diabetic patient taking metaxalone to monitor blood sugar level carefully. This drug may cause inaccurate results with urine sugar tests.

CRITICAL THINKING

APPLICATION

1. Define spasticity.
2. How do diazepam, baclofen, and dantrolene reduce spasticity?
3. Describe the origin of muscle spasms.
4. What are the characteristics of the drugs used as centrally acting agents to treat muscle spasms?

CRITICAL THINKING

1. Develop a care plan for the spastic patient beginning therapy with baclofen.
2. Develop a care plan for the spastic patient beginning therapy with dantrolene.

SECTION XIV

Drugs Affecting the Endocrine and Reproductive Systems

This section presents the pharmacology of drugs affecting the endocrine system. Chapter 58, *Introduction to Endocrinology,* defines the terms that must be mastered before the material in the subsequent chapters can be understood. This chapter also describes the concepts involved in treating endocrine diseases or in using hormones in therapy for other diseases. Knowledge of this material promotes understanding of many of the nursing assessments and actions described in later chapters.

Chapters 59 through 66 cover specific endocrine systems. In these chapters the pertinent physiology of the endocrine system is reviewed first. When appropriate, specific endocrine diseases are described so that discussion of the therapy for these diseases has a rational basis. Three classes of agents are described: natural hormones, synthetic forms of hormones, and nonhormonal drugs affecting the endocrine system. The purpose of therapy with each of these agents is clearly defined. Diagnostic tests are also described so that the student may understand the information that must be considered during patient assessment.

Some agents discussed in this section have significant medical uses outside of endocrinology. For example, synthetic adrenal steroids (Chapter 60) are widely used as antiinflammatory agents. These drugs are discussed in Chapter 36.

CHAPTER 58

Introduction to Endocrinology

OBJECTIVES

After studying this chapter, you should be able to do the following:

- *Define a hormone.*
- *Name the three uses of hormones in clinical medicine.*
- *Discuss how hormone action is regulated.*
- *Discuss the role of the nurse in hormone therapy.*

KEY TERMS

endocrine glands
hormones
prohormones
receptors
target tissues

CHAPTER OVERVIEW

This introduction to endocrinology defines important terms, introduces the classes of hormones, and illustrates the concept of hormonal regulation of body processes. Properties of individual hormones are detailed in subsequent chapters, along with the specific function of each gland and the effects of related drugs.

Therapeutic Rationale: Endocrine Diseases

Definition of the Endocrine System

A **hormone** is a substance that is synthesized by a specific cell type, is released into the circulation, and acts on target tissues elsewhere in the body to produce a physiologic or biochemical response. An example is thyrotropin, or thyroid-stimulating hormone (TSH), which is synthesized in the anterior pituitary, released into systemic circulation, and taken up by the thyroid gland, there stimulating production of thyroid hormones (Chapter 61).

Organs producing hormones that enter systemic circulation are the **endocrine glands**—pancreas, adrenal glands, thyroid, parathyroid glands, testes, ovaries, and pituitary gland. Those tissues affected by hormones from endocrine glands are designated **target tissues.** For example, TSH from the anterior pituitary has the thyroid gland as a target tissue. Other tissues do not respond to TSH.

Some compounds that have been called hormones act strictly locally, producing their effect at or near the site where they are synthesized. Examples of such compounds include prostaglandins, which are formed from membrane fatty acids at the sites of prostaglandin action. Prostaglandins are considered for their action on the uterus in Chapter 65. These locally acting substances are not discussed further in this chapter.

Types and Sources of Hormones

Hormones are of two types, based on their chemical composition. One type, the steroid hormones derived from cholesterol, includes hormones of the adrenal gland (cortisol, cortisone, aldosterone, corticosterone, and others) and hormones of the sex glands (androgens, estrogens, and progestins).

Many steroid hormones have been synthesized by organic chemists, so their production for medicinal purposes does not depend entirely on isolating them from such natural sources as bovine or porcine adrenal glands obtained from meat-packing plants. Some clinically useful steroids are obtained from natural sources, however, because the steroids are present in such high concentrations and are so easily extracted, making the procedure economically feasible. An example of such a preparation is Premarin, a mixture of conjugated estrogens extracted from the urine of pregnant mares.

The second type of hormone is formed from amino acids. This type may include amino acid derivatives and proteins. Examples of amino acid derivatives are thyroxine and triiodothyronine, formed in the thyroid by iodinating tyrosine. Other examples are catecholamines, produced from tyrosine in various tissues.

Peptides and proteins are different in size, with peptides containing fewer amino acids than proteins. Peptides and proteins are similar chemically in that both are formed by peptide bonds linking carboxyl and amino groups of adjacent amino acids. Examples of peptide hormones are releasing factors produced in the hypothalamus (e.g., thyrotropin-releasing hormone, composed of three amino acids) and the posterior pituitary hormones oxytocin and vasopressin (antidiuretic hormone [ADH]), which are each composed of eight amino acids. Protein hormones are larger. For example, insulin has 51 amino acids and a molecular weight of 6000; follicle-stimulating hormone (FSH) has a molecular weight of 41,000.

The active forms of many protein hormones are derived from larger protein molecules called **prohormones.** For example, insulin is originally released as part of a prohormone containing at least 86 amino acids. Cleavage of 35 amino acids from this larger precursor molecule releases active insulin.

The peptide and protein hormones are usually present in very small quantities in natural sources and may be difficult to isolate. For example, insulin, the protein hormone most often used medically, can be prepared in large quantities from bovine or porcine pancreas glands, but the process requires tedious and expensive extraction procedures. Growth hormone, a protein used to treat a rare endocrine disease, may be extracted from pituitary glands, but the only form that is active in humans is human or primate growth hormone. The supply of this hormone therefore was restricted by the limited source material. In the past, growth hormone was obtained postmortem from human pituitaries, but the risk of viral contamination has caused this product to be dropped.

A powerful new method for producing human protein hormones is based on genetic engineering. Genetic engineering involves taking genes from one species and placing them into an unrelated species, thereby creating new characteristics in the recipient. The human genes for insulin, growth hormone, interferons, and other proteins have been inserted into host bacteria. These altered bacteria then may be grown on a large scale in fermentation tanks to produce large quantities of the human protein. Human insulin produced in this way is now a standard clinical agent.

Genetic engineering is applicable to a variety of proteins and solves the problem of limited supply of clinically useful proteins. In addition, hormones produced by this technique are less likely to be contaminated with viruses. For this reason, human growth hormone produced by genetically engineered bacteria is now the standard preparation for human use.

Synthesis, Release, and Clearance of Hormones

Hormones are potent agents capable of exerting profound effects on metabolism. To remain healthy the body must ensure that hormones act only where and when they are needed and that they be present at the proper concentrations. The time of appearance and the concentration of a hormone in blood may be regulated by controlling its rate of synthesis, release from storage sites, degradation, and clearance from the body. Several hormones are stored after synthesis and are released from storage sites only when the proper stimulus is received. For example, thyroxine and triiodothyronine are stored complexed with thyroglobulin in the thyroid gland. Insulin is stored in granules within beta-cells of the pancreas. In these cases when the endocrine gland is stimulated to release hormone, the stored hormone is first released. Then if required, newly synthesized hormone is released into the blood.

Regulation of synthesis and release of many hormones involves interactions between the central nervous system (CNS) and the endocrine glands. For example, the hypothalamus in the brain controls the pituitary gland, which in turn regulates production of hormones by ovaries, testes, thyroid, and adrenal glands. This system is the negative feedback regulation discussed in Chapter 59.

Hormones disappear from the blood when they are taken up by various organs or when they are degraded by enzymes in blood. The kidneys degrade or excrete several hormones, including most steroids. The kidneys and the liver degrade insulin. Vasopressin, in contrast, is very rapidly destroyed by enzymes in blood. The half-life of vasopressin (i.e., the time required for half of the injected dose to disappear from the blood) is approximately 15 minutes. Other hormones persist for much longer periods. For example, thyroxine has a plasma half-life of about 7 days.

Localizing Hormone Effects

Distribution Limited to Portal Circulation

Controlling the location of action of a certain hormone is accomplished in one of two ways. The first localization mechanism is to restrict distribution of the hormone. Examples are the releasing factors synthesized in the hypothalamus and released into local portal veins carrying the hormones directly to the anterior pituitary and not into general circulation.

Hormone Receptors

A second mechanism localizes the effect of widely released hormones. These hormones interact with specific **receptors** found only in their target tissues. The specific receptor is required for hormone activity. For example, TSH receptors are found in the thyroid gland but not in most other organs. Therefore even though TSH is released into general circulation, it acts only on the thyroid.

Intracellular receptors. The receptors for hormones may be within cells. For example, steroids and thyroid hormones affect target cells by interacting with intracellular receptors (Figure 58-1). Steroid hormones are bound by specific receptors that transport the hormones through the cytoplasm of the cell and into the nucleus, where the final effect of the hormone is produced. Thyroid hormones likewise move to the nucleus where they bind to specific receptors and ultimately alter protein synthesis in cells.

Cell surface receptors. In contrast to the receptors for steroids and thyroid hormones, receptors for peptide and protein hormones exist on the external surface of cell membranes (Figure 58-1). The peptide and protein hormones therefore need not enter cells to become effective. One mechanism by which these externally bound hormones act is by releasing an internal regulator, or second messenger. Second messengers include cyclic adenosine monophos-

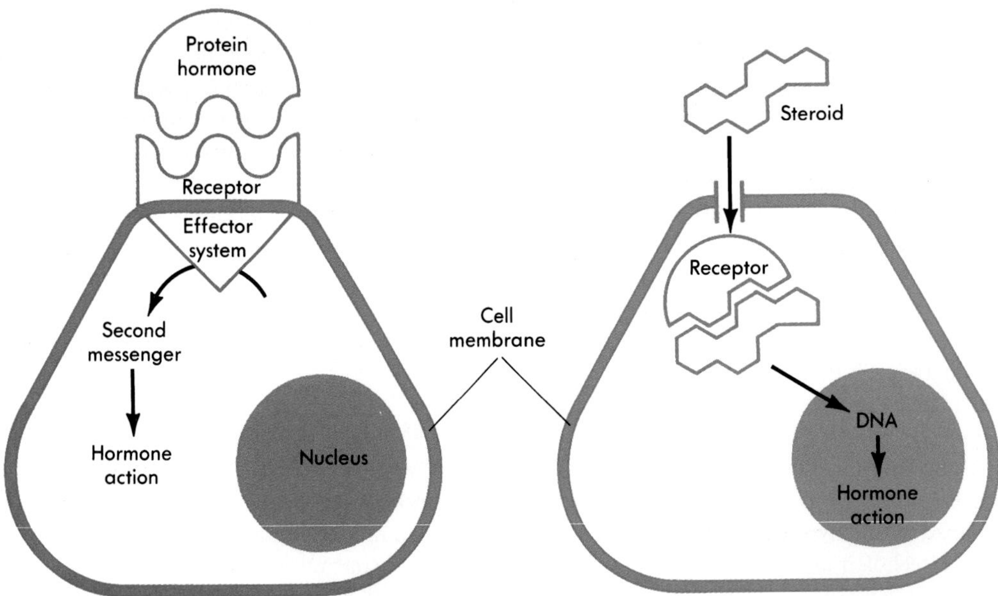

FIGURE 58-1
Sites for hormone receptors. Cell on left illustrates common mechanism for responding to protein hormones, with external receptor interacting through effector system. Cell on right illustrates mechanism shared by steroid hormones and thyroid hormones in which hormone enters cytoplasm, is bound by a receptor, and is carried to nucleus, where effect is produced.

phate (cyclic AMP), calcium ion, and inositol 1,4,5-trisphosphate (IP3).

One of the best understood second messenger systems is that involving cyclic AMP. Many hormones bind receptors that are associated with an enzyme called *adenylate cyclase.* When the hormone binds to the receptor, adenylate cyclase is stimulated to release cyclic AMP within the cell. Cyclic AMP then alters the internal processes of the cell. Hormones that act through this system include parathyroid hormone and ADH. This second messenger system is also used by beta-adrenergic receptors.

Other second messenger systems are also important for endocrine function. For example, the multiple metabolic changes produced by insulin within target cells arise from the action of the enzyme tyrosine kinase and do not depend on cyclic AMP.

Modulating Hormone Responses

The response of a target cell to a hormone depends on how many hormone receptors are available. Regulating the number of receptors is therefore another mechanism by which the body can maintain metabolic balance. An example of this type of regulation is found in obese persons with a high food intake. These persons have chronically high insulin concentrations in the bloodstream. To protect itself from the metabolic effects of this high amount of insulin, the body eliminates a certain percentage of the insulin receptors on cells. The loss of insulin receptors, called down-regulation, lowers the responsiveness of the cell to insulin.

Defining Endocrine Diseases

Understanding the role of receptors in fulfilling the metabolic role of hormones allows a clearer understanding of endocrine diseases and how they are classified. An endocrine deficiency can arise from a lack of hormone or from a lack of receptors that enables the tissue to respond to the hormone. An example is diabetes insipidus, which may be produced by a lack of ADH or by a lack of receptors in the kidney that can respond to ADH. Similarly, diabetes mellitus can be characterized by the lack of insulin in the blood or by high levels of insulin in blood but lower-than-normal numbers of active insulin receptors on cells.

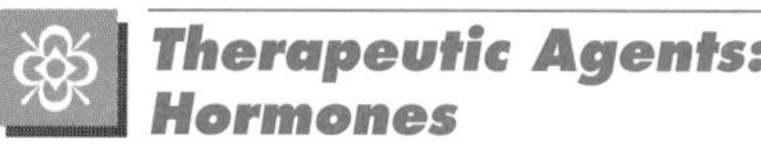

Therapeutic Agents: Hormones

Hormones are used clinically in one of three ways—as diagnostic agents, in replacement therapy, or as pharmacologic agents.

The most common diagnostic use of hormones is to assess the function of target organs of the administered hormone. For example, adrenocorticotropic hormone (ACTH) may be given to test the ability of the adrenal glands to produce steroids. Similarly, thyrotropin is used to test the capacity of the thyroid gland to synthesize thyroid hormones.

Replacement therapy is aimed at restoring normal levels of hormones, which, for some reason, a patient's body no longer produces. Physiologic doses are used in an attempt to maintain normal hormone levels without producing toxic effects from hormone excesses. The use of thyroxine to treat hypothyroidism and cortisol to treat Addison's disease (chronic adrenal insufficiency) are examples of replacement therapy. Insulin use in diabetic patients is also an example of replacement therapy.

The use of hormones as pharmacologic agents, with administered doses far in excess of those required to produce physiologic levels, makes use of some function of the compound other than the one seen at physiologic concentrations. For example, adrenal corticosteroids may be given in large doses to suppress inflammatory responses in certain diseases. This antiinflammatory effect is not obvious at physiologic concentrations of the steroid.

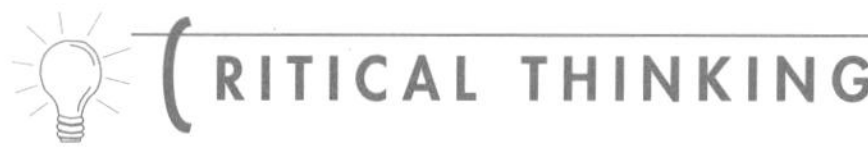

CRITICAL THINKING

APPLICATION

1. What is a hormone?
2. What is a target tissue?
3. Describe the two major chemical types of hormones.
4. What is a prohormone?
5. Name three ways in which large amounts of hormones may be obtained for clinical use.
6. What are the three primary clinical uses of hormones?
7. Describe how the amount of hormone in the body may be regulated.
8. How may the site of action of a hormone be restricted?
9. In what ways may the actions of hormones be terminated?
10. What is a releasing factor?
11. Describe the two general types of endocrine deficiency diseases.

CRITICAL THINKING

1. What are the two main types of hormone receptors? How do these receptors differ in the way they interact with hormones?

CHAPTER 59

Therapeutic Uses of Pituitary Gland Hormones

OBJECTIVES

After studying this chapter, you should be able to do the following:

- *Identify the two parts of the pituitary gland.*
- *Describe the function of the two hormones of the neurohypophysis.*
- *Describe the use of antidiuretic hormone.*
- *Identify the source and use of growth hormones.*
- *Develop a nursing care plan for the patient receiving drug therapy for diabetes insipidus, for growth hormone deficiency, or to suppress excessive release of growth hormone.*

KEY TERMS

adenohypophysis
antidiuretic hormone (ADH)
diabetes insipidus
growth hormone
nephrogenic diabetes insipidus
neurohypophysis
oxytocin
somatomedins
syndrome of inappropriate ADH (SIADH)

CHAPTER OVERVIEW

The pituitary gland, or hypophysis, lies in the sella turcica, a bony cavity at the base of the brain. Although the gland weighs less than 1 gm, it is the primary regulator of the endocrine system, controls normal growth, and regulates water balance.

The pituitary gland is divided into two portions with very different tissue compositions and embryologic origins. These two regions are the anterior pituitary, or adenohypophysis, and the posterior pituitary, or neurohypophysis. The structure and function of each of these tissues, the function and regulation of the various hormones produced, and the pathologic states resulting from abnormalities in hormone production are considered in this chapter.

Therapeutic Rationale: Neurohypophysis

The *posterior pituitary,* or **neurohypophysis,** is composed of nerve fibers embryologically derived from the hypothalamus. Close contact between the central nervous system (CNS) and the neurohypophysis is maintained by the nerve fibers that run from the hypothalamus through the hypophyseal stalk to the neurohypophysis (Figure 59-1). Two octapeptide hormones closely related in structure are released by the neurohypophysis. These are antidiuretic hormone and oxytocin. These peptide hormones are synthesized in the hypothalamus and transported in secretion granules down the axons running between the hypothalamus and the neurohypophysis. The granules accumulate at the nerve fiber terminals and are stored in the neurohypophysis, where their release into systemic circulation is regulated by nerve impulses from the hypothalamus. Damage to the hypophyseal stalk impairs transport of secretory granules to the neurohypophysis and interferes with appropriate release of the hormones.

Neurohypophyseal Hormones

Oxytocin

Oxytocin is an octapeptide hormone released by the neurohypophysis. The major target organs of oxytocin are breast myoepithelium and smooth muscle of the uterus, especially during the second and third stages of labor. The effects of oxytocin on these tissues are discussed in Chapter 65. Oxytocin also causes milk ejection by stimulating contraction of the myoepithelium of the breast.

The regulation of oxytocin release is a particularly good example of the close interaction of the CNS with pituitary function. Suckling by the infant induces afferent nerve impulses from the breast to the brain, which causes more oxytocin to be synthesized and stored hormone to be released. A similar reflex loop may operate in parturition when dilation of the cervix is thought to stimulate synthesis and release of oxytocin.

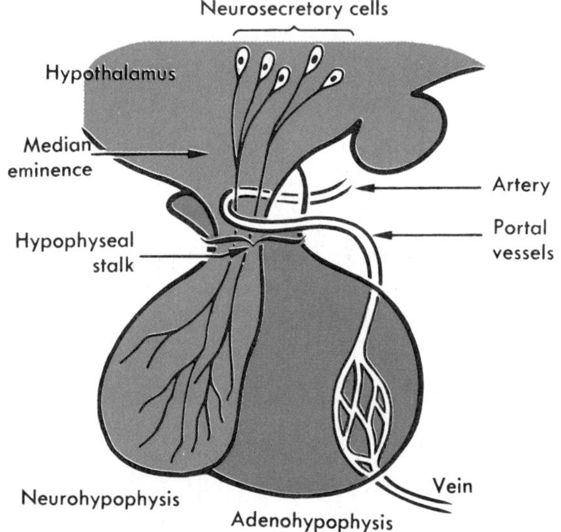

FIGURE 59-1
Anatomy of pituitary gland.

No specific syndrome resulting from abnormalities in oxytocin function has been described.

Antidiuretic hormone

Physiologic Action

Antidiuretic hormone (ADH), also called *vasopressin,* has as its primary target tissue the renal tubular epithelium. ADH increases permeability of certain sections of the renal tubules to water, allowing water to be reabsorbed from tubules and returned to the blood. This is the mechanism by which healthy kidneys concentrate urine. Other target tissues include smooth muscle of blood vessels and of the gastrointestinal (GI) tract. ADH actions on these tissues cause vasoconstriction and increased GI motility, respectively.

Regulation of Secretion

Secretion of ADH is regulated mainly in response to plasma osmolarity, the concentration of solute molecules that increase osmotic pressure (see Chapter 17). In dehydration the effective osmotic pressure of blood increases. Osmoreceptors in the hypothalamus respond to this change by stimulating the neurohypophysis to secrete ADH. ADH in turn causes the kidney to conserve body water and to prevent or slow further dehydration. Recovery from dehydration is aided further by concomitant stimulation of the thirst center, leading to increased intake of fluids. Reduction in the effective plasma volume caused by hemorrhage or reduced cardiac output stimulates ADH release and promotes antidiuresis.

In addition to these physiologic controls, certain drugs also may influence ADH secretion. Acetylcholine, barbiturates, nicotine, morphine, and bradykinin cause release of ADH in healthy subjects. Ethanol or phenytoin may promote diuresis by inhibiting ADH release.

Effects of Antidiuretic Hormone Deficiency

ADH is markedly reduced or absent when the hypothalamic region responsible for its synthesis is destroyed or when the hypophyseal stalk above the median eminence is separated (see Figure 59-1). In these cases, urinary concentration is impossible, and large volumes of dilute, sugar-free urine are produced. This condition is called **diabetes insipidus** and is not to be confused with the disease *diabetes mellitus,* which arises from the inability to use blood glucose or to release insulin.

Diabetes insipidus is not life-threatening unless severe electrolyte imbalances develop. If the patient has a functional thirst center and can balance excessive fluid losses with high fluid intakes, severe imbalances usually do not occur. When a person is unconscious and unable to take in adequate fluids, however, severe dehydration may set in before the condition is noticed. Thus, following head injuries or surgery to the hypothalamic region of the brain, it is vital that health care personnel monitor urinary specific gravity and blood sodium levels, along with fluid intake and urinary volumes, to detect excessive diuresis and resultant dehydration.

In many patients with trauma to the hypothalamus or the

hypophyseal stalk the resultant diabetes insipidus may be transitory. In patients whose condition is chronic, reversal of symptoms can be achieved by replacement therapy with a form of ADH or by therapy with pharmacologic agents that relieve the symptoms of the disease.

Therapeutic Agents: Treatment of Diabetes Insipidus

Central Diabetes Insipidus

Antidiuretic hormone

Mechanism of Action

Central diabetes insipidus is caused by a deficiency in ADH, and therefore can be treated by replacement therapy with ADH. The administered ADH has the same effect as the natural hormone.

Pharmacokinetics

Because ADH is a peptide hormone, it cannot be administered orally, and all replacement therapy with ADH involves the administration of the hormone parenterally or intranasally (Table 59-1).

Vasopressin (Pitressin), an aqueous preparation of purified ADH, is not routinely used because the half-life of ADH in the blood is short. This preparation is injected intramuscularly or subcutaneously two or three times daily for short-term management of patients. Lypressin, a synthetic form of ADH that is sprayed onto the mucous membranes of the nasal passages, is usually administered four times daily.

Desmopressin acetate (DDAVP) administered intranasally is the drug of choice in replacement therapy for chronic diabetes insipidus. DDAVP is a chemically altered form of vasopressin, differing from the natural hormone by having a long serum half-life, a more potent antidiuretic effect, and less pressor activity. It is administered only once or twice daily, unlike other ADH preparations.

Uses

The primary use for ADH is as replacement therapy for diabetes insipidus. ADH has been used as a pressor agent but now is not recommended for that use. Occasionally, the vasoconstrictor action of ADH is used to help control massive GI tract bleeding, especially from esophageal varices.

Adverse Reactions and Contraindications

ADH can promote activity of smooth muscle in the intestinal tract. During routine therapy of diabetes insipidus the action of ADH on intestinal smooth muscle may result in nausea, belching, and cramps.

ADH is a vasoconstrictor, which tends to raise blood pressure. This vasoconstrictor action prevents safe use for patients with vascular or coronary artery disease. Even small doses may cause difficulty to a patient prone to angina attacks. Side effects caused by the pressor action of vasopressin are less problematic with desmopressin than with other forms of vasopressin.

Toxicity

Overdose with ADH may produce water intoxication (see Chapter 17).

Interactions

Demeclocycline or lithium may interfere with the effects of ADH on the kidneys, with the result that diuresis continues.

Other Drugs to Treat Diabetes Insipidus

Agents other than ADH preparations have been used to treat diabetes insipidus. Paradoxically, thiazide diuretics (see Chapter 14) are effective in some cases, especially when combined with another oral agent listed in this section. The effectiveness of thiazide diuretics is based on their blockade of electrolyte reabsorption, resulting initially in increased sodium and water excretion. The kidney responds to this change by reabsorbing more water by mechanisms that do not depend on ADH. Moderate salt restriction may enhance the action of these drugs. Doses of thiazides used to treat diabetes insipidus are the same as those used for other indications. The most common side effect is potassium depletion, which in extreme cases may induce cardiac arrhythmias and impair neuromuscular, GI tract, or renal function.

TABLE 59-1 Drugs to Treat Diabetes Insipidus

GENERIC NAME	TRADE NAME	ADMINISTRATION/DOSAGE	COMMENTS
Desmopressin	DDAVP* Stimate	INTRANASAL: *Adults*—10 μg at bedtime initially; up to 40 μg for maintenance. FDA pregnancy category B. *Children 3 mo-12 yr*—5 μg initially at bedtime; up to 4 μg/kg for maintenance. INTRAVENOUS, SUBCUTANEOUS: *Adults*—1-2 μg twice daily.	Synthetic derivative of vasopressin used as replacement therapy.
Lypressin	Diapid	INTRANASAL: *Adults*—1-2 sprays in each nostril 4 times daily. FDA pregnancy category C.	Synthetic derivative of vasopressin used as replacement therapy.
Vasopressin	Pitressin*	INTRAMUSCULAR, INTRAVENOUS, SUBCUTANEOUS, INTRAARTERIAL: *Adults*—5-10 U 2-3 times daily as needed. May be given IV or intraarterially by means of infusion pump. FDA pregnancy category C. *Children*—2.5-10 U 3-4 times daily.	Synthetic vasopressin used as replacement therapy or diagnostic aid.

*Available in Canada and United States.

Chlorpropamide, a sulfonylurea used as an oral hypoglycemic agent to treat diabetes mellitus (see Chapter 63), is also used at comparable doses for diabetes insipidus. When chlorpropamide is used to treat diabetes insipidus, the action sought is a direct sensitization of the kidney to vasopressin so that lower-than-normal levels of vasopressin cause nearly normal water reabsorption. Chlorpropamide is not effective in patients who produce no vasopressin. The drug may also stimulate the pituitary to release vasopressin. Alone or with a thiazide diuretic, chlorpropamide usually reduces urine volumes. The major potential toxicity is hypoglycemia.

Clofibrate, an oral agent used to reduce serum triglyceride levels (see Chapter 21), may also be effective in treating diabetes insipidus, either alone or combined with a thiazide diuretic. It may produce nausea or rarely muscle cramps and weakness. Clofibrate increases release of ADH from the posterior pituitary.

Nephrogenic Diabetes Insipidus

The form of diabetes insipidus covered in the previous paragraphs is called central diabetes insipidus because it arises from a lack of secretion of ADH from the neurohypophysis. The symptoms of diabetes insipidus may also arise if the neurohypophysis is producing normal amounts of ADH, but the kidney is unresponsive or responds poorly to ADH. This syndrome, called **nephrogenic diabetes insipidus,** may be treated with thiazide diuretics but is resistant to therapy with ADH. Although nephrogenic diabetes insipidus may arise as a genetic disease, it also may be induced by drugs that impair the ability of the kidney to react to ADH. Drugs such as lithium used in treating mental disease (see Chapter 53) and demeclocycline, a tetracycline antibiotic (see Chapter 42), can induce nephrogenic diabetes insipidus by this mechanism.

Syndrome of Inappropriate Antidiuretic Hormone (SIADH)

The **syndrome of inappropriate ADH (SIADH)** secretion is a rare condition in which patients show symptoms of water intoxication including hyponatremia, or low sodium levels in the blood (see Chapter 17), and low serum osmolality. Despite these conditions, the kidneys continue to excrete sodium. The symptoms of SIADH are caused by release of more ADH than is appropriate, based on normal osmotic regulatory signals. In most patients with SIADH, the excess ADH is released by a tumor such as a bronchogenic carcinoma. Other less common causes of SIADH are CNS disorders, including head injuries or infections, extreme physical stress such as surgery, or extreme emotional stress. A variety of drugs occasionally may trigger SIADH, including carbamazepine, chlorpropamide, clofibrate, narcotics, cyclophosphamide, nicotine, thiazide diuretics, and vincristine.

Treatment of SIADH usually is aimed directly at removing the cause of the condition such as removing the tumor or discontinuing the drug thought to precipitate the disorder. Fluid restriction, infusion of hypotonic saline, and use of diuretics all may help control the fluid and electrolyte imbalances associated with SIADH. If the cause of excessive ADH cannot be completely removed, symptoms may be relieved by administering demeclocycline, which renders the kidneys less sensitive to ADH.

Therapeutic Rationale: Adenohypophysis

The anterior pituitary, or **adenohypophysis,** is regarded as the master gland of the entire endocrine system. The adenohypophysis secretes several peptide hormones, most of which directly stimulate secretion by the adrenal glands, the thyroid gland, and the reproductive organs (Table 59-2).

Although the adenohypophysis is true secretory tissue that synthesizes and releases its hormones, control of those secretions lies in the brain. Small polypeptides, called *neurohormones,* are synthesized in the median eminence of the hypothalamus and are released into the portal venous system (see Figure 59-1) that carries them directly to the adenohypophysis. In the adenohypophysis, these neurohormones act on the specific target cell to stimulate or to inhibit synthesis and release of the proper hormone.

Damage to the hypophysis may cause it to produce insufficient quantities of hypophyseal hormones, a condition called *panhypopituitarism.* Adults suffering from this syndrome may require replacement therapy with thyroid hormones, adrenal steroids, and appropriate sex steroids. Children with panhypopituitarism may also suffer growth stunting because of a lack of growth hormone.

Regulation of Growth

Growth hormone

Physiologic Action

Growth hormone regulates the length of the long bones of the skeleton, which determines adult stature. In addition, the hormone is a potent anabolic agent that causes many tissues to increase cell size and numbers. This anabolic action results from changes produced in protein, carbohydrate, and fat metabolism. The hormone increases amino acid transport into cells and elevates cellular protein synthesis. Growth hormone also antagonizes the action of insulin, which tends to decrease glucose uptake and carbohydrate use, thus elevating liver glycogen and blood glucose levels. Finally, growth hormone increases the mobilization of fats for energy, which leads to a rise in blood levels of free fatty acids.

Many actions of growth hormone are mediated by peptides called **somatomedins.** Growth hormone stimulates production of somatomedins by liver. The somatomedins then act on various body tissues to change metabolism. Somatomedins also have been called *insulin-like growth factors;* in addition to stimulating skeletal growth, these peptides may have insulin-like actions on other tissues.

Regulation of Secretion

The secretion of growth hormone is regulated by two factors from the hypothalamus, one stimulating and one inhibiting release. The releasing factor is a protein containing about 40

TABLE 59-2 Physiologic Action of Adenohypophyseal Hormones

DESCRIPTIVE NAME	OTHER NAMES	HYPOTHALAMIC-RELEASING FACTOR	TARGET TISSUE	TARGET TISSUE RESPONSE
Adrenocorticotropic hormone	ACTH Corticotropin	Corticotropin-releasing factor (CRF)	Adrenal cortex Pigment cells of skin	Increased steroid synthesis Increased pigmentation
Follicle-stimulating hormone	FSH	Gonadotropin-releasing hormone (GnRH); FSH-releasing hormone (FRH and FSH-RH)	Ovary Seminiferous tubules	Increased estrogen production Maturation
Growth hormone	GH Somatotropin Somatropin STH	Somatotropin or growth hormone–releasing factor (SRF or GRF); somatostatin or somatotropin-releasing inhibitory factor (SRIF)	Whole body	Increased anabolism, cell size, and cell numbers
Luteinizing hormone or interstitial cell–stimulating hormone	ICSH LH	Gonadotropin-releasing hormone (GnRH); luteinizing hormone–releasing factor or hormone (LRF, LRH, LHRF, and LH-RH)	Ovary Leydig's cells	Ovulation; formation of corpus luteum Increased androgen synthesis
Prolactin	LTH Luteotropic hormone	Prolactin-inhibiting factor (PIF); prolactin-releasing factor (PRF)	Breast	Milk formation
Thyroid-stimulating hormone	Thyrotropin TSH	Thyrotropin-releasing hormone or factor (TRH and TRF)	Thyroid gland	Increased triiodothyronine (T_3) and thyroxine (T_4) synthesis

amino acids. The inhibitory factor is a smaller, 14-amino-acid peptide called *somatostatin*. In addition to regulating growth hormone release, somatostatin may also influence thyroid-stimulating hormone (TSH) and adrenocorticotropic hormone (ACTH) release from the pituitary. Somatostatin is found in other tissues such as gut and pancreas and may have other functions in those tissues.

Effects of Growth Hormone Deficiency

Deficiency of growth hormone in childhood results in stunted growth, with adult height being well below average. Treatment of this rare condition is by replacement therapy with growth hormone.

Effects of Excessive Growth Hormone

Acromegaly and gigantism are produced by excessive growth hormone, but the age of onset causes marked differences in the manifestations of the disease. Excessive growth hormone from an early age produces the rare condition of gigantism. Growth rates of 3½ inches per year have been reported. One patient grew to be 8 feet 11 inches tall.

Acromegaly results if the onset of excessive growth hormone production is delayed until after puberty (i.e., after the plates of the long bones have joined and normal skeletal growth has halted). In this condition, only those tissues still able to grow and expand respond to growth hormone, resulting in malproportions. Typically, finger bones flare at the end, and the fingers thicken to produce a spatula-like appearance. Bones and cartilage of the face also grow and thicken, producing coarse features and a massive lower jaw.

Gigantism and acromegaly are both caused by pituitary neoplasms, which secrete excessive amounts of growth hormone. Consequently, therapy is designed to destroy or to remove the tumor. Successful treatment arrests progressive symptoms of the disease but does not erase existing deformations. When removal or destruction of the tumor is not possible or is only partially successful, the drug bromocriptine may inhibit release of growth hormone from the hypophysis. Octreotide, an analogue of somatostatin, can also help suppress excessive release of growth hormone (Table 59-3).

Regulation of Sexual Development and Function

Gonadotropic hormones

Physiologic Action

The gonadotropic hormones of the adenohypophysis are follicle-stimulating hormone (FSH), luteinizing hormone (LH), and prolactin. FSH and LH regulate maturation and function of male and female sexual organs. In women, prolactin stimulates milk formation in the estrogen- and progestin-primed breast.

In the maturing male, FSH causes the seminiferous tubules to mature. LH, which is sometimes called *interstitial cell–stimulating hormone,* increases the number of testicular interstitial cells and stimulates their secretion of androgens. These androgens are the steroid hormones that complete the maturation process, leading to the production of viable sperm and to the development of secondary male sexual characteristics.

In the maturing female, FSH and LH are produced in greater quantities at puberty and stimulate ovarian estrogen production. Estrogens, the female steroid hormones, cause the female secondary sex characteristics to develop.

Regulation of Gonadotropin Secretion in Adult Females

In addition to their role in development, FSH and LH control the menstrual cycle in mature females (Figure 59-2). Regulation of this function involves hypothalamus, adenohypoph-

TABLE 59-3 Growth Hormone and Related Drugs

GENERIC NAME	TRADE NAME	ADMINISTRATION/DOSAGE	COMMENTS
Bromocriptine	Parlodel*	ORAL: *Adults*—For acromegaly: 5-30 mg daily in divided doses. FDA pregnancy category B.	This derivative of ergot alkaloids suppresses growth hormone levels.
Octreotide	Sandostatin*	SUBCUTANEOUS: *Adults*—For acromegaly: 0.1 mg 3 times daily. FDA pregnancy category B. *Children*—0.001 to 0.01 mg/kg daily.	This analog of somatostatin suppresses intestinal peptide hormones, insulin, glucagon, and growth hormone.
Sermorelin	Geref	INTRAVENOUS: *Adults*—For diagnosis of pituitary function: 1 mg/kg.	Form of growth hormone–releasing hormone; stimulates release of growth hormone from intact pituitaries.
Somatrem	Protropin*	INTRAMUSCULAR, SUBCUTANEOUS: *Children*—For growth failure: 0.025-0.05 mg/kg every other day.	This recombinant protein differs from natural human growth hormone by one amino acid; used as replacement therapy.
Somatropin	Humatrope* Nutropin	INTRAMUSCULAR, SUBCUTANEOUS: *Children*—For growth failure: 0.025-0.05 mg/kg every other day.	This recombinant protein is identical to natural human growth hormone; used as replacement therapy.

*Available in Canada and United States.

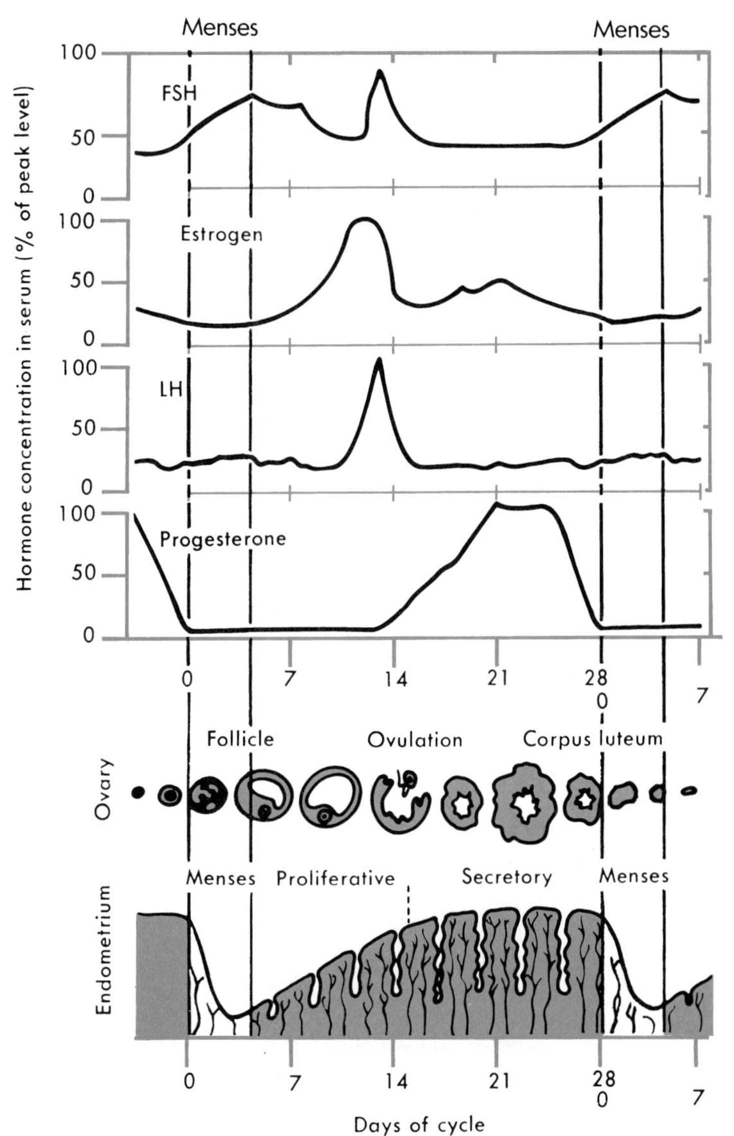

FIGURE 59-2
Pituitary regulation of menstrual cycle. Changes in circulating hormone levels are correlated with ovarian follicle and endometrial alterations.

ysis, ovaries, and endometrium (uterine lining). The first event in the cycle is a rise in the concentration of FSH in blood. In response, one of the hundreds of primordial ovarian follicles begins to develop. As the follicle matures under the influence of FSH, it begins to produce increasing amounts of estrogens, which greatly increase adenohypophyseal secretion of LH. The surge of LH at midcycle is the primary trigger for ovulation, the release of an ovum from the mature follicle.

In the second half of the menstrual cycle, LH causes the follicle from which an ovum was released to develop into a thickened, secretory tissue called *corpus luteum.* The corpus luteum secretes large quantities of progesterone, another steroid hormone. By day 21 of the cycle, the large quantities of circulating estrogen and progesterone inhibit adenohypophyseal secretion of FSH and LH (see Figure 59-2), and the corpus luteum begins to involute. Steroid hormone production falls rapidly as the corpus luteum fails and brings about the final stage in the cycle, the collapse of the endometrial lining.

During menses the inner uterine surface is denuded, and the endometrium rapidly collapses to about 65% of its former thickness. About 70 ml of blood and serum is lost along with necrotic and dissolving tissue during a typical menstrual period. Normally, this blood does not clot because of the presence of fibrinolysin in the fluid. Fibrinolysin is an enzyme that digests the fibrin matrix on which blood clots form. Despite the seemingly favorable environment for bacterial growth, the uterus during menstruation is resistant to infection, partly because many leukocytes are present in menstrual fluid.

Effects of Gonadotropin Deficiency

Alterations in hypophyseal or ovarian function can upset the interaction of these tissues. Throughout childhood, pituitary secretion of FSH and LH is low, and circulating sex steroid concentrations are also low. At puberty the adenohypophysis greatly increases its secretion of FSH and LH. If this increase does not occur, sexual development does not take place, because androgen, estrogen, and progesterone production are not induced.

Gonadotropin-releasing hormone (GnRH) may help diagnose the cause of failure of sexual development (see Chapter 64). FSH may be used clinically to help reverse female infertility (see Chapter 64). For long-term replacement therapy in patients with hypogonadism, the androgens and estrogens are usually used (see Chapters 64 and 66).

Regulation of Response to Stress

Adrenocorticotropic hormone

Physiologic Action

When ACTH is released by the adenohypophysis, it stimulates the adrenal cortex to synthesize and to release cortisol, a major adrenocortical steroid hormone, as well as other glucocorticoids and minor amounts of sex steroids (see Chapter 60).

Regulation of Secretion

Cortisol blood levels are monitored by the hypothalamus, which adjusts the rate of release of corticotropin-releasing factor (CRF) into the hypophyseal portal venous system to the adenohypophysis, thereby controlling systemic levels of ACTH. When cortisol levels become too high, the hypothalamus reduces CRF release. The adenohypophysis, lacking appropriate stimulation, reduces ACTH production, and blood levels of ACTH fall. The adrenocortical production of cortisol then falls because of the lowered ACTH levels. Blood levels of cortisol thus are prevented from exceeding an upper limit. Conversely, when cortisol levels in blood fall too low, the hypothalamus normally prevents a dangerously low level from developing. CRF is released in large amounts into the hypophyseal portal venous system; in response the adenohypophysis releases ACTH, and in response to ACTH the adrenal cortex elevates cortisol production. This intricate regulatory sequence is an example of a negative feedback loop, a regulatory mechanism in which the end product of a reaction sequence inhibits operation of the sequence, thereby keeping the concentration of the product between fixed limits (Figure 59-3).

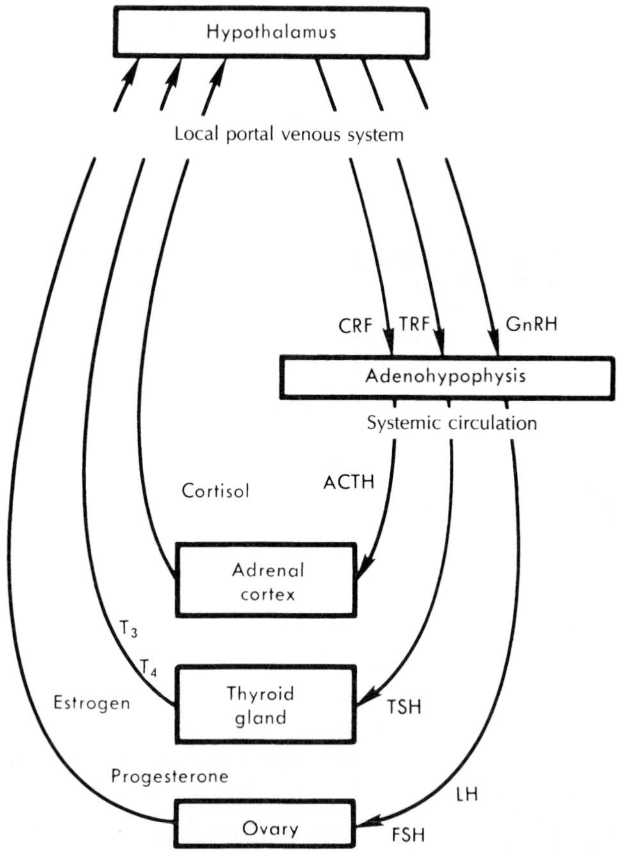

FIGURE 59-3
Regulation of hormone synthesis by negative feedback loops. Each *arrow* indicates a hormone, its source, and its target tissue. Hypothalamic synthesis of individual releasing factors is suppressed by high blood concentrations of appropriate final hormone. For example, cortisol suppresses CRF synthesis and release, thereby blocking further cortisol synthesis. Other loops are similarly regulated.

Thyroid-stimulating hormone

Negative feedback regulation applies not only to the adrenal cortex and the ovary but also to the thyroid gland (see Figure 59-3). TSH is discussed in Chapter 61.

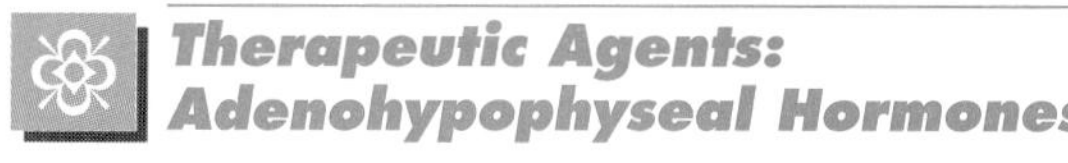

Therapeutic Agents: Adenohypophyseal Hormones

The diagnostic or therapeutic uses of most adenohypophyseal hormones are covered in the chapters devoted to the target organs. Only growth hormone is considered in this chapter because it targets the whole body.

Growth hormone

Mechanism of Action

Exogenously administered growth hormone stimulates growth by the same physiologic mechanisms as natural growth hormone.

Pharmacokinetics

Growth hormone, as a peptide, is susceptible to degradation by gastric acid and thus cannot be used orally. When given subcutaneously or intramuscularly, the hormone has a half-life in serum of 5 hours or less, but the duration of measurable metabolic effects may be as long as 2 days. Growth hormone is cleared by hepatic mechanisms.

Uses

Slow or inadequate growth may arise from many causes, but only that form caused by growth hormone deficiency is appropriately treated with growth hormone. The standard preparations for therapy are prepared by recombinant DNA techniques. Recombinant somatotropin has the same amino acid sequence as the natural hormone in the human hypophysis (see Table 59-3). Somatrem is a recombinant-derived form that has one more amino acid than natural growth hormone. Children or adolescents with pituitary dwarfism who receive growth hormone typically show an immediate increase in growth and may increase 1 foot or more in height over several years of treatment. Ultimately, resistance to the protein develops, and growth tapers off.

Adverse Reactions and Contraindications

Many actions of growth hormone antagonize those of insulin, and in predisposed individuals, prolonged treatment with growth hormone may precipitate diabetes mellitus. Thus patients receiving growth hormone are monitored to detect elevated blood glucose levels or altered glucose tolerance. In adults with established diabetes, destruction of the hypophysis with loss of growth hormone reduces their insulin requirement.

Growth hormone should not be used in adolescents whose epiphyses have sealed because stimulation of further natural growth is unlikely. These preparations should not be used to enhance size or bulk in healthy young athletes because the risks outweigh the minimal benefits.

Toxicity

No direct toxicity is expected with this agent.

Interactions

Glucocorticoids may antagonize the growth stimulation produced by growth hormone. This effect is more pronounced with long-term dosing of glucocorticoids.

NURSING PROCESS OVERVIEW

Pituitary Therapy

Assessment

In most cases patients with pituitary hormone problems have had long-term excesses or deficiencies of the hormones previously. Perform a thorough examination to obtain baseline data, paying particular attention to subjective and objective changes that the patient may indicate have occurred over an extended period.

Nursing Diagnoses

- Knowledge deficit
- Fluid volume excess related to excessive dose of vasopressin

Patient Outcomes

The patient will demonstrate correct administration technique for prescribed medication. The patient will accurately state when and how to use the medication, and when to seek medical assistance for side effects. The patient's fluid volume will return to normal.

Planning/Implementation

Monitor the patient for expected drug side effects. Before discharge, begin the teaching and emotional support required to help the patient move to self-management.

Evaluation

Before discharge, ascertain that the patient can explain why the prescribed drugs are necessary, how to administer them correctly, signs of overdosage or underdosage, side effects that might occur, and which ones should be reported immediately. If a patient does not have a medical identification tag or bracelet before leaving the hospital, the patient will state the need to obtain one.

NURSING IMPLICATIONS SUMMARY

Care of Patient With Diabetes Insipidus

Drug Administration

- Monitor fluid intake and output, serum sodium levels, and urine specific gravity. Diabetes insipidus is characterized by dilute urine, in large volume, with output often exceeding input, and with urine specific gravity of 1.000 to 1.003. This condition is often diagnosed initially by an alert nurse.
- Uncontrolled diabetes mellitus may be associated with excessive urine production. Monitor urine and blood glucose levels and urine specific gravity to help differentiate the two.
- Monitor blood pressure. Monitor serum electrolyte level.
- Read orders carefully. Vasopressin and vasopressin tannate in oil are different and have different requirements for administration.
- See the box on p. 60 for a discussion of administration of oil-based intramuscular (IM) preparations.

Intravenous Desmopressin Acetate

- Desmopressin acetate may be given undiluted in diabetes insipidus. Administer a single dose over 1 minute. Monitor blood pressure and pulse. This drug may also be administered intravenously in patients with hemophilia A and von Willebrand's disease. For these conditions, it is diluted and is administered as an infusion. Consult the manufacturer's literature.

Patient and Family Education

- Review with the patient the anticipated benefits and possible side effects of drug therapy
- If appropriate, instruct the patient to measure urine output at home. Most patients will not need to do this since they can usually tell when urine output is increasing and another dose of medication is needed.
- In preparing a patient for discharge with a drug for nasal administration, review the manufacturer's instructions. Have the patient give a return demonstration.
- Inform the patient that a severe cold, nasal surgery, or anything that interferes with the ability to sniff may necessitate a temporary switch to an injectable drug, and the patient should contact the physician.
- If GI tract distress develops, it may indicate too high a dose. If GI tract distress is severe or persistent, instruct the patient to notify the physician.
- Generally, if more than two sprays per nostril of a drug are needed, it is better to increase the frequency of dosage rather than the number of sprays for each dose.
- If a dose is missed, instruct the patient to take the dose as soon as it is remembered unless within a few hours of the next dose, in which case the patient should take a dose but omit the next scheduled dose. The patient should not double up for missed doses. Reinforce to the patient the need to consult the physician for questions about doses.
- Refer the patient to a community-based nursing agency for follow-up as appropriate.
- Instruct the patient with diabetes insipidus to wear a medical identification tag or bracelet indicating his or her diagnosis.
- Instruct the patient to avoid ingestion of alcohol unless permitted in small amounts by the physician.
- Chlorothiazide and other thiazide diuretics are discussed in Chapter 14.
- Chlorpropamide is discussed in Chapter 63.
- Clofibrate is discussed in Chapter 21.
- Oxytocin and bromocriptine are discussed in Chapter 65.

Sermorelin

Drug Administration

- Dilute each 50 μg with at least 0.5 ml of the 2 ml of normal saline provided. Administer a single dose as a bolus and follow with a normal saline flush.
- Monitor vital signs. Assess for headache, nausea/vomiting, paleness, strange taste in the mouth, and tightness in chest.

Somatrem and Somatropin

Drug Administration

- Monitor weight and height.
- Monitor blood glucose levels and thyroid function tests.
- Encourage the patient to return for regular follow-up.
- Warn the patient that pain and swelling at the injection site may occur.

Patient and Family Education

- Review the anticipated benefits and possible side effects of drug therapy. Warn the patient to take the drug only as ordered and not to increase dose unless directed to do so by the physician.
- Warn a diabetic patient to monitor blood glucose levels carefully, since changes in diet or insulin may be necessary.
- Consult with the physician, then teach the family to monitor and record the patient's weight, height, and other parameters regularly.

Octreotide

Drug Administration

- Monitor blood glucose levels.
- Preferred sites for subcutaneous administration include the hip, thigh, or abdomen. Rotate sites.
- Assess for GI tract symptoms including abdominal pain, diarrhea, and nausea and vomiting.
- Monitor serum glucose levels and thyroid function tests.

Intravenous Octreotide

- Octreotide may be given undiluted at a rate of one dose over 1 minute. Intravenous (IV) administration is usually reserved for emergency situations; the subcutaneous route is usually preferred.

NURSING IMPLICATIONS SUMMARY—cont'd

Patient and Family Education

- Review administration technique with the patient. See the patient instruction leaflet
- Instruct the patient to administer doses between meals and at bedtime to help avoid GI tract symptoms.
- Warn a diabetic patient to monitor blood glucose levels carefully since changes in diet or insulin may be necessary.

Panhypopituitarism

Drug Administration/Patient and Family Education

- The patient who loses all or nearly all pituitary function from trauma, surgery, or disease must be treated with replacement hormonal therapy to survive. Treatment with exogenous forms of cortisol usually substitutes for ACTH loss. Thyroid hormones usually replace TSH. Growth hormone is not usually replaced, except in children. ADH may or may not be replaced. Gonadotropic hormones are rarely used in replacement therapy. Estrogens and androgens are used as needed for cosmetic and comfort purposes. In females, it is difficult to recreate the monthly cyclic surges of these hormones, so this may not be attempted unless requested by the patient; she is usually sterile. Oxytocin is not replaced unless the woman has conceived and the hormone would be needed during labor and delivery. For information about individual hormones, see Chapters 60 to 66.
- Instruct the patient requiring hormonal replacement therapy to wear a medical identification tag or bracelet.

CRITICAL THINKING

APPLICATION

1. What are the two divisions of the pituitary gland (hypophysis)?
2. What is the nature of neurohypophyseal tissue?
3. What hormones are released by the neurohypophysis?
4. Where does synthesis of the hormones released by the neurohypophysis take place?
5. What is the target tissue of ADH?
6. What is the mechanism of action of ADH?
7. What physiologic conditions stimulate the release of ADH?
8. What is diabetes insipidus? How should you assess for this?
9. What two types of therapy may be used to treat diabetes insipidus?
10. What advantage does desmopressin acetate (DDAVP) have over other vasopressin preparations?
11. What are the side effects associated with vasopressin?
12. What is the mechanism of action by which thiazide diuretics control diuresis in diabetes insipidus?
13. What is the mechanism of action of chlorpropamide and clofibrate in treating diabetes insipidus?
14. What are the target tissues of oxytocin?
15. What hormones are secreted by the adenohypophysis?
16. Where does synthesis of the hormones secreted by the adenohypophysis take place?
17. What are the target tissues of growth hormone?
18. What are the anabolic effects of growth hormone?
19. What are the antiinsulin effects of growth hormone? What would the manifestations of this be in the patient?
20. What are somatomedins?
21. What is the effect of growth hormone deficiency?
22. How is growth hormone deficiency treated?
23. What is the effect of excessive growth hormone?
24. What are the gonadotropic hormones?
25. What roles do FSH and LH play in causing the development and release of a mature ovum from the ovary?
26. What are the effects of gonadotropin deficiency?
27. What is the target tissue for ACTH?
28. How is the concentration of ACTH in the blood regulated?

CRITICAL THINKING

1. Compare and contrast the symptoms of diabetes insipidus and diabetic mellitus. What are the causes of these symptoms?
2. Your preadolescent patient complains that he or she is "too short," and wants medicine "to make me grow." What factors should be considered in deciding if administration of growth hormone is good for a child?

CHAPTER 60

Drugs Affecting the Adrenal Gland

OBJECTIVES

After studying this chapter, you should be able to do the following:

- *Describe the two types of hormones produced in the adrenal glands.*
- *Describe the use of corticosteroids as replacement therapy.*
- *Distinguish mineralocorticoid effects from glucocorticoid effects.*
- *Develop a nursing care plan for a patient receiving a corticosteroid.*

KEY TERMS

acute adrenal insufficiency
Addison's disease
corticosteroids
Cushing's syndrome
glucocorticoids
mineralocorticoids
renin-angiotensin system
secondary adrenal insufficiency

CHAPTER OVERVIEW

The human adrenal gland is divided into two distinct functional units, the adrenal medulla and the adrenal cortex. These regions of the gland differ in embryologic origin, type of cells composing the tissue, and hormones produced. The structure and function of these regions of the adrenal gland, the regulation of synthesis of the various hormones produced, and the pathologic states arising from abnormalities in hormone production are discussed in this chapter. The widespread clinical uses of several of these hormones and their derivatives in diagnosis and therapy are also considered.

Therapeutic Rationale: Adrenal Cortex

The adrenal cortex is composed of lipid-rich secretory tissue. Three distinct layers within the cortex may be distinguished on the basis of histology. These regions differ not only in cellular arrangement but also in the major steroid hormone produced and in the regulation of steroid synthesis (Figure 60-1).

Adrenal Steroids

Mineralocorticoids

Physiologic Action

The outer layer, or zona glomerulosa, is where the precursor cholesterol is converted to **mineralocorticoids.** These steroids cause the kidneys to retain sodium and associated water but promote potassium loss.

Regulation of Secretion

Regulation of mineralocorticoid synthesis involves the **renin-angiotensin system** (Figure 60-2). The trigger for this feedback system is in the kidneys, where lower blood sodium levels or lower intravascular volume causes release of renin into the blood. The enzyme renin converts angiotensinogen, a protein from liver, to angiotensin I. Another enzyme found in blood and lungs rapidly converts angiotensin I to angiotensin II. Angiotensin II in turn stimulates the adrenocortical zona glomerulosa to secrete mineralocorticoids, especially aldosterone. The result of this regulatory loop is that mineralocorticoid release slows further loss of sodium and water through the kidneys. When sodium and water retention exceeds certain limits, plasma volume expands and renin release decreases. When the concentration of renin falls, production of angiotensin II slows, aldosterone secretion by the adrenal gland falls, and the kidneys begin to rid the body of accumulated sodium.

Effects of Mineralocorticoid Deficiency

When the adrenal gland fails, mineralocorticoid action is lost. As a result, salt balance becomes deranged. Survival requires replacement of the lost hormone activity.

Effects of Excessive Mineralocorticoids (Hyperaldosteronism)

Certain tumors of the adrenal gland produce excessive amounts of aldosterone or less often one of the other mineralocorticoids. In these patients, two types of symptoms appear: those associated with hypertension and those associated with hypokalemia (low blood potassium concentration). Hypertension is produced by sodium and water retention arising from excess aldosterone acting on the kidneys, whereas the muscle weakness associated with hypokalemia is a result of the potassium-wasting action of the steroid in the kidneys. Treatment ultimately involves surgical removal of the tumor.

Corticosteroids

Physiologic Action

The inner two layers of the adrenal cortex convert cholesterol to **corticosteroids,** including **glucocorticoids** and sex steroids. The primary glucocorticoid is cortisone and the primary sex steroids are androgens and progestins.

The glucocorticoids produce potent and varied effects on metabolism. The primary metabolic effect is stimulation of gluconeogenesis (the formation of new glucose) by actions on liver and peripheral tissues. In striated muscle, glucocorticoids mobilize amino acids from muscle protein. The result is an increase in circulating levels of amino acids and an over-

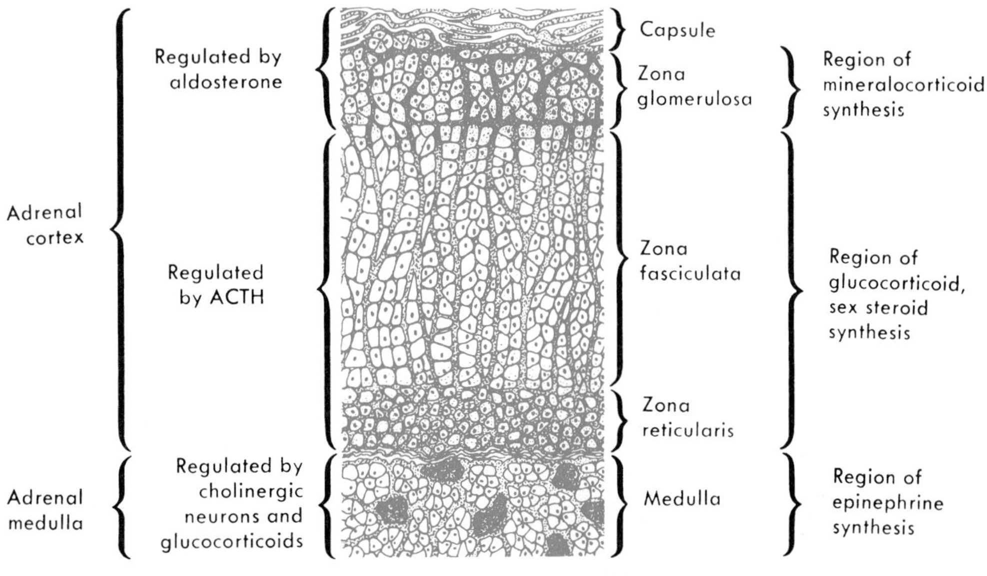

FIGURE 60-1
Regions of adrenal gland. Each histologically distinguishable zone of adrenal gland synthesizes specific hormones and is controlled by specific regulators. Medulla forms center of adrenal gland and is thicker than shown in cross section.

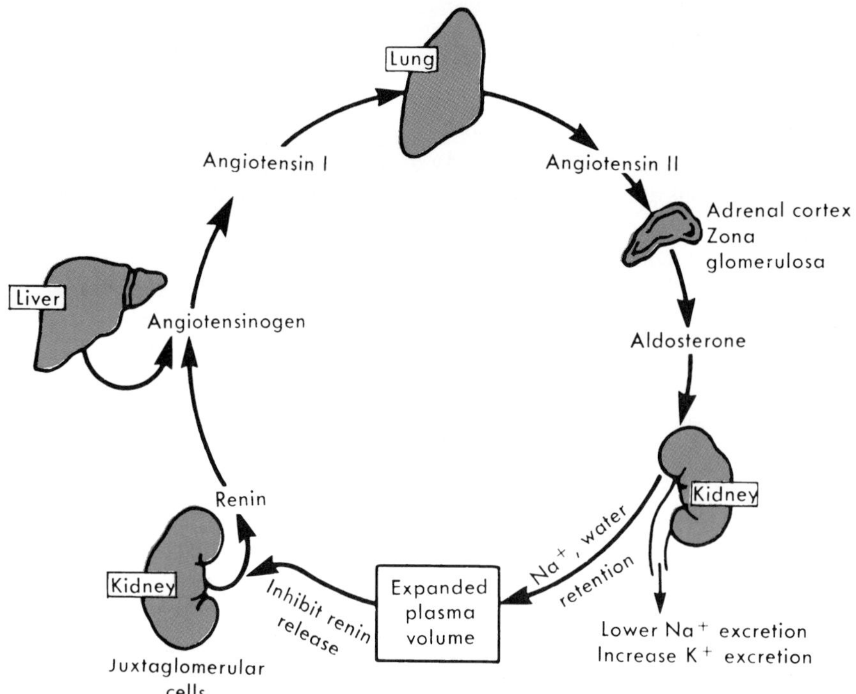

FIGURE 60-2
Negative feedback loop regulating mineralocorticoid synthesis and release. Kidney is key to regulating synthesis and release of aldosterone, primary natural mineralocorticoid. Renin is released from juxtaglomerular cells of kidney to set cascade in motion, and kidney is ultimate target of aldosterone. Expanded plasma volume, which results when kidney retains sodium ion (Na^+) and water, is regulator that halts renin release.

all depletion of muscle protein, which ultimately is expressed as a negative nitrogen balance (more nitrogen is excreted than is absorbed in the diet). In the liver, glucocorticoids increase activities of enzymes that convert amino acids to glucose. Much of this excess glucose is then stored in liver as glycogen. In addition, amino acids are the source of precursors for fat synthesis, which is also increased by glucocorticoids.

Glucocorticoids have many direct actions in the body. They maintain water diuresis by antagonizing the effects of antidiuretic hormone (ADH) in the kidney, lower the threshold for electrical excitation in the brain, and reduce the amount of new bone synthesis. In addition, glucocorticoids affect the immune system by suppressing the activity of lymphoid tissue and by reducing the numbers of circulating lymphocytes. These steroids also reduce inflammatory processes by impairing synthesis of prostaglandins and related compounds, an action that has several useful therapeutic applications (see Chapter 36).

In addition to direct effects, glucocorticoids have permissive activities that allow the body to deal successfully with stress or trauma. For example, cortisol sensitizes arterioles to norepinephrine, allowing the catecholamine to increase blood pressure. In the liver, cortisol must be present before epinephrine and glucagon can stimulate breakdown of liver glycogen to glucose, releasing the sugar as an energy source for peripheral muscle.

Regulation of Secretion

The synthesis of these steroids is regulated by the pituitary gland and the hypothalamus via the negative feedback loop described in Chapter 59. Cortisol is the major glucocorticoid produced and it is the key to regulation of steroid synthesis in the zona fasciculata and zona reticularis. Low levels of cortisol in blood stimulate and high levels suppress total steroid synthesis by respectively raising and lowering adrenocorticotropic hormone (ACTH) release from the pituitary.

Effects of Adrenal Insufficiency

Failure of the adrenal cortex is life threatening. If failure is sudden, which might occur after adrenal injury or thrombosis, death can occur within hours. Early symptoms of **acute adrenal insufficiency** include confusion, restlessness, nausea, and vomiting. Circulatory collapse, deep shock, and death may follow rapidly.

If synthesis of glucocorticoids is reduced but not halted, patients may not be in immediate danger, in the absence of stress or trauma, but they may still suffer from inadequate amounts of glucocorticoids. This chronic primary adrenal insufficiency is called **Addison's disease.** Symptoms include weakness, weight loss, dehydration, hypotension, hypoglycemia, and anemia. Most patients with Addison's disease also display increased skin pigmentation. This unusual or excessive tanning is caused by a direct effect on melanin-containing skin cells by the long-term excess of ACTH, which is secreted by the hypophysis in response to the elevated corticotropin-releasing factor (CRF) induced by chronically low blood levels of cortisol.

Symptoms similar to those of Addison's disease are produced when the adenohypophysis is diseased or destroyed and no longer produces adequate ACTH. Without ACTH, the zona reticularis and zona fasciculata do not synthesize cortisol, and over time these adrenal tissues atrophy. This condition is called **secondary adrenal insufficiency.** One characteristic that often visibly distinguishes these patients from those with Addison's disease is the absence of excessive pigmentation. In secondary adrenal insufficiency the hypophysis does not release large quantities of ACTH, and the skin is not darkened.

Effects of Excessive Glucocorticoids

Overproduction of cortisol, a condition called **Cushing's syndrome,** may be induced by a variety of factors. Some patients have high cortisol production from tumors of the adrenal cortex, which may synthesize massive amounts of the steroid. Other patients have high cortisol synthesis because of increased ACTH release into the blood, which keeps the zona fasciculata and zona reticularis maximally stimulated to produce glucocorticoids. Excess ACTH usually comes from a tumor of the hypophysis, but occasionally it comes from some unusual source such as a lung tumor, which would not ordinarily be expected to synthesize ACTH. Most often, however, Cushing's syndrome is caused by administration of high doses of glucocorticoids.

The symptoms of Cushing's syndrome can be predicted from the metabolic actions of cortisol. Certain fat stores, especially those on the face and shoulders, are increased as a result of cortisol stimulation of fat synthesis. The extremities may be weak and in more advanced cases may be thin because of the muscle-wasting effects of the hormone. The skin is fragile and easily bruised as a result of protein breakdown in that tissue. Examination of the skin on the trunk may reveal striae, or stretch marks, over areas where fat deposition is most pronounced. Many patients also have superficial fungal infections of the skin, related in part to the fragility of the skin and to the reduced host immune response caused by the excess steroid. Bone thinning occurs because of changes in calcium metabolism; compression fractures of the spine may occur relatively easily. Diabetes may be precipitated from the increased insulin demand caused by excess cortisol. Hypertension is very common in these patients, and atherosclerosis may occur. Mood changes are also common and may be extreme. Psychosis may be precipitated.

Effects of Excessive Adrenal Production of Sex Steroids

Sex steroids produced in the adrenal cortex are normally of minor importance, the adrenal output being small compared with that of the gonads, but under certain conditions sex steroid overproduction in the adrenal glands may cause a devastating endocrine imbalance. For example, a female with an androgen-producing adrenal tumor may undergo masculinization, including development of secondary male sex characteristics and suppression of the menstrual cycle. A male with an estrogen-producing tumor may develop breast tenderness or loss of libido. A child may show precocious sexual development.

Therapeutic Agents: Adrenal Steroids and Related Compounds

Compounds Used in Replacement Therapy

Glucocorticoids

Mechanism of Action

Three major activities of the adrenal steroids are metabolic effects on carbohydrate, protein, and fat metabolism; antiinflammatory and immunosuppressive activity; and sodium-retaining activity associated with potassium loss. The first two are classified as glucocorticoid actions and the third as a mineralocorticoid action.

The natural adrenal steroids, cortisol and cortisone, possess both glucocorticoid and mineralocorticoid activity, but glucocorticoid action predominates. Treatment with one of these natural compounds therefore produces multiple effects. For example, cortisol in the high doses required for antiinflammatory action (see Chapter 36) changes metabolism as expected from a glucocorticoid, but also produces excessive sodium retention and potassium loss, a mineralocorticoid effect. Synthetic glucocorticoids have been designed to have very little mineralocorticoid activity. These drugs include betamethasone, dexamethasone, methylprednisolone, and triamcinolone, which are used primarily as powerful antiinflammatory drugs (see Chapter 36).

To produce their effects, steroids must pass through the membranes of target cells, bind to soluble cytoplasmic receptors, and be carried to the cell nucleus (see Chapter 58). In the nucleus the steroid induces changes in RNA and protein synthesis, which will be expressed as some change in function of the target cell. A considerable delay may occur between uptake of the steroid into the cell and appearance of the effect in the target cell. Further time may elapse before the effect ends and the steroid is destroyed.

Pharmacokinetics

The chemical form of a steroid determines the pharmacokinetics of the preparation. In their naturally occurring forms, most corticosteroids are relatively insoluble in water. Because these drugs form suspensions but not solutions in water, these preparations are not suitable for intravenous (IV) administration. In contrast, sodium phosphate and sodium succinate derivatives of several glucocorticoids are quite water soluble; these are the forms that must be used when IV administration of an adrenal steroid is required.

Administered intramuscularly as suspensions, many glucocorticoids are dissolved and absorbed slowly from the injection site, producing a relatively long duration of action, which may be an advantage for control of certain conditions (see Chapter 36).

Uses

Corticosteroids used most often for replacement therapy are summarized in Table 60-1. Other glucocorticoids used primarily for their antiinflammatory and immunosuppressant effects are covered in Chapter 36. In addition to these indications, corticosteroids have been used in the control of certain types of cancers (see Chapter 50).

Corticosteroids are used clinically (1) at physiologic doses in replacement therapy for endocrine diseases such as pituitary deficiency or adrenal hypofunction or (2) at pharmacologic doses to treat various nonendocrine diseases.

Examples of replacement therapy include the use of cortisol to treat Addison's disease or secondary adrenal insufficiency. Doses of adrenal steroids used in replacement therapy are relatively low because they are intended only to replace amounts of the hormone normally present. Since the normal daily production of cortisol is about 15 to 25 mg, the daily replacement dose would be designed to achieve the level of activity produced by that amount of cortisol. Wide variations in dosage exist because stress and other factors affect steroid requirements. Dosage must be adjusted to each patient's needs and monitored to ensure continued success of the therapy.

Successful treatment of adrenal insufficiency often is obtained with hydrocortisone or cortisone, natural glucocorticoids with sufficient mineralocorticoid activity to maintain sodium balance for many individuals. Other patients may require additional supplementation with a mineralocorticoid such as fludrocortisone (see Table 60-1).

In pharmacologic doses the antiinflammatory action of glucocorticoids is the primary action sought. The level of steroid at the site of action must be much higher than normally would be found at that site to achieve antiinflammatory effects. In some cases, this goal may be achieved by local application of the steroid; in other cases the steroids must be administered systemically.

Adverse Reactions and Contraindications

Adverse reactions are generally mild when glucocorticoids are used in replacement therapy, where doses are usually small. Higher doses used for longer than a few days, such as those used to control inflammatory conditions (see Chapter 36), are associated with many more side effects. For example, patients receiving relatively high doses for long periods for inflammatory conditions should not be abruptly withdrawn from long-term systemic steroid therapy. All adrenal steroids suppress the normal function of the hypothalamus, adenohypophysis, and adrenal glands. If exogenous steroids are withdrawn suddenly, patients may die of acute adrenal insufficiency because their own adrenal glands cannot immediately produce the required steroids. It may require 6 to 9 months for the natural negative feedback loop that regulates adrenal steroid synthesis to regain normal function after long-term steroid therapy, apparently because some atrophy of the tissues occurs. Schedules for gradual withdrawal from steroids must be followed faithfully, with dosage adjusted only to relieve symptoms of adrenal insufficiency if they develop during withdrawal. Patients who receive corticosteroids as replacement therapy would normally continue to receive them for life.

Toxicity

Any glucocorticoid, if given in high enough doses, will produce Cushing's syndrome. This toxicity is one of the most common reactions seen with glucocorticoid therapy. For these patients the steroid dose should be reduced, if allowed by the severity of the condition being treated. Although usual replacement doses slightly exceed normal daily production of steroids, these doses would not be expected to cause Cushing's syndrome.

Other common symptoms of glucocorticoid toxicity include euphoria, glucose intolerance, osteoporosis, and muscle wasting. These effects occur after long-term use of glucocorticoids. Large doses given for a short time to control acute allergic responses or other acute conditions are seldom associated with significant signs of toxicity.

TABLE 60-1 Drugs for Adrenal Replacement Therapy

GENERIC NAME	TRADE NAME	ADMINISTRATION/DOSAGE	COMMENTS
Betamethasone	Celestone*	ORAL: *Adults*—600 μg daily or more as needed. *Children*—5.83 μg/kg 3 times daily.	Synthetic glucocorticoid with little or no mineralocorticoid action; must be used with mineralocorticoid.
Cortisone	Cortone*	ORAL: *Adults*—25 mg daily or more as needed. *Children*—0.35 mg/kg daily.	Natural hormone with both glucocorticoid and mineralocorticoid action.
Fludrocortisone	Florinef*	ORAL: *Adults*—0.1 mg daily. FDA pregnancy category C. *Children*—0.05-0.1 mg daily.	Synthetic steroid with strong mineralocorticoid action; used with glucocorticoid for replacement therapy.
Hydrocortisone	Cortef*	ORAL: *Adults*—20 mg daily or more as needed. *Children*—0.56 mg/kg daily.	Has both glucocorticoid and mineralocorticoid action.
Triamcinolone	Aristocort* Kenacort*	ORAL: *Adults*—4-12 mg daily in single or divided doses. *Children*—0.117 mg/kg in single or divided doses.	Synthetic glucocorticoid with little or no mineralocorticoid action; must be used with mineralocorticoid.

*Available in Canada and United States.

Interactions

The effect of many drugs are altered in patients receiving high doses of glucocorticoids (see Chapter 36). Interactions are unlikely with the low doses used in replacement therapy.

Mineralocorticoid

Mechanism of Action

Any mineralocorticoid could be used for replacement therapy in adrenal insufficiency, but the potent synthetic agent fludrocortisone is preferred. Fludrocortisone has the same mechanism of action as natural mineralocorticoids, increasing renal excretion of potassium and hydrogen ions while promoting sodium and water retention.

Pharmacokinetics

Fludrocortisone is the mineralocorticoid of choice because it is well absorbed orally. The duration of action of a single dose is 1 to 2 days. The drug is eliminated as inactive metabolites by the kidneys.

Uses

Fludrocortisone is used only for its mineralocorticoid action. Conditions treated include chronic primary and secondary adrenocortical insufficiency. The drug may also be effective in salt-losing forms of adrenogenital syndrome.

Adverse Reactions and Contraindications

Adverse reactions are rare with fludrocortisone. Allergic reactions are possible. Some patients may be sensitive to the effects of sodium retention caused by the drug, resulting in congestive heart failure or peripheral edema.

There is no contraindication for fludrocortisone when used for replacement therapy. Patients with heart disease or hypertension may require special precautions.

Toxicity

Excessive action of fludrocortisone leads to excessive sodium retention and potassium loss (Chapter 17).

Interactions

Interactions with fludrocortisone are often associated with the electrolyte changes caused by the drug. For example, the hypokalemia caused by fludrocortisone can increase toxicity of digitalis glycosides and increase the risk with other drugs that cause hypokalemia. Drug preparations or foods that contain high sodium may cause hypernatremia because kidneys under the influence of fludrocortisone may not be able to clear the excess sodium.

Inducers of hepatic metabolic enzymes may increase metabolism of fludrocortisone, necessitating an increase in dosage of fludrocortisone. Rifampin and phenytoin have been reported to cause this effect.

Compounds Used in Diagnosing Adrenal Disorders

Adrenocorticotropic hormone

Adrenocorticotropic hormone (ACTH, corticotropin) is discussed in Chapter 59 as part of the natural feedback regulatory cycle controlling adrenal function. ACTH directly stimulates the adrenal cortex to synthesize adrenal steroids. This action can be used diagnostically to distinguish between Addison's disease and secondary adrenal insufficiency resulting from pituitary dysfunction (Table 60-2). Normal adrenal glands respond to ACTH by synthesizing and releasing cortisol into the bloodstream, where it may be measured. In Addison's disease the adrenal gland cannot respond to ACTH, and no excess cortisol is produced. In patients who have low pituitary function the adrenal gland may be suppressed and may respond less rapidly to ACTH than would a normal gland.

TABLE 60-2 Agents Used in Diagnosing Adrenal Gland Dysfunction

GENERIC NAME	TRADE NAME	ADMINISTRATION/DOSAGE	COMMENTS
Corticotropin	Acthar*	INTRAVENOUS: *Adults*—For diagnosis of adrenal/pituitary function: 10-25 U in 500 ml of 5% dextrose, given over 8 hr. FDA pregnancy category C. INTRAVENOUS, SUBCUTANEOUS: *Children*—1.6 U/kg divided into 3 or 4 doses.	Natural ACTH, protein from pituitary.
Cosyntropin	Cortrosyn*	INTRAVENOUS, INTRAMUSCULAR, SUBCUTANEOUS: *Adults*—0.25 mg as single injection or infused over 2 min-6 hr. FDA pregnancy category C. INTRAMUSCULAR: *Children <2 yr*—0.125 mg. *Older children:* same as adult doses.	Synthetic subunit of ACTH.
Metyrapone	Metopirone*	ORAL: *Adults*—For diagnosis of secondary adrenal insufficiency: 750 mg every 4 hr for 6 doses. FDA pregnancy category C. *Children*—15 mg/kg every 4 hr for 6 doses.	Metyrapone blocks cortisol synthesis in adrenals; acute adrenal insufficiency may occur.

*Available in Canada and United States.

In the past, ACTH has been used to treat adrenal insufficiency or other diseases responding to glucocorticoids. The rationale for this therapy was that adrenal function was maintained and that a natural balance of steroids was produced. In practice, however, ACTH therapy was not as reliable or convenient as steroid therapy. ACTH must be injected because it is a peptide, whereas oral glucocorticoids are available. In addition, the response of the adrenal gland to ACTH was not easily predictable, making dosage adjustment unreliable. Finally, many patients developed antibodies to ACTH; as a result, they became unresponsive to it. For these reasons and others, ACTH is no longer widely used in therapy.

Dexamethasone

The highly potent synthetic glucocorticoid dexamethasone may be used diagnostically to test steroid suppression of cortisol synthesis. Relatively small doses of dexamethasone administered over 2 days inhibit cortisol production in a healthy person and, to a lesser extent, in a person with pituitary-induced Cushing's syndrome. Ordinarily, tumor production of cortisol is unaffected.

Metyrapone

Metyrapone blocks cortisol synthesis in the adrenal gland and may be used to test the ability of the pituitary gland to increase ACTH release (see Table 60-2). Before the test is run, it should be demonstrated that the patient's adrenal glands respond to ACTH. While metyrapone is being administered, cortisol synthesis falls dramatically. In healthy persons the fall in blood cortisol level stimulates the hypothalamus and in turn the pituitary gland, with the result that ACTH is released into the blood. Under the influence of ACTH, early steps in steroid synthesis proceed, but metyrapone prevents cortisol from being formed in normal amounts. Therefore steroid precursors accumulate and are excreted in urine. If no precursors accumulate under these conditions, it is concluded that the pituitary gland failed to produce ACTH. If the metyrapone test is administered to a person with adrenalin sufficiency, a danger exists of precipitating an adrenal crisis because in such a patient metyrapone may stop cortisol synthesis altogether.

Therapeutic Rationale: Adrenal Medulla

The adrenal medulla arises from neuroectodermal tissue during embryonic life and remains closely associated with the autonomic nervous system at maturity. The cells (pheochromocytes or chromaffin cells) can synthesize catecholamines by the same series of reactions found in nerve terminals and can release catecholamines into the bloodstream in response to sympathetic cholinergic presynaptic neurons. One major difference between the synthetic pathways is that nerve terminals form norepinephrine as the final product, whereas the adrenal medulla converts norepinephrine to epinephrine. The enzyme for this final conversion is induced by adrenal steroids, indicating that the anatomic proximity of the disparate tissues of the cortex and medulla may have functional importance.

Therapeutic Agents: Hormones of Adrenal Medulla

The hormones of the adrenal medulla are not essential to survival, but they are useful in adapting to stress. Epinephrine produces widespread effects throughout the body, mediated by the beta- and alpha-adrenergic receptors. The actions of epinephrine are discussed in Chapter 10, and the clinical uses of epinephrine are discussed in Chapter 16.

Nursing Process Overview

Drugs Affecting the Adrenal Gland

Assessment

Monitor vital signs, blood pressure, and weight. Question the patient about history of infections, energy level, and ability to perform activities of daily living.

Nursing Diagnoses

- Potential complication: electrolyte abnormalities

Patient Outcomes

The nurse will manage and minimize electrolyte disturbances.

Planning/Implementation

Many of the drugs in this chapter are used for diagnostic purposes. Keep the patient informed as tests are completed. Provide emotional support as needed. Prepare the patient for self-administration at home, if appropriate. If the drugs are used for a chronic problem, instruct the patient about side effects. Emphasize the importance of continuing therapy as prescribed and not discontinuing drug therapy without talking with physician.

Evaluation

If the drug is used for diagnostic purposes, the drug is effective if the test is completed with no side effects. If used for long-term therapy, make certain the patient can administer the drug correctly, knows the side effects of the drug, and can explain when to contact the physician.

NURSING IMPLICATIONS SUMMARY

Glucocorticoids

- Glucocorticoids are discussed in detail in Chapter 36.

Fludrocortisone and Mineralocorticoids

Drug Administration

- All glucocorticoids also have mineralocorticoid activity but in varying amounts; see Table 36-1.
- Monitor weight, blood pressure, and pulse. Auscultate lung and heart sounds.
- Monitor serum electrolyte level.
- For a discussion of intramuscular (IM) injection of oil-based medications, see p. 60.

Patient and Family Education

- Review anticipated benefits and possible side effects of drug therapy with the patient.
- Counsel the patient about sodium restriction and increasing potassium intake as needed. See the dietary consideration boxes on potassium sources (p. 170) and sodium and hypertension (p. 150).
- Encourage the patient to wear a medical identification tag or bracelet.
- Remind the patient to inform all health care providers of all drugs being used.

Corticotropin

Drug Administration/Patient and Family Education

- Emphasize the importance of continuing this drug as prescribed, and not discontinuing this drug without discussing it with the physician.
- Review administration technique with the patient.
- Reinforce the importance of dietary changes (low-salt or potassium-rich diet) if prescribed.
- Review the manufacturer's insert for administration guidelines, depending on use.

Cosyntropin

Drug Administration

- See the manufacturer's instruction sheet.
- For IV administration: Dilute with the diluent provided by manufacturer. Cosyntropin may then be given by direct IV or further diluted in 5% dextrose in water (D5W) or 0.9% saline and given as an infusion. For a single dose, administer over 2 minutes. For infusion, administer over 4 to 8 hours, depending on the volume of infusion and age and condition of patient.
- Monitor vital signs. Assess for dizziness, fever, flushing, rash, and urticaria.

Metyrapone

Drug Administration/Patient and Family Education

- Monitor blood pressure and vital signs.
- Instruct the patient that this drug may cause nausea and vomiting. Take doses with food, milk, or meals to lessen this side effect.
- Caution the patient to avoid driving or operating hazardous equipment if dizziness, drowsiness, or light-headedness occur.
- Monitor plasma or urinary cortisol and serum electrolytes.

CRITICAL THINKING

APPLICATION

1. What are the two functional units of the adrenal gland?
2. What are mineralocorticoids?
3. In which part of the adrenal cortex are mineralocorticoids synthesized?
4. What hormones regulate mineralocorticoid synthesis?
5. Where are glucocorticoids synthesized?
6. What are the main effects of glucocorticoids on metabolism?
7. What is the result of untreated adrenal insufficiency?
8. What causes Cushing's syndrome?
9. What is the effect of overproduction of mineralocorticoids?
10. What are the three major actions of corticosteroids?
11. Why should steroid therapy not be stopped suddenly in a patient who has been receiving long-term high-dose therapy?
12. Name three clinical uses of adrenal corticosteroids.
13. What is the aim of replacement therapy in treating adrenal insufficiency?
14. Which mineralocorticoid is most commonly used clinically? Why?
15. Which are the water-soluble glucocorticoid preparations, and when are they preferred over the suspensions?
16. What drug interactions commonly occur with corticosteroids?
17. How is ACTH used in diagnosis?
18. Why is ACTH not commonly used in replacement therapy?
19. What hormone is released by the adrenal medulla?

CRITICAL THINKING

1. What is Addison's disease? How would you assess for this?
2. What are the symptoms of Cushing's syndrome? How would you assess these?
3. What is the effect of long-term overdosage with glucocorticoids? What signs and symptoms would you assess?

CHAPTER 61

Drugs Affecting the Thyroid Gland

OBJECTIVES

After studying this chapter, you should be able to do the following:

- *Discuss the rationale for therapy of hypothyroidism.*
- *Describe the classes of drugs used for hypothyroidism.*
- *Discuss the rationale for therapy of hyperthyroidism.*
- *Describe the classes of drugs used for hyperthyroidism.*
- *Develop a nursing care plan for the patient receiving drug therapy for hypothyroidism or hyperthyroidism.*

KEY TERMS

follicular cells
Graves' disease
hyperthyroidism
hypothyroidism
myxedema
primary hypothyroidism
secondary hypothyroidism
thyroid storm

CHAPTER OVERVIEW

The thyroid gland is a richly vascularized, horseshoe-shaped organ lying across the trachea in the region of the larynx (Figure 61-1). The gland contains primarily two cell types differing in function and embryologic origin: follicular cells and parafollicular cells. The function of the parafollicular cells is discussed in the next chapter. Hormones produced by follicular cells and the drugs commonly used in diagnosing and treating disease states associated with deficient or excessive thyroid function are described in this chapter.

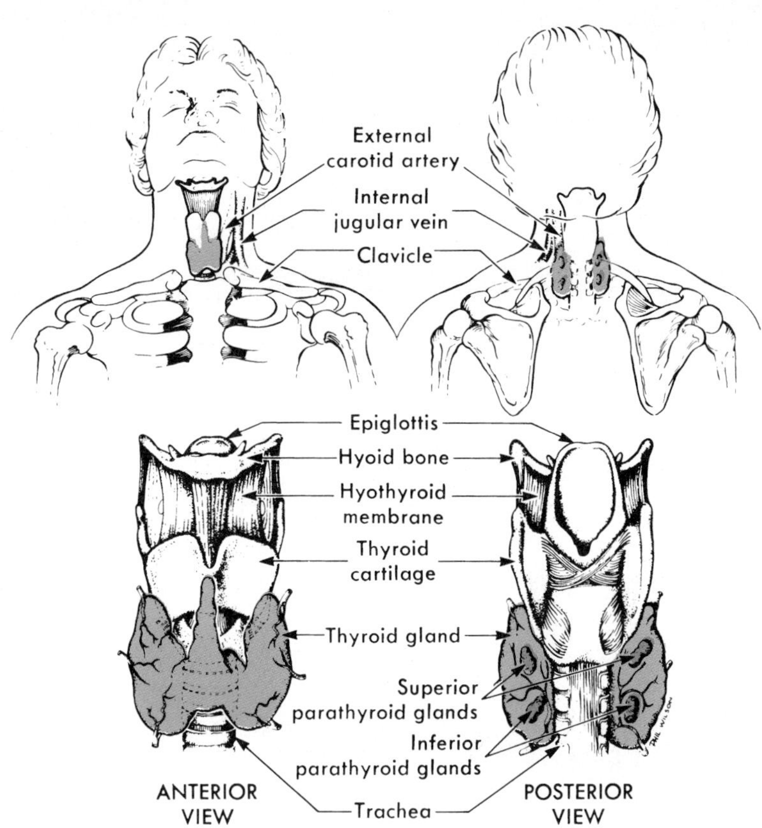

FIGURE 61-1
Anatomic location of thyroid and parathyroid glands.

Therapeutic Rationale: Thyroid Gland

Follicular Cells

The function of **follicular cells** in the thyroid is to regulate the basal metabolic rate (BMR), mainly by altering oxidative processes in target tissues. The iodine-containing hormones, thyroxine (T_4) and triiodothyronine (T_3), released by follicular cells into the general circulation, establish metabolic rates for most body tissues.

Thyroid hormones (T_4 and T_3)

Physiologic Action

Thyroid hormones bind to specific high-affinity receptors in cell nuclei. They thus regulate expression of genes and modulate the primary function of cells. Tissues especially sensitive to thyroid hormones are skeletal muscles, heart, liver, and kidneys. Basal metabolic rate in these tissues is strongly stimulated by thyroid hormones, but other organs including the brain are much less responsive. Clinically observed signs of these effects include rapid heart beat and increased cardiac output.

Regulation of Secretion

Regulation of thyroid hormone levels in the blood is accomplished in part by the negative feedback system described in Chapter 59. Thyroid-stimulating hormone (TSH) from the anterior pituitary (adenohypophysis) stimulates each step in thyroid hormone synthesis described here.

The first step in synthesizing T_4 and T_3 is iodine uptake by follicular cells (Figure 61-2). Because iodide ion levels in blood are relatively low, follicular cells must concentrate iodine to carry out the synthetic reactions required. In the normal human body the concentration of iodide ion in the thyroid is 30 to 40 times that found in plasma. In the second step in thyroid hormone synthesis, iodide ion activation is catalyzed by the peroxidase enzyme formed in follicular cells. This activation step takes place on the surface of microvilli that protrude into colloid filling the thyroid follicle.

Once activated, iodine may be attached to thyroglobulin in a process called *organification.* Thyroglobulin, a large protein synthesized in follicular cells and extruded into follicles, is the major protein component of colloid. Most iodine atoms are attached to tyrosine molecules contained within the peptide chains of thyroglobulin. A tyrosine may contain one (3-monoiodotyrosine, or MIT) or two (3,5-diiodotyrosine, or DIT) atoms of iodine.

After iodination, some tyrosine molecules may undergo a coupling reaction in which two molecules of DIT combine to produce one molecule of thyroglobulin-bound T_4. Coupling may also occur between one molecule each of DIT and MIT to yield one molecule of T_3.

Thyroglobulin serves primarily as a storage depot for thyroid hormones and the precursors MIT and DIT. In healthy persons, each molecule of thyroglobulin contains about six molecules of MIT, five molecules of DIT, and two molecules of T_4. Less T_3 is stored. A single molecule of T_3 occurs in

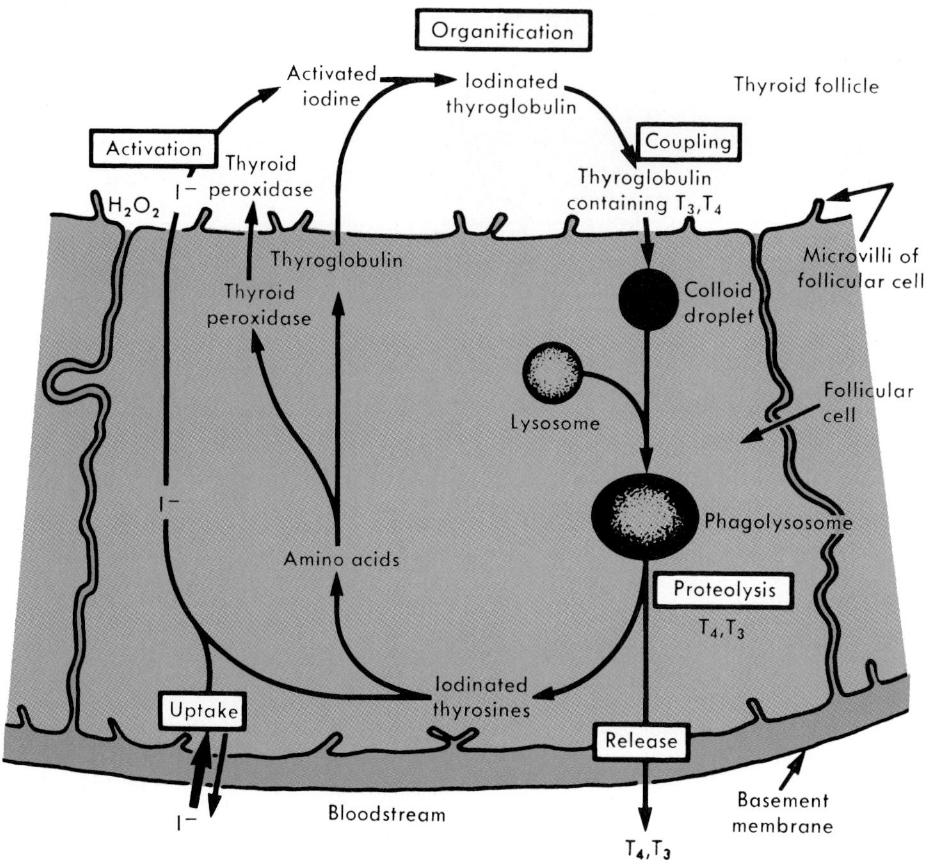

FIGURE 61-2

Synthesis of T_3 and T_4 by follicular cells within the thyroid gland. Single follicular cell is depicted. Cell base is in close contact with blood, and cell apex is in contact with colloid. These cells surround areas of colloid to form thyroid follicles. Parafollicular cells of thyroid gland do not directly contact colloid.

about one out of three molecules of thyroglobulin within the follicles. Normal thyroids thus contain a 30-day supply of T_3 and T_4 and a 20-day supply of iodine stored as MIT and DIT.

When release of thyroid hormones is required, TSH stimulates microvilli of the follicular cells to move droplets of colloid into the cell. The colloid droplets fuse with lysosomes inside the cells to form vesicles called *phagolysosomes.* The low pH and the protein-digesting enzymes from the lysosomes break thyroglobulin down to amino acids. This process releases T_3, T_4, MIT, and DIT into the cell. T_3 and T_4 are transported to the cell surface and are released into the blood. In contast, MIT and DIT are retained within the cell, and the iodine they contain is reclaimed for use in new hormone synthesis. Patients who lack the salvage pathway lose excessive iodide ion in urine and ultimately fail to produce sufficient thyroid hormones.

Once in blood, thyroid hormones are rapidly and almost completely bound to plasma proteins. Most of the hormones are bound to a special alpha-globulin called *thyroid-binding globulin* (TBG). A less important carrier is prealbumin. Very little thyroid hormone is bound to plasma albumin in normal persons because the thyroid hormones are so tightly bound to TBG. However, the amount of thyroid hormone that may be bound to TBG is limited. TBG can bind about 2.5 times more hormone than it ordinarily carries. When that limit is reached, the excess hormone is bound to albumin and prealbumin. These proteins are less avid carriers than TBG but have nearly unlimited capacity for hormones.

The relative distribution of T_3 and T_4 differs within the body. T_4 is much more abundant than T_3 in the thyroid and in blood. The thyroid gland normally releases 70 to 90 μg of T_4 daily but only 1 to 6 μg T_3. More important, because T_4 is rapidly converted to T_3 in most tissues, the most abundant form of thyroid hormone in target cells is T_3. T_3 is also the primary thyroid hormone that binds to nuclear receptors, setting off the metabolic events characteristic of thyroid action. For these reasons, T_3 may be considered to be the most important thyroid hormone.

Effects of Thyroid Hormone Deficiency

Hypothyroidism occurs when the production of thyroid hormones is insufficient to meet the body's demands. Mild hormone deficiencies produce minimum disease with vague symptoms, sometimes making the condition difficult to diagnose. Untreated patients may ultimately develop characteristic signs and symptoms related to slowed metabolic rates and changes in the central nervous system (CNS) (Table 61-1). The severe form of the disease is called **myxedema,** which may progress to a life-threatening coma with profoundly lowered metabolic rate, depressed CNS, and hypoventilation.

Hypothyroidism may develop in newborns because of an embryologic or genetic defect that arrests thyroid development or prevents its function. A child lacking adequate thyroid function during fetal development may appear nearly normal at birth since much of fetal development can proceed without fetal thyroid hormones. If the disease is not detected very soon after birth, however, irreversible brain damage and associated physical signs develop. Congenital hypothyroidism is called *cretinism.*

Hypothyroidism that develops after the neonatal period but before puberty is called juvenile hypothyroidism. The most prominent early sign of juvenile hypothyroidism is growth stunting. If not appropriately treated, juvenile hypothyroid patients suffer not only arrested growth but also other signs and symptoms associated with adult forms of the disease.

Effects of Excessive Thyroid Hormones

Hyperthyroidism occurs whenever excess thyroid hormones are released into circulation. The disease may range from mild forms displaying few of the symptoms shown in Table 61-1 to a severe condition called **thyroid storm** in which death may result from an abrupt rise in body temperature and vascular collapse. Increased thyroid hormone production may result from hyperfunction of the entire gland or from excessive output of one or more small nodules within the thyroid. A rare cause of hyperthyroidism is excess TSH, either from the pituitary gland (hypophysis) or from a tumor.

Hyperthyroidism may exist with or without thyroid nodules. The disease without nodules is the most common form and is referred to as toxic diffuse goiter, thyrotoxicosis, or **Graves' disease.** Many patients with this condition display exophthalmos (bulging eyes). Since many patients also have enlarged thyroid glands, another common name for this condition is *exophthalmic goiter.* Toxic nodular goiter produces the same general symptoms as Graves' disease, except that eye symptoms are rare in the nodular form.

Hyperthyroidism is rare in children and is most common in adults in the third or fourth decade of life. Women are af-

TABLE 61-1 Thyroid Disorders

CONDITION	SYMPTOMS	PHYSICAL APPEARANCE
Hypothyroidism, adult onset (also called *myxedema* and *Gull's disease*)	Diminished vigor and muscle weakness Reduced mental acuity Emotional changes, especially depression Slow relaxation of deep tendon reflexes Muscle cramps Constipation Decreased appetite Abnormal menses in females Slow pulse and enlarged heart Tendency to gain weight Lowered basal metabolic rate	Puffy face and eyes Thin, coarse hair and eyebrows Dry, scaly, cold, and slightly yellow skin Enlarged tongue Slow, husky speech Dull or slow-witted appearance
Hypothyroidism, congenital (cretinism)		
At birth	Absence of distal femoral and proximal tibial epiphyses Slowed brain development	Essentially normal Slightly longer and heavier than normal
At 3 months with no treatment	Lethargy Feeding difficulty Constipation Neonatal jaundice, persistent Respiratory distress Hoarse cry Intermittent cyanosis	Enlarged tongue Puffy face and thick neck Poor muscle tone Depressed nasal bridge with broad, flat nose Distended abdomen Umbilical hernia Short legs
Hyperthyroidism (also called *thyrotoxicosis* or *Graves' disease*)	Cardiac arrhythmia Enlarged thyroid gland Rapid pulse rate Increased basal metabolic rate Muscle weakness and wasting Fine tremor Heat intolerance Weight loss in most patients	Restlessness or nervousness Abrupt actions and speech Warm, moist palms Loosening of fingernails from nail beds Bulging eyes with sclera visible all around iris White, unpigmented patches on skin (vitiligo)

fected more often than men, but the reasons are not clear. Graves' disease may be precipitated in women by puberty, pregnancy, or menopause. Subacute thyroiditis can produce a reversible hyperthyroidism. This condition seems to appear sometime after recovery from viral diseases and may be caused by the infectious process.

Therapeutic Agents: Thyroid Gland

Diagnosis of Hypothyroidism

Hypothyroidism is diagnosed by the judicious use of a combination of the thyroid function tests summarized in Table 61-2. An understanding of these tests requires knowledge of normal thyroid physiology and an understanding of the negative feedback regulation of the thyroid (see Chapter 59).

In **primary hypothyroidism** the thyroid gland is defective. The diagnosis of primary hypothyroidism requires establishing that a patient has lower-than-normal thyroid hormone levels and elevated levels of TSH in the blood. Of the many tests available, TSH determinations are the most widely used. Free thyroxine (FT_4) levels are lower than normal in 80% to 90% of hypothyroid patients tested. Serum T_4 or T_3 uptake may also be measured, although these tests may be affected by conditions unrelated to thyroid disease that change the serum concentration of TBG (see Table 61-2).

Thyroidal uptake of iodine is also lowered in hypothyroidism, but this test is seldom useful in diagnosing the disease since thyroidal uptake is affected by intake of iodine, which may come in food or drugs. The patient may be unaware that iodine is being taken. For example, potassium iodide, used an an expectorant, is a constituent of several prescription cough medicines.

Hypothyroidism may arise for reasons other than primary failure of the thyroid gland. For example, if the pituitary fails to release adequate TSH, insufficient thyroid hormone is made, and **secondary hypothyroidism** develops. More rarely patients with damage to the hypothalamus fail to produce thyrotropin-releasing hormone (TRH), which is required to stimulate TSH production in the pituitary (see Chapter 59); this condition is called *tertiary hypothyroidism.*

Secondary and tertiary hypothyroidism may be distinguished from primary hypothyroidism by measuring TSH. In primary hypothyroidism TSH is elevated by the natural action of the negative feedback system attempting to elevate thyroid hormone levels, but TSH levels are low or undetectable in the other two forms of hypothyroidism. If the TSH assay is not available, a TSH test may be performed in which injected TSH is expected to stimulate T_4 formation and release in secondary or tertiary hypothyroidism but not in primary hypothyroidism (see Table 61-2).

Secondary and tertiary hypothyroidism may be distinguished from each other by the protirelin (TRH) test, which measures the ability of the hypophysis to respond to its normal regulatory hormone (see Table 61-2). If TSH rises after TRH administration, the implication is that the hypothalamus is defective, and both the anterior pituitary and the thyroid would be capable of normal function if properly stimulated.

Treatment of Hypothyroidism: Replacement Therapy

Treatment of hypothyroidism requires replacement therapy with the thyroid hormones. The goal of therapy is to produce the euthyroid state (normal thyroid hormone levels). Several preparations containing natural or synthetic forms of the hormones are available (Table 61-3).

Thyroid hormones

Mechanism of Action

Thyroid hormones used in replacement therapy have exactly the same actions as the hormones naturally produced in the body. Basal metabolic rates are increased by actions on nuclear receptors in skeletal muscle, heart, liver, and kidneys.

Pharmacokinetics

T_3 and T_4 are metabolized by the liver to glucuronide and sulfate derivatives, which then are eliminated in bile. No significant reuptake of the hormones occurs from the gut. Other hormone destruction occurs in the target tissues, where the hormones are deiodinated and transformed to inactive products. Elimination of thyroid hormones used for replacement therapy is the same as for the normal hormones.

The protein-binding properties of thyroid hormones explain some clinically important differences between these agents. T_4, being more highly protein bound, leaves the blood more slowly than does T_3. Therefore the onset of action for T_4 is about 2 days, whereas T_3 effects may be expected within 6 hours of administration (Figure 61-3). Moreover, T_4, which is bound to plasma protein, is less available for elimination, excretion, or tissue biotransformation than is T_3. Thus T_4 persists longer in the body than T_3.

The effects of a single equimolar dose (same number of molecules) of T_3 and T_4 are shown in Figure 61-3, in which the BMR was followed as an indicator of thyroid hormone action in hypothyroid subjects. When patients are switched from T_4 to T_3, or vice versa, these different time courses must be considered. For example, a patient being switched from a preparation containing primarily T_4 to T_3 alone might suffer from excessive thyroid hormone action if started on full T_3 doses immediately after T_4 administration is terminated. Therefore patients are given small doses of T_3 after T_4 is stopped, and the dose of T_3 is gradually raised as necessary to maintain the euthyroid state.

Uses

Thyroid hormones are primarily used to treat thyroid deficiency. They also have a role in control of goiter and thyroid carcinoma. They may also occasionally be used for diagnosis. Thyroid hormones should never be used in weight loss programs.

Patients with myxedemic coma must be treated aggressively with thyroid hormones, glucocorticoids, and other sup-

TABLE 61-2 Tests to Evaluate Thyroid Function

TEST	PROCEDURE	DIAGNOSTIC USE	NORMAL VALUES	COMMENTS
Serum T_4	Total serum T_4 is measured by competitive protein-binding test or radioimmunoassay.	To distinguish hyperthyroid or hypothyroid conditions from euthyroid state.	5-12 μg/100 ml serum	Conditions that elevate TBG levels (e.g., pregnancy or estrogen use) also elevate total serum T_4 levels. Lowered TBG levels in cirrhosis or nephrotic syndrome also lower total serum T_4 levels. In both situations free hormone levels are usually normal, and patient is functionally euthyroid.
Free thyroxine (FT_4)	FT_4 is measured by radioimmunoassay or equilibrium dialysis.	To distinguish hyperthyroid or hypothyroid conditions from euthyroid state.	1-2.5 ng/100 ml	Normal values may vary greatly from laboratory to laboratory.
T_3 uptake (T_3U) or resin T_3 uptake (RT_3U)	Test measures degree of saturation of patient's TBG with endogenous thyroid hormones.	To distinguish hyperthyroid or hypothyroid conditions from euthyroid state.	25-45%, or 0.82-1.35 when expressed as ratio of T_3U to normal	Hyperthyroidism elevates ratio; hypothyroidism lowers ratio. Levels of TBG and T_4 in blood affect test more than do T_3 values.
Serum T_3	Total serum T_3 is measured by specific radioimmunoassay.	To distinguish hyperthyroid conditions from euthyroid state.	0.08-0.20 μg/100 ml	Test is not useful in hypothyroidism since T_3 may be more abundant than T_4.
Serum TSH	Serum TSH is measured by specific radioimmunoassay.	To distinguish hypothyroid conditions from euthyroid state; to distinguish primary from secondary hypothyroidism.	0.5-5 μU/ml	Primary hypothyroidism shows elevated TSH levels; secondary hypothyroidism caused by pituitary failure shows little or no TSH.
Protirelin test (TRH test)	Synthetic TRH (500 μg) is given intravenously, causing peak release of TSH 30 min later in patients with normal pituitary glands.	To distinguish hypothyroidism caused by pituitary failure from other forms of hypothyroidism.	Peak levels of TSH seen in normal patients are 5-35 μU/ml serum.	No rise is usually observed in serum TSH level in hyperthyroid patients.
Thyroid uptake of radioiodine	Radioactivity in thyroid is measured 4, 6, and 24 hr after administration of tracer dose of radioactive iodine.	To distinguish hyperthyroid and hypothyroid conditions from euthyroid state.	Normal glands take up 10-35% of tracer dose in 24 hr.	This test may be affected by dietary intake of iodine or by use of iodine-containing medications or antithyroid drugs.
TSH test	Bovine TSH is given intramuscularly after which serum T_3 and T_4 or radioiodine uptake is measured.	To distinguish primary from secondary hypothyroidism.	Normal thyroids respond by increasing iodine uptake and T_4 release.	This test is rarely used when TSH levels are to be measured.
Thyroid suppression tests	T_3 (75 μg) is given daily for 7 days. Radioiodine uptake by thyroid gland is measured before and after test.	To distinguish hyperthyroid conditions from euthyroid state.	Uptake is 50% or less of pretest uptake.	This test may be dangerous for older adult patients, weakened patients, or patients with heart disease.

TABLE 61-3 Drugs for Thyroid Replacement Therapy or Diagnosis

GENERIC NAME	TRADE NAME	ADMINISTRATION/DOSAGE	COMMENTS
Thyroid Hormones			
Levothyroxine	Eltroxin† Levothroid Levoxyl Synthroid*	ORAL: *Adults*—Initially 12.5-50 μg daily; gradually increase to maintenance dose (usually 75-125 μg daily). FDA pregnancy category A. *Children:* 2-6 μg/kg daily as single dose. INTRAVENOUS: *Adults*—Up to 500 μg daily.	This chemically pure form of T_4 is preferred therapy for hypothyroidism. IV form is used for myxedema coma.
Liothyronine	Cytomel*	ORAL: *Adults*—Initially 2.5-25 μg daily; gradually increase to maintenance dose (usually 25-50 μg daily). FDA pregnancy category A.	This chemically pure form of T_3 may be used for adult hypothyroidism but is not used for cretinism because T_3 may not cross blood-brain barrier as well as T_4 does.
Liotrix	Thyrolar	ORAL: *Adults and children*—Initially 12.5 μg of T_4 with 3.1 μg of T_3 daily; gradually increase to maintenance dose (usually 50-100 μg T_4 with 12.5-25 μg T_3). FDA pregnancy category A.	This combination of chemically pure T_4 and T_3 in 4:1 ratio may be used for hypothyroidism.
Thyroid	Thyrar	ORAL: *Adults and children*—Initially 7.5-15 mg daily; gradually increase to maintenance dose (usually 60-120 mg daily). FDA pregnancy category A.	This crude preparation from thyroid glands contains variable amounts of T_4 and T_3. Dosage is difficult to adjust and maintain.
Adenohypophyseal Hormones			
Protirelin	Relefact TRH*	INTRAVENOUS: *Adults*—0.5 mg. *Children*—7 mg/kg.	This synthetic tripeptide is identical to natural hypothalimic hormone. It is used for diagnosis (Table 61-2).
Thyrotropin	Thytropar*	INTRAMUSCULAR, SUBCUTANEOUS: *Adults and children*—10 IU daily for 1-7 days. FDA pregnancy category C.	Thyrotropin is natural peptide TSH that is extracted from animals. It is used for diagnosis (Table 61-2).

*Available in Canada and United States.
†Available in Canada only.

portive measures. Rapid replacement with thyroid hormones is necessary. Since T_3 is well absorbed from the gastrointestinal (GI) tract, T_3 tablets may be crushed and given through a nasogastric tube. Alternatively, T_4 may be injected intravenously.

Adverse Reactions and Contraindications

In a newly diagnosed hypothyroid patient, thyroid hormones are started at low doses and increased at varying intervals until the euthyroid state is achieved. Thyroid USP and levothyroxine doses are doubled every 2 weeks, but liothyronine doses are doubled weekly until symptoms are controlled. These gradually increasing doses are used because a sudden return to adequate thyroid hormone levels produces acute stress on several body systems. One common and dangerous example observed occasionally even with low doses is angina pectoris, coronary occlusion, or stroke in older adult or predisposed patients (see box). Another difficulty may be relative adrenal insufficiency, which arises in patients with inadequate pituitary function who suffer secondary hypothyroidism and secondary adrenal insufficiency. If thyroid hormone therapy is started in these patients without also restoring adequate glucocorticoid levels, they may suffer a dangerous adrenal crisis.

Toxicity

Overdosage with thyroid hormones produces signs of hyperthyroidism (see Table 61-2).

Interactions

Catecholamines must sometimes be used to combat the shocklike symptoms found in myxedemic coma. Patients so treated are especially at risk for cardiac arrhythmias since catecholamines and thyroid hormones may cause this dangerous consequence.

Cholestyramine or colestipol may impede oral absorption of thyroid hormones; doses can be adjusted, based on thyroid function tests.

Coumarins or other anticoagulants may be influenced by thyroid function; doses can be adjusted, based on prothrombin times.

Specific thyroid hormone preparations

Levothyroxine

Levothyroxine is a pure synthetic form of the natural thyroid hormone T_4. It therefore has high affinity for serum proteins, long half-life in blood, and is converted to T_3 by peripheral tissues. Levothyroxine is the preferred drug for replacement therapy of hypothyroidism.

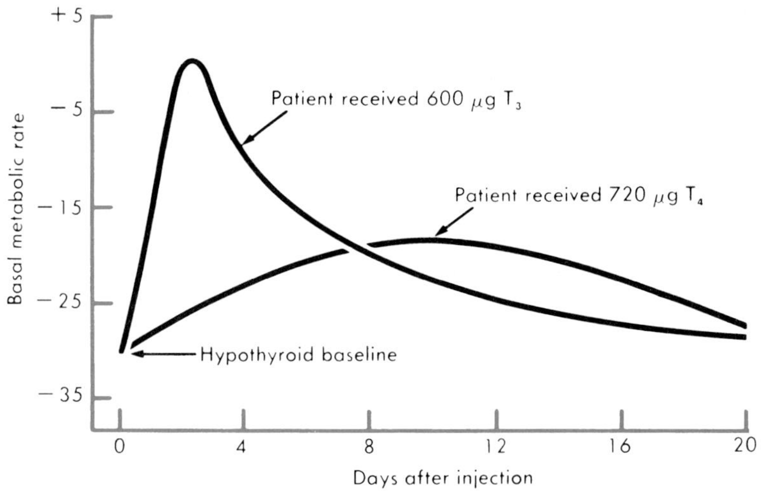

FIGURE 61-3
Time course of thyroid hormone effects. Patient in each test received single oral dose of medication indicated. Doses T_3 and T_4 administered are equimolar (contain equal number of molecules).

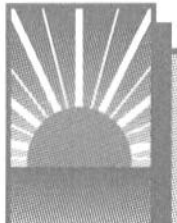

GERIATRIC CONSIDERATION

Thyroid Hormones

THE PROBLEM

Adults over the age of 60 may be more sensitive to the actions of thyroid hormones than are younger adults. This sensitivity may place older adults at risk for angina or strokes when thyroid hormone replacement is started.

THE SOLUTION

Older adults should be started on low doses of thyroid hormones initially. The doses should be increased by small amounts every 3 to 4 weeks, unless symptoms of stress appear. The initial doses for older adults may be one fourth to one half the normal dose for mildly hypothyroid younger adults. Maintenance doses are the minimum required to reverse the signs of hypothyroidism.

Liothyronine

Liothyronine is a pure synthetic form of the natural thyroid hormone T_3. It therefore has a shorter half-life in blood than T_4 and is converted to inactive products in peripheral tissues. In addition, T_3 seems to be better absorbed orally than T_4. Liothyronine is the most potent thyroid hormone, with 0.025 mg being equivalent to 1 mg of levothyroxine.

Liotrix

Liotrix is a thyroid preparation that contains both pure synthetic T_4 and T_3 in the ratio of 4:1. This mixture was designed to produce normal thyroid function tests when therapy is adequate, but there is little evidence that liotrix has any clinical advantage over levothyroxine. One tablet of liotrix containing 50 µg of T_4 and 12.5 µg of T_3 is equivalent to 1 mg of levothyroxine.

Thyroid USP

Thyroid USP is a defatted extract of whole thyroid glands. It contains T_4 and T_3 in the natural ratio of 2.5:1. The iodine content of these preparations is regulated by law in the United States, but thyroid hormone activity is not directly standardized, so variations in strength are possible. Considerable potency also may be lost on long storage or if the powder becomes moist. In terms of biologic activity, 60 mg of thyroid USP is equivalent to approximately 1 mg of levothyroxine.

Diagnosis of Hyperthyroidism

Hyperthyroidism is characterized by elevated serum T_4, serum T_3, free T_4, and free T_3 levels in most patients. Thus diagnostic tests that directly measure one of these parameters (serum T_4 and serum T_3 testing) are most often used (see Table 61-2). The T_3 resin uptake test also may be used because hyperthyroidism increases the degree of TBG saturation with thyroid hormones. Radioactive iodine uptake also may be measured and is useful in distinguishing between various forms of hyperthyroidism. These diagnostic tests form part of a larger clinical picture. Much information is gained by determining the size of the thyroid by palpation, checking for nodules in the thyroid, and conducting a thyroid scan to measure the pattern of radioactive iodine concentration in the gland.

Diagnosis of Graves' disease has been aided by the realization that the disease has an immunologic basis. In this condition the thyroid is chronically overstimulated by immunoglobulins that supplant TSH as the regulator of thyroid function. These immunoglobulins are found in the sera of nearly all patients who have Graves' disease, and the amounts of the immunoglobulins correlate with the severity of the hyperthyroidism observed.

Treatment of Hyperthyroidism

Hyperthyroidism most often is controlled with drugs or radioactive iodine. The drugs fall into two main classes, those that control the symptoms of hyperthyroidism and those that lower the production of T_3 and T_4 by the thyroid.

Propranolol

Propranolol, a beta-adrenergic blocking agent discussed in Chapters 10 and 13, represents the class of drugs that controls symptoms of hyperthyroidism but produces no significant long-term change in thyroid hormone levels. Propranolol is effective because it alters the response of peripheral tissues to high circulating levels of thyroid hormones. Blockade of beta-receptors reduces palpitation, tremor, sweating, proximal muscle weakness, mental agitation, and cardiac arrhythmias. One advantage of propranolol therapy is that clinical improvement is seen rapidly. With many other drugs, relief of symptoms may be greatly delayed. Propranolol or other blockers of beta-adrenergic receptors may be used to prepare a hyperthyroid patient for surgery.

Thioamides

Mechanism of Action

Two thioamides, methimazole and propylthiouracil, currently are used in the United States (Table 61-4). The thioamides inhibit the synthesis of thyroid hormones, blocking each step in synthesis except iodine uptake (see Figure 61-2). Propylthiouracil also inhibits the conversion of T_4 to T_3 in peripheral tissues. Since these compounds are primarily enzyme inhibitors, they do not directly destroy thyroid tissue but only prevent its excessive action.

Thioamide action on the thyroid gland is immediate, and reduced hormone synthesis occurs within hours. Observable clinical response to the drugs, however, does not appear for days or weeks, the period required for stored thyroid hormones to be depleted. A patient's condition may be maintained for months by thioamide therapy, provided the hyperthyroidism is well controlled during that time. Usually, after about 1 year, the thioamide is withdrawn and thyroid function is reevaluated. Many patients remain euthyroid after thioamides are discontinued. For this 15% to 50% of patients treated, no further therapy may ever be required.

Pharmacokinetics

Thioamides taken orally are rapidly absorbed and concentrated in the thyroid. The drugs also distribute to other tissues and cross the placenta to enter the fetus. Thioamides appear in the milk of nursing mothers, and they are metabolized and excreted in urine.

Uses

Thioamides are used only for control of hyperthyroidism.

Adverse Reactions and Contraindications

Common reactions to thioamides include fever, itching, and skin rash. Blood dyscrasias or peripheral neuropathy may occur. Propylthiouracil is especially associated with pain and swelling of joints or with a lupuslike syndrome. Methimazole may cause dizziness or alterations in taste.

Patients who have had allergic or other severe reactions to thioamides should not receive the drugs again. Patients with impaired hepatic function may require reduced doses.

TABLE 61-4 Drugs Used to Treat Hyperthyroidism

GENERIC NAME	TRADE NAME	ADMINISTRATION/DOSAGE	COMMENTS
Thioamides			
Methimazole	Tapazole*	ORAL: *Adults*—Initially 15-60 mg daily in 1 or 2 doses; maintenance: 5-30 mg daily in 1 or 2 doses. FDA pregnancy category D. *Children*—0.4 mg/kg initially in 1 or 2 doses; maintenance: 0.2 mg/kg daily.	Inhibits thyroid hormone synthesis but not release.
Propylthiouracil	Generic	ORAL: *Adults*—Initially 300-900 mg daily; maintenance: 50-600 mg daily. FDA pregnancy category D. *Children 6-10 yr*—50-150 mg daily. *Children >10 yr*—50-300 mg daily.	Inhibits thyroid hormone synthesis but not release; also inhibits conversion of T_4 to T_3 in peripheral tissues.
Beta-Adrenergic Blocker			
Propranolol	Inderal*	ORAL: *Adults*—10-40 mg 3 or 4 times daily. FDA pregnancy category C.	Controls symptoms of hyperthyroidism but does not lower T_4 and T_3 release from thyroid.
Iodine			
Potassium iodide	Pima	ORAL: *Adults*—250 mg 3 times daily as presurgical medication.	Produces short-term inhibition of thyroid hormone synthesis by direct action on thyroid.
^{131}I as NaI	Iodotope	ORAL: *Adults*—4-10 mCi (148-370 megabecquerels) as single dose for Graves' disease. For thyroid carcinoma: single doses of up to 150 mCi (5.5 gigabecquerels) may be used. Smaller doses are used for diagnosis.	This radionuclide is concentrated in thyroid and releases radiation, which destroys thyroid tissue.

*Available in Canada and United States.

Toxicity

Overdosage with thioamides results in hypothyroidism. The signs are the same as for non–drug-induced hypothyroidism (see Table 61-2).

Interactions

Any preparation containing iodine may interfere with the antithyroid action of thioamides. Such preparations may include amiodarone, iodine solution, potassium iodide, and certain contrast imaging dyes.

Coumarins or other anticoagulants may be influenced by thyroid function; doses can be adjusted, based on prothrombin times.

Digitalis dosage may be influenced by thyroid status. Doses of the cardiac glycoside may require reduction as hyperthyroidism is brought under control.

Radioactive iodine uptake may be reduced by thioamides. This action can interfere with diagnostic tests.

Iodine

Iodine is required for synthesis of thyroid hormones, but high concentrations of iodine suppress continued uptake of iodine by the thyroid gland and thus slow synthesis of thyroid hormones. Suppression of hormone synthesis is by no means complete with iodine administration, and many patients return to the hyperthyroid state even with continued high doses. Iodine is seldom used today for long-term suppression of a hyperactive thyroid gland. The most common current use of iodine is to prepare a hyperthyroid patient for surgery. Iodine not only suppresses thyroid function but also reduces vascularization of the gland, thus reducing surgical risk. Iodine pretreatment is especially important for hyperthyroid patients who have received thioamide therapy because those drugs increase vascularization of the thyroid gland. In addition, iodine may be used as part of emergency therapy for hyperthyroid crisis. In this situation, iodine is given intravenously after a thioamide has been started.

Radioactive iodine

Radioactive iodine is used to treat hyperthyroidism and for diagnosis. Therapy depends on the ability of the radioactive iodine to be concentrated in the thyroid gland, where it then destroys surrounding tissue by emitting low-energy radiation. Iodine doses are small. The use of radioactive iodine allows the thyroid to be functionally destroyed without resorting to surgery. Nearly all patients treated with radioactive iodine ultimately become hypothyroid and require replacement therapy with thyroid hormones. The incidence of hypothyroidism is about 10% of treated patients during the first year after therapy and about 3% per year thereafter. Because of the likelihood of hypothyroidism, patients should be urged to return periodically for thyroid evaluation.

NURSING PROCESS OVERVIEW

Thyroid Therapy

Assessment

The nursing process in diseases of the thyroid gland is the same, whether the problem is hyperthyroidism or hypothyroidism. In most cases the original problem develops insidiously. Obtain a complete assessment of the patient, including temperature, pulse, respiration, blood pressure, weight, history of weight changes, level of energy, mood, subjective feeling, and response to temperature. Check the height of children. Question family members to determine onset of symptoms. Check thyroid function test results and blood glucose levels.

Nursing Diagnoses

- Self-concept disturbance
- Activity intolerance related to fatigue related to excessive metabolic rate

Patient Outcomes

The patient will discuss changes in feelings about self. The patient will identify methods to increase activity while medications are being adjusted.

Planning/Implementation

Monitor the temperature, pulse, respiration, blood pressure, weight, height of children, and blood glucose level. Question about the subjective response to therapy. If weight reduction is an additional goal of therapy, teach about diet, or refer as needed. If radioactive iodine is used, follow hospital procedures for the handling of radioactive materials.

Evaluation

Before discharge, check that the patient can explain the action of the drug and how to take the prescribed dose. Other parameters the patient should monitor and record at home include pulse, weight, and height. Explain the side effects that may occur and what to do about them, adjustments needed in the treatment of other medical problems (e.g., changes in insulin or anticoagulant doses), the need for continuing the medication, and the need to wear an identification tag or bracelet. With radioactive iodine, the patient will not receive long-term drug therapy but should be able to explain what symptoms should be reported to the physician.

Nursing Implications Summary

Natural and Synthetic Thyroid Hormones

Drug Administration

- The side effects of natural and synthetic thyroid hormones are essentially the same as the symptoms of hyperthyroidism; see Table 61-1.
- Assess for headache, insomnia, nervousness, and tremor.
- Monitor blood pressure and pulse. If pulse is over 100 beats per min in an adult, withhold the dose, and notify the physician.
- Monitor the electrocardiogram (ECG) before starting therapy and at regular intervals.
- Monitor weight. Assess for edema, pallor, and fatigue.
- Monitor thyroid function tests. In children, monitor growth, bone age, and psychomotor development.

Intravenous Levothyroxine

- Read the manufacturer's instructions; different brands permit different diluents. Administer at a rate of 0.1 mg or less over 1 minute. Monitor vital signs.
- Monitor thyroid function tests.

Patient and Family Education

- Review the anticipated benefits and possible side effects of drug therapy with the patient.
- Inform the patient that several weeks to months of therapy may be required before full benefit is seen. Encourage the patient to return for regular follow-up and blood tests.
- Instruct the patient to take doses in the morning to avoid nighttime insomnia.
- Warn a diabetic patient to monitor blood glucose levels carefully since an adjustment in diet or insulin dose may be needed.
- Encourage the patient to wear a medical identification tag or bracelet stating that thyroid medication is used regularly.
- Instruct the patient not to switch brands of medication without consulting the physician or the pharmacist.
- Instruct a female patient to keep a record of menstrual periods since menstrual irregularities may occur.
- Remind the patient to inform all health care providers of all drugs being used. Regular use of thyroid replacement hormones may contribute to interactions with other drugs.

Protirelin

Drug Administration

- Have the patient fast for 6 hours before the test, or restrict the diet to low fat before the test.
- Have the patient assume the supine position before administering protirelin and maintain the supine position for at least 15 minutes after drug administration. Monitor vital signs.
- Protirelin may be administered undiluted, 1 dose over 15 to 30 seconds.

Thyrotropin

Drug Administration

- Thyrotropin is for intramuscular (IM) or subcutaneous use. Reconstitute with the diluent provided by the manufacturer.
- Assess for flushing of face, headache, nausea and vomiting, and allergic reaction. Anaphylaxis is rare. Remain with patient for 10 to 15 minutes after administering a dose. Monitor vital signs.

Methimazole and Propylthiouracil

Drug Administration

- Overdose would produce clinical hypothyroidism; see Table 61-1.
- Assess for tingling of fingers and toes. Monitor weight. Inspect for skin changes or hair loss.
- Monitor complete blood count (CBC), white blood cell (WBC) differential, and thyroid and liver function tests.

Patient and Family Education

- Review the anticipated benefits and possible side effects of drug therapy with the patient. Side effects may not appear for days to weeks after beginning therapy; remind the patient to report any new side effects. See the patient problem box on bleeding tendencies (p. 586).
- Instruct the patient to report signs of agranulocytosis such as fever, chills, sore throat, and unexplained bleeding or bruising.
- Instruct the patient to take doses with meals or a snack to lessen gastric irritation.
- The patient may take doses without meals; but however doses are taken, they should be taken the same way each time, either always with meals or always on an empty stomach.
- Encourage the patient to return as instructed for follow-up.
- Remind the patient to inform all health care providers of all drugs being used.
- If more than 1 dose per day is prescribed, it is best to space doses evenly throughout the day. Work with the patient to develop a satisfactory dosing schedule.

Iodine

Drug Administration/Patient and Family Education

- Dilute an oral iodine solution well in juice, milk, or beverage choice. The solutions may stain teeth; take with a straw.
- Signs of iodism (excessive iodine) include metallic taste in the mouth, sneezing, swollen and tender thyroid gland, vomiting, and bloody diarrhea. Concomitant excessive use of over-the-counter (OTC) preparations containing iodine (e.g., asthma or cough preparations) may contribute to iodism.
- Consult the manufacturer's literature for information about intravenous (IV) iodine.

NURSING IMPLICATIONS SUMMARY—cont'd

Radioactive Iodine

Drug Administration/Patient and Family Education

- The radiation dose of radioactive iodine is not high, but those preparing or administering the preparation should be careful to avoid spilling the mixture on themselves or on countertops. Wear rubber gloves. Follow agency protocol for handling radioactive substances.
- Side effects are rare but include soreness over the thyroid gland and, in rare cases, difficulty in swallowing and breathing because of gland enlargement. Eventually, many patients who take radioactive iodine will become hypothyroid.

CRITICAL THINKING

APPLICATION

1. What is the function of the follicular cells of the thyroid gland?
2. What hormones are produced by the follicular cells of the thyroid gland?
3. What is the function of TSH? Where is it produced?
4. What are the steps in thyroid hormone synthesis?
5. How much T_3 and T_4 is stored in the thyroid gland?
6. What is the function of thyroglobulin?
7. How are the thyroid hormones transported in blood?
8. How are thyroid hormones eliminated?
9. Which of the thyroid hormones is found most abundantly in target cells?
10. In primary hypothyroidism, how do blood concentrations of TSH and thyroid hormones differ from normal?
11. What is the difference between secondary hypothyroidism and tertiary hypothyroidism?
12. What is the treatment for all forms of hypothyroidism?
13. Which of the available preparations of thyroid hormones is the most potent?
14. How do T_3 and T_4 differ in onset and duration of action?
15. Which thyroid hormone is available as an injectable preparation?
16. How does Graves' disease differ from subacute thyroiditis?
17. What general classes of drugs are used to treat hyperthyroidism?
18. To what class of drugs does propranolol belong? Why is it useful in treating hyperthyroidism?
19. What is the mechanism of action of the thioamides?
20. How are the thioamides distributed in the body?
21. How may radioactive iodine be used in the treatment of hyperthyroidism?

CRITICAL THINKING

1. What are the characteristic signs of hypothyroidism? How should you assess for these?
2. What side effects may occur with replacement therapy of thyroid hormones? How should you assess for these?

CHAPTER 62

Drugs Affecting Calcium Metabolism

OBJECTIVES

After studying this chapter, you should be able to do the following:

- *Describe the hormones that influence calcium metabolism.*
- *Discuss the therapeutic roles for vitamin D.*
- *Describe the types of patients who should receive calcium supplements.*
- *Develop a nursing care plan for a patient receiving dialysis therapy who is receiving calcifediol.*
- *Develop a nursing care plan for a patient receiving dietary calcium supplements.*

KEY TERMS

calcitonin
parafollicular cells
parathyroid glands
parathyroid hormone
vitamin D

CHAPTER OVERVIEW

Calcium is a crucial element required for the proper function of all cells and tissues. Close control of calcium levels is required because very small changes in blood calcium levels can profoundly alter many cellular functions, with effects on many body systems (Table 62-1). Because of this fundamental role in maintaining function, calcium uptake, distribution, and elimination are very tightly controlled in the body to maintain a constant concentration of 4.7 to 5.6 mEq/L in plasma or serum. The overall interaction of parathyroid hormone, calcitonin, and vitamin D allows the body to maintain blood calcium levels within this very narrow margin. This chapter discusses the therapeutic roles of these regulators of calcium metabolism and that of calcium itself.

TABLE 62-1 Symptoms of Altered Calcium Balance

HYPERCALCEMIA	HYPOCALCEMIA
Early Symptoms	**Early Symptoms**
Central nervous system	Hyperreflexia
Depression	Muscle spasms
Headache	Paresthesias
Irritability	Positive Chvostek's sign
Tiredness or weakness	
Gastrointestinal tract	
Anorexia	
Constipation	
Dry mouth	
Other	
Increased thirst	
Metallic taste	
Late Symptoms	**Late Symptoms**
Central nervous system	Central nervous system
Confusion	Convulsions
Drowsiness	Cardiovascular
Cardiovascular	Arrhythmias
Arrhythmias	Other
Hypertension	Difficulty breathing
Gastrointestinal tract	Laryngeal spasm
Nausea	Tetany
Vomiting	
Other	
Sensitivity to light	
Large urine volume	

Therapeutic Rationale: Regulators of Calcium Metabolism

Parafollicular Cells

Parafollicular cells are found in the thyroid gland, where they constitute about 10% to 20% of total thyroid cells. Unlike most thyroid cells, parafollicular cells do not synthesize thyroxine or triiodothyronine. Instead, the parafollicular cells synthesize the peptide hormone called **calcitonin.**

Calcitonin

Physiologic Action

Calcitonin in animals is thought to prevent blood calcium levels from exceeding the normal range after meals; its physiologic role in humans has not been resolved. Nevertheless, calcitonin does have direct effects when administered exogenously. The primary effect of the hormone is to prevent the loss of calcium from bone. This action lowers the amount of calcium entering the blood.

Regulation of Secretion

Calcitonin synthesis and secretion is stimulated by high concentrations of calcium ion in plasma. The released calcitonin tends to lower plasma calcium concentrations back toward the normal range.

Effects of Calcitonin Deficiency or Excess

Calcitonin deficiency is not a well-documented condition, perhaps because some calcitonin is found in thymus and parathyroid glands, as well as in the thyroid. Calcitonin excess is uncommon but may arise from medullary carcinomas of the thyroid, which arise from parafollicular cells.

Parathyroid Glands

The **parathyroid glands** are closely associated with the thyroid. These small bodies normally lie behind the lobes of the thyroid but rarely may be found within the thyroid (see Figure 61-1).

Parathyroid hormone

Physiologic Action

The parathyroid glands synthesize **parathyroid hormone,** a peptide whose major function is to maintain blood calcium levels above the critical threshold required for body function. In many ways, parathyroid hormone acts opposite to calcitonin. For example, parathyroid hormone increases reabsorption of calcium from bones, lowers renal excretion of calcium, and along with vitamin D increases calcium absorption from the intestine; all these actions tend to raise calcium concentration in blood.

Regulation of Secretion

Parathyroid hormone secretion is regulated by calcium concentrations in the blood. As the calcium concentration falls, secretion of parathyroid hormone is stimulated, and more calcium is mobilized from bone to enter the blood. High calcium concentrations slow secretion of parathyroid hormone.

Effects of Parathyroid Hormone Deficiency: Hypoparathyroidism

Hypoparathyroidism usually results after thyroid or parathyroid surgery, but idiopathic (unknown cause) forms of the disease exist. Hypoparathyroidism is associated with hypocalcemia. This electrolyte imbalance produces symptoms such as paresthesia, muscle spasms, tetany, and convulsions (see Table 62-1). In theory, parathyroid hormone could be used to raise blood calcium levels in conditions in which blood levels are abnormally low; however, administration of one of the forms of vitamin D with or without calcium is the preferred treatment.

Effects of Parathyroid Hormone Excess: Hyperparathyroidism

Hyperparathyroidism usually arises from excess secretion of parathyroid hormone from a tumor. Many patients with this condition show decreases in bone calcification as a result of the action of parathyroid hormone. High amounts of calcium are excreted by these patients, and renal stones are common. No specific inhibitors of parathyroid release are available for clinical use; thus therapy consists primarily of surgery to remove the source of excess parathyroid hormone synthesis.

Dietary Regulators of Calcium Metabolism

Vitamin D

The term **vitamin D** refers to a group of lipid-soluble substances that may be formed or interconverted in the body. Cholecalciferol, or vitamin D_3, may be formed from cholesterol in skin when it is exposed to sunlight. The vitamin may also be taken in the diet.

Depending on what form of the vitamin is ingested, various biotransformations are possible. The liver converts vitamin D_3 to the more active 25-hydroxyvitamin D_3. The kidney converts 25-hydroxyvitamin D_3 to calcitriol, the most active metabolite of the vitamin.

Physiologic Action

Vitamin D acts like a hormone in the body, regulating calcium concentrations in concert with parathyroid hormone and calcitonin.

Specifically, vitamin D promotes the release of calcium and phosphate from bone, blocks renal excretion of these materials, and promotes their absorption from the gastrointestinal (GI) tract. All these actions increase calcium concentration in blood.

Vitamin D interacts with receptors in target cells throughout the body to produce its effects on calcium metabolism. The vitamin D receptor, like steroid receptors, is found in the cytoplasm of cells and moves to cell nuclei where the hormone-receptor complex influences gene expression.

Regulation of Secretion

Original synthesis of vitamin D_3 in skin occurs continuously, so long as exposure to sunlight is adequate. Formation of the most active form of vitamin D, calcitriol, is promoted by relative deficiencies of calcium, phosphate, or vitamin D. Active stimulation of the process occurs with parathyroid hormone, whereas very high vitamin D intake can inhibit conversion to the more active metabolite.

Effects of Vitamin D Deficiency

Vitamin D deficiency can occur in persons who are not adequately exposed to sunlight and who ingest a diet poor in the vitamin. A deficiency of the vitamin limits the amount of calcium that can be absorbed from the diet.

In children vitamin D deficiency leads to a condition called rickets in which the calcium that would normally be used to build bones is robbed to serve other life-supporting needs.

In adults a vitamin D deficiency may not produce visible signs; however, uncalcified bone matrix is produced.

Effects of Vitamin D Excess

The most common cause of vitamin D excess is overdosage with dietary supplements. The result is hypercalcemia (see Table 62-1).

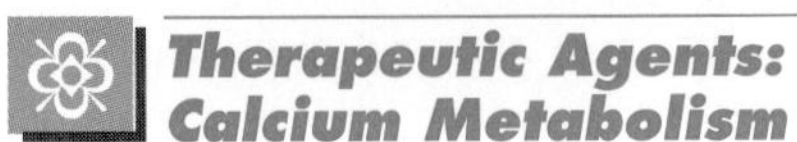

Therapeutic Agents: Calcium Metabolism

Metabolic Diseases

Calcitonin

Mechanism of Action

When calcitonin is used clinically, the effect sought is reduction of calcium release from bone.

Pharmacokinetics

As a protein, calcitonin must be administered parenterally, usually by subcutaneous or intramuscular (IM) injection. The absorbed protein is rapidly metabolized in blood, kidneys, and other tissues. The hypercalcemic effect of the hormone persists for several hours.

Uses

Calcitonin has been used to treat Paget's disease, in which excessive bone resorption leads to fragile bones. A synthetic form of salmon calcitonin (Table 62-2) is the most potent of the naturally occurring forms of the hormone. Synthetic human calcitonin is also used for Paget's disease.

Salmon calcitonin has been used to control postmenopausal osteoporosis, along with vitamin D and calcium supplements. This form of calcitonin is also occasionally used in emergencies to treat hypercalcemia.

Adverse Reactions and Contraindications

Many patients suffer nausea and vomiting, facial flushing, and occasional inflammatory reactions at the injection site. Since the hormone is a peptide and is administered in a gelatin solution, allergic reactions may occur. Synthetic human calcitonin may be less likely to cause allergic reactions than is salmon calcitonin. Allergic reactions to foreign proteins may increase the risk of reactions to calcitonin.

Toxicity

Overdosage of calcitonin may produce relative hypocalcemia, but the effect may be mild and short lived.

Interactions

Calcium or vitamin D preparations may antagonize the actions of calcitonin.

Edetate disodium

Mechanism of Action

Edetate disodium is a strong chelator of calcium, forming soluble complexes that are excreted readily by the kidneys. One gram of edetate disodium binds up to 120 mg of calcium. The effect is to rapidly lower blood calcium concentrations.

Pharmacokinetics

Edetate disodium is used by intravenous (IV) infusion with constant monitoring of serum calcium. Up to 95% of a dose

TABLE 62-2 Agents That Alter Calcium Metabolism

GENERIC NAME	TRADE NAME	ADMINISTRATION/DOSAGE	COMMENTS
Calcitonin human	Cibacalcin	SUBCUTANEOUS: *Adults*—Initially 0.5 mg daily; maintenance: 0.25 mg daily. FDA pregnancy category C.	Long-term for Paget's disease; lower risk of forming antibodies than salmon calcitonin.
Calcitonin salmon	Calcimar* Miacalcin	INTRAMUSCULAR, SUBCUTANEOUS: *Adults*—For Paget's disease: 100 IU daily initially; then 50 IU once daily or every other day. For postmenopausal osteoporosis: 100 IU once daily or every other day. For hypercalcemia: 4 IU/kg every 12 hr; increase up to 8 mg/kg every 6 hr. FDA pregnancy category C.	This most active form of calcitonin may cause formation of antibodies, which limits response over time.
Edetate disodium	Disotate Endrate	INTRAVENOUS: *Adults*—For hypercalcemia: 50 mg/kg over 24 hr for no more than 4 days; upper limit 3 gm daily. FDA pregnancy category C. *Children*—40 mg/kg in 24 hr.	This strong chelating agent removes excess calcium from system on short-term basis.
Etidronate	Didronel*	ORAL: *Adults*—For Paget's disease: 5 mg/kg daily for up to 6 mo. For heterotropic ossification: 20 mg/kg for 1 mo before and 3 mo after hip replacement. For hypercalcemia: 20 mg/kg daily, for up to 90 days. FDA pregnancy category C.	This agent interacts directly with bone to slow bone resorption; hence lower release of calcium.
Gallium nitrate	Ganite	INTRAVENOUS: *Adults*—100-200 mg/m^2 infused over 24 hr, for 5 days. FDA pregnancy category C.	For control of hypercalcemia caused by cancer.
Pamidronate	Aredia*	INTRAVENOUS: *Adults*—For hypercalcemia: 60 mg over 4-24 hr. For Paget's disease: 90-180 mg total over days to weeks. FDA pregnancy category C.	Interacts directly with bone to slow bone resorption; hence lower release of calcium.
Teriparatide	Parathar	INTRAVENOUS: *Adults*—5 U/kg infused over 10 min. FDA pregnancy category C. *Children >3 yr*—3 U/kg infused over 10 min.	For differential diagnosis of hypoparathyroidism and pseudohypoparathyroidism.
Vitamin D			
Alfacalcidol	One-Alpha†	ORAL: *Adults*—1 μg daily initially; maintenance: 0.25-1 μg daily. FDA pregnancy category C.	Used for hypoparathyroidism or chronic renal failure.
Calcifediol	Calderol	ORAL: *Adults*—0.05-0.1 mg daily. FDA pregnancy category C. Children—0.02-0.05 mg daily.	Alternate agent for vitamin D deficiency or rickets.
Calcitriol	Calcijex* Rocaltrol*	ORAL: *Adults*—0.25 μg slowly increased to maximum of 3 μg daily. FDA pregnancy category C. *Children*—0.25 μg daily gradually increased to 0.08 μg/kg. INTRAVENOUS: *Adults*—0.01 μg/kg by rapid injection 3 times weekly; may increase to 0.05 μg/kg.	Used for hypoparathyroidism or chronic renal failure.
Dihydrotachysterol	DHT Hytakerol*	ORAL: *Adults*—0.1-2.5 mg daily, as needed to maintain normal serum calcium. FDA pregnancy category C.	Used for hypoparathyroidism or tetany.
Ergocalciferol	Calciferol* Drisdol Ostoforte†	ORAL: *Adults and children*—400 U daily for replacement doses; up to 500,000 U daily for rickets or other conditions. FDA pregnancy category C.	Used to treat and prevent vitamin D deficiency and for hypoparathyroidism.

*Available in Canada and United States.
†Available in Canada only.

appears in urine within 1 day. There is no metabolism of edetate in the body.

Uses

Edetate disodium is used for emergency treatment of hypercalcemia. The drug may also be used for digitalis toxicity, but digoxin immune fab is the preferred drug.

Adverse Reactions and Contraindications

The most serious side effect with edetate disodium is thrombophlebitis at the site of injection. Dizziness may occur, as well as GI tract signs including cramps and diarrhea. Nephrotoxicity is also a problem with edetate disodium. The drug is usually avoided in patients with preexisting renal problems.

Toxicity

Acute overdoses of edetate disodium may cause hypocalcemia (see Table 62-1). Calcium ion replacement may occasionally be necessary.

Interactions

Digitalis effects are reduced when serum calcium is lowered.

Etidronate

Mechanism of Action

Etidronate is a synthetic analogue of inorganic pyrophosphate that blocks removal of calcium from bone, but the exact mechanism is unclear. The effect is to slow bone resorption and remodeling.

Pharmacokinetics

Etidronate binds to bone, concentrating at sites where bone is being remodeled. The effects on serum calcium levels develop slowly with oral doses of the drug. Therapeutic effects may persist for months after drug is discontinued. This prolonged effect may be related to persistence of drug in bone for months.

Uses

Etidronate is used to control Paget's disease, which promotes excessive remodeling of bone. The drug is also used for heterotropic ossification that may follow hip replacement surgery. Occasionally etidronate may be used to control hypercalcemia, especially when the condition arises from malignancies of the bone.

Adverse Reactions and Contraindications

Many patients with Paget's disease experience tenderness or pain weeks or months after therapy is started. The pain localizes at the site of Paget's disease lesions in bones. Some patients may suffer bone fractures caused by changes in bone mineralization. Nausea, diarrhea, and allergic reactions may also occur.

Etidronate is avoided in patients with impaired renal function (serum creatinine above 5 mg/dl) because etidronate elimination may be limited.

Toxicity

Higher doses of the drug tend to cause more severe GI tract symptoms.

Interactions

Foods or drugs that have a high content of metal ions can impair oral absorption of etidronate and prevent its action. Antacids, mineral supplements, calcium salts, or calcium-rich dairy products may all be involved.

Gallium nitrate

Mechanism of Action

Gallium nitrate blocks removal of calcium from bone, but the exact mechanism is unclear. The effect is to slow bone resorption and lower blood calcium concentrations.

Pharmacokinetics

Gallium nitrate usually shows a half-life of about a day, but the effect of the drug persists for up to 6 days.

Uses

Gallium nitrate is used to control hypercalcemia that arises from malignancies of the bone.

Adverse Reactions and Contraindications

Phosphate as well as calcium is lowered in blood; in some patients this change may cause anorexia or muscle weakness. Nephrotoxicity is also a common reaction with gallium nitrate. Nausea, vomiting, and diarrhea are also often seen.

Gallium nitrate is avoided in patients with impaired renal function (serum creatinine above 2.5 mg/dl) because gallium nitrate elimination may be limited.

Toxicity

Higher doses of gallium nitrate tend to cause more severe nephrotoxicity.

Interactions

Antacids, mineral supplements, calcium salts, or calcium-rich dairy products can impair the oral absorption of gallium nitrate and prevent its action. Nephrotoxic medications are also avoided because of the risk of additive renal damage.

Pamidronate

Mechanism of Action

Pamidronate blocks removal of calcium from bone by several mechanisms. The effect is to slow bone resorption and remodeling, as well as to prevent high blood calcium concentrations.

Pharmacokinetics

Pamidronate binds to bone, concentrating at sites where bone is being remodeled. Drug not bound to bone is excreted in urine. Effects on serum calcium levels persist after the drug is stopped.

Uses

Pamidronate is used for Paget's disease or to treat hypercalcemia, especially when it arises from malignancies of the bone.

Adverse Reactions and Contraindications

Hypocalcemia is common with pamidronate and may produce muscle spasms. Leukopenia is also common, with chills, fever, or sore throat. Nausea and pain at the injection site also occur.

Pamidronate is avoided in patients with impaired renal function (serum creatinine above 5 mg/dl) because etidronate elimination may be limited.

Toxicity

Higher doses of the drug tend to cause more severe hypocalcemia.

Interactions

No significant interactions have been noted.

Parathyroid hormone

Mechanism of Action

Parathyroid hormone directly promotes release of calcium from bone. Parathyroid hormone also has effects on kidneys that include inhibition of calcium clearance. This action is easily tested by measuring urinary excretion of cyclic adenosine monophosphate (AMP) and phosphate.

Pharmacokinetics
Parathyroid hormone, as a protein, is rapidly destroyed in blood. Effects are therefore seen quickly and disappear quickly.

Uses
A synthetic fragment of parathyroid hormone, teriparatide, retains full biologic activity and is used as a diagnostic agent. The agent is infused, and urinary cyclic AMP and phosphate are measured to detect the response of a target organ to the hormone. Hypoparathyroidism is a deficiency in parathyroid hormone production, but the target organs respond to exogenous parathyroid hormone. Pseudohypoparathyroidism is a rare condition in which the target organs fail to respond to parathyroid hormone.

Adverse Reactions and Contraindications
The adverse reactions are those of hypercalcemia (see Table 62-1). Because the effect is so short lived, hypercalcemia is usually mild. The use of teriparatide is usually safe, but the agent should be avoided in patients with allergies to gelatin or to parathyroid hormone.

Toxicity
Severe overdosage can produce arrhythmias and muscle weakness. These effects pass quickly if the drug is discontinued and fluids are administered.

Interactions
There are no significant interactions noted because the drug is cleared quickly from the body.

Calcium Deficiency (Hypocalcemia)
Mild calcium deficiencies may produce no short-term signs, but chronic deficiencies can lead to a general weakening of bone, as calcium is removed for metabolic use. This problem is especially prevalent in postmenopausal women.

Calcium supplements
Mechanism of Action
Calcium present in the diet or in dietary supplements replaces calcium that would otherwise be mobilized from bone to supply the body's metabolic needs. Maintaining an adequate intake of calcium helps prevent loss of calcium from bones and maintains their strength (see box).

Pharmacokinetics
Calcium is not well absorbed orally, with less than one third of the amount ingested being absorbed. Vitamin D can increase absorption, but certain fiber-rich foods can diminish absorption. Calcium elimination from the body is regulated by the kidneys, under the influence of parathyroid hormone and other factors.

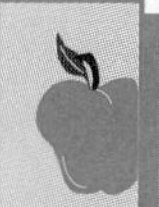

DIETARY CONSIDERATION
Calcium

Calcium is important for growth and maintenance of healthy bones and for its role in nerve and muscle function and blood clotting. Some medical conditions contribute to hypocalcemia (low blood calcium levels), including hypoparathyroidism, kidney disease, massive cellulitis, burns, and peritonitis. An extremely low level of calcium can result in tetany, a medical emergency that is treated with IV calcium. Milder cases of hypocalcemia may be treated in part by having the patient increase dietary intake of calcium. Good dietary sources of calcium include the following:

- Blackstrap molasses
- Calcium-fortified orange juice
- Cheese
- Clams
- Dark-green leafy vegetables (e.g., kale and spinach)
- Ice cream
- Milk products
- Oysters
- Salmon
- Sardines
- Tofu, if made with calcium carbonate
- Yogurt

Uses
Oral calcium supplements are designed primarily to prevent calcium deficiency and maintain bone strength. These preparations are also often used as antacids.

Adverse Reactions and Contraindications
Systemic effects are uncommon with oral calcium preparations. Constipation and loss of appetite may occur frequently.

Calcium supplements should not be used in patients with symptoms of hypercalcemia, including those with sarcoidosis or renal calculi.

Toxicity
High doses of calcium supplements can produce signs of hypercalcemia (see Table 62-1).

Interactions
Calcium preparations can diminish absorption of several drugs, including etidronate, phenytoin, and tetracyclines. Calcium also directly antagonizes the effects of drugs such as gallium nitrate and magnesium sulfate.

Vitamin D
Mechanism of Action
Vitamin D is required for proper absorption of calcium. Exogenous vitamin D has the same action as the vitamin D normally produced in the body.

Pharmacokinetics

Vitamin D is a highly lipid-soluble material that is readily absorbed orally. Once in the blood, vitamin D is bound to specific alpha-globulins that transport the material to target tissues. This lipid-soluble vitamin is concentrated in liver and other fat stores.

The metabolic fate of vitamin D depends on which form is taken. Vitamin D_3, or cholecalciferol, is therapeutically equivalent to vitamin D_2, or ergocalciferol. Both drugs are converted to calcifediol by the liver. Calcifediol and alfacalcidol are both converted by renal tissue to calcitriol (1,25-dihydroxycholecalciferol),the most active vitamin D derivative. Most vitamin D metabolites are excreted in bile.

Uses

All vitamin D derivatives may be used to control hypocalcemia or vitamin D deficiency, but certain forms are more appropriate for certain indications (see Table 62-2). Calcitriol is the most active form and is very effective for many conditions, but this drug form is expensive. Since adequate treatment is possible for most conditions with other forms of the vitamin, calcitriol is reserved for those rare patients who respond only to this drug form.

Adverse Reactions and Contraindications

Excess of vitamin D produces symptoms that are primarily those expected with high blood calcium concentrations (see Table 62-1).

Toxicity

Massive overdosages with vitamin D may be fatal, as cardiovascular and renal function is compromised. Chronic overdoses can cause deposits of calcium to appear in blood vessels, kidneys, and other tissues. High doses of vitamin D can arrest growth in children, which can persist for up to 6 months.

Interactions

Antacids or other preparations containing magnesium may be more dangerous when given with vitamin D because high magnesium concentrations in blood may occur.

NURSING PROCESS OVERVIEW

Drugs Affecting Calcium Metabolism

Assessment

Monitor vital signs. Take dietary history, if appropriate. Assess for pain, inability to perform activities of daily living. Assess exercise patterns, if appropriate. Monitor serum calcium and phosphorus, and blood urea nitrogen (BUN) and serum creatinine levels.

Nursing Diagnoses

- For patients with Paget's disease: Risk for bone fractures
- For patients with hypercalcemia: Potential complication: arrhythmias

Patient Outcomes

The patient will not have any fractures. The nurse will manage and minimize arrhythmic episodes.

Planning/Implementation

Administer medications as ordered. If concomitant dietary changes are appropriate, instruct the patient as needed or refer to a dietician. Monitor vital signs and laboratory work. If the patient is at risk for arrhythmias, monitor electrocardiographic (ECG) changes. Work with the physician to develop an appropriate treatment plan if the patient is in pain. Instruct the patient how to take medications in the home setting.

Evaluation

The drugs in this chapter vary in their use. Before discharge, verify that the patient can explain how to take medications at home, what symptoms should prompt the patient to contact the physician, and explain any prescribed dietary changes needed.

NURSING IMPLICATIONS SUMMARY

Calcitonin

Drug Administration

- Monitor weight. If vomiting or diarrhea occurs, monitor intake and output.
- Warn the patient that flushing may occur.
- Before the first dose of calcitonin salmon, a test dose may be ordered to check for allergic response. Consult the manufacturer's literature. Have drugs, equipment, and personnel available to treat acute allergic reactions in settings where salmon calcitonin is used.
- Assess for hypercalcemia or hypocalcemia (see Table 17-1).
- Monitor serum electrolyte levels and (in patients with Paget's disease) serum alkaline phosphatase and 24-hour urinary hydroxyproline concentration.

Patient and Family Education

- Review the anticipated benefits and possible side effects of drug therapy with the patient.
- Encourage the patient to return for regular follow-up visits. For home administration, instruct the patient to administer the drug subcutaneously. Review the injection technique and have the patient give a return demonstration.
- Store salmon calcitonin in the refrigerator. Store human calcitonin at a temperature below 77°F but do not refrigerate.
- Refer the patient to a community-based nursing care agency as needed.
- Inform the patient that taking ordered doses in the evening may minimize flushing.
- Encourage the patient receiving long-term therapy to wear a medical identification tag or bracelet indicating that calcitonin is being taken regularly.
- A low-calcium diet may be prescribed. Review the dietary consideration box on calcium (p. 751) for food items that should be used in limited amounts when trying to restrict calcium intake. Refer to a dietitian as needed.

Edetate Disodium

Drug Administration

- Read drug labels carefully; do not confuse this drug with edetate calcium disodium.
- To prepare dose for an adult, dissolve dose in 500 ml of 5% dextrose in water (D5W) and administer over at least 3 hours. For a child, dissolve the calculated dose in sufficient diluent (D5W or sodium chloride injection) to make a final concentration no more concentrated than 3% (30 mg/ml). Too concentrated a solution may increase the risk of thrombophlebitis. Administer the dose over at least 3 hours, and preferably 4 to 6 hours. Too rapid infusion may precipitate a sudden drop in serum calcium, resulting in hypocalcemic tetany or cardiac arrhythmias. Have calcium gluconate readily available.
- Monitor vital signs and continuous ECG during the infusion. Keep the patient supine during infusion and for a short time afterward.
- Monitor BUN and serum creatinine levels, serum electrolytes, liver function tests, and urinalysis.

Etidronate

Drug Administration

- Assess for bone pain, which may occur in patients with Paget's disease.
- Monitor serum electrolyte levels. Assess for signs of hypocalcemia (see Table 17-1).
- Monitor serum creatinine BUN levels.
- For IV etidronate, dilute in 250 ml or more of normal saline. Infuse 250 ml over at least 2 hours.

Patient and Family Education

- Review the anticipated benefits and possible side effects of drug therapy with the patient.
- Provide emotional support. Weeks to months of therapy may be required to obtain maximum drug effect. Remind the patient not to discontinue therapy without consulting the physician.
- Instruct the patient to take doses with black coffee, tea, fruit juice, or water, on an empty stomach, at least 2 hours before or after food. Suggest that patients take doses at midmorning or bedtime.
- Notify the patient not to take doses within 2 hours of ingesting milk or milk products, antacids, mineral supplements, or medicines high in calcium, magnesium, iron, or aluminum.
- Take a dietary history. Patients should continue following a well-balanced diet with adequate but not excessive amounts of calcium and vitamin D.
- Notify physician if severe or persistent diarrhea develops or bone pain worsens.

Gallium Nitrate

Drug Administration/Patient and Family Education

- Assess for bone pain, loss of appetite, muscle weakness, nausea, vomiting, or diarrhea.
- Encourage the patient to have sufficient fluid intake to maintain 24-hour output at 2000 ml or more. Encourage the patient to drink at least eight or nine 8-ounce glasses of liquid a day.
- Dilute daily dose in 1 L of 0.9% sodium chloride injection or D5W. Administer over 24 hours. Use an infusion monitoring device and/or microdrip tubing. If the patient is to administer at home, refer to a home care nursing agency.
- Monitor BUN and serum creatinine levels, serum albumin, serum calcium, and serum phosphorus.

Continued.

NURSING IMPLICATIONS SUMMARY—cont'd

Pamidronate

Drug Administration/Patient and Family Education

- Assess for symptoms of hypocalcemia: abdominal cramps, confusion, muscle spasms. Assess for fever, nausea, and pain and swelling at the injection site.
- A low-calcium diet may be prescribed. Review the dietary consideration box on calcium (p. 751) for food items that should be used in limited amounts when trying to restrict calcium intake. Refer to a dietitian as needed.
- Reconstitute each 30 mg vial with 10 ml sterile water. Further dilute in 1000 ml normal saline, 0.45% normal saline, or D5W. Administer dose over 24 hours. Use an infusion monitoring device and/or microdrip tubing.
- Monitor serum electrolytes, complete blood count (CBC) and white blood cell (WBC) differential, BUN and serum creatinine levels, and in patients with Paget's disease serum alkaline phosphatase.

Teriparatide

Drug Administration

- Review the pretest instructions with the patient. Usually, the patient may have nothing to drink after 8 PM the night before the test. Begin drinking 200 ml of water every 30 minutes, beginning 2½ hours before the scheduled time of the test. Urine and blood samples will be drawn periodically during the test.
- To prepare teriparatide, use the diluent provided. Administer the dose evenly over 10 minutes.
- Allergic reactions are possible, although rare. Have epinephrine, equipment, and personnel available to treat acute allergic reactions.

Vitamin D Preparations

Drug Administration

- The side effects are essentially those of hypercalcemia and are a result of overdosage. They include ataxia, fatigue, irritability, seizures, somnolence, tinnitus, hypertension, GI tract distress or constipation, and hypotonia in infants. Other symptoms of overdose include headache, increased thirst, metallic taste in the mouth, nausea or vomiting, and fatigue.
- Assess for central nervous system (CNS) effects. Ongoing assessment is important since some symptoms such as fatigue may be difficult to distinguish from those accompanying renal failure or chronic disease.
- Monitor blood pressure and pulse. Monitor intake and output.
- Monitor BUN and serum creatinine levels, serum calcium and phosphorus levels, serum alkaline phosphatase, and urinalysis.

Intravenous Calcitriol

- May be administered by rapid direct IV push.

Patient and Family Education

- Review the anticipated benefits and possible side effects of drug therapy with the patient. Encourage the patient to notify the physician if any new side effects occur.
- Remind the patient not to increase or decrease the dose without consulting the physician.
- Warn the patient to avoid over-the-counter preparations that contain calcium, phosphorus, or vitamin D unless approved by the physician.
- Warn the patient to avoid driving or operating hazardous equipment if fatigue, somnolence, vertigo, or weakness occurs.
- Remind the patient to inform all health care providers of all drugs being used. Avoid using any medications not previously approved by the physician.
- Instruct the patient to avoid antacids containing magnesium.
- Instruct the patient to avoid excessive amounts of substances containing vitamin D (see the dietary consideration box on vitamins, p. 215).

CRITICAL THINKING

APPLICATION

1. What is the function of parafollicular cells in the thyroid?
2. What are the metabolic effects of calcitonin?
3. What forms of calcitonin are used to treat Paget's disease? How do they differ?
4. What is the function of the parathyroid glands?
5. What are the metabolic effects of parathyroid hormone?
6. How is hypoparathyroidism treated?
7. Which metabolite of vitamin D is the most active?
8. What is the metabolic function of vitamin D?
9. What organs form metabolites of vitamin D?
10. What are the signs of vitamin D deficiency?
11. Why is edetate disodium effective treatment for hypercalcemia?
12. How may etidronate be used clinically?
13. Why is knowledge of renal function important for a patient receiving etidronate?
14. What type of patient is likely to benefit most from oral calcium supplements?
15. What side effects are common with oral calcium supplements?
16. What are the dangers associated with high doses of vitamin D?

CRITICAL THINKING

1. What are the symptoms of hypoparathyroidism? How should you assess for these?
2. What side effects are most common with edetate? How would you assess for these?

CHAPTER 63

Drugs to Treat Diabetes Mellitus

OBJECTIVES

After studying this chapter, you should be able to do the following:

- *Discuss the difference between insulin-dependent (IDDM) and non–insulin-dependent diabetes mellitus (NIDDM).*
- *Explain the advantages of the different forms of insulin.*
- *Explain the clinical uses of sulfonylureas.*
- *Develop a nursing care plan for a patient with diabetes.*
- *Develop a teaching plan for a patient with diabetes.*

KEY TERMS

diabetes mellitus
glucosuria
hyperglycemia
hypoglycemia
insulin
insulin-dependent diabetes mellitus (IDDM)
ketoacidosis
non–insulin-dependent diabetes mellitus (NIDDM)
sulfonylureas

CHAPTER OVERVIEW

The pancreas is an exocrine gland that supplies digestive juices to the small intestine. Within the gland lie discrete clusters of cells with different functions from those of most pancreatic cells. These cell clusters, called the *islets of Langerhans,* contain several types of endocrine cells. Three of these cell types release peptide hormones that affect glucose metabolism. Alpha (A) cells synthesize and release the peptide hormone glucagon, beta (B) cells synthesize and release insulin, and D cells synthesize somatostatin. This chapter includes an examination of the function of islet cells, a description of diabetes mellitus, and a description of drugs used in the diagnosis and control of that disease.

Therapeutic Rationale: Diabetes Mellitus

Normal Hormonal Regulation of Metabolism

Glucose Metabolism

One of the rules of metabolic regulation is that the body seldom relies on a single mechanism to control an important physiologic function. This rule applies to the processes by which the body regulates glucose use. The primary hormone regulating glucose metabolism is **insulin,** a peptide hormone synthesized in beta-cells of the pancreas. Insulin stimulates glucose uptake in fat and muscle cells and promotes the conversion of glucose to the storage carbohydrate glycogen in the liver.

Insulin does not work alone and its metabolic actions must always be considered in relation to the actions of other hormones. For example, the elevated blood glucose level after a meal stimulates insulin release from the pancreas. Blood glucose is thereby lowered because insulin stimulates the burning of glucose for energy in fat and muscle cells and the storage of glucose in the liver. As blood glucose levels fall in response to insulin, glucagon release from alpha-cells of the pancreas is stimulated. Glucagon in many ways directly opposes the action of insulin in glucose metabolism. Glucagon stimulates the liver to break down glycogen and amino acids so that glucose is released into the blood. Glucagon also inhibits the uptake of glucose by muscle and fat cells. By balancing the action of these hormones, the body protects itself from high blood glucose (**hyperglycemia**) and low blood glucose (**hypoglycemia**).

Even the concept of metabolic balance achieved with two antagonistic hormones does not adequately describe glucose regulation. For example, somatostatin (see Chapter 59) released from D cells inhibits release of insulin and glucagon from islet cells. Other hormones antagonize the peripheral effects of insulin. Cortisol, an adrenocortical glucocorticoid, and epinephrine, a catecholamine from the adrenal medulla, which are elevated during stress, antagonize the actions of insulin in muscle or fat cells (Table 63-1). The overall action of these two hormones is to increase blood glucose levels. Growth hormone (see Chapter 59) also increases blood glucose, primarily by lowering glucose uptake in muscle cells.

Fat and Protein Metabolism

Although insulin is most often considered as a regulator of glucose metabolism, it also regulates fat and protein metabolism. Insulin directly stimulates synthesis of storage lipid within fat cells, blocks breakdown and release of stored lipid, and promotes protein synthesis by stimulating amino acid uptake and by directly stimulating protein synthetic processes.

As in carbohydrate metabolism, the action of insulin in regulating fat and protein metabolism is opposed by other hormones (see Table 63-1). For example, epinephrine, glucagon, cortisol, and growth hormone stimulate fat breakdown in fat cells, thereby directly opposing the action of insulin in that tissue. These hormones therefore tend to raise the blood content of free fatty acids and other breakdown products of lipids. In addition, glucagon and cortisol block protein synthesis in direct opposition to insulin action. Growth hormone differs from the other insulin-opposing hormones in that growth hormone directly stimulates protein synthesis in many body tissues. An understanding of this delicate balance of hormonal actions is important to appreciate the origin of some of the metabolic derangements that occur in diabetes mellitus.

TABLE 63-1 Metabolic Actions of Insulin and Insulin-Opposing Hormones

TISSUE AND METABOLIC PROCESS	INSULIN	GLUCAGON	EPINEPHRINE	CORTISOL	GROWTH HORMONE
Liver					
Glycogen formation	Increase	Decrease	Decrease	Increase	—
Glucose formation from amino acids	Decrease	Increase	—	Increase	Decrease
Glucose formation from glycogen	Decrease	Increase	Increase	—	—
Skeletal Muscle					
Glucose uptake or use	Increase	Decrease	Decrease	Decrease	Decrease
Amino acid uptake	Increase	—	—	—	Increase
Protein synthesis	Increase	Decrease	—	Decrease	Increase
Glucose release from glycogen	Decrease	Increase	Increase	—	—
Fat Cells					
Synthesis of storage lipid	Increase	Decrease	Decrease	Decrease	Decrease
Release of free fatty acids from stored lipid	Decrease	Increase	Increase	Increase	Increase
Blood					
Glucose level	Decrease	Increase	Increase	Increase	Increase
Free fatty acid level	Decrease	Increase	Increase	Increase	Increase

Diabetes Mellitus

Types and Causes

In **diabetes mellitus,** insulin action is lost. If all insulin production ceases, the disease is referred to as **insulin-dependent diabetes mellitus (IDDM).** Other terms for this form are *type I* or *juvenile-onset* diabetes. If insulin production continues but is insufficient to meet the body's demands, the disease is referred to as **non–insulin-dependent diabetes mellitus (NIDDM),** also called *type II* or *adult-onset* diabetes; most diabetic persons have this type of disease. As the name implies, diabetes characterized by absence of insulin production primarily affects the young. NIDDM is usually a disease of persons who are over 40 years of age or who are obese. Diabetes in these patients may involve insulin resistance; insulin concentrations in the blood may be normal, but the target tissues are unresponsive to insulin.

The exact cause of diabetes mellitus has not been established, but several factors may be involved. Viruses and autoimmune mechanisms have been suggested to contribute to development of the disease. Heredity may also play a role in some types of diabetes, especially NIDDM, but it has never been proved that heredity alone determines who will or will not develop the disease.

Metabolic Derangements

Significant metabolic derangements occur when insulin action is lost. Without insulin, less glucose is used in muscle and fat cells, and more glucose is released into the circulation by the liver. Muscle cells, starved for energy sources, break down protein and release amino acids into the blood. The liver converts a portion of these amino acids into glucose and returns it to the blood. These processes contribute to the persistent elevated levels of glucose in blood. When glucose levels in blood exceed a certain threshold (about 160 mg/dl), glucose begins to appear in urine.

The most common early symptoms of diabetes mellitus result directly from osmotic and metabolic changes. Patients often first note a feeling of constant fatigue because energy production in body cells is impaired. Increased frequency of urination (polyuria), often first noticed at night, occurs because excess glucose in urine produces osmotic diuresis (i.e., more water must be excreted to carry out the high concentration of glucose). As urine output increases, most patients develop excessive thirst (polydipsia), which results from the body's efforts to maintain normal hydration despite excessive fluid losses through the kidney. Some patients develop perineal infections, made likely by the presence of glucose in urine.

The alterations in metabolism caused by insulin deficiency and the relative excess of catabolic hormones (catecholamines and steroids) ultimately result in excessive protein and fat breakdown. Protein is metabolized to amino acids and then to glucose, whereas fats are converted to free fatty acids and then to ketone bodies that are released into the circulation. These excess breakdown products may cause a patient to become ketotic or acidotic. **Ketoacidosis** is a serious acute complication of diabetes mellitus seen primarily in patients with IDDM who have little or no endogenous insulin production. These patients are sometimes called *ketosis-prone diabetics.* Patients with NIDDM who produce enough insulin to suppress lipid breakdown are resistant to ketosis. Ketoacidotic coma is associated with mortalities of 3% to 30%. Mortality is highest when treatment is delayed.

Any diabetic person may become comatose as a result of dehydration. As the plasma becomes hyperosmolar (higher solute concentration than normal for blood), water is pulled from body tissues, and severe water and electrolyte imbalances occur. Patients in this type of hyperosmolar coma tend to be older and to have an even higher mortality rate than patients in ketoacidotic coma.

Long-Term Complications

Pathologic changes in blood vessels, nerves, and kidneys occur in diabetic patients. Retinal hemorrhages may destroy sight. Other vessels may also be affected, although those changes are not so easily observed early in the disease. At later stages, circulation to the limbs may be impaired. Pathologic changes also occur in kidneys, at first affecting glomerular filtration rate, then progressing to glomerulosclerosis with thickening of capillary basement membranes. Nephrotic syndrome with protein loss in urine and frank kidney failure are late complications of diabetes. Nerve function is impaired so that late in the disease there may be loss of feeling in the limbs or other parts of the body. Sexual impotence is common among diabetic men.

Some studies suggest that many of the late pathologic changes may be delayed or reduced in severity by strict control of the blood glucose level from the earliest possible time after the appearance of diabetes.

Diagnosis

Diabetes mellitus is diagnosed by applying one or more of the following procedures.

Fasting blood sugar (FBS) is determined by obtaining 1 to 3 ml of blood after a 12-hour fast and measuring the glucose content by any of several methods approved for use in clinical laboratories. Most conveniently, the blood is taken in the early morning. The range of normal fasting plasma sugar values is 60 to 100 mg/dl for venous blood. A value above 140 mg/dl in a truly fasting individual suggests the diagnosis of diabetes mellitus. Values between 100 and 140 mg/dl may require further patient evaluation.

Glucose in urine (**glucosuria**) is conveniently tested in screening programs with commercially available pretreated test strips (Dextrostix), which develop a particular color when exposed to urine containing glucose. Glucose does not routinely appear in urine of nondiabetic persons because a blood glucose level of about 160 mg/dl is required before healthy kidneys allow glucose to spill into urine. Some diabetic persons spill glucose into urine at lower blood glucose concentrations, possibly as a result of impaired renal function.

An oral glucose tolerance test (OGTT) detects not only overt diabetes but also may reveal a prediabetic state. Fifty to

100 gm of glucose are taken orally and blood is sampled at hourly or 30-minute intervals. Glucose levels in plasma are compared with the value obtained immediately before the glucose was administered. In nondiabetic individuals plasma glucose levels rise in response to this acute glucose load and immediately trigger the release of insulin from beta-cells of the pancreas. As a result of the circulating insulin, glucose levels begin to fall within about 1 hour after the glucose load is ingested and return to normal within 2 hours (Figure 63-1). In contrast, plasma glucose levels of a diabetic person fall more slowly than those of nondiabetic individuals because insulin is not released to aid in disposition of the glucose load. Plasma glucose levels in diabetic persons remain over 200 mg/dl of plasma 2 hours after the glucose load.

Long-term hyperglycemia causes a significant fraction of the hemoglobin in the blood to be glycosylated. Glycosylated hemoglobin can be assayed to assess how well diabetic persons are controlling their glucose levels with the medications discussed in the next section.

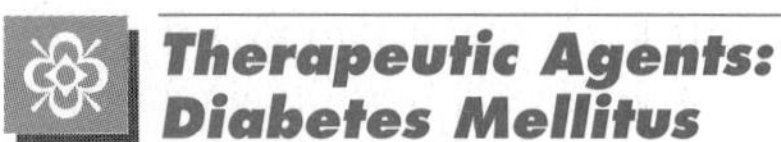

Therapeutic Agents: Diabetes Mellitus

Parenteral Agents

Insulin

Mechanism of Action

Insulin used in diabetes mellitus constitutes replacement therapy. The administered insulin restores the ability of cells to use glucose as an energy source and corrects many associated metabolic derangements.

Pharmacokinetics

Insulin must be used by injection because it is a protein and therefore would be destroyed in the gastrointestinal (GI) tract. In its natural form, insulin is relatively soluble in water and is quickly absorbed from subcutaneous injection sites. This property is reflected in the pharmacologic behavior of regular insulin for injection (Table 63-2), which is rapidly absorbed, has its peak effect within 2 to 4 hours, and is no longer active after 8 hours. The longer-acting insulin preparations are prepared by crystallizing insulin in the presence of zinc or other agents to form slowly dissolving complexes. These preparations differ from regular insulin and from each other in onset and duration of action because of differences in absorption from the injection site.

Health care professionals must be familiar with the onset and duration of insulin products. With different insulin forms, control can be adjusted to fit the lifestyle and metabolic demands of individual patients. Diabetic persons must become proficient not only in techniques of storing, preparing, and injecting their insulin, but they also must be taught proper testing procedures. To avoid complications, patients must also understand the onset and duration of action of the insulin preparations they are receiving.

As an example of the many patterns of dosage that may be used successfully, consider the following hypothetical case.

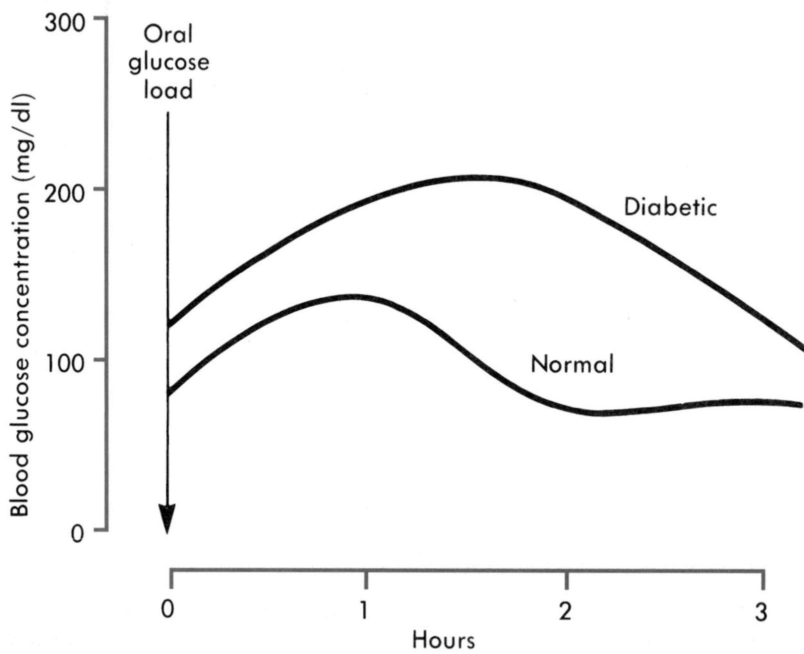

FIGURE 63-1

Typical oral glucose tolerance tests for normal and diabetic patients. Test is performed preferably in ambulatory patients in morning before eating. Oral glucose load is about 75 gm given in solution. Blood is drawn at appropriate intervals (before glucose and 60, 90, 120, and 180 minutes after glucose) and is analyzed for glucose concentration.

TABLE 63-2 Pharmacokinetics of Insulin Preparations

GENERIC NAME	CLASSIFICATION	DESCRIPTION	PHARMACOKINETICS		
			ONSET	PEAK	DURATION
Insulin injection	Rapid acting	Clear solution containing no zinc or modifying agents; IV or subcutaneous injection	Within 1 hr	2-4 hr	6-8 hr
Prompt insulin zinc suspension	Rapid acting	Cloudy suspension of amorphous insulin precipitated with zinc to slow absorption; subcutaneous only	1-2 hr	4-7 hr	12-16 hr
Isophane insulin suspension	Intermediate acting	Cloudy suspension of insulin complex for slow absorption; subcutaneous only	2-4 hr	10-16 hr	18-30 hr
Insulin zinc suspension	Intermediate acting	Cloudy suspension containing 30% semilente insulin and 70% ultralente insulin; subcutaneous only	1-2 hr	10-16 hr	18-30 hr
Extended insulin zinc suspension	Long acting	Cloudy when well mixed; large complexes of insulin with zinc to slow absorption; no protein modifiers; subcutaneous only	5-8 hr	16-24 hr	24-36 hr or longer

A person with IDDM who has been maintained on a single dose of insulin zinc suspension (Lente insulin) before breakfast each morning has started to show hyperglycemia by the next morning. To overcome this problem, the physician splits the insulin dose, giving 80% of the daily dose in the morning and the remainder before supper. The rationale for this therapy is simple. Lente insulin injected at around 7 AM reaches its peak effect around dinnertime (see Table 63-2). The small dose administered before supper helps to protect the patient from developing hyperglycemia overnight.

Many individualized schemes for insulin dosage may be devised. In all cases the principle is the same; doses of insulin must be timed so that the patient is protected from hyperglycemia at any time and from hypoglycemia during peak periods of insulin action.

Uses

Insulin is used primarily for IDDM, the condition in which beta-cell function is lost and insulin production is very low or absent. Insulin may also be used in NIDDM that cannot be controlled by diet and/or oral hypoglycemic agents.

Adverse Reactions and Contraindications

Insulin therapy is associated with two important acute side effects. If therapy is inadequate, the person may go into a coma resulting from uncontrolled metabolic derangements; blood glucose concentrations will be high, and ketoacidosis or hyperosmolar coma may result. If insulin overdosage occurs or if a patient does not eat or overexercises, the patient may lapse into coma resulting from hypoglycemia. It is critical for health care professionals to be able to differentiate between these conditions. The distinguishing symptoms are outlined in Table 63-3. Treatment of hypoglycemia consists of elevating blood glucose levels by oral administration of sugar in conscious patients or by glucagon injection or glucose intravenous (IV) infusion in unconscious patients. Treatment of diabetic coma requires insulin administration to lower blood glucose concentration and to reduce ketone body formation.

Many patients receiving insulin therapy have insulin antibodies in their blood. These antibodies may contribute to insulin resistance in some patients.

Insulin may also provoke subcutaneous fat near injection sites to atrophy. This lipoatrophy leads to the formation of hollows or depressions in the skin. Careful rotation of injection sites minimizes this effect. Lipoatrophy may be less common with the highly purified insulin preparations.

Three types of insulin are available in the United States—bovine, porcine, and human. Bovine and porcine insulin are obtained from the pancreas of animals slaughtered for food. Many commonly used preparations are mixtures of bovine and porcine insulin that also may contain proinsulin as a contaminant (Table 63-4). Highly purified insulins have a much lower level of proinsulin contamination.

Human insulin comes from two sources. Semisynthetic human insulin is prepared by converting porcine insulin to the human form by chemically changing the one differing amino acid. Human insulin is also produced by recombinant DNA techniques; human genes for insulin are inserted into bacteria, which then produce large amounts of the protein to be processed and purified.

The hypoglycemic actions of the various forms of insulin are similar; however, the preparations differ slightly in pharmacokinetics and side effects. For example, human insulin preparations have a slightly shorter duration of action than corresponding porcine preparations. Dosages may require slight adjustment when switching from one preparation to another. Human insulin and purified porcine insulin are less

TABLE 63-3 Differential Diagnosis of Diabetic Coma and Hypoglycemic Reactions

CLINICAL DATA	DIABETIC COMA	HYPOGLYCEMIC REACTIONS
Symptoms	Thirst Abdominal pain Nausea and vomiting Headache Constipation Shortness of breath (Kussmaul's respiration)	Nervousness Hunger Sweating Weakness Stupor Convulsions
Signs	Facial flushing Air hunger Soft eyeballs Normal or absent reflexes Acetone breath	Pallor Shallow respiration Normal eyeballs Babinski's reflex may be seen
Urine glucose	Positive	Negative or low
Urine acetone	Positive	Negative
Blood glucose	High (above 250 mg/dl)	Low (below 60 mg/dl)
Blood CO_2	Low	Normal
Precipitating factors	Untreated diabetes Infection or disease appearing in previously controlled diabetic patient High degree of emotional or psychologic stress	Insulin overdosage Skipping meals Excessive exercise before meals
History	Onset of symptoms usually occurs over period of days	Onset of symptoms is related to type of medication used; regular insulin overdose produces symptoms more rapidly than longer-acting insulins or oral agents

antigenic than the other types available. Patients may be switched to one of these forms to help control allergic side effects associated with insulin therapy.

Toxicity

Insulin overdose produces hypoglycemia. In severe cases, convulsions or coma may result.

Interactions

Alcohol tends to enhance the hypoglycemic action of insulin. The result can be a greater risk of hypoglycemic reactions, but the risk is usually minimal unless alcohol consumption is moderate to high and the alcohol is taken without food.

Beta-adrenergic agents or corticosteroids may antagonize the actions of insulin (see Table 63-1). Insulin doses may require adjustment.

Oral Hypoglycemic Agents

Sulfonylureas

Mechanism of Action

Most oral hypoglycemic agents used in North America are **sulfonylureas.** These drugs are useful only for patients who produce some insulin on their own (i.e., patients with NIDDM). Clinical studies of patients with NIDDM have shown that many have normal or even above-normal insulin levels in their blood. The cells of many of these patients, however, are resistant to the action of insulin. Insulin action therefore is lost not because insulin is missing but because target cells fail to respond normally.

Sulfonylureas stimulate insulin release from the pancreas. The drugs also may diminish hepatic glucose production and may directly increase tissue responsiveness to insulin. These actions tend to diminish fasting plasma glucose concentrations and to improve glucose use by fat and muscle cells. The effectiveness of sulfonylureas in obese patients with NIDDM is enhanced by caloric restriction and weight loss. This dietary manipulation also tends to increase the responsiveness of target cells to insulin.

Pharmacokinetics

Sulfonylureas are well absorbed orally and bind extensively to serum proteins. The sulfonylureas differ from one another primarily in onset and duration of action (Table 63-5), which is in turn strongly influenced by their hepatic metabolism. For example, tolbutamide is relatively short acting because it is quickly converted to an inactive product. In contrast, acetohexamide and tolazamide must be converted in the body to active products before they become effective. Hence they are intermediate in action. Chlorpropamide, the longest-acting member of the class, is tightly bound to plasma protein, slowly metabolized and excreted in urine.

Glyburide and glipizide are many times more potent than other sulfonylureas. For example, 5 mg of glyburide or glipizide has an effect equivalent to that of 250 mg of chlorpropamide or tolazamide. At the doses used in patients, clinical effects are similar. Glyburide is extensively metabolized, with the products excreted in bile and in urine. Glipizide is also converted to inactive metabolites in liver, but excretion is primarily via the kidney.

Uses

Sulfonylureas are used for NIDDM, along with diet and exercise. They are occasionally combined with insulin.

TABLE 63-4 Insulin Preparations

GENERIC NAME	TRADE NAME	SOURCE	CONCENTRATION (U/ml)
Insulin injection	Regular Iletin I, Insulin-Toronto†, Regular Iletin†	Beef/pork mixture	100
	Regular Insulin, Regular Iletin II†	Pork	100
	Regular Insulin, Regular Iletin II	Purified pork	100
	Regular Concentrated Iletin II	Purified pork	500
	Humulin R,* Novolin R, Novolin ge Toronto†	Human, biosynthetic	100
	Velosulin BR, Velosulin Human†	Human, semisynthetic (buffered)	100
Insulin zinc suspension	Lente Iletin I, Lente Iletin,† Lente Insulin†	Beef/pork mixture	100
	Lente Iletin II,* Lente L	Purified pork	100
	Humulin L,* Novolin L, Novolin ge Lente†	Human biosynthetic	100
Isophane insulin	NPH Iletin I, NPH Iletin,† NPH Insulin†	Beef/pork mixture	100
	NPH Iletin II,* NPH-N	Purified pork	100
	Humulin N,* Novolin N, Novolin ge NPH†	Human, biosynthetic	100
	Humulin 50/50,* Novolin ge 50/50†	Human, biosynthetic (50% NPH, 50% regular insulin)	100
	Humulin 70/30, Novolin 70/30	Human, biosynthetic (70% NPH, 30% regular insulin)	100
	Humulin 10/90,† Novolin ge 10/90†	Human, biosynthetic (10% regular insulin, 90% NPH)	100
	Humulin 20/80,† Novolin ge 20/80†	Human, biosynthetic (20% regular insulin, 80% NPH)	100
	Humulin 30/70,† Novolin ge 30/70†	Human, biosynthetic (30% regular insulin, 70% NPH)	100
	Humulin 40/60,† Novolin ge 40/60†	Human, biosynthetic (40% regular insulin, 60% NPH)	100
Prompt insulin zinc	Semilente Insulin†	Beef/pork mixture	100
Extended insulin zinc suspension	Ultralente Insulin†	Beef/pork mixture	100
	Humulin U Ultralente, Humulin-U,† Novolin ge Ultralente†	Human, biosynthetic	100

*Available in Canada and United States.
†Available in Canada only.

Adverse Reactions and Contraindications

Side effects of sulfonylurea therapy include GI tract distress and neurologic symptoms such as dizziness, drowsiness, or headache. Allergy to the drugs occurs in some patients, with skin reactions being the most common sign. The incidence of these types of reactions is reported to be less than 5% of patients treated.

The use of sulfonylureas in the treatment of diabetes mellitus is controversial. Some clinical studies suggest that treatment with sulfonylureas is no more effective than dietary therapy alone. Other studies have suggested that toxicity of sulfonylureas is higher than previously expected. Of special concern is the apparent increase in risk of death from cardiovascular disease in patients receiving a sulfonylurea in the large-scale study conducted by the University Group Diabetes Program (UGDP). Although these questions remain unresolved, some treatment centers avoid the use of sulfonylureas and control mild NIDDM with diet and exercise alone or, if necessary, combine diet and exercise with low doses of insulin. Even when sulfonylureas are used, careful attention to the diet is required for best results.

Toxicity

Hypoglycemia is a danger with sulfonylureas and may be caused by drug overdose, drug interactions, altered drug metabolism, or the patient failing to eat. Sulfonylureas should not be used when renal or liver function is inadequate; normal function of those organs is required for metabolism and elimination of sulfonylureas (see Table 63-5). Older adult patients also occasionally show excessive hypoglycemia reactions to these drugs.

Interactions

Sulfonylureas are implicated in drug interactions that can have serious consequences to the patient. The major interactions occur with ethyl alcohol, phenylbutazone, sulfonamides, salicylates, phenothiazines, and thiazides.

TABLE 63-5 Oral Antidiabetic Agents

GENERIC NAME	TRADE NAME	DOSAGE RANGE	DURATION OF ACTION	TIME TO PEAK EFFECT
Acetohexamide	Dimelor† Dymelor	0.25-1.5 gm daily, single or divided dose. FDA pregnancy category C.	8-24 hr	2-6 hr
Chlorpropamide	Diabinese*	0.1-0.75 gm daily, single dose. FDA pregnancy category C.	Up to 60 hr	2-4 hr
Gliclazide†	Diamicron†	40-160 mg twice daily.	24 hr	4-6 hr
Glipizide	Glucotrol	Tablets: 2.5-40 mg daily. Doses >15 mg should be divided. Extended-release tablets, 5-20mg once daily. FDA pregnancy category C.	12-24 hr	Tablets: 1-3 hr; extended-release tablets: 6-12 hr
Glyburide	Diabeta* Glynase Micronase	Nonmicronized tablets: 1.25-20 mg daily. Micronized tablets: 0.75-12 mg once daily. FDA pregnancy category B. FDA pregnancy category C (Diabeta).	16-24 hr	Nonmicronized: 3.5-4.5 hr; micronized: 2.5-3.5 hr
Metformin	Glucophage	500 mg twice daily up to 850 mg 3 times daily. FDA pregnancy category B.	6-12 hr	2.25 hr
Tolazamide	Tolinase	0.1-1 gm daily; single dose for lower range, divided dose for higher range. FDA pregnancy category C.	12-24 hr	3-4 hr
Tolbutamide	Orinase* Mobenol†	0.25-3 gm daily, divided doses. FDA pregnancy category C.	6-12 hr	3-4 hr

*Available in Canada and United States.
†Available in Canada only.

Patients receiving sulfonylureas should routinely avoid alcohol. Several interactions between alcohol and sulfonylureas are possible. Some patients receiving sulfonylureas develop a "disulfiram-like reaction" when they ingest alcohol. The most striking symptoms of this reaction are unpleasant flushing and severe headache. Other patients taking sulfonylureas become hypoglycemic when they ingest alcohol, probably because ethanol is a hypoglycemic agent in some people.

Hypoglycemia can result when one of several drugs is given to a patient taking sulfonylureas, most importantly the antiinflammatory agents, phenylbutazone and salicylates, and sulfonamide antibiotics. These three types of drugs are all tightly bound to plasma protein and may displace sulfonylureas, which tend to be highly bound to serum protein. Thus blood concentrations of free sulfonylurea are elevated. Since the free drug is the active form, the result is an enhancement of the hypoglycemic effect of the sulfonylurea. In addition to this mechanism, phenylbutazone may block excretion of the active metabolite of acetohexamide, an action that also tends to increase hypoglycemia. Sulfonamides may inhibit the metabolic breakdown of tolbutamide and thereby may enhance its hypoglycemic action.

Phenothiazines such as chlorpromazine may impair the effectiveness of sulfonylureas. Chlorpromazine inhibits the release of insulin from beta-cells in the pancreas and elevates adrenal production of epinephrine, a hormone that can raise blood glucose levels (see Table 63-1). These actions of chlorpromazine directly antagonize the hypoglycemic action of sulfonylureas.

Thiazide diuretics possess hyperglycemic activity in addition to their diuretic actions; thus they may impair diabetes control with sulfonylureas.

Metformin

Mechanism of Action

Metformin is a biguanide that is thought to increase the ability of insulin to bind to peripheral tissues, thus increasing glucose uptake by muscle and other tissues. Metformin is only effective in patients who produce insulin.

Pharmacokinetics

Metformin is slowly absorbed after oral doses. Food delays absorption and lowers the total amount of drug absorbed. Bioavailability is generally low. Absorbed drug is not significantly bound to plasma protein. Metformin is excreted unchanged primarily in urine, with a half-life of 6.2 hours.

Uses

Metformin is used only for NIDDM, alone or with a sulfonylurea.

Adverse Reactions and Contraindications

The most common side effects with metformin are gastrointestinal. Effects may include anorexia, flatulence, metallic taste, nausea, stomach pain, vomiting, or weight loss. Some of these effects are transient and may be minimized by using small doses initially and increasing dosage gradually.

Metformin is not appropriate for traumatic disease or injury in a diabetic patient; insulin is usually required. Metformin is also avoided in patients with significant cardiorespiratory insufficiency, congestive heart failure, heart attack, or severe liver or renal disease or in patients prone to lactic acidosis. In all these conditions the risk of potentially fatal lactic acidosis is increased. For the same reason, metformin is avoided in patients undergoing angiography or pyelography because the contrast medium used in these procedures may increase risk of lactic acidosis.

Toxicity

Overdoses of metformin cause hypoglycemia and lactic acidosis.

Interactions

Alcohol should be avoided while taking metformin to avoid excessive risk of hypoglycemia or lactic acidosis. Amiloride, cimetidine, digoxin, morphine, procainamide, quinidine, quinine, ranitidine, triamterene, trimethoprim, and vancomycin may block renal secretion of metformin. Furosemide may increase oral absorption of metformin. The result of both types of interaction is to increase blood concentration of metformin; doses of metformin may require reduction.

Alternatives to Drug Therapy

Diet therapy

Mechanism of Action

Obesity, or more specifically excessive caloric intake, tends to reduce the number of insulin receptors. An understanding of this disease mechanism helps in appreciating the rationale for dietary control of diabetes. Reduced caloric intake allows the insulin receptors to increase and makes the available insulin more effective. Dietary restriction may lower insulin requirements in obese diabetic persons and in many cases may be the only form of therapy required. The effectiveness of sulfonylureas in obese patients with NIDDM is enhanced by caloric restriction and weight loss.

Careful dietary control is important for all diabetic persons. Successful long-term treatment of the condition frequently involves counseling by a dietitian and supportive follow-up for the rest of the patient's life.

NURSING PROCESS OVERVIEW

Diabetes Mellitus

Assessment

Diabetes occurs in all age groups. Assess vital signs, weight, serum and urine glucose levels, and any signs associated with possible long-term effects such as decreased circulation to the lower extremities. Assess the condition of skin and nails.

Nursing Diagnoses

- Possible complication: hypoglycemia
- Knowledge deficit related to diabetes mellitus

Patient Outcomes

The nurse will minimize and manage complications of hypoglycemia. The patient will explain how or demonstrate how to measure blood or urine glucose, administer insulin, treat hypoglycemia, manage diet, or other aspects of management as needed.

Planning/Implementation

In relation to drug therapy, monitor blood glucose and examine other appropriate laboratory work such as electrolytes or arterial blood gas levels. Begin planning for discharge as soon as the patient is diagnosed. Instruct the patient about the medications that have been prescribed, their method of administration, and how to test blood glucose. Refer the patient as appropriate to the hospital or community dietitian, the local visiting nurse association, and the local diabetes association.

Evaluation

Before discharge, verify that the patient can explain why the drugs are prescribed and can demonstrate how to administer insulin or other medications correctly. Be certain that the patient can explain the symptoms of hyperglycemia and hypoglycemia and how to treat them and other prescribed aspects of care such as foot care, dietary restrictions, and any limitations in activity that have been prescribed. Check that the patient can demonstrate how to test for blood glucose levels and can state what to do based on the information obtained from this test.

Nursing Implications Summary

General Guidelines: Treatment of Diabetes Mellitus

Patient and Family Education

- Teach the patient and family the signs and symptoms of hyperglycemia and hypoglycemia (see Table 63-3).
- The development of hypoglycemia may relate to the time the insulin or the oral agent was taken (see Tables 63-2 and 63-5) . If possible, obtain a blood glucose level. Whether or not a blood glucose level is obtained, treat by administering a fast-acting carbohydrate such as ½ cup fruit juice, ½ cup cola drink (not diet forms), ½ cup regular gelatin dessert, 4 cubes or 2 packets of sugar, 2 squares of graham crackers, or 2 to 3 pieces of hard candy. A common treatment is a glassful of orange juice containing 2 or 3 teaspoonsful of sugar. Wait about 15 minutes after ingesting carbohydrate, then measure blood glucose again. Instruct the patient to carry hard candy or other sources of carbohydrate with them at all times. Glucagon may be used if the patient is unconscious. Teach family members how to use this and instruct the patient to have glucagon always available.
- If hypoglycemia is severe, repeated, or occurs without explanation, consult the physician.
- Teach about appropriate dietary restrictions or refer the patient as needed to a dietitian. Losing weight to desirable body weight is helpful in controlling diabetes.
- Encourage participation in a regular exercise program.
- Review foot care and other aspects of personal hygiene to prevent infection.
- Instruct the patient how to test blood glucose level. Review methods of testing and frequency and supervise the patient performing the test activity for accuracy. If a urine test method is being used, point out to the patient that some drugs may cause urine test results to be inaccurate. Instruct the patient to ask the physician and pharmacist if there is a possibility of drug-urine test interaction whenever new drugs are prescribed.
- Refer the patient as appropriate to the health department or other community-based nursing care agencies for follow-up.
- Refer the patient to the American Diabetes Association or local support groups for additional information and resources; examples of such resources include syringes adapted for the visually impaired, information booklets, automatic insulin injectors, and cookbooks.
- Encourage the patient with diabetes to wear a medical identification tag or bracelet.
- Instruct the patient to avoid drinking alcoholic beverages.
- Instruct the patient to avoid smoking. Patients who begin or stop smoking may require an adjustment in diet or drug.
- Warn the patient to inform all health care providers about the diabetes and the type of drug used to control it.
- Avoid taking any drug unless first approved by the physician. Many drugs cause changes in blood glucose level. Instruct the patient to monitor blood and/or urine glucose level carefully when starting or stopping a new medication.
- The specific regimen prescribed for any patient is based on many factors, including age, type of diabetes, severity of diabetes, weight, resources available, philosophy of the health care team, and other medical problems the patient may have. Although general guidelines are noted in this text, consult other nursing texts and printed resources as needed.
- Caution female patients to consult the physician before attempting to conceive since management of diabetes may be modified during pregnancy. A diabetic female who becomes pregnant should notify the physician immediately.

Insulin

Drug Administration

- Local allergic reactions involving itching, redness, swelling, or stinging at the injection site are usually transient and are not uncommon. Anaphylaxis is very rare. Insulin resistance occasionally involves antibodies to insulin. It may not be possible to eliminate local allergic reactions. Supervise insulin administration technique since scrupulous attention to technique may lessen local irritation. Record and rotate sites on a systematic basis so that accessible sites are not overused (see Chapter 5). Prepare dose of insulin as ordered and let it warm to room temperature. Cleanse the injection site carefully and allow skin surface to dry completely. Pinch skin between thumb and fingers of one hand and insert needle into the "pocket" between the subcutaneous fat and muscle; a 45- to 90-degree angle can be used, depending on the amount of subcutaneous fat and the length of the needle. Inject the insulin and withdraw the needle. Apply moderate pressure to the site but do not rub.
- If local irritation is severe or persistent, consult the physician about a change in type of insulin.
- Systemic reactions are rare and may be caused by the animal source of the insulin (bovine, porcine, or mixed bovine-porcine). Treat symptomatically and notify the physician.
- Use regular insulin for patients on "sliding scale" management.
- Consult with the physician about diabetes management when patients are permitted nothing by mouth (NPO) in preparation for surgery or are otherwise unable to maintain usual dietary intake.
- For IV use, only regular insulin can be used. Insulin adsorbs to bags, tubing, and other items made of polyvinyl chloride (PVC). To decrease the amount of insulin lost to adsorption to the PVC during continuous infusion (e.g., 100 units regular insulin in 500 ml normal saline), flush

NURSING IMPLICATIONS SUMMARY—cont'd

the system with 50 ml of the diluted insulin mixture, then store the IV for 30 minutes before connecting it to the patient. Titrate the rate of infusion to the patient response, blood glucose levels, and ordered rate of drop of blood glucose level. Also monitor serum electrolyte level, especially potassium.

- Only buffered regular insulin is used in insulin pumps. Review the manufacturer's instruction sheet with the patient. Some patients follow a regimen that includes continuous infusion of insulin via pump, with periodic subcutaneous injections of additional insulin.
- Observe agency policies regarding insulin administration. For example, many hospitals require that insulin doses be checked by two licensed nurses before administration.
- Monitor serum and urinary glucose, serum potassium, pH, urinary ketones, and glycosylated hemoglobin.

Patient and Family Education

- Review the general guidelines and the information about injection with the patient.
- Teach the patient that only syringes marked for units of insulin should be used with insulin. There are special syringes available for doses less than 50 units. Review carefully with the patient the need to obtain the correct concentration and type of insulin and correct syringe.
- To mix insulins, instruct the patient to always draw up the regular (unmodified) insulin first, then the other insulin that is ordered. If two modified insulins are to be drawn up together, either can be drawn up first, but the patient should establish a pattern and always draw the same one up first.
- Some mixtures of insulin in a syringe must be administered within a few minutes of drawing them up, although others are stable for longer periods. The patient should consult the physician or pharmacist.
- Regular insulin is clear, and modified insulins are cloudy. Instruct the patient to not use discolored insulins or ones that appear grainy. Instruct the patient to warm and resuspend insulins by rotating the vials between the hands and to avoid vigorous shaking.
- Generally, insulin injected into the abdomen is absorbed the fastest, insulin in the arm is absorbed more slowly, and insulin is absorbed slowest when injected in the thigh. However, several things may influence this. For example, a diabetic patient who jogs has faster absorption from the thigh when jogging and using the thigh muscles. Consider the daily habits of the patient in working out an appropriate plan for diabetes management.
- Insulin can be safely kept at room temperature for up to 1 month. Insulin kept at room temperature for longer than 1 month should be discarded. Insulin may be stored in the refrigerator for longer than 1 month. Instruct the patient to not freeze insulin and to check the expiration date.
- Teach the patient that when illness occurs it is important to maintain fluid intake. Consult the physician about specific guidelines for insulin dose and diet when the patient is sick. Remind the patient to contact the physician whenever a question occurs about management.
- Develop an individualized teaching plan about insulin for patients. Decisions to be made include whether patients will use disposable syringes or will sterilize and reuse glass syringes, whether the patient has the ability (vision, dexterity, and so on) to draw up and administer the insulin, and what type of glucose test method will be used.
- Disposable syringes and needles were designed for one-time use. However, some patients reuse these syringes and needles, usually for economic reasons. If the patient must reuse syringes and needles, review the importance of cleaning the needle and capping the needle between uses. A syringe and needle should be used, even repeatedly, on only one patient, never shared. Finally, the syringe and needle should be reused for a few injections only, not on a continuing basis. If skin irritation is a problem, the patient may want to use a new needle or syringe more often.
- There are many kinds of specialized insulin injectors in use, including automatic injectors, insulin "pen" devices, and spray injectors. Review the manufacturer's instructions in teaching the patient how to prepare and use these injectors.
- Instruct the patient not to switch type or source of insulin without consulting the physician since a change in dose is often necessary. Also, do not switch the brand of syringe because small variations may be sufficient to cause improper dosage.
- Remind the patient to monitor the supply of insulin and syringes on hand to avoid running out unexpectedly.
- Instruct the patient with IDDM to carry insulin and syringes with hand luggage to avoid losing them whenever traveling. For large quantities of insulin and syringes, divide them among pieces of luggage so all are not lost if a piece of luggage is lost. Some states require prescriptions for syringes, so suggest the patient carry an adequate supply for the entire trip. This is especially important in international travel. Suggest the patient carry a letter from the physician listing the need for insulin and syringes since this may help if insulin is lost in delayed baggage or in delays at Customs. Discuss in advance with the pharmacist any special considerations for insulin storage.

Oral Hypoglycemic Agents

Drug Administration

- Review the symptoms of hypoglycemia and hyperglycemia listed in Table 63-3 and teach them to the patient.
- Monitor weight.
- Monitor complete blood count (CBC) and white blood cell (WBC) differential, platelet count, liver function tests, and blood glucose.

Continued.

NURSING IMPLICATIONS SUMMARY—cont'd

Patient and Family Education

- See the general guidelines for treating diabetes mellitus.
- Instruct the patient to report any new side effects.
- See the patient problem boxes on constipation (p. 304) and photosensitivity (p. 649).
- See the patient problem box on disulfiram-like reactions (p. 635). Some patients develop disulfiram-like reactions when they ingest alcohol and are taking a sulfonylurea.
- Remind the patient to take the medication as ordered, even if not feeling well.
- Usually, the patient should take ordered doses with the first meal of the day. If a dose is missed, instruct the patient to take it as soon as remembered, unless it is almost time for the next dose, in which case skip the missed dose and resume the regular dosing schedule. The patient should not double up for missed doses.

CRITICAL THINKING

APPLICATION

1. What three peptide hormones from pancreatic islets affect glucose metabolism?
2. What effect does insulin have on glucose metabolism?
3. What effect does glucagon have on glucose metabolism?
4. What effects do cortisol, epinephrine, and growth hormone have on glucose metabolism?
5. What effect does insulin have on fat and protein metabolism?
6. What is diabetes mellitus? How should you assess for this?
7. What are the characteristics of IDDM?
8. What are the characteristics of NIDDM?
9. What effect does diabetes mellitus have on protein and fat metabolism?
10. What are the long-term complications of diabetes mellitus?
11. How is diabetes mellitus diagnosed?
12. How does insulin therapy relieve the symptoms of diabetes mellitus?
13. Why must insulin be injected?
14. What is the onset and duration of action of regular insulin?
15. What advantages do the insulin preparations containing relatively insoluble insulin complexes have over regular insulin?
16. When does peak hypoglycemic action occur after a dose of insulin injection? Semilente insulin? NPH insulin? Ultralente insulin?
17. What reaction would be expected from an overdose of insulin? What are signs and symptoms of this?
18. What type of reactions may insulin produce at the site of injection?
19. What is the mechanism of action for the sulfonylureas as hypoglycemic agents?
20. What type of diabetic patient benefits from sulfonylurea therapy?
21. How are sulfonylureas administered?
22. Which sulfonylureas are converted to active forms by the body?
23. Which is the longest-acting sulfonylurea?
24. What side effects occur with sulfonylureas?
25. Why does caloric restriction enhance effectiveness of sulfonylureas?
26. What other drugs may enhance the hypoglycemic effect of sulfonylureas?
27. What reaction may be seen in patients receiving sulfonylureas who ingest ethyl alcohol?
28. How does metformin aid in controlling diabetes mellitus?
29. What are the most common side effects with metformin?
30. What classes of patients should not receive metformin?
31. What are the expected signs of overdosage with metformin?
32. What risk is associated with alcohol use by a patient receiving metformin?

CRITICAL THINKING

1. What is the duration of action of each of the insulin preparations? What are implications of this information in teaching patients?

CHAPTER 64

Drugs Acting on the Female Reproductive System

OBJECTIVES

After studying this chapter, you should be able to do the following:

- *Describe the use of estrogens in replacement therapy.*
- *Discuss the use of progestins alone or progestins in combination with estrogens as contraceptive agents.*
- *Discuss the drugs that can increase female fertility.*
- *Develop a nursing care plan for a patient receiving a drug discussed in this chapter.*

CHAPTER OVERVIEW

The female reproductive function depends on a complex, intricately regulated interaction of endocrine tissues. The negative feedback loop that regulates the menstrual cycle involves the hypothalamus, the anterior pituitary, and the ovaries (Chapter 59). Actions of the natural female hormones, as well as clinical uses of synthetic and natural drugs that affect the female reproductive system, are considered in this chapter.

KEY TERMS

amenorrhea
estrogens
gonadotropins
human chorionic gonadotropin (HCG)
menarche
menopause
progestins

Therapeutic Rationale: Hormones Involved in Female Reproduction

Classes of Female Hormones

Hormones involved in developing and maintaining female reproductive capacity include examples of all the chemical classes of hormones. The hypothalamus supplies gonadotropin-releasing hormone (GnRH), a peptide that acts directly on the anterior pituitary, stimulating synthesis and release of follicle-stimulating hormone (FSH) and luteinizing hormone (LH). In addition, the central nervous system (CNS) neurotransmitter dopamine is the inhibitory factor that regulates the release of prolactin from the anterior pituitary. FSH, LH, and prolactin are the major **gonadotropins.** These hormones each have a different primary target tissue. FSH stimulates the ovarian cells that form follicles and nurture the maturing ovum. Under the influence of FSH, these cells synthesize the potent steroid known as estradiol. LH acts primarily on a mature follicle to cause release of the ovum. Prolactin stimulates breast tissue to promote milk production but may affect other reproductive tissues as well.

The most important steroid hormones regulating female reproduction are estrogens and progestins. **Estrogens** are compounds that stimulate female reproductive tissues; **progestins** are compounds that specifically stimulate the uterine lining. Estrogens are produced in greatest abundance by FSH-stimulated cells of the ovarian follicle. Progesterone, the most important progestin, is synthesized in cells remaining in the follicle after expulsion of the ovum. This tissue is called the corpus luteum.

All the steroids produced in the ovary are derived from cholesterol. Progestins are formed first and are the precursors of androgens. Androgens, the steroid hormones capable of producing masculinization, are primarily precursors of estrogen synthesis in females. Androstenedione is the androgen precursor of estrone, a circulating estrogen formed mostly in peripheral tissues and not in the ovary. Estradiol, the most abundant circulating estrogen, is formed in the ovary.

Hormones Affecting Female Reproductive Development

At birth the ovary is already in an advanced stage of development and contains between 2 and 4 million oocytes, cells that will form ova. The primordial follicles containing oocytes are not quiescent before puberty but undergo a process called *atresia* in which oocytes are destroyed and follicles are resorbed. At **menarche,** when menstrual cycles begin during puberty, an estimated 400,000 oocytes remain. Even after ovulation is initiated, atresia continues and is responsible for the destruction of more than 99% of the follicles present in the ovary.

As puberty begins the immature ovaries are stimulated by increasing amounts of pituitary gonadotropins. As a result, estrogen synthesis is promoted, and estrogen levels in the blood rise. The primary function of estrogens during early puberty is to promote development of the reproductive system. The uterus and fallopian tubes enlarge to adult proportions. The vagina enlarges, and the vaginal epithelium thickens and strengthens. In the breasts, estrogen promotes proliferation of tissues responsible for the production of milk.

The secondary sexual characteristics also depend on estrogens. These hormones promote increased deposition of fat, especially in the breasts and hips. Without estrogens, the typical contours of the female body do not develop.

Estrogens are also involved in regulating the start and the stop of the growth spurt that is characteristic of puberty. Along with other hormones, estrogen causes retention of calcium and phosphorus and thereby promotes bone growth. Estrogens also induce closure of the epiphyses. When this closure occurs, no further increase in height occurs.

Hormones Affecting Ovulation

Ovulation requires proper functioning of the hypothalamus, anterior pituitary, and ovaries in the negative feedback loop described in Chapter 59. FSH and LH are required to act on the developing follicle before a mature ovum may be released to begin its journey down the fallopian tube to the uterus. Estrogen synthesis is required for its action on the follicle and for its ability to trigger the midcycle surge of LH from the anterior pituitary.

Hormones Affecting Endometrial Function

The uterus is composed of smooth muscle (myometrium) and glandular epithelium (endometrium). The endometrium, which nourishes and supports the ovum during development, is controlled primarily by estrogens and progestins. Estrogens promote proliferation of the endometrium during the first half of the menstrual cycle before ovulation occurs. Progesterone, which is formed in the corpus luteum of the ovary during the second half of the menstrual cycle, acts on the endometrium and the myometrium. Progesterone reduces myometrial activity, preventing muscular contractions, and promotes development of the secretory capacity of endometrium. Actions on these two tissues aid in establishing the environment in which the fertilized ovum may implant successfully and begin development. Once implantation of the ovum has occurred, progesterone continues to alter the endometrium, ultimately changing the tissue so that a second implantation becomes impossible.

Hormones in Pregnancy

Pregnancy requires that a mature ovum be released from the ovary at the appropriate time, that the ovum be fertilized successfully within about 2 days of its release, and that the ovum be able to implant within the endometrium and to draw nourishment to support the early stages of development. The most important hormone during these first days and weeks of pregnancy is progesterone. Without adequate progesterone, the endometrium is sloughed and the fertilized ovum is lost. Luteal progesterone is produced for about the first 10 weeks of pregnancy. Control of progesterone synthesis is exercised by cells of the fetus, which develop into the placenta. A few days after implantation of the ovum in the endometrium, these fetal cells begin to produce a hormone called **human chorionic gonadotropin (HCG);** HCG takes over control of the corpus luteum and maintains its production of progesterone. By the fifth week of pregnancy the placenta has developed to where it begins to synthesize progesterone directly. Placental progesterone production increases during the remainder of the pregnancy, whereas progesterone production in the corpus luteum virtually disappears.

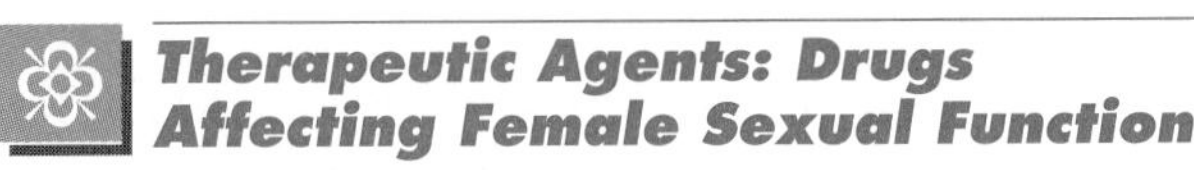

Therapeutic Agents: Drugs Affecting Female Sexual Function

Agents for Replacement Therapy

Estrogens

Mechanism of Action

Many conditions of the female reproductive tract for which women seek medical aid may be treated successfully by replacement therapy. The most common conditions are those that arise as a result of estrogen deficiency. A lack of estrogen during puberty prevents normal growth and sexual development; menarche may not occur. This endocrine malfunction is one of several abnormalities that may be responsible for **amenorrhea** (no menstrual cycles). **Menopause,** which usually occurs in the late forties or early fifties, is the state in which estrogen levels begin to decline. Lower estrogen levels may cause vasomotor symptoms (hot flashes and sweating), osteoporosis (bone loss), and atrophy of vaginal and urethral tissue. Exogenously supplied natural or synthetic estrogens have the same actions described earlier for endogenously formed estrogens and thus can effectively replace the missing natural estrogen.

Other medical problems of the female reproductive system cannot be ascribed to a specific hormone deficiency. Nevertheless, many of these conditions respond to hormones used for some pharmacologic action rather than as replacement therapy. The rationale for therapy for these conditions is listed in Table 64-1.

TABLE 64-1 Pharmacologic Therapy of Dysfunctions of Female Reproductive System

CLINICAL CONDITION	TREATMENT	RATIONALE
Hypogonadism	Cyclic estrogen-progestin or menotropins	Estrogens are required to promote secondary sex characteristics. Other hormonal support may be required for full fertility.
Amenorrhea	Bromocriptine, gonadorelin, or a progestin	Drugs are effective only for specific types of conditions producing amenorrhea.
Menopause		
Vasomotor symptoms	Estrogens	Hot flashes and sweating are relieved by estrogens.
Osteoporosis	Estrogens	Loss of calcium may be halted temporarily but not reversed.
Atrophy of vaginal and urethral tissue	Estrogens	Estrogen support is needed to maintain tissue tone.
Dysfunctional uterine bleeding	Estrogen and progestin	Combination stops bleeding; drug withdrawal induces endometrial sloughing.
Luteal phase defect (infertility)	Progestins	Infertility resulting from inadequate synthesis of progesterone from corpus luteum may be treated by progestin early in pregnancy.
Metastatic breast carcinoma	Estrogens, androgens, or progestins	Tumors show differing sensitivities to these hormones.
Metastatic endometrial carcinoma	Progestins	Natural suppressive effect of progestins on endometrium is retained in some of these tumors.
Galactorrhea	Bromocriptine	Drug suppresses prolactin release, thereby preventing excessive stimulation of breast secretory tissue.
Dysmenorrhea	Oral contraceptives or prostaglandin inhibitors	Suppression of ovulation gives relief to some patients. Drugs such as ibuprofen, indomethacin, mefenamic acid, naproxen, and ketoprofen relieve symptoms by preventing excessive production of prostaglandins.
Pelvic endometriosis	Estrogen, progestin, danazol, goserelin, leuprolide, naferelin	Suppresses proliferation of endometrial tissue. Inhibits gonadotropins, thus preventing proliferation of endometrial tissue.
Anovulation (infertility)	Bromocriptine, clomiphene citrate, menotropins, HCG, gonadorelin, or urofollitropin	Ovulatory failure may be corrected by use of agents that promote gonadotropin release (clomiphene) or supply them directly (menotropins). HCG acts as LH to trigger release of ovum.
Premenstrual tension	Ergotamine, diuretics, or antianxiety agents	Therapy is empiric and is often ineffective.

Pharmacokinetics

Many estrogens are available (Table 64-2). The two naturally occurring steroid estrogens used clinically are estradiol and estrone. As steroids, these compounds are not water soluble, but they are soluble in oil. With estradiol, slower absorption and longer duration of action may be achieved by using the cypionate or the valerate ester of the natural steroid. Estradiol is absorbed orally if the drug crystals are reduced to particles 1 to 3 μm in diameter. Estradiol is also effectively absorbed transdermally.

Estrone is not well absorbed orally in its natural form but may be used orally if it is converted to the piperazine sulfate (estropipate). Estrone is also the major component of various estrogen mixtures described as *esterified or conjugated estrogens.* These mixtures, which are isolated from the urine of pregnant mares, are relatively cheap and are effective for many purposes, and all can be taken orally, which makes them a convenient drug form for many patients.

Synthetic estrogens such as ethinyl estradiol are also available. Ethinyl estradiol is more potent than naturally occurring estrogens. This drug used orally has a relatively short duration of action but persists in the body longer than any of the natural estrogens.

Nonsteroidal estrogens such as chlorotrianisene and diethylstilbestrol (DES) are oral agents. DES, which was discovered in 1938, was once widely used to prevent spontaneous abortions, but the children who were in utero at the time of DES treatment may have suffered drug effects. As adults, female offspring have an increased incidence of vaginal adenosis and adenocarcinoma; male offspring are more prone to develop epididymal cysts. DES is currently used as an antineoplastic agent (Chapter 50). Chlorotrianisene may be used as an anticancer drug or as an estrogen.

Natural estrogens do not persist long in the body because they are rapidly metabolized by the liver and excreted by the kidney. Ethinyl estradiol is less rapidly metabolized and is therefore longer acting than natural estrogens. Nonsteroidal estrogens are not metabolized rapidly and also persist longer than natural ones.

Uses

Estrogen doses vary depending on the condition being treated. When used in replacement therapy, estrogen doses tend to be low. Higher doses treat conditions such as advanced breast cancer. Table 64-2 gives ranges for doses of the various preparations, but a drug handbook or the pharma-

TABLE 64-2 Estrogens Used Primarily for Replacement Therapy

GENERIC NAME	TRADE NAME	ADMINISTRATION/DOSAGE	COMMENTS
Chlorotrianisene	TACE	ORAL: *Adults*—12-25 mg daily.	Primarily for prostatic carcinoma.
Dienestrol	Dienestrol*	VAGINAL: *Adults*—One application twice daily, tapering to 1 dose 1 to 3 times weekly for 3 wk, then no drug for 1 wk.	For vaginal and vulval atrophy.
Estradiol	Estrace*	ORAL: *Adults*—0.5-2 mg daily. VAGINAL: *Adults*—0.1 mg 1-3 times weekly for 3 wk, then no drug for 1 wk.	For estrogen replacement.
	Estraderm	TRANSDERMAL: *Adults*—One patch delivers 0.05 or 0.1 mg daily; change twice weekly.	For estrogen replacement.
Estradiol cypionate	Depo-Estradiol Dura-Estrin	INTRAMUSCULAR: *Adults*—1-5 mg every 3 or 4 wk.	For estrogen replacement.
Estradiol valerate	Delestrogen* Femogex†	INTRAMUSCULAR: *Adults*—10-20 mg every 4 wk.	For estrogen replacement; higher doses for prostatic carcinoma.
Estrogens, conjugated	Congest† Premarin*	ORAL: *Adults*—0.3-7.5 mg daily. INTRAMUSCULAR, INTRAVENOUS: 25 mg every 6-12 hr. VAGINAL: *Adults*—1.25-2.5 mg daily for 3 wk; may repeat after 1 wk with no drug.	For estrogen replacement; IM doses for abnormal uterine bleeding.
Estrogens, esterified	Estratab Neo-estrone†	ORAL: *Adults*—0.3-7.5 mg daily.	For estrogen replacement.
Estrone	Aquest Estragyn Wehgen	INTRAMUSCULAR: *Adults*—0.1 mg-2 mg/wk.	For estrogen replacement; higher doses for abnormal uterine bleeding.
Estropipate	Ogen*	ORAL: *Adults*—0.75-9 mg daily. VAGINAL: *Adults*—3-6 mg daily for 3 wk, then no drug for 1 wk.	For estrogen replacement.
Ethinyl estradiol	Estinyl*	ORAL: *Adults*—0.05 mg 1-3 times daily.	For estrogen replacement; higher doses for breast or prostatic carcinoma.
Quinestrol	Estrovis	ORAL: *Adults*—0.1mg daily for 1 week, then 0.1 mg once weekly.	For estrogen replacement.

*Available in Canada and United States
†Available in Canada only.
NOTE: All estrogens are FDA pregnancy category X.

cist should be consulted for the dose of a specific preparation in a specific condition.

Estrogens are also used in combinations with progestins. These combinations are discussed in the section on oral contraceptive drugs.

Adverse Reactions and Contraindications

Side effects of estrogens include overreactions of certain reproductive tissues to the hormones. Breast tenderness is reported by many women who take estrogen. Estrogens stimulate endometrial proliferation, and some evidence suggests that estrogens alone may increase the risk of endometrial cancer; estrogens given cyclically with progestins do not support endometrial hyperplasia and the risk of endometrial cancer is reduced. Estrogens have not been shown to increase the risk of breast cancer in women but may do so in men.

Estrogens are often associated with acute adverse reactions such as nausea and vomiting, anorexia, and mild diarrhea. Malaise, depression, or excessive irritability are also related to estrogen therapy in some women. Estrogens promote salt and water retention and may therefore produce edema in some patients. Atherosclerosis is a definite risk for patients who take estrogens, especially if they have other high-risk factors such as smoking. Hypertension has been associated with estrogen use.

Estrogens are routinely avoided in patients with breast cancer because estrogens may promote growth of these tumors. Rarely, metastatic tumors may be treated with estrogens. Vaginal bleeding also precludes the use of estrogens because the bleeding may signal conditions such as endometrial hyperplasia or carcinoma, which would be worsened by estrogens.

Toxicity

High doses of estrogens in women may produce any of the signs noted above. Migraine headaches and vomiting may also occur. The vomiting is triggered by effects in the CNS.

Interactions

Estrogens may block the effects of bromocriptine. Estrogens also increase the risk of toxicity with hepatotoxic drugs. Both hepatotoxicity and nephrotoxicity of cyclosporine may be enhanced.

Progestins

Mechanism of Action

Progestins used as drugs promote all the actions of the naturally occurring progestins. Some preparations are most effective as progestational agents, whereas others have significant activities in other areas. For example, some progestins have detectable androgenic effects. Megesterol has a medically useful antianoretic and anticachectic action. These actions and others all arise as the progestin interacts with the steroid receptors inside target cells and alter gene expression.

Pharmacokinetics

Progestins available for medical use include the natural steroid hormone progesterone and synthetic derivatives of that compound (Table 64-3). Although progesterone is not useful orally, many derivatives are administered conveniently and effectively by that route. Injections of progesterone are painful and may produce local inflammation. Progesterone is rapidly metabolized by the liver and eliminated in urine.

TABLE 64-3 Clinical Summary of Progestins

GENERIC NAME	TRADE NAME	ADMINISTRATION/DOSAGE	COMMENTS
Hydroxyprogesterone	Hylutin	INTRAMUSCULAR: *Adults*—375 mg FDA pregnancy category D.	For amenorrhea or dysfunctional bleeding.
Levonorgestrel	NORPLANT	SUBDERMAL IMPLANT: *Adults*—6 capsules implanted; duration 5 yr. FDA pregnancy category X.	For contraception.
Medrogestone†	Colprone†	ORAL: *Adults*—5-10 mg on days 15 through 25 of cycle.	For dysfunctional uterine bleeding, menopause, or induction of menses.
Medroxyprogesterone	Cycrin Provera*	ORAL: *Adults*—5-10 mg for 5-10 days. FDA pregnancy category X.	For amenorrhea, induction of menses, or dysfunctional uterine bleeding.
Medroxyprogesterone	Depo-Provera	INTRAMUSCULAR: *Adults*—150 mg every 3 mo. FDA pregnancy category X.	For contraception; higher doses for carcinoma.
Megestrol	Megace	ORAL: *Adults*—800 mg daily for 1 mo, then 400-800 mg for 3 mo. FDA pregnancy category X.	For AIDS-associated anorexia, cachexia, and weight loss; also for breast or endometrial carcinoma.
Norethindrone acetate	Aygestin Norlutate*	ORAL: *Adults*—2.5-10 mg daily on days 5 through 25 of cycle. For endometriosis: 5-15 mg daily. FDA pregnancy category X.	For amenorrhea or dysfunctional uterine bleeding.
Progesterone	Gesterol	INTRAMUSCULAR: *Adults*—Up to 50 mg daily. VAGINAL: *Adults*—25-100 mg once or twice daily. FDA pregnancy category D.	For amenorrhea or dysfunctional uterine bleeding; vaginal suppositories for corpus luteum insufficiency.
	Progestasert	INTRAUTERINE: *Adults*—One IUD replaced yearly; contains 38 mg progesterone.	For contraception.

*Available in Canada and United States.
†Available in Canada only.
NOTE: For oral contraceptive use of progestins, see Table 64-5.

Uses

Progestins are used clinically for their effects on the endometrium. High doses suppress bleeding of the endometrium, and withdrawal induces sloughing of the tissue; thus, they may be useful for secondary amenorrhea, dysfunctional uterine bleeding, and to induce menses (see Table 64-3). Lower doses of progestins induce changes in the endometrium and cervical mucus that prevent pregnancy. This use of progestins is discussed in the section on contraceptive agents.

Adverse Reactions and Contraindications

Adverse reactions to progestins may involve several organ systems other than reproductive organs. Some of these reactions are similar to those seen with estrogens including edema, breast tenderness and swelling, gastrointestinal (GI) disturbances, depression, and weight change. Other reactions include changes in menstrual blood flow, midcycle spotting or breakthrough bleeding, cholestatic jaundice, and rashes. Medroxyprogesterone has been associated with delays in returning to fertility after the drug is withdrawn. Megestrol is associated with hyperglycemia in as many as 16% of treated patients.

Progestins should be avoided during pregnancy because many progestins have some androgenic activity and may cause masculinization of female fetuses. Patients with a history of thromboembolic disorders or thrombophlebitis should not be treated with progestins. These drugs are also normally avoided in patients with breast tumors or hepatic disease because these conditions may be worsened by progestins.

Toxicity

High doses of progestins are associated with greater risks of thromboembolitic disease. If blood clots form, patients may note sudden sharp pains, sudden and severe headaches, or sudden changes in speech, vision, or coordination. Any of these signs are reason to immediately seek medical attention. Fatalities have occurred.

Interactions

Aminoglutethimide lowers serum concentrations of medroxyprogesterone. Drugs such as carbamazepine, phenobarbital, phenytoin, rifabutin, or rifampin may induce enzymes in the liver that metabolized progestins; this action lowers the effect of progestins.

Agents That Restore Fertility

Loss of fertility in women may occur for many reasons. Therapy depends on evaluating the cause of infertility. In some women the pituitary and ovaries are normal, but the proper stimulus for follicular development is not transmitted. For these women, clomiphene may be effective (Table 64-4). This

TABLE 64-4 Fertility Agents and Agents for Endometriosis

GENERIC NAME	TRADE NAME	ADMINISTRATION/DOSAGE	COMMENTS
Bromocriptine	Parlodel*	ORAL: *Adults*—1.25 mg once at bedtime with food; increase to 2.5 mg 2 or 3 times daily. FDA pregnancy category B.	Inhibitor of prolactin release used for infertility caused by excessive prolactin; also used to suppress effects of pituitary prolactinoma.
Chorionic gonadotropin	A.P.L.* Profasi*	INTRAMUSCULAR: *Adults*—5000-10,000 U once in an appropriately primed patient. FDA pregnancy category C.	Placental hormone related to LH is used for stimulation of ovulation.
Clomiphene	Clomid*	ORAL: *Adults*—50 mg daily on days 5 through 10 of menstrual cycle. FDA pregnancy category X.	For infertility caused by anovulation. Mechanism is probably hypothalamic.
Danazol	Cyclomen†	ORAL: *Adults*—50-400 mg twice daily.	Inhibitor of pituitary gonadotropin release; used for endometriosis or fibrocystic breast disease.
Gonadorelin	Factrel*	SUBCUTANEOUS, INTRAVENOUS: *Adults*—0.1 mg once for diagnosis or repeated for infertility. FDA pregnancy category B.	Stimulates release of FSH and LH from healthy ovary; diagnostic or treatment of infertility.
Leuprolide	Lupron*	INTRAMUSCULAR: *Adults*—3.75 mg once a month. FDA pregnancy category X.	Analog of GnRH used continuously suppresses estradiol and progestins; used for endometriosis.
Menotropins	Pergonal*	INTRAMUSCULAR: *Adults*—75 U each of FSH and LH daily for 9-12 days. FDA pregnancy category X.	Human urinary menopausal gonadotropins; FSH and LH in preparation induce ovulation.
Nafarelin	Synarel*	INTRANASAL: *Adults*—0.2 mg in one nostril in morning; repeat in other nostril in evening. FDA pregnancy category X.	Peptide analog of GnRH, used continuously suppresses estradiol and progestins; used for endometriosis.
Urofollitropin	Metrodin*	INTRAMUSCULAR: *Adults*—150 U daily. FDA pregnancy category X.	Human urinary menopausal FSH used to induce ovulation.

*Available in Canada and United States.
†Available in Canada only.

drug seems to activate the pituitary by hypothalamic mechanisms, and ovarian stimulation is thus achieved. Stimulation of several follicles may be induced by clomiphene, and multiple births have occurred.

In women with pituitary glands that cannot supply sufficient gonadotropins to properly stimulate the ovaries, infertility may also occur. In this situation, menotropins may be prescribed. This mixture of compounds extracted from the urine of postmenopausal women contains FSH and LH in approximately equal amounts. When LH action alone is required, HCG may be prescribed. HCG is chemically related to LH and possesses many of the same physiologic actions, including the ability to stimulate ovulation.

Bromocriptine is a chemical relative of the ergot alkaloids, which are used as oxytocic agents. Bromocriptine is clinically useful because it can inhibit prolactin secretion. Bromocriptine is approved in the United States to control *galactorrhea* (spontaneous milk production) caused by excessive prolactin secretion usually from functional tumors. Amenorrhea (no menstrual cycles) and infertility also are produced when prolactin secretion is excessive. Bromocriptine suppression of prolactin secretion reverses these symptoms, and fertility becomes possible.

CONTRACEPTIVE AGENTS

Oral Contraceptives

Mechanism of Action

Reversible sterility induced by pharmacologic agents has been possible since the late 1950s when the oral contraceptive agents became available. These agents contain a combination of estrogen and a progestin or a progestin alone (Table 64-5). The effectiveness of oral contraceptives is very high. Most reports give estimates of 0% to 6% failure rates in a year of use for the combined estrogen-progestin agents. This pregnancy rate is in contrast to rates of 2% to 28% failures per year for mechanical devices such as diaphragms, sponges, and condoms.

Estrogen-progestin combinations suppress ovulation. In addition, these drugs induce changes in the cervical mucus, which make it difficult for sperm to enter the uterus. Changes also occur in the endometrium that make implantation difficult even if fertilization occurs. The preparations that contain progestins alone alter the cervical mucus and the endometrium as the combination products do, but they do not always suppress ovulation. The effectiveness of agents that contain only progestins is less than that of the combined preparations.

To achieve contraception and to simulate the normal menstrual cycle, the oral contraceptives usually are taken for 21 consecutive days. The increased estrogen and progestin levels suppress the hypothalamus and the hypophysis so that no LH is released at the time when ovulation would normally occur. This is the mechanism by which ovulation is suppressed. During the 7 days when hormones are not administered, the endometrium involutes and sloughs off, primarily as a result of loss of progestin activity. This withdrawal period prevents excessive proliferation of the endometrium.

Synthetic progestins are used in oral contraceptives. Progesterone, a natural progestin, is used in an intrauterine device (IUD). This device (Progestasert) was developed to administer the fertility-controlling drug directly to the target tissue. The very small amounts of progesterone released are retained within the reproductive tract rather than being systemically absorbed. The effectiveness of this device depends on the mechanical effects of the IUD and on the pharmacologic effects of progesterone.

Pharmacokinetics

The pharmacokinetics of oral contraceptives is the same as previously discussed for the estrogen or progestin components of these preparations.

Uses

The oral contraceptive preparations are intended to provide reversible prevention of pregnancy in otherwise healthy women. These preparations are also useful to control irregular or excessive menstrual cycles.

Adverse Reactions and Contraindications

Side effects produced by oral contraceptives may come from the estrogen or the progestin component. Side effects caused by estrogens may include nausea, bloating, breast fullness, edema, hypertension, and cervical discharge. Patients who report these symptoms may be given a preparation with low estrogen such as Loestrin 1/20 or Lo/Ovral. Side effects associated with progestins include hair loss, hirsutism, oily scalp, acne, increased appetite and weight gain, tiredness and depression, breast regression, and reduced menstrual blood flow. Oral contraceptives fall into FDA pregnancy category X.

Oral contraceptives are used by millions of women worldwide to prevent pregnancy. Oral contraceptives are highly effective, but questions about the safety of these agents have been raised. In particular the incidence of unexpected serious or fatal medical conditions has been studied in the relatively healthy women who take oral contraceptives. Risk of certain serious medical conditions is now shown to be increased in oral contraceptive users when they are compared with similar women who do not take these drugs (Table 64-6).

As with any medication, oral contraceptives must be considered in terms of the risk-to-benefit ratio. Of primary importance may be how much value the patient places on almost complete protection against unwanted pregnancy. Women who desire this high level of control should then consider the safety factors of the medication. Many of the dangerous complications (e.g., stroke and thromboembolytic diseases) are rare even among oral contraceptives users. The risk of these complications is greater than the risk among nonusers of oral contraceptives but much lower than the risk of these complications during pregnancy. Women should also consider the other predisposing risk factors such as smoking, obesity, and hypertension. The combination of oral contra-

TABLE 64-5 Oral Contraceptives

PROGESTIN	ESTROGEN	PROGESTIN:ESTROGEN RATIO	TRADE NAME
Desogestrel	Ethinyl estradiol	0.15 mg:30 μg	Desogen, Marvelon,† Ortho-Cept*
Ethynodiol diacetate	Ethinyl estradiol	1.0 mg:50 μg	Demulen 1/50,* Nelulen 1/50 E
		1.0 mg:35 μg	Demulen 1/35, Nelulen 1/35 E
		2.0 mg:30 μg	Demulen 30†
Levonorgestrel	Ethinyl estradiol	0.15 mg:30 μg	Nordette, Levlen
		0.05 mg:30 μg (6 tablets), and 0.075 mg:40 μg (5 tablets), and 0.125 mg:30 μg (10 tablets).	Triphasil,* Triquilar,† and Tri-Levlen
Norethindrone	None	0.35 mg	Micronor,* and Nor-QD
Norethindrone acetate	Ethinyl estradiol	1.5 mg:30 μg	Loestrin 1.5/30*
		1.0 mg:20 μg	Loestrin 1/20, Minestrin 1/20†
Norethindrone	Ethinyl estradiol	1.0 mg:50 μg	N.E.E 1/50, Ovcon-50
		1.0 mg:35 μg	Genora 1/35, N.E.E. 1/35, Nelova 1/35, Norcept-E, Norethin 1/35, Norinyl 1 + 35, and Ortho-Novum 1/35
		0.5 mg:35 μg	Brevicon,* Genora, Modicon, and Nelova 0.5/35E
		0.4 mg:35 μg	Ovcon-35
		0.5 mg:35 μg (10 tablets), and 1.0 mg:35 μg (11 tablets)	GenCept 10/11, Nelova 10/11‡ and Ortho-Novum 10/11‡
		0.5 mg:35 μg (7 tablets), and 0.75 mg:35 μg (7 tablets), and 1.0 mg:35 μg (7 tablets)	Ortho-Novum 7/7/7§
		0.5 mg:35 μg (7 tablets), and 1.0 mg:35 μg (9 tablets), and 0.5 mg:35 μg (5 tablets)	Tri-Norinyl¶
Norethindrone	Mestranol	1.0 mg:50 μg	Norinyl 1 +50, Genora 1/50, Nelova 1/50, Norethin 1/50, and Ortho-Novum 1/50*
		0.5 mg:100 μg	Ortho-Novum 0.5†
		1.0 mg:80 μg	Ortho-Novum 1/80
		2.0 mg:100 μg	Ortho-Novum 2†
Norgestimate	Ethinyl estradiol	0.25 mg:35 μg	Ortho-CyClen
		0.18 mg:35 μg (7 tablets), and 0.215 mg:35 μg (7 tablets), and 0.250 mg:35 μg (7 tablets)	Ortho Tri-Cyclen
Norgestrel	Ethinyl estradiol	0.5 mg:50 μg	Ovral*
		0.3 mg:30 μg	Lo/Ovral
Norgestrel	None	0.075 mg	Ovrette

*Available in Canada and United States.
†Triphasic preparation—0.05 mg: 30 μg pills are taken the first 6 days of the cycle, 0.075 mg: 40 μg pills the next 5 days, and 0.125 mg: 30 μg pills the next 10 days of the cycle, followed by a week of no medication or placebo.
‡Biphasic preparation—0.5 mg: 35 μg pills are taken the first 10 days of the cycle, and 1.0 mg: 35 μg pills the next 11 days of the cycle, followed by a week of no medication or placebo.
§Triphasic preparation—0.5 mg: 35 μg pills are taken the first 7 days of the cycle, 0.75 mg: 35 μg pills the next 7 days, and 1.0 mg: 35 μg the next 7 days, followed by a week of no medication or placebo.
¶Triphasic preparation—0.5 mg: 35 μg pills are taken the first 7 days of the cycle, 1.0 mg: 35 μg pills the next 9 days, and 0.5 mg: 35 μg pills the next 5 days of the cycle, followed by a week of no medication or placebo.
NOTE: All oral contraceptives are FDA pregnancy category X.

ceptives with these conditions leads to unacceptable risk for many patients. All women who take oral contraceptives should be urged to stop smoking.

Some medical conditions are improved or the symptoms are ameliorated by oral contraceptives. Many patients report a reduction in menstrual disorders and especially in dysmenorrhea. Menstrual blood flow usually is reduced, and anemia is prevented or lessened in many women. Benign breast tumors may be improved in a time-dependent fashion by oral contraceptive therapy, but patients with carcinoma of the breast, cervix, liver, uterus, or vagina should not take these drugs because these cancers may be stimulated by estrogens.

Current medical data suggest that oral contraceptives are safe in young women in whom other risk factors are minimized. Women with a history of hypertension or thromboembolytic disease probably should not receive the drugs. Women who choose to take oral contraceptives should undergo thorough physical examinations yearly. The dose of es-

TABLE 64-6 Oral Contraceptives: Adverse Reactions

ADVERSE REACTION	RELATION TO ORAL CONTRACEPTIVES	COMMENTS
Thromboembolytic diseases	Risk increased 2- to 7-fold in users over nonusers. Incidence about 100:100,000 woman years; fatalities 2:100,000 woman years.*	Obesity, family history of thromboembolytic disorders, immobility, or group A blood type may increase risk. Group O blood type females have lower risk. Directly related to estrogen dosage.
Thrombotic stroke	Risk increased 3.1- to 6-fold. Incidence about 25: 100,000 woman years; fatalities 0.5:100,000 woman years.*	Hypertension increases risk.
Hemorrhagic stroke	Risk increased at least 2-fold. Incidence about 10: 100,000 woman years.*	Hypertension and heavy smoking are strong risk factors.
Myocardial infarction	Risk increased about 2-fold over nonusers when estrogen doses exceed 50 μg daily.	Synergistic increase in risk if oral contraceptives are used by smokers.
Hypertension	Between 1% and 5% of patients show increase in blood pressure. Clinical hypertension is more rare.	Risk is increased by age, obesity, and parity.
Gallbladder disease	Risk increased an estimated 2-fold.*	Risk may be related to duration of use.
Liver disease	Up to 50% of patients show altered liver function. Incidence 10:100,000 woman years for jaundice. Tumors are rare.	Reversible. Dangerous for patients with preexisting liver disease (hepatitis or cholestasis). Liver tumors may be related specifically to mestranol.
Carbohydrate metabolism	Many patients show reduced glucose tolerance.	Important only in prediabetic women who may become insulin-dependent. Related to dose and potency of progestin.
Lipid metabolism	Many patients have increased serum triglyceride levels.	Reversible effect; relationship to coronary artery disease in these patients is unknown.
Chloasma	3%-4% of patients treated.	Increased sensitivity to sunlight also occurs. Reversible.
Headaches	Variable reports with no clear conclusion.	Chronic headache may presage stroke.
Visual disturbances	Have been associated with use of oral contraceptives.	Temporary blindness, blind spots, and changes in field of vision have been reported.
Emotional state disturbances	Variable reports with no clear conclusion.	No evidence that oral contraceptives significantly increase depression.
Endometrial cancer	No increased risk when combined estrogen-progestin agents used.	Risk is increased by estrogens alone but is reduced by progestins. Some studies suggest protection.
Cervical cancer	No relationship established.	Frequency of coitus and number of sexual partners more important risk factors.
Breast cancer	No relationship established.	Benign breast tumors are improved.
Permanent infertility	No relationship established.	Most patients quickly return to fertility when oral contraceptives are discontinued.
Outcome of later pregnancies	No increased risk to mother or fetus has been demonstrated.	Data are for pregnancies begun after oral contraceptives have been discontinued.

*Risk may be less with the lower dose estrogen products currently in use.

trogen and progestin should be the lowest dose that achieves contraception and prevents unwanted side effects such as breakthrough bleeding.

Careful history taking may reveal symptoms that the patient has not linked to oral contraceptive use. Migraine headaches, dizziness, and visual disturbances often are not related by the patient to oral contraceptive use and may not be mentioned spontaneously. Breakthrough bleeding, excessive cervical mucus formation, breast tenderness, and other changes in the reproductive tract usually are quickly connected to oral contraceptive use by patients. These symptoms may be more annoying than serious. Severe headaches or visual disturbances are often early signs of impending stroke and may be sufficient cause to discontinue the medications.

The first contraceptive agents contained relatively high amounts of estrogens, but the agents available today have lower estrogen content. These lower estrogen combinations are usually as effective as the older agents and may be associated with a lower incidence of side effects (see Table 64-6).

Toxicity

Acute overdoses with oral contraceptives often cause nausea and vomiting. Withdrawal vaginal bleeding may also occur. Higher doses over longer periods of time are associated with greater risk of thromboembolitic complications.

Interactions

Oral contraceptive agents are subject to the same interactions as the estrogen and progestin components. Hepatotoxic medications should be avoided. Hepatic enzyme inducers may impair effectiveness of the oral contraceptives and lead to unexpected pregnancy. Oral contraceptives interfere with the activity of bromocriptine and anticoagulants and increase the toxicity of tricyclic antidepressants.

Contraceptive Implants

When long-term pharmacologic contraceptive protection is desired, systemic absorption can be achieved without the need for daily oral dosing. Because most forms of the steroid hormones such as estrogens and progestins are relatively insoluble in water, they are slowly absorbed from tissue sites when injected. This property can be used to advantage by confining the drugs to insoluble polymers that can then be implanted under the skin. Small amounts of drug are continuously released over very long periods of time. One example of such an application is the contraceptive Norplant (Figure 64-1). Six slender capsules each containing 36 mg of the synthetic progestin levonorgestrel are implanted subdermally. This application affords contraceptive protection for up to 5 years.

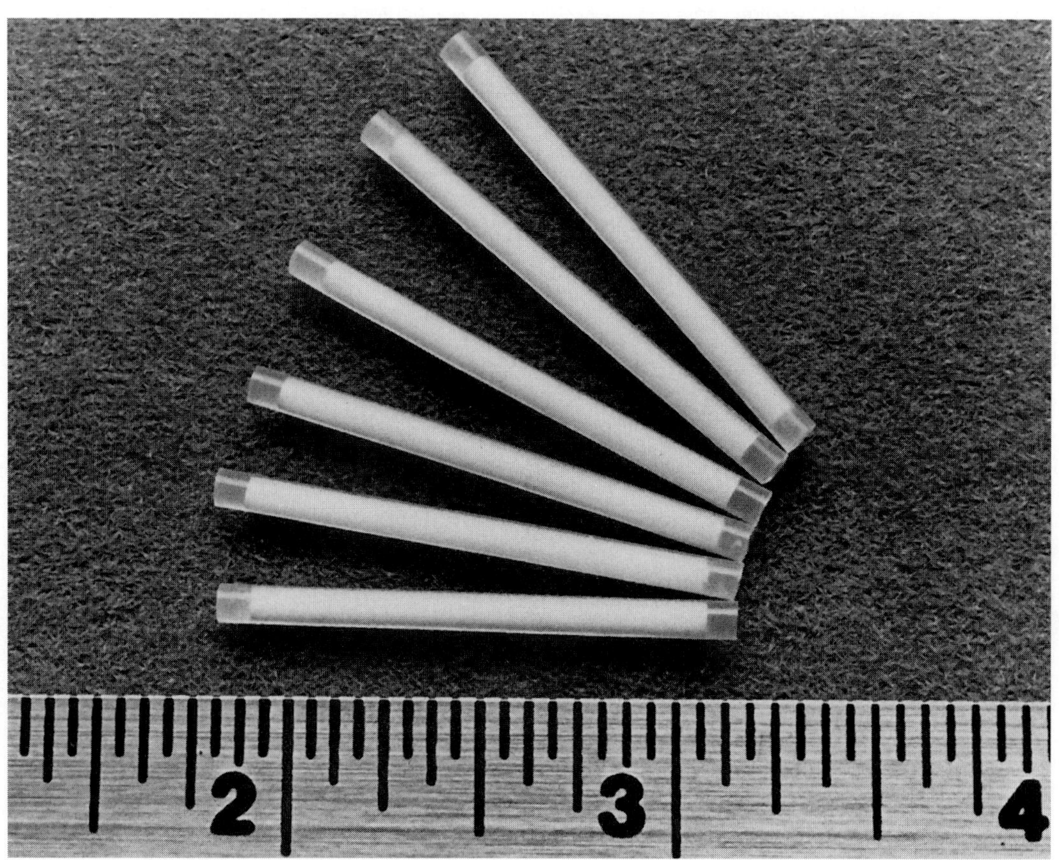

FIGURE 64-1
Contraceptive implant form called Norplant.

NURSING PROCESS OVERVIEW

Drugs Acting on Female Reproductive System

Assessment

Drugs acting on the female reproductive system provide replacement therapy, cause or inhibit ovulation and conception, and treat hormonally sensitive tumors. Obtain a complete patient assessment, focusing on the problem being addressed by the drug. Monitor the vital signs, blood pressure (BP), weight, description of the menstrual cycle; assess the patient's breasts and condition of skin.

Nursing Diagnoses

- Potential complication: vascular disorders
- Self-concept disturbance: acne and weight gain related to drug therapy

Patient Outcomes

The nurse will minimize and manage vascular complications. The patient will discuss concerns related to self-concept and will state two positive features about himself or herself.

Planning/Implementation

Continue to monitor the pulse, BP, and weight. Explain patient activities needed in detail to help ensure success. For example, activities such as using alternative birth control measures during the first month of birth control pill therapy, keeping basal temperature charts to monitor possible ovulation, and saving urine specimens to measure hormone or drug excretion need thorough explanations. Monitor calcium levels in patients being treated for cancer.

Evaluation

Before discharge, verify that the patient can explain why and how to take the drug, possible side effects that might occur, which side effects require immediate medical attention, and the risks associated with therapy.

NURSING IMPLICATIONS SUMMARY

Estrogens

Drug Administration

- Assess vital signs, blood pressure, weight, history of weight gain or loss, nausea and vomiting, breast for enlargement, complaints of breast pain, and mammogram if available. Assess dependent areas for edema.
- Monitor liver function tests, serum lipid profile. Monitor x-rays of hand and wrist in children to monitor bone age.
- Patients with metastatic bone cancer who are started on hormonal therapy may develop severe hypercalcemia. Monitor serum electrolyte levels (see Table 17-1).

Patient and Family Education

- Teach the patient to take drug as ordered even if not feeling well. Nausea may develop during the first few weeks of therapy but should diminish with regular use. Take doses with meals or food, or just after eating, to lessen GI symptoms.
- Emphasize the importance of regular follow-up visits to monitor for side effects and effectiveness.
- Notify the physician if any of the following develop: breast pain, discharge from breasts, lumps in breast, changes in vaginal bleeding such as breakthrough bleeding or amenorrhea, stomach cramps, nausea, vomiting, diarrhea, loss of appetite, headache, or jaundice.
- For men taking estrogens for breast or prostate cancer, review symptoms of possible thromboembolism: severe or sudden headache, shortness of breath, sudden slurred speech, changes in vision, weakness or numbness in the arm or leg.
- Teach the patient to perform monthly breast self-examination. Encourage regular mammograms if recommended by the physician.
- Encourage patient to have regular Pap smears.
- Drug may cause tenderness, swelling, or bleeding of gums. Encourage the patient to brush and floss teeth carefully and regularly, see a dentist regularly, and have teeth professionally cleaned periodically.
- Notify the physician immediately if pregnancy is suspected.
- Encourage the patient to avoid or limit smoking while taking this drug.
- Teach proper injection technique if patient is to administer intramuscular (IM) forms at home.
- To use *transdermal patch:* See the manufacturer's instruction leaflet. Wash and dry hands before and after handling patches. Apply patch to a clean, dry, nonoily area of abdomen or buttocks. Avoid areas with excess hair, cuts, or irritation. Avoid the waist, other areas that may be rubbed with clothing. Do not apply to breasts. Apply patch firmly for about 10 seconds. If patch falls off or comes loose, reapply or apply a new patch. Apply each new patch to a different area, so that at least a week passes before an area is used again.
- To administer *vaginal cream:* See the manufacturer's instructions. For daily application, use at bedtime. Avoid

Continued.

NURSING IMPLICATIONS SUMMARY—cont'd

tampons but wear a sanitary napkin to protect clothing. Do not use this medication as a lubricant during sexual intercourse; regular absorption by the male partner through the skin of the penis may cause side effects. This drug may also weaken diaphragms, cervical caps, or condoms; check with the physician or pharmacist.

Progestins

Drug Administration

- If drug is used in an estrogen-progestin combination product for birth control, see the section on birth control (below).
- Assess vital signs, blood pressure, menstrual history, weight, and history of weight gain or loss. Assess dependent areas for edema. Assess skin for hair loss, acne, and changes in hair growth. Perform mental status exam. Assess vision.
- Monitor liver function tests.

Patient and Family Education

- If the patient is using a combination estrogen/progestin product for birth control, see the section on birth control (below).
- Emphasize the importance of returning for regular follow-up visits to monitor for drug effectiveness and side effects.
- Spotting or breakthrough bleeding during the first 3 months of therapy is not unusual. Notify the physician of heavy or prolonged bleeding or amenorrhea.
- Instruct the patient to notify the physician of sudden or severe headache, changes in vision, pain in chest leg or groin, shortness of breath, slurred speech, increase or decrease in weight over 2 pounds per day or 5 pounds in 1 week; discharge from breasts, depression, GI pain, swelling of feet or legs, acne, or thinning of hair.
- This drug may cause tenderness, swelling, or bleeding of gums. Encourage the patient to brush and floss teeth carefully and regularly, see a dentist regularly, and have teeth professionally cleaned periodically.
- Women who are fertile and sexually active should use a birth control method while taking this drug. Notify the physician immediately if pregnancy is suspected or if 45 days have elapsed since the last menstrual period.
- Encourage the patient to have regular Pap smears.
- For IM administration: review proper injection technique with patient.
- This drug may alter lab results. Remind the patient to tell physician before having lab work performed that progestins are being used.

General Guidelines: Fertility Agents

Patient and Family Education

- Teach the patient to keep a record of basal body temperature, consistency of vaginal mucus, and 24-hour urine specimen as prescribed by the physician.
- Make certain the patient understands the best time of the month to have intercourse to attempt to get pregnant on the basis of the drugs being used.
- Provide emotional support. Treatment of infertility problems may be prolonged and discouraging.
- Encourage the patient to return as directed for blood tests, ultrasounds, examinations, additional medications, and other therapies as prescribed.
- Remind the patient to keep all drugs out of the reach of children.
- If pregnancy is suspected, notify the physician, because these drugs should usually not be continued during pregnancy.

Bromocriptine

Drug Administration

- Assess mental status. Assess for signs of depression including lack of interest in personal appearance, withdrawal, anorexia, and insomnia.
- Monitor pulse and BP. Check stools and emesis for occult blood.
- If drug is used for fertility problems, assess date of last menstrual period and other measures used to treat infertility.
- If drug is used for acromegaly: assess ring and shoe size, height, and weight.
- If drug is used for Parkinson's disease, assess other current treatments, ability to perform activities of daily living, signs of disease (mask-like facial expression, tremor, rigidity, salivation, shuffling gait). See Chapter 56.

Patient and Family Education

- Review the anticipated benefits and possible side effects of drug therapy. Tell the patient to report any new side effects.
- Suggest that the patient take the first dose while lying down or at bedtime because dizziness is more likely to occur with first dose. Take doses with meals or snack.
- See the patient problem boxes on constipation (p. 304), dry mouth (p. 300), and orthostatic hypotension (p. 157).
- When used to treat Parkinson's disease, full benefit of this drug may not be seen for several weeks. Provide emotional support. See Chapter 56.
- See the general guidelines for infertility.
- Take doses with meals or a snack to lessen gastric irritation. Warn patients to avoid driving or operating hazardous equipment if drowsiness develops
- Avoid drinking alcoholic beverages; see the patient problem box on alcohol use and disulfiram on p. 635.
- Depending on the patient's age and reason for taking bromocriptine, counsel about methods of birth control as appropriate.

NURSING IMPLICATIONS SUMMARY—cont'd

Chorionic Gonadotropin

Drug Administration/Patient and Family Education

- Review the anticipated benefits and possible side effects of drug therapy. Remind the patient to notify the physician if any unexpected side effects develop or if any side effects are severe or persistent. Instruct the patient to monitor daily basal body temperature if prescribed.
- Remind women of common side effects including breast enlargement, headache, irritability, edema, fatigue, depression, or stomach or pelvic pain.
- This drug may be used to treat cryptorchidism if no anatomic obstruction is present. Notify the physician if acne, enlargement of the penis or testes, growth of pubic hair, or rapid increase in height develops.
- Warn the patient to avoid driving or operating hazardous equipment if excessive fatigue or visual changes occur; notify the physician.
- See the general guidelines for infertility.

Clomiphene Citrate

Drug Administration/Patient and Family Education

- Review the anticipated benefits and possible side effects of drug therapy. Common side effects include breast discomfort, headache, heavy menstrual periods, and nausea or vomiting. Notify the physician if abdominal pain, blurred or double vision, or jaundice develops. Encourage the patient to notify the physician if any unexplained side effects develop.
- Typical instructions for taking this drug are to count the first day of the menstrual cycle as day 1. Begin clomiphene in the dose ordered on day 5, and continue daily until the prescribed number of doses is completed. Review instructions with the patient, and check to see that she understands the dosing schedule. In addition, the physician may want the patient to use an ovulation prediction kit; review the manufacturer's instructions with the patient.
- The drug may also be prescribed for men; review the physician's prescription with the patient.
- Warn the patient to avoid driving or operating hazardous equipment. If changes in vision occur, the patient should notify the physician.
- See the general guidelines for infertility.
- Monitor liver function tests, HCG levels, and urinary LH levels.

Danazol

Drug Administration

- This drug may be used to treat endometriosis, fibrocystic breast disease, hereditary angioedema, and hematologic disorders including idiopathic thrombocytopenic purpura (ITP). It has weak androgenic and anabolic properties (see Chapter 66).
- Assess for weight gain. Inspect for acne, edema of dependent areas, and hirsutism. Monitor BP and liver function tests.

Patient and Family Education

- Review the anticipated benefits and possible side effects of drug therapy. Encourage the patient to notify the physician if any unexpected side effects develop. Common side effects in women include reduction in breast size, hirsutism, weight gain, deepening of voice, and emotional lability. Side effects caused by the androgenic properties of the drug may be less noticeable in male patients.
- Tell the female patient that menstrual periods may diminish or cease while taking this drug (depending on dose). She should keep a record of menstrual periods. Instruct her to use birth control measures while taking danazol and for 2 months after stopping therapy but not to use birth control pills. Tell the patient to notify the physician if pregnancy is suspected.
- Side effects are dose related but may be intolerable to some patients. Remind the patient to take drugs as ordered for best effects and not to discontinue therapy without consulting the physician.
- Warn the diabetic patient to monitor blood glucose levels carefully while taking this drug; a change in diet or insulin dose may be needed.

Gonadorelin

- Except for allergic reaction, usually after multiple doses, no serious side effects have been reported with this drug. Warn the patient that itching may occur at the injection site. Consult the manufacturer's literature. See the general guidelines for infertility.
- Monitor serum LH levels.

Leuprolide

Drug Administration

- This drug is used to treat cancer of the prostate (see Chapter 50) and endometriosis.
- For endometriosis, assess menstrual history and previous treatment for infertility.
- Review the side effects with the patient: hot flashes, nausea or vomiting, weight gain, trouble sleeping. Men may experience constipation, decreased size of testicles, transient bone pain, impotence or decreased libido, and loss of appetite. Women may experience decreased libido, breast tenderness, mood changes, vaginitis, and amenorrhea or spotting. Instruct the patient to notify the physician of any unexpected sign or symptom.
- Read physician's orders carefully; there is an injectable subcutaneous form and an IM depot form. The depot form should be administered by the physician. If the patient is to self-administer at home, review the patient instruction leaflet supplied with the subcutaneous form.
- Perform a pregnancy test before treating for endometriosis, unless starting drug during menstrual period. For prostate cancer, monitor serum acid phosphatase and/or prostate-specific antigen (PSA).

Continued.

Nursing Implications Summary—cont'd

Menotropins

Drug Administration/Patient and Family Education

- Review the anticipated benefits and possible side effects of drug therapy. Tell the patient to report any new, severe, or persistent side effects.
- Teach the female patient to record basal body temperature if prescribed.
- This drug is often administered with chorionic gonadotropin. Side effects are often related to excessive ovarian stimulation and include abdominal discomfort, nausea and vomiting, diarrhea, increased weight, and hypertension.
- The drug may also be administered to men. It may cause breast enlargement.
- If the patient is to self-administer, teach IM injection technique.
- See the general guidelines for infertility.

Nafarelin

Drug Administration/Patient and Family Education

- Assess menstrual history, history of infertility.
- Review the possible side effects with the patient, including breakthrough bleeding, heavy menstrual periods, amenorrhea or spotting; pelvic pain or bloating, joint pain, headache, rash, breast pain, depression, weight changes. Instruct the patient to report new, severe, or persistent side effects to the physician.
- Administer doses as a nasal spray. Review the patient instruction leaflet supplied by manufacturer.
- The drug may cause vaginal drying. Encourage the use of a water-soluble lubricant during sexual intercourse.

Urofollitropin

Drug Administration/Patient and Family Education

- Review the anticipated benefits and possible side effects of drug therapy. Tell the patient to report any new, severe, or persistent side effects.
- Common side effects include bloating, pelvic pain, nausea and vomiting, and breast tenderness.
- See the general guidelines for drugs for infertility.
- Instruct the patient to record daily basal body temperature if prescribed.
- If the patient is to self-administer this drug, teach injection technique.

Oral Contraceptives

Drug Administration

- Monitor blood pressure, pulse, and weight. Assess for skin changes.
- Instruct the patient to report leg pain, sudden onset of chest pain, shortness of breath, coughing up blood, dizziness, changes in vision or speech, or weakness or numbness of an arm or leg because these may indicate pulmonary embolism or other thromboembolic problems.
- Assess for signs of depression including withdrawal, insomnia, anorexia, and lack of interest in personal appearance.
- Assess tactfully for changes in libido. The patient may be reluctant to discuss this problem.
- Monitor complete blood cell count (CBC) and liver function tests.
- For discussion of IM administration of oil-based suspension, see Chapter 5.

Patient and Family Education

- Review the anticipated benefits and possible side effects of drug therapy. Review Table 64-6. Tell the patient to notify the physician if any new side effects develop.
- Counsel or refer the patient as needed about stopping smoking, losing weight to achieve desirable weight, and modifying diet to decrease cholesterol and triglycerides.
- Warn the diabetic patients to monitor blood glucose levels carefully because these drugs may alter glucose levels.
- Tell the patients to take doses with meals or a snack to lessen nausea. This side effect usually lessens with continued use. The patient should try taking the dose at bedtime rather than in the morning.
- Warn the patients to avoid driving or operating hazardous equipment if changes in vision occur; notify the physician.
- Instruct the female patient to report any vaginal bleeding or menstrual irregularities. Notify the physician immediately if pregnancy is suspected.
- Remind the patients to inform all health care providers of all medications being used. It may take several months for these drugs to be completely eliminated even when the patient has stopped taking them, so the patient should be reminded to inform health care providers for up to several months after therapy has stopped.
- See instruction leaflet supplied with oral contraceptive for instruction about missed doses. The guidelines vary somewhat depending on the product being used.
- Many drugs interfere with effectiveness of birth control pills. Teach the patients to ask physician or pharmacist about this possibility whenever a new medication is taken.
- If a patient discontinues oral contraceptives to become pregnant, recommend that she use an alternative form of birth control for 2 months after stopping the pills to ensure more complete excretion of the hormonal agents before conceiving and thus reducing the potential effects of the medications on the fetus.
- Teach the patient how to do a breast self-examination and encourage them to perform this monthly.
- A patient taking estrogens may develop brown areas on the skin. See the patient problem box on photosensitivity (p. 649).
- Tell the patient taking birth control pills that the drugs work best when used regularly. Keep an additional month's supply on hand to avoid running out of pills.

NURSING IMPLICATIONS SUMMARY—cont'd

- Remind the patient to keep all medications out of the reach of children.
- For *implant* dosage form: the implants are inserted under the skin of the upper arm by a physician or trained professional. Instruct the patient to keep gauze in place on the insertion site for 24 hours, then remove it. Leave strips of tape in place for 3 days. Full contraceptive protection begins within 24 hours if the insertion is performed within 7 days of the beginning of a menstrual period. Contraceptive protection should last for 5 years. The implants should be removed and replaced if desired after 5 years.
- For medroxyprogesterone injection form: Instruct the patient to return at 3-month intervals for injection of this contraceptive. Full contraceptive protection begins immediately if the patient receives the injection within the first 5 days of a menstrual period or within 5 days of delivering a baby if the mother is not breast feeding. Emphasize the importance of returning on schedule for later injections.

CRITICAL THINKING

APPLICATION

1. What are gonadotropins?
2. How are the synthesis and release of FSH, LH, and prolactin regulated?
3. What are the major steroid hormones that affect the female reproductive tract?
4. What are the functions of estrogens during puberty?
5. What hormones regulate ovulation?
6. What effect do estrogens have on the endometrium in an adult woman?
7. What effects does progesterone have on the endometrium and myometrium?
8. What is the function of progesterone in pregnancy?
9. What is the role of HCG in pregnancy?
10. How do the steroidal estrogens differ from the nonsteroidal estrogens in duration of action and route of excretion from the body?
11. What side effects are characteristic of pharmacologic use of progestins?
12. What is the mechanism of action of clomiphene, and what is its medical use?
13. What hormones are contained within menotropins?
14. What is the mechanism of action of bromocriptine, and how is it currently used?
15. What is the mechanism of action of gonadorelin, and what is its medical use?
16. What is the mechanism of action of urofollitropin, and what is its medical use?
17. What agents are used to produce pharmacologic contraception?
18. What is the mechanism of action of the oral contraceptive agents?

CRITICAL THINKING

1. What side effects and toxic reactions are seen with the chronic use of estrogens? How should you assess for these?
2. What side effects occur with use of the oral contraceptives? What should you teach about these side effects?

CHAPTER 65

Drugs for Labor and Delivery

OBJECTIVES

After studying this chapter, you should be able to do the following:

- *Compare the actions and uses of the three classes of oxytocic drugs.*
- *Explain how ritodrine may control premature labor.*
- *Develop a nursing care plan for a patient receiving a drug discussed in this chapter.*

KEY TERMS

myometrium
oxytocin
prostaglandins

CHAPTER OVERVIEW

A successful pregnancy and postpartum period depends on the proper functioning of several systems of the body. This chapter reviews the endocrine control of pregnancy and discusses drugs used to facilitate delivery of the fetus. It discusses drugs used to protect the fetus from premature delivery and drugs used in the postpartum period to control uterine bleeding.

Therapeutic Rationale: Childbirth and Postpartum Care

Physiology of Childbirth

To understand the pharmacologic management of labor and delivery, an understanding of the physiologic processes involved is necessary.

During pregnancy, high progesterone levels are thought to aid in maintaining the pregnancy by suppressing contractions of the **myometrium,** the powerful muscle layer in the uterine wall. As the pregnancy comes to term, progesterone levels begin to decrease, allowing the uterus to begin to produce **prostaglandins.** Prostaglandins are involved in regulating myometrial activity. These derivatives of fatty acids are readily formed in their target tissues and are rapidly degraded without persisting in blood for any appreciable time. In the uterus, these hormones induce very powerful myometrial contractions. Prostaglandins, especially the E and F series (PGE_2 and PGF_2alpha), may play a role in natural induction of labor. Prostaglandin levels rise in the amniotic fluid and other pelvic reproductive tissues as term approaches. This increasing concentration of prostaglandins has been suggested to be the stimulus causing Braxton Hicks contractions, the mild myometrial contractions occurring during the final few weeks of pregnancy. **Oxytocin,** a hormone produced by the neurohypophysis, is also capable of inducing uterine contractions. The uterus increases its sensitivity to oxytocin at term and during the puerperium (period immediately after birth).

During stage I of parturition, uterine contractions begin to increase in frequency and intensity, and the cervix begins to dilate. In stage II uterine contractions occur at the rate of about one every 2 minutes. The cervix is fully dilated, and uterine contractions bring about the delivery of the infant. During stage III of labor the frequency of contractions decreases, and the placenta separates from the uterus and is expelled. Uterine contractions continue for hours to days, with the frequency and intensity of the contractions diminishing with time.

When contractions occur during labor and delivery, the myometrium compresses major blood vessels supplying oxygen to the fetus. The result is that during a contraction, the fetus is relatively anoxic. When the uterus relaxes between contractions, oxygenated blood quickly returns to the fetus. If the uterus is overstimulated and fails to relax sufficiently between contractions, the prolonged anoxia can harm the fetus. Induction of labor with one of the oxytocic drugs carries with it the risk of producing this condition. Therefore all patients in whom labor is being induced should receive continuous care, and fetal monitoring should be done when possible. Oxytocin is the drug of choice to induce or stimulate labor because it seems to allow the uterus to relax between contractions. The ergot alkaloids and other oxytocic drugs tend to increase the overall tone of the myometrium and the strength of contractions and therefore carry a greater risk of producing fetal anoxia.

Uterine contractions that occur after delivery have two beneficial effects on the mother. First, they are responsible for expulsion of the afterbirth and produce a general cleansing of the uterus. Second, these contractions aid in controlling postpartum bleeding by clamping the vessels that were ruptured by the birth process. If bleeding is a problem at this stage, the physician may use an agent with a longer and more continuous action such as one of the ergot alkaloids.

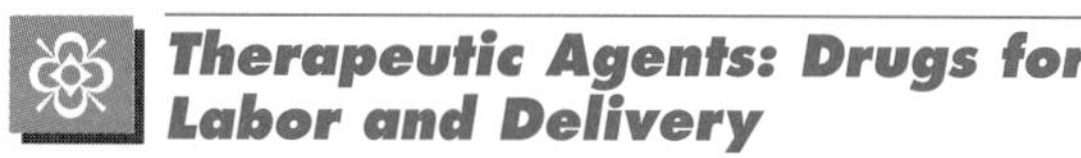

Therapeutic Agents: Drugs for Labor and Delivery

Oxytocic Drugs

Oxytocin

Mechanism of Action

Oxytocin interacts with specific receptors in the myometrium and raises the level of calcium inside these smooth muscle cells; this action induces contraction of the myometrium (Table 65-1). The uterus is relatively insensitive to the action of oxytocin until labor has started. Oxytocin also acts on breast tissue; it stimulates the myoepithelium of the breast and promotes milk letdown. Suckling by the infant sets off a reflex action in which oxytocin release is stimulated. The central nervous system (CNS) controls this process; the sight of the infant is sufficient in some women to induce oxytocin release and milk letdown. Oxytocin action is responsible for the improved uterine muscle tone in nursing mothers and for the more rapid return of the uterus to the pregravid size in these women.

Pharmacokinetics

Oxytocin is a peptide and is therefore quickly broken down by enzymes in target tissues and in plasma. Oxytocin has a quick onset of action by intranasal, intramuscular, or intravenous routes, but the effect disappears within 3 hours. Effects of intranasal doses on milk letdown are lost within 20 minutes.

Uses

Oxytocin is used to induce or augment labor. In addition, it may be used to control postpartum bleeding by inducing contraction of the myometrium. The intranasal route is used to promote milk letdown and facilitate breast feeding. Oxytocin may be used to induce or complete an abortion.

Adverse Reactions and Contraindications

Adverse reactions to oxytocin are rare. Possible reactions include allergies, arrhythmias, changes in blood pressure, uterine rupture, or water intoxication.

Oxytocin should be avoided in patients with a history of allergy to the drug. It should not be used to augment or induce labor in a patient who cannot support a vaginal delivery or in a patient with hypertonic uterine contractions.

Toxicity

High doses of oxytocin may cause hypotension. Other reactions may also be worsened.

TABLE 65-1 Oxytocic Drugs

GENERIC NAME	TRADE NAME	ADMINISTRATION/DOSAGE	COMMENTS
✤ Oxytocin	Pitocin Syntocinon*	INTRAVENOUS: *Adults*—For induction or augmentation of labor: 0.5-2 mU/min gradually increased to 10 mU/min. For postpartum hemorrhage or abortion: 10 U at 20-100 mU/min. INTRANASAL: *Adults*—Lactation stimulant: 1 spray of 40 U/ml solution before nursing. FDA pregnancy category X.	May produce uterine hypertonicity with fetal or maternal injury; monitor uterine contractions and status. Onset of action within 2-3 min; also causes nasal vasoconstriction.
Ergot Alkaloids			
Ergonovine	Ergotrate*	ORAL, SUBLINGUAL: *Adults*—To control postpartum bleeding: 0.2-0.4 mg every 6-12 hr for 48 hr. INTRAVENOUS: *Adults*—To control postpartum bleeding: 0.2 mg IV given over 1 min; repeat every 2-4 hr up to 5 doses.	Produces strong tetanic contractions; avoid use until placenta is delivered.
Methylergonovine	Methergine	ORAL: *Adults*—To control postpartum bleeding: 0.2-0.4 mg every 6-12 hr for 48 hr. INTRAVENOUS, INTRAMUSCULAR: *Adults*—To control postpartum bleeding: 0.2 mg IV given over 1 min; repeat every 2-4 hr up to 5 doses.	Produces strong tetanic contractions; avoid use until placenta is delivered.
Prostaglandins			
Carboprost	Hemabate Prostin/15M†	INTRAMUSCULAR: *Adults*—To control postpartum bleeding: 0.25 mg by deep IM injection; repeat every 15-90 min up to total dose of 2 mg. INTRAAMNIOTIC: *Adults*—To induce abortion: 2.5 mg over 5 min.	Two thirds of patients experience vomiting and diarrhea.
Dinoprost†	Prostin F_2 Alpha†	INTRAAMNIOTIC: *Adults*—To induce abortion: 5 mg at 1 mg/min; then 35 mg over 5 min. Repeat in 24 hr.	Up to 57% of patients experience vomiting or other GI symptoms.
Dinoprostone	Prepidil* Prostin E_2*	INTRACERVICAL: To induce cervical ripening: 0.5 mg in cervical canal. Maximum dose 7.5 mg in 24 hr. INTRAVAGINAL: *Adults*—For induction of labor: 1 mg repeated in 6 hr. To induce abortion: 20 mg repeated every 3-5 hr up to maximum of 240 mg in 48 hr.	Patients should remain supine for 10-30 min after dosing.

*Available in Canada and United States.
†Available in Canada only.

Interactions

Oxytocin may cause excessively strong uterine contractions if combined with other oxytocic agents or with intraamniotic urea or sodium chloride.

Ergot alkaloids: ergonovine and methylergonovine

Mechanism of Action

Ergot alkaloids are fungal products that have been known as poisons since the Middle Ages, when it was noted that people who ate grain contaminated with this fungus suffered from dry gangrene. This extreme reaction is caused by the potent vasoconstrictive effect of ergot alkaloids. Blood flow to the limbs may be reduced so severely that the tissues die, and the limbs eventually fall away with little or no bleeding. In addition, pregnant women who ate the affected grain entered an abrupt and devastating labor that expelled fetuses at any stage of development. The preparations used today have less vasoconstrictive activity but retain the ability to directly increase the force and frequency of myometrial contractions.

Pharmacokinetics

Oral doses of ergonovine or methylergonovine produce effects on uterine contractions within 15 minutes. Intramuscular doses take effect within 5 minutes. Effects are maintained for about 3 hours. Hepatic metabolism inactivates these drugs, and the metabolites are excreted in urine.

Uses

Ergot alkaloids are indicated for postpartum hemorrhage after delivery of the placenta.

Adverse Reactions and Contraindications

Reactions to ergot alkaloids include angina and bradycardia. Other cardiac arrhythmias, myocardial infarction, and severe hypertension are rare but can occur.

Ergot alkaloids are usually avoided in patients with significant cardiovascular disease, peripheral vascular disease, hypertension, eclampsia, or preeclampsia. These conditions are worsened by the vasoconstrictive effects of the drugs.

Toxicity

High doses of these drugs are associated with peripheral vasospasm or vasoconstriction, angina, miosis, confusion, respiratory depression, seizures, or unconsciousness. Uterine tetany may occur.

Interactions

Vasoconstrictors may be more potent in the presence of the ergot alkaloids, which are themselves vasoconstrictors.

Prostaglandins: carboprost, dinoprost, and dinoprostone

Mechanism of Action

Prostaglandins are potent stimulators of the myometrium and have been successfully used to induce abortion during the second trimester when the uterus is resistant to oxytocin. Carboprost also facilitates dilation of the cervix.

Pharmacokinetics

Prostaglandins are rapidly degraded in the blood and are unstable to gastric acid.

The most comfortable and safest route of administration may be transabdominal instillation into the amniotic fluid. Given this way, the drug stays primarily within the uterus and persists in action for hours. Intravaginal delivery also keeps the drug at the site of action and avoids rapid degradation carried out in maternal lung and liver.

Uses

Prostaglandins are used primarily as abortifacients. Carboprost is also used to soften the cervix to facilitate vaginal delivery.

Adverse Reactions and Contraindications

These drugs very often cause significant gastrointestinal (GI) side effects, including diarrhea, nausea, vomiting, and stomach cramps. Fever, chills, and flushing are also noted.

Less common but more serious reactions include anaphylaxis, arrhythmias, bronchoconstriction, chest pain, hypertension, and peripheral vasoconstriction.

Toxicity

Overdoses may cause the exaggerated responses noted above as well as uterine cramping or tetany.

Interactions

Prostaglandins are usually not combined with oxytocin because the risk of uterine tetany or uterine laceration is increased.

Uterine Relaxants

✣ Ritodrine

Mechanism of Action

Specific uterine relaxation in cases of hypertonicity or premature labor is not yet possible, but several types of compounds produce uterine relaxation along with other reactions. For example, premature labor is sometimes treated with agents that stimulate beta-2-adrenergic receptors, because stimulation of these receptors in the uterus causes relaxation of the myometrium. Agonists of beta-2-adrenergic receptors cause side effects throughout the body, however, as a result of beta-adrenergic receptor stimulation in other tissues. The best beta-2-adrenergic agonist for use in halting premature labor is ritodrine. This agent effectively relaxes the myometrium but also affects the peripheral vasculature and other tissues. (See Table 65-2.)

Pharmacokinetics

Ritodrine may be used orally or intravenously. Ritodrine usually is administered intravenously when premature labor begins. When contractions have been controlled for 12 to 24 hours, the patient may be started on oral ritodrine, and the intravenous (IV) infusion may be discontinued. The onset of action after oral doses is within 30 minutes. The drug is inactivated in the liver and eliminated by the kidneys.

TABLE 65-2 Drugs Used to Control Premature Labor

GENERIC NAME	TRADE NAME	ADMINISTRATION/DOSAGE	COMMENTS
Isoxsuprine	Vasodilan*	INTRAMUSCULAR: *Adults*—5-10 mg 2 or 3 times daily.	Canadian preparation; not approved for this use in the United States.
✣ Ritodrine	Yutopar*	INTRAVENOUS: *Adults*—0.05-0.1 mg/min increased by 0.05 mg every 10 min up to maximum of 0.35 mg/min. ORAL: *Adults*—10 mg 30 min before IV infusion is terminated; then 10 mg every 2 hr for 24 hr; maintain within 10-20 mg every 4-6 hr.	Ritodrine is the preferred drug to control premature labor.
Terbutaline	Bricanyl*	INTRAVENOUS: *Adults*—0.01 mg/min increasing up to 0.08 mg/min. SUBCUTANEOUS: *Adults*—0.25 mg every hr until contractions cease. ORAL: *Adults*—2.5 mg every 4-6 hr until at term.	Primary use is to control bronchospasms; alternate for control of premature labor.

*Available in Canada and United States.
†Available in Canada only.

Uses
Ritodrine is used to halt spontaneous labor when it appears after the twentieth week of pregnancy and before the thirty-sixth week. Spontaneous labor beginning before the twentieth week often is associated with a defective fetus and may not be interrupted.

Adverse Reactions and Contraindications
The heart is sensitive to stimulation by ritodrine suggesting that the drug is also an agonist with some activity on beta-1-adrenergic receptors. The major side effects noted with this drug have been heart palpitations, nausea and vomiting, trembling, flushing, and headache. These effects appear transient and rarely cause termination of therapy. Patients should be observed for undue tachycardia or signs of cardiac distress. The fetal heart may also be stimulated by ritodrine. Ritodrine increases the workload of the mother's heart and is contraindicated in patients with preexisting cardiac disease.

Toxicity
Overdoses of ritodrine may produce excessive beta-adrenergic stimulation, especially noticed as cardiovascular symptoms.

Interactions
Beta-adrenergic blockers inhibit the effects of ritodrine. Corticosteroids may increase the risk of pulmonary edema.

Other drugs to halt premature labor
CNS depressants may halt premature labor. Ethanol, which is an inhibitor of oxytocin release and a CNS depressant, has been used to halt premature labor. The levels required to relax the uterus are sufficient to produce acute alcohol intoxication. Controlled clinical trials have suggested ritodrine is more effective and less toxic.

General anesthetics may also relax the uterus. Enflurane and halothane are the preferred agents. In addition to CNS effects, these agents may act directly on the myometrium and may also slow catecholamine release from the adrenal gland, thus reducing endogenous stimulators of myometrial activity.

Progesterone is the natural steroid that normally functions as a uterine relaxant. The use of this or another progestins is not recommended in cases of uterine hypertonicity during delivery, because the hormone may not reach the uterus in sufficient quantities to relax the uterus quickly and effectively. Use of progesterone during earlier stages of pregnancy may cause undesirable effects on the developing fetus.

NURSING PROCESS OVERVIEW

Drugs for Labor and Delivery

Assessment

Assess the vital signs, blood pressure, history of previous pregnancies and deliveries, fetal heart tones, and fetal position.

Nursing Diagnoses

- Potential complication: preterm labor
- Potential complication: fetal distress

Patient Outcomes

The nurse will minimize and manage complications of preterm labor. The nurse will manage and minimize episodes of fetal distress.

Planning/Implementation

Continue to monitor vital signs and blood pressure. Assess frequency, duration, and force of contractions. With oxytocics, monitor the mother and infant closely, and use an IV monitoring device. Provide emotional support. Monitor intake, output, specific gravity. Initiate and maintain fetal monitoring, as appropriate.

Evaluation

Ideally, all pregnancies would continue to term, with successful delivery of a healthy child or children. Emphasize importance of follow-up visit.

NURSING IMPLICATIONS SUMMARY

Oxytocin

Drug Administration

- See Table 65-1. Monitor level of consciousness, weight, and intake and output. Monitor blood pressure and pulse. Auscultate lung and heart sounds. Monitor frequency, duration, and force of contractions.
- Monitor fetal heart sounds; notify the physician of significant changes in rate or rhythm; follow agency protocol.
- Monitor serum electrolyte levels and complete blood cell (CBC) and platelet counts.
- Do not leave patient unattended when IV oxytocin is being used.
- Monitor vaginal bleeding.
- Have drugs, equipment, and personnel available to treat acute allergic reactions in settings where oxytocin is administered.
- For IV use, dilute as ordered or according to agency protocol. Use a microdrip infusion set or an infusion monitoring device. Measure dose according to physician order and patient response.

Patient and Family Education

- Review the anticipated benefits and possible side effects of drug therapy. Instruct the patient to call for assistance if any new side effects develop.
- For intranasal spray, instruct patients to sit upright to use spray; for nose drops, tell the patient to tilt head back to administer drops. When intranasal use is prescribed to promote milk ejection, review with the mother other actions that may also aid in milk ejection such as relaxing, massaging breasts, staying well hydrated, getting enough sleep, and cuddling the infant before trying to nurse.

Ergot Alkaloids

Drug Administration

- See Table 65-1. Monitor level of consciousness, weight, and intake and output. Monitor blood pressure and pulse. Auscultate lung and heart sounds.
- Monitor serum electrolyte level and CBC and platelet counts.
- Monitor vaginal bleeding.
- Have drugs, equipment, and personnel available to treat acute allergic reactions in settings where ergot alkaloids are administered.
- For IV use, either drug may be administered undiluted. Administer at a rate of 0.2 mg or less over 1 minute.
- Read drug labels carefully; do not confuse ergotamine with ergonovine.

Patient and Family Education

- Review the anticipated benefits and possible side effects of drug therapy. Instruct the patient to call for assistance if any new side effects develop.
- Alert patient to avoid smoking while using ergot alkaloids.

Prostaglandins

Drug Administration

- See Table 65-1. Monitor level of consciousness, weight, and intake and output. Monitor blood pressure, pulse, and temperature. Auscultate lung and heart sounds.
- Keep siderails up. Have a suction machine available.
- Monitor serum electrolyte level and CBC and platelet counts.
- Monitor vaginal bleeding. Palpate the fundus at regular intervals.
- GI symptoms are common; antidiarrheal and antiemetic medications may be ordered concomitantly or prophylactically.
- Remain with the patient at least 30 minutes after dose is administered to monitor for anaphylaxis: shortness of breath or difficulty breathing, tachycardia, hives, tightness in chest, swelling of face.

Patient and Family Education

- Review with the patient the anticipated benefits and possible side effects of drug therapy. Instruct the patient to call if any unexpected side effects develop.
- Provide emotional support. Refer for counseling if appropriate.
- Emphasize importance of follow-up visit.

Isoxsuprine

Drug Administration

- This drug is also discussed in Chapter 15.
- Monitor blood pressure and pulse, uterine contractions, and fetal heart tones. Assess the patient and fetus frequently. Fetal monitoring may be indicated.
- Stay calm. Provide reassurance to the mother as much as possible. The drug may increase the subjective sense of anxiety and may cause tachycardia, tightness in the chest, tremor, and other symptoms.

Patient and Family Education

- Review the anticipated benefits and possible side effects of drug therapy.
- Review with the patient the limits of activity.
- Tell the patient to notify the physician if labor begins again, membranes rupture, or contractions increase in frequency or duration.

Ritodrine

Drug Administration

- Review the information about beta-2-adrenergic receptors in Chapter 12.
- Monitor blood pressure and pulse, uterine contractions, and fetal heart tones. Assess the patient and fetus every 5 minutes when initiating intravenous (IV) therapy, every 15 to 30 minutes when the patient is stable, and every 4 hours when the patient is taking oral maintenance doses

Continued.

NURSING IMPLICATIONS SUMMARY—cont'd

(or according to agency protocol). Fetal monitoring may be indicated.

- For IV administration, use a minidrip infusion set or an infusion control device.
- Stay calm. Provide reassurance to the mother as possible. The drug may increase the subjective sense of anxiety and may cause tachycardia, tightness in the chest, tremor, and other symptoms.

Patient and Family Education

- Review the anticipated benefits and possible side effects of drug therapy.
- Review with the patient the limits of activity.
- Tell the patient to notify the physician if labor begins again, membranes rupture, or contractions increase in frequency or duration.

Terbutaline

Drug Administration/Patient and Family Education

- See Table 65-2. This drug is also used as a bronchodilator; see Chapter 27.
- Monitor blood pressure and pulse, uterine contractions, and fetal heart tones. Assess the patient and fetus every 5 minutes when initiating IV therapy, every 15 to 30 minutes when the patient is stable, and every 4 hours when the patient is taking oral maintenance doses (or according to agency protocol). Fetal monitoring may be indicated.
- For IV administration, use a minidrip infusion set or an infusion control device.
- Stay calm. Provide reassurance to the mother as possible. The drug may increase the subjective sense of anxiety and may cause tachycardia, tightness in the chest, tremor, and other symptoms.

Patient and Family Education

- Review the anticipated benefits and possible side effects of drug therapy.
- Review with the patient the limits of activity.
- Tell the patient to notify the physician if labor begins again, membranes rupture, or contractions increase in frequency or duration.

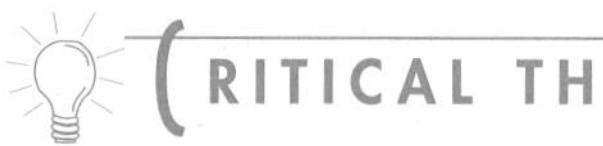

CRITICAL THINKING

APPLICATION

1. How does oxytocin stimulate uterine contractions?
2. How do the uterine contractions produced by prostaglandins differ from those produced by oxytocin?
3. What is the desired effect of intranasal administration of oxytocin?
4. What are the ergot alkaloids?
5. What is the only clinical indication for ergonovine and methylergonovine?
6. What is the other significant action of ergot alkaloids? How does this action lead to potentially serious side effects?
7. What is the source of natural prostaglandins?
8. Why are prostaglandins best administered intraamniotically or intravaginally?
9. What indication does carboprost have that is not shared by the other prostaglandins?
10. What is the most common side effect with prostaglandins?
11. What is the mechanism of action of ritodrine?
12. What is the clinical use of ritodrine?
13. Why are cardiovascular effects seen with ritodrine?

CRITICAL THINKING

1. Your patient is undergoing her first pregnancy. She is worried about premature labor. What symptoms would you teach her to watch for? How can a patient differentiate between Braxton Hicks contractions and the contractions of labor?

CHAPTER 66

Drugs Acting on the Male Reproductive System

OBJECTIVES

After studying this chapter, you should be able to do the following:

- *Describe the uses of androgens.*
- *Describe the uses and abuses of anabolic steroids.*
- *Develop a nursing care plan for the patient receiving androgens.*

KEY TERMS

anabolic steroids
androgens
testosterone

CHAPTER OVERVIEW

The major reproductive hormones in men are **androgens.** These steroids are synthesized primarily in the testes and to a lesser extent in the adrenal glands. Within the testes the status of interstitial or Leydig's cells and the seminiferous tubular cells is most important for determining male sexual potential. Leydig's cells synthesize testosterone, the primary masculinizing steroid hormone. The seminiferous tubules contain the germ cells that in the adult male produce functional sperm. The endocrine control of male sexual development and function, the actions of natural male hormones, and the clinical uses of synthetic and natural drugs acting on the male reproductive system are discussed in this chapter.

Therapeutic Rationale: Development and Regulation of Male Sexual Function

In adult males, sexual function depends on the proper interaction of the hypothalamus, anterior pituitary, and the testes. Regulation of testicular function is by a negative feedback loop (Chapter 59). The primary hormones in this cycle are testosterone from the testes; interstitial cell–stimulating hormone (ICSH), also called luteinizing hormone (LH); follicle-stimulating hormone (FSH) from the anterior pituitary; and gonadotropin-releasing hormone (GnRH) from the hypothalamus. When testosterone levels in blood are low, GnRH is released from the hypothalamus to enter the anterior pituitary through a portal venous system. Under the influence of GnRH, both ICSH and FSH are released from the pituitary into general circulation, where they act on testicular tissues.

The action of these regulatory hormones is slightly different during the three stages of life in which they act. During fetal development, Leydig's cells develop in the embryonic testes as a result of stimulation with the maternal hormone, human chorionic gonadotropin (HCG). These embryonic cells produce the small amounts of testosterone necessary for the development of the male external genitalia; without testosterone, genetically male infants are born with female genitalia. After birth, Leydig's cells regress because the stimulus of HCG is no longer available.

The second period of life when these regulatory processes are most important is puberty. In childhood, very low concentrations of gonadotropins are found in blood. With the onset of puberty the anterior pituitary begins to synthesize and release greater quantities of ICSH and FSH. The targets for ICSH in males are Leydig's cells, where ICSH stimulates testosterone production. FSH acts directly on cells in seminiferous tubules to prepare that tissue for spermatogenesis. This process cannot be completed unless testosterone from Leydig's cells is also present. With FSH and testosterone acting on the seminiferous tubules, mature sperm can be produced. Testosterone acts not only within the testes but also throughout the body at this stage of life. These actions are discussed in the next section.

The third period of life to be considered is sexual maturity. During this time, ICSH is important in the maintenance of sexual function because it is still required for the synthesis of testosterone, which maintains spermatogenesis.

A third hormone of the anterior pituitary involved in male sexual function is prolactin. The role of prolactin in men is unclear, but men with pituitary tumors that secrete large quantities of prolactin often have decreased libidos and low concentrations of ICSH, FSH, and testosterone in their blood. Prolactin seems to suppress synthesis and release of ICSH and FSH from the pituitary gland and may directly interfere with the actions of these hormones on testes.

The major steroid affecting male sexual function is **testosterone.** This hormone is synthesized in the Leydig's cells and in the adrenal cortex. Testosterone is a potent androgen, a substance that stimulates growth of the organs of the male reproductive tract. Testosterone is responsible for the enlargement and maturation of the penis, scrotum, seminal vesicles, prostate gland, and other accessory tissues of the male reproductive tract. These actions constitute the primary sexual effects on the male.

Testosterone is also responsible for the development of secondary sexual characteristics. The increased testosterone level during puberty stimulates growth of facial and pubic hair and hair on chest and armpits. Sustained levels of testosterone trigger the onset of baldness in genetically predisposed males. The other dramatic changes that occur in the pubertal male are also related to the increased testosterone levels and include lowering of the voice caused by thickening of the vocal cords, stimulation of sebaceous glands, and stimulation of the libido. Psychologists who work with primates other than humans have related aggression to high testosterone levels.

In addition to these primary and secondary sexual effects, testosterone also has profound effects on metabolism. Androgens are anabolic (i.e., they stimulate synthetic rather than degradative processes). Testosterone increases nitrogen retention, protein formation, and overall metabolic rate. This anabolic action is responsible for the increase in muscle mass associated with puberty and the distribution of this mass in the male pattern. In addition, calcium is retained, and the size and strength of bone are enhanced. Blood-forming cells are also affected so that more red blood cells may be formed.

Although testosterone is the major circulating androgen in human males, it is not the only metabolically important androgen. Testosterone is transformed within many target cells to dihydrotestosterone, which is a more potent androgen than testosterone. Small amounts of another androgen, androstenedione, may also affect various tissues of the body.

Testosterone and androstenedione are close chemical relatives of the estrogens, steroid hormones that have feminizing effects. Some tissues in the brain, breasts, and testes can convert androgens to estrogens. Low estrogen concentrations therefore are found in the blood of healthy adult men. These estrogens have no obvious influence on healthy men, but under certain circumstances estrogen concentrations may increase and produce pathologic signs such as breast development.

Therapeutic Agents: Drugs Affecting Development and Regulation of Male Sexual Function

Androgens

Fluoxymesterone, methyltestosterone, testosterone

Mechanism of Action

The androgens are steroids that diffuse into cells and bind to receptors that move to the nucleus of the cell and affect gene expression. These changes bring about a change in the proteins that are produced, and cell function is altered. The effect on the body is as described above for naturally produced androgens.

Pharmacokinetics

Testosterone in its natural form is not water soluble and therefore is used as an aqueous suspension suitable only for intramuscular (IM) injection (Table 66-1). In this form the drug has a short duration of action and produces somewhat erratic clinical responses. Testosterone can be absorbed from the gastrointestinal (GI) tract; however, this route of administration does not produce clinically useful testosterone concentrations in blood because the steroid absorbed from the intestine passes directly into portal circulation to the liver before it circulates to the rest of the body. The liver can inactivate testosterone rapidly by forming less active metabolites or by converting the steroid to a glucuronide or to sulfated derivatives.

Testosterone esters are much more useful than testosterone for producing sustained androgenic effects. Two preparations commonly used clinically are testosterone enanthate and testosterone cypionate (Table 66-1). Both are supplied in forms that are slowly absorbed from intramuscular sites and therefore are effective for 3 to 4 weeks. This increased convenience for the patient is at the cost of less flexibility in control. Another testosterone ester, testosterone propionate, has a short duration of action more similar to that of testosterone.

Orally absorbed androgens have been developed, including methyltestosterone and fluoxymesterone. These compounds are effective orally because they are resistant to the action of liver enzymes that degrade testosterone. Unfortunately, these compounds also are associated with liver toxicity of various types, including cholestatic jaundice.

Tablets of methyltestosterone are available for buccal administration. Absorption through mucous membranes in the mouth may be more effective than with oral doses because buccally absorbed materials do not directly enter portal circulation and therefore are circulated to the rest of the body before they enter the liver (Chapter 1).

Uses

Androgenic drugs are primarily used in replacement therapy for patients who have reduced endogenous androgen production. For some patients the loss of androgens occurs early and prevents the normal changes of puberty. Androgen loss after puberty may cause a loss in libido or sexual desire or may cause mild feminizing tendencies. Aging males produce

TABLE 66-1 Androgens

GENERIC NAME	TRADE NAME	ADMINISTRATION/DOSAGE	COMMENTS
Fluoxymesterone	Halotestin*	ORAL: *Adults*—Replacement therapy in males: 5-20 mg daily. For breast cancer in females: 20-50 mg daily. FDA pregnancy category X. *Children*—For delayed puberty in boys: 2.5-10 mg daily for 4-6 mo.	Relatively short-acting agent; risk of liver toxicity.
Methyltestosterone	Android Metandren† Testred Virilon	ORAL: *Adults*—Replacement therapy in males: 10-50 mg daily. For breast cancer in females: 50-200 mg daily. FDA pregnancy category X. *Children*—For delayed puberty in boys: 5-25 mg daily for 4-6 mos.	Relatively short-acting agent; risk of liver toxicity.
Methyltestosterone	Metandren† Oreton	BUCCAL: *Adults*—Replacement therapy in males: 5-25 mg daily. For breast cancer in females: 25-100 mg daily. FDA pregnancy category X. *Children*—For delayed puberty in boys: 2.5-12.5 mg daily for 4-6 mos.	Relatively short-acting agent; risk of liver toxicity.
Testosterone	Andro Histerone Malogen† Testaqua	INTRAMUSCULAR: *Adults*—Replacement therapy in males: 25-50 mg 2 or 3 times weekly. For breast cancer in females: 50-100 mg 3 times weekly. FDA pregnancy category X. *Children*—For delayed puberty in males: 100 mg monthly for 4-6 mo.	Aqueous suspension for IM use only.
Testosterone	Testoderm	TRANSDERMAL PATCH: *Adults*—4 or 6 mg patch placed on scrotal area daily.	For replacement therapy only.
Testosterone cypionate	Andro-Cyp Depotest Duratest	INTRAMUSCULAR: *Adults*—Replacement therapy in males: 50-400 mg every 2-4 wk. For breast cancer in females: 200-400 mg every 2-4 wk. FDA pregnancy category X. *Children*—For delayed puberty in males: 100 mg monthly for 4-6 mo.	Very long-acting preparation for IM use only.
Testosterone enanthate	Delatest Delatestryl* Everone Malogex†	INTRAMUSCULAR: *Adults*—Replacement therapy in males: 50-400 mg every 2-4 wk. For breast cancer in females: 200-400 mg every 2-4 wk. FDA pregnancy category X. *Children*—For delayed puberty in males: 100 mg monthly for 4-6 mos.	Very long-acting preparation for IM use only.
Testosterone propionate	Malogen† Testex	INTRAMUSCULAR: *Adults*—Replacement therapy in males: 25-50 mg 2 or 3 times weekly. For breast cancer in females: 50-100 mg 3 times weekly. FDA pregnancy category X. *Children*—For delayed puberty in males: 100 mg monthly for 4-6 mos.	For IM use only.

*Available in Canada and United States.
†Available in Canada only.

less testosterone than younger men and may suffer a loss of sexual drive. Some older men have more severe symptoms suggestive of a male climacteric or male menopause. These conditions and others related to specific malfunctions of the male sexual organs may be treated with testosterone or one of the other androgenic compounds (Table 66-1). For these patients with reduced natural testosterone production, this treatment constitutes replacement therapy.

Androgens have been used for various conditions in females such as relief of dysmenorrhea, menopausal symptoms, and postpartum breast engorgement, but other agents now are preferred (Chapter 64). Androgens are still indicated for treatment of certain advanced breast carcinomas (Chapter 50). The high doses used for this purpose exceed those required for replacement therapy and may be expected to cause masculinization (Table 66-1).

Adverse Reactions and Contraindications

The reactions experienced with androgens differs in men and women. Men frequently report urinary tract infections, bladder irritation, tender breasts, gynecomastia, or priapism. Women, who generally received higher doses than men, experience menstrual irregularities or virilism. Virilism may also be noted in boys who receive androgens.

Less common symptoms in men or women include edema, erythrocytosis, hypercalcemia, liver dysfunction, nausea, or vomiting. Acne, diarrhea, and changes in libido are also possible. Men may also experience pain in the scrotum or groin; difficulty in urination may signal changes in the prostate gland. Androgens are usually avoided in men with known prostatic or breast carcinoma because androgens often stimulate growth of these tumors.

Toxicity

The most important toxicity of androgens is directed to the liver.

Interactions

The effects of anticoagulants are increased by androgens, which may require dosage adjustment. Hepatotoxic drugs are avoided with androgens because of the risk of additive damage to the liver.

Anabolic Steroids

In addition to androgenic properties, the natural male steroids also possess anabolic properties that may be useful in certain clinical situations (Table 66-2). For example, these drugs may be used to treat conditions for which increased nitrogen retention and protein formation are desirable. Accordingly, these drugs may alleviate the catabolic state produced by severe trauma. Patients who have extensive burns or have had surgery may benefit from the action of the **anabolic steroids.** The effects of anabolic hormone on red blood cell formation make these drugs valuable in the treatment of certain forms of anemia.

Although a few anabolic compounds have relatively low androgenic potency, all anabolic steroids possess androgenic properties to some degree. These androgenic effects may be indistinguishable in healthy men, but they may become obvious when the compounds are used to treat women or children. Patients receiving these compounds may develop increased libido. Men may develop priapism (continuous erection). Women should be especially watched for androgen-induced changes such as inappropriate hair development, voice changes, or personality alterations. Children should be watched closely for precocious sexual development. These compounds, while promoting bone growth in children, also promote fusion of the epiphyses, which permanently halts skeletal growth. Therefore full adult height may be diminished, although a growth spurt may be attained when the drugs are first given. For this reason and because of the effects on sexual development, these drugs are less than ideal for therapy in children.

TABLE 66-2 Anabolic Steroids

GENERIC NAME	TRADE NAME	ADMINISTRATION/DOSAGE	COMMENTS
Nandrolone decanoate	Deca-Durabolin* Hybolin	INTRAMUSCULAR: *Adults*—For deep IM injection, 50-200 mg. Repeat doses every 3-4 wk. FDA pregnancy category X. *Children*—25-50 mg. Repeat doses every 3-4 wk.	Refractory anemias.
Nandrolone phenpropionate	Durabolin*	INTRAMUSCULAR: *Adults*—Oil solution for deep IM injection, 25-100 mg. Repeat doses every 1-4 wk. FDA pregnancy category X.	Metastatic breast cancer.
Oxandrolone	Oxandrin	ORAL: Adults—Tablets, 2.5mg 2-4 times daily. *Children*—0.25 mg/kg body weight intermittently. FDA pregnancy category X.	To produce weight gain after severe trauma.
Oxymetholone	Anadrol Anapolon†	ORAL: *Adults and Children*—Tablets, 1-5 mg/kg body weight/day up to 100 mg total daily dose. FDA pregnancy category X. Neonates: 0.175 mg/kg or 5 mg/m^2.	Anemias or hereditary angioedema.
Stanozolol	Winstrol	ORAL: *Adults*—Tablets, 2 mg 3 times daily for initial therapy. Reduce dose when response allows. FDA pregnancy category X. *Children*—1 mg twice daily with meals, only during attack.	Hereditary angioedema.

*Available in Canada and United States.
†Available in Canada only.

Anabolic steroids are inappropriate for use in athletes who seek to increase bone or muscle mass. In healthy young men the anabolic effects are minimal, but the side effects can be serious (altered liver function, reduced gonadotropin levels, lowered testosterone synthesis, and depressed spermatogenesis). In healthy young women bone and muscle mass may be increased more dramatically but at the cost of virilization and menstrual disturbances.

NURSING PROCESS OVERVIEW

Drugs and the Male Reproductive System

Assessment

Perform a complete patient assessment before initiating drug therapy. Assess the vital signs, blood pressure, weight, serum calcium level, height, and serum and urine glucose. Focus part of the assessment on the presenting problem. For example, in treatment of reduced androgen production, assess development of secondary sexual characteristics. In the patient receiving androgen therapy for its anabolic effects, assess nutritional needs, level of mobility, and intake and output.

Nursing Diagnoses

- Body image disturbance: acne related to androgen therapy
- Body image disturbance: masculinization of women related to androgen therapy

Patient Outcomes

The patient will discuss feelings related to body image changes.

Planning/Implementation

Monitor the vital signs and other data mentioned in the assessment. Review possible and probable side effects. Refer the patient receiving steroids for their anabolic effects to the hospital or community dietician.

Evaluation

Before discharge, verify that the patient can explain how and why to take the drugs, anticipated side effects, side effects that require immediate notification of the physician, how to treat side effects that may be troublesome but are not serious, and what parameters should be measured regularly at home to monitor drug effectiveness.

NURSING IMPLICATIONS SUMMARY

Androgens

Drug Administration

- Assess mental status and neurologic function.
- Assess for signs of depression including insomnia, lack of appetite, loss of interest in personal appearance, and withdrawal.
- Monitor weight, pulse, and blood pressure. Assess for edema and skin changes. Auscultate lung and heart sounds.
- Assess for signs of liver dysfunction including right upper quadrant abdominal pain, malaise, fever, jaundice, and pruritus.
- When drug is used for treatment of hypogonadism, assess for development of secondary sexual characteristics: acne, deepening of voice, growth of pubic hair, growth of penis.
- When drug is used to treat breast cancer, assess for signs of hypercalcemia: confusion, depression, nausea, increased thirst, increased urination, constipation, vomiting.
- When drug is used in women, assess for virilization: deeper voice, hoarseness, enlargement of clitoris, decreased breast size, vaginal drying, acne, changes in hair growth patterns, abnormal menstrual periods, or amenorrhea.
- When drug is prescribed for children, review the proposed long-term treatment plan. Therapy for children is often intermittent to allow drug-free periods to permit normal bone growth. The child's progress may be monitored with regular x-ray studies of wrists and hands to monitor bone maturation. Monitor weight and height.
- Do not substitute testosterone cypionate or testosterone enanthate for testosterone propionate or testosterone base because there are different durations of action.
- For a discussion of intramuscular (IM) administration of oil-based suspensions, see Chapter 5.
- For buccal tablets, instruct the patient to place tablets in the mouth between the upper or lower gum and the cheek and to allow the tablet to dissolve. While the tablet is in place, the patient should refrain from eating, drinking, chewing, or smoking. Instruct the patient to rotate sites with each administration. Remind the patient to maintain a program of good regular oral hygiene and to report any oral irritation to the physician.
- For transdermal form, instruct the patient to dry-shave a small area on scrotum and apply the patch to the scrotum once daily. Chemical hair removers should not be used.
- Monitor complete blood cell count (CBC) and differential, serum electrolyte level, and liver function tests.

Patient and Family Education

- Review the anticipated benefits and possible side effects of drug therapy. Tell the patient to report any new side effects.
- Assess the patient tactfully for side effects such as decreased ejaculatory volume, amenorrhea, menstrual irregularities,

Continued.

Nursing Implications Summary—cont'd

virilization of females, and clitoral enlargement. Children may experience premature virilization. Patients may be reluctant to discuss these problems, or children may not know how to do so. Provide emotional support. Remind the patient to take drugs as ordered for best effects and not to stop taking the drug without notifying the physician.

- Instruct the patient to notify the physician if priapism develops.
- Tell the patient to take oral doses with meals or a snack to lessen gastric irritation.
- Warn the diabetic patient to monitor blood glucose levels frequently for the first 2 weeks of therapy and after androgen therapy is completed, because a change in insulin dose or diet may be needed.
- Warn the patient using patch on scrotum that there is the possibility that testosterone from the patch may be transferred to female sexual partners. Assess female sexual partners for increases in acne or changes in body hair distribution.

Anabolic Steroids

Drug Administration

- Assess mental status. Assess for signs of depression including lack of interest in personal appearance, insomnia, loss of appetite, and withdrawal.
- Monitor weight, blood pressure, and pulse. Assess for edema and skin changes.
- When drug is used for anemia, take diet history if needed. Assess for shortness of breath, activity tolerance level, ability to perform activities of daily living, malaise, fatigability, and paleness.
- Assess prepubertal boys for darkening of skin, and development of secondary sexual characteristics.
- When drug is used for treatment of breast cancer, assess for signs of hypercalcemia: confusion, depression, nausea, increased thirst, increased urination, constipation, or vomiting.
- When drug is used in women, assess for virilization: deeper voice, hoarseness, enlargement of clitoris, decreased breast size, vaginal drying, acne, changes in hair growth patterns, abnormal menstrual periods, or amenorrhea.
- Monitor CBC, white blood cell differential, iron and total iron binding capacity, serum calcium, serum cholesterol, and liver function tests.

Patient and Family Education

- Review the anticipated benefits and possible side effects of the drug therapy. Tell the patient to take drugs only as ordered and not to share drugs with others. Anabolic steroids should not be used to change body size or function or for athletic purposes.
- Teach the patient to take oral doses with meals or a snack to lessen gastric irritation. If GI symptoms are severe or persistent, notify the physician.
- Assess tactfully for changes such as hirsutism and virilization in females or gynecomastia or decreased libido in males. Provide emotional support as needed. Remind the patient to take medications as ordered and not to stop medications without notifying the physician.
- Notify the physician if priapism develops.
- Warn the diabetic patient to monitor blood glucose levels carefully when starting or ending therapy with steroids because an adjustment in insulin dose or diet may be necessary.
- A patient who has been burned, traumatized, or immobilized should be informed that the effectiveness of anabolic steroids may be enhanced by concomitant use of a diet high in calories and protein. Continue regular physical therapy to help reduce bone demineralization.

Critical Thinking

APPLICATION

1. Which three organs produce hormones that affect male sexual development and function?
2. What is the function of GnRH in the adult male?
3. What is the function of ICSH in the adult male?
4. What is the function of FSH in the adult male?
5. What is the function of testosterone during fetal development in males?
6. What is the primary natural androgenic steroid?
7. What is the most common clinical use of androgen steroids?
8. Why is testosterone not administered by the oral route?
9. What two androgenic steroids are well absorbed orally?
10. What is the major effect of the anabolic steroids?
11. What side effect is frequently associated with anabolic steroids?

CRITICAL THINKING

1. What effect does testosterone have on metabolism? How should you assess for this?
2. What advantages do testosterone esters such as testosterone enanthate have over testosterone for long-term replacement therapy of androgen deficiency?
3. What disadvantages do the orally administered androgenic steroids possess compared with other androgenic agents?
4. What is the advantage of administering testosterone by the buccal route rather than by the oral route? What are teaching points associated with this route of administration?

Section XV

Drugs for the Patient Receiving Anesthesia

Section XV presents the drugs that have made modern surgery possible. Chapter 67, *Local Anesthetics,* reviews the surface use of local anesthetics for minor procedures and administration by injection for major surgery. Chapter 68, *General Anesthetics,* discusses inhalation and intravenous anesthetics and combinations of drugs that are currently widely used for balanced anesthesia. The limitations and desirable characteristics of each anesthetic are described. Chapter 69, *Neuromuscular Blocking Agents,* discusses the drugs that are used to provide muscle relaxation during surgery and to facilitate such procedures as endotracheal intubation and electroconvulsant therapy.

CHAPTER 67

Local Anesthetics

OBJECTIVES

After studying this chapter, you should be able to do the following:

- *Describe the mechanism of action of local anesthetics.*
- *Describe the side effects and adverse reactions of local anesthetics.*
- *Explain the differences between agents for surface anesthesia and those injected to produce local anesthesia.*
- *Differentiate among infiltration, nerve block, epidural, caudal, and spinal anesthesia.*
- *Develop a nursing care plan for a patient who has received local anesthesia.*

KEY TERMS

caudal anesthesia
epidural anesthesia
infiltration anesthesia
local anesthetic
nerve block anesthesia
saddle block
spinal anesthesia
surface anesthetics

CHAPTER OVERVIEW

Local anesthetics reversibly block nerve conduction, leading to loss of sensation and preventing muscle activity. In addition to topical anesthesia, local anesthetics can be infiltrated to various nerve sites, producing anesthesia over a wide area.

Cocaine was the first local anesthetic used clinically, after the observation in the late 1880s that when cocaine was administered orally to patients, their tongues and throats became numb. Its main use as a local anesthetic was to desensitize the cornea to allow local surgery without a general anesthetic. It was quickly recognized that cocaine had a high potential for abuse, and it was replaced by procaine (Novocain) in 1905. Today lidocaine (Xylocaine), introduced in the 1940s, is the most versatile and widely used local anesthetic. More than 15 local anesthetics are available, but they vary in their suitability for different applications.

Therapeutic Rationale: Local Anesthesia

Many medical and dental procedures require only anesthesia of only a portion of the body. Local anesthesia is achieved by drugs that reversibly inhibit nerve conduction to produce both a loss of sensation and a loss of muscle activity. The **local anesthetic** is administered at the desired site of action. The inhibition of nerve conduction persists until the drug diffuses and enters the circulation for subsequent degradation and excretion. All neurons in the area of administration, whether pain, motor, or autonomic, are affected, so in addition to the loss of pain, loss of sensory, motor, and autonomic activities occurs. The size of the nerve fiber determines its sensitivity to local anesthetics; smaller fibers are the most sensitive. Since sensory fibers are smaller than motor fibers, loss of sensation precedes loss of motor activity and, conversely, motor activity is regained before sensory function.

The choice of local anesthetic depends on the route of administration and the desired duration of action.

Therapeutic Agents: Local Anesthetics

Local Anesthetics: General Characteristics

Mechanism of Action

Chemically, most local anesthetics are weak bases, being secondary or tertiary amines. This means that under physiologic conditions most molecules carry a positive charge and are not lipid soluble. However, it is the uncharged form that diffuses across the nerve membrane and then reequilibrates to charged and uncharged forms. Within the neuron the positively charged form blocks nerve conduction. The positively charged form displaces calcium bound to the inner membrane and thus prevents the inward flow of sodium ions. Since the action potential is generated by the influx of sodium ions, the local anesthetic depresses the action potential so that it is not propagated. The resting potential of neurons is not affected by local anesthetics.

Pharmacokinetics

Local anesthetics eventually enter the systemic circulation and can affect other organs, limiting their safety. The relative safety of procaine and chloroprocaine results from their rapid hydrolysis in the plasma by pseudocholinesterases. Other local anesthetics are slowly degraded by the liver and have a longer plasma half-life.

The rate at which local anesthetic is removed from the infiltrated area depends largely on the degree of vascularization. The duration can be increased by 50% to 100% with the inclusion of epinephrine, 1:200,000, or phenylephrine to cause vasoconstriction and thereby restrict systemic absorption. However, epinephrine is contraindicated for infiltration of areas with end arteries (fingers, toes, ears, nose, and penis) since the resultant ischemia may lead to tissue death. Similarly, the addition of a vasoconstrictor is contraindicated in epidural anesthesia in labor because of the potential vasoconstriction of the uterine blood vessels with a resultant decrease in placental circulation. Epinephrine is also contraindicated for patients with severe cardiovascular disease or thyrotoxicosis, in whom cardiac function would be compromised by added vasoconstrictors.

Uses

In general, local anesthetics can be divided into those applied topically to provide surface anesthesia and those injected into an area to produce local anesthesia. Only lidocaine (Xylocaine), dibucaine (Nupercaine), and tetracaine (Pontocaine) are used both topically and by injection.

Surface anesthesia. Those local anesthetics applied as drops, sprays, lotions, creams, or ointments, also called **surface anesthetics,** are listed in Table 67-1. Distinction is made between those drugs safely applied to the eyes, skin, and mucosal areas. Only tetracaine (Pontocaine) is suitable for application to all three sites.

Most drugs for surface anesthesia are effective when applied to the skin. These drugs are poorly soluble, so little systemic absorption occurs when they are applied to the skin to relieve itching or the pain of mild burns. The main potential toxicity of local anesthetics applied to the skin is allergy, usually contact dermatitis. Since several chemical classes are represented by local anesthetics, a drug from a different chemical group can be substituted if an allergy develops.

Mucosal membranes of the nose, mouth, and throat (bronchotracheal mucosa) and of the urethra, rectum, and vagina are highly vascular and allow ready absorption of the local anesthetic into systemic circulation. Application of excessive amounts of local anesthetics to mucosal surfaces is the most common cause of systemic toxicity with local anesthetics. A local anesthetic is often used to eliminate the gag reflex when inserting an endotracheal tube or to limit the discomfort of endoscopic procedures. The lowest concentration possible of the local anesthetic should be used on mucosal surfaces to avoid systemic toxicity, and the total amount of drug should be recorded and matched against recommended total doses.

Local anesthetics administered by injection. Local anesthetics used by injection are listed in Table 67-2. The potency and the duration of action increase together with the lipid solubility of the drug. The onset of anesthesia is determined by the concentration of drug and the size of the nerve. Before infiltrating an area with a local anesthetic, the syringe should first be aspirated to ensure that a blood vessel has not been entered. This step is necessary because the concentration of drug is high and could prove fatal if injected systemically.

The area affected by a local anesthetic depends on how and where it is injected. The anesthesia produced is described by the technique of injection—infiltration, nerve block, epidural, and spinal. These techniques are described with their potential for producing toxic side effects.

TABLE 67-1 Local Anesthetics for Surface Anesthesia

GENERIC NAME	TRADE NAME	EYES*	MUCOUS MEMBRANES*†	SKIN*	COMMENTS
Benzocaine	Americaine	0	0	+	Widely used. Included in many nonprescription preparations to relieve sunburn, itching, and mild burns. Long acting and poorly absorbed.
Butamben picrate		0	0	+	Nonprescription ointment to relieve itching and burning. Contains benzocaine and tetracaine.
Cocaine hydrochloride		+	+	0	Schedule II drug. Medically used in ear, nose, and throat procedures when vasoconstriction and shrinking of mucous membranes are desired. Ophthalmic preparations anesthetize cornea and conjunctiva.
Dibucaine hydrochloride	Nupercaine‡	0	0	+	Nonprescription skin ointment or cream.
Dyclonine hydrochloride	Dyclone Sucrets	0	+	+	Suppresses gag reflex and lessens discomfort of genitourinary endoscopy. Precipitated by iodine of contrast media used in pyelography and should not be used.
Lidocaine Lidocaine hydrochloride	Xylocaine‡ Xylocaine hydrochloride‡	0 0	+ +	+ +	Widely used for topical anesthesia in ear, nose, and throat procedures; upper digestive tract procedures; and genitourinary procedures. Rapid onset and intermediate duration. Not irritating and low incidence of hypersensitivity.
Pramoxine hydrochloride	Tronothane‡	0	+§	+	Nonprescription cream or ointment primarily used to relieve pain of itching, burns, and hemorrhoids.
Proparacaine hydrochloride	Ophthaine‡	+	0	0	Applied topically to eye to anesthetize cornea and conjunctiva.
Tetracaine hydrochloride	Pontocaine‡	+	+	+	Topically, onset is 5 min, and duration is 45 min. Usual topical dose is 20 mg; maximum, 50 mg because of toxicity and slow degradation. Ophthalmic preparations are dilute solutions for instillation.

*+ indicates suitable site for application; 0 indicates site not suitable for application.
†Mucous membranes include the bronchotracheal mucosa and the mucosa of the urethra, rectum, and vagina.
‡Available in Canada and United States.
§ Not for application to the bronchotracheal mucosa.

Infiltration anesthesia refers to the superficial application of a local anesthetic. To suture a cut or to perform dental procedures, local anesthetic is injected superficially in small amounts to block the small nerves and to numb the area. To work on the scalp or to make an incision in the skin, the anesthetic is infused around the area. Small incisions require a small volume and a low concentration of drug, so little toxicity is associated with these uses. However, systemic toxicity from local anesthetics is frequently seen in the emergency room when large cuts are infiltrated with local anesthetic.

Nerve block anesthesia refers to the injection of a local anesthetic along a nerve before it reaches the surgical site. The volume and concentration of a local anesthetic for a nerve block must be larger than in infiltration anesthesia to penetrate the larger nerve.

The most extensive field of local anesthesia is achieved by applying the local anesthetic around the nerve roots near the spinal cord to produce epidural or spinal anesthesia. As shown in Figure 67-1, the spinal cord proper ends at the lumbar region. The spinal cord is surrounded by three membranes—first the pia mater, then the arachnoid, and finally the outer membrane, the dura mater. These membranes extend below the spinal cord proper to form a sac in the lumbar and sacral region. The dura mater and arachnoid membranes are close together, and the subarachnoid space is between the arachnoid and pia mater. Cerebrospinal fluid fills the subarachnoid space throughout the spinal cord.

For **epidural anesthesia,** the local anesthetic is administered outside the dura mater (see Figure 67-1) so that the nerve roots are blocked at the point after they emerge from the dura mater. The extent of anesthesia depends on the volume and concentration of local anesthetic used. **Caudal anesthesia** is another form of epidural anesthesia and is achieved by administering the local anesthetic epidurally at the base of the spine (see Figure 67-1). The extent of anesthesia affects only the pelvic region and legs. Caudal anesthesia is used for obstetrics and for surgery on the rectum, anus, and prostate gland.

Spinal anesthesia is achieved by injecting local anesthetic into the subarachnoid space between the arachnoid and pia mater membranes in the lumbar area, usually between the second lumbar and first sacral vertebrae and well below the spinal cord proper. This method blocks the nerve roots for the entire lower body. If the solution containing local anes-

TABLE 67-2 Local Anesthetics for Injection

GENERIC NAME	TRADE NAME	LOCAL INFILTRATION OR NERVE BLOCK OR EPIDURAL BLOCK*	SPINAL BLOCK (SUBARACHNOID)*	DURATION†	COMMENTS
Bupivacaine hydrochloride	Marcaine‡	+	Investigational	Long§	Provides long-acting epidural anesthesia in labor with no reported effects on fetus. Maximum dose, 200 mg.
Chloroprocaine hydrochloride	Nesacaine†	+	Investigational	Short	Little systemic toxicity because of rapid hydrolysis in plasma. No effects reported on fetus after epidural anesthesia in mother. Maximum dose, 800 mg.
Etidocaine hydrochloride	Duranest	+	0	Long	Highly lipid soluble. Onset for epidural block, 5 min. Profound muscle relaxation is desirable for abdominal surgery but not for labor.
Lidocaine	Xylocaine‡	+	+	Intermediate	Widely used local anesthetic. Maximum dose, 300 mg (4.5 mg/kg body weight). Can cause drowsiness, fatigue, and amnesia.
Mepivacaine	Carbocaine‡	+	0	Intermediate	Chemically related to lidocaine. Maximum dose, 400 mg (7 mg/kg body weight).
Prilocaine	Citanest‡	+	0	Intermediate	Maximum dose, 600 mg (8 mg/kg body weight). Useful for outpatient surgery because of low incidence of drowsiness or fatigue as side effects. Metabolites can cause methemoglobinemia.
Procaine hydrochloride	Novocain‡	+	+	Short	Noted for its safety because of its rapid hydrolysis in plasma. Maximum dose, 600 mg (10 mg/kg body weight). Duration of epidural block is unreliable.
Tetracaine	Pontocaine‡	0	+	Long	Most widely used drug for spinal anesthesia. Onset, 5 min. Dose for spinal anesthesia, 2-15 mg. Available in hyperbaric, isobaric, and hypobaric solutions.

*+ indicates suitable use; 0 indicates use not suitable.
†Duration without epinephrine: short, 1 hr; intermediate, 2 hr; long, 3 hr (approximations).
‡Available in Canada and United States.
§Duration of bupivacaine in nerve block is 6-13 hr.

thetic has the same density (isobaric) as cerebrospinal fluid and is administered slowly, it will stay where it is injected and will only slowly diffuse into the rest of the cerebrospinal fluid. The solution of local anesthetic can be made more dense (hyperbaric) by diluting the local anesthetic into 5% dextrose. The solution will then move downward (toward the ground). If the patient is on a tilt bed with feet high and head low, the hyperbaric solution will travel up the spinal cord toward the head and anesthetize more of the body. The solution of local anesthetic also can be diluted with distilled water to be less dense (hypobaric). In patients positioned on the tilt bed, this solution would move to the end of the dura mater and anesthetize only the lower part of the body. Procedures using hypobaric and hyperbaric solutions of local anesthetic require skill in positioning patients. If the level of anesthesia is adjusted to block more of the spinal cord than just the lumbar and sacral regions, there is danger of paralyzing the intercostal and phrenic nerves, thereby paralyzing spontaneous respiration.

If the patient is seated when the local anesthetic is administered as a low spinal anesthetic, only those nerves affecting the parts of the body that would be in contact with a saddle are affected; hence the name **saddle block.** This procedure is used principally in obstetrics for vaginal delivery. With spinal anesthesia the patient is awake, breathing and cardiovascular function are not immediately affected, and good muscle re-

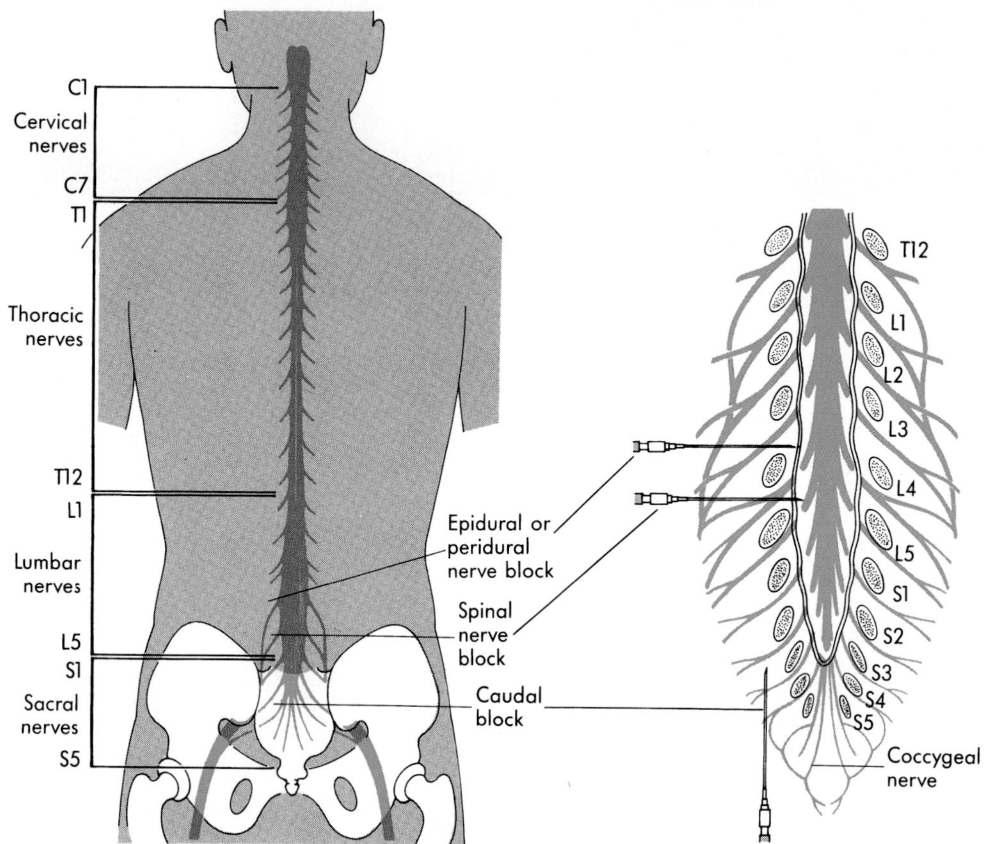

FIGURE 67-1
Sites for injection of local anesthetic to achieve spinal, epidural, and caudal anesthesia.

laxation is present. These are advantages for patients with heart and lung disease or for older adults. However, the sympathetic fibers to the blood vessels are blocked, so vasodilation with hypotension is a frequent side effect of spinal anesthesia. Spinal anesthesia is therefore considered hazardous for abdominal surgery in poor-risk patients because of the potential for sudden vasodilation and hypotension. Spinal anesthesia is widely used in obstetrics, particularly for cesarean sections.

Adverse Reactions, Toxicity, and Contraindications

Although cocaine is unique in causing euphoria, all local anesthetics act as central nervous system (CNS) stimulants if absorbed systemically, producing symptoms such as anxiety, tingling (paresthesia), tremors, and ringing in the ears (tinnitus). This CNS stimulation may ultimately result in convulsions. Intravenous (IV) diazepam (Valium) in 2.5 mg increments or small doses of an ultrashort-acting barbiturate such as thiopental (Pentothal), thiamylal (Surital), or methohexital (Brevital) are given to stop these convulsions.

A high plasma concentration of a local anesthetic causes CNS depression, with or without prior symptoms of CNS stimulation. Depression of CNS function is serious, since vasomotor control is lost, and results in profound hypotension, respiratory depression, and coma.

In addition to the CNS effects, direct cardiovascular effects of local anesthetics are important. Local anesthetics cause direct vasodilation, increasing blood flow and favoring removal of the drug. Thus epinephrine is sometimes added to the local anesthetic since it causes vasoconstriction and prolongs the time the local anesthetic remains at the injection site. Cocaine is unique among the local anesthetics in being a potent vasoconstrictor. Prolonged abuse of cocaine by insufflation (sniffing) can cause loss of nasal septa caused by tissue death after ischemia (insufficient blood flow). Local anesthetics are cardiac depressants. Lidocaine is used to depress cardiac arrhythmias (see Chapter 19).

Local anesthetics that are esters (chloroprocaine, procaine, and tetracaine) can cause an allergic response. Anaphylaxis is rare, and more commonly the topical use of a local anesthetic with an ester bond leads to skin rash (contact dermatitis).

Spinal anesthesia can cause variable hypotension because the neurons controlling vasomotor tone are in the spinal tract. A severe headache may be experienced after spinal anesthesia and may last for hours or days after the anesthetic has worn off. This postspinal headache is believed to reflect a drop in the pressure of the cerebrospinal fluid caused by a leak where the dura mater was penetrated. Incidence of a spinal headache is reduced when patients are kept flat on their backs and instructed not to raise their heads for 12 hours after spinal anesthesia. This minimizes the hydrostatic pressure of the cerebrospinal fluid on the head.

NURSING PROCESS OVERVIEW

Local Anesthesia

Assessment

Assess vital signs and temperature, history of allergies, response to previous surgery, and overall condition.

Nursing Diagnoses

- Risk for urinary retention and inability to void related to spinal anesthesia
- Impaired swallowing and loss of gag reflex related to local anesthesia

Patient Outcomes

The patient will void completely, without difficulty. The patient will not aspirate because of the effects of local anesthetics.

Planning/Implementation

For minor or brief procedures such as suturing or dental work, careful observation of the patient may be sufficient. For longer procedures or when spinal anesthesia is used, monitor vital signs and other parameters of patient function. With spinal anesthesia, position the lower extremities carefully. Insert a Foley catheter to allow urinary output. Monitor the level of consciousness. Allergic responses are possible when local anesthetics are used by any route; have epinephrine and equipment for resuscitation available to treat possible anaphylaxis.

Evaluation

All anesthetics require time to wear off, and specific nursing care depends on the area that has been anesthetized. For example, if the throat has been anesthetized for bronchoscopy, evaluate ability to swallow, position the patient on the side to reduce the possibility of aspiration, restrict oral intake until the patient can swallow, and have a suction machine available at the bedside. After spinal anesthesia, keep the patient flat for 12 to 24 hours. Check the position of the lower extremities to prevent pressure areas, and keep the patient in bed until sensation returns to the lower extremities. Monitor vital signs and intake and output.

If the patient is still under the effects of the local anesthetic at discharge, verify that the patient can explain any restrictions in activity or diet to be followed until the anesthesia wears off. If analgesic medications are prescribed for use after the anesthesia wears off, the patient should be able to explain their use (see Chapter 31). If a local anesthetic is prescribed for outpatient use, determine that the patient can explain how and with what frequency to use the medication and what to do if it is ineffective.

NURSING IMPLICATIONS SUMMARY

General Guidelines: Local Anesthesia

Drug Administration

- Obtain a careful history of previous response to local anesthetics. Remember that the term *Novocain* is often used by patients to refer to any local anesthetic, regardless of the specific drug. Monitor the blood pressure and pulse. If epidural, nerve block, or spinal anesthesia is used, monitor respirations. If anesthesia is used during labor and delivery, assess fetal heart tones.
- Keep the patient flat up to 12 hours after spinal anesthesia. Transfer the patient flat from the stretcher to the bed. Use a thin pillow.
- Assess the patient who has had epidural, nerve block, or spinal anesthesia for ability to void or for a distended bladder. Monitor intake and output. If the patient has not voided in 8 hours after surgery or delivery, notify the physician.
- Assist the patient who has received epidural, nerve block, or spinal anesthesia when ambulating for the first time.
- Position the patient carefully in bed after epidural, nerve block, or spinal anesthesia since the patient has no sensation to warn of wrinkles, tight sheets, or other skin irritants.
- Apply heat or cold to anesthetized area with extreme caution since the patient will be unable to indicate if irritation or burning occurs. If applying heat or cold is necessary, shield the skin well from the heat or cold source and check the patient and the skin surfaces every 5 to 15 minutes. This applies after oral or dental anesthesia also.
- Although serious systemic reactions are rare with local anesthetics, have drugs, equipment, and personnel available to treat acute allergic reactions in settings where these drugs are used.
- A patient in the operating or delivery rooms who is receiving local anesthesia may be drowsy from preoperative medications but will usually be alert and able to understand conversation in the room. Keep conversation and noise to a minimum. Avoid discussing other patients, complications, pathology reports, or other topics that might alarm the patient.
- After bronchoscopy or other procedures in which surface anesthesia may have been applied to the back of the throat, assess the gag reflex and ability to swallow. Do not leave the patient unattended until the patient can safely handle secretions.

Continued.

Nursing Implications Summary—cont'd

Patient and Family Education

- After dental work or injection of anesthetics into tongue, lips, and gums, caution the patient to avoid eating or chewing until sensation returns. A patient may inadvertently bite his or her tongue or cheek.
- Tell the patient to report any rash or skin irritation occurring as a result of application of a local anesthetic.
- If the patient develops an allergic or untoward response to a local anesthetic, instruct the patient to wear a medical identification tag or bracelet indicating the causative agent.
- Instruct the patient to use surface anesthetics as instructed and not to increase the frequency of application or to use the preparation on skin surfaces for which it was not designed. Before discharge, review any limitations the patient may have until the effects of the anesthetic wear off. For example, a patient who has had local anesthesia to a joint may be instructed to avoid use of the joint for a certain number of hours or until the anesthesia has worn off.
- *Dental paste:* See manufacturer's instructions. Instruct the patient to use an applicator to apply small amounts to the sore areas and not to rub with fingers while applying because the medication will crumble.
- *Anesthetic lozenges:* Instruct the patient to allow the lozenge to dissolve in the mouth and not to bite, swallow whole, or chew. Warn family to make certain the child understands how to use a lozenge correctly before giving a lozenge to a child.
- *Benzocaine film-forming gel:* Review manufacturer's instructions. Instruct the patient to dry the area with a swab where the medication is to be applied, apply gel to a second swab, then roll gel over the specified area. Instruct the patient to try to keep mouth open and dry for 30 to 60 minutes after applying gel. The gel will form a film that should not be removed; it will slowly disappear over several hours.
- *Viscous lidocaine or other thick liquid form:* Follow physician's instructions. The drug may be applied to specific areas in the mouth with an applicator, or a specified amount may be poured into a medicine cup and swished around in the mouth and throat. Remind the patient to use only the amount prescribed and measure dose carefully. The patient should not swallow the liquid unless instructed to do so by physician.
- *Aerosol forms sprayed in the mouth:* Instruct the patient to avoid inhaling the spray and avoid spraying the back of the throat unless specifically instructed to do so.
- *Gel or liquid forms of dental anesthetics:* Unless otherwise instructed, the patient should apply medication with fingertip, applicator, or piece of gauze to sore area. Instruct the patient to wait until tenderness or pain disappears before putting dentures or appliances in mouth and not to apply directly to dentures or oral appliances.
- *Ophthalmic forms:* Instruct the patient to apply ointment or solution as directed and not to rub the eye until the anesthetic has worn off because inadvertent eye injury may occur.
- *Rectal forms:* Read the manufacturer's instructions carefully. For creams or ointments that are to be inserted into rectum, instruct the patient to use applicators provided by the manufacturer and to be careful not to insert the cap into the rectum. For rectal aerosol form, instruct the patient to not insert the container itself into the rectum and to use the applicator provided by the manufacturer.
- *Topical application to the skin:* Instruct the patient to use only as directed and to read the product label carefully: some products contain alcohol. Caution the patient to not use products containing alcohol while smoking or near flame to avoid possible fire hazard. Caution the patient to avoid using any product near eyes, nose, or mouth.
- *Butamben ointment:* This ointment may stain clothing permanently and discolor hair. Instruct the patient to avoid touching clothing or hair while applying medication and to cover the area when medication has been applied with a loose bandage.

Critical Thinking

APPLICATION

1. What is the mechanism of action of local anesthetics?
2. What property of procaine and chloroprocaine makes them relatively safe?
3. What are toxic effects of systemic absorption of local anesthetics?
4. To what three types of surfaces are local anesthetics applied?
5. Describe the areas of anesthesia achieved by infiltration, nerve block, epidural, and spinal anesthesia.

CRITICAL THINKING

1. What hazards are associated with spinal anesthesia?
2. How is the duration of local anesthetics prolonged?

CHAPTER 68

General Anesthetics

OBJECTIVES

After studying this chapter, you should be able to do the following:

- *Describe the characteristics of inhalation anesthetics, intravenous anesthetics, balanced anesthesia, and neuroleptanesthesia.*
- *Explain minimum alveolar concentration.*
- *Outline the characteristics of the different agents described in the chapter.*
- *Develop a nursing care plan for the patient receiving a specific general anesthetic agent or a combination of agents.*

KEY TERMS

balanced anesthesia
dissociative anesthesia
emergence
inhalation anesthetics
intravenous (IV) anesthetics
minimum alveolar concentration (MAC)
neuroleptanesthesia

CHAPTER OVERVIEW

Modern surgery did not begin until the introduction of nitrous oxide, ether, and chloroform as general anesthetics in the late 1800s. The agents used today as general anesthetics include gases (nitrous oxide), volatile liquids (diethyl ether, halothane, methoxyflurane, enflurane, and isoflurane), and intravenous agents (ketamine and opioids). The ultrashort-acting barbiturates, benzodiazepines, and etomidate are used intravenously for induction of anesthesia.

Therapeutic Rationale: General Anesthesia

General anesthetics act on the central nervous system (CNS) to abolish the perception of pain and the reaction to painful stimuli. The use of general anesthetics requires specifically trained personnel to monitor the level of anesthesia and the patient's vital signs while under anesthesia.

Therapeutic Agents: General Anesthetics

Inhalation Anesthetics: General Characteristics

Mechanism of Action

Inhalation anesthetics are gases or volatile liquids administered as gases. They are unusual in their mechanism of action because they do not appear to act by a receptor mechanism. Instead, inhalation anesthetics are believed to alter the lipid structure of cell membranes so that physiologic functions are impaired. The network of neurons making up the CNS is especially vulnerable because alteration of membrane structure interrupts the complex intercommunication necessary for function. The most sensitive system to such alterations is the ascending reticular activating system, the neuronal formation monitoring incoming stimuli and determining what information is to be sent to the brain for processing and response. Consciousness is lost when the ascending reticular activating system ceases to transmit information effectively.

Pharmacokinetics

The effective concentration of an inhalation anesthetic in the brain does not depend on the solubility of the anesthetic in blood or tissue. Rather, effective concentration depends on the partial pressure of the anesthetic or effective pressure of the gas in the atmosphere. If a constant partial pressure of anesthetic is inhaled, partial pressure in the alveoli rises toward the inhaled level. If the gas is not soluble in blood, little gas is removed by the blood circulating around the alveoli, and the partial pressure of the gas in the blood quickly reaches the inhaled partial pressure. This anesthetic has a rapid onset of action. If the gas is soluble in blood, however, partial pressure of the gas in the alveoli quickly drops since the gas is being removed more rapidly by the blood than can be replenished by breathing. A long time is required to equilibrate the blood with the gas to where the partial pressure matches that coming into the alveoli. To shorten the time to reach this steady state, anesthesia is induced using a high partial pressure of the gas and then lowering the partial pressure to maintain anesthesia.

The potency of an inhalation anesthetic is determined by the **minimum alveolar concentration (MAC)** that produces insensitivity to a skin incision (anesthesia) in 50% of patients. For instance, MAC of 10% is equivalent to a partial pressure of 0.1 atmosphere or 76 millimeters of mercury (mm Hg) at standard conditions (sea level). MAC of 10% means that when air in the alveoli has equilibrated with the body and incoming air, all of which are 10% anesthetic gas, the patient has a 50-50 chance of being unreactive to a skin incision. Surgery is conducted at about 1.4 times the MAC value of the anesthetic chosen.

The distribution of the anesthetic is determined by the blood flow; thus the brain, liver, and kidneys reach equilibrium first. Excretion of the inhalation anesthetics is largely through the lungs. The anesthetic that is in solution is metabolized by the liver to a variable degree. Certain halogenated hydrocarbons (e.g., enflurane, halothane, and methoxyflurane) are metabolized to products that may damage the liver and kidney.

Emergence is the time during which the patient regains consciousness after the anesthetic has been discontinued. The duration of emergence from the inhaled anesthetics depends on the same factors as induction. The patient's vital signs are carefully monitored in a recovery room, and symptoms of pain or nausea and vomiting must be watched for and treated appropriately. Table 68-1 lists specific inhalation anesthetics and their properties.

Specific Inhalation Anesthetics

Diethyl Ether

Diethyl ether is a volatile liquid that is flammable and explosive. The MAC is 1.92%. A long time is required for induction and emergence when ether alone is used because it is highly soluble in blood. In addition, ether is unpleasant to inhale because it has a noxious and pungent odor, irritates the respiratory tract, and stimulates secretions. An anticholinergic drug may be administered to minimize these secretions. The explosive hazard and the noxious, pungent odor account for the rare use of ether in modern surgery. Nevertheless, ether is used in areas of the world where sophisticated equipment is unavailable for monitoring the patient. Ether has a wide margin of safety and has few effects on the cardiovascular system, allowing it to be administered without sophisticated control of concentration. Ether produces good analgesia and muscle relaxation, making extra medication unnecessary.

Desflurane

Desflurane (Suprane) is the first new inhalation anesthetic in 20 years. It is a halogenated hydrocarbon and chemically related to isoflurane. Desflurane is a nonflammable liquid that is administered with a special heated vaporizor. The MAC is 7.3%, but this decreases when combined with benzodiazepines or opioids. The sensitivity to desflurane also increases with age. One drawback of desflurane is that it irritates the respiratory tract to produce coughing, apnea, laryngospasm, and increased secretions. Induction is therefore usually accomplished with an intravenous drug. However, induction and emergence are rapid, 5 to 7 minutes. Cardiac output tends to remain stable, although the heart rate may increase and blood pressure decrease.

TABLE 68-1 Properties of Inhalation Anesthetics

DRUG	PHYSICAL PROPERTIES	ONSET	MAC	CARDIOVASCULAR EFFECTS	MUSCLE RELAXATION	ELIMINATION	OTHER PROPERTIES
Diethyl ether	Flammable liquid	Slow	1.92%	Minimum	Excellent	Lungs	Excellent analgesia. Nausea and vomiting on emergence. Secretions stimulated.
Desflurane (Suprane)	Nonflammable liquid	Rapid	7.3%	Minimum	Good	Lungs Little metabolism by liver	Rapidly acting. New anesthetic.
Enflurane (Ethrane)	Nonflammable liquid	Rapid	1.68%	Decreased blood pressure May sensitize heart to catecholamines	Good	Lungs 2-5% metabolized by liver	Causes low body temperature, hypothermia, and shivering.
Halothane (Fluothane)	Nonflammable liquid	Rapid	0.77%	Decreased blood pressure Sensitizes heart to catecholamines	Fair	Lungs 20% metabolized by liver	Poor analgesia.
Isoflurane (Forane)	Nonflammable liquid	Rapid	1.30%	Minimum	Good	Lungs Little metabolism by liver	Excellent analgesia.
Methoxyflurane (Penthrane)	Nonflammable liquid	Slow	0.16%	Decreased blood pressure	Good	Lungs 70% metabolized by liver	Excellent analgesia.
Nitrous oxide	Nonflammable gas	Very rapid	101%	Minimum	—	Lungs	Widely used with other drugs for anesthesia. Good analgesia.

Enflurane

Enflurane (Ethrane) is a halogenated hydrocarbon and a nonflammable liquid. MAC is 1.68%, and induction is fairly rapid. Enflurane is one of the stimulant anesthetics that produce muscle contractions and seizurelike brain wave patterns at high concentrations. Enflurane is usually administered with nitrous oxide to avoid high concentrations, which can cause CNS stimulation and cardiovascular depression. Enflurane causes a decrease in blood pressure resulting from depressed cardiac output and decreased peripheral resistance. Emergence is usually uneventful except for shivering. About 2.5% of enflurane is metabolized to release a low concentration of fluoride ion. The amount of fluoride ion is not harmful, except in patients with preexisting kidney damage.

Halothane

Halothane (Fluothane) is a nonflammable liquid halogenated hydrocarbon and currently is the most widely used volatile liquid anesthetic. MAC is 0.77%, and induction is fairly rapid. Postoperative nausea and vomiting are not problems. Halothane is a direct myocardial depressant and causes a dose-dependent reduction in cardiac output with no change in heart rate, a combination of effects that lowers blood pressure. Halothane also sensitizes the myocardium to exogenously administered catecholamines. This sensitization means that a sympathomimetic drug must be used cautiously during surgery to maintain blood pressure since sympathomimetic drugs may precipitate arrhythmias. Catecholamines may be used topically such as on the brain or in irrigation of the bladder to stop bleeding. Halothane does not give adequate muscle relaxation; a separate muscle relaxant must be used.

Rarely (1:800,000 patients) halothane is responsible for fatal hepatitis. Current theory is that free radical metabolites, which are very reactive compounds, may be produced by the liver and may damage liver cells.

Isoflurane

Isoflurane (Forane) is a chemical isomer of enflurane, but unlike enflurane, isoflurane is a depressant anesthetic similar to halothane. MAC is 1.3%. Induction is smooth and rapid, and muscle relaxation is adequate. The heart is not sensitized to catecholamines, but the blood pressure falls because of a decrease in the peripheral resistance of blood vessels. Only 0.25% of isoflurane is metabolized. Isoflurane is a more recent anesthetic that many anesthesiologists believe will be widely used in the future.

Methoxyflurane

Methoxyflurane (Penthrane) is a nonflammable liquid halogenated hydrocarbon. It produces analgesia adequate for obstetrics. MAC is 0.16%. Methoxyflurane depresses the cardiovascular system but does not sensitize the heart to catecholamines. Methoxyflurane that is not exhaled is metabolized extensively (70%) by the liver to fluoride ion. Prolonged anesthesia with methoxyflurane may result in high-output renal failure because in the presence of the fluoride ion, the kidney loses its concentrating ability so that urine volume is high. This renal failure is usually reversible.

Nitrous Oxide

Nitrous oxide is a nonexplosive gas that is widely used. The major limitation of nitrous oxide is that the maximum concentration allowable, 65% to 70% N_2O and 30% to 35% O_2, does not produce surgical anesthesia because MAC is 101%. Nevertheless, nitrous oxide produces good analgesia and is used for this purpose in dental and obstetric procedures. In addition, nitrous oxide is widely used with other anesthetics to produce surgical anesthesia. Its effect is additive with other anesthetics, so a 50% MAC concentration of nitrous oxide and a 50% MAC concentration of another inhalation anesthetic produces surgical anesthesia. In addition, nitrous oxide is widely used as one component of **balanced anesthesia,** in which an opioid, a skeletal muscle relaxant, and nitrous oxide are used together to produce surgical anesthesia.

Nitrous oxide has been shown to increase the incidence of spontaneous abortions in women and to decrease spermatogenesis in men who work in operating rooms. Scavenging equipment must now be used in the operating room to remove nitrous oxide. The gas is much more soluble (34 times) than nitrogen in the blood so that pockets of trapped gas in the patient expand as nitrogen leaves and is replaced by larger amounts of nitrous oxide. Locations where trapped gas is common include a blocked middle ear, pneumothorax, loops of intestine, lungs, renal cysts, and in the skull after a pneumoencephalogram. These conditions represent contraindications for nitrous oxide since the large increases in pressure or volumes that may result after its administration may cause serious damage.

Intravenous Anesthetics: General Characteristics

For a summary of information on intravenous anesthetics; see Table 68-2.

Intravenous (IV) anesthetics include the ultrashort-acting barbiturates: thiopental (Pentothal) and methohexital (Brevital); two benzodiazepines: diazepam (Valium) and midazolam (Versed); and the agents ketamine (Ketaject), etomidate (Amidate), and propofol (Diprivan). In addition, the development of two short-acting opioids, fentanyl citrate (Sublimaze) and sufentanil citrate (Sufenta), for use as IV agents has extended the use of multiple drugs for anesthesia. Two widely used types of combinations are *balanced anesthesia* and *neuroleptanesthsia.*

Only ketamine is a true anesthetic, abolishing the perception of and the reaction to pain. The barbiturates and benzodiazepines do not abolish reflex reaction to pain even when they are administered in doses large enough to render the patient unconscious. These drugs are used primarily as induction agents. The advantage of the IV agents is that they are effective seconds after administration.

TABLE 68-2 Injectable Drugs for Anesthesia

GENERIC NAME	TRADE NAME	ADMINISTRATION/DOSAGE	COMMENTS
Barbiturates			
Methohexital sodium	Brevital Sodium Brietal Sodium†	INTRAVENOUS: *Adults*—For induction: 5-12 ml of 1% solution no faster than 1 ml every 5 sec. Maintenance 2-4 ml of 1% solution as required. FDA pregnancy category C.	Shortest duration of action (5-7 min) of barbiturates. Some patients develop hiccups after rapid injection. Schedule IV substance.
Thiopental sodium	Pentothal*	INTRAVENOUS: *Adults*—For induction: 50-100 mg (2-4 ml) in 2.5% solution every 30-40 sec or 3-5 mg/kg body weight. Maintenance 2-4 ml of 2.5% solution as required. *Children*—3-5 mg/kg as described for adults. FDA pregnancy category C.	Duration of action about 15 min. May cause yawning, coughing, or laryngospasm. Schedule III substance.
Benzodiazepines			
Diazepam	Valium*	INTRAVENOUS: *Adults*—0.1-0.2 mg/kg body weight to induce sleep; maximum dose 10-20 mg. Basal sedation requires only 5-30 mg, so 2.5-5 mg is injected every 30 sec until light sleep or slurred speech is produced.	Do not mix with other liquids. Local anesthetic may be required for IV injection.
Midazolam	Versed*	INTRAMUSCULAR: *Adults*—For preoperative sedation: 70-80 μg/kg, 30-60 min before surgery. FDA pregnancy category D. *Children*—80-200 μg/kg. INTRAVENOUS: *Adults*—For conscious sedation: 2.5 mg administered over 2 min just before procedure. For general anesthesia: 200-350 μg/kg administered over 5-30 sec. *Children*—50-200 μg/kg.	Schedule IV substance. Older or debilitated patients should be administered smaller dose.
Miscellaneous			
Alfentanil	Alfenta*	INTRAVENOUS: *Adults*—For induction of anesthesia: 130 ug/kg body weight. FDA pregnancy category C.	Schedule II substance. Potent, short-acting narcotic analgesic. Very short-acting (30-45 min) drug.
Droperidol	Inapsine*	INTRAVENOUS: *Adults and children >2 yr*—0.15 mg/kg body weight. Onset: 10-15 min. Duration: 3-6 hr.	Antipsychotic drug. Used with fentanyl citrate and nitrous oxide to produce neuroleptanesthesia. May cause extrapyramidal symptoms.
Etomidate	Amidate Hypnomidate	INTRAVENOUS: *Adults and children >10 yr*—For induction: 0.3 mg/kg body weight injected over 30-60 sec; may vary between 0.2 and 0.6 mg/kg. FDA pregnancy category C.	Nonbarbiturate agent used for induction and sometimes maintenance of anesthesia.
Fentanyl	Duragesic	TRANSDERMAL: *Adults*—Apply to skin of upper torso every 72 hr. Initially, one 2.5 mg transdermal system. For maintenance, dosage may be adjusted every 3 days, according to patient response. Some patients require application every 48 hr.	Patients tolerant to opioids may require higher dosages. First opioid analgesic available in a transdermal system. Not for short-term relief of acute pain.
Fentanyl citrate	Sublimaze*	INTRAVENOUS: *Adults and children >2 yr*—0.002-0.003 mg/kg body weight in divided doses over 6-8 min. Maintenance 0.05-0.1 mg every 30-60 min. Onset: 1-2 min. FDA pregnancy category C.	Potent, short-acting narcotic analgesic. Used with droperidol and nitrous oxide for neuroleptic anesthesia and with nitrous oxide for balanced anesthesia.
Ketamine	Ketaject Ketalar*	INTRAVENOUS: *Adults and children*—1-4.5 mg/kg body weight over 60 sec, ½ of initial dose used for maintenance as needed. INTRAMUSCULAR: *Adults and children*—6.5-13 mg/kg body weight, ½ of initial dose for maintenance as needed.	Produces cataleptic anesthesia with good analgesia. Not a scheduled drug.

*Available in Canada and United States.
†Available in Canada only.

Continued

TABLE 68-2 Injectable Drugs for Anesthesia—cont'd

GENERIC NAME	TRADE NAME	ADMINISTRATION/DOSAGE	COMMENTS
Miscellaneous—cont'd			
Propofol	Diprivan*	INTRAVENOUS: *Adults* (up to 55 yr)—For induction of anesthesia, increments of approximately 40 mg every 10 sec until adequate anesthesia is achieved. usual total dose is 2-2.5 mg/kg. For maintenance, 25-50 mg as required is given by intermittent bolus, or 0.1-0.2 mg/kg/min is infused. For older adult, debilitated, or hypovolemic patients, dose is reduced by ½.	New IV anesthetic. Rapid onset and recovery. Causes hypotension and respiratory depression.
Sufentanil citrate	Sufenta*	INTRAVENOUS: *Adults*—Initial dose is 1-8 μg/kg with nitrous oxide and oxygen. Additional doses are 10-25 μg/kg. Doses depend on severity of pain associated with surgery. *Children >2 yr*—For cardiovascular surgery: 10-25 μg/kg with oxygen and muscular relaxant. Additional doses are 25-50 μg (1-2 μg/kg). FDA pregnancy category C.	Potent, short-acting narcotic analgesic used with nitrous oxide for balanced anesthesia or alone with oxygen and muscle relaxant.

It may seem paradoxical that an IV anesthetic would be so short acting when it must be metabolized to be excreted. The explanation is that the IV anesthetics are lipid soluble. Initially, they are distributed to the brain, liver, and kidneys, the organs with the largest blood flow, but later the drug is redistributed to body fat and skeletal muscle, which are less well perfused. This redistribution lowers the circulating concentration to that which no longer maintains anesthesia. This redistribution is responsible for the short duration of action. Metabolism of the drug proceeds as the drug passes through the liver.

Barbiturates

Thiopental (Pentothal) and methohexital (Brevital) are ultrashort-acting barbiturates used primarily to induce anesthesia. Loss of consciousness occurs within 60 seconds. Thiopental is effective as the sole anesthetic for about 15 minutes. Methohexital is even shorter acting. Barbiturates provide no analgesia and can cause excitement or delirium in the presence of pain in an awake patient. Changes in blood pressure or cardiac output are not common unless the injection is made rapidly. Respiration is markedly depressed, and yawning, coughing, or laryngospasm may occur. Methohexital can cause hiccups.

Solutions of barbiturates should be injected only into veins. Arterial injections can cause inflammation and clotting. The barbiturate solution damages tissue if it leaks around the injection site, and this situation can lead to gangrene.

Benzodiazepines

Diazepam (Valium) is used occasionally as an induction agent but more frequently to sedate patients undergoing cardioversion or endoscopic or dental procedures. IV diazepam takes 60 seconds to become effective. Sedation, sleep, and amnesia are achieved with little depression of cardiovascular or respiratory functions. Unlike barbiturates, diazepam is metabolized to active products and has a long duration of action (see Chapter 51).

Midazolam (Versed) is a relatively short-acting benzodiazepine used as an IV anesthetic. It should be used only in hospital or ambulatory care settings where respiratory and cardiac functions can be monitored. Midazolam may be administered intravenously or intramuscularly to induce sedation or amnesia.

Droperidol

Neuroleptanesthesia refers to the combination of droperidol (Inapsine), an antipsychotic drug of the butyrophenone class; an opioid (usually fentanyl); and nitrous oxide. A skeletal muscle relaxant may be used if needed. A fixed combination of the opioid fentanyl and droperidol is available as Innovar. Nitrous oxide produces loss of consciousness, and if it is discontinued, the patient becomes conscious but in an altered state of awareness. Neuroleptanesthesia is useful for older adult and poor-risk patients and for bronchoscopy and carotid arteriography. Innovar alone greatly facilitates intubation in awake patients.

Side effects of neuroleptanalgesia or neuroleptanesthesia are hypotension, a slow heart rate (bradycardia), and respiratory depression. The action of droperidol persists for 3 to 6 hours, whereas the analgesic effect of fentanyl persists for only 30 minutes. Droperidol has adrenergic-receptor blocking, antifibrillatory, antiemetic, and anticonvulsant actions. About 1% of patients who receive droperidol may have extrapyramidal muscle movements (see Chapter 52) for as long as 12 hours after administration of the drug. These movements may be controlled by administration of atropine or benztropine.

Etomidate

Etomidate (Amidate) is an IV anesthetic for the induction of surgical anesthesia. Etomidate produces minimum cardiovascular or respiratory changes. Since etomidate does not produce analgesia, the short-acting narcotic-analgesic fentanyl citrate also may be infused for total IV anesthesia. The most frequent side effects of etomidate are pain at the injection site and transient, myoclonic skeletal muscle movements.

Ketamine

Ketamine (Ketalar) is neither a barbiturate nor a benzodiazepine. Unlike those drug classes, ketamine produces a cataleptic anesthesia in which the patient appears to be awake but neither responds to pain nor remembers the procedure. This is sometimes referred to as **dissociative anesthesia.** Ketamine is not a controlled substance and is readily available in emergency rooms. Ketamine is rapidly effective when administered intramuscularly and intravenously. Ketamine alone provides anesthesia for 5 to 10 minutes when given intravenously and for 10 to 20 minutes when given intramuscularly.

Ketamine enhances muscle tone and increases blood pressure, heart rate, and respiratory secretions. The major side effect is seen in the recovery period, when patients may experience vivid, unpleasant dreams or hallucinations. Adults are more prone than children to these experiences. It may also cause vomiting and shivering. It is chemically related to phencyclidine (PCP), an illicit hallucinogen.

Ketamine should be used cautiously in patients with convulsive disorders, psychosis, or mild hypertension or who are undergoing eye surgery and is contraindicated for patients with coronary artery disease, severe hypertension, cerebrovascular accident (stroke), or treated hypothyroidism.

Opioids

The ideal anesthetic would produce analgesia, unconsciousness, muscle relaxation, and reduction of reflex activity. This anesthetic would act promptly and would be rapidly eliminated, remaining unmetabolized and producing no unwanted effects in body tissues. Since no anesthetic has all these desirable properties, several drugs are used in combination to achieve these goals. For surgical anesthesia, one widely used combination of agents is refered to as **balanced anesthesia.** This combines an opioid, nitrous oxide, and a skeletal muscle relaxant. Anesthesia is induced, generally with a short-acting barbiturate or occasionally with diazepam or other agents, and then the opioid, nitrous oxide, and skeletal muscle relaxant are administered. Respiration must be controlled since the opioids are potent respiratory depressants, and patients are usually paralyzed by a skeletal muscle relaxant. Nitrous oxide is effective at a 60% concentration because of its synergism with the opioid. The skeletal muscle relaxant is necessary because neither the opioid nor the nitrous oxide provides the muscular relaxation necessary for surgery.

The choice of the opioid is determined by the anticipated length of surgery. Alfentanil (Alfenta), fentanyl citrate (Sublimaze), and sufentanil citrate (Sufenta) are short-acting opioids primarily used for surgery. Meperidine (Demerol) is widely used for longer surgeries. Morphine is used as an alternate to meperidine, and it is also preferred for cardiac and poor-risk patients.

The advantage of balanced anesthesia is that the cardiovascular system is neither depressed nor sensitized to catecholamines. Respiration is depressed, but controlled ventilation is readily available. The incidence of postoperative nausea, vomiting, and pain is low.

Propofol

Propofol (Diprivan) is a new IV anesthetic for induction and maintenance of general anesthesia. It is also used with opioids and nitrous oxide in balanced anesthesia. Propofol can cause hypotension, and this is potentiated by opioid analgesics. Propofol is also a respiratory depressant. Recovery from anesthesia is rapid, with minimal psychomotor impairment. The drug is inactivated in the liver.

NURSING PROCESS OVERVIEW

General Anesthesia

Assessment

Perform a complete physical assessment, with focus on vital signs and respiratory system, laboratory data, and studies specific to known medical problems (e.g., coagulation studies in patients with liver disease or pulmonary function studies in patients with severe chronic obstructive pulmonary disease [COPD]).

Nursing Diagnoses

- Altered comfort: nausea and vomiting related to general anesthesia
- Ineffective airway clearance: inability to remove airway secretions related to general anesthesia

Patient Outcomes

The patient will experience no vomiting following general anesthesia, and any nausea will be treated. The patient will recover from surgery without aspiration or pneumonia.

Planning/Implementation

Delivery of general anesthesia requires knowledge and facility with management of the respiratory and cardiovascular systems, multiple drugs, and the immobilized unconscious patient. For further information, consult appropriate textbooks of nursing, medicine, and anesthesiology.

Evaluation

Perform frequent evaluations of vital signs, respiratory and cardiovascular status, level of consciousness, and ability to handle secretions. Assess degree of postoperative pain and medicate if appropriate. Assess wound, drainage, intake and output, and other parameters as indicated by the type of surgery performed.

Nursing Implications Summary

General Anesthesia

Drug Administration/Patient and Family Education

- Techniques of administration of general anesthesia are beyond the scope of this book; for further information consult appropriate textbooks of anesthesia.
- Obtain a careful drug history before surgery. Assess for allergic or unusual responses to previous anesthetic agents and for any current medications the patient is taking.
- Preoperative medications are an integral part of planned anesthesia. Administer them as ordered and on time.
- To prepare the patient for surgery, inform the patient and family about the surgical procedure and what to expect postoperatively. Have the patient give a return demonstration of any exercises or activities required such as coughing and deep breathing. Provide the patient with an opportunity to ask questions of the anesthesiologist or nurse anesthetist. Schedule a visit to the intensive care unit, if appropriate. Provide emotional support.
- Malignant hyperthermia is a rare but potentially fatal syndrome that can develop in genetically susceptible patients, even if patients have had previous uneventful surgeries. It can develop when any volatile anesthetic is used, but the onset is usually more abrupt when succinylcholine is used. Symptoms include tachycardia or tachyarrhythmias, tachypnea, labile blood pressure, and flushing followed by cyanotic mottling. Blood pH may fall and serum potassium levels rise. Some patients develop muscle rigidity. Elevated temperature is a late sign, but the temperature rises to high levels (110°F [42°C]). Treatment includes discontinuing anesthesia, administering 100% oxygen and IV dantrolene, correcting acid-base imbalances, and cooling the patient. A similar syndrome in appearance is neuroleptic malignant syndrome (see Chapter 52). Teach patients who develop this syndrome to wear a medical identification tag or bracelet and to inform all health care providers that this syndrome has occurred.

Postoperative Care

- Monitor temperature, pulse, respirations, blood pressure, and pulse oximetry frequently. With the exception of temperature, this may be every 5 minutes initially, progressing to every 15 minutes, then every 30 minutes and longer. Auscultate lung sounds and check neurologic status. Do not leave the patient unattended unless the patient can call for assistance and can handle secretions safely.
- Position the patient on the side initially, if possible, to prevent aspiration if vomiting should occur. Keep a suction machine at the bedside and keep siderails up.
- Evaluate the patient for pain medication in the immediate postoperative period (first 2 to 4 hours after surgery). Factors to consider include the nature and location of surgery, vital signs, age, weight, level of consciousness, what anesthetic was used, and whether analgesics were administered during surgery. The initial dose of analgesics may be one half to one fourth the ordered dose of analgesic, but make reductions in dose only after consultation with the physician.
- When Innovar is used, the first dose of postoperative analgesic should be low.
- Begin nursing measures to prevent atelectasis and pneumonia as soon as the patient is able. This may include turning and deep breathing, coughing, and early ambulation.
- Effects of anesthesia persist even after the patient appears to be alert and awake. If it is necessary to give instructions about activity, diet, or medications, as in the outpatient or day-surgery setting, do so verbally and in writing to the patient and have at least one family member present.
- Do not permit patients in the outpatient setting to drive themselves home if they have received general anesthesia, IV barbiturates or benzodiazepines, or any drug that may alter response time or level of consciousness.
- Warn a patient who has a severe reaction or response to any anesthetic to carry the name of the agent at all times. If surgery is ever again needed, instruct the patient to tell the anesthetist of the previous severe response. Suggest that the patient wear a medical identification tag or bracelet indicating the severe reaction.
- See the nursing implications summary for narcotic analgesics in Chapter 31 (p. 391). Patients perform needed postoperative activities better if they are adequately medicated for pain.

Ketamine

- Ketamine is associated with unpleasant dreams, emergence delirium, irrational behavior, disorientation, and hallucinations. These side effects may be lessened by providing the patient with a quiet wake-up period, perhaps in the quietest corner of the postanesthesia recovery room. Avoid excessive stimulation, although vital signs must be monitored. If psychic effects occur, provide calm reassurance and reorientation. Do not leave the patient unattended.

  Once the patient is returned to the room, keep it dimly lit and keep noise and stimulation to a minimum. Inform family members of the probable cause of the behavior and enlist their aid in patient reorientation and reassurance.

CRITICAL THINKING

APPLICATION

1. What is MAC?
2. What factors determine induction and emergence? Outline your responsibilities during the emergence period.
3. Why is diethyl ether seldom used in the United States?
4. Which inhalation anesthetics sensitize the heart to catecholamines?
5. Which inhalation anesthetics are metabolized to some degree?
6. Which inhalation anesthetics lower blood pressure during surgery?
7. What factor limits the use of nitrous oxide alone as an anesthetic? How is this limitation overcome?
8. What are the hazards of nitrous oxide to patients and to operating room personnel?
9. Which barbiturates are used as IV induction agents for anesthesia? How is their action effectively terminated?
10. Which benzodiazepines are used as IV induction agents for anesthesia?
11. Describe balanced anesthesia.
12. Describe neuroleptanesthesia.

CRITICAL THINKING

1. How are general anesthetics believed to work?
2. What measurement determines the effective concentration of an inhalation anesthetic? How does this differ from the concentration based on total solubility?
3. Which inhalation anesthetics are halogenated hydrocarbons? What should you monitor in a patient who has received a halogenated hydrocarbon?
4. What is the nature of anesthesia with ketamine? What nursing care activities might be needed with a patient who has received ketamine?
5. What are the properties of an ideal anesthetic?

CHAPTER 69

Neuromuscular Blocking Agents

OBJECTIVES

After studying this chapter, you should be able to do the following:

- *Discuss the action of neuromuscular blocking drugs.*
- *Differentiate between nondepolarizing and depolarizing neuromuscular blocking drugs.*
- *Develop a nursing care plan for patients receiving neuromuscular blocking drugs.*

KEY TERMS

depolarizing neuromuscular blocking drug
neuromuscular blocking drugs
nondepolarizing or competitive blocking drugs

CHAPTER OVERVIEW

Motor neurons are single neurons originating in the spinal cord and terminating on the muscle. The **neuromuscular blocking drugs** occupy the receptors for acetylcholine on muscles, thus preventing muscle contraction. These drugs produce muscular relaxation for intubation and surgical procedures.

Therapeutic Rationale: Neuromuscular Blockade

As seen in Figure 69-1, neuromuscular blocking drugs produce complete muscle relaxation by preventing muscular contraction. Since neuromuscular blockers can produce complete paralysis, they are administered only to anesthetized patients. Assisted ventilation should be available for short-acting succinylcholine and is mandatory when administering long-acting neuromuscular blockers. Skeletal muscle relaxants do not inhibit pain.

Neuromuscular blocking drugs provide muscle relaxation during surgery, particularly relaxation of the abdominal muscles, without using deep general anesthesia, which would relax abdominal muscles by depressing the spinal cord. Neuromuscular blockers are also used with light anesthesia to allow a tube to be passed down easily to the trachea (endotracheal intubation), to relieve spasm of the larynx, to prevent convulsive muscle spasms during electroconvulsive therapy for depression, and to allow breathing to be controlled totally by a respirator (controlled ventilation) during surgery.

Therapeutic Agents: Neuromuscular Blockers

Nondepolarizing Neuromuscular Blockers

Neuromuscular blocking drugs produce complete muscle relaxation by binding to the receptor for acetylcholine at the neuromuscular junction. The **nondepolarizing or competitive blocking drugs** bind to the receptor without initiating depolarization of the muscle membrane.

Table 69-1 summarizes neuromuscular blocking drugs and their administration.

Tubocurarine

Mechanism of Action

Tubocurarine (curare) was originally isolated as the active principle of the South American arrow poison. An animal hit with an arrow containing curare falls paralyzed a short time later. Curare is the classic acetylcholine blocker for the neuromuscular junction (see Chapter 11).

Pharmacokinetics

Curare is administered by slow (60 to 90 seconds) intravenous (IV) injection. Maximal paralysis occurs within 5 minutes and persists for 60 minutes (range: 25 to 90 minutes). The progression of paralysis begins with the eyelids, then the face, the extremities, and finally the diaphragm, resulting in the cessation of spontaneous breathing. Recovery from neuromuscular blockade can be assisted by injecting edrophonium, neostigmine, or pyridostigmine to increase the amount of acetylcholine at the neuromuscular junction.

About 40% of tubocurarine is excreted unchanged in the urine. Patients with renal failure or acidosis excrete tubocurarine less rapidly and require a smaller dose.

Uses

Tubocurarine produces muscle relaxation during surgery or electroconvulsive shock therapy, reduces muscle spasm in tetanus, and allows controlled ventilation.

Adverse Reactions, Contraindications, and Toxicity

Tubocurarine can cause release of histamine, which causes hypotension or bronchospasm (see Chapter 28). Hypotension can arise from ganglionic blockade by tubocurarine. Tubocurarine does not cross the placenta or blood-brain barrier.

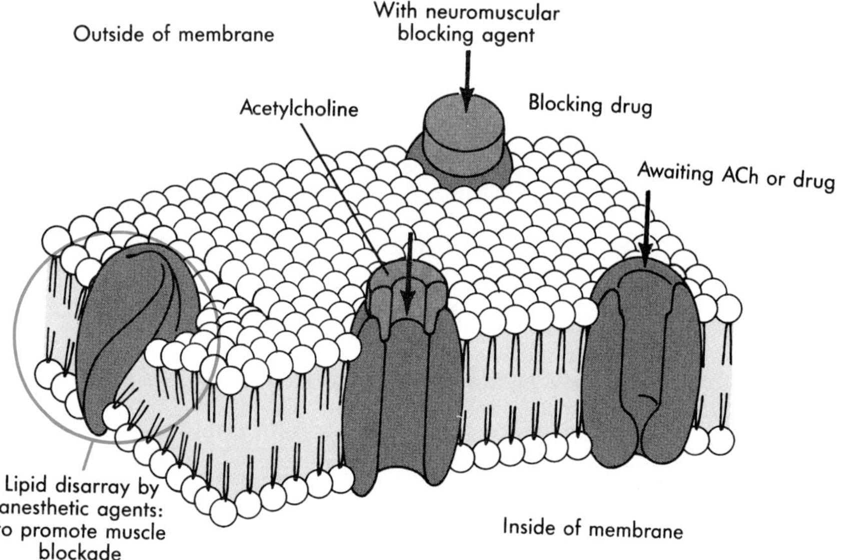

FIGURE 69-1
Neuromuscular blocking drugs block receptor, preventing acetylcholine from binding to receptor and opening channel. Anesthesia caused by neuromuscular blocking drugs differs from lipid disarray caused by general anesthetic drugs.

TABLE 69-1 Neuromuscular Blocking Drugs

GENERIC NAME	TRADE NAME	ADMINISTRATION/DOSAGE	COMMENTS
Nondepolarizing (Competitive) Drugs			
Atracurium	Tracrium*	INTRAVENOUS: *Adults*—0.3-0.6 mg/kg body weight; subsequent doses 0.05-0.1 mg/kg.	Drug is not affected by renal or hepatic impairment and is relatively free of cardiovascular side effects. Doses given are for use with nitrous oxide. Other inhalation anesthetics may require smaller doses.
Doxacurium chloride	Nuromax	INTRAVENOUS: *Adults*—Endotracheal intubation: 0.05 mg/kg body weight will provide 100 min relaxation. After succinylcholine-assisted endotracheal intubation: 0.025 mg/kg body weight to provide 60 min relaxation; maintenance requires 0.005 mg/kg body weight for relaxation. *Children*—0.03 mg/kg body weight initially for halothane anesthesia to provide 30 min relaxation.	Drug does not increase heart rate. Adult doses must be decreased by ⅓ if used with enflurane, halothane, or isoflurane anesthesia. Doses for older adult patients or patients with hepatic or renal disease may need to be reduced. Ideal body weight should be used for obese patients.
Gallamine triethiodide	Flaxedil*	INTRAVENOUS: *Adults*—1-1.15 mg/kg body weight. Supplemental doses 0.3-1.2 mg/kg. *Children*—2.5 mg/kg initially with 0.3-1.2 mg/kg supplemental doses. *Newborns up to age 1 mo:* 0.25-0.75 mg/kg initially, with 0.1-0.5 mg/kg supplemental doses.	Drug may cause increased heart rate. Drug is not used for patients in renal failure. Doses given are for use with nitrous oxide. Other inhalation anesthetics may require smaller doses.
Metocurine iodide	Metubine*	INTRAVENOUS: *Adults*—0.1-0.3 mg/kg body weight. Supplemental doses 0.02-0.03 mg/kg.	See tubocurarine chloride. Doses given are for use with nitrous oxide. Other inhalation anesthetics may require smaller doses. Drug is not for use in patients with renal failure.
Mivacurium	Mivacron	INTRAVENOUS: *Adults*—Endotracheal intubation and surgical relaxation: 0.15-0.2 mg/kg body weight administered over 5-15 sec initially; maintenance 0.1 mg/kg body weight. *Children 2-12 yr*—0.2-0.25 mg/kg body weight administered over 5-15 sec.	Drug has negligible direct effect on cardiovascular system. Metabolized by plasma cholinesterases. Renal and biliary elimination of inactive metabolites. Effective dose not affected by impaired hepatic or renal function.
Pancuronium bromide	Pavulon*	INTRAVENOUS: *Adults and children*—0.04-0.1 mg/kg body weight initially with 0.01-0.02 mg/kg supplemental doses. Newborns may be very sensitive; use test dose of 0.02 mg.	Drug does not cause hypotension. Drug may stimulate heart rate and cardiac output. Doses given are for use with nitrous oxide. Other inhalation anesthetics may require smaller doses.
Pipecuronium bromide	Arduan	INTRAVENOUS: *Adults*—Endotracheal intubation: 0.07-0.085 mg/kg ideal body weight. After succinylcholine-facilitated endotracheal intubation: 0.05 mg/kg ideal body weight for 45 min muscle relaxation or 0.07-0.085 mg/kg ideal body weight for 1-2 hr muscle relaxation. Maintenance during surgery: 0.01-0.015 mg/kg ideal body weight. *Children 1-14 yr*—0.057 mg/kg body weight.	Drug has negligible direct effect on cardiovascular system. Metabolite has some activity; most of drug is excreted unchanged in urine; doses must be reduced for patients with renal function impairment.
✣ Tubocurarine chloride (curare)	Tubarine† Tubocurarine chloride*	INTRAVENOUS: *Adults and children*—0.2-0.4 mg/kg body weight initially. Supplemental doses 0.04-0.2 mg/kg. Diagnosis of myasthenia gravis: ⅟₁₅-⅕ of above dose.	IV injection should be slow (1-1½ min). Do not combine with alkaline IV barbiturate solutions. Doses given are for use with nitrous oxide. Other inhalation anesthetics may require smaller doses.
Vercuronium	Norcuron*	INTRAVENOUS: *Adults*—0.07-0.14 mg/kg body weight for intubation; 0.04-0.1 mg/kg initially, followed by 0.015-0.02 mg/kg as needed for surgery.	Drug related to pancuronium but shorter (by ⅓ to ½) in duration. Drug is relatively free of cardiovascular side effects. Doses given are for use with nitrous oxide. Other inhalation anesthetics may require smaller doses.

*Available in Canada and United States.
†Available in Canada only.

TABLE 69-1 Neuromuscular Blocking Drugs—cont'd

GENERIC NAME	TRADE NAME	ADMINISTRATION/DOSAGE	COMMENTS
Depolarizing Drugs			
✣ Succinylcholine chloride	Anectine* Quelicin* Sucostrin	INTRAVENOUS: *Adults*—0.6-1.1 mg/kg body weight initially. Continuous infusion: 0.1% or 0.2% solution at rate of 0.5-10 mg/min. *Children*—1.1 mg/kg body weight initially with 0.3-0.6 mg/kg supplemental doses. *Newborns*—2 mg/kg. Continuous infusion is not recommended for children and newborns.	Duration is only 5 min because of hydrolysis by plasma cholinesterase. This enzyme is missing genetically in some patients, and prolonged action is seen. Drug may cause cardiac arrhythmias. Doses given are for use with nitrous oxide. Other inhalation anesthetics require smaller doses.

Interactions

Many anesthetics potentiate the action of tubocurarine, including halothane, ether, methoxyflurane, and enflurane. Antibiotics potentiating the action of tubocurarine include the aminoglycosides and the polymyxins (see Chapter 43), bacitracin, lincomycin, and clindamycin. Other drugs that potentiate the action of tubocurarine are the antiarrhythmic drugs, quinidine, ganglionic blocker drugs, trimethaphan, and magnesium sulfate. Since patients with myasthenia gravis have an exaggerated response to tubocurarine, very small doses of tubocurarine can be used to diagnose myasthenia gravis if tests with edrophonium or neostigmine are inconclusive.

Atracurium

Atracurium (Tracrium) is a nondepolarizing muscle relaxant. It is shorter in duration than tubocurarine, producing adequate relaxation for 15 to 20 minutes. Atracurium is inactivated by hydrolysis. At usual doses, atracurium does not produce cardiovascular side effects.

Doxacurium

Doxacurium (Nuromax) is a long-acting drug with minimal cardiovascular effects, desirable features for use in patients with coronary disease. It is used to facilitate endotracheal intubation in procedures lasting 90 minutes or longer and to induce skeletal muscle relaxation during surgical procedures. Doxacurium is excreted unchanged in the urine and should be used with caution in patients with renal failure.

Gallamine triethiodide

Gallamine triethiodide (Flaxedil) is a synthetic drug similar in action to tubocurarine but with a shorter duration of action. Gallamine does not cause histamine release or ganglionic blockade. The major side effect of gallamine is an increase in heart rate (tachycardia), which is seen a few minutes after injection and then declines. Gallamine is excreted unchanged in the urine and should not be used in patients with renal failure.

Metocurine (dimethyl tubocurarine) iodide

Metocurine iodide (Metubine), a semisynthetic derivative of tubocurarine, is two to three times as potent as tubocurarine but otherwise similar. Metocurine is excreted unchanged in the urine and should not be used in patients with renal failure.

Mivacurium

Mivacurium (Mivacron) has a fast onset of action and is short acting. It does not accumulate since it is rapidly broken down by cholinesterases in the plasma.

Pancuronium bromide

Pancuronium bromide (Pavulon) has a faster onset of action than tubocurarine, although the duration of action is similar. Pancuronium does not cause the histamine release or ganglionic blockade characteristic of tubocurarine. Heart rate, cardiac output, and atrial pressure are increased by pancuronium, effects that may be desired in cardiac surgery. Pancuronium is excreted in the urine, and doses must be decreased for patients with renal failure.

Pipecuronium bromide

Pipecuronium bromide (Arduan) has a long duration of action and is used for procedures lasting 90 minutes or longer. Pipecuronium has no vagal blocking action to cause tachycardia, so it can be used in the presence of coronary artery disease in which tachycardia can be dangerous. Pipecuronium is also used to facilitate the management of patients undergoing mechanical ventilation.

Vecuronium

Vecuronium (Norcuron) is a nondepolarizing muscle relaxant chemically related to pancuronium. Vecuronium is shorter acting than pancuronium, and its effects are not cumulative with repeated administration. Unlike tubocurarine, the cardiovascular side effects arising from ganglionic or vagal blockade, interference with norepinephrine reuptake, or release of histamine are minimal with vecuronium. Vecuronium's intensity and duration of action are affected significantly by liver damage and modestly by renal failure.

Depolarizing Neuromuscular Blocking Drug

Succinylcholine chloride

Mechanism of Action

Succinylcholine (Anectine and others) is the only **depolarizing neuromuscular blocking drug** in use. It binds to the receptor for acetylcholine and causes depolarization of the muscle membrane.

Pharmacokinetics

Succinylcholine chloride has the briefest duration of action (5 minutes) of the neuromuscular blocking drugs since plasma cholinesterases readily degrade succinylcholine. Longer action requires continuous infusion of succinylcholine, but then care must be taken to avoid desensitizing the muscle. The duration of action is increased by drugs that inhibit cholinesterases. Some patients have abnormal plasma cholinesterases that do not readily degrade succinylcholine. In these patients, the action of succinylcholine is prolonged. Conditions that elevate plasma potassium concentration, such as burns, tetanus, massive trauma, or brain or spinal cord injury, prolong the action of succinylcholine.

Uses

Succinylcholine's short duration of action makes it a drug of choice for endoscopy, terminating laryngospasm, endotracheal intubation, orthopedic procedures, and electroconvulsive shock therapy.

Adverse Reactions, Contraindications, and Toxicity

Children are not as sensitive to succinylcholine on a weight basis as adults and require higher doses. Children are more apt to show side effects of succinylcholine resulting from parasympathetic stimulation such as slow heart rate (bradycardia) and cardiac arrhythmias. Succinylcholine does not cross the blood-brain barrier or the placenta.

Succinylcholine initially causes fasciculations before the muscles are paralyzed. This effect is believed to cause the stiffness and soreness many patients experience 12 to 24 hours after they have received succinylcholine. Succinylcholine also transiently raises intraocular pressure and must be administered before eye surgery.

NURSING PROCESS OVERVIEW

Neuromuscular Blocking Drugs

Patients receive neuromuscular blocking drugs when undergoing anesthesia, undergoing diagnostic studies that necessitate brief muscle relaxation, "bucking" ventilators, and undergoing electroconvulsive therapy.

Assessment

Monitor the patient's pulse, respiratory rate, and blood pressure. Assess the patient, focusing on the major problems being treated and the diagnostic or therapeutic procedure to be carried out.

Nursing Diagnoses

- Ineffective airway clearance related to drug effect
- Anxiety related to inability to swallow, ineffective airway clearance, and weakness

Patient Outcomes

The patient will recover from paralysis without aspiration or development of pneumonia. The patient will state reduced anxiety as the procedures are explained or as the drug wears off.

Planning/Implementation

Observe the rate, quality, and depth of respirations and ventilate the patient's airway as needed. Have equipment for intubation and suctioning at the bedside. Use an infusion monitoring device for IV administration. Neuromuscular blockade agents alone do not produce anesthesia; medicate the patient for pain if necessary. Position the patient carefully and check to see that instruments and bed linens are not causing unnecessary pressure on the patient's body. After the drug has been administered, it may take minutes to hours for the effect of the neuromuscular blocking agents to wear off. Continue to assess the patient's ability to breathe unassisted, to cough, and to handle secretions. Use a peripheral nerve stimulator to monitor for drug effectiveness and to avoid overdose. Position the patient on his or her side and keep the siderails up. Do not leave the patient unattended until he or she can adequately cough, handle secretions, and call for help.

Evaluation

These agents are successful if they produce sufficient muscle relaxation to allow the procedure or activity to proceed. These are all short-acting drugs and are not prescribed for use outside a hospital setting.

NURSING IMPLICATIONS SUMMARY

General Guidelines: Neuromuscular Blockers

Drug Administration

- Neuromuscular blockers produce apnea. Monitor blood pressure, pulse, and respirations and auscultate lungs. Monitor arterial blood gases and electrocardiogram. Use these drugs only in a setting where personnel and equipment are available to provide immediate intubation. Have available a suction machine, oxygen, mechanical ventilator or resuscitation bag, and resuscitation equipment and drugs.
- Use a peripheral nerve stimulator to monitor effectiveness of the drug.
- Remember that neuromuscular blockers cause paralysis but not anesthesia. Unless a patient is also anesthetized, the patient can still hear, feel, and see if the eyelids are opened. Remember to remain professional in discussions within the patient's hearing, to explain sounds in the environment, to describe anticipated nursing care activities, and to use television or radio judiciously. Arrange for uninterrupted periods so the patient can sleep.
- Avoid rough handling, position the patient in a comfortable position, offer backrubs if possible, and medicate for pain if appropriate. Keep the reversing agent or antagonist readily available. When administering these drugs via constant infusion, use a microdrip tubing set and an infusion controlling device.
- Consult the manufacturer's literature for specific guidelines regarding calculation of dosages. In many institutions, induction with a neuromuscular blocking agent must be done by the anesthesiologist or nurse anesthetist; follow agency guidelines.
- When discontinuing therapy, do not leave the patient unattended until sufficient muscle tone has returned so the patient can breathe, handle secretions, and call for assistance if needed. In infants, assess for the ability to hold up the legs. Keep the siderails up and the call bell within reach.
- Usually these drugs are not used for home management. Keep the patient and family informed of the patient's condition.

CRITICAL THINKING

APPLICATION

1. Make a list of the nondepolarizing neuromuscular blocking drugs.
2. List the depolarizing neuromuscular blocking drugs.

CRITICAL THINKING

1. Describe the uses of tubocurarine.
2. What genetic alteration do some patients have that prolongs the action of succinylcholine? What supportive actions would you take?
3. How would you assess the patient's ability to handle secretions?

SECTION XVI

Ophthalmic Drugs

CHAPTER 70 *Drugs to Treat Glaucoma* reviews the pathology behind glaucoma and the various agents used to control this condition.

CHAPTER 71 *Drugs Affecting the Eye* discusses the anticholinergic agents, adrenergic agents, and prostaglandin inhibitors used for examination of the eye and eye surgery.

CHAPTER 70

Drugs to Treat Glaucoma

OBJECTIVES

After studying this chapter, you should be able to do the following:

- *Differentiate between chronic and acute glaucoma.*
- *Discuss the categories of drugs to treat glaucoma, including cholinomimetic drugs, adrenergic drugs, beta-blockers, carbonic anhydrase inhibitors, and osmotic agents.*
- *From a list of drugs used in the treatment of glaucoma, develop a teaching plan to prepare patients for discharge.*

KEY TERMS

acute (closed-angle) glaucoma
chronic (open-angle) glaucoma
glaucoma

CHAPTER OVERVIEW

The key functions of the eye are controlled by the autonomic nervous system. Selected drugs with autonomic actions are used to treat glaucoma. These drugs are presented in this chapter.

Therapeutic Rationale: Glaucoma

Glaucoma is the leading cause of adult blindness in the United States. Blindness results from damage to the optic nerve cause by an increased intraocular pressure. The detection and treatment of glaucoma is important. About 3 million people in the United States are estimated to have glaucoma, half being unaware of their condition. The risk factors for glaucoma are indicated in the box. An estimated 120,000 people in the United States are estimated to be blind as a consequence of glaucoma.

The increase in intraocular pressure is caused by the accumulation of aqueous humor in the space between the lens and cornea. Aqueous humor is a protein-poor fluid formed by the ciliary body. As illustrated in Figure 70-1, this fluid is normally reabsorbed through the trabecular spaces into Schlemm's canal in a region of the cornea called the *anterior chamber.* If the aqueous humor cannot be reabsorbed through the anterior chamber, the fluid accumulates and intraocular pressure increases. If the intraocular pressure is not relieved, the optic nerve becomes damaged, resulting in blindness.

Chronic (open-angle) glaucoma is the more common form of glaucoma and is very gradual in its onset. The defect is a slow degeneration of the anterior chamber that impairs the uptake of aqueous humor (see Figure 70-1). Traditionally, drug therapy, applied as eyedrops, has been used to improve the uptake of aqueous humor and thereby lower intraocular pressure. The most commonly prescribed drugs are beta-blockers, epinephrine, and miotics.

Laser surgery is an effective method for treating the drainage area to improve fluid outflow. In the United States laser surgery is used when drug therapy fails. Laser treatment properly performed has minimal side effects. The need for medication is usually greatly reduced. Current studies are examining whether laser treatment may be the preferred first treatment for glaucoma. There is also filtration surgery for treating glaucoma in which conventional surgical instruments are used to open a passage for draining of excess aqueous humor.

RISK FACTORS FOR GLAUCOMA

Advancing age (>40 years old)
Intraocular pressure >20 mm Hg
Family history of glaucoma
African-American background
Diabetes mellitus
High myopia
Systemic vascular disease

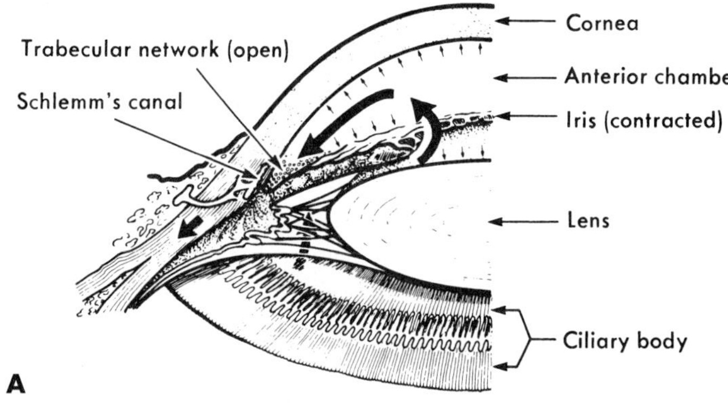

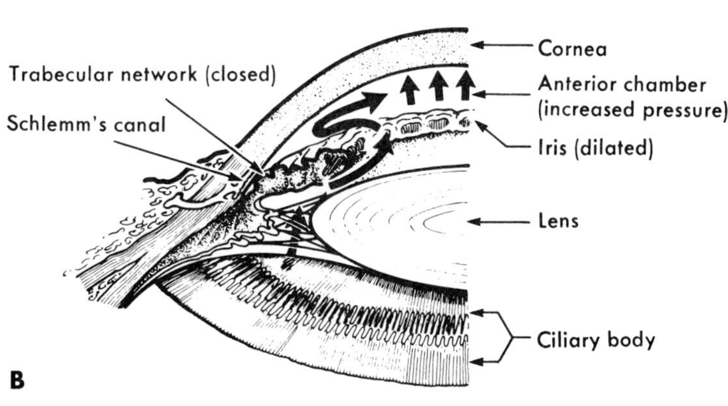

FIGURE 70-1
A, Normal eye or eye with chronic glaucoma. Flow of aqueous humor is shown from ciliary body and around iris. Aqueous humor is normally absorbed into body through trabecular network into Schlemm's canal. In chronic glaucoma, aqueous humor accumulates because trabecular network degenerates. **B,** Eye in acute glaucoma. Flow of aqueous humor is stopped because iris has blocked trabecular network and Schlemm's canal. Aqueous humor can accumulate quickly to cause marked rise in ocular pressure that may damage optic nerve.

Acute (closed-angle) glaucoma is characterized by the iris bulging up to shut off access of the aqueous humor to the anterior chamber (see Figure 70-1). This creates an emergency because the buildup of intraocular pressure may rapidly become severe, damaging the optic nerve and causing blindness. Emergency treatment consists of a cholinomimetic drug, a carbonic anhydrase inhibitor, epinephrine, and an osmotic diuretic. This drug regimen provides transient treatment while the patient is being prepared for eye surgery in which the iris is cut to allow fluid access to the anterior chamber once again.

Therapeutic Agents: Glaucoma

For a summary of the drugs commonly used to treat glaucoma, see Table 70-1.

The adrenergic drug epinephrine is the alternative drug to initiate therapy or the next drug added when the miotic drug alone is inadequate. Epinephrine stimulates alpha- and beta-receptors. In the eye, stimulation of alpha-receptors reduces resistance to the outflow of aqueous humor, whereas stimulation of the beta-receptors decreases production of aqueous humor.

The adrenergic beta-blocking drug timolol may also be used initially to treat chronic glaucoma or may be applied in addition to the miotic and epinephrine. The mechanism by which blockade of the beta-receptors of the eye decreases intraocular pressure is not clear, particularly since stimulation of the beta-receptor also causes reduction of intraocular pressure.

The drugs discussed previously are all applied directly to the eye. In resistant cases of glaucoma, systemic drugs are added. A carbonic anhydrase inhibitor is the next drug added because, aside from being weak diuretics, carbonic anhydrase inhibitors are also effective in decreasing the production of aqueous humor.

Osmotic agents such as glycerin, isosorbide, urea, or mannitol provide an immediate but short-term reduction in intraocular pressure by drawing fluid from the eyeball to the hyperosmotic blood.

✣ Pilocarpine

Mechanism of Action

Pilocarpine (PV Carpine, Ocusert Pilo-20/Pilo-40 Systems, Pilopine HS Gel) is a direct-acting cholinomimetic drug. These drugs mimic the action of the neurotransmitter, acetylcholine (see Chapter 11). In the eye, cholinomimetic drugs produce contraction of the sphincter (circular) muscles, which constricts the pupil, a process called *miosis.* Therapeutic effectiveness results from the spread of the trabecular spaces of the anterior chamber when the sphincter muscles contract. The larger area allows improved uptake of the aqueous humor, which relieves intraocular pressure.

Pharmacokinetics

Pilocarpine administered as drops of a 1% or 2% solution produces miosis in 15 to 30 minutes and lasts for 2 to 4 hours. To increase the duration of action, pilocarpine may also be administered as a gel, which lasts 18 to 24 hours. A more sophisticated delivery system is the Ocusert system (see Figure 70-2). This drug delivery system is placed in the upper or lower cul-de-sac of the eye and allows pilocarpine to slowly diffuse out. The system is designed to deliver pilocarpine over 7 days, but the duration varies with the individual.

Uses

Beta-blockers are now more commonly prescribed for the initial therapy for glaucoma, but pilocarpine is still widely used alone or in combination with beta-blockers and other agents to control glaucoma. Pilocarpine is also used in the emergency treatment of acute-angle glaucoma, both before and after surgery. Pilocarpine is also used to counteract the effects of cycloplegics and mydriatics following ophthalmoscopic examinations.

Adverse Reactions, Contraindications, and Toxicity

Pilocarpine is well tolerated; because it is applied in small amounts directly to the eye, systemic effects are uncommon. The most common reaction is some stinging and local irritation. Ciliary spasm and miosis may be troublesome when starting therapy. Miosis makes vision in dim light poor, so patients should be cautioned against night driving.

The Ocusert system may migrate and produce pain, but this is not common. Patients with loose lids may not be able to retain the system and may need to check for its presence each morning.

Patients with acute iritis or other conditions in which pupillary constriction is undesirable should not take pilocarpine.

Interactions

Pilocarpine can be administered with carbonic anhydrase inhibitors, epinephrine, or beta-blockers to control glaucoma, as the mechanisms of actions vary and are therefore synergistic when combined. Pilocarpine counteracts the anticholinergic effects of atropine and other anticholinergics.

Carbachol

Carbachol (Isopto Carbachol) is a direct-acting cholinomimetic agent like pilocarpine. It is more potent and slightly longer acting than pilocarpine. However, it does not penetrate the eye as well as pilocarpine and must be used with a wetting agent.

Anticholinesterase Miotics

Demecarium, echothiophate, and isoflurophate

Mechanism of Action

The anticholinesterase miotics inhibit the degradation of acetylcholine. The increased amount of acetylcholine then causes miosis. As with the direct-acting miotic, pilocarpine, therapeutic effectiveness results from the spread of the tra-

TABLE 70-1 Drugs to Treat Glaucoma

GENERIC NAME	TRADE NAME	ADMINISTRATION/DOSAGE	COMMENTS
Cholinomimetic Drugs (Weak Miotics)			
Carbachol	Isopto Carbachol* Miostat*	TOPICAL: 1 drop 0.75%-3% solution every 8 hr. Onset: 15-30 min.	Carbachol is direct-acting cholinomimetic and miotic for treating chronic glaucoma.
Physostigmine salicylate Physostigmine sulfate	Isopto-Eserine Eserine Sulfate	TOPICAL: 1 drop of 0.25%-1% every 4-6 hr. Ointment for night use primarily. Onset: 30 min.	Physostigmine salicylate and sulfate are acetylcholinesterase inhibitors and miotics for chronic glaucoma; conjunctivitis and allergic reactions are common if use is prolonged.
✣ Pilocarpine hydrochloride	Isopto Carpine* Pilocar Various others	TOPICAL: 1 drop, 1%-2% every 6-8 hr. Onset: 15-30 min. Ocular insert: 1 system inserted every 7 days.	Pilocarpine hydrochloride is direct-acting cholinomimetic and miotic; it is drug of choice for acute and chronic glaucoma.
✣ Pilocarpine nitrate	PV Carpine† Pilofrin Liquifilm Pilagan	TOPICAL: 1 drop, 1%-2% every 6-8 hr. Onset: 15-30 min.	Pilocarpine nitrate is direct-acting cholinomimetic and miotic; it is drug of choice for acute and chronic glaucoma.
Cholinomimetic Drugs (Strong Miotics)			
Demecarium bromide	Humorsol	TOPICAL: 1 drop 0.125%-0.25% solution every 12-48 hr. Onset: 12 hr.	Demecarium bromide is irreversible acetylcholinesterase inhibitor; it is potent miotic for resistant chronic glaucoma. Cataracts can develop with long-term administration.
Echothiophate iodide	Phosphaline iodide*	TOPICAL: 1 drop 0.03%-0.06% every 12-48 hr. Onset: 12 hr.	Same as for demecarium.
Isoflurophate	Floropryl	TOPICAL: ¼ in strip of 0.025% ointment every 12-72 hr. Onset 12 hr.	Same as for demecarium.
Adrenergic Drugs			
Apraclonidine hydrochloride	Iopidine	Instillation of 1 drop in affected eye 1 hr before laser surgery; repeated immediately before surgery.	Apraclonidine hydrochloride controls or prevents acute transient spikes in intraocular pressure after laser surgery for glaucoma.
Dipivefrin hydrochloride	Propine*	TOPICAL: 1 drop into conjunctival sac every 12 hr for glaucoma.	Dipivefrin is converted to epinephrine by esterases in cornea and anterior chamber.
Epinephrine borate	Epinal* Eppy	TOPICAL: 1 drop of 0.25%-2.0% solution 1 or 2 times daily.	Persons with darkly pigmented irises may require higher concentration of solution.
Epinephrine hydrochloride	Epifrin* Glaucon*	Same as epinephrine borate.	
Beta-Blockers			
Betaxolol hydrochloride	Betoptic*	TOPICAL: 1 drop of 0.5% solution twice daily.	Cardioselective (beta-1) beta-adrenergic antagonist.
Carteolol hydrochloride	Ocupress	TOPICAL: 1 drop of 1% solution 2 times/day.	Nonselective beta-adrenergic antagonist.
Levobunolol	Betagan*	TOPICAL: 1 drop of 0.5% solution once or twice daily.	Nonselective beta-adrenergic antagonist.
Metipranolol	OptiPranolol	TOPICAL: 1 drop 2 times/day.	Nonselective beta-adrenergic antagonist.
Timolol maleate	Timoptic* Apo-Timop†	TOPICAL: 1 drop of 0.25% solution twice daily; if not sufficient, 0.5% solution is used.	Nonselective beta-adrenergic antagonist
Carbonic Anhydrase Inhibitors			
Acetazolamide	Acetazolam† AK-Zol Apo-Acetazolamide† Diamox* Others	ORAL: *Adults*—250 mg every 6 hr. *Children*—10-15 mg/kg body weight daily in divided doses; timed-release capsules taken every 12-24 hr but may not be as effective.	Acetazolamide is weak diuretic.

*Available in Canada and United States.
†Available in Canada only.

Continued.

TABLE 70-1 Drugs to Treat Glaucoma—cont'd

GENERIC NAME	TRADE NAME	ADMINISTRATION/DOSAGE	COMMENTS
Carbonic Anhydrase Inhibitors—cont'd			
Acetazolamide sodium	Diamox, Parenteral*	INTRAVENOUS, INTRAMUSCULAR: *Adults*—500 mg repeated in 2-4 hr if necessary. *Children*—5-10 mg/kg body weight every 6 hr.	
Dichlorphenamide	Daranide	ORAL: *Adults*—50-200 mg every 6-8 hr.	
Methazolamide	Neptazane*	ORAL: *Adults*—25-100 mg every 8 hr.	
Osmotic Agents			
Glycerin	Glyrol Osmoglyn	ORAL: *Adults and children*—1-1.5 gm/kg body weight as 50% or 75% solution once or twice daily.	Nurse may flavor glycerin with instant coffee or lemon juice to increase palatability. Nurse may chill it with chipped ice. Glycerin may cause hyperglycemia in diabetic patients.
Isosorbide dinitrate	Iso-Bid Isordil* Others	ORAL: *Adults*—1.5 gm/kg body weight up to 4 times daily.	Nurse may chill it with chipped ice.
Mannitol	Osmitrol*	INTRAVENOUS: *Adults and children*—0.5-2 gm/kg body weight as 20% solution infused over 30-60 min.	Nurse may discontinue it when intraocular pressure is decreased, even though full dose has not been given.
Urea	Ureaphil	INTRAVENOUS: *Adults*—0.5-2 gm/kg body weight as 30% solution infused at 60 drops/min. *Children*—0.5-1.5 gm/kg body weight of 30% solution infused over 30 min.	Urea should be infused carefully. patients with hereditary fructose intolerance should not be given urea made up in invert sugar.

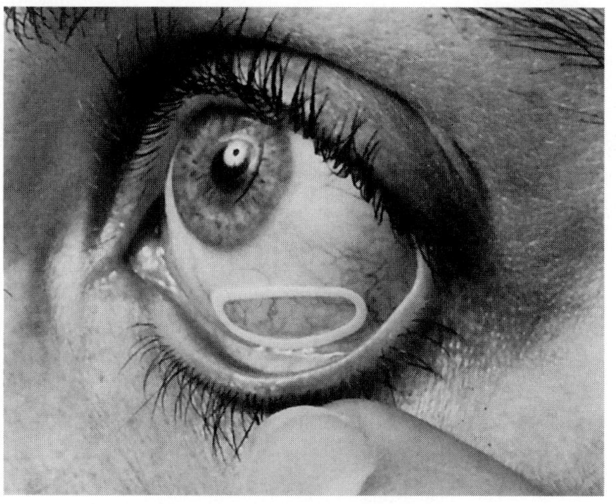

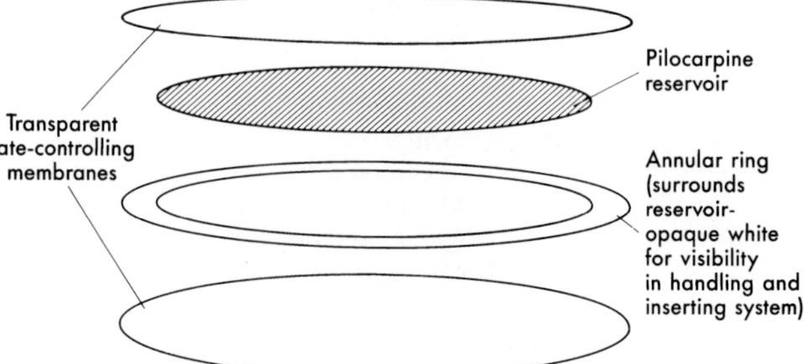

FIGURE 70-2
Ocusert ocular therapeutic system for delivery of pilocarpine for treatment of glaucoma. Flexible wafer is placed under eyelid and provides drug for week. Eyelid is shown displaced to expose device. Expanded view denotes purpose of each component. *(Courtesy ALZA Corp.)*

becular spaces of the anterior chamber when the sphincter muscles contract. The larger area allows improved uptake of the aqueous humor, which relieves intraocular pressure.

Pharmacokinetics

The anticholinesterase miotics are applied directly to the eye and are very long acting. Miosis begins in about an hour and lasts for up to 1 month after the drug is discontinued. Reduction in intraocular pressure begins in 4 hours and lasts about 1 to 2 days after the drug is discontinued.

Uses

Demecarium (Humorsol), echothiophate (Phospholine Iodide), and isoflurophate (Floropryl) are potent miotics. They are generally used only for patients with chronic glaucoma that is not well controlled by other agents.

Adverse Reactions and Contraindications

Miotics inhibit accommodation so that patients taking these drugs have poor vision in dim light. Other common local effects can include browache, ocular pain, ciliary and conjunctival congestions, tearing, and twitching of the eyebrows. In patients over 60 years old, the development of cataracts can be accelerated.

The anticholinesterase inhibitors, especially echothiophate and demecarium, do occasionally cause systemic cholinergic effects, including muscle weakness, hypersalivation, sweating, nausea, vomiting, abdominal pain, urinary incontinence, diarrhea, bradycardia, severe hypotension, and bronchospasm.

The anticholinesterase inhibitors are contraindicated during pregnancy. They are contraindicated for patients with retinal detachment or uveitis or for patients with glaucoma associated with iridocyclitis. Patients with myasthenia gravis are not good candidates for treatment with anticholinesterase miotics.

Toxicity

Symptoms of systemic toxicity include ataxia, confusion, seizures, coma, and muscle paralysis. The most common symptoms in children are abdominal cramps and diarrhea, with a runny nose and tearing.

Interactions

Other agents with anticholinesterase activity should be avoided when an anticholinesterase miotic is taken because of the additive toxicity. This includes atropine, anticholinesterases for treatment of myasthenia gravis, and pesticides with anticholinesterase activity.

Demecarium, echothiophate, and isoflurophate can decrease plasma concentrations of plasma cholinesterases, thereby enhancing the neuromuscular blockade of succinylcholine. This effect can be present for several weeks or months after the anticholinesterase has been discontinued.

Epinephrine

Mechanism of Action

Epinephrine (Epifrin, Epinal, Epitrate, Glaucon) is an adrenergic agonist that stimulates alpha- and beta-adrenergic receptors (see Chapter 12). The stimulation of ocular alpha-receptors increases the outflow of aqueous humor while the stimulation of ocular beta-receptors decreases the production of aqueous humor. These actions result in a decrease in intraoptic pressure. Epinephrine dilates the pupil (mydriasis) by stimulating the dilator muscles.

Pharmacokinetics

Ophthalmic solutions of epinephrine are available as bitartrate, hydrochloride, or borate salts. The onset of action is in 1 hour and persists for 12 to 24 hours. Epinephrine is taken up by nerve endings.

Uses

Epinephrine is used to treat chronic glaucoma, commonly given with pilocarpine or a carbonic anhydrase inhibitors. It may also be combined with a beta-blocker or hyperosmotic agent. Epinephrine is also applied to the eye during eye surgery to reduce hemorrhaging and conjunctival congestion.

Adverse Reactions and Contraindications

When applied to the eye, epinephrine can produce a burning or stinging sensation and watering of the eyes. Epinephrine can also cause a headache or browache. With repeated use, a reactive redness of the eye, allergic conjunctivitis, or contact dermatitis may develop, requiring discontinuance in about 20% of patients taking epinephrine.

Although systemic effects are not common, care should be used when a patient has a history of hypertension, arrhythmias, hyperthyroidism, or a recent heart attack.

Interactions

Additive reduction in intraocular pressure is seen when epinephrine is administered with topical miotics, topical beta-blockers, or systemically administered carbonic anhydrase inhibitors. Epinephrine may sensitize the heart to arrhythmias when used with halogenated hydrocarbon anesthetics or digitalis glycosides.

Dipivefrin Hydrochloride

Dipivefrin (dipivalyl epinephrine) is another form of epinephrine for the treatment of chronic glaucoma. Dipivefrin (Propine) is a prodrug that is inactive but is converted to epinephrine by esterases in the cornea and anterior chamber of the eye. Dipivefrin is more lipid soluble than epinephrine and therefore concentrates in the eye more readily than epinephrine. It produces less burning and irritation than epinephrine and may cause fewer allergic reactions.

Apraclonidine

Apraclonidine (Iopidine) is an alpha-adrenergic agonist that acts by reducing intraocular aqueous formation. Apraclonidine prevents acute, transient spikes in intraocular pressure after laser surgery for glaucoma. The drug is administered 1 hour before surgery and again just before surgery. Side effects can include upper lid elevation, conjunctival blanching, and mydriasis.

Beta-Blockers: General Characteristics

Mechanism of Action

Beta-adrenergic blockers act in the eye to decrease the production of aqueous humor. This action lowers intraocular pressure.

Pharmacokinetics

The beta-blockers are applied as ophthalmic solutions directly to the eye. The onset of action is 30 to 60 minutes, and the duration of action varies with the beta-blocker used. The drug is removed by gradual systemic uptake and excretion.

Uses

An ophthalmic preparation of one of the beta-blockers is the drug of choice for the initial treatment of chronic glaucoma. The major advantage of beta-blockers is that neither pupil size nor reactivity to light is altered. This is of particular benefit for young patients with active accommodation and for older adult patients with opaque lens who cannot tolerate miotics. Some irritation and blurred vision may occur at the start of therapy, but these effects usually disappear with continued administration.

Adverse Reactions and Contraindications

Beta-blockers applied to the eye may cause ocular pain, dizziness, or headache. The eyes may be red, and occasionally the irritation can be severe. Other occasional side effects include blurred vision, different size of pupils, discoloration of pupil, or double vision.

Systemic concentrations of beta-blockers administered to the eye are seldom significant. Nevertheless, patients with severe cardiovascular disease or severe asthma should not take these drugs. The systemic absorption of beta-blockers may worsen asthma or may mask signs of hyperthyroidism or hypoglycemia in diabetic patients taking insulin.

Interactions

Beta-blockers provide an additive reduction in intraocular pressure when administered with topical miotics or systemically administered carbonic anhydrase inhibitors.

Specific Beta-Blockers for Ophthalmic Use

Betaxolol

Betaxolol (Betoptic) is a selective beta-1 blocker and is preferred for patients with pulmonary problems (especially asthma) being treated for glaucoma. Betaxolol is effective for about 12 hours. The ophthalmic suspension form appears to be less irritating than the ophthalmic solution form. In general, betaxolol produces more eye irritation than the other beta-blockers.

Carteolol

Carteolol (Ocupress) is effective for 6 to 8 hours after administration. Decreased night vision has been reported for carteolol.

Levobunolol

Levobunolol (Betagan) has a longer onset of action (60 minutes) than the other beta-blockers. It is effective for up to 24 hours after a single dose.

Metipranolol

Metipranolol (Optipranolol) is effective for up to 24 hours after administration.

Timolol

Timolol (Timoptic) is used not only in treating chronic glaucoma, but also for treating glaucoma related to specific causes. It is as effective as pilocarpine or epinephrine in lowering intraocular pressure and, in general, is better tolerated.

Carbonic Anhydrase Inhibitors: Acetazolamide

Mechanism of Action

Carbonic anhydrase inhibitors decrease the formation of aqueous humor by 50% to 60% by blocking ocular carbonic anhydrase. A fall in intraocular pressure is seen only in individuals with glaucoma. The fall in intraocular pressure is negligible in individuals with normal ocular pressure.

Pharmacokinetics

Carbonic anhydrase inhibitors are given orally and distribute throughout the body. Acetazolaminde (Diamox) formulated in tablets has an onset of action in about an hour with a duration of action of 8 to 12 hours. The bioavailability of acetazolamide varies significantly with some brands. Formulated in extended-release capsules, acetazolamide has an onset of action of 2 hours and a duration of action of 18 to 24 hours. The drug is excreted unchanged in the urine.

Uses

Acetazolamide is used principally as an adjunct in the treatment of chronic glaucoma when other drugs alone do not control intraocular pressure. Acetazolamide is also used with osmotic agents, miotics, and beta-blockers for the emergency treatment of acute (closed-angle) glaucoma on a short-term basis only. Acetazolamide is also used as an anticonvulsant and in the treatment of altitude sickness. Carbonic anhydrase inhibitors are weak diuretics but are no longer used for this purpose.

Adverse Reactions and Contraindications

Acetazolamide is not well tolerated in general for prolonged therapy. Malaise, weight loss, fatigue, headache, nervousness, loss of libido, impotence, and tingling sensations are all common side effects. Infants show a failure to thrive. Infrequently, acetazolamide causes confusion, ataxia, tremor, and tinnitus. Diuresis is common initially but usually subsides. Hypokalemia is a problem if other drugs are taken that lower body potassium.

Acetazolamide may precipitate acute pulmonary failure in patients with chronic obstructive lung disease. Gout may also be precipitated in patients with a history of this disease. Acetazolamide is also teratogenic and should be avoided in pregnancy. Patients with renal failure develop excessively high concentrations of the drug.

Interactions

Acetazolamide is highly bound to plasma protein. Diflunisal, a nonsteroidal antiinflammatory drug (NSAID), has been reported to displace bound acetazolamide, thereby increasing side effects.

Acetazolamide increases the pH of the urine to the alkaline range, which decreases the excretion of several drugs, including amphetamines, anticholinergics, mecamylamine, and quinidine. These drugs may reach toxic levels if their dose is not adjusted down. The bacteriostatic activity of methenamine is decreased in an alkaline urine.

Other Carbonic Anhydrase Inhibitors

Dichlorphenamide

Dichlorphenamide (Daranide) has an onset of action of 30 to 60 minutes and a duration of action of 6 to 12 hours.

Methazolamide

Methazolamide (Neptazane) has an onset of action of 2 to 4 hours and a duration of action of 10 to 18 hours. It is not as highly protein bound as acetazolamide. Only 25% of the drug is excreted unchanged in the urine.

Specific Osmotic Agents

The osmotic agents are used as short-term treatment only to lower the intraocular pressure of glaucoma before surgery or as an emergency treatment of acute (closed-angle) glaucoma. Glycerin and isosorbide are administered orally, whereas mannitol and urea are administered intravenously.

Glycerin

Glycerin (Glyrol, Osmoglyn) lowers intraocular pressure 1 hour after ingestion, and the effect lasts 5 hours. Since glycerin is metabolized, it does not cause diuresis; however, glycerin can cause hyperglycemia in patients who have diabetes. Headache, nausea, and vomiting are additional side effects of glycerin.

Isosorbide

Isosorbide (Iso-Bid) is used sometimes in the emergency treatment of acute (closed-angle) glaucoma. Isosorbide produces diuresis but otherwise has few side effects.

Mannitol

Mannitol (Osmitrol) is effective in lowering intraocular pressure in 30 to 60 minutes, with the effect lasting 6 to 8 hours. Mannitol produces a pronounced diuresis and often causes headache, nausea and vomiting, and dehydration.

Urea

Urea (Ureaphil) is less satisfactory than mannitol because it can penetrate the eye and cause a rebound increase in intraocular pressure when the systemic osmotic effect is over, 8 to 12 hours after administration. Urea is also highly irritating on injection.

NURSING PROCESS OVERVIEW

Drugs to Treat Glaucoma

Assessment

Patients requiring treatment of glaucoma may have no visible signs of their condition. Assess the patient, focusing on symptoms related to the eye. Check peripheral vision and test visual acuity using a Snellen chart. Question patients about recent difficulties driving or ambulating. Examine the eyes for signs of infection, exudate, excessive tearing or dryness, or other deviations.

Nursing Diagnoses

- Risk for injury related to impaired vision related to specific eye problem

Patient Outcomes

The patient will suffer no injury related to impaired vision.

Planning/Implementation

The drugs discussed in this chapter are used to treat glaucoma. Other eye medications include antibiotics, glucocorticoids, and lubricants. Caution the patient about side effects, particularly those related to vision. Inform the patient about possible systemic side effects (see box).

Evaluation

Drugs used to treat glaucoma are successful if the intraocular pressure is lowered to within safe limits. Before discharge, check that the patient can explain why the drug is being used, demonstrate how to administer the drug correctly, explain potential local and systemic side effects, list the signs and symptoms requiring medical evaluation, and explain the need for continuing therapy as ordered.

NURSING IMPLICATIONS SUMMARY

General Guidelines: Drugs to Treat Glaucoma

Drug Administration

- Wash hands carefully before administering eye medications to avoid contaminating the eye or applicator. Wash hands after administering eye medications to rinse off any residue that might accidentally be rubbed into your eye. Use a separate bottle or tube of medication for each patient to avoid accidental cross-contamination; wash hands between patients.
- Place ordered dose of eye medication in the lower conjunctival sac, never directly onto the cornea. Avoid touching any part of the eye with the dropper or applicator. For additional information on administration, see Chapter 5.
- To prevent overflow of medication into nasal and pharyngeal passages, thus reducing systemic absorption, occlude (or teach the patient to occlude) the nasolacrimal duct with one finger for 1 to 2 minutes after instilling the medication.
- When two or more eye medications are administered, wait at least 3 minutes between drugs. Administer drops or liquid preparations before ointments. Administer glucocorticoid preparations before other drugs. If in doubt, consult the physician.
- Monitor the pulse of a patient receiving beta-blockers and instruct the patient to do the same. If the pulse is below 50 to 60 beats per minute in an adult, withhold the next dose of medication and notify the physician. Reassess whether the patient is occluding the nasolacrimal duct correctly after administration of each dose. Use 1 drop of a 1% or 2% epinephrine solution to reverse the redness caused by potent acetylcholinesterase inhibitors; consult the physician.
- Use pralidoxime (PAM), 0.1 to 0.2 ml of a 5% solution, to reverse the action of the irreversible acetylcholinesterase inhibitors. PAM must be injected subconjunctivally to be effective in the eye (see Chapter 11).
- Glycerin may cause hyperglycemia. Monitor blood glucose levels, especially in diabetic persons.
- See Chapter 14 for additional information about carbonic anhydrase inhibitors, mannitol, and urea.

Patient and Family Education

- Teach the patient how to instill medication correctly and supervise instillation until the patient can do it safely (see section on drug administration and Chapter 5). Instruct the patient to read labels carefully to ensure administration of correct drug and correct strength. Remind the patient to keep these drugs out of the reach of children.
- Warn the patient to avoid driving or operating hazardous equipment if vision is blurred. If the patient is using eye medications that cause pupillary constriction, caution the patient to be careful driving at night or doing any potentially dangerous activities in dim light because vision may be impaired.
- If photophobia occurs, instruct the patient to wear sunglasses and avoid bright lights. Instruct the patient not to wear sunglasses after dusk.
- Instruct the patient to administer missed doses as soon as they are remembered, unless within 1 to 2 hours of the next dose. Instruct the patient not to double up for missed doses.
- Instruct the patient to lie down if headache occurs after doses of glycerin. To make doses of glycerin or isosorbide more palatable, encourage the patient to chill them over crushed ice and to flavor glycerin with instant coffee or lemon juice.
- Inform a diabetic patient that beta-blockers may affect blood glucose levels. Instruct the patient to monitor blood glucose levels. Observe the patient's drug administration technique. Occluding the nasolacrimal duct may decrease drug absorption.
- Inform a patient with glaucoma that it cannot be cured, only controlled. Reinforce the importance of using medications to treat glaucoma as prescribed and not to discontinue these medications without consulting the physician. Drugs used to treat glaucoma may cause pain and blurred vision, especially when therapy is begun. Inform the patient that this may diminish with time. Encourage the patient to try cold compresses to relieve painful eye spasm.
- Instruct the patient to report the development of any eye irritation.
- Instruct a patient using *eye gel* to store the gel at room temperature or in the refrigerator but not to freeze it. Discard unused gel kept at room temperature after 8 weeks. After each use, wipe the tip of the tube with tissue and replace the cap tightly.
- Soft contact lenses may absorb certain eye medications, and preservatives in eye medications may discolor the contact lenses. Encourage a patient wearing contact lenses to question the physician carefully about special precautions to observe.
- For *sustained-release forms:* Instruct the patient to review carefully the instruction sheet provided by the manufacturer. The eye system is inserted into the upper or lower cul-de-sac of the eye, and the drug is released slowly; it should be replaced weekly. Instruct the patient to check each morning and evening to make sure the system is still in place. If the unit does not seem to be working, is damaged, or is releasing too much medication, instruct the patient to remove it and insert a new one. Since vision may change in the first few hours after the eye system is inserted, advise the patient to replace it at bedtime. Instruct the patient to store the eye system in the refrigerator but to avoid freezing it.
- For patients using anticholinesterase miotics (cholinomimetics): see Interactions. Caution patients who are farmers, gardeners, or residents of areas where pesticides or insecticides are sprayed to avoid contact with these sprays and to wear a mask over the nose and mouth if they must be in the area when spraying occurs.

CRITICAL THINKING

APPLICATION

1. Describe glaucoma and the role of aqueous humor.
2. Differentiate between chronic and acute glaucoma.
3. How are carbonic anhydrase inhibitors and osmotic agents used to treat glaucoma?
4. When two or more eye medications are ordered to be given at the same time, what are the guidelines for the sequence of administrations?
5. What are the abbreviations for left eye, right eye, and both eyes that may be used when eye medications are ordered? (See Chapter 5.)

CRITICAL THINKING

1. How are cholinomimetic drugs used to treat glaucoma? Which drugs might a nurse administer in the treatment of glaucoma?
2. What role do drugs acting at adrenergic receptors play in the treatment of glaucoma? Describe the actions of epinephrine and timolol.
3. How would you determine whether a patient is administering ordered eye medications correctly?

CHAPTER 71

Drugs Affecting the Eye

OBJECTIVES

After studying this chapter, you should be able to do the following:

- *Define miosis, mydriasis, and cycloplegia, and give examples of when they are therapeutically produced.*
- *Discuss the use of anticholinergic drugs for the eye.*
- *Discuss the use of nonsteroidal antiinflammatory drugs (NSAIDs) for the eye.*

CHAPTER OVERVIEW

The key functions of the eye are controlled by the autonomic nervous system. Selected drugs with autonomic actions are used in eye examinations, eye surgery, and glaucoma treatment. These ophthalmic drugs are presented in this chapter.

KEY TERMS

autonomic nervous system
cycloplegia
miosis
mydriasis
prostaglandins

Therapeutic Rationale: Examining the Eye

An internal examination of the eye requires dilation of the pupil (mydriasis) and paralysis of accommodation (cycloplegia). These actions require the use of parasympathetic and sympathetic drugs.

The **autonomic nervous system** controls the amount of light entering the eye and in focusing images. The amount of light penetrating the eye is controlled by the size of the pigmented iris, which contains two sets of muscles, the sphincter and dilator muscles. The sphincter muscles are circular muscles with muscarinic receptors innervated by the parasympathetic nervous system. As shown in Figure 71-1, the pupil is constricted when the sphincter muscles contract so that only a small surface on the eye transmits light. The dilator muscles contain alpha-receptors innervated by the sympathetic nervous system. **Miosis** refers to a constricted pupil and is achieved primarily by stimulating the muscarinic receptors of the sphincter muscles. **Mydriasis** refers to a dilated pupil and is achieved by blocking the muscarinic receptors of the sphincter muscles or by stimulating the alpha-receptors of the dilator muscles.

The cornea and the lens determine the focus of images onto the retina. The cornea accomplishes the coarse focusing, but the fine focusing for sharp images and near vision is accomplished by the lens. The shape of the lens is controlled by muscarinic receptors of the parasympathetic nervous system. As diagramed in Figure 71-1, the accommodation for near vision requires the contraction of ciliary muscles to change the shape of the lens. Ligaments normally pull the lens to keep it relatively flat. Contraction of the ciliary muscles relaxes the ligaments so that the lens becomes rounder as required for near vision. **Cycloplegia** refers to the paralysis of the ciliary muscles by drugs that block muscarinic receptors. Cycloplegia causes blurred vision since the shape of the lens can no longer be adjusted to near vision.

Therapeutic Agents: Mydriatics

Mydriasis is achieved with anticholinergic drugs or with adrenergic drugs. Anticholinergic drugs also cause cycloplegia. Prostaglandin inhibitors prevent miosis related to prostaglandin synthesis. Drugs from all these classes are listed in Table 71-1.

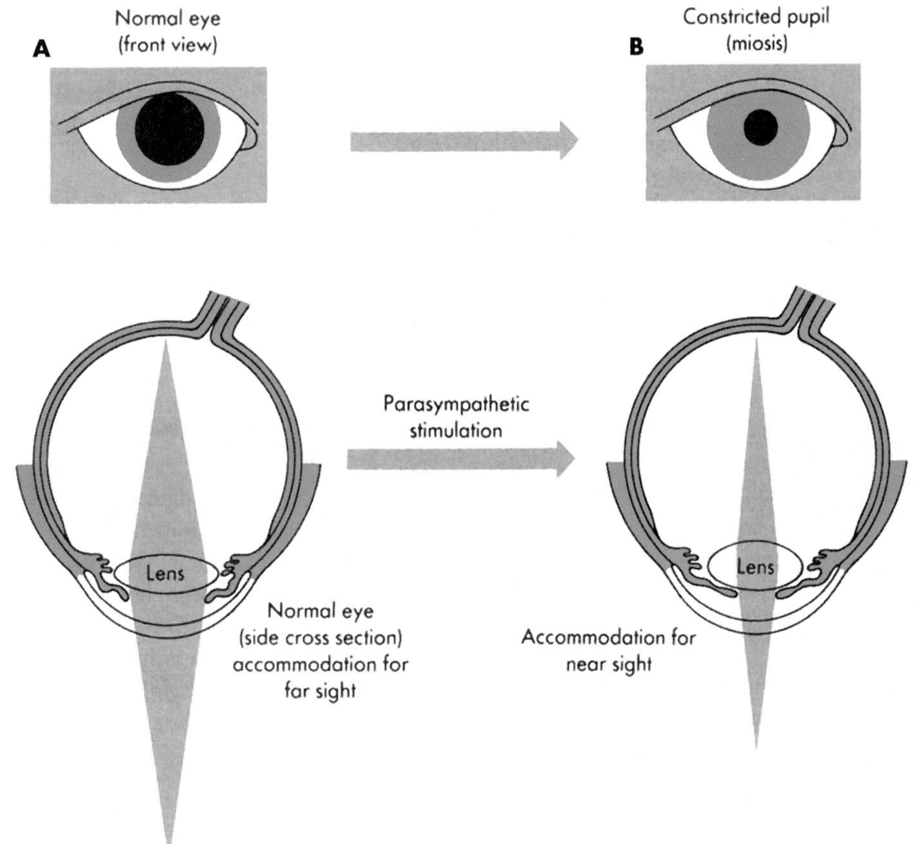

FIGURE 71-1

A, Normal eye. Effects of parasympathetic nervous system on eye are mediated through muscarinic receptors. **B,** Pupil is made smaller because circular muscles contract. Accommodation is made by contracting muscles to thicken lens.

TABLE 71-1 Drugs for Mydriasis and Cycloplegia

DRUG	TRADE NAME	ADMINISTRATION/DOSAGE	COMMENTS
Anticholinergic Drugs for Mydriasis and Cycloplegia			
✥ Atropine sulfate	Atropair Atropisol* Isopto-Atropine* Minims Atropine† Ocu-Tropine Others	Topical solutions: 0.5-3%. *Adults*—1 drop of 1-3% solution to each eye. Frequency of administration depends on condition being treated. *Children <8 yr*—1drop of 0.125-0.5% solution. *Children >8 yr*—0.25-1% solution 3 times daily for 3 days before and once on morning of day refraction is measured. Duration: 6 days.	For children, for refraction measurements. For adults, to relax eye muscles during surgery or treatment of eye inflammation, to aid in eye surgery or treatment of eye inflammation.
Cyclopentolate hydrochloride	AK-Pentolate* Cyclogyl* I-Pentolate Minims Cyclopentolate† Pentolair Others	Topical solutions: 0.5%, 1%, and 2%. *Adults*—1 drop of solution in each eye, repeated after 5 min. Darker irises or children require stronger solutions. *Children*—1 drop of solution in eye, repeated after 10 min. Onset: 25-75 min. Duration: 6-24 hr.	To aid in measuring refraction.
Homatropine hydrobromide	AK-Homatropine Isopto Homatrine* I-Homatrine† Spectro-Homatrine	Topical solutions: 2% and 5%. *Adults*—For refraction: 1 drop of 5% solution every 10 min 2 or 3 times. Duration: 2 days.	To aid in refraction measurements in adults; to aid in treating mild eye inflammation.
Scopolamine hydrobromide	Isopto Hyoscine	Topical solutions: 0.2-0.3%. *Adults*—1 drop of solution or ointment to each eye. 1 or more times daily, depending on condition being treated. *Children*—1 drop of 0.2-0.25% solution or ointment twice daily for 2 days before refraction measurement. Duration: 3 days.	For children, to measure refraction. For adults, to treat eye inflammation.
Tropicamide	I-Picamide Mydriacyl* Minims Tropicamide† Tropicacyl Others	Topical solutions: 0.5% and 1%. 1 drop in each eye; repeated in 5 min. Onset: 20-35 min. Duration: 2-6 hr.	To aid in measuring refraction.
Adrenergic Drugs for Mydriasis Only			
Phenylephrine hydrochloride	AK-Dilate Dilatair Mydfrin Ocu-Phrin Others	Topical use: 1 drop of 2.5% solution.	To obtain maximum mydriasis in 60-90 min. To obtain recovery in 6 hr.
Alpha-Adrenergic Blocker			
Dapiprazole hydrochloride	Rev-Eyes	Topical: 1 drop to the conjunctiva after completion of the retinal examination, followed by another drop in 5 min.	To counteract mydriasis induced by phenylephrine and to a lesser degree, by tropicamide.
Prostaglandin Inhibitors			
Flurbiprofen sodium	Ocufen	Topical: 1 drop instilled every 30 min beginning 2 hr before surgery; total dose 4 drops.	To prevent miosis during surgery. (Nonsteroidal antiinflammatory drug is applied topically.)
Suprofen	Profenal	Topical: 2 drops are applied 3, 2, and 1 hr before surgery; 2 drops may be applied every 4 hr during waking hours day before surgery.	To prevent miosis during surgery. (Nonsteroidal antiinflammatory drug is applied topically.)

*Available in Canada and United States.
†Available in Canada only.

Anticholinergics: General Characteristics

Mechanism of Action

Classic anticholinergic actions include dilated pupils (mydriasis) and blurred vision (cycloplegia). Anticholinergic drugs block the muscarinic receptors of the sphincter muscles so that the pupil cannot contract (see Figure 71-1). The ciliary muscles controlling the shape of the lens are also paralyzed so that the eye can no longer accommodate and produce focused images.

Pharmacokinetics

These agents are solutions or ointments instilled in the eye. The onset and duration of action depend on the agent and the strength of the solution. The drug is gradually removed through systemic circulation.

Uses

The major use of the anticholinergic drugs is to induce mydriasis and cycloplegia for examination of the eye. Accurate measurement of lens refraction requires both actions. Some anticholinergics are used in the treatment of inflammation of the eye (uveitis). The relaxation of sphincter and ciliary muscles hastens healing of inflammatory conditions, especially after eye surgery.

Adverse Reactions and Contraindications

Systemic reactions may occur when the anticholinergic drug is absorbed into the body, particularly with atropine. Systemic reactions are associated with anticholinergic effects such as dry mouth and dry skin, fever, thirst, confusion, and hyperactivity. Children are the most prone to systemic toxicity from ophthalmic drugs.

Acute (closed-angle) glaucoma may occur in certain patients when the iris crowds the anterior chamber. Patients with keratoconus (protrusion of the central cornea) or Down syndrome are especially sensitive to the mydriatic effect of anticholinergic drugs.

Interactions

Physostigmine salicylate, an indirect-acting cholinergic drug, is an effective antidote to reverse systemic anticholinergic toxicity but not for hypotensive reactions.

Specific Anticholinergic Drugs

✣ Atropine

Atropine (Atropair, Ocu-Tropine, others) is the drug of choice for use in children because it is potent and long acting and children have an active accommodation. Mydriasis may last 12 days, although accommodation usually returns in 6 days. Since atropine is applied for 3 days, the child should be watched for systemic reactions and application discontinued if any reactions appear. The child will also require protection from bright light.

Atropine is also used before surgery (often with phenylephrine) to produce mydriasis and for other conditions requiring prolonged mydriasis. Atropine may cause contact dermatitis of the eyelids.

Cyclopentolate

Cyclopentolate (Cyclogyl) is a rapidly acting mydriatic and cycloplegic drug. It is effective in 25 to 75 minutes, and accommodation returns in 6 to 24 hours. Cyclopentolate is used as for aiding refraction, for ophthalmoscopy, and for preoperative mydriasis. Systemic reactions have been reported. A combination of cyclopentolate and phenylephrine (Cyclomydril) is used and is the combination of choice for use with premature infants.

Homatropine

Homatropine (AK-Homatropine) is applied 2 or 3 times at 10-minute intervals to produce mydriasis and cycloplegia, which are achieved in 60 minutes. Recovery may take 2 days.

Scopolamine

Scopolamine (Isopto Hyoscine) is a potent mydriatic and is used like atropine, but cycloplegia lasts for only 3 instead of 6 days. Scopolamine can be used in patients who are allergic to atropine.

Tropicamide

Tropicamide (Mydriacyl) acts rapidly, taking effect in 20 to 35 minutes. Accommodation returns in 2 to 6 hours. Systemic side effects are rare. This is the agent most commonly used for routine eye examinations.

Adrenergic Drugs

The adrenergic drug phenylephrine is used as a mydriatic when only the interior structures of the eye are examined and cycloplegia is not required. The alpha-adrenergic blocker dapirazole is used to reverse the mydriasis produced by phenylephrine.

Phenylephrine

Phenylephrine (AK-Dilate, Dilatair, Mydfrin, Ocu-Phrin) acts on the alpha-receptors of the dilator muscles to produce mydriasis without cycloplegia. Dilation is maximal in 60 to 90 minutes, and recovery occurs in 6 hours. Cyclomydril is a combination of cyclopentolate and phenylephrine used when maximal dilation is required.

Phenylephrine is also used in the treatment of uveitis and postoperative inflammation. Dilute solutions of phenylephrine are used to bring temporary relief of the redness of the eyes caused by minor eye irritations.

Dapiprazole

Dapiprazole (Rev-Eyes) is an alpha-adrenergic blocking agent used to reverse the mydriasis produced by phenylephrine and to a lesser degree tropicamide. Dapiprazole acts rapidly but is slower acting in more heavily pigmented brown eyes than in blue or green eyes. About 50% of patients experience a burning sensation when the drops are applied. About 80% have a redness of the eye (conjunctival injection) lasting about 20 minutes.

Prostaglandin Inhibitors

Flurbiprofen (Ocufen) and Suprofen (Profenal) are NSAIDs specifically for ophthalmic use (see Table 71-1). Ophthalmic surgery may stimulate the synthesis of prostaglandins in the eye. **Prostaglandins** are chemical transmitters synthesized in response to stimulation, locally in tissues. In the eye, newly synthesized prostaglandins cause a miosis that resists the mydriatic action of atropine. The locally applied NSAIDs prevent miosis during surgery.

NURSING PROCESS OVERVIEW

Drugs to Treat Eye Conditions

Assessment

Patients requiring treatment of eye conditions may have no visible signs of their condition. Assess the patient, focusing on symptoms related to the eye. Check peripheral vision and test visual acuity using a Snellen chart. Question the patient about recent difficulties driving or ambulating at home; such difficulties might include tripping or bumping into objects. Examine the eyes for signs of infection, exudate, excessive tearing or dryness, or other deviations.

Nursing Diagnoses

- Risk for injury related to impaired vision related to specific eye problem
- Altered home maintenance management related to insufficient knowledge about eye medications, their use, or their instillation

Patient Outcomes

The patient will suffer no injury related to impaired vision. The patient will demonstrate correct use of eye medications

Planning/Implementation

The drugs discussed in this chapter are used to assist evaluation of eye problems or to treat specific problems. Other eye medications include antibiotics, glucocorticoids, and lubricants. Caution the patient about side effects, particularly those related to vision. Blurred vision, photophobia, and other symptoms can be frightening when they occur without warning. Teach the patient about possible systemic side effects.

Evaluation

Drugs used to assist in diagnostic evaluation of the eye are successful if they aid in the examination without producing serious side effects. Before discharge, check that the patient can explain why the drug is being used, demonstrate how to administer the drug correctly, explain potential local and systemic side effects, list the signs and symptoms requiring medical evaluation, and explain the need for continuing therapy as ordered.

NURSING IMPLICATIONS SUMMARY

Drugs Affecting the Eye

Drug Administration

- Wash hands carefully before administering eye medications to avoid contaminating the eye or applicator. Wash hands after administering eye medications to rinse off any residue that might accidentally be rubbed into your eye. Use a separate bottle or tube of medication for each patient to avoid accidental cross-contamination; wash hands between patients.
- Place ordered dose of eye medication in the lower conjunctival sac, never directly onto the cornea. Avoid touching any part of the eye with the dropper or applicator. For additional information on administration, see Chapter 5.
- To prevent overflow of medication into nasal and pharyngeal passages, thus reducing systemic absorption, occlude (or teach the patient to occlude) the nasolacrimal duct with one finger for 1 to 2 minutes after instilling the medication.
- When two or more eye medications are administered, wait at least 3 minutes between drugs. Administer drops or liquid preparations before ointments. Administer glucocorticoid preparations before other drugs. If in doubt, consult the physician.
- Use atropine and the belladonna alkaloids cautiously in older adult patients since these drugs may precipitate an acute attack of glaucoma.

Patient and Family Education

- Teach the patient how to instill medication correctly and supervise instillation until the patient can do it safely (see Drug Administration and Chapter 5). Instruct the patient to read labels carefully to ensure administration of correct drug and correct strength. Remind the patient to keep drugs out of the reach of children.
- Warn the patient to avoid driving or operating hazardous equipment if vision is blurred. Caution adults that they may be unable to drive home after eye examinations in which medications to dilate the pupil (mydriatics) or drugs to paralyze the ciliary muscle (cycloplegics) were used; a friend or family member should drive until the effects of the medication wear off.
- If photophobia occurs, instruct the patient to wear sunglasses and avoid bright lights. Instruct the patient not to wear sunglasses after dusk.
- Instruct the patient to administer missed doses as soon as they are remembered, unless within 1 to 2 hours of the next dose. Instruct the patient not to double up for missed doses.
- In infants, atropine eyedrops may contribute to abdominal distension. Instruct caregivers to keep a record of bowel movements of infants. In the health care setting, auscultate bowel sounds of infants and children receiving atropine eyedrops.
- Instruct the patient to report the development of any eye irritation.
- Soft contact lenses may absorb certain eye medications, and preservatives in eye medications may discolor the contact lenses. Encourage a patient wearing contact lenses to question the physician carefully about special precautions to observe.
- See Chapter 70 for information about *eye gel* and *sustained-release forms.*

CRITICAL THINKING

APPLICATION

1. Which anticholinergic drugs might you administer in the eye?
2. When two or more eye medications are ordered to be given at the same time, what are the guidelines for the sequence of administrations?
3. What are the abbreviations for left eye, right eye, and both eyes that may be used when eye medications are ordered? (See Chapter 5.)

CRITICAL THINKING

1. Explain what you would observe in a patient given a drug to produce miosis, mydriasis, or cycloplegia.
2. What would you observe when anticholinergic drugs are applied to the eye? How are these actions medically useful?
3. What action is mediated by the alpha-adrenergic receptor in the eye? Which drugs might you administer for this effect?
4. How would you determine whether a patient is administering ordered eye medications correctly?

Disorders Index

(i) = illustration
(t) = table

Comprehensive Index

Generic drugs are in *lower case italics.*
Trade names are in SMALL CAPS.
(i) = illustration
(t) = table

H

Q

Compatibility Chart for Drugs in Syringe

	Atropine	Benzquinamide	Butorphanol	Chlorpromazine	Dimenhydrinate	Diphenhydramine	Droperidol	Fentanyl	Glycopyrrolate	Hydroxyzine	Meperidine	Metoclopramide	Midazolam	Morphine	Nalbuphine	Pentazocine	Pentobarbital	Perphenazine	Prochlorperazine	Promazine	Promethazine	Scopolamine Hbr	Secobarbital	Thiethylperazine	Trimethobenzamide
Atropine		C	C	C	C	C	C	C	C	C	C	C	C	C	C	C	I	C	C	C	C	C	I		
Benzquinamide	C								C	C	C		C	C		C	I					C	I		
Butorphanol	C				I	C	C	C		C	C	C	C	C		C	I	C	C		C				
Chlorpromazine	C				I	C	C	C	C	C	C	C	C	C		C	I	C	C	C	C	C	I		
Dimenhydrinate	C		I	I		C	C	C	I	I	C	C	I	C		C	I	C	I	I	I	C			
Diphenhydramine	C		C	C	C		C	C	C	C	C	C	C	C	C	C	I	C	C	C	C	C	I		
Droperidol	C		C	C	C	C		C	C	C	C	C	C	C	C	C	I	C	C	C	C	C	I		
Fentanyl	C		C	C	C	C	C			C	C	C	C	C		C	I	C	C	C	C	C			
Glycopyrrolate	C	C		C	I	C	C			C	C		C	C	C	I	I		C	C	C	C	I		C
Hydroxyzine	C	C	C	C	I	C	C	C	C		C	C	C	C	C	C	I		C	C	C	C			
Meperidine	C	C	C	C	C	C	C	C	C	C		C	C	I		C	I	C	C	C	C	C			
Metoclopramide	C		C	C	C	C	C	C		C	C		C	C		C		C	C	C	C	C	I		
Midazolam	C	C	C	C	I	C	C	C	C	C	C	C		C	C		I	I	I	C	C	C		C	C
Morphine	C	C	C	C	C	C	C	C	C	C	I	C	C			C	#	C	#	C	#	C			
Nalbuphine	C					C	C		C	C			C				I		C	#	#	C			C
Pentazocine	C	C	C	C	C	C	C	C	I	C	C	C		C			I	C	C	C	C	C	I		
Pentobarbital	I	I	I	I	I	I	I	I	I	I	I		I	#	I	I		I	I	I	I	C			
Perphenazine	C		C	C	C	C	C	C			C	C	I	C		C	I		C		C	C		I	
Prochlorperazine	C		C	C	I	C	C	C	C	C	C	C	I	#	C	C	I	C		C	C	C	I		
Promazine	C			C	I	C	C	C	C	C	C	C	C	C	#	C	I		C		C	C	I		
Promethazine	C		C	C	I	C	C	C	C	C	C	C	C	#	#	C	I	C	C	C		C			
Scopolamine Hbr	C	I		C	C	C	C	C	C	C	C	C	C	C	C	C	C	C	C	C	C				
Secobarbital	I	I		I		I	I		I		I					I			I	I					
Thiethylperazine													C					I							
Trimethobenzamide									C				C		C										

C, Compatible if used within 15 minutes; I, incompatible; #, compatibility varies with brand and dilution (check with pharmacist); M , no documented information.

DRUG CLASSIFICATIONS AT-A-GLANCE

Drug class	Function/major uses
ACE inhibitors	Agents that prevent the synthesis of angiotensin II, a potent vasoconstrictor; used to treat hypertension and congestive heart failure
Acetylcholinesterase inhibitors	Agents that promote the accumulation of acetylcholine
Alpha blockers	Agents that inhibit the activity of the sympathetic neurotransmitter, norepinephrine
Anabolic steroids	Agents that stimulate nitrogen retention and protein synthesis; may be abused for purpose of body building
Analgesics	Agents that relieve pain
Androgens	Steroids that cause masculinizing effects
Anesthetics, local	Agents that reversibly block nerve conduction to cause loss of sensation
Anesthetics, general	Agents that act on the central nervous system to abolish perception of pain and reaction to painful stimuli
Anorexiants	Agents that suppress appetite
Antacids	Weak bases that neutralize stomach acid
Antianxiety agents	Agents that relieve anxiety without marked drowsiness
Antiarrhythmics	Agents that convert any unusual heart rate or rhythm back to normal sinus rhythm
Antibiotics	Agents used to treat infections caused by pathogenic microbes; term is often used interchangeably with antimicrobial agents
Anticholinergics	Agents that block the action of cholinergic neurotransmitters and acetylcholine
Anticoagulants	Agents that prevent clot formation
Anticonvulsants	Agents used to control seizures
Antidepressants	Agents that relieve depression
Antidiarrheals	Agents used to treat diarrhea
Antidyskinetics	Anticholinergic agents that work in the central nervous system to reduce Parkinson's symptoms
Antiemetics	Agents used to prevent nausea or to control vomiting
Antifungals	Agents used to treat infections caused by pathogenic fungi
Antihelminthics	Agents used to treat worm infestations
Antihistamines	Agents that block the action of histamines, principally to control allergic reactions
Antihypertensives	Agents that control chronic hypertension
Antiplatelets	Agents that block platelet aggregation, thereby decreasing clot formation; used for preventive therapy for strokes and myocardial infarction
Antipsychotics	Agents that reduce psychotic symptoms
Antipyretics	Agents used to lower a fever
Antispasmodics	Agents that decrease gastrointestinal tone and motility
Antitussives	Agents that suppress coughs by depressing the cough center in the central nervous system
Antivirals	Agents used to treat infections caused by pathogenic viruses
Beta-adrenergic bronchodilators	Agents that stimulate beta-2 receptors to promote bronchodilation
Beta-blockers	Agents that inhibit the activity of sympathetic transmitters, norepinephrine, and epinephrine; used to treat angina, arrhythmias, hypertension, and glaucoma
Beta-lactams	Penicillin, cephalosporins, and related antibiotics
Bile acid sequestrants	Resins that bind bile acids to promote the lowering of cholesterol
Bronchodilators	Agents that dilate the bronchioles
Calcium channel blockers	Agents that decrease the entry of calcium into smooth muscle and depress cardiac nodal conduction; used for treating angina, hypertension, and tachycardia
Carbonic anhydrase inhibitors	Weak diuretics; agents also used to block the production of aqueous humor, thus reducing intraocular pressure in glaucoma
Cell-stimulating agents	Agents that improve immune function by stimulating the activity of various immune cells
Colony-stimulating factors	Agents that stimulate progenitor cells in bone marrow to increase numbers of leukocytes, thereby improving immune function
Cough suppressants	Agents that suppress the cough reflex center in the brain
Cycloplegics	Anticholinergic agents that paralyze accommodation
Cytotoxics	Agents that cause direct cell death; often used for cancer chemotherapy
Decongestants	Agents that cause vasoconstriction in the nasal passages to relieve symptoms of the common cold or allergies
Digitalis glycosides	Agents that improve cardiac function by increasing the force of contraction and slowing the heart rate
Diuretics	Agents that increase urine output
Emetics	Agents used to induce vomiting
Estrogens	Steroids that cause feminizing effects
Expectorants	Agents that promote respiratory secretions to keep mucus liquefied
Fibric acid derivatives	Triglyceride-lowering agents
Gastrointestinal stimulants	Agents that stimulate intestinal motility by acting on muscarinic or serotonergic receptors
Glucocorticoids	Antiinflammatory agents related to the adrenal hormone, cortisol
Gonadotropic hormones	Pituitary hormones that regulate the maturation and function of reproductive organs

Drug class	Function/major uses
H_2-receptor antagonists	Agents that block histamine receptors in the stomach to inhibit acid secretion; used to treat ulcers and acid reflux
HAART	High activity antiretroviral therapy, involves combinations of anti-HIV agents that may be much more effective than single or dual drug combinations
Hemostatics	Systemic or local agents used to control excessive bleeding
Herbals	Plant products usually sold as food supplements; may have pharmacologic effects that are not evaluated or regulated by the FDA
Hypnotics	Agents used to promote sleep
Hypoglycemics	Agents that lower blood glucose levels
Immunostimulants	Agents that activate T and B cells, promoting an immune reaction
Inotropics	Agents that increase the strength of heart contractions
Insulins	Hormones required for glucose transport into cells; used as replacement therapy for insulin-dependent diabetes mellitus
Laxatives	Agents that produce soft stools
Macrolides	Erythromycin, azithromycin, and related antibiotics
MAO inhibitors	Agents that block monoamine oxidase, thereby preventing the degradation of norepinephrine and serotonin
Mineralocorticoids	Steroids that cause the kidneys to retain sodium and water
Minoglycosides	Gentamicin, amikacin, and related antibiotics; noted for potentially dangerous toxicity
Miotics	Cholinomimetic agents used to constrict the pupil
Muscle relaxants	Centrally acting agents used to reduce muscle spasms
Mydriatics	Anticholinergic or adrenergic agents used to dilate the pupil
Neuromuscular blockers	Agents that block the action of acetylcholine at the muscle receptor, temporarily paralyzing muscle
Nitrates	Agents that degrade to nitric oxide, a potent vasodilator used to treat angina
NSAIDs	Nonsteroidal, antiinflammatory agents, that inhibit prostaglandin synthesis; aspirin-like drugs with analgesic, antipyretic, and antiinflammatory activity
Opioids	Centrally acting analgesic agents related to morphine
Oral contraceptives	Agents that block ovulation or implantation, thus preventing pregnancy
Oral hypoglycemics	Agents used in noninsulin dependent (type 1) diabetes mellitus to improve glucose metabolism and lower blood glucose levels
Osmotic diuretics	Urea or mannitol; retained in the renal tubules and used to promote the excretion of water; also move water from tissues into plasma
Oxytocics	Agents that stimulate uterine contraction; may be used to hasten delivery or to control postpartum bleeding
Plasma expanders	Given intravenously, these large proteins or complex carbohydrates remain in the vasculature and cause water to move into the vessels
Progestins	Steroids regulating endometrial and myometrial function; used alone or in combination with estrogen for oral contraception
Protease inhibitors	Saquinavir, ritonavir, indinavir, and related drugs that block the maturation of HIV; used for HIV infections
Reverse transcriptase inhibitors	Zidovudine and related drugs that block the action of an enzyme needed for HIV replication; used for HIV infections
Saline (osmotic) cathartics	Poorly absorbed salts that attract water into the lumen of the large intestine to promote defecation
Sedatives	Agents used to calm an anxious person, often promoting drowsiness
Selective serotonin reuptake inhibitors (SSRIs)	Antidepressants that act by specifically blocking the reuptake of serotonin
Statins (HMG-CoA reductase inhibitors)	Agents that block the synthesis of cholesterol
Stimulant cathartics	Agents that act in the large intestine to inhibit water resorption and promote defecation
Stool softeners (wetting agents)	Detergents that inhibit the absorption of water to keep the fecal mass large and soft
Sympatholytics	Agents that interfere with the storage and release of norepinephrine
Sympathomimetics	Agents that mimic the action of dopamine, norepinephrine, and epinephrine
Thrombolytics	Agents that dissolve thrombi by promoting the digestion of fibrin
Thyroid hormones	Hormones needed to regulate the basal metabolic rate; used for replacement therapy when normal hormone production is insufficient
Topicals	Agents used on the surface of the body
Tricyclics	Antidepressants that inhibit the reuptake of norepinephrine and serotonin
Urinary antiseptics	Substances concentrated in urine to a level required for clearing bacterial infection
Uterine relaxants	Agents used to limit myometrial contractions and prevent preterm labor and delivery
Vaccines	Immunostimulants that promote immunity to specific diseases
Vasodilators	Agents that relax the arteriolar smooth muscle